Pharmacologic Basis of Nursing Practice

Pharmacologic Basis of Nursing Practice

JULIA B. FREEMAN CLARK, Ph.D.

Health Scientist Administrator,
National Institutes of Health,
Bethesda, Maryland

SHERRY F. QUEENER, Ph.D.

Professor of Pharmacology,
Indiana University School of Medicine,
Indianapolis, Indiana

VIRGINIA BURKE KARB, R.N., Ph.D.

Assistant Dean and Associate Professor,
School of Nursing,
University of North Carolina at Greensboro,
Greensboro, North Carolina

FOURTH EDITION

with 89 illustrations

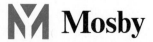

St. Louis Baltimore Boston Chicago London Philadelphia Sydney Toronto

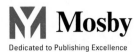

Mosby

Dedicated to Publishing Excellence

Editor: Robin Carter
Project Manager: Carol Sullivan Wiseman
Production Editor: Shannon Canty
Designer: Gail Morey Hudson
Illustrator: Mark Swindle

The cover image "Asuras Spires" is reproduced courtesy of fiber artist Jennifer Moore
and Style Works, St. Louis, Missouri.

FOURTH EDITION

Printed in the United States of America

Mosby–Year Book, Inc.
11830 Westline Industrial Drive, St. Louis, Missouri 63146

Library of Congress Cataloging in Publication Data

Freeman, Julia B.
    Pharmacologic basis of nursing practice / Julia B. Freeman Clark,
Sherry F. Queener, Virginia Burke Karb.—4th ed.
        p.   cm.
    Rev. ed. of: Pharmacological basis of nursing practice. 3rd ed.
1990.
    Includes bibliographical references and index.
    ISBN 0-8016-6673-2 : $45.95
    1. Pharmacology. 2. Nursing. I. Freeman, Julia B.
Pharmacological basis of nursing practice. II. Queener, Sherry F.
III. Karb, Virginia Burke. IV. Title.
    [DNLM: 1. Drug Therapy—nurses' instruction. 2. Pharmacology—
—nurses' instruction.   QV 4 F855p]
RM300.F72 1992
615'.1'024613—dc20
DNLC/DLC
for Library of Congress   92-49911
                                                              CIP

        94 95 96 97 GW/VH 9 8 7 6 5 4 3 2

Preface

Pharmacology is a rapidly changing field. Newly acquired knowledge about the molecular basis of medicine has expanded the therapeutic strategies available. The role of the nurse is increasingly sophisticated as new drugs and new strategies are applied to patient care.

CONTENT AND FEATURES

This fourth edition of *Pharmacologic Basis of Nursing Practice* contains information on **over 70 new drugs** that have appeared in the 3 years since the last edition. We have thoroughly revised the appropriate portions of the book, including the addition of new drugs in tables and integration of these agents into the text. The entire text has been reviewed, revised, and, in many cases, entirely reformatted to keep up with current knowledge on drug mechanisms and therapeutic uses of agents. The rapidly developing area of immunopharmacology, first added in the third edition, has been updated extensively, as have antihypertensive agents, antianginal agents, antibiotics, and others.

The fourth edition also contains the following new features to facilitate use of the book and to integrate more fully the nursing-related aspects of pharmacology into the text:

- **Learning Objectives** now appear at the beginning of each chapter to guide students in their study. These objectives specifically highlight the nursing relevance of the drugs presented within each chapter.

- **Chapter Overviews** describe the range of material to provide a focus and to allow the student to place individual drug and drug-group content into a nursing practice context. These brief overviews follow the learning objectives. Together, the learning objectives and chapter overviews provide a solid nursing-oriented approach to content in each chapter.

- **Nursing Process Overviews** introduce each therapeutic segment or drug-group discussion. This content is subdivided into a nursing process framework: Assessment, Nursing Diagnoses, Management, and Evaluation. Included under the management heading are the planning and implementation steps of the nursing process. This approach is a highly practical one in that it eliminates unnecessary repetition of content that applies to both the planning and evaluation steps of the nursing process and thus enables us to keep the book to a more manageable length.

- **Nursing Implications Summaries,** which were formerly called *Patient Care Implications,* have been moved to the end of each chapter and highlighted with color to draw attention to them. These summaries serve two functions. First, they present general guidelines on the nursing implications for drug groups or specific therapies covered in each chapter. Second, they provide detailed, specific nursing implications for each therapeutic agent. This is the focal content for nursing students; it builds on the foundational content that is presented within each chapter. These extensive summaries can also be used by the student as a quick yet thorough review before each assignment in the clinical setting.

- **Chapter Review** sections have been added to the end of each chapter to facilitate review of key content and encourage comprehension. These reviews include **key terms,** which are bold-faced in the text where introduced, and **review questions,** which have been thoroughly revised to reflect a stronger nursing focus. Summaries that formerly appeared at the end of each chapter have been moved to the *Instructor's Resource Manual* to aid in preparing lecture content.

- To facilitate use of the book in programs where pharmacology is integrated into the curriculum and not offered as a separate course, we have included a separate **Disorder Index** at the beginning of the comprehensive index. The disorder index presents all disorders discussed in the book to permit students to locate and read all disorder-specific content more readily. The comprehensive index also includes this information should the student desire to locate material in traditional index form.

Several content features have been retained from the previous edition and, in some cases, retitled to clarify their content.

♦ **Geriatric Considerations** are boxed for emphasis and included wherever there are significant implications of specific agents among elderly patients. These boxes are cross-referenced if pertinent to other chapters and, as are the features noted below, listed on the endpapers with page-number references to facilitate retrieval.

♦ **Pediatric Considerations** are also boxed and included where important. These life-span boxes are set off to allow the student to identify them readily and to locate age-related content.

♦ **Drug Abuse Alerts** are boxed to bring attention to this increasingly timely topic and to make the nursing student more aware of the nurse's responsibility in this area.

♦ **Dietary Considerations** feature information on drug-food interactions or health maintenance and promotion.

♦ **Patient Problem** boxes highlight patient problems that occur as side effects of drug therapy or otherwise present nursing challenges. These problems are emphasized because they are relatively common yet highly treatable, and, therefore, the nurse will encounter them frequently in practice.

♦ **Over 50 two-color illustrations** have been redrawn for better presentation and several new ones have been added. Illustrations have been enlarged, wherever possible, for clarity and visual appeal.

GOALS

Our goal remains to provide an up-to-date, scientifically based pharmacology book that assists nursing students studying drugs. Specifically, we seek to present clearly the concepts of pharmacology that guide all drug use; to discuss the major drug classes with an emphasis on mechanisms of action; and to detail the nursing implications for drug administration throughout the nursing process.

Our approach is to emphasize the rationale for drug therapy by relating the physiologic factors of disease processes to drug mechanisms. Although more thorough in describing the scientific basis of drug action than most textbooks for nursing students, this book carefully reviews pertinent physiologic facts so students can readily see how drugs modify physiologic processes and apply this to nursing practice.

Students of nursing look forward to pharmacology as one of the important background courses for their professional education, but they often express frustration about trying to remember the large number of drugs they must learn. We seek to minimize that difficulty by dealing with drug classes first and then by emphasizing the similarities among drugs of a single drug class. Chapters are focused on the grouping of drugs according to their mechanism of action.

For the instructor, our goal is to provide a book that can be adapted to varied curricula. The book is divided into twelve sections. Each section contains three or more chapters, and a chapter has distinct segments for different therapeutic situations. For example, antianginal drugs are covered in a section of the chapter on drugs to improve circulation; the chapter is one of nine chapters in the section on drugs affecting the cardiovascular and renal systems. This organization allows the instructor to rearrange the order in which material is presented and also gives students succinct sections to master.

ORGANIZATION

Sections I through III contain introductory material on the general principles of pharmacology, patient care, and neuropharmacology. These areas are the cornerstones of pharmacology. The goal of these chapters is to provide the background information for discussing drug actions and use. These concepts provide a guide for study of the drug classes presented later in the text. It has been our experience as teachers that basic concepts need to be reinforced throughout the study of pharmacology. We refer students to these early chapters at logical points throughout the text to assist the student in recalling basic concepts.

Sections IV through XII present drug classes by broad categories grouped on body systems or processes. Each section consists of three or more chapters with each chapter targeted to a general therapeutic goal. A chapter may contain several therapeutic segments, and a segment covers one or more drug classes.

Each chapter follows a consistent and logical format. The student is first presented the Learning Objectives for the chapter. The Chapter Overview describes the range of material covered in the chapter and is followed by the Nursing Process Overview, a section on the application of nursing process to content in that chapter or section. A therapeutic goal is then introduced, and the student is presented with the physiology and cell biology required as background. Disease processes are discussed briefly to explain the aberrant physiologic processes involved. Illustrations are used to clarify the biologic processes reviewed. Specific drug classes are presented, with the mechanisms of action of the particular class discussed first, followed by pharmacokinetics, side effects, toxicity, drug interactions, and special comments on clinical use of the drugs. Each drug group is also listed in a table that gives both the generic and trade names, information on administration, and comments about the drug. Each chapter closes with an extensive Nursing Implications Summary, Key Terms, Review Questions, and Selected Readings, a list of suggested readings primarily from the nursing literature.

NURSING CONTENT

Much attention is given to emphasizing the relevant nursing information for the drugs discussed.

The Nursing Process Overview guides the nursing student in relating knowledge of medications to the overall plan of care for the patient. It is not meant to supplant the use of additional textbooks of nursing or current literature. Focus is on the pharmacologic factors rather than on the disease process itself. As mentioned previously, each Nursing Process Overview is divided into four parts. The first, Assessment, briefly summarizes key aspects of the assessment database. The second part, Nursing Diagnoses, gives examples of appropriate nursing diagnoses. The third part, Management, encompasses the planning and implementation phase of the nursing process. It identifies the type of data that should be monitored throughout therapy and some of the nursing activities needed to promote the drug activity or to foster patient well-being. The fourth part, Evaluation, describes the desired outcome of drug therapy.

The Nursing Implications Summary section supplements the Nursing Process Overview in assisting new practitioners and nursing students in translating knowledge of a drug action into appropriate nursing interventions. The specific clinical details of drug administration and of patient and family education are purposely separated from the body of the text and detailed in the Nursing Implications Summary section. The Nursing Implications Summary section does presuppose familiarity with the drug being discussed. A person using this section for reference on a completely unfamiliar drug would be well advised to first read the appropriate material on the drug in the body of the text.

We believe the presentation we have used to integrate basic pharmacology with nursing practice enables students to use the book effectively. Students can first master the scientific basis of the action of a particular drug. General comments on nursing assessment and management of patients are made in the text and are summarized and brought into focus in the Nursing Process Overview and in Alert boxes. However, when students enter the clinical setting, they require much more specific information than can be effectively included in the body of the text. By gathering this information in the Nursing Implications Summary and in the drug tables, we provide students concrete material for clinical use.

ACKNOWLEDGMENTS

The production of this textbook has involved several able and experienced members of the editorial staff at Mosby–Year Book. We wish to thank Robin Carter and Don Ladig for their special editorial contributions. We also thank Linda Wendling for the Instructor's Resource Manual; Shannon Canty and Carol Sullivan Wiseman for production; and Gail Morey Hudson for design.

Henry R. Besch, Jr., Ph.D., Chairman of the Department of Pharmacology and Toxicology at Indiana University School of Medicine, deserves special mention for the support and help he has given us during the continued development of all editions of this book. Mrs. Janie Siccardi, Administration Assistant in the Department of Pharmacology and Toxicology, has greatly aided us in this effort. Thanks also for the support of Lynne Goodykoontz, Ph.D., R.N., Dean of the School of Nursing, University of North Carolina at Greensboro. The continued contributions of Dr. Lynn R. Willis, Professor of Pharmacology, Indiana University School of Medicine, and Dr. Stephen Hatfield, Research Scientist, Eli Lilly and Company, are much appreciated. Illustrations in several chapters were rendered by Mark Swindle, Phil Wilson Artcraft, and Sylvia Eidam.

We would also like to thank two special colleagues who have lived with the book as long as we have. They are Dr. Stephen W. Queener, Research Scientist, Department of Antibiotic Culture Development, Eli Lilly and Company; and Dr. Kenneth S. Karb, Medical Oncologist, Greensboro, North Carolina.

Julia B. Freeman

Sherry L. Queener

Virginia Burke Karb

Contents

SECTION I

PRINCIPLES OF PHARMACOLOGY

Chapter 1, General Principles of Drug Action, covers the principles that govern the action of all drugs in the body. These basic concepts and terms recur repeatedly throughout the study of pharmacology. Initial study of these concepts will help the student approach the study of individual drugs and rationalize the manner in which they are used clinically.

Chapter 2, Legal Implications of Drug Therapy, places the legal status of modern drugs in perspective. This chapter also introduces the Schedule of Controlled Substances and the Drug Efficacy Study Implementation (DESI) rating—topics that recur at appropriate places throughout the text. Canadian drug classifications are covered in this chapter and referred to elsewhere in the text.

Chapter 3, Application of the Nursing Process to Drug Therapy, discusses the use of the nursing process with patients receiving drug therapy. The chapter also discusses patient education; medication errors; the roles of the nurse, physician, and pharmacist; and patient compliance.

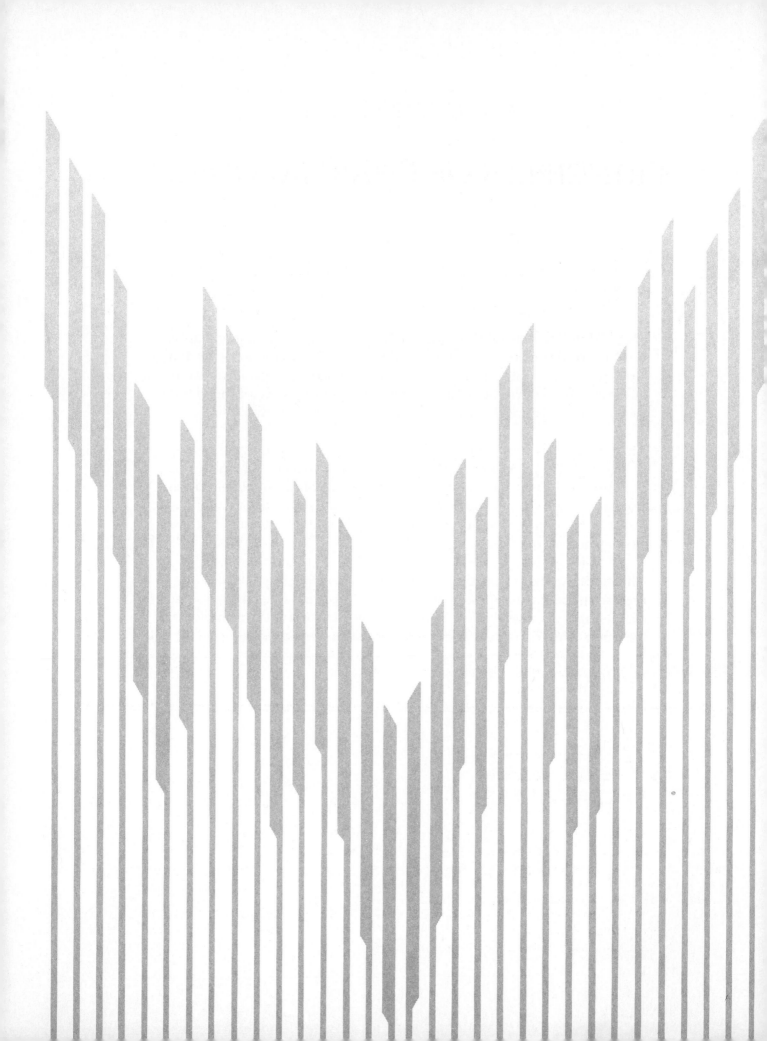

CHAPTER 1

General Principles of Drug Action

LEARNING OBJECTIVES

After studying this chapter, you should be able to:

- Describe the three principles of drug action.
- Describe three ways in which drugs interact with the body.
- Discuss the mechanisms producing unwanted drug reactions.
- Describe four types of allergic responses.
- Explain how drug dissolution, the lipid solubility of the drug, and the presence of gastric contents can influence absorption of drugs by enteral routes.
- Discuss factors influencing persistence, distribution, metabolism, and excretion of drugs from the body.
- Discuss advantages and disadvantages to common routes of administration.
- Explain how the elimination half-life of a drug influences the time required to attain a steady-state concentration of drug given at fixed intervals.
- Give examples of kinds of drug interactions.
- Suggest three possible explanations for biologic variation in patients' responses to drugs.

CHAPTER OVERVIEW

◆ Pharmacology is the study of the interaction of chemicals with living organisms to produce biologic effects. This book presents those chemicals that produce therapeutically useful effects, chemicals referred to as *drugs*. This chapter reviews the general principles of drug action that form the basis for understanding the actions of specific drugs.

◆ Most drugs produce biologic effects by interacting with specific receptors at the drug's site of action. The magnitude of the biologic effect produced by a drug is related to the concentration of the drug present at the site of action. Drugs differ not only in their intrinsic ability to produce an effect, but also in their ability to penetrate to the site of action and in their rates of removal from that site. **Pharmacokinetics** is the study of how drugs enter the body, reach their site of action, and are removed from the body. **Pharmacodynamics** is the study of drug action at the biochemical and physiologic level. Both the pharmacokinetics and the pharmacodynamics of a drug determine how a drug is administered, how often it is given, and what the dose is.

Nursing Process Overview
GENERAL PRINCIPLES OF PHARMACOLOGY

Assessment

The material presented in this chapter forms the framework on which subsequent specific information about drugs may be placed.

Study the mechanism of action of each drug class presented. Does this drug operate through specific receptors? Does it alter a body fluid or cell membranes? What are the anticipated effects? How does the typical patient manifest these effects? How does the patient's age influence drug administration?

Management

Consider the possible side effects of the action of the drug in tissues. For example, does the drug affect receptors in more than one organ or tissue? Note whether experience has indicated that allergies or idiosyncratic reactions are common with the drug. How might the drug's half-life influence the patient's response? What is the drug's dosing schedule?

Evaluation

Consider the balance between the positive effects of the drug and the negative reactions to understand what place a drug has in clinical practice. For example, some very effective drugs have limited clinical use because the side effects that they produce are unacceptable for most patients. Understanding the pharmacology of individual drugs thus becomes a more rational process and is much more easily accomplished. Chapter 3 deals with the application of the nursing process to drug therapy.

MECHANISMS OF DRUG ACTIONS
Drug Action is Determined by How a Drug Interacts with the Body

Drugs may chemically alter body fluids

Drugs that chemically alter body fluids directly enter a body fluid or compartment. An example is an antacid, which enters the stomach and neutralizes excess stomach acid. Alteration of the pH of stomach fluid is the only intended action of these drugs. Other examples are drugs that accumulate in the urine and alter the pH of that fluid. By acidifying the urine with ammonium chloride or alkalinizing the urine with sodium bicarbonate, the ion flow in the kidney is altered, and drug excretion patterns are changed.

Drugs may chemically alter cell membranes

Drugs that chemically alter cell membranes interact nonspecifically. The interaction involves a chemical attraction and is usually based on the lipid nature of the cell membrane and the lipid attraction of the drugs. General anesthetic gases act in this way. These agents dissolve in lipid-containing membranes and thereby alter the properties of the cells involved.

Drugs may act through specific receptors

The biologic activity of most drugs is determined by the ability of the drug to bind to a specific receptor; this is in turn determined by the chemical structure of the drug. The interaction of a drug with a specific receptor is similar to a lock-and-key fit (Figure 1-1). Only a certain critical portion of the drug is usually involved in binding, not the entire molecule. Drugs that have similar critical regions but differ in other parts of the molecule might also be expected to have similar biologic activity (*drugs D, E,* and *F* in Figure 1-1).

The ability to bind to the receptor and the capability of stimulating an action by the receptor are two different aspects of drug action. The ability to bind to the receptor is known as **affinity**. Drugs with high affinities have a high attraction to the receptor. The capability of stimulating the receptor to some action is called **efficacy**.

When receptors are highly specific and have high affinities for the compounds that bind to them, very low concentrations of these compounds may show biologic activity. For example, hormones naturally found in the body act through specific receptors. Some of these hormones are found in the bloodstream at concentrations of less than 1 picomole, or less than one part per trillion. Nevertheless, these tiny amounts are biologically effective because the hormone is detected and bound by the specific receptor.

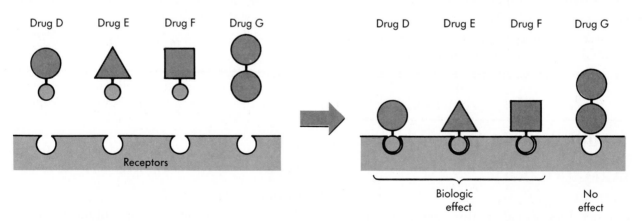

FIGURE 1-1

Lock-and-key fit between drugs and receptors through which they act. Site on receptor that interacts with drug has definite shape. Those drugs conforming to that shape can bind and produce biologic response. In example, only shape along lower surface of drug molecule is important in determining whether drug will bind to receptor.

Receptors also allow localization of drug effects to certain tissues. Each tissue or cell type possesses a unique array of specific receptors. For example, certain cells in the kidney possess specific receptors for antidiuretic hormone (see Chapter 50). These cells therefore have the capacity to respond to this hormone. Cells in other tissues that lack these receptors cannot respond to antidiuretic hormone.

The concept of drug receptors is one of the major concepts in pharmacology. The specific receptors called *drug receptors* are actually natural components of the body intended to respond to some chemical normally present in blood or tissues. For example, specific receptors within the brain respond to morphine and related compounds from the opium poppy, but the natural function of these receptors was not known until 1975 when endogenous morphine-like substances were discovered. It is now known that the brain and other tissues contain compounds called *enkephalins* and *endorphins*. These natural compounds bind to the so-called morphine receptor and are more potent than morphine in producing analgesia (see Chapter 44).

Any compound, either natural or synthetic, that binds to a specific receptor and produces a biologic effect by stimulating that receptor is called an **agonist.** For example, the hormone norepinephrine binds to specific sites in the heart called *beta-1 adrenergic receptors.* Stimulation of these receptors causes the heart to beat faster. The synthetic drug isoproterenol acts on the same receptors in the heart and produces the same effects. Both norepinephrine and isoproterenol are therefore called *agonists* for the beta-1 adrenergic receptor (see Chapter 10). Agonists have both affinity for receptors and efficacy because they cause some action by the receptor.

Some drugs produce their action not by stimulating receptors but by preventing natural substances from stimulating receptors. These drugs are called **antagonists.** For example, the drug propranolol blocks beta-1 adrenergic receptors and prevents agonists such as norepinephrine from stimulating the receptor normally. Propranolol therefore is classed as an antagonist of the action of norepinephrine. Antagonists have affinity for receptors but lack efficacy. When the receptor is occupied by an antagonist, the receptor cannot carry out its normal function.

Drugs do not Create Functions but Modify Existing Functions Within the Body

This principle explains the necessity for understanding the physiology of healthy humans and the changes caused by disease as a background for pharmacology. Drugs must always be considered in terms of the physiologic functions they alter in the body.

In no case do drugs *create* a function in a tissue or organ. For example, digitalis is a drug used to strengthen the action of the heart. Digitalis produces this effect by altering the existing pattern of ion flow into and out of heart cells; it does not create a new way for the heart to contract. Digitalis simply alters the natural process.

To emphasize this principle, subsequent chapters on drug families start with a brief description of the normal physiology influenced by that group of drugs.

No Drug Has a Single Action

The **desired action** of a drug is an expected, predictable response. Ideally, each drug would have the desired effect on one physiologic process and produce no other effect. However, all drugs have the potential for altering more than one function in the body. These unwanted actions are known as **side effects** or drug reactions. For example, digitalis strengthens the failing heart; this is the desired clinical effect of the drug. At the same time, however, it may cause erratic heartbeats. This action is an undesirable side effect.

Predictable reactions arising from the known pharmacologic action of a drug account for between 70% and 80% of all drug reactions. For example, barbiturates put a patient to sleep because they depress the central nervous system. However, excessive depression of the central nervous system is lethal because the brain centers that control breathing will be depressed. Respiratory depression would therefore be an expected toxic reaction when barbiturates are used at doses that allow the drug to accumulate in the body. This type of toxic reaction to excessive amounts of the drug may be distinguished from predictable side effects seen at normal doses of the drug. These predictable side effects are related to the secondary actions of the drug. For example, at normal therapeutic doses, barbiturates increase the drug-metabolizing activity of the liver. This ability is unrelated to the therapeutically desired activity of these drugs and, in fact, is the mechanism by which barbiturates cause a number of reactions with other drugs.

Unpredictable reactions to drugs account for between 20% and 30% of all drug reactions. Although experience shows that a certain percentage of the population may be expected to react to a drug in an unusual manner, it is often not possible to predict which individual will show the reaction. The unpredictable drug reactions are of two types: idiosyncratic and allergic.

Idiosyncratic reactions are unusual, unexpected reactions to a drug that are most often explained by a genetic difference between the patient and the normal population. For example, a small percentage of the population lacks the enzyme pseudocholinesterase, which is usually found in the bloodstream. Persons lacking this enzyme show no signs of this abnormality until they are exposed to drugs such as succinylcholine. Succinylcholine is a paralyzing agent used before surgery to relax the muscles and allow easy tracheal intubation. In most persons the drug is very short acting because it is destroyed by pseudocholinesterase. In persons lacking this enzyme, succinylcholine stays in the bloodstream, and the drug is very long acting. These patients require artificial ventilation until the paralyzing effects of succinylcholine wear off, whereas normally, people recover within a minute or so and require no assistance. This prolonged reaction to succinylcholine is one example of an idiosyncratic reaction.

Allergic reactions to drugs account for between 6% and 10% of all drug reactions. The allergic reaction may be triggered by the drug in its original form or by a metabolite of the drug formed in the body. Most drugs are not very allergenic, but others are very efficient at stimulating reactions from the immune system.

Drug allergies can be divided into four types, based on the mechanism of the immune reaction. Type I reactions occur soon after exposure and commonly produce **urticaria,** also called *hives*. These raised, irregularly shaped patches on the skin are frequently accompanied by severe itching. Although allergic reactions involving the skin are annoying, they are not usually serious; they can, however, progress to a severe acute allergic reaction that involves the cardiovascular and respiratory systems. This dangerous reaction is called **anaphylaxis** or anaphylactic shock. Anaphylaxis is marked by sudden contraction of the bronchiolar muscles and frequently by edema of the mouth and throat. These reactions may completely cut off air flow to the lungs. In addition, blood pressure falls, and the patient may go into shock. These violent reactions may occur within a very short time, and aggressive therapy is required to save the patient's life. Few people react to drugs in this way. All symptoms of type I reactions are caused by immunoglobulin E (IgE) antibodies, which are released in response to the drug and prompt target cells to discharge immune modulators such as histamine (see Chapter 24). Drugs associated with type I reactions include penicillins, cephalosporins, and iodides.

Type II reactions to drugs involve immunoglobulin M (IgM) or immunoglobulin G (IgG) antibodies, which can trigger lysis of specific blood cells under the appropriate conditions. These delayed reactions are sometimes called *autoimmune responses*. Examples include hemolytic anemia induced by methyldopa and thrombocytopenic purpura induced by quinidine. Procainamide and hydralazine can induce a con-

dition resembling systemic lupus erythematosus.

Type III reactions are frequently described as serum sickness, but symptoms include urticaria, pain in the joints, swollen lymph nodes, and fever. Penicillins, iodides, sulfonamides, and phenytoin can cause this type of delayed reaction, which may involve IgE, IgM, or IgG antibodies.

The type IV reaction is contact dermatitis, caused by topical application of drugs.

Any patient can suffer an allergic reaction in response to any drug, but certain drugs are more prone to cause reactions. Patients receiving these agents should be closely monitored to detect early signs of allergic responses and thereby protected from injury.

Allergic reactions do not occur during the first exposure to a drug because time is required for the immune system to develop the antibodies that cause these reactions. In theory, this should help predict which patients are at risk of allergic reactions; however, documenting prior exposure to a drug is not always easy. Patients do not always know the names of drugs they have received and are not always reliable sources of information on prior reactions to drugs. Moreover, persons may be unknowingly exposed to antibiotics or other drugs through food or milk, if the drugs are improperly used in animal medicine.

PRINCIPLES RELATING DRUG DOSE TO DRUG ACTION
Pharmacokinetics

Factors controlling drug absorption by enteral routes

To be effective systemically, a drug must be present in the blood in a free or available form. For most medications, less than the total amount of administered drug is ultimately available to produce effects on target tissues. The term **bioavailability** describes what proportion of the administered drug is available to produce systemic effects. With a drug having low bioavailability, most of the administered dose of the drug is lost or destroyed, never reaching the blood in a form that can be effective. Drugs that are freely and rapidly absorbed have a high bioavailability. The many factors that can influence bioavailability are discussed in the following sections.

Drug dissolution. About 80% of drugs used in clinical practice are administered orally, primarily because of the ease and convenience of administration by this route. The drug may be given in liquid form, but most often it is given in a solid form such as a pill, tablet, or capsule (Table 1-1). To achieve this solid form, the drug is usually mixed with other compounds that serve various functions. Starches and other compounds may be added as inert fillers, especially when the actual amount of drug required per

Table 1-1   Forms of Medications

Form	Description	Form	Description
Capsules	Solid dosage forms for oral use in which medication is enclosed in gelatin shell that dissolves in stomach or intestine. Gelatin of capsules is colored to aid in product identification. Manufacturers use distinctive shapes for identifying their capsules.	Suspension	Finely divided drug particles that are suspended in suitable liquid medium before being injected or taken orally. Suspensions must not be injected intravenously.
Douche	Aqueous solution used as cleansing or antiseptic agent for part of body or body cavity. Douches are usually sold as powder or liquid concentrate to be dissolved or diluted before use.	Sustained action drug	Form of medication that is altered so that dissolution is slow and continuous for extended period. Total dosage in sustained action medication is greater than for regular formulations because drug is not all released at once.
Elixirs	Clear fluids for oral use that contain primarily water and alcohol with glycerin and sorbitol or another sweetener sometimes added. Alcohol content of these preparations varies.	Syrups	Medication dissolved in concentrated solution of sugar such as sucrose. Flavors may be added to mask unpleasant taste of certain medications.
Glycerites	Solutions of drugs in glycerin for external use. Solution must be at least 50% glycerin.	Tablets	Solid dosage forms, frequently shaped like disks or cylinders, that contain, in addition to drug, one or more of following ingredients: binder (adhesive substance that allows tablet to stick together), disintegrators (substances promoting tablet dissolution in body fluids), lubricants (required for efficient manufacturing), and fillers (inert ingredients to make tablet size convenient).
Patches	Inner surface of the patch contacts skin and allows transdermal absorption of lipid-soluble drugs. The total amount of drug on the patch is very large, but typically only a small fraction is absorbed.		
Pills	Solid dosage forms for oral use in which drug and various vehicles are formed into small globules or ovoids. True pills are rare; most have been replaced by compressed tablets.	Enteric-coated drugs	Solid dosage forms for oral use. Medication in tablet form is coated with materials designed not to dissolve in stomach. Coatings dissolve in intestine, where medication may be absorbed.
Solution	Liquid preparations, usually in water, containing one or more dissolved compounds. Solutions for oral use may contain flavoring and coloring agents. Solutions for intravenous injection must be sterile and particle free. Other injectable solutions must be sterile. Solutions of certain drugs may also be used externally.	Press-coated or layered drugs	Preformed tablet that has another layer of material pressed on or around it. This practice allows incompatible ingredients to be separated and causes them to be dissolved at slightly different rates.
		Tincture	Alcoholic or water-alcohol solutions of drugs.
		Transdermal creams	Relatively lipid-soluble drugs that may be absorbed transdermally. Dosage is usually measured in inches of cream extruded from tube.
Suppositories	Solid dosage forms to be inserted into body cavity where medication is released as solid melts or dissolves. Suppositories frequently contain cocoa butter (cacao butter or theobroma oil), which is solid at room temperature but liquid at body temperature, or glycerin, polyethylene glycol, or gelatin, which dissolves in secretions from mucous membranes.	Troches (also called *lozenges* or *pastilles*)	Solid dosage forms, frequently shaped like disks or cylinders, that contain drug, flavor, sugar, and mucilage. Troches dissolve or disintegrate in mouth, releasing medication such as antiseptic or anesthetic for action in mouth or throat. Troches dissolve more slowly than tablets.

dose is too small to be conveniently handled. Adhesive substances called *binders* may also be added to allow the tablet to hold together after it is compressed in manufacture. Other compounds called *disintegrators* may be required to allow the tablet to absorb water and to break apart. Lubricants are frequently added to prevent the tablet from sticking to machinery during manufacture. These other additions to the dosage form may make up the bulk of the tablet. For

example, in tablets containing 100,000 units of penicillin the active ingredient, potassium penicillin, makes up only 11% of the tablet mass.

To be effective, the solid dose of a drug must break apart in the gastrointestinal tract and allow the drug to go into solution. Only the dissolved drug is absorbed from the gastrointestinal tract into the blood. Breakdown of the solid dosage form is the required first step in absorption of the drug; therefore any variability in this process can affect how rapidly and completely the drug is absorbed. The formulation of a tablet or capsule obviously affects dissolution rates. Tablets from different manufacturers that contain the same amount of active ingredient but different types and amounts of inert ingredients may not be identical in clinical action because each formulation may have different dissolution properties. Tablets may also change with age and conditions of storage. Older tablets tend to dry out and become more difficult to disintegrate, leading to reduced bioavailability of the drug.

The gastrointestinal tract. Food may interefere with dissolution and absorption of certain drugs. However, some drugs are so irritating to the stomach that food may be useful to dilute high local concentrations of the drug. There is considerable variation from person to person in gastric emptying times and, therefore, in the length of time the drug spends in the acid environment of the stomach. In addition, the amount of acid in the stomach varies with the individual and the time of day. The very young and the elderly have less stomach acid than middle-aged persons. Lower acidity may mean less drug is degraded and more is available for absorption.

Chemical properties of the drug. In addition to the physical state of the drug, its chemical nature determines how satisfactory oral administration will be. First, to pass through the membrane lining the gastrointestinal tract, a drug must be relatively **lipid soluble** because the membranes themselves contain a high concentration of lipid. Ionic (charged) forms of drugs do not easily pass through these membranes. Many drugs can exist in an ionic state or in an uncharged lipid-soluble state, depending on the chemical environment (pH) in which the drug is found. This environment changes along the gastrointestinal tract (Figure 1-2). The stomach fluid is highly acidic. A drug such as aspirin, which is a weak acid, is converted from a charged to an uncharged form by the strong acid in the stomach. Because the uncharged form of the drug can readily diffuse through the lipid membranes of the stomach cells, the drug is rapidly absorbed. In contrast, drugs such as penicillins are not stable in the acid of the stomach, and part of the dose is destroyed rather than absorbed.

Enteric coatings on tablets or capsules protect some drugs that are sensitive to the acid in the stomach (see Table 1-1). These coatings are inert at low (acidic) pH but soluble at higher (alkaline) pH. Therefore the drug passes through the stomach and is released in the intestine. Enteric coatings are also used for drugs that are highly irritating to the gastric mucosa.

The fluids in the small intestine are slightly alkaline.

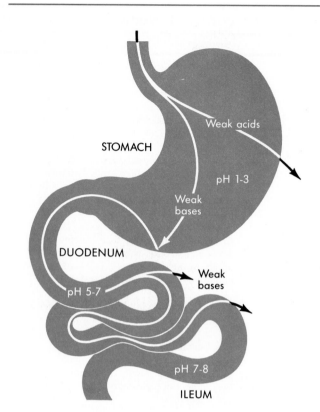

FIGURE 1-2

Effect of pH on ability of drugs to cross gastrointestinal membranes. Strongly acidic environment of stomach (pH 1 to 3) maintains weak acids in uncharged form, which is more easily absorbed. Weak bases remain charged in stomach but are converted to uncharged forms as pH approaches neutrality (pH 7) or becomes slightly alkaline (pH 7 to 8).

This higher pH favors the absorption of weakly basic drugs because at this pH range weak bases are uncharged (Figure 1-2). The small intestine also has an enormous surface area for drug absorption, which makes it a major site of absorption. However, some drugs, particularly proteins such as insulin or growth hormone, are destroyed in the small intestine by the action of digestive enzymes from the pancreas.

Drugs that are absorbed from the small intestine are transported by the portal circulation directly to the liver before entering the circulation to the rest of the body (Figure 1-3). The liver metabolizes a significant proportion of certain drugs before they can enter the general circulation. The term **first-pass phenomenon** refers to the process of absorption of a drug into the portal circulation, with metabolism of the drug in the liver before it reaches systemic circulation. Liver metabolism often inactivates drugs

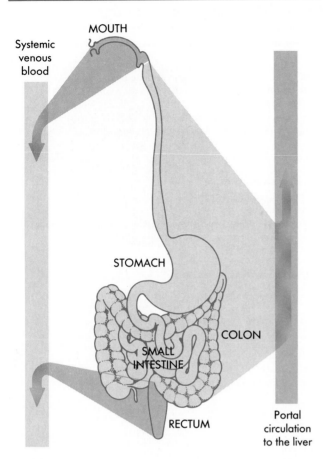

FIGURE 1-3

Two circulatory pathways for materials absorbed from gastrointestinal tract. Materials absorbed from stomach, small intestine, or colon enter portal circulation, which perfuses liver before returning to heart. Materials absorbed from these sites are exposed first to action of liver microsomal enzymes and then are circulated to rest of body. In contrast, absorption through membranes lining mouth or rectum deliver material directly to systemic circulation.

and, in this case, the first-pass phenomenon lowers the amount of active drug released into the systemic circulation. For example, morphine is very rapidly extracted from the blood and metabolized by the liver; therefore to achieve the same level of pain relief, it is necessary to administer six times more morphine orally than intramuscularly. In contrast, the related drug codeine is much less affected by the first-pass effect; therefore it takes only two times more codeine orally than intramuscularly to produce the same degree of pain relief. In these examples, the larger oral doses compensate for the drug lost through inactivation by the liver.

The first-pass phenomenon may be avoided by using other routes of administration, such as sublingual (drug dissolved under the tongue), buccal (drug dissolved between the cheek and gum), and rectal routes (Figure 1-3). Drugs administered by these routes are absorbed directly across the mucous membranes and rapidly enter the systemic circulation. The sublingual and buccal routes are useful when a palatable, very lipid-soluble drug is involved. The rectal route is useful, especially when a patient is unconscious. The best physical form for a drug intended for rectal use is a suppository that will melt in the rectum and release the drug for absorption (Table 1-2).

Factors controlling drug absorption by parenteral routes

The *parenteral routes* of drug administration are those that require injection of the drug into the skin, muscle, or blood (see Chapter 6). Injection necessarily involves breaking the skin, and sterile technique must be used to prevent bacteria from gaining entry (Table 1-2). Special precautions often must be taken to avoid producing undue tissue damage with irritating drugs. Sometimes these precautions involve preventing the drug from contacting the skin; other drugs require dilution before administration.

Subcutaneous injection (under the skin) is appropriate for small drug volumes and for drugs intended to be slowly absorbed. Insulin is an example of such a drug. When very slow absorption is desired, drugs may be formulated as solid inserts that release drug over prolonged periods. Examples include the inserts that release hormones and provide birth control for several years (see Chapter 53).

Intramuscular injection (into a muscle) is appropriate when larger volumes of a drug must be injected. Absorption from intramuscular sites is faster than from subcutaneous sites because muscles are better supplied with blood vessels than is skin. Absorption from subcutaneous or intramuscular sites can be speeded somewhat by applying heat or massage to the site to accelerate blood flow. Absorption can be slowed by decreasing blood flow to the injection site by applying ice packs or by the simultaneous injection of a drug such as epinephrine, which constricts blood vessels.

The forms of drugs intended for intramuscular or subcutaneous injection may be relatively insoluble. Some drugs are formulated specifically to dissolve slowly and therefore to be absorbed slowly from injection sites. These dosage forms are called *depot injections*.

Intravenous injection (directly into a vein) requires special precautions. Drugs that are to be used intravenously must always be in solution and can contain no particulate matter. Some drugs irritate the veins and cause thrombophlebitis if administered at too

Table 1-2   Summary of Major Routes for Systemic Administration of Drugs

Description	Advantages	Disadvantages
ORAL		
Drug swallowed, absorbed from stomach and/or small intestine	Route is convenient. Procedure is not sterile. Route is economical.	Unpleasant taste may cause patient to discontinue medication. Irritation to gastric mucosa may induce nausea and vomiting. Patient must be conscious. Drug may be partly or completely destroyed by digestive juices. Absorbed drug enters portal circulation to liver, where drug may be destroyed.
SUBLINGUAL		
Drug dissolved under tongue, absorbed across mucous membranes of mouth	Route is convenient. Procedure is not sterile. Drug enters general circulation before passing through liver.	Route is not useful for drugs that taste bad. Irritation to oral mucosa may occur. Patient must be conscious. Only very lipid-soluble drugs are absorbed rapidly enough to be administered by this route.
BUCCAL		
Drug dissolved between cheek and gum, absorbed across mucous membrane of mouth	Same as sublingual.	Same as sublingual.
TRANSDERMAL		
Drug absorbed directly through skin	Dosage is continuous. Procedure is not sterile. Drug enters general circulation before passing through liver.	Route is effective only for lipid-soluble drugs. Local irritation can occur. Discarded patches may pose danger of poisoning.
RECTAL		
Drug inserted into rectum, absorbed through mucous membranes of rectum	Route may be used for unconscious or vomiting patient. Drug enters general circulation before passing through liver.	Route is inconvenient. Drug may irritate rectal mucosa. Drug must be made as suppository.
INHALATION		
Drug inhaled as gas or aerosol	Route is for drugs intended to act directly on lung. Route is useful for drugs that are gases at room temperature and are very lipid soluble (i.e., inhalation anesthetics).	Irritation of lung mucosa may occur.
SUBCUTANEOUS		
Drug injected under skin	Route is useful for drugs in soluble or relatively insoluble forms. Route may be used in unconscious or uncooperative patients.	Sterile procedures are necessary. Pain and irritation at site may occur.

Table 1-2   Summary of Major Routes for Systemic Administration of Drugs—cont'd

Description	Advantages	Disadvantages
INTRAMUSCULAR		
Drug injected into muscle mass	Relatively rapid absorption occurs because blood supply is good in muscles. Route is useful for drugs in soluble or relatively insoluble forms. Route may be used in unconscious or uncooperative patients.	Sterile procedures are necessary. Minor pain is common. Irritation and local reactions may occur.
INTRAVENOUS		
Drug injected directly into vein	Route allows direct control of blood concentration of drug. Route allows most rapid attainment of effective blood levels.	Sterile procedures are necessary. Too-rapid injection may produce transient, dangerously high blood concentrations of drug.

high a concentration. Other drugs must be injected slowly to avoid toxic concentrations of the drug reaching the heart or other vital organs. The intravenous route is valuable when drug concentrations must be maintained continuously, but potential harm to the patient is greater by this route.

Special injection routes may be employed in certain circumstances. For example, local anesthetics may be injected into the spinal column to produce certain types of anesthesia. Other drugs may be injected directly into body cavities or joints. Such routes are employed when conventional routes of injection do not allow high enough drug concentrations to be achieved at the desired site of drug action.

Factors controlling drug persistence in the blood

After a drug has entered the blood, its ultimate fate is determined by the chemical propeties of the drug and the way it is affected by the blood and tissues it contacts. Some drugs are metabolized by enzymes in the blood. An example is succinylcholine. Drugs that persist in the blood for any length of time are usually bound to proteins in the blood rather than being simply dissolved directly in plasma.

The most important carrier protein is albumin, which is formed in the liver and released into the blood. Drugs bound to albumin or other carrier proteins remain in the blood because these proteins as a rule do not diffuse through capillary walls. Drug binding to albumin is a reversible process, and an

equilibrium is established in the blood between drug bound to the protein and drug that is free in solution. Only free drug is able to diffuse into tissues, interact with receptors, and produce biologic effects. The same proportion of bound and free drug is maintained in the blood at all times. Thus when free drug leaves the blood, some drug is released from protein binding to reestablish the proper ratio between bound and free drug.

The anticoagulant dicumarol is an example of a drug that binds to plasma protein. In the blood, 99% of this drug is bound to plasma albumin. Therefore only 1% of the blood content of the dicumarol is free to diffuse to its site of action or to its sites of elimination. The net effect of binding to albumin is to create a reservoir of the drug that is released to replenish free drug removed to other sites. In general, drugs that do not bind to plasma albumin remain in the body for shorter periods than drugs that are tightly bound. A drug such as dicumarol, which is very strongly bound to albumin, remains in the body for up to 3 days. Drugs that are bound to plasma proteins are thus characterized by longer duration of action.

Factors controlling drug distribution throughout the body

High lipid solubility and low protein binding favor diffusion of a drug through membranes. All transport into tissues involves passing through lipid-containing membranes, a process that is difficult for water-soluble compounds but easy for lipid-soluble agents. High concentrations of free drug in the blood also favors diffusion into tissues; high protein binding lowers free drug concentrations in blood and impedes diffusion into tissues.

Factors controlling drug metabolism in the body

Biotransformation is the ability of living organisms to modify the chemical structure of drugs. Most drugs are metabolized in the body by the liver, specifically by the microsomal enzyme system. These enzymes allow the body to metabolize potentially toxic compounds. Many types of chemical transformations are carried out, but in general these reactions create water-soluble compounds that are more easily eliminated from the body by the kidneys. These enzymes have two important properties. First, the enzymes are relatively nonspecific. Therefore many drugs may be metabolized by the same enzyme system. Second, the liver can synthesize more enzyme in response to being exposed to higher-than-normal concentrations of certain drugs. This property means that the liver can increase its capacity to destroy a drug over a period of a few days. This increase in microsomal enzyme content in the liver is called *enzyme induction.*

Biotransformation often inactivates drugs, but biotransformation does not always produce inactive products. For example, drugs such as codeine, diazepam, and amitriptyline are all converted by the liver into metabolites that are also active. A few drugs are not active until they are biotransformed by the liver. For example, the anticancer drug cyclophosphamide is inactive, but one of its metabolites produced in the liver is a highly reactive alkylating agent that is effective against cancer cells.

The liver is by far the most important site for biotransformation of drugs, but it is not the only one. For example, systemically administered prostaglandins are destroyed almost instantaneously in the lung. The kidney is another important site for biotransformation of certain types of drugs.

Biotransformation may be carried out by bacteria within the colon. This process may limit absorption of the drug from the bowel after oral administration, or it may be a mechanism by which the drug is eliminated from the blood after administration by parenteral routes.

Factors controlling drug elimination

The three main routes by which drugs may be eliminated from the body involve the liver, kidney, and bowel.

Elimination in the feces. The first route involves uptake of the drug by the liver, release into bile, and elimination in the feces. For some drugs, such as erythromycin and certain penicillins, the concentration of drug in the bile may be much higher than its concentration in the blood. Because between 600 and 1000 ml of bile is formed each day, this route of elimination may dispose of significant amounts of drug. However, drugs in the bile enter the small intestine, where they may be reabsorbed into the blood, returned to the liver, and again secreted into bile. This secretion and reabsorption process is called **enterohepatic circulation.** Drugs that are extensively reabsorbed from the intestinal tract after biliary secretion obviously persist in the body much longer than drugs that remain in the lumen of the intestine and pass out with the feces. If the reabsorbed drug is in an active form, the duration of action of the drug is prolonged.

Elimination in urine after metabolism by the liver. The second route of elimination involves the liver and the kidney. Common biotransformations of drugs by the liver include formation of glucuronides, hydroxylations, and acetylations. The kidney is also capable of forming glucuronides and sulfates. All these reactions tend to form more polar compounds, which can be more efficiently excreted by the kidney. For example, a drug such as the antibiotic chloramphenicol normally enters glomerular fluid by passive diffusion but is reabsorbed from the tubules and reenters the blood. In the liver, however, chloramphenicol is transformed into chloramphenicol glucuronide. In this form the drug enters glomerular fluid, cannot be reabsorbed from the tubules, and hence is excreted in the urine.

Various factors may influence the ability of the liver to metabolize drugs. For example, premature infants and neonates have immature livers that are incapable of carrying out certain biotransformations. Therefore these patients may accumulate drugs that must be metabolized in the liver before they can be excreted by the kidney. Patients who have suffered hepatic damage, such as those who suffer from chronic alcoholism, may also accumulate drugs normally excreted by this route.

Elimination in the urine without metabolism by the liver. Some drugs are not extensively metabolized anywhere in the body and are excreted unchanged in the urine. This excretion may take place in one of two ways. Some drugs are excreted by passive diffusion into glomerular fluid and are not extensively reabsorbed; hence these drugs enter the urine. Other drugs are actively secreted by specific systems in the renal tubule. These active processes lead to more rapid drug elimination and allow much higher urinary concentrations of drug to be achieved. The antibiotic penicillin G is a good example of a drug that is actively secreted by the renal tubule. Half of an intravenous dose of penicillin G can be eliminated in about 20 minutes by active tubular secretion. In contrast, an antibiotic such as tetracycline, which is eliminated primarily by passive diffusion in the kidney, persists in the body for several hours.

Drugs that are normally eliminated unchanged in the urine accumulate in the body when there is a loss of kidney function. Patients with kidney disease must frequently have drug dosages lowered to compensate for the reduced ability of the kidney to excrete various substances. Kidney function declines with age even in healthy persons, and elderly patients may show a reduced ability to excrete drugs in their urine. Certain drugs such as aminoglycoside antibiotics are themselves nephrotoxic and may directly damage the kidneys and thereby interfere with their own excretion.

Pharmacodynamics

Dose-response curve

The relationship between the dose of drug administered and the response produced is described by an S-shaped (sigmoid) curve called the *dose-response curve* (Figure 1-4). This curve is obtained by plotting the observed response (on a linear scale) against the dose of the drug used to elicit that response (on a logarithmic scale) and illustrates several important quantitative properties about drugs. First, there is a threshold for each drug-induced response. Doses of drug below that threshold will produce no observable effect. Second, the drug-induced response will reach a plateau rather than increase indefinitely. For example,

the drug shown in Figure 1-4 produces its maximum response at a dose of about 512 units. Doubling the dose produces no detectable further effect. Even beginning at lower drug concentrations, doubling the dose still does not double the effect. In this example the 50% maximum response to this drug is produced by a dose of 16 units, but at double that dose (32 units), only about 70%, not 100%, of the maximum response is produced. In summary, the dose-response curve demonstrates that a finite dose is required to see a response and that the intensity of the response produced is not linearly related to the dose.

The dose-response curve in Figure 1-4 shows the effect of a drug on an individual (or average responses from several individuals). The same type of curve is produced when the drug response is instead defined as an all-or-none phenomenon (such as asleep versus awake) and the logarithm of the drug dose is plotted against the percentage of patients who show the drug effect at that given dose. The plateau for this curve is the drug dose at which all patients respond, and the threshold is the drug dose below which no patients respond. The recommended therapeutic dose of the drug is a dose at which most patients respond to the drug. Figure 1-5 shows this second type of dose-response curve.

Drugs produce multiple predictable biologic effects, and for each of these effects a dose-response curve may be drawn. For example, the drug digitalis, although increasing the force of contraction of the

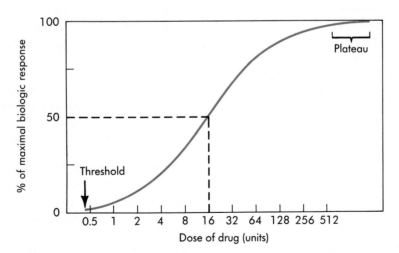

FIGURE 1-4

Log dose-response curve. Percent of maximum biologic response is plotted on linear scale on vertical axis. Dose of drug is plotted on logarithmic scale on horizontal axis. Threshold is dose of drug required to cause measurable response. Plateau is region of curve where increasing drug dose does not increase biologic response.

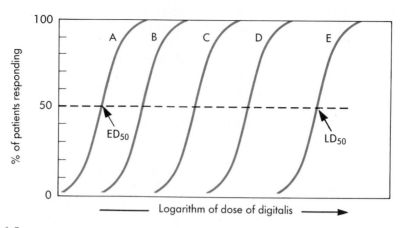

FIGURE 1-5

Log dose-response curves for effects of digitalis. Percent of patients responding to digitalis is plotted on vertical axis, and dose of digitalis is plotted on logarithmic scale on horizontal axis. These undesirable effects are all dose-related responses to digitalis. *Curve A,* strengthened force of contraction of the heart produced by digitalis; *curve B,* nausea; *curve C,* visual disturbances; *curve D,* cardiac arrhythmias; *curve E,* ventricular fibrillation and death.

failing heart, also produces nausea, causes neurologic symptoms such as headaches and visual disturbances, induces cardiac arrhythmias, and ultimately triggers ventricular fibrillation. Each of these responses can be plotted as a dose-response curve (see Figure 1-5). When the dose-response curves for these other reactions to the curve for the principal therapeutic effect are compared, nausea is seen as an effect observed in a significant number of patients receiving therapeutic doses of digitalis. With increasing doses of the drug, more and more patients suffer visual disturbances and arrhythmias. At drug concentrations well above normal therapeutic doses, ventricular fibrillation occurs. These predictable drug reactions become an important part of patient care. For digitalis, the visual disturbances are a warning that the concentration of digitalis in the patient is approaching concentrations that can cause cardiac arrhythmias and ventricular fibrillation.

Each drug may be described as relatively safe or relatively dangerous, based on consideration of dose-response curves such as those in Figure 1-5. For example, nausea is frequently associated with the use of digitalis because doses that produce nausea are only slightly greater than those that increase the force of contraction of the heart. Doses of digitalis that produce more serious reactions are only slightly higher than those that cause nausea. Digitalis therefore is a drug with a narrow margin of safety; doses must be rigorously controlled, and great care must be taken

to keep blood levels of the drug within a very narrow range. In contrast, a drug with a wide margin of safety, such as penicillin G, may be given in doses greatly exceeding normal therapeutic doses without much danger of producing direct toxic effects.

Therapeutic index. The relative safety of drugs is also sometimes expressed as the therapeutic index. The therapeutic index (TI) is the ratio of the dose of the drug lethal in 50% of the tested population (LD_{50}) to the dose of the drug therapeutically effective in 50% of the tested population (ED_{50}), or $TI = LD_{50}/ED_{50}$. Obviously, these figures come from tests conducted in animals. A drug with a high therapeutic index has a wide safety margin; the lethal dose is greatly in excess of the therapeutic dose. A drug with a low therapeutic index is more dangerous for the patient because small increases over normal doses may be sufficient to induce toxic reactions.

Time course of drug action

Drugs may enter the body by a number of routes, but except for the intravenous route, some time will be required for the drug to enter the blood after administration. There is also a delay between the time the drug enters the blood and the time the drug reaches its site of action. If the response to a single dose of a drug is measured as a function of time, the pattern shown in Figure 1-6 is observed. The time for the **onset** of drug action is the time it takes after the drug is administered to reach a concentration that

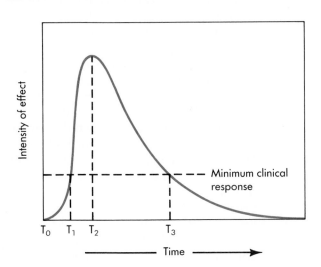

FIGURE 1-6

Time course of action of single dose of drug. Drug is administered at T_0. Time interval between T_0 and T_1 represents time of onset of action of drug. Peak action occurs at T_2. Time interval between T_0 and T_2 represents time for peak action. At T_3, drug response falls below minimum required for clinical effectiveness. Time interval between T_1 and T_3 represents duration of action of drug.

given repeatedly for a course of therapy. The drug **half-life** or elimination half-time is how long it takes for elimination processes to reduce the blood concentration of the drug by half. For example, the peak concentration of penicillin G in the blood occurs a few moments after the drug is administered intravenously. Thereafter penicillin is rapidly excreted by the kidney and disappears from the blood. The length of time required for these processes to decrease the blood concentration of penicillin by 50% is the drug half-life or elimination half-time, which for penicillin G is about 20 minutes. Therefore 20 minutes after the intravenous dose of penicillin, only half of the initial concentration of the drug remains in the blood. After 40 minutes only a quarter of the initial concentration remains, and after 60 minutes only an eighth remains. During each succeeding 20-minute period the remaining concentration decreases by half.

When drug absorption is not instantaneous, the elimination processes compete with the absorptive processes, delaying the appearance of peak blood concentrations of the drug. The example shown in Figure 1-7 is for a drug with a half-life of 1 hour. When the drug is given intravenously, the highest concentration

produces a response. As drug continues to be absorbed, higher concentrations of the drug reach the site of action, and the response increases. As the drug is being absorbed, it is also subject to the influences that tend to eliminate it from the body. Ultimately elimination dominates, and the concentration of the drug in the body begins to fall. As a result, the response will also begin to diminish. The **time to peak effect** is the time it takes for the drug to reach its highest effective concentration. The **duration** of action of a drug is the time during which the drug is present in a concentration large enough to produce a response and is determined by the rates of absorption and elimination.

Insulins are good examples of drugs for which an understanding of onset and duration of action is critical for successful drug therapy. Insulin lowers blood sugar levels, and the peak drug action must be planned to coincide with the absorptive period after meals when blood sugar levels rise rapidly if no insulin is present. If insulin is injected at the proper dose but at the wrong time, a serious hypoglycemic (low blood sugar) reaction may endanger the patient.

Half-life. The concepts of onset and duration of drug action are also important for understanding the proper timing of administration of drugs that are

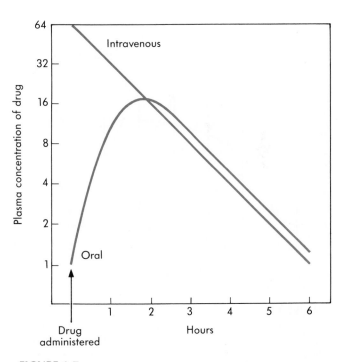

FIGURE 1-7

Absorption and elimination rates for drug administered by oral or intravenous route. Plasma concentration of drug is plotted on logarithmic scale on vertical axis.

is achieved on administration and decreases thereafter because of the elimination processes. When the same dose is given orally, the drug is absorbed relatively slowly so that drug elimination is responsible for lowering the peak drug concentration that can be achieved. Once in general circulation, however, the drug is eliminated in the same way, no matter what the initial route of administration.

Plateau principle. When a drug is given repeatedly for therapy at fixed dosage intervals, its concentration in the blood reaches a plateau and is maintained at that level until the dose or the frequency of administration is changed. An example is shown in Figure 1-8, in which a rapidly absorbed drug is administered at fixed intervals. The concentration of the drug in the blood fluctuates around a mean value, which approaches a plateau value after four elimination half-times have passed; this happens regardless of the dose or frequency of administration, as long as they are constant. The actual dose of the drug and the frequency of dosage determine the plateau concentration of drug in the blood, but they do not determine how long it will take to reach that plateau.

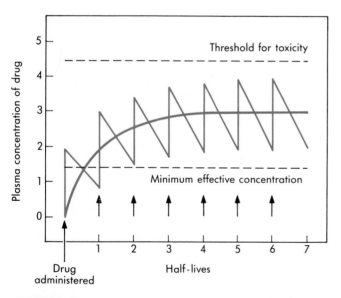

FIGURE 1-8

Plateau principle. In example, drug is administered once every elimination half-time for drug. Plasma concentration of drug rises and falls as drug doses are rapidly absorbed and slowly eliminated. Drug accumulates over time so that after four elimination half-times average plasma concentration of drug has reached steady state. By adjusting dose, average plasma concentration of drug may be adjusted.

As an example of this plateau principle, consider a patient who is given a drug with a half-life of 24 hours. The patient takes one tablet at 8 AM every day. In 4 days the amount of drug being taken in each dose roughly equals the amount of drug being eliminated each day; the plateau has been reached (Figure 1-9, *patient A*). The dose in this case is sufficient to produce clinically effective blood levels but is below the level that produces toxicity. On day 6 the patient decides to take two tablets instead of one tablet each morning. As a result, the mean concentration of the drug in the blood rises, and after 4 days (four elimination half-times) a new plateau concentration is reached. At this new higher level, some drug toxicity is seen. When the patient returns to the old dosage schedule of one tablet daily, the mean drug concentration returns to the original plateau concentration after 4 days (4 elimination half-times) and is maintained until the dosage amount or intervals change.

Patient B in Figure 1-9 receives the same drug as patient A, but patient B takes one tablet every 12 hours instead of once daily. As a result, the plateau concentration of drug in the blood is higher in patient B than in patient A taking 1 tablet every 24 hours; it is the same as for patient A taking 2 tablets daily. Note, however, that it still takes 4 days (four elimination half-times) to reach the plateau concentration. After 3 days of therapy, patient B mentions some unusual symptoms, which the nurse recognizes as toxic reactions to the drug. On the basis of this report the physician reduces the frequency of drug administration to 1 tablet daily. After 5 days on this dosage schedule the patient complains that the medication effect wears off by the early morning hours. The physician therefore advises the patient to take half a tablet every 12 hours. This dosage regimen minimizes the fluctuations in drug concentration in the blood; the mean plateau concentration is ultimately the same.

These examples illustrate the importance of maintaining regular dosage schedules and adhering to prescribed doses and dosage intervals. If the total dose of drug administered each drug half-life is held constant, the average concentration of the drug in the blood stays constant. Timing of the dose (single dose or divided doses) affects the peak concentration and the minimal concentration of the drug in the blood. For some drugs, these variations may not be critical, but for many drugs the difference between a safe dose and a toxic dose is not very great.

Monitoring levels of certain drugs in the blood has become a routine part of patient care in many settings. Direct assays for drugs allow physicians to adjust doses to ensure safe and effective blood levels of such drugs as gentamicin, amikacin, digitoxin, and phenytoin, which have a low therapeutic index.

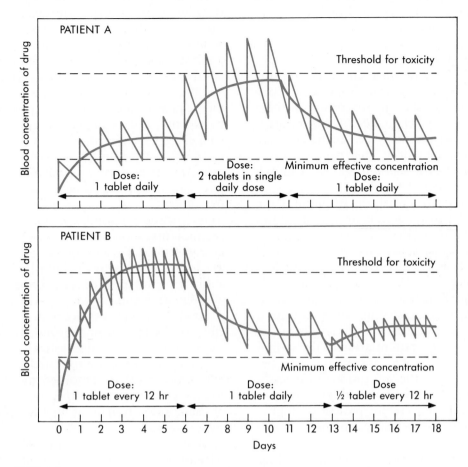

FIGURE 1-9

Plateau principle in practice. Patient A receives drug with half-time of 24 hr. Increasing dose of drug from one to two tablets in single daily dose increases plateau concentration of drug. In contrast, patient B illustrates that, by dividing dose (taking half a tablet every 12 hr rather than 1 tablet once daily), fluctuations in drug concentration are minimized.

The nurse's responsibility in dealing with patients being monitored in this way may include drawing blood samples at specific times or adjusting the dosage or timing of doses in response to the physician's instructions.

Drug Interactions

Definition of a drug interaction

A **drug interaction** is any modification of the action of one drug by another drug. Drug interactions may either potentiate or diminish the action of the drugs involved. **Synergism** is a special drug interaction in which the effect of two drugs combined is greater than the effect expected if the individual effects of the two drugs independently were added together.

Drug interactions are commonly encountered in clinical practice and are sometimes actively sought as part of a therapeutic program. An excellent example is the treatment of chronic moderate hypertension, which frequently involves several drugs, each amplifying the action of the others to lower the blood pressure.

The negative side of drug interaction is that the therapeutic result expected from a drug can be greatly distorted by other drugs. This negative side can be diminished when health care personnel are aware of the major drug interactions; are thorough in determining which drugs a patient is taking, including over-the-counter drugs, alcohol, and tobacco; and give careful instruction to patients about drugs that interact with their prescribed medication.

Comprehensive lists of drug interactions have been published and may be referred to if necessary when information about rare or unlikely interactions is sought. Clinically important common interactions are discussed with each drug class in this text and are summarized in the Appendix.

Origin of drug interactions

Drug interactions may arise when one drug alters the pharmacokinetics of another drug. For example, one drug may alter the dissolution, absorption, protein binding, metabolism, or elimination of another drug. Drug interactions of the pharmacokinetic type are generally one sided. One drug alters the pharmacokinetics of a second drug without its own pharmacokinetics being altered. The effect of the drug interaction is to change the actual concentration of the second drug in the blood and at its site of action. For instance, if one drug decreases the absorption of a second drug, the actual concentration of the second drug is diminished, and therefore the usual dose does not give the expected result. The same effect is produced if the metabolism or elimination of the second drug is increased by the first drug. Alternatively, if one drug increases the actual concentration of the second drug, the result is **potentiation** of the second drug. Pharmacokinetic potentiation may arise because one drug increases the absorption or decreases the protein binding, metabolism, or elimination of a second drug, which is therefore present in higher actual concentration than would be anticipated at that dose.

Drug interactions may also arise when one drug alters the pharmacodynamics of a second drug. If two drugs have the same action, drug potentiation results. An example is seen with vasodilators, which can lower blood pressure. A vasodilator such as hydralazine might be part of a therapeutic program to control hypertension. Nitroglycerin is another vasodilator that is taken to relieve angina. Patients who take hydralazine for hypertension and also take nitroglycerin for angina can anticipate a severe hypotensive response to nitroglycerin; they may need to lie down when taking nitroglycerin to avoid fainting.

Drugs that are antagonists often produce pharmacodynamic interactions that diminish the response of both drugs at the usual therapeutic doses. An example is the beta-receptor antagonist propranolol, often prescribed for patients with hypertension. If such a patient developed asthma, a beta-receptor agonist such as albuterol would be indicated. Although in this example the therapeutic target for propranolol is the heart and that for albuterol is the bronchioles, these drugs would antagonize each other at all organs with beta-adrenergic receptors, and neither drug would give the desired therapeutic effect. (In fact, propranolol on its own would make the asthma worse and could not be used.)

Alcohol is a frequent cause of pharmacodynamic drug interactions. As a central nervous system depressant, alcohol acts synergistically with the other drug classes that depress the central nervous system: antihistamines, sedative-hypnotics, antianxiety drugs, antidepressants, antipsychotics, general anesthetics, and the narcotic analgesics. At low doses the drowsiness characteristic of these drug classes is exaggerated by alcohol, but at higher doses respiration can be dangerously depressed.

Alcohol may also interact with certain drugs to cause an intense reaction, including flushing of the face, palpitations, rapid heart rate (tachycardia), and low blood pressure (hypotension). This set of symptoms is called the *disulfiram reaction,* named for the chemical first shown to cause the reaction in persons taking alcohol. This reaction is occasionally observed in patients who ingest alcohol while receiving certain antibiotics, the sedative chloral hydrate, and oral hypoglycemic agents, as well as other drugs.

Foods may also interact with drugs and alter the effect of therapy, most obviously by altering the absorption of an orally administered drug. A few drugs are better absorbed or tolerated on a full stomach, but most drugs are absorbed more slowly or less completely when taken with food (see box). A few of these interactions may significantly diminish the clinical usefulness of the drug. For example, the antibiotic tetracycline forms insoluble precipitates with calcium and magnesium in food. This interaction lowers absorption of the drug so that insufficient amounts of the antibiotic enter the blood and therapy fails.

Some food-drug interactions directly antagonize the action of the drug in the body. For example, patients receiving a coumarin anticoagulant may lose the action of the drug if they ingest large amounts of leafy green vegetables and other foods high in vitamin K. Vitamin K directly antagonizes the action of the coumarins.

Conversely, chronic administration of a drug may interfere with normal vitamin metabolism (Table 1-3). For example, long-term use of the antituberculosis drug isoniazid can deplete vitamin B_6 and cause neuritis. This complication can be prevented by administering vitamin B_6 supplement during isoniazid therapy.

Other food-drug interactions may arise when drugs interfere with normal mechanisms for removing noxious compounds from the body. For example, patients receiving monoamine oxidase inhibitors have a diminished ability to metabolize catecholamines and related compounds such as tyramine. When these patients eat foods with high concentrations of tyramine, such as aged cheese, red wine, or other foods, they

---

ORAL ADMINISTRATION OF SELECTED DRUGS

DRUGS NORMALLY BEST TAKEN ON AN EMPTY STOMACH WITH A FULL GLASS OF WATER

Acetaminophen
Aspirin
Cephalosporins
Erythromycin*
Isoniazid
Penicillins
Propantheline
Quinidine*
Rifampin
Sulfonamides
Tetracyclines*
Theophylline*

DRUGS NORMALLY TAKEN WITH FOOD TO IMPROVE ABSORPTION

Carbamazepine
Cimetidine
Griseofulvin†
Hydralazine
Indomethacin*
Lithium
Nitrofurantoin*
Propranolol
Spironolactone

---

*Gastric irritation may require that the drug be taken with food, but absorption is delayed or diminished.
†This drug is taken with foods rich in fat for best absorption.

Table 1-3 Drug Effects on Vitamin Metabolism

Effect	Drugs
Interferes with absorption or action of folic acid, which can cause folate deficiency	Aminopterin, antibiotics, anticonvulsants, aspirin, clofibrate, cycloserine, ethanol, methotrexate, oral contraceptives
Depletes vitamin B₆	Hydralazine, isoniazid, oral contraceptives
Interferes with absorption or action of vitamin B₁₂	Aminopterin, antibiotics, anticonvulsants, clofibrate, colchicine, ethanol, oral hypoglycemic agents
Interferes with absorption or action of vitamin D	Antacids, anticonvulsants, mineral oil
Interferes with synthesis or absorption of vitamin K	Antibiotics, mineral oil

cannot eliminate the tyramine rapidly and it may accumulate, causing headache and hypertension.

In addition to foods and medications, environmental chemicals increasingly are being recognized as agents causing significant drug interactions in some patients. For example, polycyclic hydrocarbons in cigarette smoke and the chlorinated hydrocarbons in pesticides are active inducers of liver microsomal enzymes. Persons chronically exposed to these chemicals metabolize drugs such as the antiasthmatic medication theophylline more rapidly than normal. In these persons the blood concentration of theophylline may be lower than desired unless dosage adjustments are made (see Chapter 25).

Biologic Variation

Not all patients respond to a set drug dosage in the same way. Moreover, it is not possible to predict in most cases which patients will be more or less sensitive to a drug than normal. The term *normal* in this context really means average for the population.

Biologic variability is based on subtle differences in physiologic functions among people. For example, absorption of oral drug doses can be greatly influenced by stomach acidity, gastrointestinal motility, pancreatic function, and gastrointestinal microbiologic flora. Yet these parameters vary greatly in most people. Likewise, people vary in the sensitivity of certain tissues to drugs. This variability may be the result of differences in the numbers of drug receptors, differences in permeability barriers, and many other factors. These factors are all difficult to assess and yet greatly influence the magnitude of drug effects in patients.

In the clinical setting the causes of biologic variation are not usually known with any degree of certainty. Patients are observed for the proper response to a drug, and dosages are usually adjusted on the basis of clinical assessment of progress. Although the exact causes of biologic variation are not known for an individual, some general factors are known to influence patient responses to medications. These include age, sex, overall health status, and genetic background.

Effect of age on drug response

The fetus. Developing embryos and fetuses are unintended targets of drugs and chemicals taken by their mothers. The effects of many drugs are benign or at least cannot be proved to be harmful, but a few drugs pose grave risks to the unborn. The degree of damage may be related to dose and length of exposure, but it is often also related to the developmental stage of the fetus at the time of exposure. Table 1-4 summarizes potential adverse effects of representative drugs.

Table 1-4 Adverse Drug Effects During Pregnancy*

Effect of Drug	Drugs known to produce the effect in humans
FIRST-TRIMESTER EFFECTS ON EMBRYONIC DEVELOPMENT	
Abortion	Isotretinoin, quinine
Multiple anomalies involving craniofacial development	Dicumarol, ethanol, isotretinoin, methotrexate, paramethadione, phenytoin, quinine, trimethadione
Neural tube defects	Valproate
Goiter	Iodide, methimazole, propylthiouracil
Abnormalities or reproductive organs	Androgens, diethylstilbestrol, estrogens, progestins
Inhibition of growth	Methotrexate, tetracycline, tobacco smoke
SECOND- AND THIRD-TRIMESTER EFFECTS ON FETAL DEVELOPMENT	
Abortion, mortality	Heroin, isotretinoin, tobacco smoke
Mental retardation	Dicumarol, ethanol
Altered cardiovascular function	Anticholinergic drugs, propranolol, terbutaline
Hearing loss and loss of balance	Aminoglycoside antibiotics
Hyperbilirubinemia	Nitrofurantoin, sulfonamides
Hemolytic anemia	Nitrofurantoin
Goiter	Iodide, methimazole, propylthiouracil
Abnormalities of reproductive organs	Androgens, diethylstilbestrol, estrogens, progestins
Inhibition of growth	Dicumarol, ethanol, heroin, methotrexate, tetracycline, tobacco smoke
LABOR, DELIVERY, AND PERINATAL PERIOD	
Increased mortality	Tobacco smoking, cocaine abuse
Altered cardiovascular function	Anticholinergic agents, caffeine, heroin, lidocaine, meperidine, propranolol, terbutaline
Gray-baby syndrome	Chloramphenicol
Respiratory depression	Diazepam, meperidine, morphine, phenobarbital, ethanol, tobacco smoking
Respiratory distress	Reserpine
Bleeding	Aspirin, dicumarol, indomethacin
Hypoglycemia	Chlorpropamide, propranolol, tolbutamide
Hyperbilirubinemia	Nitrofurantoin, sulfonamides
Hemolytic anemia	Nitrofurantoin
Hyperirritability	Cocaine

*This list does not include all drugs that affect fetal and neonatal function but is intended to give representative examples. The nurse should check sources of specific information about individual agents when drugs are administered to pregnant patients.

Table 1-5   FDA Pregnancy Categories

Category	Level of risk with drug exposure	Examples
A	Controlled studies in women fail to demonstrate risk in the first trimester (and there is no evidence of risk in later trimesters), and possibility of fetal harm appears remote.	Thyroid hormones
B	Animal reproduction studies have not demonstrated fetal risk, but there are no controlled studies in pregnant women. Animal reproduction studies have shown adverse effect (other than decreased fertility) that was not confirmed in controlled studies on women in first trimester. There is no evidence of risk in later trimesters.	Amoxicillin, buspirone, cimetidine, fluoxetine, hydrochlorothiazide, metronidazole, piperacillin
C	Studies in animals have revealed adverse effects on fetus, and there are no controlled studies in women. In some cases, studies in women and animals are not available. Drugs in this category should be given only if potential benefit justifies risk to fetus.	Alteplase, captopril, ciprofloxacin, codeine, enalapril, gentamicin, isoproterenol, lisinopril, morphine, nizatidine, reserpine, tubocurarine
D	There is positive evidence of human fetal risk, but the benefits for pregnant women may be acceptable despite the risk, as in life-threatening diseases for which safer drugs cannot be used or are ineffective. An appropriate statement must appear in the "warnings" section of the labeling of drugs in this category.	Amikacin, midazolam, netilmicin, tobramycin
X	Studies in animals or humans have demonstrated fetal abnormalities, there is evidence of fetal risk based on human experience, or both. The risk of using the drug in pregnant women clearly outweighs any possible benefit. The drug is contraindicated in women who are or may become pregnant. An appropriate statement must appear in the "contraindications" section of the labeling of drugs in this category.	Isotretinoin, lovastatin, methotrexate

Drugs that are absorbed systemically have been categorized by the Food and Drug Administration (FDA) according to the level of risk to the fetus. These FDA pregnancy categories are summarized in Table 1-5, along with examples of drugs in each category. Discussions of individual drugs throughout the text also refer to the FDA pregnancy category, when appropriate.

The neonate. Premature infants and neonates may respond to medications quite differently from adults or even older children. Many of these different responses are caused by immaturity of the liver and kidneys in infants. At birth the liver lacks many of the metabolizing enzymes that enable the adult liver to biotransform certain types of compounds. Both microsomal and nonmicrosomal enzyme systems may be reduced. Before these activities increase to normal levels during the first weeks or months of life, neonates are more vulnerable than adults to chemicals requiring detoxification in the liver.

The kidney is also less efficient at birth than in adult life. Therefore excretion of many compounds takes longer in the neonate than in the adult. Failure to take into account this reduced excretory capacity when calculating drug dosage can be important when certain drugs are administered to a neonate.

The antibiotic chloramphenicol illustrates the clinical effect of reduced detoxification and excretion in neonates. This potentially toxic drug is detoxified in the adult liver by the formation of chloramphenicol glucuronide, a metabolite that is efficiently excreted by adult kidneys. Unable to form the glucuronide or excrete the drug efficiently, neonates quickly accumulate chloramphenicol and suffer potentially lethal toxicity. This deadly outcome is prevented by reducing the dose of drug administered to take into account the reduced routes of elimination. The result is that less drug is required per kilogram of body weight to maintain effective concentrations of chloramphenicol in neonates than in adults.

The elderly. Elderly patients are also a group especially at risk from many drugs. Several factors may be involved, including altered central nervous system function and reduced renal function. Elderly patients are also more likely to be malnourished and suffer from chronic diseases for which they may be receiving more than one drug. For these reasons, they may need special attention to detect early signs of drug interactions or drug toxicity related to diminished excretory capacity or altered drug sensitivity.

The aminoglycoside antibiotic gentamicin is an example of the type of drug likely to cause troublesome reactions in elderly patients. The aminoglycosides are excreted almost exclusively by the kidney. Therefore in elderly patients whose normal renal function is significantly lower than that of younger adults, aminoglycosides are excreted at reduced rates. If physicians do not reduce doses to take this effect into account, aminoglycosides accumulate. One of the early signs of toxicity may be some loss of hearing or equilibrium. However, loss of hearing or an unstable gait in elderly patients may be mistaken for normal signs of aging. Therefore the older patient may suffer toxicity for a longer time than a younger patient because in the latter the same signs would be recognized immediately as **iatrogenic** (caused by a drug).

Genetic traits

Some drug reactions are clearly linked to a particular genetic trait that may be more prevalent in certain ethnic groups. For example, the enzyme glucose 6-phosphate dehydrogenase is abundant in the tissues of most people. In red blood cells, this enzyme plays a role in generating reduced nicotinamide adenine dinucleotide phosphate (NADPH), a compound required to maintain active hemoglobin. As a result of a genetic alteration, some individuals lack adequate concentrations of this enzyme in their red blood cells. Therefore NADPH is generated slowly. Under normal circumstances, this alteration would not be critical. However, if a person with this trait is exposed to chemicals that enhance the conversion of hemoglobin to methemoglobin (a relatively inactive form of hemoglobin), serious problems can arise. Because of the lack of glucose 6-phosphate dehydrogenase, too little NADPH is present to fully reform active hemoglobin. When too much methemoglobin accumulates, the red blood cell is destroyed.

Glucose 6-phosphate dehydrogenase deficiency is important for pharmacology because many drugs accelerate methemoglobin formation. Sulfonamides, antimalarial medications, and analgesic-antipyretic drugs (including aspirin) fall into this category. In a person lacking adequate glucose 6-phosphate dehydrogenase activity, these drugs can cause life-threatening hemolysis (rupture of the red blood cells). The same drugs are relatively innocuous in most people who possess adequate glucose 6-phosphate dehydrogenase activity.

Certain populations have a high proportion of the gene that causes glucose 6-phosphate dehydrogenase deficiency. For example, 13% of black American men and 20% of black American women may carry this gene. Sardinians also have an incidence of approximately 14%. More than half of Kurdish Jewish populations show glucose 6-phosphate dehydrogenase deficiencies. This genetic difference from the bulk of

the American population places patients from these special populations at greater risk for serious reactions with drugs such as those mentioned earlier. When these patients receive medications, they should be watched carefully for signs of toxicity.

The rate of drug acetylation in the liver is another genetically determined trait that may affect the incidence of certain drug reactions. About half of Americans, both black and white, possess liver enzyme systems that acetylate drugs and other chemicals slowly, at rates less than half of those of the rest of the population. In contrast, slow acetylation is very rare in Eskimos and persons of Japanese ancestry.

Isoniazid, a drug used to treat tuberculosis, illustrates how the genetically determined ability to acetylate the drug can influence unwanted reactions. Isoniazid is inactivated primarily by acetylation and is eliminated by the kidney entirely as metabolites. In slow acetylators the half-life of the drug is about 3 hours, but in rapid acetylators, it is only about 1 hour. Liver damage may be more common in rapid acetylators because the concentration of a hepatotoxic acetylated metabolite is high. Slow acetylation may be more closely associated with dose-related toxicity (neuropathy, depression of liver biotransformation enzymes) because the untransformed drug may accumulate in persons with this trait.

CHAPTER REVIEW

◆ **KEY TERMS**

affinity, p. 4
agonist, p. 5
anaphylaxis, p. 6
antagonists, p. 5
bioavailability, p. 6
biotransformation, p. 12
desired action, p. 5
drug interaction, p. 17
duration, p. 15
efficacy, p. 4
enterohepatic circulation, p. 12
first-pass phenomenon, p. 8
half-life, p. 15
iatrogenic, p. 22
lipid soluble, p. 8
onset, p. 14
pharmacodynamics, p. 3
pharmacokinetics, p. 3
potentiation, p. 18
side effects, p. 5
synergism, p. 17
time to peak effect, p. 15
urticaria, p. 6

◆ **REVIEW QUESTIONS**

1. What is the difference between a drug action and a side effect?
2. What are two major types of unpredictable reactions to drugs that nurses may encounter?
3. What are the four types of allergic reactions to drugs that nurses may encounter?
4. What are the three general mechanisms by which drugs interact with a patient's body to produce a biologic effect?
5. What is an agonist?
6. What is a drug antagonist?
7. How does affinity differ from efficacy?
8. How are pharmacodynamics and pharmacokinetics helpful to the nurse in understanding the clinical use of drugs?
9. Describe how a drug in tablet form enters the blood after oral administration. What factors may influence absorption?
10. What is the first-pass phenomenon? Does it affect all routes of administration?
11. What are the advantages and disadvantages of subcutaneous, intramuscular, and intravenous routes of drug administration?
12. How does the binding of drugs to proteins in the blood influence the effect of the drug?
13. What is biotransformation?
14. What is enterohepatic circulation?
15. What information is expressed in a log dose-response curve?
16. What is the therapeutic index of a drug?
17. What is the onset time for a drug, and how does it differ from the duration of action of a drug? What is the elimination half-time of a drug?
18. What is the plateau principle?
19. What are drug interactions? What are the two major mechanisms by which they occur?
20. Do drug interactions increase or decrease the action of the drugs involved?
21. Which type of drug interaction may actually change the concentration of one of the drugs involved?
22. Why must biologic variability be considered in drug therapy?
23. What are some of the possible reasons for the observed differences in drug response seen among patients?
24. How may smoking, environmental chemical exposure, or dietary patterns influence the response of a patient to a drug?
25. What consideration should the nurse be aware of in administering drugs requiring hepatic detoxification to a premature infant?
26. What major organ system involved in drug elimination is likely to have diminished function in normal elderly people? In chronic alcoholics?
27. Why are persons of African and Mediterranean ancestry more likely to suffer drug-induced hemolysis than most other American populations?

SUGGESTED READING

General principles of pharmacology

Clark WG, Brater DC, Johnson AR, editors: *Drug-receptor interactions*. In *Goth's medical pharmacology*, ed 13, St Louis, 1991, Mosby–Year Book.

Levine RR: *How drugs act on the living organism*. In *Pharmacology: drug actions and reactions*, ed 3, Boston, 1983, Little, Brown.

Pharmacokinetics and drug disposition

Brater DC: The pharmacological role of the kidney, *Drugs* 19(1):31, 1980.

Brentin L, Sieh A: Caring for the morbidly obese, *Am J Nurs* 91(8):40, 1991.

Vesell ES: On the significance of host factors that affect drug disposition, *Clin Pharmacol Ther* 31(1):1, 1982.

Weinshilboum RM: Human pharmacogenetics, *Fed Proc* 43(8):2295, 1984.

Drug interactions

D'Arcy PF: Tobacco smoking and drugs: a clinically important interaction? *Drug Intell Clin Pharm* 18(4):302, 1984.

McInnes GT, Brodie MJ: Drug interactions that matter, *Drugs* 36:83, 1988.

Todd B: Cigarettes and caffeine in drug interactions, *Geriatr Nurs* 8(2):97, 1987.

Drug-food interactions

Cerrato PL: Drugs and food: when the dangers increase, *RN* 51(11):65, 1988.

Hathcock JN: When drugs compromise good nutrition, *Drug Therapy* 16(8):71, 1986.

Osis M: Scheduling drug administration: drug and food interactions, *Gerontion* 1(5):8, 1986.

Drugs and the fetus or neonate

Ferrar HC, Blumer JL: Fetal effects of maternal drug exposure, *Ann Rev Pharmacol Toxicol* 31:525, 1991.

Hill LM: Effects of drugs and chemicals on the fetus and newborn, *Mayo Clin Proc* 59(10):707, 1984.

Nice FJ: Can a breast-feeding mother take medication without harming her infant? *MCN* 14(1):27, 1989.

Drugs and the elderly

Delafuente JS: Perspectives on geriatric pharmacotherapy, *Pharmacotherapy* 11(3):222, 1991.

Greenblatt DJ, Sellers EM, Shader RI: Drug disposition in old age, *N Engl J Med* 306(18):1081, 1982.

MacIsaac AM, Rivers R, Adamson CB: Multiple medications: is your elderly patient caught in the storm? *Nurs 89* 19(7):60, 1989.

Matteson MA, McConnell ES: *Gerontological nursing concepts and practice*, Philadelphia, 1988, WB Saunders.

Nesbitt B: Nursing diagnosis in age-related changes, *J Gerontol Nurs* 14(7):7, 1988.

Ramsey R: Adjusting drug dosages for critically ill elderly patients, *Nurs 88* 18(7):47, 1988.

Sellers EM, Frecker RC, Romach MK: Drug metabolism in the elderly: confounding of age, smoking, and ethanol effects, *Drug Metab Rev* 14(2);225, 1983.

Westfall LK and others: Why the elderly are so vulnerable to drug reactions, *RN* 50(11):39, 1987.

CHAPTER 2

Legal Implications of Drug Therapy

LEARNING OBJECTIVES

After studying this chapter, you should be able to do the following:

- Discuss how drugs are tested for safety.
- Explain how a drug is determined to be effective for use in patients.
- Explain what controlled substances are.
- Discuss the role of the nurse in drug testing.

CHAPTER OVERVIEW

◆ This chapter discusses the legal implications of drug therapy for the nurse. Patients receiving medications have always faced certain risks, which include the possibility that (1) the medication will not produce the beneficial effect claimed by those who make and sell the drug, (2) the medication may be directly harmful, or (3) the medication may be improperly administered. Modern drug legislation is designed to reduce or to eliminate these risks to patients.

Nursing Process Overview

NURSES, DRUGS, AND THE LAW

Countries vary in the laws governing the role of the nurse in practice and in drug testing. In the United States, each state has a nurse practice act regulating nursing practice for that state. Each nurse is responsible for knowing the appropriate laws governing practice in that state, province, or country.

Assessment

Assess all patients in a thorough, individualized manner.

Management

Provide safe, individualized care as defined by law and as expected by the health care agency. Work with others on the health care team to achieve common goals in consultation with the patient. Stay informed about medications being administered. Serve as patient advocate, and ask questions of the health care team as needed.

Evaluation

Regularly determine whether the patient goals are being met. Involve the patient in all aspects of care. Document patient status and nursing care provided in a consistent manner.

ESTABLISHING SAFETY AND EFFICACY OF DRUGS

History of Drug Development

The earliest form of medical practice involved the use of various natural products that were discovered by trial and error to have certain effects on the body. For example, parts of the poppy plant were known by the ancient Egyptians to relieve pain. This remedy was already ancient when it was recorded in the Ebers papyrus in 1500 BC. Equally ancient is the use of parts of the ephedra shrub by the Chinese, who called the preparation *ma huang*. In the New World, South American Indians used the bark of the cinchona tree to relieve the symptoms of malaria. Even in more recent times natural products have been introduced for medical practice. For example, in 1785 a British physician named Withering described the use of the leaf of the foxglove plant to relieve edema of a certain type, which had previously resisted all therapy.

Until very recently, natural products such as those listed above were the only medicinal agents, or materia medica, available. The most common medications, made from plants or parts of plants, were called *botanicals*. Some botanicals continue to be used in medical practice, but most have been replaced as chemists have analyzed these crude products and identified active ingredients. The active ingredients are the chemicals found in the crude preparation that are responsible for producing the biologic effect of the medicinal agent. For example, the poppy plant relieves pain because the plant contains opium. *Ma huang* produces its effects on the heart, lungs, and other organs because it contains ephedrine, an agent that stimulates the sympathetic nervous system. Similarly, the quinine in cinchona bark relieves the symptoms of malaria, and the digitalis in foxglove leaves relieves the edema associated with heart failure.

Identification of the active ingredient in a crude medicinal agent has two benefits. First, the active ingredient may be measured (or assayed) in the crude preparation and the dose adjusted for the content of the active ingredient. For example, the digitalis content of the foxglove leaf may vary from plant to plant. Therefore a dosage based on the amount of the leaf administered may actually contain a variable amount of digitalis and may therefore have variable biologic effects. Because the biologic activity of a drug is related to the actual dose of the active ingredient, dosages based on the weight of pure digitalis should have a more predictable biologic effect.

The second benefit of identifying the active ingredient of a medicinal agent is that the chemical structure and properties of the active drug are revealed. This knowledge can lead to better ways of isolating the active material from natural sources. Digitalis is an example of a drug that is still prepared by extraction from its plant source. Alternatively, after the structure of an active agent is known, chemists may be able to synthesize the material. Ephedrine is an example of a drug now chemically synthesized in a simple, economical process that has replaced the procedure of isolating the drug from plant materials.

Standardization of Agents

Recognizing the relationship between drug dose and biologic effect produced, most nations of the world have attempted to adopt codes for standardizing the content of medicinal agents. Drugs sold in the United States must comply with the standards established in *The United States Pharmacopeia (USP)* and the *National Formulary (NF)* or the *United States Homeopathic Pharmacopeia*. The *USP* contains chemical, physical, and biologic information on all active ingredients used in medications. To qualify as a standard, or official, medication, the preparation must conform to the information listed in this source. The *NF* was originally independent of the USP, but the fourteenth edition, published in 1975, was the last to be published separately. The latest edition, *USP XXIII* and *NF XVIII,* published as a single volume, became official January 1, 1990. The volume is updated continuously by way of published supplements.

As an example of the type of information found in the USP, we may consider aspirin. The USP classifies aspirin as an antipyretic (fever-reducing) analgesic (pain-reducing) agent. In the USP, aspirin powder is listed separately from aspirin tablets. A variety of tablet sizes are described, containing amounts of aspirin ranging from 65 to 650 mg (approximately 1 to 10 gr). To meet USP standards, tablets must actually contain between 95% and 105% of the amount of aspirin indicated on the label. For example, an aspirin tablet labeled 500 mg must contain between 475 and 525 mg of aspirin. The aspirin used in these tablets must meet the chemical and physical standards listed for that compound in the USP. Although drug doses for adults and children are listed, the USP is less useful for clinical personnel than for persons in pharmaceutical manufacture or pharmacy.

Some drugs used in medical practice cannot be standardized easily by chemical analysis because the drug preparations are relatively complex mixtures of compounds. Standardization of these products may be obtained by measuring a biologic effect. For example, insulin isolated from porcine or bovine pancreas glands is standardized on the basis of the amount of the preparation required to reduce the blood sugar of a test animal a certain amount. Antibiotics may be standardized on the basis of the amount of the preparation required to kill 99.9% of a certain sensitive strain of bacteria in a rigidly controlled laboratory test. Other complex pharmaceutical preparations, such as serums, vaccines, and human blood products, are tested and licensed by the Food and Drug Administration (FDA) Center for Biologic Evaluation and Research.

Standards for medicinal agents vary somewhat from country to country. Several pharmacopeias and other references may apply. In Canada, the current *Compendium of Pharmaceuticals and Specialties (CPS)* indexes agents available and contains monographs on specific drugs. The *British Pharmacopoeia 1988* is the current standard reference for the United Kingdom but also includes a significant amount of information from the *European Pharmacopoeia*. It is updated yearly with published addenda. The *International Pharmacopoeia* is published by the World Health Organization (WHO) and includes drug methods and standardizations for reference use in any country.

The information in these references is often indexed by **generic** or nonproprietary names. The generic name applies to the drug, no matter who manufactures or markets it. The proprietary or **trade name** is the property of a specific drug company. For example, cefuroxime sodium is the nonproprietary name for a specific antibiotic; this single compound is sold under the trade names of Zinacef by Glaxo, Inc., and Kefurox by Eli Lilly & Co.

Legislation

Drug manufacturing and sale are regulated by state and federal agencies. For federal laws to apply, a drug must enter interstate commerce. A drug totally manufactured within a single state and sold only in that state would not be subject to the federal drug laws. Very few drugs fall into this category.

The first effective federal law concerning drugs in the United States was passed in 1906 (Table 2-1). This law was intended to protect citizens from adulterated medicines and medications that contained harmful ingredients but failed to list these ingredients on the label. Each new law passed since that time has been intended to overcome specific problems that have arisen. For example, in the early 1900s a certain patent medicine was advertised as a cure for cancer. The federal government sought to force this company to halt the false advertisement. However, the drug label as it appeared on the bottle was accurate in naming the contents of the medicine. Under the 1906 law, accurate labeling of the contents was all the government could require. When the Sherley Amendment was added in 1912, the federal government gained the ability to control advertising claims, as well as the contents of the drug label.

The next major piece of drug legislation, passed in 1938, added the requirement that a drug sold in the United States had to be shown as safe before it could be marketed. Before this law a pharmaceutical company was not responsible for the safety of the drugs it manufactured and sold. For example, in 1937 over 100 people died from taking a product that was sold as "elixir of sulfanilamide." Investigations revealed that the cause of death was not the sulfanilamide but the propylene glycol used to dissolve the drug. The amazing fact is that no one had tested the toxicity of propylene glycol before using it in this medication. Under the law in 1937, however, the company responsible for this disaster could be charged only with mislabeling the drug because an elixir is by definition an alcohol solution.

One of the major provisions of the legislation currently controlling drug marketing and use in the United States is that a drug must be effective in treating the medical condition for which it is recommended (Table 2-1). The requirement for proving effectiveness and safety has greatly increased the amount of drug testing done by private companies who develop new drugs. As a result, the number of new drugs entering the market has been sharply reduced, and the time and money required to get a drug on the market have increased. On the other hand, drugs that do enter the market are much more reliable medications than they were in the past.

One class of drugs especially affected by the great cost of drug development is the group known as orphans. **Orphan drugs** are medicines that have not been profitable to develop and market, either because the market is too small (e.g., drugs used for rare diseases) or because patent protection has expired on the drug. Under the provisions of the Orphan Drug Act (1983), companies can recover a substantial portion of their development costs for orphan drugs. Companies that develop and market nonpatentable orphan drugs are also protected from competition by a FDA policy that limits approval for an orphan drug to one company for the first 7 years. To further support development of orphan drugs, the FDA established an Orphan Products Development Office, the Pharmaceutical Manufacturers Association created a Commission on Drugs for Rare Diseases, and the Generic Pharmaceutical Industry Association formed an Institute for Orphan Drugs. These efforts have resulted in the approval of an increasing number of orphan drugs since 1983.

Another current provision of drug legislation is that pharmaceuticals be produced by what are termed *good manufacturing practices*. Under this provision of the Food and Drug Act, the FDA inspects manufacturing facilities and oversees the general production of medications. Good manufacturing practices are general procedures, not specific processes. Indeed, the methods employed to produce the same medication can vary widely from company to company. Such variation is perfectly acceptable, as long as both procedures are in accordance with good manufacturing practices.

Legislation adopted in 1984 established guidelines for bioequivalence of drugs and streamlined application processes so that approval of generic drugs was facilitated. When a drug is first introduced, it is sold only by the company that developed it or by others licensed to sell it. The developer's control of the drug is protected for 17 years by patents. After that time, other companies can choose to manufacture the drug and sell it after they have satisfied FDA requirements for good manufacturing processes and have met bioequivalence standards. For example, the antibiotic clindamycin was discovered by Upjohn and sold under the trade name Cleocin. Sales were protected by Upjohn's patent rights to the compound, but recently, when the patent expired, several other companies applied for the right to manufacture and market the drug. These companies cannot use the trade name Cleocin but can sell the generic compound clindamycin. These generic preparations of clindamycin now share the market with the original drug.

Under the existing drug laws, a number of federal

Table 2-1   Federal Drug Legislation in the United States

Date	Title of law	Major provisions
1906	Pure Food and Drug Act	Established *USP* and *NF* as official standards Set standards for proper drug labeling
1912	Sherley Amendment	Prohibited fraudulent claims for therapeutic effects of drugs.
1914	Harrison Narcotic Act	Legally defined term *narcotic* Regulated and restricted importation, manufacture, sale, or use of opium, cocaine, marijuana, and other drugs likely to produce dependence
1938	Food, Drug, and Cosmetic Act	Maintained major provisions of previous laws Required that a drug be demonstrated to be safe before it was marketed Added *Homeopathic Pharmacopoeia of the United States* as a third standard for drugs
1941-1945	Amendments to Pure Food and Drug Act	Required that biologic products used as drugs (e.g., insulin or antibiotics) be certified on a batch-by-batch basis by a government agency
1952	Durham-Humphrey Amendment	Designated certain drugs as legend drugs (must be marked "Caution: Federal Law prohibits dispensing without prescription") Restricted right of pharmacist to distribute legend drugs
1962	Kefauver-Harris Amendment	Required proof of efficacy for a drug to remain on market Authorized FDA to establish official names for drugs
1970	Comprehensive Drug Abuse Prevention and Control Act (or Controlled Substances Act)	Defined *drug dependency* and *drug addiction* Classified drugs according to abuse potential and medical usefulness Established methods for regulating manufacture, distribution, and sale of controlled substances Established education and treatment programs for drug abuse
1983	Orphan Drug Act	Offered tax relief to companies marketing orphan drugs Protected companies for 7 years against competition on nonpatentable orphan drugs
1984	Drug Price Competition and Patent Term Restoration Act	Drugs first marketed after 1962 are eligible for abbreviated new drug application Generic drugs are more easily introduced Established guidelines for bioequivalence Restored up to 5 years of patent protection for time used in drug development
1986, 1988	National Childhood Vaccine Injury Act	Private health care providers are required to keep records on adverse events following immunization Covers diphtheria, measles, mumps, pertussis, poliomyelitis, rubella, and tetanus toxoids or vaccines
1987	Prescription Drug Marketing Act	Bans diversion of prescription drugs from legitimate channels Restricts reimportation of drugs from other countries
1988	Food and Drug Administration Act	Establishes the FDA within the Department of Health and Human Services Sets mechanism for appointing the Commissioner of Food and Drugs

Table 2-2   Organizations Involved in Drug Regulation in the United States

Name	Common abbreviation	Function
Department of Health and Human Services	HHS	The secretary of HHS is a cabinet-level officer whose duties include designating the official names for drugs sold in the United States and overseeing the Public Health Service.
Drug Enforcement Administration	DEA	This agency within the Department of Justice is the sole drug enforcement arm of the U.S. government, under the Controlled Substances Act of 1970.
Federal Trade Commission	FTC	This federal agency regulates the advertisement of medications aimed at the general public (not medical personnel).
Food and Drug Administration	FDA	This federal agency is responsible for guaranteeing the safety, purity, effectiveness, and reliability of drugs sold in the United States. In addition, this agency regulates the advertising of medications to medical personnel.
National Academy of Sciences–National Research Council	NAS–NRC	The NAS is a private organization composed of outstanding scientists in the United States. The NRC is the research arm of the NAS and is involved in evaluating the efficacy of drugs for the FDA in the Drug Efficacy Study Implementation.
Public Health Service	PHS	This federal agency not only funds extensive clinical research but also is responsible for maintaining basic research programs under the National Institutes of Health. Biologicals used as drugs are also certified by this agency.
Pharmaceutical Manufacturers Association	PMA	This private organization represents the pharmaceutical houses where most drugs are developed. This group functions as an advisory group to the FDA on occasion and as a lobbying group to Congress.
United States Adopted Names Council	USAN	This private group contains members from government, private industry, the medical profession, and research institutions whose function is to advise the secretary of HHS as to the appropriate official name for each new drug introduced.
United States Pharmacopeial Convention	USP	This group of experts sets standards for medications (published in the *USP*) and establishes consensus on drug uses (published in the USP Drug Information volumes).

agencies are involved in regulating drug trade. In addition to the official government agencies, a number of private organizations contribute advice or expertise to the government on matters concerning medicines. These organizations are listed and described in Table 2-2.

DRUG TESTING

The development of new drugs and biologicals is a major industry in the United States. To meet the current standards set by drug legislation, a detailed format is followed to test drugs as they are developed for market. This format is described in this section. The final stage of this drug development is testing in human beings. Nurses play an important role in drug testing trials.

Nursing Process Overview

NURSES AND DRUG TESTING

Laws governing the role of the nurse in drug testing vary among countries. In the United States, each state's nurse practice act regulates all aspects of nursing practice for that state. Examine the appropriate laws governing practice to determine the extent to which nurses are allowed to participate in drug testing in your state, province, or country.

Assessment

Assess all patients in a thorough, individualized manner, whether or not the patients are involved in a drug testing program.

Nursing Diagnosis

Nursing diagnoses are based on individualized patient assessment. In the early stages of drug testing, the major focus may be to identify and describe frequently encountered drug side effects.

Management

Patient management in a drug testing study may differ from that in a normal clinical situation. For example, the nurse should be certain that the institution where the study is taking place permits the nurse to administer investigational drugs. Some institutions require that the person conducting the experiment (study) actually administer the experimental drugs. The nurse should also determine whether a nurse is legally allowed to obtain informed consent. Some institutions do not permit anyone but the principal investigator to obtain informed consent from the patient.

Evaluation

Evaluation of the patients receiving experimental drugs may be a major component of the research aspect of the drug testing program. In many cases, detailed evaluation is carried out by the physician or researcher, including detailed patient histories, laboratory tests, and radiographic evaluation. Nevertheless, the nurse should continue to evaluate the patients in a manner consistent with good nursing practice. The extent to which the nursing evaluations become part of the permanent record of the experiment depends on the institution and the protocol established by the investigator.

Assessing the Safety of Drugs

All medications intended for human use must undergo extensive toxicity testing in at least two species of animals. The toxicity tests must include acute and chronic studies. Acute toxicity tests assess the short-term effects of extreme doses of the drug. The intent of these tests is to identify organs or tissues that may be sensitive to an action of the drug. These acute tests also allow researchers to determine how dangerous the drug might be in cases of overdose in human beings.

Chronic toxicity tests assess the effects of prolonged dosage with the experimental agent. Several exposure levels are usually tested, with at least one group of animals receiving doses far in excess of those expected to be received by human patients. After prolonged exposure to the test drug, the animals are sacrificed and extensive pathologic and histologic examinations are performed. Again, any pathologic effects on organs or tissues, if present, must be noted.

Significant toxicity observed in animals is usually sufficient cause for abandoning development of a drug.

Chronic toxicity tests are carried out in both males and females because the sensitivity of the reproductive systems may differ. Certain other organs may differ between the sexes as well. For example, many chemicals induce bladder cancer more easily in males than females.

Chronic toxicity tests are also the point at which a drug is usually tested for carcinogenic (cancer-inducing) effects. The carcinogenic effects of compounds may also be assessed by the Ames test, which is based on the fact that mutagenic chemicals (chemicals that induce genetic mutations) accelerate the rate at which mutant bacteria revert to normal. Because many chemicals that are mutagens are also carcinogens, this test can help predict which drugs may be carcinogenic. This bacterial test is less expensive and faster than chronic toxicity tests in animals, which may run months or years.

Drugs are also tested for their effects on pregnant animals and on fetuses. Drugs that cause fetal abnormalities are called *teratogens*. Some drugs are very dangerous to fetuses at certain stages in embryonic development but relatively harmless to adult animals or more mature fetuses. The stage of fetal development most sensitive to drugs or toxins is approximately the first third of fetal life. A tragic example of this principle occurred with the drug thalidomide. Thalidomide is a sleep medication that was widely marketed in Europe during the 1960s. The drug was not dangerous to adults, but when used by women in the early stages of pregnancy, the drug inhibited the proper development of fetal limb buds. The result was a number of babies born with tiny nonfunctional limbs—a tragedy that could have been prevented by more extensive drug testing. Thalidomide was, in fact, never marketed in the United States because insufficient information was available to satisfy the FDA guidelines for new drugs.

Efficacy of Drugs

After an experimental drug has been thoroughly tested for toxicity in animals, the manufacturer may be ready to file with the FDA a "notice of claimed investigational exemption for a new drug (IND)." Included in this notice must be information on the chemical structure of the new drug, partly to aid in establishing that the drug is, in fact, new. All the toxicity data in animals, data on drug absorption and metabolism, and data on the expected biologic activity of the drug must be included. The manufacturer or licenser must outline in great detail the tests that will be run in human subjects.

Phase I, the first testing of a drug in human beings,

is carried out on a small number of healthy volunteers. The purpose of this phase is to identify a safe dosage range for the drug in most persons and to establish how well the animal studies correlate with the results in humans. For example, drug absorption in humans may be quite different from that observed in certain animal species. Therefore it may be necessary to repeat certain studies in humans. Occasionally an unexpected side effect may show up at this stage of testing. For example, alterations of mood may not be easily recognized in experimental animals and yet may be severe enough in humans to prevent further development of an experimental drug.

Phase II, the second stage of testing in human beings, involves clinical trials on patients. Clinical trials may take many forms, but all are designed to answer the question, "Is this drug an effective treatment for a defined medical condition?" To answer this question, a relatively large number of patients must be studied, and the results must be analyzed in an objective manner, usually with statistical methods.

The **double-blind design** is one very effective format for a clinical trial. In this type of study patients are randomly assigned to treatment groups or are assigned so that groups have the same average age, the same proportion of men and women, or some other desired characteristic. One group receives the drug to be tested. Another group receives a placebo (a dosage form containing no pharmacologically active ingredient). The drug and the placebo should be in the same form so that they are indistinguishable by sight or taste. The placebo-treated group of patients serves as a control and allows the researcher to assess the percentage of patients that would improve without therapy. The term *double-blind* refers to the fact that during the experiment neither the patient nor the medical personnel dispensing medication know which patients are receiving the test drug and which are receiving the placebo. In some studies the control group receives the therapy that is currently accepted as the best available for the condition being tested, rather than a placebo. This type of control allows the researchers to compare the efficacy of the new drug to existing therapy.

Patients who receive placebo in clinical trials and show clinical improvement may be of two types. The first type includes patients whose disease has gone into spontaneous remission during the course of the clinical trial. For example, spontaneous remission is commonly observed in certain types of depressive diseases and in certain types of arthritis. The second type of patient who improves while receiving placebo does so simply as a result of receiving medical attention rather than an effective drug. For example, as many as **30%** of a group of patients suffering mild pain report significant pain relief when they are given a placebo. With drugs affecting mood, the response to placebo is observed in an even higher percentage of patients.

The **placebo effect** (clinical improvement in response to placebo) is a complication in clinical trials and makes the task of clearly evaluating the role of a particular drug in therapy more difficult. The existence of such an effect, however, emphasizes the importance of sympathetic human contact in relieving the suffering of a patient. A patient who responds to a placebo should by no means be considered to have originally been suffering from an imaginary complaint. We now understand the normal mechanisms by which the body produces analgesia (endogenous morphine like compounds, or endorphins; see Chapter 44) and realize that these internal mechanisms may be regulated by the central nervous system and affected by emotional states. Therefore the attention and support given to patients may alter their emotional state and allow the natural mechanisms of the body to improve the patients' clinical condition.

After a drug has been proved effective in controlled clinical trials, the manufacturer may file a request with the FDA to release the drug into limited circulation so that it can be tested in several medical centers on large numbers of patients. This is *phase III* of the evaluation process. During the first round of clinical trials the total number of patients tested may be only a few hundred. When the drug is released into limited circulation, it may be tested in a few thousand patients. This larger number of patients allows assessment of rare complications of drug therapy that could not be predicted from more limited trials. Before a tested drug is finally released for interstate marketing, its developer must file with the FDA a new drug application (NDA). The NDA includes all information available on toxicity of the new drug, its use in patients, and the results of the clinical trials. If the FDA rules that the drug has been proved safe and effective, and that the claims made for the drug in the package insert and other professional advertising are supported by the results of the clinical trials, the drug may be released for sale in interstate commerce.

The procedure as outlined above for testing drugs was a careful, conservative approach that often took many years to complete. In 1985, the FDA took steps to streamline its procedures and thereby bring drugs into the marketplace more rapidly. The agency reduced the number of individual case reports required in the application, but increased requirements for postmarketing surveillance. All serious adverse effects must be reported to the FDA within 15 days; all adverse effects must be reported every 3 months for the first 3 years and yearly thereafter. Forms for reporting these reactions are published regularly as part of the *FDA Drug Bulletin.*

Further pressure for more rapid movement of drugs into clinical tests arose as the acquired immunodeficiency syndrome (AIDS) epidemic broke out. Without treatment, AIDS patients have a very short life expectancy. For these patients and for others with conditions for which no effective therapy exists, a new procedure was created to allow experimental agents to be used on a wider scale than was previously possible. This treatment with investigational new drug (IND) process releases drugs for use in patients who meet certain criteria, even though the drug is not yet on the market. For example, while didanosine was an investigational drug being tested for activity against human immunodeficiency virus (HIV), it was available under the treatment IND, even though the drug was not yet on the market, for treatment of AIDS patients over the age of 12 years who had symptomatic HIV infection, had developed intolerance to the standard drug zidovudine, and were unable to enroll in a phase II trial because of geographic location. Examples of drugs currently available on treatment IND status include alglucrase for nonneuropathic Gaucher's disease, baclofen for severe spasticity of spinal cord origin, beractant for hyaline membrane disease in premature infants, fludarabine phosphate for refractory B-cell chronic lymphocytic leukemia, pentostatin for hairy cell leukemia insensitive to alpha-interferon, tenoposide for unresponsive acute lymphoblastic leukemia, and trimetrexate for *Pneumocystis carinii* pneumonia.

Drug Efficacy Study Implementation

All drugs introduced after the Kefauver-Harris Amendment in 1962 are required to go through the extensive testing just described and must be proved effective and safe before they can be marketed. However, drugs already on the market in 1962 posed a special problem because they had been tested primarily for safety and not efficacy. To bring all drugs up to the same standard, the FDA contracted the National Research Council of the National Academy of Sciences to evaluate all medications being sold in the United States. This project was the Drug Efficacy Study Implementation (DESI). To carry out this project, scientific and clinical experts were called to study data from clinical trials. Based on this information, drugs were rated according to the scale shown in Table 2-3. Drugs rated as ineffective were removed from the market. Drugs listed as possibly effective or probably effective required reformulation or retesting to stay on the market. Over-the-counter drugs were originally included in the DESI review, but the vast number of these drugs overwhelmed the review process. In 1972 evaluation of over-the-counter drugs was assigned to the FDA advisory panels (see Chapter 4).

Table 2-3   DESI Rating System

Rating	Description
Effective	Substantial evidence exists to demonstrate that drug is effective treatment for defined medical condition.
Probably effective	Some evidence exists, but more will be required to prove drug effective.
Possibly effective	Minimum evidence exists to suggest that drug may be effective.
Ineffective	Controlled trials have failed to show that drug is more effective than placebo.
Ineffective as a fixed combination	Individual components of medication might be effective alone at appropriate doses, but no evidence suggests that all components of medication are necessary to effect.
Effective but	Qualification to use of drug is made, which must be added to labeling.

Rights of the Patient in Drug Testing

Anyone involved in assessing the clinical usefulness of a new drug is bound by certain moral and legal constraints. No one may be coerced into receiving a drug that is under investigation. All drug studies must be done on volunteers who have read, understood, and signed informed consent forms. The law requires that all potential hazards associated with the use of the drug be clearly explained to the patient. The patient or volunteer must not be promised unrealistic benefits from therapy. The patient must also be free to withdraw from the study at any time without fear that the level of medical care received will be compromised.

Although compliance with the constraints just mentioned seems a simple matter, there are complications in practice. For example, some people believe that experimental drugs are always better than currently used drugs. These people may not have realistic expectations, in spite of having been told the properties of the drug being tested. Another problem concerns patients who are intimidated by medical personnel and who are afraid to refuse to participate in a drug study. These patients may confide their fears to an accessible and sympathetic nurse. It is the duty of the nurse to assist such patients in making their true feelings known.

Nurses play several roles in assisting the patient with drug testing. Nurses working in settings where drug protocols are being tested may help identify potential candidates for drug testing. These individuals may be knowledgable about their medical problems, interested in trying new therapy, or even willing to do anything to achieve a possible improvement.

Another role of the nurse is to serve as advocate for the patient. The nurse assesses whether the patient seems to understand the possible benefits and limitations of the drugs being tested and the testing protocol. Also, the nurse assesses the patient throughout the testing period about benefits, fears, drug side effects, and changes in the underlying health problem.

Finally, the nurse supports the patient in the decisions made regarding participation in drug testing. This may be difficult because the nurse may disagree with the patient's decision but must support it.

CONTROLLED SUBSTANCES

Certain substances can alter the normal function of the human body so profoundly that the body becomes dependent on that substance and suffers physical harm if it is withdrawn. This condition is **physical addiction** or *dependence*. Other substances, although not producing clear evidence of physical addiction, cause profound changes in the psychologic makeup of the user and produce psychologic addiction. Examples of types of compounds producing each of these types of addiction are listed in Table 2-4.

Table 2-4 Compounds that Produce Dependence with Continued Use

Type of dependence	Drug category	Specific drugs
Physical and psychologic	Narcotic analgesics	Morphine, heroin, codeine, paregoric, methadone
Physical and psychologic	General depressants	Ethanol, barbiturates, glutethimide, methaqualone
Psychologic	Psychomotor stimulants*	Amphetamines, cocaine, methylphenidate
Psychologic	Hallucinogens	Lysergic acid diethylamide (LSD), mescaline (peyote), NN-dimethyltryptamine (DMT), 2,5-dimethoxy-4-methyl amphetamine (STP), phencyclidine
Psychologic	Cannabis	Marijuana, hashish

*Physical dependence has been suggested for certain of these drugs but remains controversial.

Nursing Process Overview
CONTROLLED SUBSTANCES

Because of the addictive potential of many controlled substances, legal restraints have been placed on the use of these drugs in medical practice. These regulations, as well as the special nature of the drugs, add a special burden and responsibility to the nurse.

Assessment

Observe whether an individual displays signs and symptoms that make the use of the controlled substance appropriate. Be alert to signs of drug abuse in patients. Patients may have obtained prescriptions from several physicians to acquire excessive amounts of controlled substances. Be alert not only to physical signs of excessive drug use, but also to the psychologic signs pointing to this problem. For example, a patient who is dependent on drugs obtained under false pretenses may be reluctant to enter the hospital for even the most routine testing, fearing that the drug dependency will be discovered in the closely regulated hospital environment.

Nursing Diagnoses

Altered bowel elimination: constipation secondary to frequent use of narcotic analgesics
Altered comfort: nausea secondary to narcotic use

Management

When dealing with controlled substances, the nurse has legal and nursing responsibilities. The legal responsibilities include ensuring that controlled substances (schedules II through IV, United States) are kept under lock and key. These substances are available only to authorized personnel. All of the material must be accounted for, so records on the use of these substances must be kept. Any unauthorized use of controlled substances must be reported to the proper authority.

The nurse must also be aware of institutional policies regarding use of these drugs, such as standing orders for controlled substances. For example, for schedule II drugs (United States), the physician's order may require renewal every 48 hours. A nurse who administers the drug after the 48-hour period without obtaining a renewal order is in violation of institutional policy. There are comparable national and institutional restrictions related to Canadian narcotics and schedule G drugs. On the other hand, patients with a legitimate need for controlled substances should not be refused the medications they need. See Chapter 44 for guidelines for patient requiring narcotics for pain relief. Patients receiving controlled substances may express concern about possible drug dependence. The use of the medication should be explained in terms of the patient's own condition, and the patient may be appropriately reassured.

Evaluation

Patient evaluation is a two-level process for controlled substances. First, the patient evaluation should be performed as for any other type of drug. Ascertain whether the medication is successfully controlling the signs and symptoms for which it was given. Second, evaluate the patient for psychological response to addictive drugs. Note signs of drug dependence and excessive fears of addiction. These observations may dictate changes in the therapeutic program.

REGULATION OF CONTROLLED SUBSTANCES

Because substances that produce physical or psychological addiction clearly have the capacity to harm their users, they have been regulated extensively in the United States and Canada, as well as throughout the world. The original legislation in the United States was the Harrison Narcotic Act of 1914. This law restricted the importation of many of these addictive substances. One of the major aims of the Pure

Food and Drug Act of 1906 and the Harrison Act was to prevent the sale of patent medicines that contained no active ingredient except one of these addicting agents.

The Harrison Act did not eliminate the problem of illicit drug use and addiction. The existing law was also clearly limited in dealing with certain synthetic agents that were useful clinically but also highly addictive. This legislation was replaced by a more comprehensive law in 1970, the Controlled Substances Act. In addition to supplying guidelines for the definition of drug dependency and establishing education and treatment programs, this law clearly classifies drugs based on abuse potential and clinical usefulness and specifies the restrictions that apply to each type of controlled drug. The drug schedules are described in Table 2-5.

Drugs in each of the schedules defined by the Controlled Substances Act are regulated by rules appropriate to them. For example, schedule I substances have no approved medical uses and are therefore simply banned. Schedule II drugs are controlled at every stage from initial manufacture through distribution and final use. By law, no prescription for a schedule II drug may be refilled. Physicians must be licensed to prescribe these medications and must keep accurate records to ensure that drugs are used strictly for legitimate purposes. Likewise, pharmacies must be specially licensed and keep accurate records for schedule II drugs.

Drugs in schedules III, IV, and V are considered less dangerous than those in schedule II. For the most part, this greater safety is a result of the inherent properties of the chemicals that appear in these schedules. However, some chemicals appear in more than

Table 2-5   Classification of Controlled Substances

Classification	Description	Specific substances
Schedule I	Drugs that have high potential for abuse and no accepted medical use. Containers are marked C-1.	Heroin, LSD, peyote, marijuana
Schedule II	Drugs that have high potential for abuse but have accepted medical use. Dependence may include strong physical and psychologic dependence. Containers are marked C-II.	Amobarbital, amphetamine, codeine, dextroamphetamine, meperidine, methadone, hydromorphone, morphine, opium, pentobarbital, phenazocine, methylphenidate, secobarbital
Schedule III	Medically accepted drugs that may cause dependence but are less prone to abuse than drugs in Schedules I and II. Containers are marked C-III.	Codeine-containing medications, butabarbital, paregoric
Schedule IV	Medically accepted drugs that may cause mild physical or psychologic dependence. Containers are marked C-IV.	Chloral hydrate, chlordiazepoxide, diazepam, meprobamate, phenobarbital
Schedule V	Medically accepted drugs with very limited potential for causing mild physical or psychologic dependence. Containers are marked C-V.	Drug mixtures containing small quantities of narcotics, such as over-the-counter cough syrups containing codeine

one schedule. For example, codeine used alone as an antitussive is a schedule II drug. However, medications containing codeine compounded with aspirin, acetaminophen, or other agents are schedule III drugs, even when the total dose of codeine is the same as that used in the schedule II preparations. One reason that these compounded forms of codeine are considered less likely to be abused is that adverse symptoms from overdoses of the other ingredients in the compounds discourage abuse of these forms of codeine. Codeine also appears in several cough syrups that are schedule V drugs. The recommended single dose of codeine for adults in these schedule V medications is 5 or 10 mg, whereas the doses found in schedule II or III forms are 15 to 60 mg. This lower dose in the cough medications is responsible for the schedule V classification.

CANADIAN DRUG LEGISLATION
Food and Drugs Act

Drug regulation is carried out through the Health Protection Branch of the Canadian government. Under this branch the Drugs Directorate oversees the various bureaus that deal with specific areas of regulation. For example, the Bureau of Human Prescription Drugs deals with new drugs intended for human use. Separate bureaus deal with veterinary products, nonprescription drugs, biologicals, drug research, and control of drug quality.

Under the Food and Drugs Act of 1953, drugs are divided into various categories (Table 2-6). When approved for sale, all Canadian drugs are assigned a six-digit number preceded by the letters GP (proprietary drug) or DIN (over-the-counter drug). In addition, all prescription drugs must be well marked with the appropriate symbol to identify the schedule to which they belong. Regulations covering the various schedules of drugs differ, making the clear identification system important. Drugs listed in schedule F are sold only by prescription, with refills limited to 6 months. Drugs in Schedule G are called *controlled drugs* and have more stringent controls regulating the number and timing of refills for the prescription. Certain controlled drugs are called *designated drugs* because their use is restricted to specific conditions described by law. For example, amphetamines, phenmetrazine, and phendimetrazine are designated for use in conditions such as narcolepsy, hyperkinesis in children, or minimum brain dysfunction, but they must not be used without special permission for conditions not listed in the regulations.

The Food and Drugs Act in Canada also protects citizens from contaminated, adulterated, or unsafe drugs. To ensure drug quality the law requires in-

Table 2-6   Canadian Drug Classifications

Classification	Description	Specific substances
NONPRESCRIPTION DRUGS		
Proprietary medicines	Drugs that may be widely purchased for self-treatment of symptoms of minor self-limiting diseases; identified by six-digit code preceded by letters *GP*	Cough drops, medicated shampoos, minor pain relievers
Over-the-counter drugs	Drugs available through a pharmacy and used on advice of a health professional for control of symptoms of minor self-limiting diseases, identified by six-digit code preceded by letters *DIN*	Laxatives, cough syrups, cold remedies, sinus preparations, certain vitamins
PRESCRIPTION DRUGS		
Schedule F	Over 200 drugs that may not be used except after professional consultation; identified by symbol *Pr* on label	Hormones, antibiotics, tranquilizers
Schedule G	Drugs that affect central nervous system (e.g., stimulants, sedatives); identified by symbol *C* on label	Amphetamines, barbiturates
Narcotics	Drugs used primarily for relief of pain but also possessing significant psychotropic activity; identified by letter *N* on label	Cannabis (marijuana), cocaine, codeine, morphine, opium, phencyclidine
RESTRICTED DRUGS		
Schedule H	Drugs with no recognized medical use and significant danger of physiologic and psychologic side effects; available only to institutions for research	Lysergic acid diethylamide (LSD), *N,N*-diethyltryptamine (DET), *N,N*-dimethyltryptamine (DMT), 4-methyl-2, 5-dimethoxyamphetamine (STP, DOM)

spection of manufacturing facilities, calls for analysis of drug samples by government laboratories, and maintains an active monitoring system to detect adverse reactions to drugs. Drug labeling is also closely controlled so that false, misleading, or deceptive labels are prohibited. Drugs may not be advertised to the general public as cures for alcoholism, cancer, heart disease, infectious diseases, and other specific conditions. No prescription drug may be advertised to the general public.

Narcotic Control Act

The Narcotic Control Act (1961) regulates the manufacture, distribution, and sale of narcotic drugs, establishing this group as separate from drugs regulated under the Food and Drugs Act. Regulations, which have the force of law, spell out specific provisions of this act and are frequently revised in response to changing needs.

All steps in the manufacturing, distribution, and sale of drugs on schedules G and H, as well as narcotics, are subject to stringent regulation. Possession of these drugs for any reason other than those related to medical use as described in the legislation is an offense subject to severe penalties. Dispensers of these drugs must be licensed by the government and must maintain extensive records documenting sources and recipients for all drugs, as well as amounts and dates for all transactions. As in the United States, nurses may be in possession of narcotics or controlled and restricted drugs only when authorized by a physician's order to administer the drug to a patient or when authorized to act as official custodian of drugs for a specific unit of a health care facility.

Development of New Drugs in Canada

New drugs are evaluated in Canada by a sequence of tests similar to those used in the United States. Promising drugs undergo preclinical testing in three mammalian species, including one nonrodent species, to determine threshold doses that produce toxicity or death. The next stage of evaluation is the clinical pharmacology trial, which is analogous to phase I trials in the United States. During the clinical pharmacology trial the drug is administered to healthy human volunteers to establish the safety of doses that might be required for clinical applications. If the drug proves safe and if manufacturing processes have been developed to allow the production of a pure and uniform preparation for human use, the manufacturer may apply for permission to distribute the drug to qualified investigators who will test the use of the drug in patients. This stage of testing is analogous to phase II in the United States. Before the drug may be released for general use, extensive documentation must be filed and evaluated concerning the chemical properties of the drug, its formulation, labeling, and packaging, as well as all the clinical data on humans and the test data on animals. All new drugs are monitored after being placed on the market. Only after extensive information has been accumulated to document the safety of a new drug when used in normal medical practice is the drug released from the controls required by the designation new drug.

NURSING IMPLICATIONS SUMMARY

General Guidelines

◆ Be familiar with the nurse practice acts that govern practice in your setting. As these acts are written in legislative language, ask questions as needed to clarify thmeaning of all components.

◆ Stay informed of agency policies related to dispensing, administering, and accounting for drugs. Observe deadlines and expiration dates of orders. Maintain vigilance in working with controlled and scheduled drugs.

◆ Consult the current literature, the pharmacist, and the physician to learn about new drug preparations. Ask questions as needed to clarify changes in protocols for administration of drugs.

◆ Assess each patient individually, and ask, "Is this the right drug in the right dose for this patient?" See Chapter 3 for additional information.

◆ Be familiar with policies regarding the role of the nurse with investigational drugs. Serve as the patient's advocate in working with patients involved in drug studies.

CHAPTER REVIEW

◆ **KEY TERMS**

double-blind design, p. 30
generic, p. 25
orphan drugs, p. 26
physical addiction, p. 32
placebo effect, p. 30
trade name, p. 25

◆ **REVIEW QUESTIONS**

1. What is the "active ingredient" of a medicinal preparation?
2. What is the purpose of the *United States Pharmacopeia* and the *National Formulary*?
3. Outline the steps involved in getting a new drug approved in the United States or Canada.
4. What is a clinical trial? Describe a clinical trial following the double-blind design.
5. What is the placebo effect?
6. Suggest two explanations for the placebo effect observed in drug trials. How might the nurse use knowledge of the placebo effect to possibly improve the patient's response to a medication?
7. What is the purpose of the informed consent form?
8. What is a treatment IND?
9. What is the purpose of the Drug Efficacy Study Implementation?
10. What are controlled substances? What are some nursing implications related to administering a controlled substance?
11. What special precautions are required in handling controlled substances?

SUGGESTED READING

Current drug information

British pharmacopoeia 1988 and Addendum for each year following, London, 1988, Her Majesty's Stationery Office.
Compendium of pharmaceuticals and specialties, ed 28, Ottawa, 1988, Canadian Pharmaceutical Association.
Drug evaluations annual, Chicago, 1991, American Medical Association.
Drug information, Bethesda, MD, American Hospital Formulary Service, published yearly.
Drug information for the health care provider, Rockville, MD, United States Pharmacopeial Convention, published yearly.
Facts and comparisons, St Louis, Facts and Comparisons, updated monthly.
FDA drug bulletin, Rockville, MD, Department of Health and Human Services, published three times a year.
Gahart BL: *Intravenous medications*, ed 8, St Louis, 1992, Mosby–Year Book, published yearly.
The international pharmacopoeia, ed 3, 1988, World Health Organization.
Karb VB, Queener SF, Freeman JB: *Handbook of drugs for nursing practice*, St Louis, 1989, Mosby–Year Book.
Nursing 92 I.V. drug handbook, Springhouse, Pa, Springhouse published yearly.
Physician's desk reference, Ordell, NJ, Medical Economics, published yearly.
Skidmore-Roth L: *Mosby's 1992 nursing drug reference*, St Louis, 1991, Mosby–Year Book, published yearly.

Drug regulation

Food and Drug Administration: Investigational new drug, antibiotic, and biological drug product regulations; treatment use and sale; final rule, *Federal Register* 52(99):19466, 1987.
Hodges LC, Patterson R, Rapp CG: Clinical trials: the role of the neuroscience nurse, *J Neurosci Nurs* 22(3):195, 1990.
Investigational new drug regulations, *AORN J* 47(6):1473, 1988.
Nielsen JR: *Handbook of federal drug law*, Philadelphia, 1986, Lea & Febiger.
Parks BR Jr: Orphan drugs . . . pharmaceutical products that may be commercially available in other countries but not in the United States, *Pediatr Nurs* 14(2):152, 1988.
US Department of Justice: Regulations implementing the comprehensive Drug Abuse Prevention and Control Act of 1970, *Federal Register* 36(80):1, 1971.
Weinstein SM: Use of investigational drugs, *NITA* 10(5):336, 1987.
Young FE and others: The FDA's new procedures for the use of investigational drugs in treatment, *JAMA* 259:2267, 1988.

CHAPTER 3

Application of the Nursing Process to Drug Therapy

LEARNING OBJECTIVES

After studying this chapter, you should be able to do the following:

- Discuss the use of the nursing process with patients receiving medications.
- Explain the rights of drug administration.
- Describe factors that influence patient compliance.
- Discuss legal constraints on the administration of drugs.
- Describe the nurse's role when medication errors occur.

CHAPTER OVERVIEW

- The focus of this chapter is on the use of the nursing process in administering drugs. This includes a discussion of the classic steps in the nursing process but then elaborates on some of the steps the nurse should consider in preparing and administering drugs. This chapter complements Chapter 2 on regulations, Chapter 4 on over-the-counter medications, and Chapter 6 on drug administration techniques.

Nursing Process Overview

THE NURSING PROCESS AND DRUG THERAPY

Assessment

Assessment includes gathering all of the subjective and objective pertinent data about a patient, physically assessing the patient, and evaluating laboratory, radiographic, and other data. Throughout assessment the nurse analyzes the data and formulates nursing diagnoses.

Nursing Diagnoses

Nursing diagnoses are derived from the assessment data. With the possible exception of "knowledge deficit," no single nursing diagnosis fits all situations related to drug therapy.

Management

Management includes the planning and implementation phases. The nurse develops the plan in response to the assessment of patient needs and the knowledge of the treatment plan. The plan should include goals and specific steps to reach the goals. The patient or family is included in the plan development. Implementation involves carrying out the plan. Planning and implementation should include individualizing the approach to fit unique patient needs.

Evaluation

Evaluation involves determining the success of the plan and the implementation of the plan, as well as determining whether the goals have been reached for the patient. It involves deciding whether the goals were appropriate for the patient. Finally, evaluation involves revising the overall plan.

THE NURSING PROCESS AND PHARMACOLOGY

Assessment

Assessment involves gathering data about the patient or client. This data base is important in the treatment of the patient. It forms the baseline against which changes will be compared. It also allows the nurse to develop an individualized plan for the patient.

The physical assessment should be complete, yet tailored to the patient's needs and the severity of the presenting health problems. The history of the present health problems includes a drug history (Figure 3-1). Information from the drug history helps the nurse better understand the patient's previous drug

Name _____

Age _____ Date _____

Major health problems: _____

_____

Other health problems requiring medications: _____

_____

1. Medications used for major health problems

   These questions are only a guide. The patient's comments may lead the examiner to pursue certain topics in more detail.

   What medicines are you currently taking?

Medicine	Dose	Frequency	Comments

   Are you having problems with any of these medicines? *Go through each medicine, asking the following questions.*

   a. Are you able to take this drug the way it is ordered? What time(s) each day do you take it?
   b. Are you having any side effects? *Use words that the patient can understand, such as "Are there reasons you cannot take this medicine?" or "Are there any problems with taking this medicine?"*
   c. Do you think this drug is helping? *For example, "Is your blood pressure pill helping your blood pressure?"*
   d. If appropriate, ask about cost. *"Some patients find that this medicine is very expensive. Has the cost of this drug been a problem?"*
   e. If appropriate, ask about ability to obtain refills. *"Do you have any problems getting refills for this drug?" "Do you have any problems picking up your refills at the drugstore?"*

   Note anything that might be important in teaching this patient about medications: drugs that should be refrigerated or left at room temperature, dangers of putting drugs in unlabeled containers, importance of storing drugs out of reach of small children, etc.

2. General drug use

   How do you take care of the following problems/conditions? What medicines do you use for them? *"How often do you take the medicine?" "Does it work?" "When did you last take it?"*

   a. Pain: headache, muscle pains, toothaches? *Expand as needed for each patient.*
   b. Gastrointestinal system: constipation, diarrhea, upset stomach, heartburn?
   c. Skin conditions: psoriasis, athlete's foot, dry skin? *Ask about special shampoos and creams.*
   d. Nervous, mental, or emotional disorders: nervousness, being unable to sleep, upset?
   e. Reproductive system: birth control pills, female hormones, menstrual pain, backache?
   f. Nutritional deficiencies: iron, vitamins, bran, yeast, etc.?
   g. Upper respiratory tract, eye, and nose: What do you do for a cold? Cough? Stuffy nose? Sinus problem? Do you take nose drops? Use nasal spray? Eye drops?
   h. Other: special teas, liniments, plasters, soda, drugs made from roots? *Knowledge of local custom is helpful in this category.*

3. General health habits

   a. Do you smoke? How much?
   b. How much whiskey (beer, wine) do you drink? (Response may not be accurate)
   c. How often do you do drugs on a recreational basis? (Response may not be accurate. Remain nonjudgmental.)
   d. Do you follow any special diet (low salt, diabetic, low protein, etc.)? Are you a vegetarian? *In some cases a complete diet history might be warranted.*
   e. Where do you work? What kinds of work have you done in the past? Have you lived anywhere else in the country?
   f. Are you allergic to anything? Are there any medicines you cannot take? Why?
   g. Which immunizations have you received? When did you last have a tetanus shot?

FIGURE 3-1

Sample drug history.

use, attitudes about drugs, and knowledge about drugs.

Another component of the assessment comes from the laboratory results, radiology reports, and results of other diagnostic testing. These results may confirm existing health problems or provide a baseline against which the nurse can later check for deviations or improvement, possibly related to drugs administered.

Nursing Diagnoses

A **nursing diagnosis** is a statement of a health problem or potential problem that a nurse is licensed and competent to treat. The nurse derives nursing diagnoses by analyzing the data obtained in the patient assessment. There are no nursing diagnoses that apply only to drug administration. The diagnoses reflect analysis of the entire patient and the patient's needs, and these may include aspects of drug administration.

The wording of the nursing diagnoses is specific, and comes from the North American Nursing Diagnoses Association (NANDA). NANDA has met regularly since 1973 to refine the list of NANDA-approved nursing diagnoses. The most recent listing is published when updated (see reference list).

With regard to medication administration, several points related to nursing diagnoses should be made. The only nursing diagnosis that possibly could be applied in all situations of drug administration is the "knowledge deficit." Most patients who are to receive new drug therapy have some knowledge deficit, but it may be minimal. Careful assessment may reveal that other diagnoses are more appropriate.

Some nursing diagnoses that encompass an entire health problem may be more appropriate than a diagnosis that focuses on the drug therapy alone. For example, for the diabetic patient who must take insulin, a nursing diagnosis of "high risk for altered health maintenance related to lack of knowledge of diabetes mellitus, management, and signs and symptoms of complications" would allow for a more detailed plan than a diagnosis that focuses on insulin alone.

Side effects that are frequently encountered or are very serious may form the basis for some nursing diagnoses. For example, the narcotic analgesics cause constipation. When the narcotics are used for 2 or 3 days, the constipation may be minimal. When narcotics are used in high doses for extensive periods, as they may be for some patients with cancer, it may be appropriate to have a nursing diagnosis in the plan that comes from this knowledge. Thus for a patient with cancer who is receiving frequent or high doses of narcotics, a nursing diagnosis of "High risk for constipation related to narcotic use for pain relief" may be appropriate. For a patient on a diuretic known to contribute to potassium loss, "high risk for electrolyte abnormalities (hypokalemia) related to furosemide therapy" may be appropriate.

Nursing diagnoses may describe a problem for which additional data are needed. Consider the patient who is to take moderate to large doses of corticosteroids. These drugs have side effects of weight gain and development of a characteristic round face (moon face). A nursing diagnosis might be "possible self-concept disturbance related to physical changes secondary to prednisone therapy."

It could be easy to develop extensive lists of "high risk" and "possible" diagnoses related to any known side effect of drug therapy. It is more prudent to use these for serious or frequently encountered problems. Remember that each patient is unique, and a problem for one patient will not necessarily be the same for another.

Planning

Planning involves developing an outline of nursing interventions needed to treat the nursing diagnoses. Usually, the steps in the plan should direct the nurses toward common goals, so it is often helpful to develop the goals first. These goals should be developed with the patient and family. The goals should be specific enough to allow the nurse and patient to know whether the goal is being reached. The patient newly diagnosed as diabetic provides an example. A measurable goal might be "Mr. Hayes will demonstrate correct technique in administering insulin injections to himself." Correct technique may be spelled out on the care plan also but should include maintaining aseptic technique, drawing up the dose accurately, locating the injection site correctly, administering the injection correctly, and recording the injection site.

The plan should then spell out nursing interventions that should be used by members of the team. These interventions may be carried out on a daily timetable, or deadlines for accomplishing components of the plan may be identified. Thus an intervention to "check the stool for occult blood" should be done each time a patient has a bowel movement. Another intervention might be "increase ambulation by walking 10 feet more each time the patient is up; by Tuesday the patient should be able to walk to the end of the hall and back." This intervention includes a goal within the intervention.

Implementation

The **implementation** phase is the carrying out of the plan. In this phase, the nurse must incorporate the steps on the plan within the daily routine for the patient. It is often during this phase that the nurse or patient begins to identify changes that need to be made (e.g., the plan is unreasonable, or the patient is not ready for such detailed instruction).

Evaluation

Evaluation, although listed as the final step of the nursing process, takes the nurse back to the first step of assessment. During evaluation, the nurse determines whether the plan is working. Has the patient reached the desired goals? What should be modified in the plan? What additional data are needed? Are the drugs working as planned? Are side effects developing? What new problems are there?

The nursing process is often presented in a linear fashion: assessing → diagnosing → planning → implementing → evaluating. However, it often also occurs in a circular fashion. The nurse working closely with the patient may assess the patient and begin to develop nursing diagnoses. Finding a need for more information, the nurse obtains more assessment data. In developing the plan and implementing it, the nurse constantly evaluates its feasibility and success. While evaluating the plan, the nurse continues to assess. The **nursing process** is a systematic, organized way of approaching the patient and developing a plan for health care.

THE RIGHTS OF DRUG ADMINISTRATION

Traditionally, the teaching of principles of drug administration has centered around the **five rights of drug administration** (see box): the right drug, via the right route, in the right dose, at the right time, and to the right patient. Although at first glance it might seem that these rights should be easy to achieve, the day-to-day practice of nursing requires thoughtful attention to these rights at all times.

The right drug suggests not only that the patient receives the prescribed drug, but also the right drug for the particular health problem. The nurse must pay careful attention to drug orders and medication labels while preparing drugs and be familiar with each

---

THE FIVE RIGHTS OF DRUG ADMINISTRATION

The right *drug*

The right *route*

The right *dose*

The right *time*

The right *patient*

---

patient and his or her health care problems. To know if a prescribed drug is appropriate the nurse must know and understand the patient's health problems and be current in pharmacologic knowledge. The rest of this book provides basic material about drugs, but the nurse in practice must also regularly consult printed materials and other health care professionals for additional information. Some of these sources are discussed in Chapters 2 and 4.

To ensure that the patient receives prescribed medications via the right route, the nurse must know each medication that is administered. The student may have difficulty understanding how or why a nurse could administer a medication via the wrong route, but in a busy nurse's day errors can occur easily. For example, an experienced nurse who usually works in the coronary care setting is asked to work for a day in the surgical intensive care unit. The nurse, accustomed to administering morphine intravenously for cardiac pain, administers all parenteral pain medications in the surgical intensive care setting intravenously also, even those ordered via the intramuscular (IM) route. Fortunately, in this true incident the nurse discovered the errors and reported them, and no harm came to the patients.

Administering the right dose of medication is extremely important. Not only must the nurse double check calculations for mathematical accuracy, the nurse also must ask, "Is this dose appropriate for the size and age of the patient?" This responsibility emphasizes the need for current knowledge about drugs and usual dosage ranges. Although the administration of an incorrect dose is serious for any patient, it can be especially serious in the pediatric patient, for whom prescribed doses are often small. A review of dosage calculations can be found in Chapter 7.

Ensuring that the patient receives drugs at the right time may be difficult. Often the health care team must weigh the information available about the pharmacokinetics and pharmacodynamics of drugs (see Chapter 1) against the patient's lifestyle and potential for compliance. In the critical care setting, where one nurse may care for one or two patients, drugs are administered at evenly spaced intervals throughout a 24-hour period. The nurse, although usually very busy, can concentrate on administering medications to a few patients. On a busy general care unit, the nurse may have 20 or more patients who must receive drugs, and these patients may be coming and going to the radiology department, therapy, or surgery. In addition, most patients would prefer not to be wakened at night to receive medications. In the home, it is even easier for the patient to forget a dose or be less careful about intervals between doses. Another factor in the home setting is general lifestyle. For example, patients who work a night shift and sleep during the day may need help determining the right times to take drugs.

Other factors that influence the right dosage time include whether the patient is receiving multiple drugs, whether a drug can be taken on an empty or full stomach, or whether a prescribed drug can be taken with other medications. To ensure that patients receive drugs at the right time, the nurse must know about the patient, the health care problems, and the drugs.

Finally, the right patient must receive the drug. The nurse must check the patient's identity each time drugs are administered. Not only should the patient be Ms. Smith, but it must be the right Ms. Smith. The right patient also means that the right drugs were prescribed for the right patient, and thus the nurse is back to the first of the five rights of drug administration.

PATIENT EDUCATION AND MEDICATIONS

One of the major goals of nursing care in drug administration is preparing the patient and family for return to independent function in the home or community. The patient, when able, will take over the role of self-administration of medications. No one can guarantee that the patient will take a medication exactly as directed and derive the expected benefits of drug therapy. However, careful patient assessment, planning, and teaching by the nurse can help the patient to better understand prescribed medications and how to use them safely.

Attitudes about Medications

All patients come to the health care system with preexisting ideas and attitudes about who should take medications, whether or not they are generally helpful, what the meaning of sickness and health is, and what to expect of the health care team. Additional factors include personally held beliefs, attitudes and opinions of family and friends, religious and cultural beliefs, and influence of the media about certain kinds of medications. The public may not even use the same vocabulary as the health care team. For example, a nurse or physician may use the words *drug, medicine,* or *medication* interchangeably; but these words may have different connotations to the patient.

To be successful in preparing the patient for self-management, assess the patient's attitudes about medicines. Do this by asking questions or developing an assessment tool, by remaining attuned to the patient's response to medications in the health care setting, and by attempting to validate these impressions with the patient. The nurse in the hospital or insti-

tution is generally in control of the medication situation, and the patient can avoid becoming very involved in the self-medication plans. The nurse in the home is given many more clues about patient attitudes regarding medication administration. Any plan for teaching patients about drugs will be more successful if it is compatible with the patient's existing beliefs and attitudes. It is possible to change attitudes and beliefs, but this requires careful planning, and it is difficult.

General Principles to Teach about All Medications

Regardless of the specific drugs prescribed for a patient, there are some general principles about drugs to teach all patients (see box). Keep all drugs out of reach of children, and keep the drugs in the original labeled containers. Decorative pill boxes are attractive, but many patients fill them with several drugs simultaneously. This practice provides great potential for error and may hasten decomposition of some drugs. Use child-proof caps unless the patient cannot independently remove them. Even so, children must be protected from access to drugs. Ideally, keep all drugs in a locked container, out of the reach of children.

Take medications only as ordered. Patients should not double up to catch up when doses have been missed. Do not share drugs with family or friends. Warn patients that altering the dose size does not improve the effect; two is not better than one. If any medication is left after a health problem has been treated, discard it. Treat drugs purchased over the counter with the same degree of respect as other medications; they are not to be considered less seriously just because they have not been prescribed by a physician or dispensed by a pharmacist.

Instruct patients to keep all health care providers informed of all drugs they are taking. Patients taking multiple drugs should keep a list of drugs and dosages, preferably with them at all times, and check it regularly to see if it is current. Encourage patients with chronic conditions or severe allergies to wear a medical identification bracelet or necklace listing the allergy, medical condition, or type of medication used.

Teach all individuals, especially parents of small children, to keep the number of the local poison control center near the phone in the event of ingestion of or exposure to toxic kinds or amounts of drugs. Teach children that drugs are not for playing; they are not candy. This rule applies to all drugs, including vitamins, birth control pills, laxatives, and other prescription and nonprescription substances.

SAFE MEDICATION USE: POINTS TO REVIEW WITH ALL PATIENTS

Take drugs prescribed for you; do not borrow drugs from others or share your drugs with others.

Take only the dose prescribed. If you feel the dose is too high or too low, check with the physician before adjusting the dose or frequency of doses.

When a new drug is prescribed, find out what to do if a dose is missed. Usually, do not double-up for missed doses. Take a missed dose as soon as it is remembered, unless it is within 2 hr of the next regularly scheduled dose. Resume the regular dose schedule.

When a new drug is prescribed, find out how to take it in relation to meals or other drugs you may be taking. Some drugs should be taken with meals or food, whereas others should be taken on an empty stomach.

Each time a new drug is prescribed, find out why you are taking it and what the common side effects are. Never hesitate to call the doctor if an unexpected sign or symptom develops; it may be related to the medications you are taking.

Store your medications properly. Usually, this means in a dry place, but not in the bathroom, where there may be steam and moisture, since these may cause medicines to deteriorate and lose strength. Do not mix different pills in the same container, such as a pill box for your pocket or purse. This may cause the medicines to lose their strength, and without labels, you may take the wrong drug by accident.

Write down the names of the drugs you are taking, and take this list whenever you visit the doctor, nurse, dentist, podiatrist, ophthalmologist, osteopathic physician, chiropractor, or clinic. Keep all your health care providers informed of all the drugs you are taking, even those you purchase over the counter.

Keep drugs out of the reach of children. Use child-proof caps if there are children in your home. Never refer to medications as candy.

Read the label each time you take a dose of medicine to make sure you are taking the drug you think you are taking; sometimes two different drugs may look alike.

Wear a medical identification tag, bracelet, or necklace listing chronic health problems and medication allergies.

Keep track of your prescription drugs. Try not to run out of them on the weekend or during holidays, when it may be difficult to get a prescription refilled. If your drug supply is getting low, call the physician's office. Be prepared to give the nurse the name of the drug and dose and the name of the pharmacy and its telephone number where you wish to have the prescription filled.

Keep the telephone number of the local poison control center near your telephone. Keep ipecac in your home but out of the reach of children. This drug can be used to make a person vomit if a drug was taken that should not have been. Never use ipecac unless the poison control center or your doctor says you should.

Information about a Specific Drug

When teaching a patient about a specific drug, tailor the instructional approach to the needs and abilities of the patient. Careful patient assessment and analysis is the foundation of the teaching plan. Figure 3-1 illustrates a sample drug history that may provide data for use in developing a teaching plan. It could also be incorporated into the general health history done for all patients. It should be modified as needed.

Teach the patient what the name and dosage of the prescribed drug is, why it is being used, and what the anticipated benefits of the drug are. Discuss the potential side effects in sufficient detail so that the patient will be able to list the most frequently encountered side effects. Whether the more serious (sometimes fatal, but also more rare) side effects should be discussed in detail depends on the patient and the situation. Instruct all patients and caregivers about whom to call (e.g., physician or nurse practitioner) if anything unexpected occurs.

If there are any management decisions that the patient must make, review them carefully with the patient. Examples include changes in dose strength or frequency, depending on the patient's response to the medication, or home treatment of frequently en-

countered side effects. Have the patient practice any measurements that would be made at home (e.g., taking and recording pulse and checking blood sugar).

Inform the patient of any special considerations related to the dose, such as whether to take a drug on an empty or full stomach, whether to avoid milk, or whether to avoid taking two particular drugs simultaneously. If a new drug administration technique is involved, ascertain that the patient can demonstrate how to do this safely and accurately. Include appropriate general principles related to drug use.

Finally, provide the patient with information about how and when follow-up will occur and how to call for help or additional information. It is often advisable and helpful to have additional family members present if the instruction is lengthy and complicated. Provide written instructions whenever possible. It also may be helpful to refer the patient to a community-based nursing agency for follow-up in the home.

Patient Compliance

Even when the nurse has developed and implemented what seems to be a complete and individualized teaching plan, patient compliance may be poor. The many possible reasons for this include the following:

◆ The patient or family misunderstands the directions.

◆ Poor vision or hearing leads to errors in understanding or reading labels.

◆ The patient cannot afford the drug (see box on p. 80).

◆ The patient cannot get the prescription refilled.

◆ The patient becomes confused with the number of medications taken, taking the drugs in incorrect amounts and at wrong times.

◆ The patient cannot manage the new route of administration in the home without help (e.g., self-injection).

◆ The patient is unable to accept a particular diagnosis (e.g., the teenager who does not check blood for glucose in the morning before insulin administration or who injects insulin too late in the day.)

◆ Intolerable side effects occur, and the patient is too embarrassed to mention them to anyone (e.g., sexual impotence).

◆ Side effects that cause the patient to feel worse than the health problem occur, a common problem with some antihypertensive drugs.

The nurse who is in the patient's home may find clues to noncompliance. For example, too many pills may remain in the bottle at the end of the month, or the patient cannot describe how to take the prescribed medications. In the office or hospital, it may be more difficult for the nurse to find these clues; only the lack of congruence between objective data and subjective response (e.g., the patient describes taking the antihypertensive, but the blood pressure remains high) may give the nurse a clue. The nurse must use careful nonjudgmental questioning to find out if there is a problem and to help the patient find a way to better manage the health problem (i.e., by taking the drug).

The nurse must be creative in finding ways to help patients. Some frequently tried methods include making a special calendar with items the patient must check off when the dose is taken or putting the pills into color-coded cups or containers, with each color corresponding to a specific mealtime. The doses of a medication may be prepared for 7 days and left with the patient who has difficulty preparing the dosage form. Pill containers with an alarm are also available; these can be set to go off each time a patient is to take a dose of drug. In other situations, compliance can be improved by changing the dose, the time the drug is to be taken, or even the drug; consult the physician. Finally, remember that patients have the right to choose whether and how they will take their medications; some simply choose to not comply.

REGULATIONS AND DRUG ADMINISTRATION
Personnel: Who Does What

Many people may be involved in the prescription, preparation, and administration of a drug to a patient. Generally, physicians prescribe drugs. Their authorization to prescribe is granted through licensing and medical practice acts. Other individuals do prescribe, including dentists and oral surgeons, osteopathic physicians, podiatrists, nurse practitioners, midwives, and physician's assistants. However, the degree of independence of practice that these and other health care practitioners may exercise varies with laws of the state, province, or nation. This introduces the first of many points that the nurse must consider before administering a drug. Who has prescribed the drug, and does that person have the legal right to do so in that setting?

In the institutional setting, safeguards are often created to prevent unauthorized prescription of drugs. For example, to be granted privileges to practice in a hospital, a physician must present appropriate credentials, proof of licensure, and other documents required by that hospital. After a nurse has worked on a nursing unit for several weeks, the physicians will become known to the nurse, which also helps reduce the chance of errors in who may prescribe. Even in the hospital, the nurse ascertains the role of each person on the health care team. For example, in some teaching hospitals it is customary for medical students to have rotations as acting interns (they may have other titles also). These individuals are not yet licensed, yet they may be caring for patients under the supervision of licensed preceptors (physicians). The nurse must be clear about the legal ramifications of administering drugs prescribed by a nonlicensed individual.

When looking for guidance about who may prescribe and whose prescriptions must be administered, the nurse can consult the nurse practice act (or comparable professional practice act) for that state, province, or country. The written policies of the employing agency or institution also provide guidance. Finally, nurses must consider their own moral and ethical codes of conduct in deciding whether to administer a specific drug to a patient. The nurse always has the personal right to refuse to administer a medication. For example, a nurse may refuse to give an ordered medication if professional judgment indicates the dose is excessively high. The nurse must notify the physician and the nurse in charge of the decision not to administer the medication.

It is important to remember that the legal constraints the nurse must consider may have less meaning to the patient. This situation is faced more often in the home, where the patient may wish to have the nurse administer a medication or home remedy prescribed or recommended by someone not recognized by the nurse practice act.

Pharmacists, who usually dispense medication, are licensed to do so and are governed by legal statutes. Pharmacies often employ aides or technicians to help fill prescriptions, but these individuals function under the supervision of the registered pharmacist. The pharmacist is an excellent source of information about drugs for the nurse or the patient but is often underutilized in this role.

Registered nurses can administer medications within the legal framework of the nurse practice act. Licensed practical nurses and licensed vocational nurses also have practice acts that regulate the role they play in drug administration. In some areas, pharmacists, medication technicians, medical students, emergency medical technicians, or others may administer drugs as employees of an institution or agency. Various students may be permitted to administer drugs in an agency, institution, or other setting if supervised. This includes students in nursing, medical, physician assistant, emergency medical technician, and other educational programs. In the home the patient and family administer drugs.

Institutional Policies and Practices

The nurse practices not only within the legal framework of the practice act but also within the policies and procedures of the employing agency. The nurse is responsible for reading carefully any written information that defines restrictions or expectations of practice within the employing agency structure. The nurse should not blindly adhere to policy that is in direct conflict with legal guidelines or reasonable ethical and moral standards, but neither should the nurse practice outside the role defined by the agency.

In some agencies, verbal orders for drugs may be taken only by registered nurses. Students, licensed practical nurses, and others may not take these orders (see the box on p. 78). Some institutions prohibit the nurse from obtaining the patient's informed consent for investigational drugs; this consent may be obtained only by the physician. In other settings the physician alone may administer investigational drugs. Medication orders written by medical students may be administered only after they are cosigned by a licensed physician. Such policies often develop as an interpretation of the law or to prevent anticipated problems.

Other procedures developed in an agency often respond to previous problems or errors that have occurred. Examples include all heparin and insulin doses being checked by two nurses before they may be administered, any parenteral drugs administered

to pediatric patients being checked by two nurses before being administered, and narcotics being counted at the end of each shift by two nurses, one from the ending shift and one from the beginning shift.

It is not necessary for the nurse to know exactly why a policy or procedure has developed. It is important for the nurse to practice within policy and procedure guidelines and, if the guidelines need to be changed, to work through the appropriate channels to change them. The beginning nurse may view these do's and dont's as time consuming, and some probably are not as important as others. However, all were designed to ensure safe patient care. Remember that sloppy or careless nursing practice can result in harm to the patient and malpractice suits. Failure to adhere to stated policies and procedures may weigh against the nurse in determination of legal liability.

Medication Errors

All medications are ordered, prepared, and administered with the best intentions. Errors do occur with surprising frequency.

What is an error

Defining an error is not always easy. It is clear that an error has occurred if a patient receives the wrong drug, if a patient is overmedicated, or if a prescribed drug is omitted. Other situations may be called an error. Consider the following examples. The patient receives tetracycline with a glass of milk (tetracycline should not be administered with milk); a patient in the radiology department receives the 10 AM drugs at noon; through an error in calculation, the patient receives the correct drug at the correct time but in half the ordered dose.

Some institutions differentiate between an error and an incident. Others define any deviation from policy and procedure as an *error*. This variability emphasizes the need for the nurse to know and adhere to the standards of practice defined by the nurse practice act, the policies and procedures of the employing agency and institution, and common sense.

The times at which drugs are administered in a hospital or institution are established by that setting; they are usually part of the policies and procedures. In addition, there is usually a definition of what is meant by administering a drug on time. For example, a drug to be administered at 10 AM is considered to be on time if administered any time between 9:30 AM and 10:30 AM. The way in which a particular patient unit or entire institution handles deviations from the "half hour before to half hour after" rule influences whether the time at which a particular drug is administered is called an error. Since the times for q.i.d., b.i.d., and q.d. are set by custom or policy, they also can be readjusted. Another factor that affects the time is the drug itself and how frequently it is ordered. Consider the following situations. A vitamin ordered q.d., customarily given at 10 AM, is forgotten and given at 2 PM. Most agencies would not consider this an error and would not notify the physician. Insulin ordered for q.d. is administered at 10 AM instead of before breakfast, when it should be given; this would be an error. Another drug is ordered to be given q.i.d. On a particular unit, that is customarily 10 AM, 2 PM, 6 PM, and 10 PM. A nurse misreads the medications record and administers it at 8 AM. Depending on the medication, this may not be considered an error, since the dosage times could be readjusted to 8 AM, 12 noon, 4 PM, and 8 PM.

The causes of errors

There are many causes of errors that have occurred in the process of administering medications. A few situations involving errors are listed below:

◆ A drug is ordered for the wrong patient (i.e., written on the wrong patient's chart).
◆ The wrong dose is ordered.
◆ The correct drug or dose is ordered, but because of poor penmanship the wrong drug or dosage is dispensed.
◆ An error in calculating the dose is made, so the patient receives the wrong dose.
◆ Drugs are given via the wrong route.
◆ The patient's identity is not checked, and the wrong patient receives the drug.
◆ The first person administering a drug fails to record it immediately afterward. A second person, seeing that the drug has not been administered, also does so; the patient has received a double dose.

What to do if an error occurs

A professional should accept responsibility for his or her actions. First, check the patient. Obtain any subjective or objective data appropriate to the patient's condition. If the patient received the wrong drug or the wrong dose, assess the individual for the effects of the drug. For example, if too large a dose of antihypertensive was administered, take the blood pressure, then put the patient to bed. Notify the nurse in charge and the physician. Fill out any error forms required by the institution. Continue to monitor the patient. Modify personal nursing practice, if needed, to help avoid the error in the future.

Two points need to be emphasized. The student or beginning practitioner may lack experience in handling an error or in deciding what is an error. If unsure, the practitioner should always report to the nurse in charge and to the physician any problem associated with drug administration. There are students and nurses in practice who want to avoid filling out incident forms or medication error forms because they think that admitting that an error has occurred will be detrimental to their employment or student status with the institution or agency. Records of errors help institutions develop new policies, procedures, and systems that will reduce the overall incidence of errors. No hospital or agency wants to continue to employ nurses who make repeated errors, especially of a careless nature, but most institutions recognize that anyone can make an occasional error.

How to avoid medication errors

Much of avoiding errors is using and acting on common sense. Read and adhere to institutional policies and procedures; do not try shortcuts. Read each order carefully, asking whether this drug makes sense for this patient in this dose. Look up any drug or dosage that seems questionable. Never assume that the physician was right, the pharmacist was right, or the previous nurse who administered the drugs was right if there is any question. Be especially careful in taking verbal or telephone orders because it is easy to misunderstand what is said; (see the box on p. 78).

Double-check calculations. If still uneasy, have a colleague or the pharmacy double check. If a dose seems incredibly large or small, double-check it. For example, if the order was for 10 grains of aspirin, but, through an error in recording, it is noted at 100 grains, it would require 20 aspirin tablets, an unusually large dose for a patient. The other extreme would be through error; the dose of ferrous sulfate (an iron preparation) for an adult is listed as 30 mg; to administer that dose would require $\frac{1}{10}$ tablet, an impossible task.

If possible, avoid distractions while preparing medications. Check each label 3 times: when taking the drug out of the drawer or cabinet, when checking the Kardex for the dose and time, and again at the bedside just before administering the drug. Leave medications in their labeled containers until at the bedside. Always check the patient's identity carefully. If the patient asks any questions that indicate a possible error, assume the patient is right, and double-check. Examples include statements like "That doesn't look like my usual morning pill," "I already took that—the other nurse gave it to me earlier today," or "The doctor said I would have a different pill today."

Ask about a history of allergies before administering any new drug. Finally, check each patient within a short period after administering medications. Administering medications is just one of many nursing responsibilities, but it can be one of the most dangerous if done carelessly.

NURSING IMPLICATIONS SUMMARY

◆ Perform a thorough assessment on each patient.

◆ Take a drug history if appropriate for the patient.

◆ Monitor laboratory data appropriate to the health problems, while keeping in mind drug therapy; what laboratory data should be monitored to determine drug effectiveness or side effects?

◆ Develop nursing diagnoses after analysis of all data.

◆ Develop the nursing care plan with the patient. Include appropriate teaching about the medication therapy as a part of the plan.

◆ As a part of the teaching plan, include the name of the drug; what its desired effects, common side effects, and symptoms that warrant consulting the physician are; how to administer the drug; and what to do if a dose is missed.

◆ Have patients demonstrate correct drug administration technique as needed to monitor for effectiveness of drug teaching.

◆ Emphasize the importance of all aspects of the health care plan such as exercise, lifestyle changes, dietary changes, other medications.

◆ Evaluate the patient's progress toward the goals of the nursing care plan and the success of the plan itself. What should be changed? Does the patient have suggestions?

◆ Pay attention when administering drugs (right patient, right drug, right dose, right time, right route of administration). Pause to reflect as needed. Do you need to double-check anything?

◆ Keep accurate, current records.

◆ If an error in drug administration occurs, check the patient and notify the nurse in charge and the physician. Complete error reports as indicated. Examine your own nursing care. Do you need to be more careful, slow down, ask questions, or was this error unavoidable?

CHAPTER REVIEW

◆ KEY TERMS

◆ REVIEW QUESTIONS

1. What are the steps of the nursing process?
2. Discuss how medication administration fits into the nursing process.
3. What are the five rights of drug administration?
4. List some teaching points about safe medication use that should be taught to all patients.
5. What kinds of information about drugs should be included in the patient teaching plan?
6. What are some factors that influence patient compliance?
7. In the settings where you practice, who may prescribe drugs? Who prepares them? Who administers them?
8. What is the difference between the nurse practice act, or other legal statues, and institutional policies and procedures?
9. When the nurse discovers that a medication error has occurred, what should be done?
10. What are some examples of medication errors?

SUGGESTED READING

Carpenito LJ: *Nursing diagnosis: application to clinical practice,* ed 4, Philadelphia, 1992, JB Lippincott.

Carr DS: New strategies for avoiding medication errors, *Nurs 89* 19(8):38, 1989.

Cohen MR: Avoiding errors caused by drug suffixes, *Nurs 91* 21(2):48, 1991.

Dziedzicki RE, Kerber K: Computerized drug dosing, *Crit Care Nurse* 11(2):12, 1991.

Gibson J: A new approach to better medication compliance, *Nurs 89* 19(4):49, 1989.

Karb VB: Drug information sources for practicing nurses, *J Neurosci Nurs* 21(4):261, 1989.

Kim MJ, McFarland GK, McLane AM: *Pocket guide to nursing diagnoses,* ed 4, St Louis, 1991, Mosby–Year Book.

McGovern K: 10 golden rules for administering drugs safely, *Nurs 91* 21(3):49, 1992.

Smith LS: Those medication error dilemmas! *Adv Clin Care* 5(5):50, 1990.

Wolf ZR: Medication errors and nursing responsibility, *Holistic Nurs Pract* 4(1):8, 1989.

SECTION II

GENERAL PRINCIPLES OF PATIENT CARE

This section introduces the basic nursing activities involved in administering drugs to patients. Chapter 4, Over-the-Counter Drugs and Self-Medication, emphasizes the importance of these agents in nursing practice. The legal status of over-the-counter agents, their properties, and drug interactions are discussed. The material is a ready reference for the nurse in assessing the use of nonprescription medication. Chapter 5, Care of the Poisoned Patient, introduces the study of adverse effects of chemicals, including drugs, on people. Chapters 6 and 7 focus on the basic nursing activities involved in administering drugs. Chapter 6, Drug Administration, presents information and techniques that can assist the nurse in properly administering drugs to provide safe, individualized patient care. Chapter 7, Calculating Drug Dosages, helps the student achieve proficiency and develop confidence in this basic skill. Drug dosage calculations are presented as a guide to the level of proficiency expected of practicing nurses. Whereas students with good arithmetic skills can readily acquire the ability to solve problems of the level included in this chapter, many students initially experience difficulty because they have forgotten basic rules of arithmetic and algebra. Such students should review these rules before attempting the drug dosage calculations.

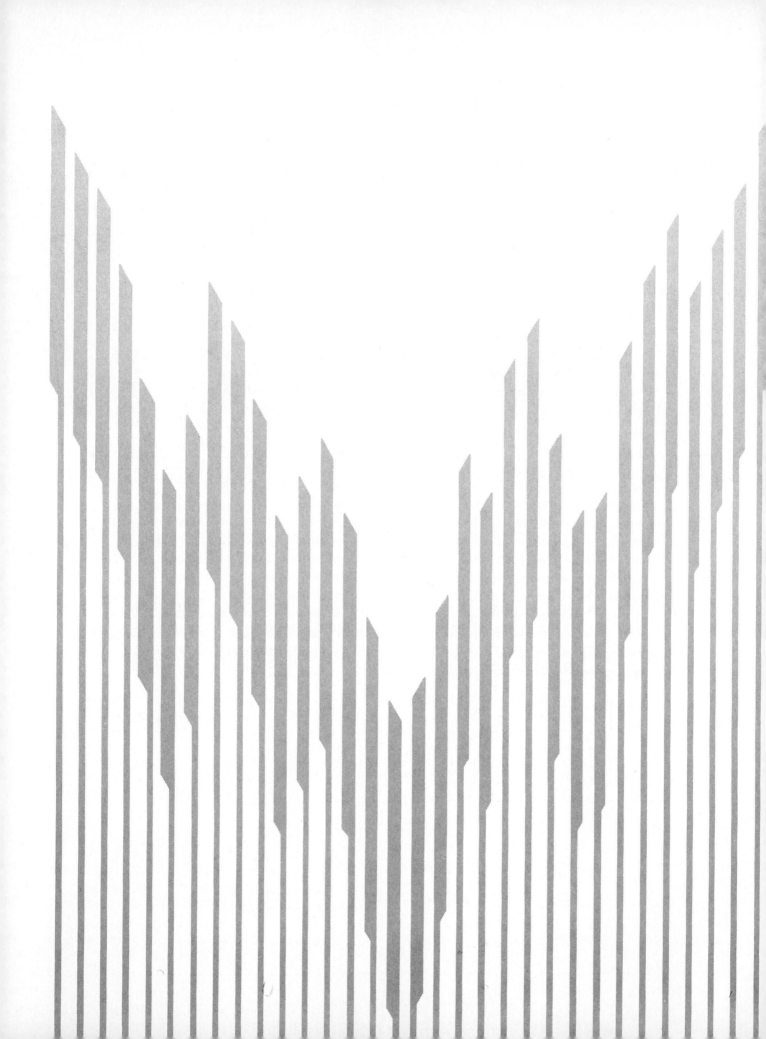

CHAPTER 4

Over-the-Counter Drugs and Self-Medication

LYNN ROGER WILLIS

LEARNING OBJECTIVES

After studying this chapter, you should be able to do the following:

- Explain the difference between over-the-counter medications and prescription drugs.
- Describe the advantages and disadvantages of fixed combinations of active ingredients.
- Explain the proper use of effective classes of over-the-counter agents.
- Discuss the dangers associated with continuous use of over-the-counter agents such as weight-loss products, laxatives, or sleeping medications.

CHAPTER OVERVIEW

◆ As medical professionals, we focus on medications ordered for the patient by the physician. It is important to remember that patients also self-medicate, using a wide array of over-the-counter medications. In certain circumstances, over-the-counter medications may significantly influence the effects of prescribed agents. This chapter summarizes the properties of most classes of over-the-counter agents. In later chapters, prescription drugs influencing the same body systems will be discussed.

Nursing Process Overview

OVER-THE-COUNTER DRUGS

Over-the-counter, or nonprescription, drugs will not form a major part of the clinical responsibilities of the practicing nurse. Nevertheless, the nurse is frequently sought to provide information on these agents.

Assessment

Since the patient is involved in self-care, assist the individual to clearly state what condition or symptoms are to be treated. For example, if the individual is seeking a medication to treat the symptoms of a cold, lead the person to consider exactly what symptoms require treatment. For some persons a cough might be the most outstanding symptom, whereas for others it might be nasal congestion or headache.

Nursing Diagnosis

Knowledge deficit related to lack of experience with self-medication for minor health problems

Management

After leading the patient to define exactly what symptoms are to be treated, teach the patient what types of medications are available to treat these symptoms. Suggest that fixed combinations of ingredients are more difficult to use, since dosages are impossible to regulate for each component of the combination. More control may be gained by using single agents at appropriate doses as necessary for defined symptoms. Suggest other sources of information about nonprescription drugs, such as the pharmacist.

Evaluation

Evaluation would be carried out by the patient involved in self-care. If the patient seeks advice because therapy is unsuccessful, have the patient consider whether the proper medication was administered for the symptom to be controlled and if the right dose was used.

LEGISLATION OF OVER-THE-COUNTER DRUGS

Over-the-counter (OTC) medications are medicinal agents deemed safe enough for sale without a prescription. Products intended for the self-medication of a variety of illnesses have been sold in the United States since colonial times. Until the early twentieth century no restrictions governed the contents, potency, purity, safety, efficacy, sale, or advertising of these products, which came to be known as *nostrums* or *patent medicines*. Consequently, some were of marginal safety at best, and most provided no obvious therapeutic benefit. Most patent medicines were harmless and ineffective, but many contained alcohol, narcotics, or other dangerous drugs in unspecified quantities.

Some control of the patent medicine industry was achieved with passage of the first Pure Food and Drug Act of 1906 (see Chapter 2). This act required that package labels accurately list the ingredients of medicinal products. Any substance present but not listed on the label was deemed an adulterant. A later amendment to the act, the Sherley Amendment (1912), forbade false and fraudulent labeling claims. In 1938, a new Food and Drug Act was enacted. It required proof of safety for all medicinal products intended for sale. In 1952, the Durham-Humphrey Amendment to the 1938 act specified (1) drugs safe enough for sale without a prescription (over the counter, or OTC) and (2) drugs deemed sufficiently dangerous or unsuitable for self-medication to require sale by prescription only.

Present control of OTC drugs stems from the Kefauver-Harris Amendment of 1962, which required proof of efficacy, as well as safety and lack of teratogenicity (the ability to cause birth defects). This amendment affected all drugs introduced after 1962 and all drugs that had entered the market since 1938. For several years after the adoption of this amendment, the Food and Drug Administration (FDA) concentrated primarily on prescription-only drugs in its assessment of efficacy, largely because the agency lacked the resources to evaluate OTC drugs at the same time. In the mid-1970s, however, the FDA began to include OTC drugs in its evaluations. Several panels of experts were convened and began reviewing the classes of OTC drugs, assigning each to one of the following categories:

Category I: Recognized as safe and effective for the claimed therapeutic indication

Category II: Not recognized as safe and effective

Category III: Additional data needed to decide safety or effectiveness

Drugs assigned to category I can be sold to the general public. Those in category II cannot. Drugs in category III, if generally recognized as safe, may be sold even though the evaluation of their safety and effectiveness has not been completed.

Since this review process began, many unsafe or ineffective OTC drugs and products have disappeared from the market. Others have undergone labeling changes or have been redesigned. However, since manufacturers are not required to indicate whether the drugs in their products are in category I or III, OTC products cannot be assumed to be effective simply because they are sold. Some consumer interest groups have objected to the sale of drugs in category III, apparently in the belief that a drug should be considered unsafe and ineffective unless proven otherwise. Such groups have also challenged the assignment of other drugs to category I. Until the FDA review panels have completed their work, the therapeutic benefit of some OTC drugs will remain questionable.

COMMON PROPERTIES OF OTC MEDICATIONS

Low Doses

Today's manufacturers of OTC products are concerned with safety. The toxicity of a drug varies in direct proportion to the dose administered; that is, the higher the dose, the greater the risk of toxicity. Thus most OTC products contain low, sometimes less-than-therapeutic, amounts of active ingredient. As such, they may serve as little more than **placebos** (inactive substances usually presented in the guise of an active medicine), especially for such subjective complaints as minor pain, itch, and sleeplessness. For such indications, proof that a drug is effective may be difficult to establish, even when adequate dosage is provided.

Combination of Ingredients

Many OTC products contain several drugs. The drugs may be totally different, or they may be of the same or similar pharmacologic classification. When drugs are combined, adverse interactions may occur. Although the risk of interactions is low for the drugs in a given product, it is not so low when other drugs are taken simultaneously.

OTC products with several ingredients are termed **fixed combination products;** that is, the doses of the drugs in the product are fixed within the tablet or other dosage form and cannot be altered. For example, if a tablet contains 4 mg of antihistamine and 60 mg of decongestant, a patient who needed to increase the antihistamine dosage would also have to take more of the decongestant. Many single-drug OTC products are also available. These products include antihistamines, analgesic-antipyretic drugs, decongestants, cough suppressants, and antifungal drugs. Complete control of drug dosage is possible with single-drug products, and such products can often be purchased less expensively than the heavily advertised combination products. By understanding the pharmacology of the drugs in OTC products and the specific needs of the patient, the nurse can advise a rational method of product selection.

MAJOR CLASSES OF OTC DRUGS

The classes of OTC drugs* chosen for discussion in this chapter include analgesic drugs, cold and cough remedies, weight-control products, and sleep aids; their component drugs are discussed in other chapters. Also discussed are vitamin C, ophthalmic products, acne treatments, sunscreens, topical antiinfectives, and hemorrhoidal products.

Analgesics

Aspirin, acetaminophen and ibuprofen are the most effective OTC analgesic drugs available. Nearly all OTC analgesic products intended for internal consumption contain one of these drugs. Aspirin and ibuprofen are the only OTC members of a larger class of drugs known as *nonsteroidal antiinflammatory drugs (NSAID)*. Both inhibit the synthesis of prostaglandins by inhibiting cyclooxygenase. This action may be related to the mechanism by which they produce analgesia. Acetaminophen is chemically unrelated to aspirin or ibuprofen. Its mechanism of action differs from that of NSAID, and it can be used by people who cannot tolerate NSAID. The complex pharmacology of these drugs is discussed in detail in Chapter 23.

Aspirin and acetaminophen are equally effective at relieving minor aches and pains and reducing fever. Maximum analgesic and antipyretic effectiveness are achieved in most adults with 650 mg of either drug. Higher doses (as in the extra-strength products) provide little, if any, additional relief for most people, but they appear to be more effective than usual doses in some people. Aspirin, but not acetaminophen, also relieves the pain and inflammation of arthritic disorders, but this effect requires higher than usual doses and medical supervision.

Aspirin produces numerous side effects. Although it normally presents no problem for individuals who take the drug only occasionally, it may be troublesome for those who take it regularly or are particularly sensitive to it. For example, aspirin inhibits platelet aggregation. As little as one 650 mg dose of aspirin

---

*For an exhaustive review of all OTC drugs, refer to American Pharmaceutical Association: *Handbook of Nonprescription Drugs*, ed 9, Washington, DC, 1990, The Association.

may double the bleeding time for several days. Aspirin also irritates the stomach lining, sometimes causing pain, discomfort, and, on occasion, bleeding, which can cause the loss of 5 to 10 ml of blood in the stool each day. The bleeding is ordinarily of no consequence with occasional use of the drug, but those who take it frequently may develop iron-deficiency anemia. Individuals with a history of peptic ulcer or intestinal bleeding or those who are taking anticoagulant drugs should not take aspirin.

Acetaminophen (Tylenol, Datril, and other brands) is remarkably free of side effects. It does not affect blood-clotting mechanisms, nor does it irritate the stomach lining. Rarely, acetaminophen causes an allergic reaction, often a skin rash. It may also damage the liver but only in association with overdosage.

Various dosage forms for aspirin are available, reflecting efforts by manufacturers to overcome some of the problems it causes. Aspirin is available in buffered, effervescent, and enteric-coated tablets to minimize gastric irritation. Timed-release tablets are available for persons who must take aspirin regularly. Since aspirin is unstable in aqueous solution, liquid forms are not available. Acetaminophen is stable in solution and is available in a variety of pleasant-tasting syrups. Both drugs are available in inexpensive but reliable generic forms.

Ibuprofen (Advil and Nuprin) has been available OTC since 1984. Until then, it could be obtained by prescription. It is one of several NSAID, such as indomethacin, naproxen, and sulindac (see Chapter 23), and was approved for OTC sale largely because it has a somewhat wider margin of safety than either aspirin or acetaminophen, especially in cases of overdose. In addition, ibuprofen appears to be more effective than aspirin or acetaminophen against menstrual cramps and is effective against pain that aspirin or acetaminophen are not always able to relieve. The recommended OTC dosage of ibuprofen is 200 to 400 mg every 4 hr in persons over the age of 12 yr, to a maximum of 1200 mg in 24 hr. Many people may find that a single 200-mg tablet of ibuprofen gives them the same level of pain relief that they get from two tablets of aspirin or acetaminophen.

Ibuprofen is recommended for people who cannot tolerate aspirin, but this recommendation requires rather narrow interpretation. People who are allergic to aspirin are also likely to be allergic to ibuprofen. Similarly, ibuprofen irritates the gastric mucosa and interferes with platelet function, but the incidence of gastrointestinal (GI) bleeding may be less with ibuprofen than with aspirin. Gastric irritation caused by these drugs can often be lessened by taking them with milk, food, or antacids, but some people find ibuprofen as troublesome as aspirin. For such people, acetaminophen remains the reasonable alternative. No therapeutic advantage is gained by taking any of these drugs together; aspirin may diminish the effectiveness of ibuprofen.

Probably the most serious hazard associated with OTC use of ibuprofen is reduced renal blood flow leading to possible renal failure in some patients. Patients who are elderly, who are taking diuretic drugs for the treatment of hypertension or digitalis for the treatment of congestive heart failure, or who have otherwise impaired renal or cardiac function should not take ibuprofen except under the direction of a physician.

Although ibuprofen is usually superior to aspirin or acetaminophen for relieving certain types of pain, such as that associated with menstrual cramps, dental work, and severe muscle strains, it is no more effective than aspirin or acetaminophen against most other types of mild pain and is generally more expensive. Consequently, nurses should exercise discretion and judgment when recommending it.

Cold Remedies

Most of the available OTC cold remedies (e.g., Contac, Novahistine, Dristan) contain a sympathomimetic drug to relieve nasal and sinus congestion, an antihistamine to dry excessive nasal secretions, or an analgesic drug to relieve minor aches and pains. Some products contain caffeine, vitamins, a laxative, or other substances. A few products contain only a single drug, usually a sympathomimetic (see later section and Chapter 14) or an antihistamine (see later section and Chapter 24), but most cold remedies are sold as combination products.

Sympathomimetic drugs relieve nasal stuffiness and congestion by constricting the blood vessels in swollen nasal membranes, decreasing local blood flow and swelling. When the swelling is relieved, the breathing passages open.

The sympathomimetic drugs commonly included in OTC cold remedies as decongestants are phenylephrine, phenylpropanolamine, and pseudoephedrine. These drugs are available in many products, and their pharmacologic characteristics are discussed in Chapter 14. Phenylephrine is the least reliable of the three because stomach acid reduces its activity, and its absorption into the blood is often erratic. For adults, safe and effective decongestant dosages of these drugs are as follows: phenylephrine, 10 mg every 4 hr; phenylpropanolamine, 25 mg every 4 hr; and pseudoephedrine, 60 mg every 4 hr. Half of the adult dose is considered safe and effective for children from ages 6 to 12 yr. Children from 2 to 6 yr should receive a quarter of the adult dose. Children under 2 yr of age should not be given these drugs except on the advice of a physician.

Sympathomimetic drugs can cause stimulation of the central nervous system (CNS) and generalized vasoconstriction. As a result, side effects of irritability, nervousness, insomnia, headache, and hypertension can occur. Individuals with high blood pressure, thyroid disease, or heart disease are cautioned against taking these drugs unless directed to do so by their physician.

The vasoconstrictive effects of sympathomimetics are intensified by monoamine oxidase inhibitors (e.g., Marplan, Nardil), which may be prescribed to treat depression (see Chapter 14) and may cause alarming and dangerous elevations of blood pressure and threat of stroke.

The rationale for including an antihistamine in a product intended to treat the symptoms of the common cold is not based on antagonism of histamine receptors. Unless the cold is associated with conditions of increased histamine release, such as allergic rhinitis, antagonism of histamine receptors will be of no use. (See Chapter 24 for a detailed discussion of antihistamines.) Instead, the justification for including antihistamines in OTC cold remedies rests largely on their anticholinergic action, which reduces the secretion of mucus by the nasal and bronchial mucosa and produces a drying effect. This effect, however, is not impressive, especially at approved OTC doses of the antihistamines.

The therapeutic index of antihistamines is high, and little risk of serious toxicity exists for adults. Thus antihistamines may relieve mild rhinorrhea in susceptible patients with little risk of adverse effects.

The most prominent side effects of antihistamines are drowsiness and sedation. These effects occur with all OTC antihistamines and doses. They pose a potentially serious threat to operators of motor vehicles or persons in hazardous occupations. Such persons should not take cold remedies containing antihistamines. Cold remedies that are promoted as "nondrowsiness formulas" generally do not contain an antihistamine.

The analgesic-antipyretic ingredients most often found in OTC cold remedies are aspirin and acetaminophen. None of the currently available products contains ibuprofen. Although aspirin and acetaminophen relieve the aches, pains, and feverishness associated with the common cold, one need never purchase a cold remedy that contains an analgesic. If analgesia is desired, aspirin or acetaminophen can be obtained at considerable savings and should be taken only as necessary.

No clear rationale exists for including caffeine, vitamins, laxatives, or other drugs in OTC cold remedies. The dose of caffeine provided in OTC cold remedies is generally far less than that contained in a cup of coffee. Vitamins are necessary only for correction of a vitamin deficiency and provide no therapeutic benefits for a cold sufferer. Laxatives, likewise, are of no known value for treatment of a cold.

Vitamin C Preparations

Vitamin C, or ascorbic acid, is necessary for a number of important biochemical reactions in the body, such as synthesis of collagen and adrenal steroids. Collagen provides the supporting framework for tooth, bone, and capillary structures. Vitamin C deficiency manifests as scurvy, diminished rate of wound healing, and other conditions.

Ascorbic acid is present in a variety of foods but especially in citrus fruits and vegetables. It is readily absorbed from the intestine and, when taken in recommended minimum daily amounts (60 mg daily in adults), most of it is converted metabolically to oxalate. Little ascorbate appears in the urine. However, when the daily intake of ascorbic acid exceeds 100 mg and the plasma ascorbate concentration exceeds 1.5 mg/dl, ascorbate appears in the urine.

Nobel laureate Dr. Linus Pauling proposed that vitamin C might be effective in treating and preventing the common cold. At that time the proposal was controversial and remains so today. Proponents of Dr. Pauling's theory assert that large doses, or megadoses, of ascorbic acid are necessary to saturate the body stores of vitamin C and to ease the drain on these stores when a cold virus attacks. They recommend a daily intake of 1 to 5 g of vitamin C to prevent, and as much as 15 g per day to treat, a cold. Many studies have been conducted to test these ideas. Although none has been negative, none has shown convincingly that the vitamin alters the severity, occurrence, or duration of the common cold. Megadoses of the vitamin do not saturate tissues any better than the minimum recommended daily dose.

There are disadvantages to the use of large doses of vitamin C. Diarrhea is a common, though not serious, side effect. In addition, oxalate stones may precipitate in the urinary tract of susceptible individuals, causing serious medical problems. Fortunately, this hazard occurs only in individuals who have an underlying disorder of oxalate metabolism. Finally, increased urinary excretion of vitamin C and the resulting acidification of the urine may alter the rate of excretion of certain other drugs. If attuned to the controversy surrounding megadose therapy with vitamin C, the nurse can provide a rational, objective evaluation of its use for patients.

Cough Remedies

If a cough accompanies the common cold, it may be productive or nonproductive. A productive cough removes phlegm from the lower respiratory tract and, unless it becomes nonproductive and excessive, should not be suppressed. A nonproductive cough is generally dry and discomforting and, because of local irritation caused by the rapid movement of air, may be self-perpetuating. Nonproductive coughs can be safely suppressed and relieved with an OTC cough suppressant (antitussive) drug. Expectorants are also included in many OTC cough remedies. Their antitussive effectiveness is questionable. The detailed pharmacologic properties of expectorants and antitussives are discussed in Chapter 26.

Expectorants

The use of expectorants in clinical medicine is controversial. The controversy stems partly from a lack of objective evidence that expectorant drugs are effective and partly from confusion concerning the effect expected of an expectorant drug. By one definition, an expectorant should promote the expulsion of mucus, phlegm, and fluid from the lungs and bronchial passages; that is, it should enhance the productiveness of a cough. By another, it should relieve a dry, irritating cough by causing the secretion of soothing and protective mucus in the airway. There is little evidence to suggest that expectorant drugs are any better than placebo for promoting the expulsion of phlegm or relieving a cough.

Guaifenesin recently became the only expectorant approved for use in OTC cough remedies. It stimulates the reflex production of bronchial secretion by irritating the gastric mucosa. In higher dosage, it causes emesis.

Cough suppressants

Three antitussives have been designated by the FDA as category I drugs. They are codeine, dextromethorphan, and diphenhydramine.

Codeine (see Chapter 44) suppresses the cough reflex center in the brain. Because it is an opium alkaloid and therefore a narcotic drug, it can cause psychologic and physical dependence. The liability for dependence with codeine is less than that for morphine, however, and it is virtually nonexistent when the drug is used in recommended doses for short periods (10 to 20 mg every 4 to 6 hr for 1 or 2 days). Larger doses may cause nausea, constipation, and drowsiness. Drowsiness is caused by depression of the CNS and is intensified by other CNS depressant drugs (e.g., barbiturates, alcohol, and antihistamines). Codeine should not be taken with any of them. Poisoning with codeine causes respiratory depression.

Abuse of OTC cough preparations that contain codeine has been a problem in the United States, and varying restrictions on their sale have been enacted by state legislatures. These restrictions range from a limit on the quantity that can be purchased by an individual to complete prohibition of sale without a prescription.

Dextromethorphan is a nonnarcotic cough suppressant with approximately the same antitussive potency and efficacy as codeine. As with codeine, dextromethorphan suppresses the cough reflex center in the brain, but it does not cause dependence or respiratory depression. Side effects are uncommon and generally mild, consisting largely of drowsiness and GI upset. Overall, dextromethorphan is the best choice for cough suppression and the great majority of OTC antitussive products contain it.

Diphenhydramine, an antihistamine, is also an effective cough suppressant. It is nonnarcotic and therefore does not cause dependence. In adults the drug suppresses coughs at a dosage of 25 mg every 4 hr. Drowsiness commonly occurs at this dosage, however, and severely limits the usefulness of this drug for many people. Paradoxically, diphenhydramine may cause stimulation, not sedation, in small children. This effect and its high propensity to cause drowsiness in adults makes it the least useful of the approved antitussive drugs.

Antitussive combinations

Some cough-suppressant products consist only of the antitussive drug in a flavored base. Others combine an antitussive drug with an expectorant. Either is suitable for suppressing coughs.

There are several reasons to avoid multidrug cough-and-cold formulas, even though they are numerous and heavily promoted by manufacturers. Not all coughs should be suppressed. In addition, a cough that accompanies a cold may be caused by irritation of the airway by an annoying trickle of mucus from swollen nasal membranes into the throat (postnasal drip). Stopping the flow of mucus with a decongestant drug should alleviate the cough and eliminate the need for an antitussive drug. If the cough is caused by irritation, low humidity, or "smoker's cough," a decongestant or antihistamine is of no value. A cough suppressant alone should be sufficient in such a case.

Decongestant nose drops and sprays

Several sympathomimetic drugs are available OTC as nose drops and sprays for the symptomatic and temporary relief of nasal congestion. These drugs include phenylephrine, ephedrine, and naphazoline, which are short-acting decongestants, to be used as frequently as every 3 or 4 hr, and xylometazoline and oxymetazoline, which are long-acting decongestants that are used only 2 or 3 times a day.

Topical decongestants have advantages over the oral decongestants, but there are some serious disadvantages, too. Since the drops and sprays apply the drugs directly to the congested nasal membranes, the onset of action and relief of congestion occur rapidly. In addition, only small amounts of the drugs need be administered, since they are applied locally. Therefore the incidence and severity of systemic side effects (e.g., elevated blood pressure) are reduced.

On the other hand, the intense localized vasoconstriction in the nasal mucosa can cause "rebound congestion," in which the congestion that returns when the effect of the drug has worn off may be worse than the congestion that existed in the first place. A vicious cycle can then develop in which the drug that originally relieved the congestion now becomes the cause of it. If unrecognized, this cycle of futile treatment can lead to chronic nasal stuffiness that will no longer respond to the decongestant drugs. Rebound congestion probably cannot be totally avoided when topical decongestants are used, but it can be minimized if the drugs are used only sparingly and strictly according to directions.

Nasal sprays are most convenient for adults and older children, and nose drops are often preferable for use in young children. Topical decongestants should not be given to children under the age of 2 years except as directed by a physician.

Weight-Control Products

Obesity is most frequently defined as a condition in which body weight is more than 20% greater than the ideal body weight. It is a complex problem that requires complex treatment. Drug treatment of obesity is of limited value at best. Amphetamines (see Chapter 43) have been prescribed for weight control. They, and related drugs, suppress appetite via a central mechanism, but the appetite remains suppressed only as long as sufficient levels of the drug are present in the brain. When the effect of the drug wears off, hunger returns. Unless the patient willfully resists the temptation to overeat, drug treatment will be of no value. Moreover, tolerance to the appetite-suppressing action of these drugs develops quickly, and they may produce dependence. Amphetamines are not available without a prescription.

Weight loss occurs if the rate at which calories are expended exceeds the rate at which they are obtained in the diet. No available OTC product enhances the rate at which calories are expended. They can aid only in reducing caloric intake. To that end, it matters little if a dietary aid possesses true pharmacologic activity. A placebo can be totally effective in some persons if they consume fewer calories while taking it.

OTC drugs for promoting weight loss consist mainly of phenylpropranolamine, bulk-producing agents, and benzocaine.

Phenylpropanolamine is structurally related to ephedrine and amphetamine. Its pharmacologic characteristics are similar to those of amphetamine, yet this drug is less potent than amphetamine. Phenylpropanolamine is clearly effective as an appetite suppressant in experimental animals, but its effectiveness in people is questionable. The drug has been assigned to category I because in controlled clinical trials human subjects who took the drug lost more weight by the end of the study than did untreated control subjects. The problem with these results is that the weight losses, and the differences between treated and untreated groups in these studies, were small. People who did not receive phenylpropanolamine often lost nearly as much weight as did those who had received the drug.

Amphetaminelike side effects can occur with phenylpropanolamine, although they are generally less intense than those associated with amphetamine. The most common of these are nervousness, insomnia, headache, nausea, and elevated blood pressure. Persons with diabetes mellitus, heart disease, hypertension, or thyroid disease should not take phenylpropanolamine, except on the advice of a physician. Persons taking the drug should be aware of its potential for interaction with other adrenergic drugs (see Chapter 10). To avoid these side effects and other problems with phenylpropanolamine, the FDA recommends that no more than 75 mg of the drug be taken in any 24-hr period, and for no more than 3 months at a time.

Phenylpropanolamine is potentially harmful. Since 1985, there have been 11 reported instances of cerebral hemorrhage in people who had taken this drug. Ten of the eleven cases involved women, and several apparently occurred after the recommended dosage had been taken.

When recommending a dietary aid containing phenylpropanolamine, the nurse should emphasize the questionable value of the drug if caloric intake is not also reduced, the tolerance after long-term use of the drug, and the side effects if the recommended daily dosage is exceeded.

A variety of bulk producers are sold as aids to weight reduction. When taken with 1 or 2 glasses of water, they tend to expand and swell in the stomach, thereby producing a feeling of fullness and a loss of appetite. Examples of OTC bulk producers are methylcellulose, carboxymethylcellulose, agar, psyllium hydrophilic mucilloid, and karaya gum. Unfortunately, the swollen bulk spends little time in the stomach, moving rapidly into the intestine, where it stimulates peristalsis and may exert a laxative effect. Some bulk producers are also marketed as laxatives and stool softeners (see Chapter 13). Bulk producers are probably no more effective at suppressing appetite and caloric intake than is drinking 2 or 3 glasses of water before meals; yet the FDA has approved bulk-producing agents for dietary use.

Several OTC weight-control products contain the local anesthetic drug, benzocaine, in tablets or as chewing gum. Presumably, the benzocaine anesthetizes the gastric mucosa or the mucous membranes in the mouth, thereby reducing appetite or removing the pleasurable sensation of taste. There is no conclusive evidence that either effect promotes weight loss.

When an OTC weight-control product is selected or recommended, the importance of a practical, balanced, and nutritious diet plan, preferably supervised by a family member, friend, nurse, registered dietitian, or physician, cannot be emphasized too strongly. By themselves, OTC products certainly do not produce weight loss. The success of a weight-loss program depends on faithful maintenance of diminished caloric intake.

Sleeping Aids

Insomnia disrupts the restful nights of nearly everyone from time to time. Some people have difficulty falling asleep; others may awaken in the middle of the night and be unable to go back to sleep. The cause of sleep difficulties may be physiologic or psychologic. In most cases the difficulties are temporary.

A wide variety of common remedies for sleeplessness may be tried. They include warm baths, a dull book, and a glass of warm milk or wine. In severe cases of insomnia the assistance of a physician may be sought, and a powerful sedative-hypnotic drug may be prescribed (see Chapter 40). Many people fear the addictive properties of these drugs, but they find little or no relief from home remedies. Between these extremes lies the OTC sleep aid.

The FDA has severely restricted the number of drugs that can be sold as OTC sleep aids. Before 1979, OTC sleep aids contained bromides, scopolamine, vitamins, or combinations of antihistamines. Since 1979, OTC sleep aids may contain an antihistamine alone or an antihistamine with aspirin or acetaminophen. The antihistamines that have been approved for use as sleep aids are pyrilamine maleate (25 to 50 mg at bedtime), doxylamine succinate (25 mg at bedtime), and diphenhydramine hydrochloride (HCl) (25 to 50 mg at bedtime).

Antihistamines are OTC sleep aids because of their tendency to cause drowsiness. This tendency, plus a wide margin of safety, lends credence to marketing claims for the effectiveness of antihistamines in the treatment of occasional insomnia. An analgesic drug is included in some preparations on the assumption that mild nighttime pain may contribute to sleeplessness. Clinical comparisons of antihistamines with placebo in sleep laboratories tend to reinforce the claims of effectiveness, but some authorities remain doubtful.

The most common side effects produced by antihistamines are drowsiness or dizziness, although young children, the elderly, and patients with CNS dysfunction may exhibit signs of stimulation at therapeutic doses. The sedating effects of these drugs are additive with ethanol and other CNS depressants, and the potential for poisoning exists when an acute overdose of the antihistamine is taken with another depressant drug. Other side effects of antihistamines include blurred vision, tinnitus, and dry mouth.

Product selection in this category of drugs is relatively simple because of the limited number of available active ingredients. It is very important for the nurse to assess the cause of the sleeplessness and the need for a sleeping aid. If mild pain is keeping someone awake, relief of the pain with aspirin or acetaminophen will often be sufficient to allow sleep to occur. If anxiety is the cause, antihistamine-induced drowsiness may be helpful, but it may also be no more effective than a glass of warm milk or a warm bath, although more expensive. Wise nursing counsel may be the most effective remedy for patients with mild insomnia.

Ophthalmic Products

OTC ophthalmic products are intended only for the symptomatic, short-term relief of mild self-limiting conditions such as eye fatigue, tearing, redness, or the itching and stinging associated with allergic or chemical conjunctivitis. The products are sold as eye washes, artificial tears, and decongestants. Conditions involving marked eye pain or blurred vision require attention by a physician.

All OTC ophthalmic products must be clear, odorless, colorless, and sterile solutions with a pH and tonicity approximating that of natural tears. They must also contain preservatives to maintain sterility. Sterility cannot be maintained indefinitely, however, and bacterial contamination may be transferred to the eye. Thus cloudy or discolored solutions should be discarded. All ophthalmic products carry an expiration date for the unopened package and a warning that they should be discarded within 3 months of the opening date.

OTC ophthalmic products contain a variety of nonmedicinal ingredients. Tonicity adjusters (e.g., dextran, glycerin) prevent excessive tearing that can dilute and wash away active ingredients. Antioxidants and stabilizers (sodium bisulfite, metabisulfite) prevent the chemical alteration of the ingredients. Buffers (e.g., boric acid) maintain the pH of the solution within a range of 6.0 to 8.0. Solutions of higher or lower pH may irritate the eyes. Wetting agents (polysorbate 80) reduce surface tension. Preservatives (e.g., benzalkonium chloride) prevent bacterial growth. Viscosity-increasing agents (gelatin, polyethylene glycol) spread the solution over the eye.

Decongestant ophthalmic products contain a sympathomimetic drug (ephedrine HCl, naphazoline HCl, phenylephrine HCl, or tetrahydrozoline). Local application of one of these drugs to the eye promptly relieves the symptoms of allergic conjunctivitis. By constricting dilated blood vessels in the white of the eye, they also relieve the bloodshot look and restore the normal white color to the eyes. Sympathomimetic drugs also stimulate the adrenergic receptors affecting pupillary size and may cause dilation of pupils (mydriasis). For this reason, these products should not be used by persons with narrow-angle glaucoma.

Problems may occur with decongestant ophthalmic products. Rebound congestion can occur by the same mechanism as described for topical nasal decongestants. It can be minimized or avoided by using the medicine only occasionally and strictly according to directions. In addition, these products will be ineffective if the cause of the symptoms is within the eyeball. The medicine may mask a bacterial infection.

Other medicinal agents contained in decongestant and other OTC ophthalmic products include antipruritics (antipyrine, camphor, and menthol) and astringents (zinc sulfate). Antipruritics produce mild local anesthesia and a cooling sensation. They are considered unsafe because they can mask the presence of foreign abrasive substances in the eye that may damage the cornea. Zinc sulfate is the only acceptable astringent in OTC ophthalmic preparations.

Acne Products

Acne and its treatment

Acne vulgaris frequently affects adolescents. For them, prevention and treatment of even mild attacks of the disease, with its unsightly pimples and scars, are given high priority.

The pimples and skin eruptions of acne are called comedones. They consist of a mixture of sebum, produced by the sebaceous glands of the hair follicles, and epithelial cells shed by the infundibulum of the follicle.

Acne is associated with excessive production of sebum, which impairs the normal washout of infundibular cells as they are shed. The cells become compacted and plug the follicle, which then becomes distended with accumulated sebum and cells. The condition is relieved by removal of the plug by lancing the comedone or by the natural growth of the hair, which brings the plug to the surface. This form of acne, termed *noninflammatory,* is not usually associated with scarring.

Scarring is more likely to occur with the inflammatory form of the disease, which is characterized by pustule formation and local inflammation. In the inflammatory form, comedones do not open at the skin surface to relieve the pressure within the hair follicle. An inflamed follicle may rupture beneath the skin surface and spread sebum, cells, and bacteria to surrounding tissues. Whereas noninflammatory acne can be treated with OTC products, cases of inflammatory acne should be referred to a physician.

External factors may contribute to the development of acne. These factors include personal hygiene, diet, and self-image.

Personal hygiene combats excessive skin oiliness, but compulsive and vigorous cleansing of the skin has not proved to be more effective in preventing acne than normal washing. Since bacterial infection is not ordinarily associated with acne, the use of antibacterial soaps and antiseptic solutions is neither necessary nor recommended.

The role of diet in acne is controversial. Chocolate has long been condemned as a causative factor, but there is no evidence of a cause-and-effect relationship between chocolate and acne. Similarly, evidence does not support the need for dietary restrictions of sweets, nuts, and greasy foods. Until a clearer understanding of acne and its cause emerges, individual trial and error with diet, hygiene, and other factors should neither be excluded nor discouraged.

Noninflammatory acne is treated symptomatically. Treatment consists of removing excess sebum from the skin by washing and promoting the production and turnover of new skin to prevent closure of the pilosebaceous orifices of the hair follicle. The skin should be washed with warm water, mild soap, and a soft washcloth, no more than 3 times daily. The washing and rubbing will produce some drying and peeling of the skin. Closure of the pilosebaceous orifices can be prevented by the topical application of mildly irritating agents, which will promote desquamation (peeling) and stimulate growth of new skin cells.

The most common OTC desquamating agents are sulfur (2% to 10%), resorcinol (1% to 4%), and salicylic acid (0.5% to 2%). Resorcinol and salicylic acid often appear in alcoholic solutions that dry quickly and do not leave a visible film. Some products contain all three agents.

Dosage forms of these drugs include creams, lotions, gels, and liquids. Ointment bases tend to be greasy and messy. Some soaps include desquamating agents, but this formulation is irrational because rinsing and drying will remove the agents from the skin. Benzoyl peroxide is a stronger irritant and desquamating agent than are sulfur, resorcinol, or salicylic acid. Used in concentrations of 5% to 10%, it generally produces mild stinging and warming of the skin. For most acne problems, benzoyl peroxide is probably no more effective than the milder agents and should be used only after the milder irritants and faithful adherence to a regular skin-washing schedule have been unsuccessful. Benzoyl peroxide is highly irritating and should not contact the eyelids, neck, or lips. Its use should be discontinued if severe and prolonged stinging or irritation occurs.

More serious forms of acne require treatment with medications available only by prescription. Antibiotics may be used topically or orally in low doses. Isotretinoin may be effective in severe cases when the patient is unresponsive to other therapy.

Sunscreen Products

The sun emits principally two types of ultraviolet radiation, UV-A and UV-B. UV-A radiation causes darkening, or tanning, of the skin. UV-B radiation causes sunburn.

Sunburn occurs when UV-B radiation damages small blood vessels in the skin, causing them to become leaky and congested. Many people incorrectly consider sunburns harmless, although painful, and a small price to pay for a seasonal tan.

UV-A radiation tans the skin by stimulating the production of the dark pigment, *melanin*. The darkness of the tan depends on how much melanin is produced. People who do not tan easily simply do not produce enough melanin. Melanin absorbs UV-A and UV-B radiation and protects the skin from the harmful effects of ultraviolet radiation. Naturally dark skin contains more melanin than pale skin and is correspondingly better protected.

The harmful effects of ultraviolet radiation can be serious, permanent, and, in some cases, life threatening. These effects include premature aging and wrinkling of the skin and skin cancer. They occur after years of repeated exposure to the sun's radiation and may occur without significant episodes of sunburn.

Sunscreens diminish the harmful consequences of ultraviolet radiation by absorbing or reflecting it. Used correctly, they prevent sunburn and premature aging of the skin, permit tanning, and reduce the risk of skin cancer.

Chemical sunscreens selectively absorb and screen out most of the harmful burning radiation, but permit tanning radiation to reach the skin. Physical sunscreens scatter and reflect all ultraviolet radiation. They prevent sunburn well, but they also prevent tanning.

Twenty-one chemical sunscreens have been approved by the FDA. Those most commonly available include aminobenzoic acid, cinoxate, homosalate, menthyl anthranilate, oxybenzone, and padimate O. Sunscreen products may contain one or several of these agents. Physical sunscreens include titanium oxide and zinc oxide in ointments and creams. They are intended for complete coverage of small areas of sunburn-prone skin such as the nose and lips.

Not all suntan products contain sunscreens. Some contain cosmetically appealing but otherwise inactive ingredients such as cocoa butter, mineral oil, and lanolin. None of these ingredients prevent sunburn or promote tanning.

Some drugs, cosmetics, and soaps sensitize a person's skin to ultraviolet radiation and cause it to burn more easily than usual. Examples of such photosensitizing drugs include tetracycline antibiotics (see Chapter 32) and diuretics (see Chapter 16). Photosensitivity reactions are triggered by UV-A radiation. Most sunscreens absorb little, if any, of this radiation and will not prevent it. Those that do include menthyl anthranilate and oxybenzone.

The effectiveness of sunscreens is rated by the **sun protection factor (SPF),** which is listed on the product label. The SPF relates the amount of time it takes a person to get a mild sunburn without sunscreen protection to the time required after a sunscreen has been applied to the exposed skin. For example, skin that ordinarily burns after 30 min of exposure to the sun will, if treated with a sunscreen with an SPF of 4, be able to stay in the sun for 2 hr (4 times as long) before it will burn to the same degree. A sunscreen with an SPF of 8 will protect 8 times as long (4 hr).

Products with SPFs greater than 8 screen out tanning and burning radiation. Therefore persons who desire a tan should not use a sunscreen with an SPF higher than 8. Those with higher SPF values (some go as high as 50) screen out virtually all of the tanning and burning radiation. These products offer approximately equal protection from the radiation and differ only in the length of time that they allow a person to stay exposed to the sun. In some cases, the higher SPF will be of marginal value at best. For example, a sunscreen with an SPF of 15 would let someone who normally burns in 60 min stay in the sun for 15 hr. This

would extend their time of protection into the night. Someone who burns after 15 min could expect to be protected for 7½ hr by a product with an SPF of 30.

The choice of SPF depends on how easily a person burns and tans. The FDA recommends products with an SPF of 8 or more for people who always burn and never tan, 6 to 7 for people who always burn and minimally tan, 4 to 5 for people who burn moderately and tan gradually, 2 to 3 for people who burn minimally and always tan well, and 2 for people who rarely burn and tan profusely.

Sunscreens should be applied at least 30 min before each exposure to the sun. The chemicals need at least that much time to penetrate the skin. Some, such as aminobenzoic acid, should be applied 1 to 2 hr before exposure. No sunscreen or suntan product will promote a deeper tan than a person's skin can naturally produce. If skin does not readily produce melanin, it will never tan as well as skin that readily produces the pigment.

Topical Antiinfective Drugs
Antifungal products

Several common tineal (fungal) infections of the skin generally respond to self-medication with OTC products, although responsiveness depends on the strain of fungus, the site of the infection, and the severity and duration of the infection. The microorganisms most often responsible for superficial tineal infections in humans are found in *Trichophyton, Microsporum, Epidermophyton,* and *Candida* genera. All but *Candida* infections can be treated with OTC antifungal products (see Chapter 36). Moreover, the products are effective only for acute superficial infections. Chronic and extensive infections respond slowly, if at all, and often require the attention of a physician. Fungal infections of the toenails or fingernails and those that have penetrated the hair shafts will also generally respond poorly to OTC antifungal products. The nurse should exercise care in selecting or recommending OTC antifungal medications. If the condition involves an apparent tineal infection of the foot (athlete's foot), groin, or scalp, reasonably rapid results can be expected from OTC products. Patients with suspected fungal infections of other body regions should be referred to a physician.

OTC antifungal preparations include keratolytic agents, fungistatic agents, and fungicides.

Keratolytic preparations include selenium sulfide and Whitfield's ointment (containing benzoic acid, 6%, and salicylic acid, 3%). These agents irritate the skin and cause peeling of the superficial layers to expose deeper sites of infection to other antifungal compounds. Selenium sulfide stops cellular growth when it is applied in concentrations of 1% to 2%. It is a common and effective ingredient in antidandruff preparations.

Fungistatic agents include fatty acids and salicylanilide. Sodium propionate and undecylenic acid are fungistatic fatty acids. Sodium propionate is effective in 1% solution and 5% ointment. Undecylenate is effective as the acid (5%) and as the zinc salt (20%). It is commonly used as an ointment, powder, or spray for the relief of athlete's foot.

The fungicidal drug tolnaftate is effective against the majority of superficial fungal infections except *Candida* species. Tolnaftate is sold in powder, liquid, cream, spray, or gel (all 1%). Relief of itching occurs within several days, but complete suppression of the infection generally requires 2 to 3 weeks of treatment. If the skin is rough and scaly, prior treatment with a keratolytic agent to remove the scale improves the effectiveness of tolnaftate.

Antibacterial products

The antibiotic drugs available without a prescription include bacitracin, neomycin, polymyxin B sulfate, tetracycline HCl, chlortetracycline HCl, and oxytetracycline HCl. The FDA OTC Panel on Antimicrobial Drugs recognizes skin-wound antibiotics and skin-wound protectants. The former includes products for the treatment of overt skin infections; the latter refers to products with antibiotics added to prevent the subsequent infection of a wound and the growth of organisms in the product. As of 1979, all OTC antibiotics sold as skin-wound antibiotics were classified in category III. All but neomycin sulfate were classified in category I for use as skin-wound protectants (see Chapters 32 and 33).

When used as directed, the OTC topical antibiotics are generally safe. However, their low concentration in the available products makes their effectiveness against skin wound infections questionable. Bacitracin, neomycin, and polymyxin B sulfate are nephrotoxic if absorbed systemically. With ordinary topical use, such toxicity is rare. In view of the questionable topical efficacy of the drugs and their potential toxicity, their use is not recommended.

Hemorrhoidal Products

People, as the result of environment, heredity, and posture, suffer from a number of painful anorectal disorders, the most prevalent of which is hemorrhoids. Hemorrhoids are varicosities produced by increased pressure in the hemorrhoidal veins. In addition to upright posture, hypertension, coughing, pregnancy and labor, physical exertion, straining during defecation, and rectal carcinoma can contribute to hemorrhoids. These varicosities, which can occur within or outside the anorectal line, are associated with itching, burning, inflammation, and swelling. Mild pain and discomfort are common, but bleeding, prolapse of an internal hemorrhoid, and severe chronic pain require the attention of a physician.

OTC products for the treatment of anorectal disorders are intended for the symptomatic relief of pain, itching, and burning. They contain a variety of pharmacologic agents, including local anesthetics, vasoconstrictors, antiseptics, astringents, emollients or lubricants, keratolytics, anticholinergics, and a variety of miscellaneous agents such as counterirritants and wound-healing agents.

The FDA OTC Panel on Hemorrhoidal Drug Products has ruled on the efficacy of these agents. Antiseptics, wound healers, and anticholinergics have all been classified as category II hemorrhoidal products.

Local anesthetics have been judged effective for relief of the itching and burning of hemorrhoids. Of the many local anesthetics available, only two are safe and effective, benzocaine (5% to 20%) and pramoxine HCl (1%).

Ephedrine sulfate, epinephrine HCl, and phenylephrine HCl are vasoconstrictor drugs that have been judged effective for the symptomatic relief of hemorrhoidal itching and swelling, although conclusive evidence of effectiveness on swollen hemorrhoidal tissue itself is lacking. Presumably, the vasoconstrictor drugs directly constrict the vascular smooth muscle in the anorectal area.

A variety of emollients or lubricants (protectants) have been recommended for use in hemorrhoidal preparations. These include calamine, cocoa butter, cod liver oil, glycerin, mineral oil, petrolatum, shark liver oil, and zinc oxide. All can be administered to the rectum externally and internally except glycerin, which is intended for external use only. Petrolatum may be the most effective of these agents. To be effective, the total protectant concentration of an OTC hemorrhoidal product should be 50%.

Mildly keratolytic agents such as aluminum chlorhydroxy allantoinate relieve the itching and burning of hemorrhoids. Their usefulness is confined to the external anal tissues, but stronger agents, such as resorcinol and sulfur, are not recommended.

Astringents coagulate skin cell protein, thereby protecting underlying skin cells from dehydration and irritation. Calamine zinc oxide and hamamelis water (witch hazel), have been judged effective for the relief of hemorrhoidal itching, irritation, and pain. Calamine and zinc oxide may be applied externally and internally to anorectal tissue, whereas hamamelis water is intended for external use only. Antiseptics are no more effective than washing with soap and water for the prevention of anorectal infections. Antiseptics may adversely alter the normal bacterial flora in that region.

Anticholinergic drugs (e.g., atropine; see Chapter 9) are of dubious value in OTC hemorrhoidal preparations. These drugs are not absorbed through the skin and, if applied to the external anal tissues, do not relieve itching or pain. They can be absorbed across the rectal mucosa, however, and in sufficient dosage can interfere with autonomic nerve function throughout the body. There is no evidence that a local or systemic anticholinergic effect is of any value in treating hemorrhoids.

A counterirritant drug distracts from the discomfort of itching, irritation, and pain by stimulating local nerve endings to provide a sensation of warmth, tingling, or coolness. Counterirritation forms the therapeutic basis for the relief of minor muscle aches and pain by OTC remedies that provide deep-heating and penetrating warmth. These remedies do not directly affect muscles. Instead, their effects are localized to the skin, where they stimulate local sensory nerve endings. However, since no sensory nerves occur in the rectal mucosa, there is no rational basis for including a counterirritant in an internal hemorrhoidal preparation. A counterirritant may provide temporary relief of pain and itching if applied externally to the anorectal region. Menthol is the only recommended counterirritant for external hemorrhoidal preparations. Camphor, oil of turpentine, and hydrastis have been included in various products, but they are considered to be too toxic even for external use or of unproven efficacy.

Wound-healing agents include an extract of brewer's yeast, skin respiratory factor (SRF), cod liver oil, and vitamins A and D. No convincing evidence of their effectiveness as wound healers has been found, and until such evidence emerges, their value in the treatment of hemorrhoids is questionable.

OTC products for the treatment of hemorrhoids and other mild anorectal disorders are provided in a variety of dosage forms including ointments, creams, suppositories, pads, and foams. Ointments (oil base), creams (water soluble), and gels are equally effective in delivering active ingredients to the affected areas. Devices such as the *pile pipe,* a tube having lateral exit ports, are useful for applying the medication directly into the rectum. Suppositories are not particularly useful for the treatment of hemorrhoids. They may slip beyond the affected site, releasing their active ingredients in contact with healthy mucosa. In addition, with suppositories the degree of coverage of the affected area may be erratic and cannot be controlled. Finally, because suppositories must melt to release their active ingredients, relief of painful symptoms is delayed. Foams provide no advantages over ointments and creams; moreover, they are messy.

Personal hygiene and normal bowel habits are important in the successful treatment of hemorrhoids. Many physicians recommend taking sitz baths or soaking with astringent solutions as an adjunct to the use of OTC products for the relief of mild itching and burning sensations. In addition, the diet should be adjusted to avoid either excessively loose or compact stools.

NURSING IMPLICATIONS SUMMARY

General Guidelines

- If asked about over-the-counter remedies, first assess the patient. What symptoms or problems need treatment? What has the patient used successfully in the past?
- Remember that many patients do not consider drugs purchased over the counter as true drugs; that is, if questioned about medications they are taking, they may not think to include over-the-counter preparations.
- As a part of assessment, ask specifically about medicine purchased at the drugstore or health-food store. It may be helpful to include some leading questions such as "Do you take any cold medicines, cough syrups, vitamins, or other medicines that you can buy without a prescription?" It may also help to know of local health problems or habits. For example, in an area where there are frequent high pollen counts, causing frequent allergy problems, ask questions about allergies and what the patient uses to relieve symptoms.
- In asking how a patient uses over-the-counter drugs, try to frame questions in a nonjudgmental way to learn about actual use patterns. Most patients want to use medications correctly and will welcome instruction about drug use but not if they feel defensive about their current practices.

Patient and family education

- Point out to patients that many over-the-counter preparations contain multiple drugs. Encourage the patient to consider purchasing products that contain only the drug needed. This may be difficult for the patient, since the ingredients for a product may be listed in generic names, which are not familiar to the patient.
- Ideally, the nurse could accompany the patient to the drugstore and review product labeling during the instruction. In the absence of this possibility, suggest that the patient talk over the medication needs with the pharmacist. In addition, the pharmacist can help the patient choose the least expensive but most effective product available at that store.
- Talking about over-the-counter drug use may provide the ideal opportunity to review general safe practices regarding drug use. Refer to the box on p. 42.
- Suggest that the patient look over all the medications in the house periodically and discard those that look discolored or crumbled or that have passed the expiration date. Emphasize to patients the need to discard medications in a way that children or animals cannot find them and take them. Small amounts of liquids can be poured down the sink or toilet, and a few remaining tablets or capsules can be flushed also. If there is a large quantity of medication, consider checking with a local pharmacy or poison control center for guidance about proper disposal.
- Encourage patients who are not obtaining relief from appropriate over-the-counter medications to seek medical care for the problem.

CHAPTER REVIEW

◆ KEY TERMS

fixed combination products, p. 50
over-the-counter (OTC) medications, p. 50
placebo, p. 50
sun protection factor (SPF), p. 58

◆ REVIEW QUESTIONS

1. The present laws that regulate the OTC drug industry have evolved from which law?
2. What classes of drugs did Durham-Humphrey Amendment to the 1938 law create?
3. What does the Kefauver-Harris amendment to the 1938 law require?
4. What are the categories used by FDA review panels on OTC drugs to classify drugs?
5. List the advantages and disadvantages of fixed-ratio combination drug products.
6. Name the ingredients of OTC cold remedies.
7. What are the major side effects of antihistaminic drugs?
8. List the OTC expectorant drugs.
9. Name the available OTC cough suppressants.
10. Which drugs are used in OTC products for the treatment of obesity and weight control? What should you teach patients who wish to control their weight?

11. Phenylpropanolamine is related to which drugs? What are its side effects? How can you assess them?

12. What is the rationale for the use of a bulk-producing agent in a weight-control product? How might you counsel patients about these?

13. What drugs are available in OTC sleep aids?

14. List the classes of ingredients in OTC ophthalmic products.

15. What precautions should be exercised in the use of OTC ophthalmic products? How might you teach patients about these precautions?

16. List the commonly available OTC drugs for treatment of acne.

17. Distinguish between chemical and physical sunscreens.

18. Define *sun protection factor*.

19. OTC antifungal products include which drugs?

20. Distinguish between keratolytic, fungistatic, and fungicidal drugs.

21. Which antibiotics are available in OTC preparations?

22. List the ingredients of OTC hemorrhoidal products and describe their actions.

SUGGESTED READING

American Pharmaceutical Association: *Handbook of nonprescription drugs,* ed 9, Washington, DC, 1990, The Association.

Carruth AK, Boss, BJ: More than they bargained for: adverse drug effects, *J Gerontol Nurs* 16(7):27, 1990.

Cowley G, Hager M: Some counter intelligence: consumer drugs aren't as friendly as they look, *Newsweek,* 115(11):82, 1990.

Johnson JE, Moore J: The drug-taking practices of the rural elderly, *Appl Nurs Res* 1(3):128, 1988.

Trainor PA: Over-the-counter drugs: count them in, *Geriatr Nurs* 9(5):298, 1988.

CHAPTER 5

Care of the Poisoned Patient

LEARNING OBJECTIVES

After studying this chapter, you should be able to:

◆ Discuss the importance of the field of clinical toxicology.

◆ Differentiate between toxicodynamics and toxicokinetics.

◆ Explain the rationale for nonspecific antidotes to poisons, including decontamination, emesis and lavage, activated charcoal, and cathartics.

◆ Describe the basis for specific antidote categories, including competitive antidotes, chelates, antibodies, and agents that produce metabolic alterations.

◆ Differentiate between diuresis and dialysis.

◆ Summarize nursing implications for drugs discussed in this chapter.

CHAPTER OVERVIEW

◆ **Toxicology** is the study of poisons. A poison is a chemical substance that causes injury or death when introduced into the body. There are literally thousands of potential poisons. Drugs, household and industrial chemicals, plants, pesticides, carbon monoxide, and heavy metals are the major agents of poisoning seen in clinical practice.

◆ Poison control centers, located throughout the United States, are usually identified in local telephone books. These centers provide the public and health professionals with information on the appropriate first aid and clinical management of suspected poisoning. Poisondex is a computerized database of more than 650,000 substances and includes information on most medicines and consumer products. Large poison control centers may also offer specialized poison treatment and consultation. Educational services such as professional training and poison prevention education for the public may also be offered.

◆ Each year, approximately 1.5 million cases are handled by poison control centers. More than 90% occur at home. Children under age 3 are the most frequent victims. These statistics highlight the tendency of young children to ingest pills, cleaning agents, and plants. Pills particularly attractive and troublesome to children include chocolate-flavored laxatives and vitamins (particularly those with iron given to pregnant women).

◆ The annual U.S. mortality rate from poisoning of all types has been reported to be approximately 12,000 deaths. Of these, about half are suicides and half are accidental. Less than 50 poisoning deaths per year are considered homicides.

◆ **Clinical toxicology** is the study of care of the poisoned patient. Poisoning can be acute, subacute, or chronic, depending on the dose, length of exposure, and extent of tissue injury. In this chapter the primary emphasis is on the acutely poisoned patient. Acute poisoning is usually the immediate and direct result of a single excessive dose. Acute poisoning in children is most commonly caused by ingestion of plants, drugs, or household products. In adults, acute poisoning is often the result of drug overdose. About 70% of adult drug overdose cases involve a central nervous system (CNS) depressant, commonly alcohol (23%) or a benzodiazepine (24%). Alcohol and benzodiazepines greatly potentiate the toxic effects of each other or other CNS depressants.

Nursing Process Overview
TREATMENT OF POISONING
Assessment

Patients who have been exposed to poisons or have ingested poisons may enter the health care system in any condition. Patients may range from the child who is alert, oriented, and feeling fine after ingesting a handful of children's vitamins to the person who requires resuscitation or is comatose and unable to provide any information about the toxic substances ingested. Obtain a complete baseline assessment, including vital signs, blood pressure, weight, serum electrolyte levels, liver and renal function studies, blood gas studies, and an electrocardiogram (ECG). The health history should include information about the poison ingested (how much, when, what treatment efforts have been tried) and preexisting health problems.

Nursing Diagnoses

Anxiety related to the treatment or possible outcome of treatment

Altered comfort: nausea and vomiting from use of ipecac syrup

Ineffective airway clearance related to drug overdose with potential for aspiration

Management

Establish and maintain a patent airway with adequate ventilation. Other measures include supportive care of the unconscious patient, administration of nonspecific or specific antidotes, and hospitalization for further observation or treatment. Monitor vital signs and ECG as needed. Initiate and maintain intravenous (IV) therapy, monitor intake and output, laboratory work (blood gas analysis, liver and renal function studies, serum levels of suspected toxins or antidotes), insert a nasogastric or orogastric tube for gastric lavage, or induce vomiting as ordered. Keep the patient and family informed of actions taken and their effect.

Evaluation

Effective treatment for overdose or exposure to toxins occurs when the poisonous substance is eliminated and the patient returns to normal health without experiencing side effects associated with the poison or treatment. Most antidotes are not administered on an outpatient basis. Before discharge, instruct the patient and the family about continuing care or observations required. If appropriate, give instructions about removing toxic substances from the home or work place. Refer the client to social services or a community-based nursing care agency if appropriate.

TOXICODYNAMICS AND TOXICOKINETICS

The general principles of toxicology are those of pharmacology extended to excessive doses. (The principles relating drug dosage to drug action are discussed in Chapter 1.) The same factors that govern pharmacokinetics and pharmacodynamics also apply to toxicology.

Toxicodynamics describes the harmful effects that a poison produces on the body. The graded dose-response curves described in Chapter 1 relate to toxic and therapeutic effects. Therefore the symptoms of poisoning reflect the dose of the poison. Treating the poisoned patient is frequently complicated because the dose of the poison is seldom known with any accuracy and the identity of the poison may not be known. Therefore a thorough assessment of the patient is especially important in cases of poisoning. If the nature of the poison is known, the severity of the symptoms shown by the patient is important in monitoring the course of treatment. When the nature of the poison is not known, the symptoms become vital in suggesting it. The application of toxicodynamics to the poisoned patient is demonstrated in Table 5-1, which lists symptoms and gives the common poisons that can cause them.

Toxicokinetics deals with the action of a poison in the patient as a function of time. This encompasses its absorption, distribution, localization, biotransformation, and elimination. The kinetics of a drug overdose, however, is not necessarily that of the therapeutic dose. This is so because a large dose of drug may saturate and overwhelm one or more of the mechanisms controlling absorption, distribution, biotransformation, and elimination of therapeutic concentrations. Moreover, normal physiologic processes such as heart rate, blood pressure, or respiration may be compromised and thereby alter the disposition of the drug overdose. In this chapter, toxicokinetics is shown to embody the major steps in the care of the acutely poisoned patient. These steps include nonspecific antidotes to remove poison not yet absorbed, specific antidotes to counteract a few select poisons, and occasionally diuresis or dialysis.

CARE OF THE ACUTELY POISONED PATIENT
Nonspecific Antidotes
Decontamination

Decontamination is the removal or neutralization of a toxin. If the toxin is on the clothing, skin, or eyes (e.g., insecticide spray), the clothing should be removed and the skin scrubbed well with soap and water. The eyes should be washed copiously with warm water. If a noxious gas has been inhaled, the individual should be given fresh air or oxygen to

Table 5-1   Physical Symptoms Produced by Common Poisons

Symptoms	Poisoning agent	Symptoms	Poisoning agent
MENTAL AND MOTOR SYMPTOMS		Hypotension	Alcohols
Drowsiness, coma	Acetaminophen		Aminophylline
	Alcohols		Aspirin
	Antihistamines		Muscarine
	Carbon monoxide		Nitrates, nitrites
	Insulin		Opioids
	Opioids (codeine, others)		Sedative-hypnotics
	Salicylates		Tranquilizers
	Scopolamine	Oliguria, anuria	Carbon tetrachloride
	Sedative-hypnotic drugs		Ethylene glycol
	Tranquilizers		Heavy metals
	Tricyclic antidepressants		Methanol
			Mushrooms
Excitation, twitching, convulsions	Aminophylline		Petroleum distillates
	Atropine		
	CNS stimulants	**ORAL AND GASTROINTESTINAL SYMPTOMS**	
	Carbon monoxide	Acetone odor	
	Cyanide	Acetone	
	Local anesthetics	Alcohol	
	Organophosphate insecticides	Salicylates	
	Phenothiazines		
		Almond odor	Cyanide
Agitation, delirium	Alcohols		
	Aminophylline	Garlic odor	Arsenic
	Atropine		Dimethyl sulfoxide
	Lysergic acid diethylamide (LSD)		Phosphorus
	Lead		Organophosphate insecticides
	Marijuana		
	Phencyclidine (PCP)	Dry mouth	Amphetamine
	Physostigmine		Antihistamines
			Atropine
Paralysis	Foods containing *Clostridium botulinum* (botulism)		Opioids
	Heavy metals		Phenothiazines
Ataxia (motor incoordination)	Alcohols	Excessive salivation	Arsenic
	Anticonvulsants		Corrosives
	Carbon monoxide		Mercury
	Hallucinogens		Mushrooms
	Heavy metals		Organophosphate insecticides
	Hydrocarbons		
	Sedative-hypnotics	Heavy vomiting	Aminophylline
	Tranquilizers		Corrosives
			Food poisoning
CARDIOVASCULAR AND RENAL SYMPTOMS			Heavy metals
Increased pulse rate	Alcohols		Salicylates
	Amphetamine		
	Aspirin	**PUPILLARY SYMPTOMS**	
	Atropine	Dilated pupils	Alcohols
	Cocaine		Anticholinergics
	Parasympatholytics		Antihistamines
	Sympathomimetics		CNS depressants
			CNS stimulants
Decreased pulse rate	Digitalis	Constricted pupils	Mushrooms
	Opioids		Organophosphate insecticides
	Parasympathomimetics		Opioids
Hypertension	Amphetamine		
	Sympathomimetics	Nystagmus	Sedative-hypnotics

Continued.

Table 5-1 Physical Symptoms Produced by Common Poisons—cont'd

Symptoms	Poisoning agent	Symptoms	Poisoning agent
DERMATOLOGIC SYMPTOMS		**PULMONARY SYMPTOMS**	
Jaundiced skin	Arsenic Carbon tetrachloride Mushrooms Naphthalene	Rapid breathing	Amphetamine Carbon monoxide Methanol Petroleum distillates Salicylates
Flushed skin	Alcohol Antihistamines Anticholinergics	Depressed respiration	Alcohol Opioids Sedative-hypnotics Tranquilizers
Cherry red skin	Carbon monoxide Cyanide Nitrites	Wheezing	Mushrooms Opioids Organophosphate insecticides Petroleum distillates

breathe. When a poison or drug overdose has been swallowed, much of it usually remains unabsorbed for some time. In treating poisoned patients, it is common to flush the poison from the gastrointestinal tract. Such techniques as induced vomiting (emesis), gastric lavage, administration of activated charcoal, and catharsis are appropriate to help eliminate a drug overdose that has been swallowed. The doses for these nonspecific antidotes are listed in Table 5-2.

Emesis and lavage

The stomach is emptied by emesis or gastric lavage. There are three major points that determine whether vomiting or gastric lavage should be used. First, induction of vomiting is not appropriate when the patient might aspirate the vomitus. Therefore this method is contraindicated when the patient lacks normal reflex control of gagging and vomiting or is unconscious or having seizures. Second, vomiting is not indicated when the regurgitated material can be damaging to the esophagus or lungs. Such material includes acids, bases, and nonaromatic or nonhalogenated hydrocarbons (oils and solvents). Third, induction of vomiting can take 20 to 30 minutes and therefore should not be used when time is critical.

The emetic of choice is **ipecac syrup,** which induces vomiting within 30 minutes in 90% of treated patients (see box). With this agent, 20% to 60% of the stomach contents can be emptied. Apomorphine is another emetic, but it must be prepared at the time of use and it causes respiratory depression. Apomorphine is usually effective within 1 to 15 minutes of administration. Emetics such as salt water (sodium

chloride), mustard water, and copper sulfate are considered dangerous and ineffective. When vomiting is induced, the vomitus should be saved for analysis.

Gastric lavage is the preferred method of emptying the stomach in adults. The airway is first protected by an endotracheal tube. Use of a large-bore tube such as an Ewald or Burke tube allows tablets

---

DRUG ABUSE ALERT: IPECAC SYRUP

BACKGROUND

Normally ipecac syrup is administered to induce vomiting in an acute poisoning. Ipecac syrup is readily obtained in a drugstore. Chronic administration of ipecac is abuse and is seen in some child abuse cases and in some cases of eating disorders. In eating disorders, ipecac syrup may be taken to purge ingested food.

PHARMACOLOGY

Emetine HCl (Ipecac alkaloid) is a safe drug for inducing vomiting in emergency home use. Administered chronically, however, it can produce many chronic symptoms. These may not be readily associated with abuse. Most of these symptoms relate to distorted electrolyte imbalances that arise from continual vomiting and loss of gastric fluids. The active alkaloid of ipecac also has a direct depressive action on heart and skeletal muscle.

HEALTH HAZARDS

Symptoms of continued ipecac administration include chronic diarrhea and vomiting, muscle weakness, colitis, cardiomyopathy, fever, edema, and electrolyte disturbances. Therapy for ipecac abuse is supportive while ipecac is discontinued.

Table 5-2 Nonspecific Antidotes

Antidote	Trade name	Administration/dosage	Comments
EMETICS			
Ipecac	Ipecac syrup*	ORAL, in 8 oz water: *Children 6 mo-1 yr*—5–10 ml. *Children 1–12 yr*—15 ml. *Adults*—30 ml. Vomiting in 30 min in 90% of patients. May repeat dose after 20-30 min if no vomiting has occurred.	Give only to conscious patients who have gag reflex and are not likely to aspirate vomitus. Do not give when vomitus will itself be injurious (acids, bases, hydrocarbons). Encourage patients to drink water. Water distends stomach and makes it more susceptible to action of ipecac syrup. Walking also helps to induce vomiting. Average return of stomach contents is 20%-60%. Keep vomitus for analysis.
Apomorphine	Apomorphine HCl	SUBCUTANEOUS: *Children*—0.07-0.1 mg/kg. *Adults*—5-6 mg.	May cause CNS and respiratory depression or protracted vomiting, which are treated with 0.005 mg/kg naloxone HCl. Keep vomitus for analysis.
GASTRIC LAVAGE			
Water: 0.45% saline 0.9% saline		BY GASTRIC TUBE: *Small children*—10 ml/kg. *Adults*—300 ml.	If patient is in deteriorating condition, unconscious, prone to seizures, or lacking a gag reflex, nasotracheal intubation is necessary before lavage to protect airway. Use large-bore (28-40 French Ewald or Burke orogastric lavacutor) tubing to allow aspiration of tablets. Keep first wash for analysis. Continue washings until return is clear (2-20 L). Administering more than recommended volume distends stomach and may induce vomiting.
Activated charcoal	Acta-Char Charcoaid Charcodate† Insta-Char* Liqui-Char	ORAL OR BY GASTRIC TUBE: *Children*—15-30 gm in 4-8 oz water. *Adults*—25-50 gm in 8-16 oz water.	Administer as slurry within first hours of poisoning, after induced vomiting (charcoal will inactivate ipecac) or gastric lavage. Do not use with acetylcysteine in management of acetaminophen poisoning. Do not use magnesium sulfate as cathartic.
CATHARTICS			
Magnesium sulfate (Epsom salts), 10% solution		ORAL: *Children*—1-2 ml/kg. *Adults*—150-250 ml.	Do not use magnesium salts if patient has renal failure. Do not use citrate if activated charcoal has been given.
Magnesium citrate, 10% solution.		ORAL: *Children*—1-2 ml/kg *Adults*—150-250 ml	Do not use magnesium salts if patient has renal failure. Do not use citrate if activated charcoal has been given.

*Available in Canada and United States.
†Available in Canada only.

to be retrieved. Gastric lavage is less successful in children because a small-bore tube must be used. Tablets from some drug formulations partially deteriorate and then coalesce in the stomach to form a mass of undissolved drug that is too large to be washed out and yet is poorly soluble. Continue lavage until the return is clear. Save the first wash for analysis.

Activated charcoal

After emesis or lavage a slurry of activated charcoal may be administered through the lavage tube or a nasogastric tube, or it may be given orally. Because activated charcoal absorbs and inactivates ipecac syrup, do not give it until after vomiting has occurred. **Activated charcoal** absorbs a number of drugs and chemicals and thereby prevents their absorption into the body. The charcoal itself, with absorbed chemicals, is eliminated in the feces. Administration of activated charcoal is most effective if given within the first few hours of poisoning. If the poisoning is known to be caused by acetaminophen, activated charcoal should not be given. The antidote for acetaminophen is acetylcysteine, which is absorbed by activated charcoal.

Cathartics

Cathartics are the final common treatment to reduce absorption of poisons from the gastrointestinal tract by hastening their elimination. The preferred cathartics are sodium sulfate, magnesium sulfate, or magnesium citrate. However, magnesium citrate should not be used after charcoal administration because the citrate can displace poisons from charcoal. Oil-based cathartics such as mineral oil and castor oil are not used in treating poisoned patients because these oils can speed systemic absorption of some poisons. Cathartics especially are indicated under the following circumstances: when enteric-coated tablets have been ingested, when poisoning occurred 1 hour or more previously, or when hydrocarbons have been ingested.

Specific Antidotes

A **specific antidote** is one that directly reverses the toxic action of the poison. There is a specific antidote in only 5% of poisoning cases (see Table 5-3).

Competitive antidotes

A specific antidote may compete at the receptor for the toxin. Naloxone displaces narcotics (opioids) at the opioid receptor. Unlike other opioids, naloxone does not depress the respiratory center; therefore the occupation of the opioid receptor by naloxone protects against respiratory depression. Oxygen in high concentration competes with carbon monoxide in binding to hemoglobin to restore oxygenation. Atropine blocks the muscarinic receptor from the acetylcholine accumulated in anticholinesterase poisoning.

Table 5-3 Specific Antidotes

Antidote	Poison	Administration/dosage	Comments
Atropine	Anticholinesterase Organophosphates Physostigmine	INTRAVENOUS: *Children*—0.02 mg/kg. *Adults*—1-2 mg. This is initial dose. Repeat every 20 min until copious secretions are controlled.	Blocks muscarinic receptors to prevent peripheral actions of excessive concentrations of neurotransmitter, acetylocholine. See Chapter 9 for more information on actions of acetylcholine and how atropine blocks actions of acetylcholine. Muscarinic symptoms for which atropine is given include nausea, vomiting, diarrhea, sweat, increased bronchial and salivary secretions, and slow heart rate (bradycardia).
Pralidoxime chloride (PAM)	Anticholinesterase Organophosphates	Organophosate poisoning: BY INFUSION in 100 ml saline over 15–30 min: *Children*—20-40 mg/kg. *Adults*—1-2 gm. A second dose can be given in 1 hr. Carbamate (neostigmine, pyridostigmine) poisoning: INTRAVENOUS: *Adults*—1-2 gm initially, followed by 250 mg every 5 min as necessary to reverse cholinergic crisis.	Reactivates enzyme acetylcholinesterase after inactivation by irreversible anticholinesterases or organophosphates. This allows acetylcholine to be degraded and relieves paralysis (overstimulation) caused by accumulated acetylcholine. Pralidoxime acts mainly outside CNS. In organophosphate poisoning, pralidoxime is given to restore neuromuscular function, especially to relieve paralysis of respiratory muscles. Atropine is given concurrently (see above) to relieve depression of respiratory center and to reverse muscarinic stimulation. In overdose by carbamate anticholinesterases (neostigmine, pyridostigmine and ambenonium, drugs for myasthenia gravis), pralidoxime antagonizes effects of these drugs on neuromuscular junction.
Physostigmine salicylate (Antilirium)	Antimuscarinic anticholinergic	INTRAVENOUS OR INTRAMUSCULAR: *Adults*—0.5-2 mg. INTRAVENOUS: *Children*—0.5 mg by slow (1 min) infusion. Repeat if needed at 5-10 min intervals until desired effect, or 2 mg total dose, is reached.	Reversible anticholinesterase that increases concentration of acetylcholine at its receptor sites. Reverses both CNS and peripheral anticholinergic effects. Useful for reversing toxic anticholinergic effects due to overdose of atropine and other belladonna alkaloids, tricyclic antidepressants, phenothiazines, and antihistamines. Central anticholinergic effects include anxiety, delirium, disorientation, hallucinations, hyperactivity, seizures, and—in the extreme—coma, medullary paralysis, and death. Peripheral anticholinergic toxic effects include fast heart rate (tachycardia), fever, mydriasis (dilated pupils), vasodilation, urinary retention, decreased secretions, and decreased gastrointestinal motility.

Table 5-3 Specific Antidotes—cont'd

Antidote	Poison	Administration/dosage	Comments
Naloxone (Narcan)	Narcotics (opioids), including pentazocine, propoxyphene, diphenoxylate	INTRAVENOUS: *Adults*—0.4-2 mg. Additional doses are repeated at 2-3 min intervals until patient responds or until 10 mg is given. INTRAVENOUS: *Children*—0.01 mg/kg with 0.1 mg/kg as subsequent dose. May also give INTRAMUSCULARLY or SUBCUTANEOUSLY.	Reversible antagonist of opioid receptor. Useful for reversing narcotic depression, including respiratory depression. Naloxone is preferred because it is pure opioid antagonist and causes no respiratory depression of its own. Naloxone is effective within 2 min and has duration of action of 1-4 hr. Because most opioids have a longer duration of action, effects of naloxone may wear off and patient may relapse, requiring additional naloxone.
Ethanol	Methanol Ethylene glycol	INTRAVENOUS: *Adults*—0.6 gm/kg + 7-10 gm over 1 hr; then 10 gm/hr maintenance. *Children*—0.6 gm/kg + 4-5 gm over 1 hr; 5 gm/hr maintenance.	All three alcohols are metabolized by aldehyde dehydrogenase. Ethanol is preferred substrate and thereby blocks metabolism of methanol and ethylene glycol to toxins formaldehyde and formic acid (both alcohols) and oxylate (ethylene glycol). Ethanol is given in additional loading dose to achieve blood level of 100 mg/dl.
Amyl nitrite Sodium nitrite Sodium thiosulfate (Cyanide Antidote Package)	Cyanide	Amyl nitrite: Crush ampule on gauze and have patient inhale vapor. Sodium nitrite: Inject 10 ml of 3% solution after IV line is established. Sodium thiosulfate: Inject 50 ml of 25% solution after administration of sodium nitrite.	Cyanide has almond odor. Toxicity of cyanide is caused by its blockage of enzymes using oxygen in mitochondria (cytochrome oxidase), thereby depressing cellular respiration. Inhibition of cytochrome oxidase depends on binding of cyanide to ferric iron in cytochrome oxidase. Nitrite converts ferrous iron in hemoglobin to ferric iron, producing methemoglobin. This large pool of ferric iron in blood competes with cytochrome oxidase for cyanide, thereby restoring cellular respiration. Thiosulfate accelerates conversion of cyanide to relatively nontoxic thiocyanate, which is readily excreted in urine.
Acetylcysteine (Mucomyst)	Acetaminophen	ORAL: 140 mg/kg as 5% solution mixed with soda, water, or grapefruit juice. Follow with 17 maintenance doses of 70 mg/kg every 4 hr.	Acetylcysteine restores sulfhydryl groups depleted by acetaminophen metabolism. This prevents toxicity to liver produced by metabolites of acetaminophen. Acetylcysteine should not be given with activated charcoal because charcoal absorbs it.
Deferoxamine mesylate (Desferal)	Iron	INTRAMUSCULAR, CONTINUOUS SUBCUTANEOUS, or SLOW INTRAVENOUS: *Adults*—1 gm initially, 0.5 gm at 4 and 8 hr. Further doses if needed, up to 6 gm daily. For IV, do not give at rate greater than 15 mg/kg/hr. Administer IM if possible. *Children*—50 mg/kg IM or IV every 6 hr up to 15 mg/kg/hr by continuous IV. Maximum dosage: 6 gm/24 hr or 2-gm/dose.	Chelates iron and thereby prevents iron from entering cells and inhibiting chemical reactions. Chelate of iron and deferoxamine is rapidly excreted in urine, removing iron from body.
Dimercaprol (BAL)	Arsenic Gold Mercury Lead	INTRAMUSCULAR: Because dimercaprol is oil, give deep intramuscularly only. Mild arsenic or gold poisoning: 2.5 mg/kg 4 times daily, 2 days; 2 times, day 3; once daily, 10 days. Severe arsenic or gold poisoning: 3 mg/kg every 4 hr for 2 days, 4 times day 3; twice daily 10 days.	Dimercaprol is a sulfhydryl compound that chelates arsenic, gold, and mercury and promotes their excretion in urine. Dimercaprol also reactivates affected sulfhydryl enzymes. Peak plasma concentrations occur 30-60 min after administration. Excretion is complete in 4 hr. Dimercaprol is not very effective for poisoning caused by antimony and bismuth. It is contraindicated in iron, cadmium, and selenium poisoning because chelates are more toxic, especially to kidney, than metal alone. Alkalinization of urine protects kidney from breakdown of dimercaprol-metal complex in acid urine.

Continued.

Table 5-3   Specific Antidotes—cont'd

Antidote	Poison	Administration/dosage	Comments
Dimercaprol—cont'd		Mercury poisoning: 5 mg/kg initially; 2.5 mg/kg 1.2 times daily for 10 days. Acute lead poisoning: 4 mg/kg alone initially, then at 4-hr intervals with calcium disodium edetate (administered at separate site) Maintain for 2-7 days.	Common side effects of dimercaprol are rise in blood pressure with tachycardia (fast heart rate) and burning sensation of lips, mouth, and throat.
Edetate calcium disodium (calcium disodium versenate)	Lead	INTRAVENOUS: 50-75 mg/kg/day in 3-6 doses, each dose administered over at least 1 hr. Can continue for up to 5 days. Wait 2 days before resuming therapy for additional 5 days. INTRAMUSCULAR: Preferred route for children. Give 35 mg/kg twice daily. After 3-5 days discontinue for 4 or more days.	Calcium-bound to EDTA is displaced by lead and resulting chelate is excreted in urine (50% in 1 hr: 95% in 24 hr). EDTA can produce toxic effects, including renal damage and irregularities in cardiac rhythm. Doses must be carefully monitored.
Penicillamine (cuprimine, Depen)	Copper Lead Zinc Mercury	ORAL: *Adults*—1-1.5 gm daily in 4 divided doses on empty stomach for 1-2 months. *Children*—30-40 mg/kg daily or 600-750 mg/m² daily for 1-6 months.	Penicillamine chelates copper, lead, zinc, or mercury, promoting their excretion in urine. Side effects include allergic reactions (principally rashes) and loss of sweet and salt tastes. Severe side effects include bone marrow depression and renal toxicity.

Chelates

Another category of specific antidotes is chelates, compounds that form a nontoxic complex with the toxin. Poisoning by heavy metals in particular is treated with chelates, which form a nontoxic complex with the metal; this complex is quickly eliminated, usually in the urine. Accumulation of the heavy metal is thereby reversed. Dimercaprol complexes arsenic, copper, lead, and mercury. Penicillamine is used to complex copper, lead, and mercury (see Chapter 23). Deferoxamine is a specific chelate for iron (see Chapter 22). Ethylenediamine tetraacetate (EDTA) is the chelate used for lead or cadmium intoxication.

Antibodies

In a few instances, treatment with specific antibodies to the poison is possible. Antibodies to digoxin are available to counteract toxic levels of this important cardiac drug. These antibodies reverse the cardiac toxicity by complexing the digoxin and lowering the large pool of digoxin that is bound to plasma albumin. The digoxin then is not free to act. Antivenoms are antibodies for certain snake and spider venoms.

Metabolic alterations

Specific antidotes may alter the metabolism of a toxin. Ethanol inhibits the biotransformation of methanol and ethylene glycol to toxic metabolites, particularly formic acid. Thiosulfate enhances the transformation of cyanide to the relatively nontoxic thiocyanate. Acetylcysteine restores the sulfhydryl groups of the liver after depletion by acetaminophen metabolism. Sulfhydryl groups protect the liver from toxic metabolites of acetaminophen. Physostigmine inhibits acetylcholinesterase, the enzyme that normally degrades acetylcholine. This action allows acetylcholine concentrations to rise at the synapses and compete with anticholinergic drugs blocking these receptors. This reversal by acetylcholine restores function in anticholinergic poisoning by drugs that are anticholinergic, such as atropine or scopolamine, or that have anticholinergic actions, such as antihistamines, tricyclic antidepressants, and antipsychotic drugs. Used as an antidote, pralidoxime reactivates acetylcholinesterase after it has been inactivated by an anticholinesterase poison. The poison is freed in an inactive form that is eliminated.

Diuresis and Dialysis

Diuresis

Diuresis can be used to hasten elimination of poisons excreted primarily by the kidneys. **Diuresis** is used when the level of poison in the blood is at a potentially fatal concentration, when the patient is in a coma, and when the patient has otherwise stable cardiovascular, respiratory, and renal function. Fluid diuresis, achieved with a potent loop diuretic such as furosemide, increases the glomerular filtration rate and thereby decreases the renal tubular reabsorption of the poison. Osmotic diuresis with mannitol or urea prevents reabsorption of the poison in the kidney by creating an osmotic load that effectively flushes the kidney tubule. Alkalinization of the urine with sodium bicarbonate enhances the excretion of weak acids such as aspirin and phenobarbital by maintaining them in their ionized form, which is not reabsorbed readily. Similarly, acidification of the urine with ammonium chloride or ascorbic acid aids the excretion of weak bases such as amphetamine or phencyclidine by maintaining them in their ionized form, which is not reabsorbed. Diuretics are discussed fully in Chapter 16.

Dialysis

Dialysis is indicated in cases of extreme poisoning or renal failure when the poison is dialyzable. For instance, the anticoagulant warfarin and the cardiac glycoside digitoxin are tightly protein bound in the blood and therefore are not successfully removed by dialysis. Hemodialysis is a highly technical and complex procedure in which the blood is shunted from the body and through tubing immersed in physiologic buffer. Any chemical present in the blood but not in the buffer diffuses into the buffer because of the concentration gradient. The dialyzed, or "washed," blood is returned continuously to the body. Salicylate, methanol, and ethylene glycol are removed effectively by hemodialysis. Hemoperfusion is a relatively new technique in which the blood is pumped from a venous catheter through a column of absorbent material and returned to the patient. Anticoagulation with heparin is necessary to prevent the patient's blood from clotting in the cartridge. Hemoperfusion is effective for high-molecular-weight poisons with poor water solubility because the cartridge has a large surface area for absorption. Peritoneal dialysis is the simplest dialysis technique, but unfortunately, it is the most inefficient way to remove the majority of drugs. In peritoneal dialysis, physiologic buffer is introduced into the abdomen and left there for several hours before being drained and replaced. Because the gastrointestinal tract has a rich blood supply, the blood is dialyzed as it flows through the normal gastrointestinal network.

NURSING IMPLICATIONS SUMMARY

General Guidelines

◆ Thoroughly assess any patient suspected of having ingested a toxic substance or a toxic amount of a generally nontoxic substance. If the patient's condition requires emergency treatment, abbreviate the initial assessment until the patient is stabilized, and then perform further assessment. Assess blood pressure and vital signs, neurologic signs, level of respiratory effort, presence of cyanosis, breath sounds, ECG, patient's appearance (including nose and mouth), blood gases, serum electrolyte levels, renal and liver function tests, and weight. Obtain a detailed history from the patient and family about the suspected toxic agents, including the amount, time the substance was ingested, efforts to induce vomiting or dilute the substance, patient's age, and any medical problems. Save samples of the toxic substance, vomitus, or stool; label them carefully and send to the laboratory for analysis.

◆ Work quickly and efficiently to administer prescribed antagonists or other treatments, but remain calm. Reassure the patient and family that everything possible will be done. Families of children may be especially upset. Nurses who work in settings where overdoses or toxic ingestions commonly are seen (e.g., emergency departments and some occupational health settings) should know the location of emergency equipment for intubation, assisted ventilation, and resuscitation; the telephone number of the nearest poison control center; the location of reference guides to emergency treatment of overdoses; the location of antidotes, antagonists, and equipment (e.g., lavage tubes) used in that setting; and general procedures to be followed in treating overdose.

◆ Prevention is preferable to treatment for overdose; however, preventive health teaching is usually not appropriate during treatment of

Continued.

NURSING IMPLICATIONS SUMMARY—cont'd

acute overdose. When working with patients or families in situations involving drugs or toxic chemicals, review general safety measures regularly. Teaching points to review include keeping medications and household products out of the reach of children and mentally impaired or confused patients; keeping medications in a locked cabinet; keeping drugs and chemicals in clearly and correctly labeled containers; using safety latches on cabinets and drawers; never referring to medicines as *candy*; treating all medicines with respect; using child-proof caps when children are in the environment; using drugs only as prescribed; and never doubling or increasing the dose of any drug unless specifically directed to do so by the physician. Teach patients never to borrow medications prescribed for another person.

◆ Ipecac syrup is available in small quantities without a prescription and should be kept in the home (out of the reach of children) for emergency treatment of overdose. However, teach families to call the poison control center before administering ipecac syrup to ascertain that inducing vomiting is appropriate for the ingested substance. Teach patients to keep the number of the poison control center near the telephone.

◆ Instruct patients or families calling for emergency help to bring a sample of the drug or toxic substance and any vomitus to the emergency department when they bring the patient.

Ipecac Syrup

Drug administration and patient and family education

◆ Ipecac syrup may be purchased without prescription and may be kept in the home. Do not administer ipecac syrup until directed to do so by the physician or poison control center. Any ipecac syrup remaining after a dose has been administered should be discarded. Check expiration dates.

◆ Have the patient drink a full glass of water (8 oz) after taking the ordered dose (½ to 1 full glass for a child). A frightened child may do better if the water is administered before the ipecac syrup. Avoid milk products. Generally, if vomiting does not occur after the first dose, the dose is repeated in about 20 minutes. If vomiting does not occur after the

second dose, take the patient to the emergency department. Do not give ipecac syrup to infants under 6 months of age. Children 6 months to 1 year old should be treated in the emergency room.

◆ If the physician has also prescribed activated charcoal, give ipecac syrup first and administer the activated charcoal after vomiting has ceased. Do not induce vomiting in anyone who is drowsy because this may predispose to aspiration. Save vomitus and send it to the laboratory for analysis.

Apomorphine Hydrochloride

Drug administration

◆ Amorphine is more effective if the stomach is full. Before administering the dose, have the patient drink a full glass of water (8 oz for an adult and ½ to 1 glass for a child). Bouncing a small child gently may also help stimulate vomiting.

◆ If the physician has also prescribed activated charcoal, administer the apomorphine first, and use the activated charcoal after vomiting has ceased.

◆ Apomorphine is related to morphine, so it produces many of the same side effects, including drowsiness and CNS depression. As with morphine, the antagonist in the event of overdose is naloxone; keep naloxone readily available. Apomorphine is contraindicated in anyone allergic to morphine.

◆ Do not administer the solution if its color is green or brown.

◆ Save vomitus and send it to the laboratory for analysis.

Gastric Lavage

Drug administration

◆ Review the information presented in Table 5-2. Follow agency policy and procedure for insertion of an orogastric or nasogastric tube. Insert a large-bore tube to permit tablets or precipitated material to be recovered. Verify correct placement of the tube before any fluid is introduced. Use a syringe to aspirate for stomach contents; auscultate over the stomach as a small amount of air (5 to 10 ml) is injected through the tube. A popping or gurgling noise is heard as the air is forced into the stomach.

◆ Place the patient in a sitting or semi-Fowler's

NURSING IMPLICATIONS SUMMARY—cont'd

position during lavage. Slowly inject a large quantity of fluid (300 to 500 ml in an adult), then slowly aspirate the fluid. Alternate injection and aspiration until the return is clear. Tap water may be used as an irrigant in adults, but 0.9% or 0.45% saline should be used in young children. Provide mouth care at the completion of the procedure.

Activated Charcoal

Drug administration

◆ Activated charcoal is most effective when administered within 30 minutes of ingestion of the poison. The mixture is unattractive. Put it into an empty soft-drink can to administer to children. Mix charcoal with water or a small amount of fruit juice. Do not mix with ice cream or milk, because these foods decrease the ability of the charcoal to absorb the toxin. Activated charcoal absorbs ipecac syrup; do not administer these simultaneously. Inform patients that activated charcoal may cause feces to turn black.

Cathartics

Drug administration

◆ See Chapter 13 for additional information about saline cathartics. Do not use sodium salts if the patient has a history of heart disease. Do not use magnesium salts if the patient has a history of renal failure. Do not use magnesium sulfate if activated charcoal has been administered.

Atropine

◆ See Chapter 9 for additional information about atropine.

Pralidoxime Chloride

Drug administration

◆ Review the information presented in Table 5-3. Keep a suction machine and intubation equipment readily available when using pralidoxime chloride. See Chapter 11 for a discussion of myasthenia gravis. Keep edrophonium, atropine, syringes, and a tourniquet handy when working with patients with myasthenia gravis. Monitor patients carefully. Side effects of pralidoxime may mimic effects of ingested substances; side effects include dizziness, blurred vision, diplopia, drowsiness, nausea, tachycardia, hyperventilation, and muscle weakness.

Physostigmine Salicylate

Drug administration

◆ Review the information presented in Table 5-3. Monitor vital signs and blood pressure. Treat an overdose with atropine, which should be kept at the bedside. Because the drug has a short duration of action (30 to 60 minutes), it may be necessary to repeat doses; monitor the patient carefully. Atropine may be administered intravenously undiluted. Administer at a rate of 1 mg or less over 1 to 3 minutes (adult) or 0.5 mg/min (child).

Naloxone

Drug administration

◆ Monitor respirations. Naloxone should promptly increase the respiratory rate and volume. If it does not, the respiratory depression is probably not the result of narcotic overdose, or multiple agents were consumed or injected. Keep intubation and resuscitation equipment and drugs readily available when patients manifest respiratory depression.

◆ Monitor vital signs and blood pressure. Naloxone has a relatively short half-life, and you may need to repeat the dose. Remember that in narcotic addicts, this drug may precipitate withdrawal symptoms. Monitor neonates carefully. Naloxone may be used to treat neonatal respiratory depression, which may be present if narcotic analgesics were administered in large doses during labor and delivery or if the mother is a narcotic addict. If the mother is an addict, naloxone will precipitate withdrawal symptoms in the infant.

Ethanol

Drug administration

◆ Ethanol can be administered intravenously or via orogastric or nasogastric tube. Orally, a 20% solution is preferred to reduce the risk of gastritis, but if needed, any blended whiskey can be used. If the patient's condition warrants it, oral administration is preferred because the IV route is limited to 5% to 10% solutions. Monitor blood ethanol levels during therapy. Monitor vital signs and ECG. When using ethanol for treatment of overdose, keep a suction machine and equipment for intubation and resuscitation at the bedside.

Continued.

Cyanide Antidote Package

Drug administration

◆ This combination of drugs (amyl nitrite, sodium nitrite, and sodium triosulfate) is recommended for cyanide poisoning and also for treatment of overdose with sodium nitroprusside (see Table 5-3 and Chapter 15). Side effects are rare. Monitor vital signs and blood pressure.

Acetylcysteine

Drug administration

◆ Review Table 5-3 and see Chapter 26. Monitor vital signs. Side effects are rare with acetylcysteine and include nausea, vomiting, and increase in blood pressure. Acetylcysteine has a very unpleasant odor. Try having patient take doses through a straw placed in a cup or container that is tightly capped.

Deferoxamine Mesylate

Drug administration

◆ Monitor vital signs, fluid intake and output, and serum iron levels. Rapid IV administration may cause hypotension, tachycardia, erythema, and urticaria. Anaphylactic reactions are rare, but keep epinephrine and intubation and resuscitation equipment handy. In acute iron poisoning, treat patient with deferoxamine, as well as lavage or induction of emesis, and maintain a patent airway, control shock (IV fluids, vasopressors), and correct acidosis (administer sodium bicarbonate or other drugs).

◆ Intramuscular injection is the preferred parenteral route. Reconstitute powder with 2 ml of sterile water for injection; dissolve all powder before injecting dose. After subcutaneous injection, some patients experience a local histaminelike reaction. Reserve IV injection for patients exhibiting signs of shock. Reconstitute powder as above, then further dilute with a compatible IV solution. Administer at a rate not exceeding 15 mg/kg/hr.

Patient and family education

◆ Advise patients on long-term therapy to have regular ophthalmic examinations.

◆ Usually discontinue chelation therapy during pregnancy.

◆ Advise women considering pregnancy to consult their physicians. Inform patients that deferoxamine may turn urine red.

Dimercaprol

Drug administration

◆ Review Table 5-3. Monitor vital signs and intake and output. Do not administer medicinal iron to patients receiving dimercaprol.

◆ Avoid skin contact with the drug when preparing doses; wear gloves. Keep the urine alkaline to facilitate chelation, and monitor the urine pH. For detailed instructions in preparing oil-based suspensions, see Chapter 6.

Patient and family education

◆ Inform patients that the drug may produce a garliclike odor on breath. Inform parents that some children develop fever during therapy.

Edetate Calcium Disodium

Drug administration

◆ Read orders carefully. Do not confuse edetate calcium disodium, used to treat lead poisoning, with edetate disodium, used to treat hypercalcemia. Assess urine output before administering. Because the chelate is excreted in the urine, patients with oliguria or renal disease may be unable to tolerate this drug. Monitor vital signs, blood urea nitrogen level, urinalysis, serum electrolyte and creatinine levels, intake and output, and ECG. Edetate calcium disodium interferes with the duration of action of zinc insulin preparations. Diabetics who receive zinc insulin may need a change in dose or drug while taking edetate calcium disodium.

◆ Intramuscular injection is the preferred route of administration in children and in individuals with lead encephalopathy. Procaine may be added to the reconstituted solution to help prevent pain at the injection site. Assess the mouth and gums for development of sores. These should subside after drug therapy. Zinc replacement may be necessary between courses of therapy with edetate calcium disodium.

Penicillamine

◆ Review Table 5-3. Penicillamine is also used to treat rheumatoid arthritis, as discussed in Chapter 23.

CHAPTER REVIEW

◆ **KEY TERMS**

activated charcoal, p. 67

cathartics, p. 68

clinical toxicology, p. 63

decontamination, p. 64

diuresis, p. 71

gastric lavage, p. 66

ipecac syrup, p. 66

specific antidote, p. 68

toxicodynamics, p. 64

toxicokinetics, p. 64

toxicology, p. 63

◆ **REVIEW QUESTIONS**

1. What do the terms *toxicology* and *clinical toxicology* mean?

2. Determine whether your community has a poison control center. What services are offered by this center? Where is the number in the telephone directory?

3. What is toxicodynamics and why is it important clinically? Why is patient assessment so important in treating poisoning?

4. What is toxicokinetics and why is it important clinically? How does this differ from pharmacokinetics?

5. How does the health professional use nonspecific antidotes in treatment of acute poisoning?

6. Contrast the uses of emesis and gastric lavage in emptying the stomach. What is the drug of choice for inducing vomiting? Why?

7. It is recommended that households with children have on hand a small quantity of ipecac syrup. What are important teaching points about this drug?

8. When is the administration of activated charcoal indicated?

9. What is the role of cathartics in treating acute poisoning? Which drugs are recommended? Why?

10. Describe specific antidotes that the health professional would consider for each of the following categories: competitive, chelate, antibody, and metabolic.

11. When is diuresis indicated in treating acute poisoning? Describe fluid and osmotic diuresis and alkalinization and acidification of the urine and when these processes may be helpful.

12. When is dialysis indicated in treating acute poisoning? Describe hemodialysis, hemoperfusion, and peritoneal dialysis.

13. What are important teaching points to promote safety and decrease the possibility of poisoning in the household?

SUGGESTED READING

Carlton FB Jr: General management of the poisoned patient, *Emerg Care Q* 6(3):1, 1990.

Cooper K: Drug overdose, *Am J Nurs* 89(9):1146, 1989.

Cooper K, Albrezzi B: Emergency! It's cyanide, *Am J Nurs* 90(11):42, 1990.

Davis NM, Cohen MR: Today's poisons: how to keep them from killing your patients, *Nurs 89* 19(1):49, 1989.

Dubiel D: Action stat! Cocaine overdose, *Nurs 90* 20(3):33, 1990.

Hathaway BK: Toxicology: an overview, *AAOHN J* 34(11):518, 1986.

Hernandez P, Johnson CA: Deferoxamine for aluminum toxicity in dialysis patients, *AANA J* 17(3):224, 1990.

House MA: Cocaine, *Am J Nurs* 90(4):41, 1990.

Huston CJ: Action stat! Caustic chemical ingestion, *Nurs 90* 20(7):33, 1990.

Joubert DW: Use of emetics, adsorbents, and cathartic agents in acute drug overdose, *J Emerg Nurs* 13(1):49, 1987.

Miller M: Combating caustic substance poisoning, *Nurs 87* 17(6):32BB, 1987.

Milstein MJ and others: Efficacy of oral N-acetylcysteine in the treatment of acetaminophen overdose, *New Engl J Med* 319(24):1557, 1988.

Newton M and others: Specific treatments of poisoning by household products and medications, *J Emerg Nurs* 13(1):16, 1987.

Povenmire KI, House MA: Recognizing the cocaine addict, *Nurs 90* 20(5):46, 1990.

Ratko JE: Action stat! Pesticide poisoning, *Nurs 91* 21(5):33, 1991.

Senanayake N, Karalliedde L: Neurotoxic effects of organophosphorous insecticides, *New Engl J Med* 316(13):761, 1987.

Snyder DS: Digoxin immune Fab ovine, *Crit Care Nurse* 8(8):10, 1988.

Thurkauf GE: Acetaminophen overdose, *Crit Care Nurse* 7(1):20, 1987.

CHAPTER 6

Drug Administration

LEARNING OBJECTIVES

After studying this chapter, you should be able to do the following:

◆ Explain differences between the unit dose system and the stock drug system.

◆ Give examples of information about drug administration that must be recorded on the patient's record.

◆ Give examples of how administration of drugs to children or the elderly may require more individualized planning.

◆ Describe how to administer drugs via a variety of routes.

CHAPTER OVERVIEW

◆ This chapter emphasizes drug administration. Drug therapy is only a part of total patient care, but for drug therapy to be successful it must be carried out properly. The patient has the right to receive the right drug, in the right dose, at the right time, via the right route of administration.

◆ The administration of drugs to patients is an opportunity for the nurse to add to the database through additional patient assessment, to teach the patient in preparation for self-management of the health condition, to participate in discharge planning with the patient, and to evaluate the effectiveness of the care plan being implemented by the health care team. The reader should also study Chapter 3 carefully for information about the application of the nursing process to drug therapy.

Nursing Process Overview

DRUG ADMINISTRATION

Assessment

When assessing a patient, the nurse should ask why this patient might need a particular drug. Identifying the reason for medications being prescribed helps the nurse detect inadvertent errors in which the wrong drug may be administered.

Obtain objective and subjective data from the patient to aid in determining the need and effectiveness of drug use. Determine any patient preferences regarding drug use and incorporate these if possible. Determine the developmental level, especially for children, to aid in planning nursing care approaches.

Nursing Diagnoses

Not all patients require the formulation of nursing diagnoses as a result of drug therapy. Most patients are not knowledgeable about a specific drug at the start of drug therapy. Other diagnoses may develop as the patient develops side effects, is unable to manage self-administration, or has collaborative problems as potential complications.

Management

Implementing the therapeutic plan involves proper administration of the prescribed medication. The nurse should seek information about specific drugs from a variety of sources, including the physician, the pharmacist, and current printed materials. For a student nurse, the prospect of learning about all the medications to be administered is likely to be overwhelming. After you are in practice, however, repeated administration of medications facilitates development of a basic understanding of frequently used drug categories.

Not only must you know about the prescribed medication, but also exercise caution that the prescribed medication is what the patient actually receives. Thus medications should remain in labeled

76

packages or containers until they are administered.

The patient has a right to receive the medication in the correct dose. Regardless of how drugs are supplied to the patient care unit, check labels carefully and double-check all dosage calculations. Some nurses have difficulty with the mathematic calculations necessary for determining correct doses; have a colleague verify dosage calculations rather than possibly subjecting the patient to an incorrect dose of medication. Consult the pharmacy for additional help. Successful drug therapy may depend on the proper timing of drug doses, as discussed in Chapter 1. To ensure that the patient receives each drug via the right route of administration, check that routes are appropriate for a specific drug and know how to administer drugs via that route.

Develop a sense of suspicion whenever a medication order seems to be out of the ordinary. Double-check a dose of medication that seems unusually large or small. When at the bedside, if the patient seems hesitant to take the medication, stating that it is new or not what is usually taken, double-check the physician's orders before administering the medication. Record that a patient has received a medication as soon as possible after administration to avoid inadvertent duplicate administration by other members of the health care team.

Evaluation

The major question during evaluation is whether the medication is working as expected. The nurse must know what was expected of the medication, have initial baseline data about the patient, and know what parameters to assess to determine whether the drug is working as desired. Determine whether there were any problems associated with the route, time, or dose of medication, and make appropriate notations on the kardex or care plan.

DRUG ADMINISTRATION SYSTEMS

The two major drug administration systems in common use today are the unit dose system and the stock drug system. In the **unit dose system,** each dose of medication is individually wrapped, labeled, and supplied to the patient's unit in sufficient quantity to last 24 hours. On the unit each patient has a designated drawer, box, or container, and the exact number of ordered doses of medications for a 24-hour period are placed in that container by the pharmacy daily. When the nurse prepares to administer a drug, the patient's container is checked for the dose. The labeled medication is taken to the bedside, and after the nurse verifies the patient's identity, the dose package is opened and the nurse administers the dose to the patient. This system has several advantages.

1. The medication remains in a labeled container until the nurse is at the bedside, thus reducing the chance of getting drugs mixed up.
2. Patients can be billed by exactly the number of medication doses that are taken.
3. Unauthorized use of medications is decreased.

Disadvantages include the increased cost for the pharmacy in setting up this system; the need for additional pharmacists or pharmacy technicians to resupply the patient units each 24 hours and to fill orders for stat and new orders; and often a need for increased space in the pharmacy for storage of drugs in the unit dose packages. The system builds in at least two opportunities to check the medication order, including when the physician's written order for drugs goes to the pharmacy to be filled and when the pharmacy stocks the patient's supply. The nurse then checks the drug when administering it.

In the **stock system** each patient unit is supplied with large-quantity stock containers of the drugs commonly used in that setting or institution. The nurse administering a drug takes the order sheet, Kardex, or medication card to the medication room and prepares the dose of drug from the stock supply, usually putting the dose into a small medicine cup. The nurse then takes the drugs, now unlabeled, to the bedside, and after checking the patient's identity administers the prepared drugs. The advantages to this system are that the pharmacy need not restock the floor stock daily; calculation and preparation of doses requires fewer pharmacy personnel, because it is done by the nurses; and stat and new orders can be filled immediately because the stock drugs are on the unit. Disadvantages are that the system is usually more time consuming for the nursing staff; billing patients for exact drug use may be difficult; significant waste and inappropriate use of the stock drugs may occur (e.g., nurses and physicians using drugs for their own ailments); and medication errors are more common.

Most institutions combine the two systems. A hospital might supply all nonliquid oral forms in unit-dose packages but have the liquid forms in multiple-dose bottles, one bottle per patient. The nurse must learn as much as possible about the drug administration system so that valuable time is not lost in searching the patient unit for a drug that is available only in the pharmacy, or conversely, in calling the pharmacy for a drug already available on the patient unit (see box on p. 78).

RECORDING DRUG-RELATED INFORMATION

Recording drug administration is an important responsibility of the nurse. Forms for recording drug

---

VERBAL MEDICATION ORDERS

Steps you should follow when taking a verbal medication order include the following:

1. If possible, have the patient's chart and medication records at hand.
2. Write down the order as it is dictated by the physician. (This may be done on scrap paper.)
3. Have the physician spell any unclear words.
4. Clarify any unclear part of the order.
5. Read the order back to the physician, including the patient's name and room number; the drug, dose, frequency, route of administration, and any other information given in the order; and the physician's name.
6. Glance at the other medications that the patient is receiving. If a question arises about the new medication ordered and the other medications the patient is currently receiving, ask the physician at that time.
7. Transcribe the order to the patient's chart, noting the physician's name, your name, the date, and the time of day. Also note whether the order was given in person or by telephone.

---

administration vary among agencies or institutions, but some general points usually do apply. The nurse should record that a dose was given as soon after administering the dose as possible. If a dose of medication is omitted, the reason must be noted, usually in the nurses' notes or on the form designated by the agency. Most institutions also require that doses given significantly early or late be accompanied by a notation explaining why. These forms are legal documents, and information recorded on them should be legible and accurate.

Information related to the route of administration or to the drug itself may need to be recorded. Examples include the full-minute apical pulse, taken before a cardiotonic is administered; the blood-glucose level before a sliding-scale insulin dose is administered; the site of an injection; and the location of a topical nitroglycerin preparation. Such information is often recorded on the same form for recording that the dose was administered.

Another important kind of information relates to individualized patient care; this includes the assessment, management, or evaluation of a specific patient. Assessment data might include the subjective and objective information that led the nurse to conclude that a p.r.n. drug was needed; the oral temperature was 102° F, and the patient was shivering and complaining of generalized achiness. These data led the nurse to administer aspirin, an available p.r.n. option for that patient. Depending on the forms in use in that institution, such data might be recorded on the nurses' notes or patient progress notes. Information

related to the management of a patient, such as the patient tolerating physical therapy best when a p.r.n. analgesic is administered 1 hr before therapy becomes part of the care plan. Another kind of management information relates to the actual techniques of administration. This information might be part of the care plan, or there might be adequate room on the medication record to include this information. An example of this kind of information is that the patient will take the drug if it is crushed and mixed with applesauce.

Information related to the patient's response to the medication and the effectiveness of the drug (evaluation) should also be recorded. This may include subjective or objective data; it is usually recorded in the nurses' notes or patient progress notes. Most of the forms in the patient's record are legal documents; therefore information recorded must be accurate, complete, and signed by the nurse.

ADMINISTERING DRUGS TO CHILDREN

Administering drugs to children presents unique challenges. Not only may the physiologic activity of the drug be altered (see Chapter 1), but the child may be unable or unwilling to take prescribed medications. For infants and toddlers, doses may be very small, requiring special care in calculation and preparation.

Use a developmental approach in administering drugs to children. Prepare a tentative plan for drug administration based on knowledge of growth and development for different age groups. The plan is initially tentative because the child's chronologic age may not match the developmental age. As the nurse and the health care system get to know the child, note effective individualized approaches in the care plan.

To give an example of a developmental approach, consider a 2-year-old who is to receive an injection and an oral medication. First, consider available information about the child's general level of functioning, motor ability, interactions with other children, vocabulary, and ability to conceptualize. Then consider theories of child development such as those of Erikson, Freud, and Piaget for guidance. The 2-year-old, in Erikson's framework, is in the stage of autonomy versus shame and doubt. Behaviors characteristic of this stage include negativism, difficulty making choices, separation anxiety, and ritual. The child shows pride in performing well, is able to feed self, and has a limited understanding of time.

A few nursing approaches that follow from this include giving simple directions; describing honestly what will occur but not until shortly before administering the medications; and asking the child to administer the oral drug. Do not ask, "Do you want to take your medicine?" because the answer frequently is "No!". If possible, give the child a choice of beverage to accompany taking the oral drug, but limit the choice (e.g, milk or apple juice). Follow the same pattern each time drugs are administered. Use firmness and consistency. Be prepared with adequate but nonthreatening assistance to restrain the child for the injection. Give positive feedback when the child cooperates and assists, provide comfort as needed, and encourage family members to do the same. Children of this age often want to assist or cooperate but need guidance in how to do so.

Remember that children vary, and although a developmental approach provides guidance, it does not replace individualized assessment and planning. Children also differ from adults in their ability to understand and accept the intrusive nature of many of the routes of drug administration. The young child may be terrified of receiving ear drops because the child cannot see what the nurse is doing to the ears. Injections are painful, and young children may have unrealistic fears (e.g., that their insides will come out of the hole created by the needle). Simply applying a bandage over the injection site may eliminate this fear. These examples may be difficult for the adult caregiver to understand, but adults have learned how to reason. Adults may also dislike injections, even fear them, but they understand that the injection is fast and for their overall benefit.

Remember that children's level of comprehension is very concrete until the early teens. Thus children may have difficulty understanding why an injection in the thigh could help their earache. Children also have trouble understanding time relationships and thinking about long-term consequences. Thus long-term drug therapy for treating a tuberculosis, seizures, or rheumatic fever may be difficult for the young child to understand.

A few additional guidelines related to techniques of administration are included. Do not dilute medications in a large volume of liquid or food; if the child does not finish eating all of it, the nurse does not know how much medication has been consumed. Do not disguise medications in a favorite or essential food; the child may be unwilling to eat that food again. Do not try to trick the patient into taking medications; be honest but caring in approaching children.

Use drawings, simple stories, coloring books, and toys dealing with medications and hospitalization; explain what is happening to preschool and young school-age children. Allow children to play out their feelings. In a setting where children are frequently treated, have a toy box available containing items such as small dolls, medicine cups, and plastic syringes without needles to allow children to pretend, before or after medications are administered.

Do not underestimate the child's ability to understand or adjust to medication administration. At early ages, many children can begin to accept responsibility for medication administration, especially for chronic health problems. For example, children 6 to 8 years old can be taught to self-administer insulin correctly.

ADMINISTERING DRUGS TO THE ELDERLY

Elderly patients can also present special problems for the nurse. As mentioned in Chapter 1, the physiologic changes that accompany aging influence the patient's response to medications. In addition, many older patients have accumulated a long list of prescribed drugs, making the act of taking drugs time consuming.

Individualized assessment and planning are important when working with the elderly. The nurse can make certain that all medications ordered for a particular patient are still necessary. As side effects to one drug develop, an additional drug is sometimes prescribed to treat them. Side effects to the second drug develop, and these are treated by a third drug. It may be difficult for the physician, the nurse, and the patient to understand what the drug regimen is designed to do.

Another problem occasionally encountered with the elderly is the use of several health care providers, who may not be communicating with one another about the patient. Thus a patient may have an ophthalmologist, a cardiologist, a podiatrist, and a urologist, each prescribing treatments and drugs for various problems. This can result in too many drugs being taken, some of which may be antagonistic to each other or contraindicated with the others.

Some patients have failing vision or hearing. This can lead to many kinds of errors in self-medication. Patients may not hear directions clearly and may not be able to read finely printed instructions or the label on the drug bottle. Some patients may not be able to afford the drug in the dosing frequency prescribed, so they may only take doses half as often (see box on p. 80).

Another problem is generalization by members of the health care team. Assuming that confusion or lack of memory is to be expected with aging, may result in symptoms being overlooked as possible drug side effects or manifestations of drug toxicity.

Elderly patients must be approached as adults. Elderly individuals who have taken many drugs over the years may have established elaborate rituals as-

---

---

sociated with taking drugs. The ritual may involve the time of day, the order in which the drugs are taken, the fluid used to swallow drugs, and so on. Ask the patient about the usual practices before rushing in at 10 AM to administer a handful of drugs. When possible, allow the patient to continue the usual routine. The elderly may also be more sensitive to nausea as a side effect. This sensitivity combined with the potential interaction of a large quantity of drugs may compound the nausea. It may be necessary to readjust the dosage schedule to spread out the prescribed medications over the course of the day.

MEDICATION ADMINISTRATION SCHEDULES

The nurse must consider factors that can influence the administration of oral medications. Schedule medications to reflect whether the drug is best taken on an empty or a full stomach. Consider whether a patient should avoid a specific liquid when taking a certain drug. For example, tetracyclines should not be taken with milk.

Patients with multiple chronic health problems may need to take several drugs simultaneously. The combination of drugs, or the total amount of fluid needed by the patient to swallow the drugs, may be nauseating. If the patient refuses to take all the medications, tires before all the drugs are taken, or becomes too nauseated to take all the drugs, you must ensure that the more necessary drugs are taken first and the less necessary ones are left until last. Consider

a patient receiving a cardiotonic, an antihypertensive, a diuretic, a potassium replacement, a vitamin, and an iron supplement at 10 AM. It is presumed that all these drugs are necessary for management of the patient's condition. However, the nurse may decide that the cardiotonic, the antihypertensive, the diuretic, and the potassium replacement are of greater priority. This is not to suggest that the nurse can simply decide not to administer certain medications but rather that the nurse is frequently required to exercise judgment and make decisions on short notice. A better long-term solution to this multiple drug problem might be to schedule the vitamin and the iron supplement at a time when the patient is taking fewer drugs and will then have less difficulty in taking all that are ordered. See Chapter 3 for additional discussion of medication scheduling.

TECHNIQUES FOR ADMINISTERING DRUGS BY SPECIFIC ROUTES

The box on p. 81 lists the steps to be followed in administering any drugs. For more detailed descriptions or additional illustrations, review the sources listed at the end of the chapter.

Stay informed about agency policies regarding infection control and guidelines from the Centers for Disease Control. Wear gloves when administering medications if there is a chance of exposure to body fluids. Follow agency guidelines for disposing of contaminated needles, and always be vigilant in working with needles. Keep up to date on immunization (e.g., hepatitis B immunization), and follow agency guidelines if a needlestick occurs.

Oral Route

Drugs are most frequently administered via the oral route. It is safe, convenient, and acceptable for most patients and medications.

After carefully checking and preparing the medications ordered, identify the patient, help the patient sit upright (if possible), then hand the medications and a glass of water or other preferred liquid to the patient. The patient then puts the pills, tablets, or capsules in the mouth and swallows them with the offered fluid. The patient should drink enough fluid to ensure that the medication reaches the stomach; drugs that lodge in the esophagus can cause irritation and burning and may result in poor absorption. Approximately 4 oz of fluid is usually sufficient, but encourage the patient to drink more unless contraindicated. Patients who are not sitting upright may need additional fluid to ensure that the medication has reached the stomach.

Ensure that the medication was swallowed and is not being hidden in the patient's mouth. Although

GENERAL STEPS IN DRUG ADMINISTRATION

1. At the start of the workday, review each patient's record, noting the medical and nursing diagnoses, current problems, relevant laboratory findings, and plan of health care.
2. Compare the physician's original order against the working tools (may be medication Kardex, medication cards, computer printout—whatever is used in that setting to guide the nurse in preparing drugs).
   a. Check for accuracy of transcription: Drug name? Drug dose? Route of administration? Frequency of administration?
   b. Check for appropriateness of the order. Does this drug make sense for this patient? Is this dose in the usual range for a patient of this age and weight?
   c. Other: Have any automatic expiration dates passed? Are there new laboratory values to be considered, such as serum electrolyte levels, serum drug levels, culture reports, renal or liver function studies?
3. Look up any new drugs or check any drug information that is unclear.
4. Check the medication supply.
   a. Is stock bottle supply adequate for the shift? If not, reorder from the pharmacy.
   b. Check each patient's drawer or box of drugs. Are the drugs present?
   c. Are any missing drugs in the refrigerator, on the back of medication cart, at the bedside? Where else?
   d. Are there sufficient supplies to prepare and administer the drugs (straws, water cups, medication cups, spoons, mortar and pestle, syringes)?
5. Review the specific drugs. Are there any special assessments to be made or data to check before any drug is administered? Examples might include measurement of apical pulse, blood pressure, temperature, weight, urine, or blood test.
   a. Organize equipment that might be needed.
   b. Make a list if necessary.
6. Check care plans (if not already done) to note personal preferences, previous problems, and nursing care approaches. Make a list of items to remember, such as: applesauce, juices, coffee, crackers, yogurt, jelly sandwich, ice cream, or other foods to disguise flavors.
7. Just before preparing the drugs, wash hands.
8. Check the working tool and obtain the medication. Read the label carefully, checking the drug, the dose, and the route of administration.*
9. Pour or prepare the dose. If from a stock bottle, read the label again before replacing the bottle. If from a unit dose, check the label; do not remove the drug from the package.
10. Prepare all medications for that patient. If preparing medications in the medication room, prepare the medications for all the patients who are to receive them.
11. Go to the bedside, and identify the patient (if possible, use all three methods):
    a. Call the patient by name. (Be especially careful if there is more than one patient on the unit with the same last name.)
    b. Ask the patient to state his or her full name.
    c. Check the patient identification band. (This may be the only possible way to identify the infant, small child, or confused adult.)
12. Assess the patient.
    a. Note any changes since you last saw the patient.
    b. Obtain any objective data needed before administering the drugs such as apical pulse, blood pressure, or breath sounds.
    c. Obtain any appropriate subjective information.
    d. If you did not previously know the patient or if new drugs are being administered, check on history of allergy.
13. If the data obtained in step 12 were not acceptable, withhold the corresponding drugs. For example, if the apical pulse is 50, do not administer the cardiotonic drug (use agency policies as guides). Other drugs may be given if the patient's condition is satisfactory.
14. Draw the curtain or otherwise ensure privacy, if needed.
15. Administer the medications, helping the patient as needed. If the medicines are in unit dose packages, open the packages. Make certain the patient takes the medication. Do not leave any medications at the bedside unless authorized by a physician's order or written institutional policy.
16. Assist the patient to resume a comfortable position.
17. Wash hands.
18. If using a medication cart, and the medication record is kept with the cart, immediately record that the drugs were given. If using a different system, administer all medications, then return to the medication record and record that the drugs were given.
19. Depending on the drug, the patient, and the usual policies and procedures, notify appropriate individuals (e.g., nurse in charge, physician) about doses that were withheld.
20. Record other appropriate information such as data obtained during assessment, drugs withheld and why, or changes in patient condition.
21. Make appropriate additions to the care plan.
22. Check on patients at appropriate intervals to evaluate the response to drug therapy.

*The next few steps vary slightly, depending on whether the drugs are prepared in the medication room, such as with a stock drug system, or in the patient's room, such as with a medication cart and unit dose system.

this situation is rare, it does occur, especially with confused individuals or those with certain psychiatric problems. After the patient swallows the drug, record that the medication has been taken.

Many patients have difficulty swallowing whole tablets or capsules. Break scored tablets along the lines indicated. It may be possible to separate the halves of capsules and pour out the powdered drug into another liquid or applesauce. Crush tablets and mix with water or food. Especially with children, use as little applesauce, or other food, as possible. Otherwise, the child may feel full or refuse the rest of the applesauce; then the nurse has no way of knowing how much of the prescribed dose was actually consumed. See the box below for a list of drug forms that should not be crushed. If in doubt, consult the pharmacist before crushing tablets or breaking open capsules.

Children sometimes take medications wrapped in a jelly sandwich. Another way to encourage the child is to give the medication in a cup and follow it with a chaser of water, milk, or carbonated beverage in another medication cup; children like the small cups and are not overwhelmed with a large volume of fluid. When choosing a food or fluid to give a child to help disguise or take medications, do not choose items with high sugar content if the medication must be taken on a regular basis because the item may contribute to dental caries. For diabetic children, use sugar-free vehicles.

Although in some institutions the pharmacy sends crushed dosage forms to the nursing unit, it is usually the nurse's responsibility to crush the medication. There are several ways to do this. Some agencies have pill crushers available in the nursing unit. A mortar and pestle may be used; be sure they are clean before use, and wash away any remaining drug residue and dry them after preparing the dose. It may be possible to place the tablet inside a plastic or paper medication cup and then place a second cup over the pill. Any

handy blunt instrument can then be used to crush the tablet between the layers of the cups. Alternatively, place the pill between two metal spoons and crush it. Also, some unit dose packages are sturdy enough to allow the pill or tablet to be crushed in the package. Regardless of how the drug is crushed, be careful to check that all of the powdered drug is brushed into the cup that you give the patient.

As an alternative to crushing medications, obtain a liquid form of the drug. Many drugs are available in liquid forms as suspensions or solutions. Make substitutions carefully; be sure to consult the physician and pharmacist. For example, a sustained-release form of a drug might be available in tablet form, but the only liquid preparation available may not be a sustained-release form, so dosage frequency may need to be adjusted.

It is generally easy to measure the prescribed dose in a capsule or tablet form, but liquid preparations require more care. If the drug is in **suspension** form, shake the container thoroughly before pouring the dose. Inadequate shaking of suspensions can result in the patient receiving a weaker dose from the top of the bottle, then a stronger dose near the bottom of the bottle, as the unsuspended particles of drug collect. In the institutional setting, medication cups are usually provided for measuring the prescribed dose, unless the drug is supplied in the unit dose from the pharmacy. Place the medication cup on a flat surface or hold it upright at eye level to check that the correct dose has been poured. The base of the meniscus should be at the level of the desired dose (Figure 6-1). For small amounts of liquids or odd quantities, measure the dose with a syringe. It is not acceptable to estimate 2 ml or 12.5 ml of a drug.

In the home, patients usually use household table-

DRUG FORMS THAT SHOULD NOT BE CRUSHED OR CHEWED

◆ Enteric-coated tablets
◆ Sustained-release forms. These often have the following suffixes attached to the drug name:
  ◆ Dur (*Dur*ation)
  ◆ SR (*S*ustained *R*elease)
  ◆ CR (*C*ontrolled or *C*ontinuous *R*elease)
  ◆ SA (*S*ustained *A*ction)
  ◆ Contin (*Contin*uous)
  ◆ LA (*L*ong *A*cting)
◆ Trade names that imply sustained release such as spansules, extentabs, extencaps
◆ Trade names with the b.i.d. (twice a day) abbreviation in the name, such as Theobid, Lithobid, Cardabid.
◆ Liquid-containing capsules, although occasionally it may be acceptable to puncture the capsule and squeeze out the contents; consult the pharmacist or manufacturer.

The name alone may not provide enough information. Consult the pharmacist if in doubt. Some forms that look like sustained forms are not, and vice versa. Some capsules containing small, slow-release pellets may be opened, and the pellets sprinkled on applesauce, or gently mixed into liquid or food, but they should not be crushed or dissolved.

Scored tablets may be broken along the scored line, but should not be chewed or crushed.

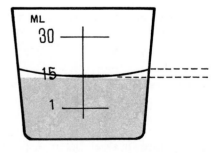

FIGURE 6-1
Reading meniscus. Meniscus is caused by surface tension of solution against container walls. Surface tension causes formation of concave or hollowed curvature on solution surface. Read level at lowest point of concave curve.

spoons and teaspoons for measuring dosages. Encourage patients to use the same spoon, since household spoons are not standardized and switching spoons may result in varying dosages. Tell patients to read the pharmacy label to see whether liquid forms must be stored in the refrigerator.

The availability of a liquid form of a drug does not necessarily ensure patient cooperation in taking the drug. Many liquid forms, especially tinctures and elixirs, may be very unpleasant tasting. Patients may be more willing to take a crushed tablet in food than to take the drug in the liquid form. Some patients may take liquid forms better through a straw placed near the back of the mouth. If the preparation can stain teeth, ensure that a straw is used so that the medication is delivered to the back of the throat, bypassing contact with the teeth. Cutting the straw in half may make it easier for children to manage.

A factor influencing the sequence of oral drug administration is the use or particular property of a drug. For example, Xylocaine Viscous, an oral preparation of lidocaine hydrochloride, is sometimes prescribed to produce relief of oral discomfort in stomatitis; it accomplishes this by producing local anesthesia. Administer this drug last if several drugs are being administered simultaneously because this drug may interfere with swallowing. In addition, an antitussive should usually be taken last because it generally should not be followed with water. Not all oral drugs are to be swallowed; sublingual or buccal tablets should dissolve in the mouth. Administer drugs to be taken via the sublingual or buccal route last, after drugs that are to be swallowed have been consumed.

Regardless of specific problems and their solutions, the quality of nursing care can be improved and much time saved if you record on the patient medication Kardex or care plan anything unique about the administration of medications to each patient.

Sublingual, buccal, troche, lozenge, and spray forms

Sublingual drugs are in tablet form placed under the tongue to dissolve. The most frequently prescribed sublingual drugs are the nitrates and nitrites for anginal heart pain. Instruct the patient to let the tablet dissolve under the tongue. Tell the patient not to drink any fluid while the drug is dissolving. This route of administration may be new to the patient, so make certain that the patient understands how to use drugs taken sublingually. Teach family members to administer drugs via this route when the patient is unable to do so, if appropriate for the patient's situation.

Teach patients to hold **buccal tablets** between the cheek and the gum and allow them to dissolve. Tell them to alternate cheeks with each dose of medication to minimize the chance for irritation of the mucosa. Report any oral irritation to the physician. Dissolve troches and lozenges in the mouth. These drug forms are usually designed to allow for slow release of the drug (i.e., over several minutes). Tell patients to avoid drinking or smoking until troches, lozenges, sublingual tablets, or buccal tablets have dissolved.

Another oral form is the sublingual spray. Teach patients to spray one or two jets from a small canister into the mouth, under the tongue (as prescribed). The canister delivers a specific dose with each jet.

Administration through Feeding Tubes

Most medications that can be administered orally also can be administered via feeding tubes. Liquid preparations are preferred, but some medications can be finely crushed and mixed with sufficient water to ensure complete passage of the drug to the stomach (see the box on p. 82). Before administering any drug via a tube, verify that the tube is in the correct place. Refer to appropriate texts of nursing fundamentals for details about the care of patients with feeding tubes. If the drugs do not form a solid precipitate, mix them together and administer. Otherwise, administer the drugs one at a time, followed by a small amount of water (about 30 ml) to flush the drug through the tube, to help maintain the patency of the tube, and to ensure that subsequent drugs do not precipitate with residue remaining in the tube from an earlier drug. Do not mix the drugs with the tube feeding itself for administration. After the final drug is administered, clear the tube with water. Remember to include the amount of fluid used to flush the tubing in the totals for the patient's fluid intake.

Parenteral Medications: Injections

The word **parenteral** means outside the intestines, but in common usage it is usually limited to injections. There are many kinds of injections, which are named by indicating the site at which the medication is deposited. Intradermal, intramuscular, intravenous, and subcutaneous injections are all commonly used in everyday practice. Other injection sites used, usually by the physician, include intracardiac (usually reserved for resuscitation efforts), intrathecal (into the subarachnoid space via lumbar or ventricular puncture), and intraarticular (into a joint). The term *hypodermic* is being replaced gradually by *subcutaneous*.

There are advantages and disadvantages associated with parenteral administration. This route is used in patients who have aphagia, who are not alert, or who lack an adequate gag reflex. It can be used for a patient unwilling or unable to take other, usually oral, medications. (If multiple doses are required, intravenous administration is usually preferred in children because it is less intrusive). Insulin, heparin, and some other medications may only be administered parenterally. On the other hand, drugs administered via this route are generally considered irretrievable. A slight chance of infection exists because the integrity of the skin is broken. Inadvertent administration into the vascular space is also possible, although rare. Damage to muscles and nerves can also occur. Parenteral injections are also uncomfortable.

Carefully calculate and prepare the prescribed dose. Many injectable medications are dry powders and must be reconstituted before administration. Although the pharmacy can do this, frequently the nurse must accomplish the task. Carefully read the manufacturer's information regarding reconstitution of dry medication. There may be restrictions on what fluids may be used for this purpose, or a specific diluent may be supplied by the manufacturer.

Not only must you obtain the appropriate diluent, but also the correct amount of diluent must be added to the dry powder. Beginning practitioners and students often find it difficult to understand the instructions related to reconstitution. For example, one form of penicillin states that certain amounts of diluent may be added to the 1,000,000-unit vial to provide the dilutions listed, stating, "add 9.6 ml, 4.6 ml, or 3.6 ml, to provide 100,000 units, 200,000 units, or 250,000 U/ml, respectively." Another vial used for some drugs combines the diluent and powder in a single glass vessel containing two compartments (Figure 6-2). Mix the diluent and powder in the closed vial before withdrawing the dose. Consult the pharmacist or a colleague if you have questions about reconstituting a powder for injection.

Write the date, time of reconstitution, and concentration on the vial of reconstituted medication. Many institutions also require that the nurse initial the vial and put the patient's name on it. Reconstituted medications must often be stored in the refrigerator. Many vials are provided in single-dose concentrations, but in pediatric settings, where the prescribed dose may be quite small, the nurse may use only a portion of the contents of a medication vial. Remember to read the label before using stored medications, and observe expiration dates. Once reconstituted, many medications may be safely used for a short period.

Not all medications for injection are supplied in vials. Many come in small glass ampules, from which a single dose is withdrawn, and the ampule is discarded (Figure 6-3). Ampules may be supplied with a small metal saw. If supplied, use the saw and make two to three passes across the neck of the ampule. Do not saw through the glass, but make a scored line as a guide for breaking the ampule. Wrap the ampule in a piece of gauze or paper towel before opening to protect your fingers from getting cut. Sharply snap the top off the ampule. Use a filter needle on the syringe, if one is available, to prevent small slivers of glass from entering the syringe. After withdrawing

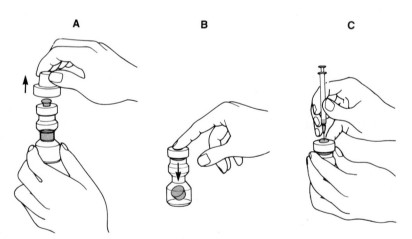

A   B   C

FIGURE 6-2

Mix-o-vial. **A,** Remove protective cap from vial. **B,** Push rubber plunger on top of vial. This forces small rubber plug between upper and lower compartment into lower compartment, which allows powder and diluent to mix. Rotate vial between hands to speed mixing. Clean off top of plunger with alcohol. **C,** Insert needle of syringe into plunger and withdraw dose. For best results, needle must go straight into plunger.

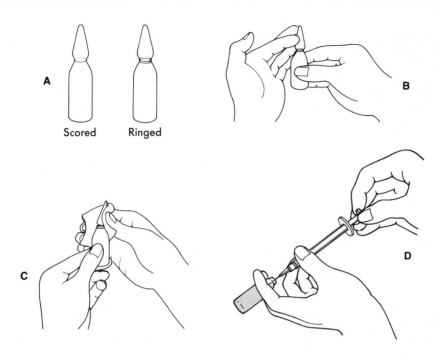

FIGURE 6-3

A, Examples of scored and ringed glass ampules. **B,** Hold ampule upright and gently flick top to shake medication into bottom of ampule. **C,** Hold vial with alcohol wipe or gauze and snap off top. **D,** Withdraw medication from bottom half of ampule.

the dose, replace the filter needle with the needle for the injection.

Other medications are provided in prefilled syringes. The advantages of these syringes are fast and easy preparation. However, they are also more expensive. Most agencies stock prefilled syringes for narcotics and for selected other situations when drugs need to be immediately available, such as the emergency drug box or resuscitation cart. Several manufacturers produce prefilled syringes and techniques for activating and using the products vary. Consult the agency or institution for information about devices used in any individual setting. See Figure 6-4 for an illustration of one kind of holder for prefilled syringes.

The choice of syringe and needle to be used for any specific medication depends on the information obtained from assessment of the patient, the route of administration to be used, the characteristics of the fluid to be injected (e.g., waterlike or oil based), and the volume of medication to be delivered. Sample syringe sizes include 1-ml tuberculin and insulin syringes and 2.5-, 5-, and 10-ml syringes. Larger syringes are available but are rarely used for medication administration via the parenteral route. Use tuberculin syringes, marked in 0.01-ml gradations, when

the volume to be administered is small. Insulin syringes are available in 0.5- or 1-ml volumes, although some institutions stock an insulin syringe with a maximum volume of 25 or 35 units. Do not substitute tuberculin and insulin syringes for each other.

Needles vary in length and gauge, from ⅜ in to 3 or more inches in length and from 14 gauge (large lumen) to 28 gauge (small lumen). Most institutions limit the variety of needles and syringes in stock, so the nurse may have a choice of five syringes and five needle sizes on the nursing unit. The smaller-lumen (larger-gauge) needles are usually used for intradermal injections. Subcutaneous injections are usually given with a ½- or ⅝-in, 23- or 25-gauge needle. Intramuscular injections are usually given with a 19- or 21-gauge, 1½- to 2-inch needle; a 16- or 18-gauge needle may also be used (see box on p. 87).

After preparing the ordered dose and choosing the appropriate needle and syringe, go to the patient's bedside to administer the injection. Check the patient's nameband to verify identity, draw the curtain or otherwise ensure privacy, explain what is going to happen, and assist the patient to assume the necessary position. If the patient is unable or unwilling to assist in positioning, bring adequate assistance. Assess the injection site, locate anatomical landmarks, and

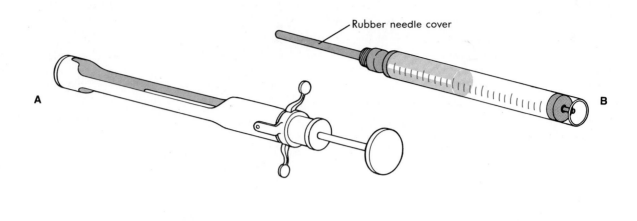

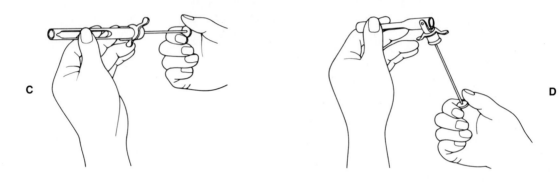

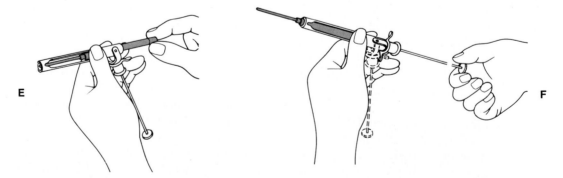

FIGURE 6-4

Prefilled medication cartridge and holder. **A,** Reusable stainless steel cartridge holder. **B,** Disposable, prefilled medication cartridge. Note rubber needle cover. Also note threads just below needle and on rubber plug. **C,** Pull back on plunger, and **D,** open holder at hinge. **E,** Insert medication cartridge and rotate it clockwise to screw cartridge into holder. **F,** Swing plunger back in place and turn plunger to secure it to small screw in rubber plug.

PREPARATION OF OIL-BASED MEDICINES FOR INTRAMUSCULAR ADMINISTRATION

Oil-based medicines are released more slowly because it takes the oil longer to be absorbed from the muscle than aqueous solutions. Administer oil-based medicines via the intramuscular route only, never intravenously.

Heat the unopened vial or ampule in warm water for several minutes to decrease oil viscosity.

Roll the vial vigorously between the hands to resuspend the medication, which is usually an inconspicuous film on the side of the ampule. Resuspension is adequate when no particles of medication remain on the bottom or sides of the vial. Failure to shake or roll the vial sufficiently results in inaccurate dosage and erratic absorption.

Draw up the correct dose into a syringe fitted with a large-bore (19- to 21-gauge), 1½-in needle (for an adult), and administer the dose immediately, before the oil cools.

Inject the medicine, exerting slow, even pressure on the plunger. Attempting to inject too rapidly can cause pressure to increase within the syringe, and the needle and syringe may separate, causing loss of medication.

Use large muscle masses, such as the buttock, thigh, or ventrogluteal site. In infants and small children, use the vastus lateralis.

The oil base can produce palpable lumps because it is absorbed slowly. Record injection sites, rotate them, and avoid the deltoid muscle.

smoothly administer the injection. Help the patient return to a comfortable position. Dispose of the syringe and needle according to the procedures of the agency. Record that the medication has been given, noting the location, so that injection sites can be rotated. Check the patient again to make certain no untoward effects have occurred and to evaluate whether the drug is working as anticipated.

Record any aspects of the injection that are unique to the patient on the medication Kardex or patient care plan to assist other nurses in providing individualized care. More detailed information about drawing up medications, handling equipment, and administering injections can be found in fundamental nursing texts. Practice in giving injections is important in helping students become accurate, efficient, and confident.

Intradermal injection

An **intradermal injection** is made just below the epidermis or outer layer of skin (Figure 6-5). Such an injection is used for allergy testing and for administration of local anesthetics. Use a small-bore needle and a small-volume syringe, such as a 1-ml tuberculin syringe. The volume injected is usually small, less than 0.5 ml. The most frequently used sites for allergy testing are the medial surface of the forearm and the back.

When preparing for the injection, clean the chosen skin surface with alcohol. Allow the surface to dry or

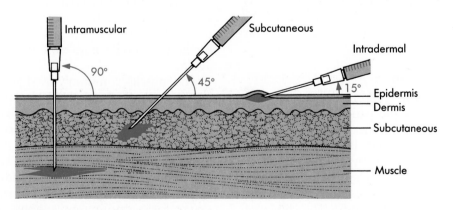

FIGURE 6-5

Comparison of angle of injection and location of deposition of medication for intramuscular, subcutaneous, and intradermal injections.

wipe off the alcohol with a sterile sponge. Hold the skin taut with one hand. With the other hand, hold the syringe with the needle bevel up, at a 10- to 15-degree angle, and gently but smoothly puncture the skin until the bevel is completely under the skin surface. Inject the prescribed amount or an amount that creates a raised wheal resembling a mosquito bite. If a wheal is not produced or the site bleeds, you probably made too deep an injection and should repeat it. If several injections are given in the same site (e.g., on the same forearm), label them with a pen, especially if the reaction is to be checked at 48 hr.

Subcutaneous injection

Subcutaneous injection is used to place medication below the skin into the subcutaneous layer (see Figure 6-5). The volume of a subcutaneous injection is usually less than 1 ml, and usually a ½- or ⅝-inch, 23- or 25-gauge needle is used. Insert the needle at a 45-degree angle, although it may be inserted at a 90-degree angle if the patient has heavy subcutaneous tissue or the nurse has pinched the subcutaneous tissue between thumb and fingers, holding it up from the underlying muscle tissue. The usual injection technique is used; choose the site, cleanse it with alcohol, let the alcohol dry or wipe it off with a sterile sponge, hold the skin taut, insert the needle, and aspirate for blood. If no blood is present, gently but smoothly inject the medication. Alternatively, cleanse the skin as described, then gently pinch the subcutaneous tissue between the thumb and the other fingers, and insert the needle, aiming it for the pocket created between the subcutaneous tissue being pinched and the tissue below. The two medications most frequently administered via this route are heparin and insulin, and controversy continues about specific aspects of their administration. For additional discussion about the administration of these two drugs, consult Chapter 20 (heparin) and Chapter 55 (insulin). The usual sites for subcutaneous injection are illustrated in Figure 6-6.

Intramuscular injection

Intramuscular injection is probably the method most familiar to students and patients. Most people have received medication via this route in the form of antibiotics or immunizations. Because the muscle layer is below the subcutaneous layer of skin, a longer needle is used, usually 1½ inches, often of larger lumen size, such as 19 or 21 gauge. Insert the needle at a 90-degree angle (see Figure 6-5). The choice of needle is influenced by the viscosity of the medication to be injected, the muscle to be used, and the size and age of the patient. A frequent error of beginning students is to choose too short a needle for admin-

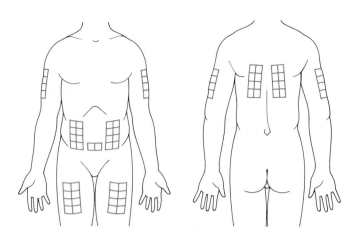

FIGURE 6-6
Commonly used subcutaneous injection sites.

istration of a medication to an overweight adult via a large muscle mass such as the vastus lateralis or dorsogluteal area.

The intramuscular technique is the same as other injection techniques previously outlined. Carefully prepare the ordered medication, take the syringe to the bedside, check the nameband and verify the patient's identity, draw the curtain or otherwise ensure privacy, assist the patient to assume the necessary position, identify appropriate anatomic landmarks to help define the injection site, cleanse the skin, and let it dry. Hold the skin taut or gently pinch the skin, swiftly insert the needle at a 90-degree angle, aspirate for blood, and, if no blood is present, gently but smoothly inject the medication. If blood oozes after you withdraw the needle, apply gentle pressure and a bandage if needed. Help the patient assume a comfortable position. Dispose of needle and syringe as directed by agency policy, and then record that the medication has been given. Finally, check the patient again.

The muscles commonly used for intramuscular injection include the **deltoid muscle,** located on the upper arm. It forms a triangular shape, with the base of the triangle along the acromion process and its peak ending about one third of the way down the upper arm (Figure 6-7). In muscular patients, the deltoid may be clearly visible. In other patients it may be necessary to palpate it. This muscle is seldom used except for certain immunizations. It is small in children, many smaller-than-average patients, and the elderly, so it can accommodate only small volumes of injected fluid (e.g., 1 ml). Bruises or needle marks may be visible, depending on the patient's clothing,

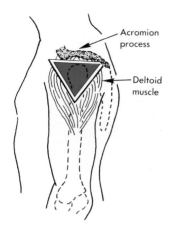

FIGURE 6-7
Deltoid muscle injection site roughly forms inverted triangle, with acromion process as base. Muscle may be visible in muscular patients.

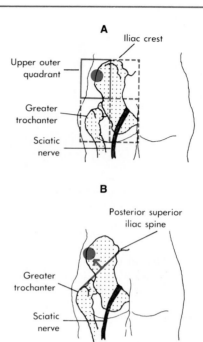

FIGURE 6-8
Two accepted methods for defining dorsogluteal injection site. **A,** Patient's buttocks can be divided on one side into imaginary quadrants. Center of upper outer quadrant should be used as injection site. **B,** Nurse locates by palpation posterior superior iliac spine and greater trochanter, then draws imaginary line between them. Injection site up and out from that line should be used.

so this may be unacceptable to the patient. The radial nerve is nearby. The advantage of the deltoid muscle is that it is easily accessible.

The **dorsogluteal site** is made up of several gluteal muscles, although the gluteus medius is the muscle used for injections most often. As indicated in Figure 6-8, there are two ways to define this site. You can divide the buttocks on one side into imaginary quadrants, and administer the injection in the upper outer quadrant or locate the posterior superior iliac spine and the greater trochanter of the femur, and then draw an imaginary line between them. Give the injection up and to the side of this line. It is important to have a clear view of the area to help define the landmarks. Have the patient lie down, with the toes pointed inward, which helps foster muscle relaxation and thus decreases discomfort. Do not use this site for children under 3 years of age because the muscles are not yet well developed and because of the proximity of the sciatic nerve. In most ambulatory adults the dorsogluteal muscles are well developed and can accommodate an injection volume up to 5 ml if necessary, although any volume over 3 ml may be uncomfortable to the patient.

The **Z-track technique** can be used with any intramuscular injection. However, it was first described for administration of an iron preparation that stains the skin if it leaks out. The dorsogluteal site is most frequently used for injections requiring the Z-track technique. When you prepare the drug to be administered, measure the ordered amount of drug into the syringe, then draw 0.1 to 0.3 ml of air into the syringe and change the needle. When administering drugs via the Z-track method, pull the skin taut to one side,

causing the layers of skin to slide sideways. While the skin is pulled laterally, insert the needle, then inject the medication and the small amount of air smoothly and slowly. Pause for 10 seconds before removing the needle. Withdraw the needle, then allow the skin to relax (Figure 6-9). This process disrupts the track created by the needle, preventing seepage, as well as possible skin discoloration caused by the medication. Do not massage or rub the site.

Both the **vastus lateralis muscle** and the **rectus femoris muscle** are found in the thigh. As shown in Figure 6-10, the two muscles lie side by side. Place one hand on the patient's upper thigh and one hand on the lower thigh. The area between your hands should represent the middle third of the thigh and the middle third of the underlying muscle. The vastus lateralis is lateral to midline, whereas the rectus femoris is in the midline. The vastus lateralis is the preferred injection site for children because it is well developed and has few major nerves that could be injured. This site is also satisfactory for adults. The rectus femoris is most often the muscle chosen by adults who self-administer intramuscular injections

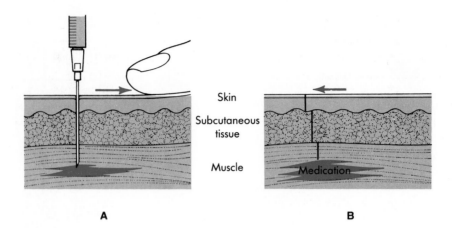

FIGURE 6-9

A, In Z-tract intramuscular injection, skin is pulled laterally, then injection is administered. **B,** After needle is withdrawn, skin is released. Technique helps prevent medication from leaking.

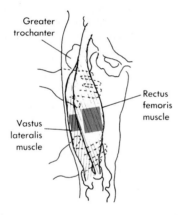

FIGURE 6-10

To define vastus lateralis and rectus femoris muscle sites, place one hand below patient's greater trochanter and one hand above knee. Space between two hands defines middle third of underlying muscle. Rectus femoris is on anterior thigh; vastus lateralis is on lateral thigh.

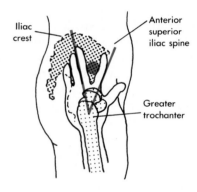

FIGURE 6-11

To locate ventrogluteal muscle injection site, place palm of hand on greater trochanter of femur. Make V with fingers, with one side running from greater trochanter to anterosuperior iliac spine and other side running from greater trochanter to iliac crest.

because it is easily accessible. The acceptable volume for injection in these sites varies with the age of the patient and the size of the muscle, but up to 5 ml may be administered in one injection to the well-developed adult.

To define the **ventrogluteal muscle,** create a V between the index finger and the remaining three fingers. Place the palm on the greater trochanter of the femur, with one side of the V extending from the greater trochanter to the iliac crest and the other side running from the greater trochanter to the anterior superior iliac spine (Figure 6-11). This muscle may accommodate up to 5 ml of drug in adults.

Intravenous injection

The administration of drugs directly into the vascular system via the intravenous route is widely used today for a variety of reasons. If an intravenous infusion line is already in place, IV infusion is easy. Drugs begin to take immediate effect. Intravenous injection avoids side effects caused by intramuscular injection. On the other hand, errors can be serious, even fatal, since medications administered via this route take effect quickly. The possibility of infection resulting from direct access to the vascular system is also present.

In many settings the technique of venipuncture is done only by members of the IV team or comparable group. If no designated team exists, many agencies or state nurse practice acts require special instruction, classes, and supervised practice in venipuncture techniques before nurses are permitted to perform this technique in their usual setting. Become familiar with the specific practices and policies of your agency or institution.

First inspect the forearms and choose the venipuncture site. Figure 6-12 illustrates the location of veins commonly used in the forearm. Figure 6-13 illustrates the location of veins on the dorsal aspect of the hand. Other veins, such as those in the feet, are used only if absolutely necessary; some agencies may require a specific physician order if they are used. Problems associated with thrombophlebitis are more common with venipuncture of the lower extremities. Scalp veins are used in infants. If the patient is to have repeated venipunctures, choose a distal site rather than a proximal one. The rationale is that with each subsequent venipuncture the site should be moved more proximal (that is, closer to the major vessels of the chest).

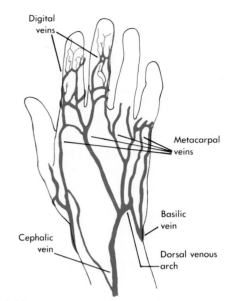

FIGURE 6-13
Major veins of dorsum of hand.

After choosing a site and preparing the necessary equipment (needle, intracatheter, heparin well, tubing, blood collection devices, medication, and tape), apply a tourniquet several inches above the expected insertion site. Put on gloves, palpate the vein to further define its location, then cleanse the skin with alcohol, povidone-iodine solution, or other cleansing substance. Allow the area to dry or wipe it with a sterile sponge. With one hand, stabilize the extremity and the vein, and with the other hold the venipuncture needle bevel up. Approach the insertion site at a slight angle, about 10 degrees. Puncture the skin and then the vein. Experienced nurses can feel the vein wall being punctured. If blood appears in the tubing or syringe, release the tourniquet. Slowly inject the medication into the vein, draw the blood, or secure the infusion device to the forearm, depending on the reason for the venipuncture.

To remove any needle or tubing from a vein, put on gloves, carefully remove any securing tapes and dressing, place a sterile sponge over the insertion site, and apply gentle pressure. With the other hand, swiftly withdraw the needle or catheter, pulling straight back from the angle of insertion; then apply firm pressure for 2 to 5 min to prevent bleeding or bruising. Apply a bandage over the insertion site. Dispose of any needles and syringes following agency procedures. Record any medication that has been administered, and check the patient again. Further elaboration of these techniques can be found in funda-

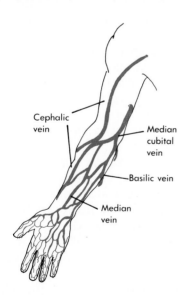

FIGURE 6-12
Veins of medial aspect of forearm commonly used for venipuncture.

mental nursing texts and agency procedure manuals. In addition, the Centers for Disease Control in Atlanta have guidelines for preventing infections in venipuncture and intravenous infusions.

Heparin lock. Nurses may administer intravenous medications via a **heparin well** or **heparin lock.** This device consists of a needle attached to a short length of tubing capped by a piece of resealable rubber. The needle is placed in the vein; the device is then secured to the forearm. Its advantage is that medication can be administered via the intravenous route, but the patient does not have to be attached to continuous intravenous infusions or have repeated venipunctures for each dose of medication. Heparin wells are particularly helpful in children needing intravenous medications but not additional fluids; they also permit children to be up and around since they are not attached to long intravenous tubing.

Heparin may be administered via heparin well, as described in Chapter 20. One method for administering other medications by intermittent infusion via heparin well is to insert and secure the heparin well, and then prime it with 1 ml of a 10 U/ml heparin solution. Solutions of 10 U/ml are available in prepackaged syringes or multiple-dose vials, or they can be prepared by the pharmacy or the nurse mixing the heparin with normal saline solution to achieve the desired concentration. Each time a drug is administered, the procedure is to cleanse the rubber insertion site with alcohol or other cleansing agent; flush the well with 1 to 2 ml of normal saline solution (this step may be omitted if the drug to be administered is compatible with heparin); administer the prescribed medication via push or infusion; flush the well with 1 to 2 ml of normal saline solution; and administer 1 ml of the solution containing 10 U/ml heparin. The purpose of leaving the heparinized solution in the well is to prevent blood from clotting in the needle. Follow your institution's policies and procedures.

Intravenous tubing. Another way to administer intravenous medications is via tubing in place for the patient who is receiving constant intravenous fluids. At least two variations should be noted. The nurse must frequently administer a small amount, usually less than 5 ml, of drug. This is often called *IV push* drug. Prepare the drug, verify the patient's identity, and then locate an injection site on the IV tubing. Cleanse the site with alcohol or another solution; then inject 2 ml of normal saline (this step may be omitted if the IV push drug is compatible with the fluids infusing); administer the ordered drug, and then administer another 2 ml of normal saline. Readjust the ongoing infusion to provide the ordered rate. Most commercially available IV tubings have check valves, or one-way valves, as part of the tubing (Fig-

ure 6-14). If one is not present, however, clamp the tubing above the injection site before administering the drug, and proceed as outlined above. If there is no check valve or if the tubing is not clamped, the injected medication will go in the direction of lower pressure, which may be up toward the bag or bottle of fluid instead of down toward the patient. Avoid this situation. When the medication goes toward the large bag or bottle of fluid the patient does not receive the complete dose until the bag is empty, and drugs administered after that dose may not be compatible with the drug remaining in the fluid line.

The second method of giving intravenous fluids is to administer a bolus of medication. The drug is prepared and diluted in a larger volume of fluid, at least 50 to 100 ml in adults, which is usually administered over 20 to 60 min. This volume can then be administered in several ways. One method is to add the drug to an in-line device such as a burette or Volutrol, and then fill the device with 50 to 100 ml of the infusing IV fluid. The ongoing fluids are temporarily stopped, the bolus is allowed to infuse, and then the ongoing fluids are continued. Commercially available infusion tubing that has two ports for hanging IV bags or bottles may also be used. These tubing systems have an identified port for attaching the primary fluids and a secondary port for attaching the intermittently administered bolus containing the drugs (see Figure 6-14).

The third method of administering intravenous fluids is to prepare the drug in a small volume of fluid and then attach IV tubing and a needle. Prime the tubing by running sufficient fluid through the tube to eliminate any air. Insert the needle into an identified insertion site on the tubing of the ongoing infusion after the site has been cleansed. The ongoing infusion is clamped, the bolus containing the drug is allowed to infuse, and the continuous fluids are restarted. You may then discard the secondary infusion tubing and needle. To be effective and efficient, become familiar with the equipment and procedures used in your agency.

Central venous catheters and multilumen catheters. Many patients, even those outside of intensive care settings, have **central venous catheters** inserted for venous access. The catheters may be inserted into a peripheral vein and threaded into a large vein closer to the heart (a more "central" vein, thus the name *central venous catheter*); more commonly, they are inserted by the physician directly into a large central vein, with the insertion site near the clavicle. The distal end of the catheter may be in the subclavian or jugular vein or the superior vena cava near the junction with the right atrium (Figure 6-15). Once in place, the catheter is sutured to the skin at the insertion site. Catheters in use include the Hickman, Hick-

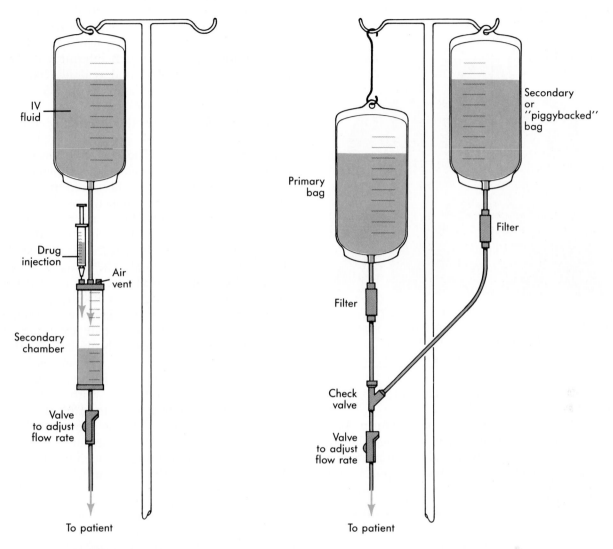

FIGURE 6-14

Example setups for intermittent drug infusion. **A,** Drug is injected into secondary chamber, where it may be further diluted with IV fluid. Upper fluid reservoir may be temporarily closed off while drug infuses. **B,** Secondary or "piggybacked" bag containing drug diluted in 50 to 100 ml of fluid is hung at level higher than primary bag. Contents of higher bag will infuse first, then contents of lower bag resume infusing. Check valve prevents medication from flowing into primary bag. There is a filter on both lines.

man-Broviac, and Groshong catheters. The catheters may have one, two, or more ports. They may be used for constant or intermittent infusion; one, two, or all ports may be in use at any time, depending on the patient's needs and condition. Some patients are discharged with the catheter in place; before discharge, teach patients how to clean the catheter and insert it daily.

Because the distal end of the catheter is in an area of high blood flow and volume, it permits infusion of large volumes of fluids. Also, central venous catheters allow administration of more irritating fluids

and drugs than can be administered via peripheral intravenous lines. There is always the risk of infection or of introducing air with such catheters, especially when those with multiple ports are used. Usually, care for the catheter and the insertion site is more rigorous for a centrally placed catheter than for a peripherally placed catheter. For example, cleansing of an injection port on a peripheral catheter may be done with an alcohol swab, whereas the port on a central line may require cleansing with a povidone-iodine solution. Follow agency procedures. Monitor the patient for signs of infection such as fever, redness

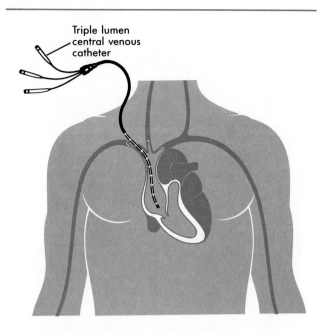

FIGURE 6-15

Triple-lumen central venous catheter in place.

at the insertion site, and increased white blood cell count.

Care of the ports not in use is important to keep the lumens patent; follow agency procedure. Different types of catheters may require different protocols. One protocol is to change the cap on each port weekly or when it appears worn. Wear sterile gloves during cap changes, and discard contaminated caps carefully. Irrigate the ports not in use with 2.5 ml of heparinized solution (10 U/ml of heparin) every 12 to 24 hr. Irrigate a port after each intermittent infusion given via that port. If blood is drawn via a port, irrigate the port after the sample is obtained. Cleanse the insertion site every 48 hr.

Implantable ports. Another form of venous access device is the implantable port, such as the Port-a-Cath or S.E.A. Port. The device is surgically implanted, with the distal end of the catheter inserted into a large central vein. The injection end of the device is implanted subcutaneously, often on the chest wall. The injection end has a self-sealing septum over a small chamber or reservoir, and the tubing extends from the side of the reservoir or chamber to the venous insertion point. The system's advantage is that after implantation, the port is available for long-term use up to 1 to 2 years. Each time the patient must receive medication, the skin must be punctured with a needle, but there is no daily cleansing procedure as there is with the partially implanted catheters.

To use an implanted device, put on sterile gloves and cleanse the site with a povidone-iodine solution (or as agency protocol directs). With one hand, palpate and locate the injection site. After the device is defined and stabilized with one hand, use the other hand to puncture the skin and septum with a Huber needle attached to a syringe containing sterile saline (Figure 6-16). Push the needle in far enough to feel

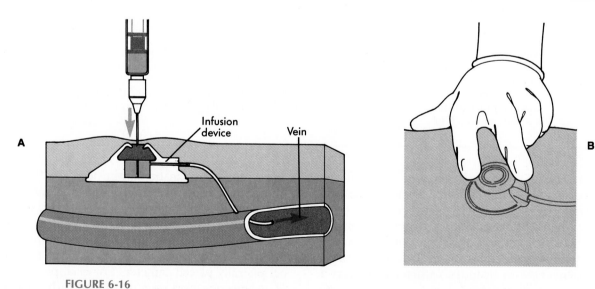

FIGURE 6-16

Implanted infusion device. **A,** Side view illustrating needle inserted through skin and top of infusion device. Distal end of device is in vein. **B,** Use one hand to secure device before inserting needle.

it touch the back of the device. Aspirate blood to help determine patency and then inject saline to flush the system. The device may be used to obtain blood samples, administer constant or intermittent infusions, or inject medications. After use, flush the device with a heparinized solution. Review the manufacturer's directions and request guidance in using these devices until comfortable with their use and operation.

Drug pumps. Several devices for slowly injecting a medication are now available for patients' home use. Cancer chemotherapy, narcotic infusion for severe pain, or insulin therapy are the most common uses of drug pumps. One such device is the auto-syringe pump, which consists of a syringe with a battery attachment for slow injection. It injects the medication subcutaneously or attaches to an implanted infusion port such as the Port-A-Cath or a partially implanted catheter such as a Hickman catheter. Follow the manufacturer's instructions when preparing and using a drug pump, and have the patient give a return demonstration before discharge.

Information about calculation of infusion rates is included in Chapter 7. Additional general guidelines for care of the patient receiving an intravenous infusion are given in Chapter 17.

Rectal Medications

Administering medications via the rectal route is an alternative for patients who are nauseated or unable to swallow. Drugs administered via this route are usually in the form of a suppository or enema.

The procedure for administering medication by enema is the same as that for any enema. The goal is to have the patient retain the medication for as long as possible; therefore a small-volume retention enema is administered. After preparing the medication and any other necessary equipment, go to the bedside, verify the patient's identity, explain briefly what will be done, and then draw the curtain or otherwise ensure privacy. Position the patient on the left side, place adequate protective covering on the bed, put on gloves, and lubricate the applicator or tubing tip with water-soluble jelly or lubricant (Figure 6-17). Separate the patient's buttocks with one hand, and ask the patient to take a deep breath. Use the other hand to insert the tubing or tip the desired distance. Administer the medication slowly to avoid stimulation and immediate expulsion. Withdraw the applicator, and gently hold the buttocks together until the patient's immediate urge to defecate has subsided. Wash the patient's buttocks, and assist the patient in returning to a comfortable position. Instruct the patient to try to hold the medication at least 30 min (or as indicated by the nature of the medication).

Suppositories are medications that have been mixed with cocoa butter, glycerin, or other substances that allow them to remain solid at room temperature but permit them to melt and release the medication when they contact the warm rectal mucosa. Suppositories are stored in the refrigerator to keep them firm. If a suppository is too soft to insert easily, run it under cold water (if foil wrapped) or place it in the refrigerator to help harden it before administering. The general procedure for administration is similar to that for the enema. Wear a finger cot or glove for inserting the suppository, which you

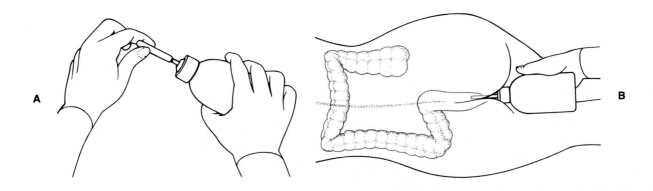

FIGURE 6-17

Administering single-dose enema. Position patient on left side and place protective covering on bed. **A,** After donning gloves, remove cover from tip. Apply water-soluble lubricant if tip is not already lubricated. **B,** Gently insert applicator tip and squeeze bottle to propel medication into the patient's rectum.

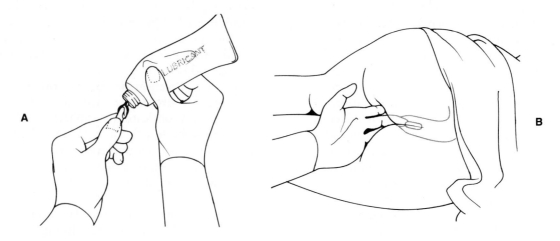

FIGURE 6-18

Inserting suppository. After positioning patient and removing suppository from package, nurse dons nonsterile gloves. **A,** Lubricate suppository with a water-soluble lubricant. **B,** Insert suppository past anal sphincter.

would previously moisten with a water-soluble lubricant. Insert the suppository about a finger's distance into the rectum in adults, past the anal sphincter (Figure 6-18). Inserting the suppository blunt end first may help the patient retain the suppository, since the rectal muscles close gently over the tapered end. If the suppository is not inserted far enough, it will be uncomfortable to the patient and will be quickly expelled. It may be necessary to place a small gauze pad over the anus to absorb oozing medication after the suppository has been inserted. If the suppository was intended to cause defecation, the patient may defecate as soon as the urge occurs. Unless the medication was prescribed to stimulate defecation, instruct the patient to retain the suppository as long as possible and to report when it is expelled.

Vaginal Medications

Vaginal medications can take the form of douches or irrigations, creams, or suppositories. The patient may be able to choose the form she prefers.

Many women are familiar with over-the-counter douche preparations and may feel comfortable with their use. For best effect, administer douches with the patient lying down. Moisten the tip of the tubing or applicator with water or a water-soluble lubricant. Insert the applicator or end of the tubing about 2 inches initially, then advance it another 1 to 2 inches as the fluid is allowed to run in by gravity. A text on fundamentals of nursing offers more complete information about douching.

Insert vaginal suppositories by pushing them in with your finger or with an applicator supplied by the manufacturer. The suppository may be lubricated with water or a water-soluble lubricant before being administered. It is important to place the suppository high in the vaginal vault, or the patient will expel it rapidly.

If the patient is taking a dose once daily, insert the vaginal suppository just before the patient goes to sleep, so that it will remain in the vaginal vault all night and not drain out or be expelled. If the dose is given more than once daily, instruct the patient to remain lying down for a short period after administration so that the medication will not be quickly lost. Instruct the patient to continue the medication even during the menstrual period and to avoid the use of tampons while taking vaginal medications. It is usually necessary for the patient to wear a sanitary napkin during the course of therapy.

Insert vaginal creams with the applicator supplied by the manufacturer. The same guidelines outlined under vaginal suppositories apply. Creams are generally messier than suppositories, and patients may not accept them as well.

Skin Applications

Many medications are applied to the skin, but it is such an easy and common route of administration that the nurse or patient may inadvertently become too casual about it. Some topical preparations, such as emollients for dry skin, may be applied liberally,

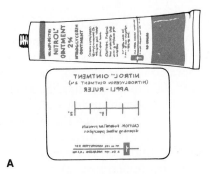

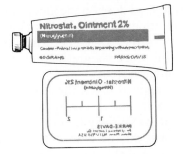

A

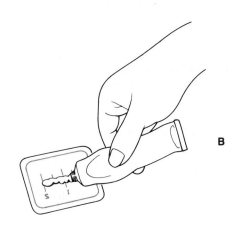

B

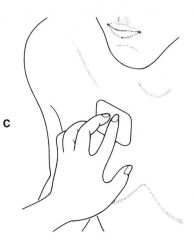

C

FIGURE 6-19

A, Nitroglycerin and papers for measuring doses. **B,** Gently squeeze out line of ointment along paper guide for prescribed length. **C,** Apply ointment to patient's skin. Clear plastic wrap may be applied over site to increase absorption and keep ointment from staining clothing.

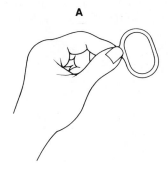

A

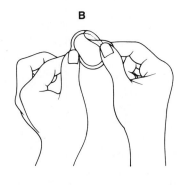

B

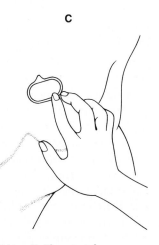

C

FIGURE 6-20

Transdermal patch. **A,** Hold patch by small wing. **B,** Remove protective backing. **C,** Place patch on chosen skin site and press into place. Sites should be changed or alternated with each successive dose.

as needed. Most skin medications, however, must be measured and applied as ordered to prevent the patient from receiving too large a dose. Avoid direct contact with the medication to prevent sensitization and to avoid the effects of the medication. Wear gloves and apply the medication with applicators, gauze, or cotton balls, or make certain that the medication is applied directly from the measuring guide, as is done with topical nitroglycerin preparations (see Chapter 14). Depending on the medication, rotate application sites, and avoid applying the medicine to abrasions, cuts, or other areas where the skin is no longer intact. Some topical preparations require dressings. If in doubt, ask the physician about the goals of therapy, and consult the pharmacist to determine the most effective method of administering the drug.

Nitroglycerin ointment is one type of skin application (Figure 6-19). The dose is ordered in inches, and the ointment is supplied with small papers printed with a 2-inch measuring guide. Squeeze out an even line of ointment of the prescribed length. Place the paper ointment-side down on the patient. Avoid rubbing in the ointment, although it is usually permissible to press the paper guide sufficiently to spread out the dose. Clear plastic wrap may be ordered to be placed over the paper and ointment to facilitate absorption and prevent staining of clothing.

A recent development in topical application is the single-dose, adhesive-backed delivery system (Figure 6-20). Examples include several types of nitroglycerin preparations and a scopolamine preparation. Refer to the manufacturer's literature for guidelines about a specific product. Review instruction sheets with the patient; these provide illustrations and additional information. Information includes the preferred location for application of the delivery system, frequency of changing, and the effect of contact with water while swimming or bathing on the delivery system.

Eye Medications

Eye medications are usually in the form of drops or ointments. Eyedrops are supplied in small volumes, since each dose contains only a few drops. Avoid contaminating the dropper; each patient in an institutional setting should have a separate bottle of eyedrops. Before administering eyedrops, be certain which eye is to be medicated (if not both). A frequent source of errors is confusion about the abbreviations for left eye (o.s.), right eye (o.d.), and both eyes (o.u.). Have the patient lie down or sit with the head tilted back. With the hand holding the dropper, place the hand on the cheek or forehead to stabilize the hand and help prevent injury to the eye. Use the thumb (or fingers) of the other hand to gently pull

down the lower lid; it may be necessary to use a small gauze sponge or cotton ball to help do this and avoid contaminating the eye. Drop the dose into the lower conjunctival sac, never onto the eyeball.

Nurses may find the following modification of technique helpful when administering eyedrops to patients who blink very easily. Place the patient in the supine position, with the head turned to one side, about 45 degrees from midline. The eye to receive the eyedrops should be uppermost. With the eye closed, drop the prescribed dose on the inner canthus of the eye. Have the patient slowly turn from the side to midline, then toward the other side, while blinking. The eyedrops will move via gravity and surface tension into the conjunctival sac.

Eye ointments are applied much the same way as eyedrops. Squeeze a thin line of ointment onto the lower conjunctival sac, close the eye, and gently rub the eyelid to help distribute the dose (Figure 6-21).

A newer drug form available for eye medications is the sustained release-insert, such as the Ocusert Pilo-20 or Pilo-40 systems. This form of pilocarpine was designed for patients with a poor history of compliance or with conditions that make accurate instillation of eyedrops difficult, such as poor vision or arthritis. Place the insert into the upper or lower conjunctival sac; the medication is released slowly, over several days. Instruct patients to make sure that the insert is in place every morning, since the unit may fall out at night. The unit is designed to be replaced weekly, but occasionally one will be effective

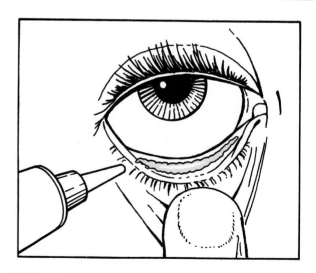

FIGURE 6-21

Administering ophthalmic ointment. To instill ointment, gently pull lower lid down as patient looks upward. Squeeze ophthalmic ointment into lower sac. Avoid touching tube to eyelid.

for only a few days before needing replacement. Other drugs may become available in this form or in other new forms. Consult the manufacturer's literature and patient instruction sheet for specific guidelines to new drug forms, both to update your personal knowledge and to teach patients and their families.

Caution patients to read labels carefully, especially on refilled prescriptions. Only medications labeled for ophthalmic use should be put into the eye. Keep eye drops in a safe place, away from other similarly shaped containers. Occasionally patients have inadvertently put glue or other toxic substances in their eyes because they did not read the label or depended on feel to select the bottle or tube of medications. Many medications cause patients to experience blurry vision briefly, so warn patients not to drive or engage in other dangerous activities immediately after using eye medications. Finally, instruct patients that the use and misuse of eye medications can have serious consequences, so eye medications should only be used as prescribed.

Nose Drops and Sprays

To instill nose drops, have the patient lie down with the head over the edge of the bed (Figure 6-22). Support the patient's head with one hand while instilling the drops with the other. When the patient's head is in the midline, the nose drops primarily reach

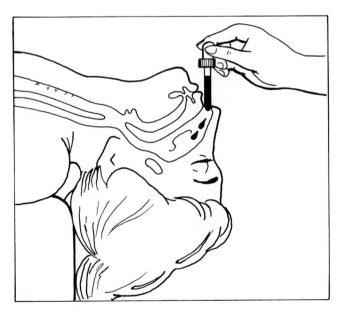

FIGURE 6-22

Administering nose drops. Have patient gently blow nose; open medication and draw up to calibration on dropper; instill medication. Have patient remain in position for 2 to 3 min. Repeat on other side if necessary.

the ethmoid and sphenoid sinuses; turning the head toward the side will facilitate having the drops reach the maxillary and frontal sinuses. Have the patient remain in this position briefly and then if possible, bend over into a head-down position to help distribute the drug. Tell patients to avoid blowing the nose for several minutes so that the medication will not be expelled.

Administering nose spray requires that the patient inhale via one nostril while occluding the other and squeezing a spray applicator. Remove the applicator from the nares before releasing the pressure to avoid pulling sensitive nasal mucosa to the applicator opening. Have the patient keep the head upright or tilted slightly back. Many nose sprays are available over the counter, especially nasal decongestants (see Chapter 4). Caution patients to use these sprays only as needed, for as short a period as possible, and only as directed.

Ear Medications

Most ear medications are in the form of drops. Have the patient lie down with the affected ear up. Keep the medication at body temperature. In adults or children over 3 years, pull the top of the ear up and back to straighten the ear canal, then gently instill the prescribed number of drops. If the patient is a child under 3 years, pull the ear down and straight back (Figure 6-23). Have the patient remain with the affected ear up for 10 min to allow the medicine to disperse. A medication-soaked cotton ball plug may be gently and loosely placed in the ear to prevent oozing; a dry cotton ball will absorb the medication. If it is necessary to treat the other ear, repeat the procedure with the other ear after the 10 min waiting period.

Drugs Administered via Endotracheal Tube

Occasionally it is necessary to administer drugs via the endotracheal tube. Use this route only if necessary and only if specified by the physician. Drugs typically administered via this route include epinephrine, atropine, lidocaine, and the new surfactants. Dilute the prescribed dose in 5 to 10 ml of sterile water and saline. Attach a long needle or soft catheter to the syringe. Auscultate the lungs to verify placement of the endotracheal tube. Keep the patient supine. Instruct patients to hyperventilate for three to five breaths, remove the ventilator or resuscitation bag, and inject the medication through the endotracheal tube as deeply as the catheter or needle permits; do not puncture the tube with the needle. Reattach the resuscitation bag or ventilator and tell the patient again to hyperventilate for three to five breaths. Assess the patient's response to the medication.

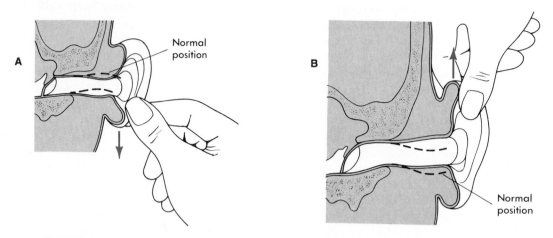

FIGURE 6-23

Straightening ear canal for administration of ear medication. Patient is lying on side with ear up. **A,** For child under 3, ear is pulled down and straight back. **B,** For all others, pull top of ear up and back.

Intraosseous Infusions

Intraosseous infusion may be used in emergency situations in children when an intravenous infusion cannot be started. In this technique a special needle is inserted into a large bone, and after verification of placement through aspiration of bone marrow, drugs, fluids, or blood can be infused. Although establishing an intraosseous infusion is easier than starting an intravenous infusion on small children and infants, several potential hazards are associated with this technique, including infection. If this technique is used in your agency, request instruction in its use, and carefully review the protocol and procedure. For additional information, see Suggested Readings at the end of this chapter.

Implanted Tablets

Some drugs may be delivered by being implanted subcutaneously. Some male hormones and a female contraceptive (Norplant) are administered this way; see Figure 53-1 for an illustration of this form. The advantage is that the drug is slowly released over months to years, so the patient does not have to try to remember to take daily or more frequent doses. Disadvantages include the need for a minor surgical procedure to administer new doses, the possibility of small scar formation, and the possibility that the patient may forget to return for subsequent doses.

Drugs Administered via Inhalation

Only a few drugs are administered via inhalation, one of the most difficult routes of administration. For best results, this method requires a cooperative patient who can inhale deeply and can manage the psychomotor tasks of using the equipment and preparing the medication. Often, though, the patient is a child or anxious or hypoxic because of the condition being treated, such as asthma.

In the hospital or institutional setting, inhalation therapy is fairly common, in the form of oxygen therapy via nasal cannula, nasal catheter, or some form of face mask. Other drugs may also be administered via intermittent positive-pressure breathing machines (IPPB). Trained respiratory therapists are often available to provide assistance. The nurse faces the greatest challenge in ensuring correct use of inhalation therapy in the outpatient setting.

Several inhalation drug delivery systems such as metered-dose inhalers and turbo-inhalers, are available. Each system has advantages and disadvantages. Carefully review the literature supplied by the manufacturer, including the patient instruction sheet. Do not attempt to teach patients how to use the delivery system if they are short of breath or anxious. Make certain that patients show a satisfactory return demonstration before concluding that they can use the prescribed drug correctly. Remind patients to keep hand-held nebulizers and other equipment clean to prevent contamination and infection. Instruct patients to use the product only as ordered to prevent side effects, drug overdose, and drug dependency. See Chapter 25 for an illustration of a metered dose inhaler. Figure 6-24 illustrates how the patient can estimate the amount of drug remaining in a canister.

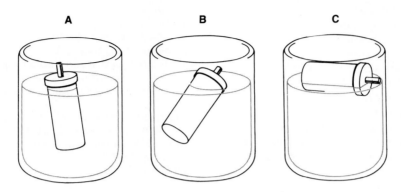

FIGURE 6-24
Checking canister for medication. This could be for metered-dose inhaler (see Chapter 25) or canister with nitroglycerin spray. **A,** Canister is full. **B,** Canister is partially full. **C,** Canister is nearly empty.

This is helpful for patients using metered dose inhalers or nitroglycerin spray forms.

Other Drug Delivery Systems

New delivery systems are a response to a problem in patient compliance, either an inability or an unwillingness of patients to comply. Frequently they respond to a problem in patient compliance with the prescribed dosage regimen, which may be unwillingness or inability. This might occur with limited vision, severe arthritis, or other medical conditions. The nurse faced with an unfamiliar delivery system should consult the manufacturer's literature and patient instruction sheet that often accompanies the dosage form.

CHAPTER REVIEW

◆ KEY TERMS

buccal tablets, p. 83
central venous catheter, p. 92
deltoid muscle, p. 88
dorsogluteal site, p. 89
heparin lock, p. 92
intradermal injection, p. 87
intramuscular injection, p. 88
IV push, p. 92
parenteral, p. 83
rectus femoris muscle, p. 89
stock system, p. 77
subcutaneous injection, p. 88
sublingual drugs, p. 83
suppositories, p. 95
suspension, p. 82
unit dose system, p. 77
vastus lateralis muscle, p. 89
ventrogluteal muscle, p. 90
Z-track technique, p. 89

◆ REVIEW QUESTIONS

1. Describe the differences between a unit dose system and a stock medication system. Which system is used in your practice settings?
2. In your practice settings, where is information about medications recorded?
3. How can you use theories of Erickson, Freud, or Piaget as a guide in administering medications to children?
4. What are some problems you may encounter in administering drugs to elderly patients?
5. For each of the routes of medication administration listed below, answer the following questions:
   - ◆ What are advantages and disadvantages of this route?
   - ◆ Are there considerations unique to elderly patients or children with this route of administration?
   - ◆ How is a drug administered via this route?
     a. Oral route—pills, capsules, tablets
     b. Oral route—suspensions, tinctures, elixirs, syrups, and solutions
     c. Oral route—sublingual, buccal, troche, spray, and lozenge forms

d. Oral drugs through feeding tubes
e. Intradermal injections
f. Subcutaneous injections
g. Intramuscular injections
h. Intravenous injections
i. Z-track intramuscular injections
j. Rectal enemas
k. Rectal suppositories
l. Vaginal douches
m. Vaginal creams and suppositories
n. Skin applications—creams, ointments that must be measured, and transdermal patches
o. Eyedrops and eye ointments
p. Nose drops and sprays
q. Ear drops
r. Drugs via inhalation

SUGGESTED READING

For more information on intravenous therapy, see the readings at the end of Chapter 17.

Allen AM: *Food medication interactions,* Pottstown, PA, 1991, AM Allen.

Bindler RM, Howry LB: *Pediatric drugs and nursing implications,* Norwalk, CT, 1991, Appleton & Lange.

Byington KC: Your guide to pediatric drug administration, *Nursing 91* 21(8):82, 1991.

Camp D, Otten N: How to insert and remove nasogastric tubes quickly and easily, *Nursing 90* 20(9):59, 1990.

Cushing M: Hazards of the infiltrated IV, *Am J Nurs* 90(9):31, 1990.

Hahn K: Brush up on your injection techniques, *Nursing 90* 20(9):54, 1990.

Heiney S: Helping children through painful procedures, *Am J Nurs* 91(11):20, 1991.

Hensley JR: Continuous SC morphine for cancer pain, *Am J Nurs* 91(3):98, 1991.

Holder C, Alexander J: A new and improved guide to IV therapy, *Am J Nurs* 90(1):43, 1990.

IV therapy, Springhouse, PA, 1990, Springhouse.

Korth-Bradley, JM: A pharmacokinetic primer for intravenous nurses, *J Intravenous Nurs* 14(1):16, 1991.

Lenox AC: IV therapy: reducing the risk of infection, *Nursing 90* 20(2):60, 1990.

Lindell KO, Mazzocco MC: Breaking bronchospasm's grip with MDIs, *Am J Nurs* 90(3):34, 1990.

Madda MA: Helping ostomy patients manage medications, *Nurs 91* 21(3):47, 1991.

McAfee T, Garland LR, McNabb TS: How to safely draw blood from a vascular access device, *Nurs 90* 20(11):42,1990.

McConnell EA: How to irrigate the eye, *Nurs 91* 21(3):28, 1991.

McLaughlin-Hagan M: Continuous subcutaneous infusions: new use for an old route, *Nurs 91* 21(7):58, 1991.

Negron SB: A smart way to secure an IV, *Am J Nurs* 89(5):687, 1989.

Newman LN: A side-by-side look at two venous access devices, *Am J Nurs* 89(6):826, 1989.

Rountree D: The PIC catheter: a different approach, *Am J Nurs* 91(8):22, 1991.

Southern JP: How to access an epidural implanted port, *Nurs 90* 20(7):48, 1990.

Taylor N, and others: Comparison of normal versus heparinized saline for flushing infusion devices, *J Nurs Qual Assur* 3(4):49, 1989.

Thomason SS: Using a Groshong central venous catheter, *Nurs 91* 21(10):58, 1991.

Tietjen SD: Starting an infant's IV, *Am J Nurs* 90(5):44, 1990.

Viall CD: Your complete guide to central venous catheters, *Nurs 90* 20(2):34, 1990.

Whitney RD: Comparing long-term central venous catheters, *Nurs 91* 21(4):70, 1991.

Wiggins MS, Sesin P: Guidelines for administering IV drugs, *Nurs 90* 20(4):145, 1990.

Wink DM: Is that needle long enough for that infant? *Am J Nurs* 90(4):28, 1990.

CHAPTER 7

Calculating Drug Dosages

LEARNING OBJECTIVES

After studying this chapter, you should be able to do the following:

- Define common abbreviations used in drug orders, such as q. 4h., gtt., p.r.n., and p.o.
- Convert units of volume or mass between the household or apothecary systems and the metric system.
- Perform calculations based on the strength of solutions of drugs.
- Calculate drug dosages, based on the patient's body weight.
- Calculate infusion rates for drugs administered intravenously.
- Calculate pediatric drug dosages.

CHAPTER OVERVIEW

◆ In Chapters 1 and 6 we discussed the various routes by which a drug may be administered and the importance of careful control of drug levels in the body. Administering the proper drug dose by the appropriate route is the obvious first step in ensuring that the desired drug concentration appears in the bloodstream. In this chapter, we consider how to calculate drug dosages.

Nursing Process Overview
CALCULATING DRUG DOSES

Assessment
The patient and ordered medications should be assessed individually. Is the drug appropriate? What is the usual dose, and is the dose ordered within the normal range? Is there anything about this patient that would indicate that an ordered dose is too large or too small?

Management
Calculate dosages systematically. Have a colleague check calculations if the dose seems unusual or if the mathematic calculations are difficult. Do a "commonsense" check also: 2 tablets might make sense but 20 tablets? If an intramuscular (IM) dose is calculated at 7 ml, is there an error? Most IM doses do not exceed 2 ml. A dose can be too small, for example, should an intravenous (IV) dose of 0.02 ml be 2.0 ml?

Evaluation
Is the patient achieving the desired result? Are there side effects? Are they severe? What data do you have that indicate a prescribed dose is too high or too low? What should be recorded?

ROLE OF THE NURSE
The nurse shares moral and legal responsibility with the physician and the pharmacist in administering drugs. In many hospitals the pharmacist calculates and prepares the drug for administration to the patient, based on the physician's order. This practice does not remove responsibility from the nurse who administers the drug to the patient. The nurse must verify that the correct drug at the proper dose has been prepared (see Chapter 6). For this reason the nurse should be familiar with the forms of drugs and be able to recognize common medications.

The nurse should also question a physician's order for a drug when that order seems inappropriate. For example, the nurse should question the physician about a drug dose outside normal clinical dosage range. The nurse has access to several sources of information about specific drugs, including the pharmacist, and the package insert supplied by the manufacturer. Other sources of information are listed in the Suggested Readings at the end of Chapter 2.

READING DRUG ORDERS

Physicians and pharmacists sometimes employ a system of abbreviations in writing orders or prescriptions. These abbreviations are derived from Latin phrases and, although Latin is no longer used in med-

ical communication, their use persists through custom. For this reason the nurse must be familiar with the common abbreviations listed in Table 7-1. Many of the abbreviations designate how to administer the drug. For example, a physician's order might read Penicillin G 100,000 U q. 3h., p.o. This order would be translated to 100,000 units (U) of penicillin G are to be administered every 3 hours (q. 3h.) by mouth (p.o.).

These abbreviations can be confusing, and the nurse must be certain that the physician's intent is clearly understood. Among the most troublesome are the abbreviations ad lib. and p.r.n. A drug given p.r.n. should be taken at the prescribed interval if the patient requires the drug. For example, after surgery a patient might have the following order on the chart: morphine 10 mg q. 4h., p.r.n. Every 4 hours the nurse should assess whether the patient requires the morphine for pain relief. If the patient is sleeping or is comfortable, the nurse may postpone administering the dose. According to the drug order, morphine may be given less frequently than every 4 hours but not more frequently. In contrast, a medication prescribed ad lib. is given whenever the patient needs it.

Such abbreviations are used as medical shorthand to save time in communicating between medical personnel. If the use of an abbreviation creates any uncertainty, the physician or the pharmacist should be consulted for clarification.

UNITS OF DRUG DOSAGE

In clinical practice, nurses encounter situations in which they must translate a physician's order for a certain drug dosage into the proper number of tablets or the proper volume of drug for an individual patient. This section is intended to prepare the student nurse to handle these problems with skill and confidence.

Before turning to the simple arithmetic required to solve dosage problems, we must be familiar with the three systems of units commonly used in the United States today. These are the metric system, the apothecary system, and the common household system (Table 7-2). Within each system we are concerned with the primary units of mass and volume

Table 7-1   Pharmaceutical Abbreviations

Abbreviation	Latin phrase	Translation
ad lib.	ad libitum	freely; as much or as often as wanted
aa. (or a̅a̅)	ana	of each
a.c.	ante cibum	before meals
b.i.d.	bis in die	twice daily
c̄	cum	with
gtt.	guttae	drops
h.s.	hora somni	at bedtime
non rep.	non repetatur	do not repeat
o.d.	oculus dexter	right eye
o.s.	oculus sinister	left eye
o.u.	oculus uterque	both eyes
p.c.	post cibum	after meals
p.o.	per os	by mouth
p.r.	per rectum	by rectal route
p.r.n.	pro re nata	according to circumstances
q.s.	quantum sufficit	as much as is necessary
q.d.	quaque die	every day
q.h.	quaque hora	every hr
q. 4 h		every 4 hr
q.i.d.	quarter in die	four times daily
ss. (or s̄s̄)	semis	one half
stat.	statim	immediately
t.i.d.	ter in die	three times daily

Table 7-2   Common Systems of Units

System	Unit of mass	Unit of volume
Metric	Gram (gm)	Liter (L)
Apothecary	Grain (gr)	Minim (m)
Household	Pound (lb)	Pint (pt)

because all of the problems we will solve are expressed in units of drug mass and drug volume.

The primary unit of mass within the metric system is the **gram** (gm). Using prefixes, this unit can be adjusted to express thousands of grams (1 kilogram [kg] = 1000 gm) or thousandths of grams (1 milligram [mg] = 0.001 gm). The prefixes *deci-* and *centi-*, meaning 1/10 and 1/100, respectively, are used less often. The primary unit of volume within the metric system is the **liter** (L). With prefixes, the liter is commonly divided into thousandths (1 L = 1000 milliliters [ml]) and less commonly into millionths (1 L = 1,000,000 microliters [μl]) or hundredths (1 L = 10 deciliters [dl]).

The milliliter (ml) is the metric unit equivalent to the unit of gas volume commonly encountered in the clinic, the cubic centimeter (cc).

The primary unit of mass in the apothecary system is the **grain** (gr). It must be remembered that 60 gr constitutes 1 dram and that 8 drams is equivalent to 1 ounce (oz). The primary unit of volume in the apothecary system is the minim. The equivalent of 60 minims is 1 fluid dram (f dr); 8 f dr = 1 f oz.

Equivalents within the household system may be familiar from your home. Table 7-3 lists the equivalents for all three systems.

Any of the three systems of units may be used by a physician to order drugs. The metric system possesses many advantages in terms of ease of calculation and convenience of units, but the older systems still persist in some situations. You may be asked to convert drug doses from one system to another. Unfortunately, the exact equivalents result in awkward and unwieldy values. For example, 1 L = 0.26418 gal; 1 qt = 0.9643 L; 1 gr = 0.0648 gm; 1 f oz = 29.57 ml; 1 oz (apothecary system) = 31.1 gm. Obviously

these numbers are not convenient in calculations. For this reason, certain approximations have been agreed on and are employed in ordinary circumstances for converting between systems. These conversions are listed in Table 7-4.

Abbreviations for the various units are not entirely standardized in the medical literature. For example, gram may be abbreviated *Gm*, *gm*, or *g*. One set of abbreviations has been adopted for use throughout this book. Table 7-5 summarizes the abbreviations in use for various units.

The apothecary system also has some unusual expressions that require explanation. Unlike any other system, apothecary units frequently are used with small Roman numerals rather than Arabic numerals. Moreover, in this system the units precede the numeral. For example, 5 gr may be written gr v, *gr* being the abbreviation for grain and *v*, the Roman numeral for 5. In this system the abbreviation *ss* designates "half". For example, *gr iss* is translated 1½

Table 7-3   Equivalents within Systems

System	Equivalents
Metric	1.0 gm = 0.001 kg
	1.0 gm = 1000 mg
	1.0 L = 1000 ml
Apothecary	1.0 gr = 1/60 dram (dr or L) = 1/480 oz
	60 gr = 1 dr
	8 dr = 1 oz (or K)
	1.0 minim (m) = 1/60 f dr = 1/480 f oz
	60 m = 1 f dr (or f L)
	8 f dr = 1 f oz (or f K)
Household	1.0 lb = 16 oz
	1.0 pt = ½ quart (qt) = ⅛ gallon (gal)
	1.0 pt = 16 f oz = 32 tablespoonsful (T)
	1.0 T = 3 teaspoonsful (t)

Table 7-4   Conversion Between Systems

Apothecary	Metric
15 gr	= 1 gm*
1 dr	= 4 gm
1 oz	= 32 gm
15 m	= 1 ml
1 f dr	= 4 ml
1 f oz	= 30 ml†

Household	Metric
1 t	= 5 ml
1 T	= 14 ml
1 pt	= 480 ml (or 500 ml)
1 qt	= 960 ml (or 1000 ml)
1 gal	= 3.84 L (or 4 L)
1 lb (avoirdupois)	= 0.46 kg or 1 kg = 2.2 lb

*Two factors have been used for converting grams to milligrams. The older conversion factor is 65 mg = 1 gr. This factor is the basis for aspirin and acetaminophen formulations (i.e., a 5-gr aspirin tablet contains 325 mg of aspirin). The newer conversion factor agreed on is 60 mg = 1 gr. This new conversion factor is easier to use for drugs, such as morphine, that are frequently administered in small doses (fractions of grains). For example, ¼ gr of morphine equals 15 mg, using the new conversion factor. The student should remember that these factors are simply agreed on for ease of calculation. All the problems presented in this book use the conversion 15 gr = 1000 mg.
†30 ml has been agreed on as the equivalent for 1 f oz, rather than the more exact approximation of 32 ml, since 30 ml is more conveniently and accurately estimated in most clinical glassware.

Table 7-5 Abbreviation Summary

Unit	Abbreviation used in this text	Other acceptable abbreviations
Gram	gm	Gm, g
Milligram	mg	mgm
Microgram	μg	mcg
Liter	L	l
Milliliter	ml	cc*

*Used for gases only.

gr. Smaller fractions of grains are written out in Arabic numerals. For example, a quarter-grain would be written gr ¼.

The nurse in practice deals with solutions of drugs on a daily basis. A solution is a given mass of solid substance dissolved in a known volume of fluid (weight/volume or w/v) or as a given volume of a liquid substance dissolved in a known volume of another fluid (volume/volume or v/v). The concentration of a w/v solution is always expressed as units of mass per units of volume. Common concentration units are gm/ml, gm/L, mg/ml, gr/m, and dr/f oz. Concentrations are also commonly expressed as percentages, based on the definition of a 1% solution as 1 gm of solid/100 ml of solution. Proportions are also used as expressions of concentrations. For example, 1:1000 designates a solution containing 1 gm/1000 ml of solution. Blood levels of certain metabolites are frequently expressed as mg% (mg/100 ml) of solution. Mg/100 ml is equivalent to mg/deciliter; that is, a 1 mg% solution is the same as a 1 mg/deciliter solution.

The relationship between the various expressions of concentration is illustrated in Table 7-6.

CALCULATIONS
Calculating the Strength of Drug Solutions

To calculate the concentration of a drug solution, use the following equation:

$$\text{Concentration} = \frac{\text{Mass of drug}}{\text{Volume of solution}}$$

If you know any two of these quantities, you can solve directly for the third, provided all the quantities are expressed in the same system of units. Therefore as a first step in the solution of any problem, it is frequently necessary to convert units from one system to another, as we see in Example 1.

Example 1: Prepare 1 L of a 5% solution.
You know:
1. Volume of solution (1 L)
2. Concentration (5%)

To solve:
1. Convert all quantities to the same system of units:

$$5\% = 5 \text{ gm}/100 \text{ ml}; 1 \text{ L} = 1000 \text{ ml}$$

2. Substitute the known quantities into the equation:

$$5 \text{ gm}/100 \text{ ml} = \text{Mass of drug}/1000 \text{ ml}$$

3. Solve for mass or drug:

$$\text{Mass} = \frac{1000 \text{ ml} \times 5 \text{ gm}}{100 \text{ ml}} = 50 \text{ gm}$$

Example 2: What is the strength of a 2-L solution containing 10 gm of drug?
You know:
1. Mass of drug (10 gm)
2. Volume of solution (2 L)

To solve, substitute the known quantities into the equation:

Table 7-6 Equivalents of Concentration Expressions

%	Ratio	gm/L	mg/ml	mg/dl	μg/ml
10.0	1:10	100	100	10,000	100,000
1.0	1:100	10	10	1,000	10,000
0.1	1:1000	1.0	1.0	100	1,000
0.01	1:10,000	0.1	0.1	10	100
0.001	1:100,000	0.01	0.01	1.0	10
0.0001	1:1,000,000	0.001	0.001	0.1	1.0

$$\text{Concentration} = \frac{10 \text{ gm}}{2 \text{ L}} =$$

$$\frac{5 \text{ gm}}{\text{L}} = \frac{0.5 \text{ gm}}{100 \text{ ml}} = 0.5\% = 1:200$$

Example 3: *How much of a 2% solution can be prepared with 6 gm of drug?*

You know:

1. Concentration (2%)
2. Mass of drug (6 gm)

To solve:

1. Convert all quantities to the same system of units:

$$2\% = \frac{2 \text{ gm}}{100 \text{ ml}}$$

2. Substitute the known quantities into the equation:

$$2 \text{ gm}/100 \text{ ml} = 6 \text{ gm}/\text{Volume of solution}$$

3. Solve for volume of solution:

$$\text{Volume} = \frac{6 \text{ gm} \times 100 \text{ ml}}{2 \text{ gm}} = 300 \text{ ml}$$

Example 4: *Prepare 4 oz of a 0.5% solution from tablets gr v each.*

You know:

1. Volume of solution required (4 oz)
2. Concentration of solution (0.5%)

To solve:

1. Convert all quantities to the same system of units:

$$0.5\% = 0.5 \text{ gm}/100 \text{ ml}$$
$$4 \text{ oz} = 4 \times 32 \text{ ml} = 128 \text{ ml}$$
$$\text{gr v} = 5 \text{ gr} = 0.333 \text{ gm}$$

2. Substitute the known quantities in the equation:

$$0.5 \text{ gm}/100 \text{ ml} = \text{Mass of drug}/128 \text{ ml}$$

3. Solve for mass of drug:

$$\text{Mass} = \frac{128 \text{ ml} \times 0.5 \text{ gm}}{100 \text{ ml}} = 0.64 \text{ gm}$$

4. Determine the number of tablets required to total 0.64 gm:

$$\frac{0.64 \text{ gm}}{0.33 \text{ gm/tablet}} = 2 \text{ tablets}$$

As shown, 2 tablets would be dissolved in 4 oz to prepare the desired solution. Note that the conversion was not exact but was very close to a value of 2 and was rounded off. In dealing with scored tablets, you may calculate to the nearest half-tablet.

Self-test for proficiency in drug calculations

After thorough study of the previous system, the student should be able to work the following problems. Check your answers and see the calculations worked out in the answers at the end of this chapter.

SET 1: *Conversions of units and expressions of concentration*

1. A solution is $\frac{1}{50}$ gr/m. Express this concentration in the following units:
    a. gm/L _____
    b. mg/ml _____
    c. % _____
    d. mg% _____
    e. ratio _____
    f. μg/ml _____

SET 2: *Conversion of units used in calculations*

1. The tablets on hand are 0.9 mg each. The order is for gr $\frac{1}{150}$. How many tablets should you give?
2. A drug in liquid form contains gr iiss in 1 t. What is the drug concentration in gm/L?
3. Prepare 3 f oz of a 0.1% solution from tablets gr iss each.
4. How would you prepare 15 gal of a 1:6000 solution from a powder?
5. The tablets on hand are marked 0.1 mg each. The order is for gr $\frac{1}{300}$. How should you proceed?
6. What is the strength of 100 ml of solvent containing gr v?

Calculating the Strength of Diluted Solutions

The examples just given have all dealt with w/v problems. In examining v/v problems, the basic equation can be modified slightly and the problems solved in much the same way as before. The equation then becomes:

(Concentration of solution) × (Volume of solution) = (Concentration of stock) × (Volume of stock)

Stock or stock solution is a concentrated, storage form of a drug, which must ordinarily be diluted before use. Using this equation, calculations are performed much as before, as shown in the following examples.

Example 5: *Prepare 1 quart of a 1:5000 solution from a 10% solution.*

You know:

1. Volume of solution (1 qt)
2. Concentration of solution (1:5000)
3. Concentration of stock (10%)

To solve:

1. Convert all quantities to the same system of units:

$$1 \text{ qt} \cong 1L = 1000 \text{ ml}$$
$$1:5000 = 1 \text{ gm}/5000 \text{ ml}$$
$$10\% = 10 \text{ gm}/100 \text{ ml}$$

2. Substitute in the equation:

$$1 \text{ gm}/5000 \text{ ml} \times 1000 \text{ ml} =$$
$$10 \text{ gm}/100 \text{ ml} \times \text{Volume of stock}$$

3. Solve for the unknown:

$$\text{Volume of stock} = \frac{1 \text{ gm} \times 1000 \text{ ml}}{5000 \text{ ml}} \times \frac{100 \text{ ml}}{10 \text{ gm}} = 2 \text{ ml}$$

Example 6: *Prepare 500 ml of a 1% solution from a 1:25 stock.*
You know:
  1. Volume of solution (500 ml)
  2. Concentration of solution (1%)
  3. Concentration of stock (1:25)
To solve:
  1. Convert all quantities to the same system of units:

$$1\% = 1 \text{ gm}/100 \text{ ml}$$
$$1:25 = 4 \text{ gm}/100 \text{ ml}$$

  2. Substitute in the equation:

$$\frac{500 \text{ ml} \times \text{gm}}{100 \text{ ml}} = \frac{4 \text{ gm}}{100 \text{ ml}} \times \text{Volume of stock}$$

  3. Solve for the unknown:

$$\frac{500 \text{ ml} \times 1 \text{ gm}}{100 \text{ ml}} \times \frac{100 \text{ ml}}{4 \text{ gm}} = 125 \text{ ml}$$

Example 7: *How much of a 0.5% solution can be prepared from 10 ml of a 20% solution?*
You know:
  1. Concentration of solution (0.5%)
  2. Volume of stock (10 ml)
  3. Concentration of stock (20%)
To solve:
  1. Convert all quantities to the same system of units:

$$0.5\% = 0.5 \text{ gm}/100 \text{ ml}$$
$$20\% = 20 \text{ gm}/100 \text{ ml}$$

  2. Substitute in the equation:

$$\frac{0.5 \text{ gm}}{100 \text{ ml}} \times \text{Volume of solution} = \frac{20 \text{ gm}}{100 \text{ ml}} \times 10 \text{ ml}$$

  3. Solve for the unknown:

$$\text{Volume of solution} = \frac{20 \text{ gm}}{100 \text{ ml}} \times 10 \text{ ml} \times \frac{100 \text{ ml}}{0.5 \text{ gm}} = 400 \text{ ml}$$

Self-test for proficiency in drug calculations

After thorough study of the previous section, you should be able to work the following problems. Check your answers and see the calculations worked out in the answers at the end of this chapter.

SET 3: Dilution of stock solutions
  1. A stock solution of a drug contains 10,000 units/ml.
     a. Calculate the amount of stock needed to include in 500 ml of infusion fluid if a 150-lb patient is to receive 20,000 units of drug in this volume.
     b. Calculate the concentration of the diluted drug.
  2. Prepare 1 qt of a 2% solution from a 1:10 stock.
  3. How would you prepare 1 gal of a 5% solution from a 50% solution?
  4. The attending physician has left orders for infusion with 25,000 units of a drug in 0.5 L of normal saline solution. The drug is supplied as 50,000 units/ml stock solution. What volume of the drug stock would you use to make up the 0.5 L drug solution for administration?

Calculating Drug Dosages

All the examples thus far have dealt with the preparation of a drug for administration. We now turn to the next step: the use of those materials to fulfill the physician's drug order for a patient. The equation is:

Body weight × Dosage =
Volume of drug × Drug concentration

A drug dosage is expressed as units or mass of drug per body weight of patient. For example, 0.1 gm of drug/kg body weight is a drug dosage expression, but 0.1 gm of drug is not. Occasionally a physician may order a dose of, for example, 500 mg of an antibiotic to be taken every 4 hours. Technically this form does not constitute a drug dosage, but in practice it is understood that 500 mg is the appropriate dose for an average-size patient; that is, the intended dosage is 500 mg/70 kg body weight. More accurate dosages, of course, must be calculated for persons who deviate greatly from the normal weight range or when highly toxic drugs are involved. Common types of problems in drug dosage are presented in the following examples.

Example 8: *A 100-kg patient is to receive a dose of 4 units/kg body weight. How many milliters of the supplied drug at 100 units/ml are required?*
You know:
  1. Drug dosage (4 units/kg body weight)
  2. Patient body weight (100 kg)

3. Concentration of the drug to be administered (100 units/ml)

To solve:

1. Substitute in the equation:

$$100 \text{ kg} \times \frac{4 \text{ units}}{\text{kg}} = \text{Volume of drug} \times 100 \text{ units/ml}$$

2. Solve for volume of drug:

$$\text{Volume of drug} = 100 \text{ kg} \times \frac{4 \text{ units}}{\text{kg}} \times \frac{\text{ml}}{100 \text{ units}} = 4 \text{ ml}$$

Example 9: *The physician orders 0.2 gm of drug for a patient. How many capsules at gr iss each will you administer?*

To solve:

1. Convert 0.2 gm to 3 gr.
2. Convert gr iss to 1.5 gr.

Therefore,

$$\frac{3 \text{ gr}}{1.5 \text{ gr/capsule}} = 2 \text{ capsules}$$

Self-test for proficiency in drug calculations

After thorough study of the previous section, the student should be able to work the following problems. You can check your answers and see the calculations worked out in the answers at the end of this chapter.

SET 4: Drug dosages

1. A 70-kg patient is to receive 1.2 gm of a drug administered in a 3-ml volume. What is the concentration of the drug solution administered to the patient, and what is the drug dosage?

2. A 60-kg patient is to receive 600 mg of a drug administered in a 2-ml volume. What is the drug dosage?

3. A certain drug is dispensed in tablets marked 250 mg. The drug package insert says that the dose of the drug is not to exceed 10 mg/kg. If a 60-kg adult patient receives 2 tablets, will the dosage exceed what the manufacturer considers safe?

4. A certain patient is to receive a drug at a dose 5 mg/kg. The drug is supplied in a vial marked 500 mg/ml. What volume of drug from the vial should be administered to a 70-kg patient?

5. A certain drug is known to cause thrombophlebitis when given intravenously at high concentrations. For this reason the package insert says the drug must be infused at a concentration of less than 10 mg/ml. A 50-kg patient is to receive 500 mg of the drug by IV infusion. What is the drug dosage, and what volume will have to be infused?

Calculating Infusion Rates

Many drugs must be administered intravenously by slow infusion rather than as a rapid bolus injection. Large volumes of fluids of various types are also given by IV infusion. Disposable infusion sets are available from several manufacturers. These sets are commonly calibrated to deliver 10, 12, 15, 20, 50, or 60 drops/ml of fluid. The nurse in practice can find the calibration, or drop factor, for any particular infusion set by examining the package in which it is supplied. Usually a hospital has only two sizes available to minimize confusion: one regular, or macrodrip, set of 10, 12, 15 drops/ml (abbreviated gtt/ml), and one pediatric, or microdrip, set of 50 or 60 gtt/ml.

Calculations of infusion rates can be carried out with the following equation:

$$\text{gtt/min} = \frac{\text{gtt/ml calibration}}{60 \text{ min/hr}} \times \frac{\text{Total ml to be administered}}{\text{Total hours of infusion}}$$

The use of this formula can be illustrated with the following examples.

Example 10: *A physician's order reads "3500 ml %5 dextrose in water IV in 24 hours." What is the correct infusion rate if the infusion set delivers 60 gtt/ml?*

You know:

1. gtt/ml calibration (60 gtt/ml)
2. Total amount to be administered (3500 ml)
3. Total length of infusion (24 hr)

To solve, substitute in the equation:

$$\text{gtt/min} = \frac{60 \text{ gtt/ml}}{60 \text{ min/hr}} \times \frac{3500 \text{ ml}}{24 \text{ hr}}$$
$$= 145 \text{ to } 146 \text{ gtt/min}$$

Example 11: *To give 50 ml of antibiotic solution IV in 30 min, what should the infusion rate be in drops per min? The infusion set is calibrated for 60 gtt/ml.*

You know:

1. Total amount to be administered (50 ml)
2. Total length of infusion (0.5 hr)

To solve, substitute in the formula:

$$\text{gtt/min} = \frac{60 \text{ gtt/ml}}{60 \text{ min/hr}} \times \frac{50 \text{ ml}}{0.5 \text{ hr}} = 100 \text{ gtt/min}$$

Example 12: *If an infusion set calibrated for 15 gtt/ml is running at a rate of 45 gtt/min, how much time will be required to infuse 1 L of fluid?*

You know:

1. gtt/ml calibration (15 gtt/ml)
2. Total volume to be administered (1000 ml = 1 L)
3. Flow rate (45 gtt/min)

To solve, substitute in the equation:

$$45 \text{ gtt/min} = \frac{15 \text{ gtt/ml}}{60 \text{ min/hr}} \times \frac{1000 \text{ ml}}{\text{Hours of infusion}}$$

The formula can be rearranged to solve for the number of hours:

$$\text{Hours of infusion} = \frac{15 \text{ gtt/ml}}{60 \text{ min/hr}} \times \frac{1000 \text{ ml}}{45 \text{ gtt/min}} = 5.55 \text{ hr}$$

Self-test for proficiency in drug calculations

After thorough study of the previous section, you should be able to solve the following problems. You can check your answers and see the calculations worked out in the answers at the end of this chapter.

SET 5: Calculating IV infusion rates

1. The physician's order reads "1000 ml of D5W IV in 8 hours." What is the correct infusion rate if the administration set delivers 10 gtt/ml?
2. To give 50 ml of antibiotic solution IV in 30 minutes, what should the infusion rate be in drops per minute if the infusion set is calibrated to deliver 10 gtt/ml?
3. Half a liter of normal saline solution is to be infused over a 5-hour period. The infusion set delivers 20 gtt/ml. What should the rate of infusion be?
4. The physician's order reads "1000 ml D5W in 24 hours." If the infusion set calibration is 60 gtt/ml, how many drops per minute should be administered?
5. An infusion of 500 ml of IV fluid is to be carried out over 3 hours. What infusion rate must be used with an infusion set delivering 10 gtt/ml?

Calculating Pediatric Dosages

Calculation of pediatric dosages requires special knowledge of each drug and how it interacts with the unique metabolism of the infant. Some drugs may be given to children and infants in doses that are in the same porportion to body weight as the doses used in adults. Other drugs must be given in greatly reduced doses because the infant is more sensitive or is incapable of metabolizing the drug as rapidly as an adult. Physicians take these considerations into account when determining recommended pediatric doses. For many drugs the pediatric doses listed in various drug reference publications include a statement indicating that the dosage may be calculated for children according to their body weight, for example, but should not exceed a stated upper limit.

Several methods for calculating pediatric dosages exist. Three methods are presented here. The first method, called **Young's rule,** is based on the age of the child and applies to children between 1 and 12 years of age. The equation is:

$$\text{Child's dose} = \frac{\text{Age of child in years}}{\text{Age of child in years} + 12} \times \text{Adult dose}$$

The use of Young's rule is illustrated in the following example.

Example 13: *What is the appropriate dose of aspirin for a 3-year-old child? A normal adult dose is gr v.*

You know:

1. Adult dose (gr v)

To solve, substitute the known quantities in the equation:

$$\text{Child's dose} = \frac{3 \text{ years}}{3 + 12} \times 5 \text{ gr}$$
$$= \frac{1}{5} \times 5 \text{ gr} = 1 \text{ gr, or gr i}$$

A second method for calculating pediatric dosages is based on a comparison of the child's weight to the average weight of an adult. This formula, which applies to all ages of children, is called **Clark's rule.** The equation is:

$$\text{Child's dose} = \frac{\text{Weight of child in pounds}}{150 \text{ lb}} \times \text{Adult dose}$$

The use of Clark's rule is illustrated in the following example.

Example 14: *What is the appropriate dose of aspirin for a 30 lb child, if the normal adult dose is gr v?*

You know:

1. Weight of the child (30 lb)
2. Adult dose (5 gr)

To solve, substitute the known quantities in the equation:

$$\text{Child's dose} = \frac{30 \text{ lb}}{150 \text{ lb}} \times 5 \text{ gr} = 1 \text{ gr}$$

Note that Clark's rule and Young's rule give the same answer when the child is not much lighter or heavier than the normal weight for age. The 3-year-old child used in examples 14 and 15, at 30 lb, is near the normal weight for that age. Clark's rule is considered the more accurate of the two rules, since it will adjust dosage for a child who does deviate from normal weight.

The most accurate method of calculating pediatric dosage is based on the **body surface area** of the child's body relative to that of an adult. Surface area is obviously more difficult to measure than age or weight. Measurements under laboratory conditions yield 1.7 square meters (M^2) as the average body surface area for an adult. Measurements under similar conditions with children have enabled us to construct charts and nomograms that relate the child's body weight to surface area. An example of such a chart is shown in Table 7-7. The equation used for the drug dose calculation is:

Table 7-7 Body Surface Area as a Function of Weight

Weight kg	Weight lb	Surface area (m²)	Approximate age of patient	Weight kg	Weight lb	Surface area (m²)	Approximate age of patient
4.0	8.8	0.25	3 weeks	19	41	0.73	5 years
5.7	12.5	0.29	3 months	21	47	0.82	6 years
7.4	16	0.36	6 months	24	53	0.90	7 years
10	22	0.46	1 year	27	59	0.97	8 years
12	27	0.54	2 years	32	71	1.12	10 years
14	31	0.60	3 years	39	86	1.28	12 years
16	36	0.68	4 years	70	150	1.7	Adult

$$\text{Child's dose} = \frac{\text{Surface area of child in M}^2}{1.7 \text{ M}^2} \times \text{Adult dose}$$

The use of the formula is illustrated in the following example:

Example 15: *What dose of Demerol does a child weighing 10 kg require?* The adult dose of Demerol is 50 mg. To calculate the dosage on the basis of body surface area, determine from Table 7-7 the surface area that corresponds to a body weight of 10 kg. That value is 0.46 M². With that information, you can solve the problem.

You know:

1. Suface area of child (0.46 M²)
2. Adult dose (50 mg)

To solve, substitute these values in the equation:

$$\text{Child's dose} = \frac{0.46 \text{ M}^2}{1.7 \text{ M}^2} \times 50 \text{ mg} = 13.5 \text{ mg}$$

Self-test for proficiency in drug calculations

After thorough study of the previous section, you should be able to work the following problems. Check your answers and see the calculations worked out in the answers at the end of this chapter.

SET 6: Calculating pediatric doses

1. A physician orders the antibiotic cephalexin for a 25-lb child. The normal adult dose for this drug is 250 mg q.i.d. Using Clark's rule, calculate the appropriate dose for this child. Does the prescribed dose fall within the recommended dose of 6 to 12 mg/kg listed in the package insert?
2. You are to give a 5-year-old child phenobarbital. The adult dose is 60 mg. Using Young's rule, calculate the appropriate dose for the child.
3. A 10-year-old child requires codeine sulfate. The normal adult dose is 30 mg. Using body surface area, calculate the appropriate dose for this child.
4. You must give aspirin to a 4-year-old child. Adults take 5 or 10 gr of aspirin, depending on the severity of the pain to be relieved. Using Young's rule, calculate the appropriate dose for the child, based on the maximum adult dose.
5. A 9-kg infant is to receive atropine. The normal adult dose is gr 1/150. What is the appropriate dose for this infant, based on body surface area?
6. You are to give penicillin G to a 40-lb child. The adult dose is 300,000 units. Using Clark's rule, calculate the child's dose.

ANSWERS TO SELF-TESTS FOR PROFICIENCY IN DRUG CALCULATIONS

The correct answer for each question is given first, followed by the calculation.

Solution to SET 1

1/50 gr/m = 0.02 grains per minim (1 ÷ 50). Remember 15 gr = 1 gm and 15 m = 1 ml. You know therefore that

$$1 \text{ gr/m} = 1 \text{ gm/ml} \left(\frac{15 \text{ gr}}{15 \text{ m}} = \frac{1 \text{ gm}}{1 \text{ ml}} \right).$$

Hence 0.02 gr/m = 0.02 gm/ml. You have now converted the expression of concentration from the apothecary system to the metric. You may now readily carry out the other conversions required. The answers are given first, followed by the calculation.

a. *20 gm/L:* 1 ml = 0.001 L. Therefore 0.02 gm/ml = 0.02 gm/0.001 L or 20 gm/L.
b. *20 mg/ml:* 1 gm = 1000 mg. Therefore 0.02 gm = 20 mg and 0.02 gm/ml = 20 mg/ml.
c. *2%:% is defined as gm/100 ml. Solving by pro-

portion, $\dfrac{0.02 \text{ gm}}{1 \text{ ml}} = \dfrac{? \text{ gm}}{100 \text{ ml}'}$? gm =

$\dfrac{(0.02 \text{ gm})(100 \text{ ml})}{1 \text{ ml}} = 2$ gm. Therefore 0.02

gm/ml = 2 gm/100 ml, or 2%.

d. *2000 mg%:* mg% is defined as mg/100 ml. 0.02 gm = 20 mg; therefore 0.02 gm/ml = 20 mg/ml, 20 mg/ml = ? mg/100 ml, ? = 2000 mg; therefore 20 mg/ml = 2000 mg%.

e. *1:50:* Ratio is defined as gm:ml, with both usually expressed as whole numbers. $\dfrac{0.02 \text{ gm}}{1 \text{ ml}} = \dfrac{1 \text{ gm}}{? \text{ ml}'}$? ml = $\dfrac{1 \text{ gm}}{0.02 \text{ gm/ml}} =$ 50 ml. Therefore 0.02 gm/ml = 1 gm/50 ml, or 1:50.

f. *20,000 µg/ml:* 1 gm = 1,000,000 µg. Therefore 0.02 gm = 0.02 (1,000,000) = 20,000 µg.

Solution to SET 2

1. *0.5 tablet:* 15 gr = 1 gm = 1000 mg.

   $1 \text{ gr} = \dfrac{1000 \text{ mg}}{15}$ and $\dfrac{1}{150} \text{ gr} = \dfrac{1000 \text{ mg}}{(150)(15)} =$

   0.44 mg. $\dfrac{0.44 \text{ mg}}{0.9 \text{ mg/tablet}} = 0.5$ tablet.

2. *33.3 gm/L:* gr iiss = 2½ (ii = 2; ss = ½) gr. Solving by proportion, $\dfrac{15 \text{ gr}}{1 \text{ gm}} = \dfrac{2.5 \text{ gr}}{? \text{ gm}}$ and

   ? gm = $\dfrac{(1 \text{ gm})(2.5 \text{ gr})}{15 \text{ gr}} = 0.167$ gm.

   l t = 5 ml = 0.005 L, so the drug concentration is $\dfrac{0.167 \text{ gm}}{0.005 \text{ L}} = 33.3$ gm/L.

3. *Add 1 tablet to 90 ml of water:* gr iss = 1.5. Solving by proportion, $\dfrac{15 \text{ gr}}{1 \text{ gm}} = \dfrac{1.5 \text{ gr}}{? \text{ gm}}$.

   ? gm = $\dfrac{(1 \text{ gm})(1.5 \text{ gr})}{15 \text{ gr}} = 0.1$ gm. 1 f oz =

   30 ml, so 3 f oz = 90 ml. 0.1% = $\dfrac{0.1 \text{ gm}}{100 \text{ ml}}$ and

   since you want 90 ml, solving by proportion, $\dfrac{0.1 \text{ gm}}{100 \text{ ml}} = \dfrac{? \text{ gm}}{90 \text{ ml}}$ and ? gm = 0.09 gm. Each

   tablet is 0.1 Gm: $\dfrac{0.09 \text{ gm}}{0.1 \text{ gm/tablet}} = 0.9$ tablet, rounding off to 1 tablet.

4. *10 gm of drug is added to 15 gal of water:* 15 gal = 60 L, and a 1:6000 solution = 1 gm/6 L. Therefore, (1 gm/6 L) × 60 L = 10 gm.

5. *Administer 2 tablets:* gr ½₃₀₀ = 0.0033 gr, and 0.1 mg = 0.0015 gr; therefore the number of tablets required = gr 0.0033/(gr 0.0015/tablet) = 2 tablets.

6. *0.33%:* gr v = 0.33 gm; therefore the strength = 0.33 gm/100 ml = 0.33%.

Solution to SET 3

1. a. *2 ml:* Calculate the *amount of stock* that contains 20,000 units. Solving by proportion, $\dfrac{10,000 \text{ units}}{1 \text{ ml}} = \dfrac{20,000 \text{ units}}{? \text{ ml}}$.

   ? ml = $\dfrac{(1 \text{ ml})(20,000 \text{ units})}{10,000 \text{ units}} = 2$ ml.

   b. *40 units/ml:* Diluted drug is 20,000 units in 500 ml, so $\dfrac{20,000 \text{ units}}{500 \text{ ml}} = 40$ units/ml.

2. *Dilute 200 ml of 1:10 stock to 1 qt (1000 ml):* 1:10 stock = $\dfrac{1 \text{ gm}}{10 \text{ ml}}$; 1 qt = 1000 ml; 2% solution = $\dfrac{2 \text{ gm}}{100 \text{ ml}}$. To make 1 qt of 2% would require: $\dfrac{2 \text{ gm}}{100 \text{ ml}} = \dfrac{? \text{ gm}}{1000 \text{ ml}}$. ? gm = $\dfrac{(2 \text{ gm})(1000 \text{ ml})}{100 \text{ ml}} = 20$ gm. To get 20 gm from the 1:10 stock: $\dfrac{1 \text{ gm}}{10 \text{ ml}} = \dfrac{20 \text{ gm}}{? \text{ ml}}$.

   ? ml = $\dfrac{(20 \text{ gm})(10 \text{ ml})}{1 \text{ gm}} = 200$ ml.

3. *Add 400 ml of the 50% stock solution to 3600 ml of water:* 1 gal = 4000 ml, a 5% solution = 5 gm/100 ml, and a 50% solution = 50 gm/100 ml; therefore the volume of stock solution to be added = $\dfrac{(5 \text{ gm/100 ml}) \times 4000 \text{ ml}}{(50 \text{ gm/100 ml})} =$ 400 ml. Note that this volume is to be mixed with 3600 ml of water for the final volume of the solution to be 1 gal.

4. *0.5 ml:* You require 25,000 units from a stock solution of 50,000 units/ml; therefore the volume to be used = 25,000 × units/(50,000 units/ml) = 0.5 ml.

Solution to SET 4

1. *The concentration is 0.4 gm/ml, and the dosage is 17 mg/kg:* Concentration = $\dfrac{1.2 \text{ gm}}{3 \text{ ml}} = 0.4$ gm/ml.

   Dosage = $\dfrac{1.2 \text{ gm}}{70 \text{ kg}} = \dfrac{0.017 \text{ gm}}{\text{kg}} = 17$ mg/kg.

2. *Dosage is 10 mg/kg:* Dosage = $\dfrac{600 \text{ mg}}{60 \text{ kg}} = 10$ mg/kg.

3. *Dosage = 8.33 mg/kg. Therefore the dose as prescribed should be within the accepted safety limits:*

$$\frac{2 \text{ tablets}}{\text{dose}} \times \frac{250 \text{ mg}}{\text{tablet}} = \frac{500 \text{ mg}}{\text{dose}}.$$

$$\frac{500 \text{ mg}}{60 \text{ kg}} = 8.33 \text{ mg/kg}.$$

4. *0.7 ml:* $\dfrac{5 \text{ mg}}{\text{kg}} \times 70 \text{ kg} = 350$ mg drug in each

dose. $\dfrac{350 \text{ mg}}{500 \text{ mg/ml}} = 0.7$ ml volume from the vial.

5. *Dosage = 10 mg/kg and the minimum infusion volume is 50 ml:* Dosage $= \dfrac{500 \text{ mg}}{50 \text{ mg}} = 10$ mg/

kg. Minimum infusion volume $= \dfrac{500 \text{ mg}}{10 \text{ mg/ml}}$

$= 50$ ml.

Solution to SET 5

1. *20 to 21 gtt/min:* gtt/min =
$\dfrac{10 \text{ gtt/ml}}{60 \text{ min/hr}} \times \dfrac{1000 \text{ ml}}{8 \text{ hr}} = 20$ to 21 gtt/min.

2. *16 to 17 gtt/min:* gtt/min =
$\dfrac{10 \text{ gtt/ml}}{60 \text{ min/hr}} \times \dfrac{50 \text{ ml}}{0.5 \text{ hr}} = 16$ to 17 gtt/min.

3. *33 to 34 gtt/min:* gtt/min =
$\dfrac{20 \text{ gtt/ml}}{60 \text{ min/hr}} \times \dfrac{500 \text{ ml}}{5 \text{ hr}} = 33$ to 34 gtt/min.

4. *41 to 42 gtt/min:* gtt/min =
$\dfrac{60 \text{ gtt/ml}}{60 \text{ min/hr}} \times \dfrac{1000 \text{ ml}}{24 \text{ hr}} = 41$ to 42 gtt/min.

5. *27 to 28 gtt/min:* gtt/min =
$\dfrac{10 \text{ gtt/ml}}{60 \text{ min/hr}} \times \dfrac{500 \text{ ml}}{3 \text{ hr}} = 27$ to 28 gtt/min.

Solution for SET 6

1. *Dosage prescribed = 3.8 mg/kg, which is less than the suggested lower limit of 6 mg/kg:* Child's dose $= \dfrac{25 \text{ lb}}{150 \text{ lb}} \times 250$ mg $= 42$ mg. 25 lb $= 11$ kg. Dosage $= 42$ mg/11 kg $= 3.8$ mg/kg.

2. *17.6 mg:* Child's dose $= \dfrac{5 \text{ years}}{5 + 12} \times 60$ mg $= 17.6$ mg.

3. *19.8 mg:* Body surface area of 10-year-old child from Table 7-7 = 1.12 M². Child's dose = $\dfrac{1.12 \text{ M}^2}{1.7 \text{ M}^2} \times 30$ mg $= 19.8$ mg.

4. *2.5 gr:* Child's dose $= \dfrac{4 \text{ years}}{4 + 12} \times 10$ gr $= 2.5$ gr.

5. *0.11 mg:* Body surface area of 9 kg infant from Table 7-7 = 0.41 M². Child's dose =

$$\frac{0.41 \text{ M}^2}{1.7 \text{ M}^2} \times (^1/_{150} \text{ gr}) = 0.24 \, (0.44 \text{ mg}) = 0.11$$
mg.

6. *80,000 units:* Child's dose $= \dfrac{40 \text{ lb}}{150 \text{ lb}} \times 300{,}000$

$= 80{,}000$ units.

CHAPTER REVIEW

◆ KEY TERMS

body surface area, p. 110
Clark's rule, p. 110
grain, p. 105
gram, p. 105
liter, p. 105
stock, p. 107
Young's rule, p. 110

SUGGESTED READING

Specific information about individual drugs

AMA drug evaluations annual, Chicago, 1991, American Medical Association.

Clark WG, Brater DC, Johnson AR, editors: *Goth's medical pharmacology: principles and concepts,* ed 12, St Louis, 1988, Mosby–Year Book.

Facts and comparisons, St Louis, 1990, Facts & Comparisons.

Gilman AG and others, editors: *The pharmacological basis of therapeutics,* ed 8, New York, 1990, Macmillan.

Karb VB, Queener SF, Freeman JB: *Handbook of drugs for nursing practice,* St Louis, 1989, Mosby–Year Book.

USP Drug information for the health care professional, Rockville, MD, 1992, United States Pharmacopeial Convention.

Dosage calculations

Aurigemma A, Bohny BJ: *Dosage calculation method and workbook,* ed 3, New York, 1987, National League for Nursing (NLN publication #20-2197).

Boyer MJ: *Math for nurses: a pocket guide to dosage calculation and drug preparation,* Philadelphia, 1987, JB Lippincott.

Brown M, Mulholland JL: *Basic drug calculations,* ed 3, St Louis, 1988, Mosby–Year Book.

Deglin JH: *Dosage calculations manual,* Springhouse, PA, 1988, Springhouse Publishing.

Dison N: *Simplified drugs and solutions for nurses, including mathematics,* ed 9, St Louis, 1987, Mosby–Year Book.

Fulton WH, O'Neil P: Mathematics anxiety and its effect on drug dose calculation, *J Nurs Educ* 28(8):343, 1989.

Hart LK: *The arithmetic of dosages and solutions: a programmed presentation,* ed 7, St Louis, 1989, Mosby–Year Book.

Murphy MA, Gravely EA: The use of hand-held calculators for solving pharmacology problems, *Nurse Educ* 15(1):35, 1990.

Radcliff RK, Ogden SJ: *Calculation of drug dosages: a workbook,* ed 3, St Louis, 1987, Mosby–Year Book.

Scott MA: *Calculations of medications: using the proportion,* Norwalk, CT, 1988, Appleton & Lange.

Self test: clinical calculations, *Nurs 91* 21(6):77, 1991.

Smith AJ: *Dosage and solutions calculations,* St Louis, 1989, Mosby–Year Book.

Weinstein SM: Math calculations for intravenous nurses, *J Intravenous Nurs* 13(4):231, 1990.

SECTION III

PRINCIPLES OF NEUROPHARMACOLOGY

A separate introductory section on neuropharmacology is unique in pharmacology texts for nursing students. We have chosen this format to provide an introduction to key concepts in neuropharmacology and to allow the student to concentrate first on mechanisms and effects before moving to drugs and therapeutics.

The autonomic and motor nervous systems provide the prototypes for our knowledge of neuropharmacology. Chapter 8 reviews these systems and the function and regulation of the neurotransmitters acetylcholine and norepinephrine. Chapter 9 reviews cholinergic drugs, and Chapter 10 reviews adrenergic drugs. Chapters 9 and 10 introduce the student to the spectrum of mechanisms and therapeutic uses for drugs that affect these two neurotransmitters. Do not be concerned initially with actual drugs listed because these drugs, their therapeutic uses, and their nursing implications are discussed in detail in later drug chapters. The detailed classification of drugs by mechanism will be useful as a review later in the course of study.

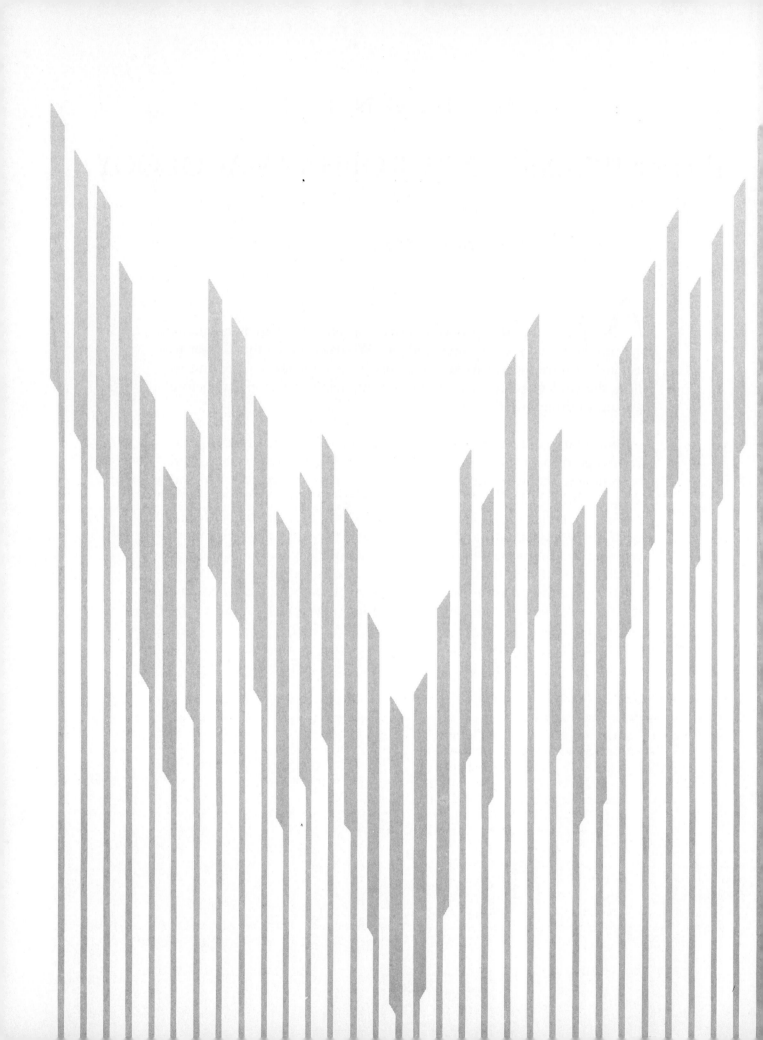

CHAPTER 8

Introduction to Neuropharmacology

LEARNING OBJECTIVES

After studying this chapter, you should be able to do the following:

- Differentiate between the motor nervous system and the autonomic nervous system.
- Distinguish among acetylcholine, norepinephrine, and epinephrine.
- Describe the sympathetic and parasympathetic divisions of the autonomic nervous system.
- List the effects of sympathetic (adrenergic) stimulation and parasympathetic (cholinergic or muscarinic) stimulation on tissues.
- Describe the "fight or flight" response.

CHAPTER OVERVIEW

- Many different classes of drugs, used for a variety of therapeutic purposes, affect the nervous system. Some of these drugs alter the function of some portion of the nervous system, whereas others alter functions of the nervous system as a side effect. A review of the anatomy and biochemical function of the nervous system is necessary to understand the mechanisms of these drugs and the side effects they produce.
- The **central nervous system** includes the brain and spinal cord. These structures have two functions. First, they monitor, convey, and process signals from sensory receptors throughout the body by way of ascending neuronal pathways. Second, they sequence information and convey signals that initiate or modify body actions.
- The neurons that relay information from the central nervous system to the rest of the body are called **efferent neurons.** The a ending sensory neurons and the efferent neurons form the peripheral nervous system. The peripheral nervous system is subdivided into the motor nervous system and the autonomic nervous system.

NEUROTRANSMITTERS

Neurotransmitters and Receptors

All neurons use neurotransmitters to contact neurons and other cells. A **neurotransmitter** is a chemical that is synthesized in the nerve cell and stored inside vesicles (sacs) in the terminal. Most neurons appear to make only one kind of neurotransmitter. When the neuron is stimulated, some of the vesicles merge with the nerve terminal membrane and quantities of neurotransmitters are released. A space exists between the neuron and the cell with which the neuron is communicating. This space is the synaptic cleft. The neurotransmitter molecules diffuse across the synapse and occupy specific receptors on the next cell. The function of the receptor is to recognize only one specific neurotransmitter and to initiate a cellular re-sponse to that neurotransmitter. The binding of the neurotransmitter to its receptor is reversible. When the neurotransmitter diffuses away from the receptor, the stimulation of the cell is terminated.

Two neurotransmitters, acetylcholine and norepinephrine, are used in the peripheral nervous system. A given class of neurons, however, uses only one of these neurotransmitters. We will first discuss the synthesis and degradation of each neurotransmitter. A description of where each neurotransmitter is found in the peripheral nervous system and the responses produced will follow.

The Neurotransmitter Acetylcholine

Acetylcholine is synthesized in the nerve terminal by the enzyme choline acetylase from choline and an

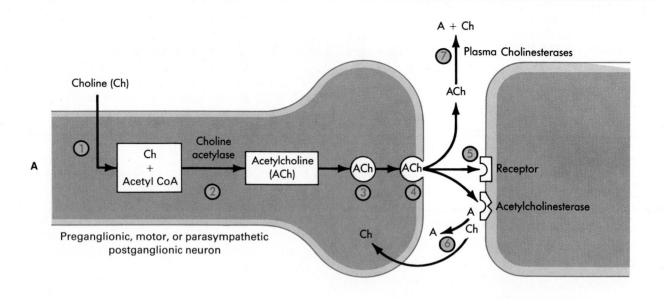

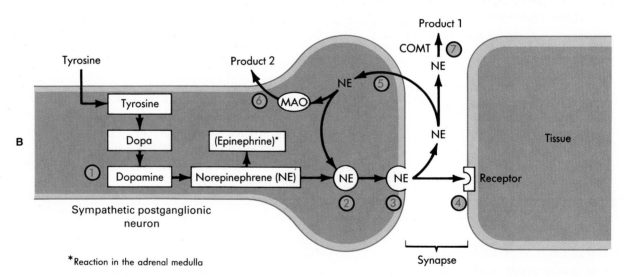

*Reaction in the adrenal medulla

FIGURE 8-1

A, Acetylcholine. *(1)* Choline is taken up by neuron, and *(2)* used to synthesize acetylcholine, which *(3)* is stored in vesicles. On stimulation of neuron *(4),* some vesicles merge with membrane to discharge acetylcholine into synapse, where acetylcholine diffuses to *(5)* its receptor to activate cell, or to *(6)* acetylcholinesterase, enzyme that degrades acetylcholine. Plasma cholinesterases can also degrade acetylcholine. **B,** Norepinephrine. *(1)* Tyrosine is taken into neuron and in three reactions is converted to norepinephrine, which is *(2)* stored in vesicles. On stimulation of neuron *(3),* some vesicles merge with membrane to discharge norepinephrine into synapse, where it diffuses to *(4)* its receptor to activate cell. Most of norepinephrine is *(5)* taken up by neuron and reused. Some norepinephrine is degraded by *(6)* mitochondrial enzyme monoamine oxidase (MAO) or *(7)* enzyme catechol-O-methyl transferase (COMT) found in most body tissues.

acetate molecule activated by coenzyme A (Figure 8-1). This acetylcholine is packaged in vesicles. On stimulation of the nerve, some of the vesicles release acetylcholine into the synapse, where the acetylcholine diffuses to the opposing membrane and binds at acetylcholine–specific receptors. In addition, the membrane contains the enzyme acetylcholinesterase, which degrades acetylcholine to acetate and choline. The acetylcholinesterase is very active, and the half-life of the acetylcholine released is only a few milliseconds. Any acetylcholine that diffuses from the synapse into the blood is degraded by nonspecific cholinesterases in the blood or tissues. Thus when released, acetylcholine produces a response in the next cell by way of the acetylcholine receptor or is rapidly degraded by the membrane-bound enzyme acetylcholinesterase or by nonspecific cholinesterases in plasma.

The Neurotransmitter Norepinephrine and the Neurohormone Epinephrine

Norepinephrine is synthesized in the nerve terminal from the amino acid tyrosine (Figure 8-1). Norepinephrine is a neurotransmitter because it is released from a neuron to act on an adjacent cell. The chromaffin cells of the adrenal medulla also synthesize norepinephrine but convert 80% to 85% of the norepinephrine to epinephrine. These adrenal stores of epinephrine and norepinephrine are released into the blood on stimulation of the adrenal medulla in response to stress. Epinephrine is called a neurohormone because it is released into the blood to produce effects at distant sites.

Most norepinephrine is *not* degraded after release. Instead, norepinephrine is taken back up into the neuron from which it was released and stored again in granules. This process is called *reuptake*. Two enzymes can degrade norepinephrine and epinephrine. Monoamine oxidase (MAO) is located in the mitochondria of most cells, including nerve terminals that release norepinephrine. Catechol-O-methyltransferase (COMT) is found in the cytoplasm of most cells. MAO and COMT are found in large concentrations in the liver and kidney. Any norepinephrine or epinephrine that diffuses into the blood is quickly degraded by the liver or kidney. No drugs that interfere with COMT are used clinically, but in later chapters we see that drugs inhibiting MAO are used for depression, hypertension, and parkinsonism.

Epinephrine and norepinephrine are metabolized to the common product vanillylmandelic acid (VMA). Since VMA is excreted in the urine, the measurement of VMA in collected urine is used as an index of sympathetic activity.

We will review the main features of the peripheral nervous system and its neurotransmitters acetylcholine and norepinephrine to prepare for discussing drugs that act by modifying neurotransmitter action within the peripheral nervous system.

MOTOR NERVOUS SYSTEM

The motor or somatic nervous system initiates muscle contraction by both conscious and unconscious control (Figure 8-2). A motor neuron has a cell body in the spinal cord and contacts a striated muscle at a specialized region, the neuromuscular junction. Motor neurons are found in several cranial nerves and in all spinal nerves. Stimulation of a motor neuron releases acetylcholine at the neuromuscular junction, and the muscle cell reacts to acetylcholine by contracting. Stimulation of a motor neuron may occur as a result of a willed impulse originating in the brain and transmitted to the appropriate neuron in the spinal cord or, unconsciously, as a reflex. A reflex is initiated by sensory input (i.e., heat, touch, pressure, and pain), which is transmitted to the spinal cord and then to the motor neurons without processing by the brain.

AUTONOMIC NERVOUS SYSTEM
Divisions

The role of the **autonomic nervous system** is to monitor and control internal body functions such as cardiac output, blood volume, blood composition, blood pressure, and digestive processes, primarily by modifying the tone of smooth muscle tissue and the quantity of tissue secretions (Figure 8-2). The autonomic nervous system has two distinct efferent divisions, the parasympathetic (cholinergic) nervous system and the sympathetic (adrenergic) nervous system. Both divisions commonly act on a given organ but produce opposite responses. This opposition is highlighted in Table 8-1, in which the prominent effects of the two divisions on key tissues are summarized. For example, the parasympathetic division slows the heart rate, whereas the sympathetic division increases the heart rate. This dual antagonistic innervation is a hallmark of the autonomic nervous system, allowing full control of organ function according to bodily requirements. This antagonism is a result of two distinct kinds of receptors, adrenergic receptors and cholinergic receptors, coexisting on the same organ. In general, activation of the cholinergic receptor produces the opposite cellular response from activation of the adrenergic receptor.

Autonomic Tone

The concept of autonomic tone is also important. Although a minimal but constant release of each neu-

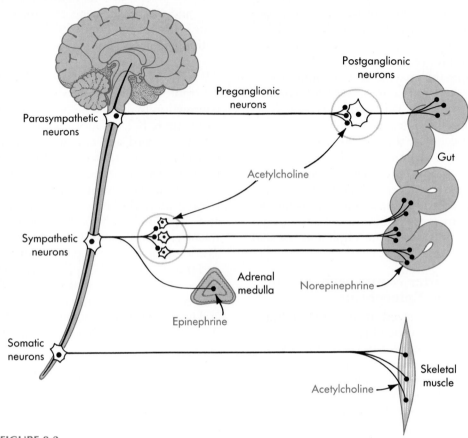

FIGURE 8-2

Neurotransmitters of autonomic nervous system. Acetylcholine and norepinephrine are released from neurons as indicated on adjacent cells. Epinephrine is released from adrenal medulla into blood to act throughout body.

rotransmitter affects each tissue, one branch of the autonomic nervous system dominates and sets the tone of that tissue to coordinate with other tissues. The sympathetic nervous system provides the dominant tone for the cardiovascular system so that the magnitude of cardiac and blood pressure responses reflects predominantly the degree of sympathetic tone, which is itself determined and coordinated within the central nervous system. Parasympathetic control of the cardiovascular system is primarily that of a reflex decelerator system to protect against rapid rises in cardiovascular function. On the other hand, parasympathetic tone is coordinated within certain brain centers to dominate visual, digestive, and eliminatory functions and to determine the intensity of these responses. The sympathetic nervous system acts primarily as an override system to depress these functions in times of stress.

Preganglionic and Postganglionic Neurons

Each efferent division of the autonomic nervous system is a two-neuron system. The cell body of the first neuron (preganglionic neuron) is in the brain stem or spinal cord; the neuron terminates outside the spinal cord in a special nervous tissue, a ganglion (Figure 8-2). The first neuron sends a projection out of the spinal cord (preganglionic fiber), which contacts a second neuron (postganglionic neuron) within the ganglion. The neurotransmitter for the synapse in the ganglion is acetylcholine. The cell body of the second neuron is in the ganglion, and by means of a postganglionic fiber, the neuron innervates an internal organ, usually modifying the action of involuntary muscle such as smooth or cardiac muscle.

Table 8-1 Autonomic Nervous System Actions

Tissue	Parasympathetic (cholinergic or muscarinic) response	Sympathetic (adrenergic) response
Eye	Constriction (miosis) Accommodation (focus on near objects)	Dilation (mydriasis)
Glands	Increased salivation (copious, watery) Increased tears and secretions of respiratory and gastro-intestinal tract	Increased sweating* Increased salivation (thick, contains proteins)
Heart	Decreased rate (negative chronotropy) Decreased strength of contraction (negative inotropy) Decreased conduction velocity through the atrioventricular node (negative dromotropy)	Increased rate (positive chronotropy) Increased strength of contraction (increased contractility or positive inotropy) Increased conduction velocity through the atrioventricular node (positive dromotropy)
Bronchioles	Smooth muscle constriction (restricts airways)	Smooth muscle relaxation (opens airways)
Blood vessels	Constriction of vessels in heart (not a prominent effect in humans) Dilation of vessels in salivary gland and erectile tissues	Dilation of vessels in heart and skeletal muscle Constriction of vessels in skin, viscera, salivary gland, erectile tissues, kidney

Gastrointestinal tract
  Smooth muscle
  Sphincters
	
	Contraction
	Relaxation
		
		Relaxation
		Contraction

Urinary bladder
  Fundus
  Trigone and sphincter
	
	Contraction
	Relaxation
		
		Relaxation
		Contraction

Uterus		Contraction
Liver		Glycogenolysis

*Acetylcholine is the neurotransmitter for this sympathetic response. This is the exception to the rule that norepinephrine is the postganglionic neurotransmitter.

Role of Acetylcholine, Norepinephrine, and Epinephrine

The most important pharmacologic difference between the parasympathetic and sympathetic nervous systems is that the final postganglionic transmitter is different for the two divisions. The preganglionic neurotransmitter at the synapses within the ganglia for both divisions is acetylcholine. However, the parasympathetic nervous system also uses acetylcholine as a postganglionic neurotransmitter. For this reason the parasympathetic nervous system is often called the *cholinergic nervous system*. The sympathetic nervous system uses norepinephrine as the postganglionic transmitter. The sympathetic nervous system has another component, the neurohormone epinephrine. Epinephrine is released from the adrenal medulla as a reaction to stress. The adrenal medulla acts like a postganglionic neuron because it is innervated by a preganglionic fiber and on stimulation releases epinephrine. Epinephrine is carried by the blood throughout the body where it not only activates tissue receptors for norepinephrine but also activates ad-

ditional receptors more specific for epinephrine itself. The sympathetic nervous system is also called the *adrenergic nervous system*. The term *adrenergic* comes from the British word for epinephrine, *adrenaline*. (Norepinephrine is called *noradrenaline*.) The identity of the neurotransmitter at the various sites of the peripheral nervous system is diagrammed in Figure 8-2.

Functional Characteristics

Certain characteristics distinguish the parasympathetic and sympathetic nervous systems functionally. These characteristic functions are listed in Table 8-1. The **parasympathetic nervous system** has dominant control over "regulatory" processes of the body, whereas the **sympathetic nervous system** provides immediate adaptation for "fight or flight." The easiest way to remember the actions of the sympathetic nervous system (and by contrast the parasympathetic nervous system) is to review the "fight or flight" adaptations: the eyes dilate so that vision is improved even in dim light, the bronchioles dilate to let air flow to and from the lungs more readily, the heart beats faster and with greater strength to get blood to muscle, the visceral blood vessels are constricted, but muscle blood vessels are dilated so that the increased blood flow can meet demands of cardiac and skeletal muscle for oxygen and nutrients, digestive and excretory processes are slowed, and the liver breaks down stored glycogen to provide glucose for fuel. All of these responses represent actions of the sympathetic nervous system.

Anatomic Characteristics

The anatomic structures of the parasympathetic and the sympathetic nervous systems also differ. The postganglionic neurons of the two systems derive from distinct areas of the spinal cord. The efferent neurons for part of the parasympathetic nervous system arise in the lower area of the brain. These parasympathetic cell bodies include the respiratory and circulatory centers of the medulla, which control cardiovascular and gastrointestinal processes. The remainder of the preganglionic neurons of the parasympathetic nervous system arise from the sacral portion of the spinal cord and allow parasympathetic control of digestive, excretory, and reproductive processes. In contrast, the preganglionic neurons of the sympathetic nervous system arise from the thoracic and lumbar regions of the spinal cord. Also, the ratio of postganglionic to preganglionic neurons is highly characteristic of each division. In the parasympathetic nervous system, each preganglionic neuron contacts one or two postganglionic neurons so that there is discrete neuronal control over organ function. In contrast, in keeping with the "alarm" nature of the sympathetic nervous system, 20 or more postganglionic neurons may be in contact with each preganglionic neuron so that the action on stimulation of preganglionic neurons is diffuse.

CENTRAL NERVOUS SYSTEM

The brain and spinal cord are more complex in their neuronal organization than the peripheral nervous system. This is because information must be processed rather than just transmitted. This processing is accomplished in two ways. First, a given neuron may send out many axonal projections and form synaptic junctions with many different neurons. Thus a flow of information is sent to several areas for further processing. Second, a given neuron can receive information from more than one neuron. Dendrites from a given neuron may have synaptic junctions with axons from many neurons. Thereby information is collected from different sources.

Neurotransmitters of the Central Nervous System

An important difference between the central nervous system and the peripheral nervous system is the number of neurotransmitters that exist. In addition to acetylcholine and norepinephrine, the central neurotransmitters we will encounter in later chapters discussing central nervous system pharmacology include dopamine, serotonin, epinephrine, histamine, gamma-aminobutyric acid (GABA), glycine, and enkephalins. Some neurotransmitters, in particular GABA and glycine, are inhibitory rather than excitatory. Neurons respond to these neurotransmitters by developing a more negative resting potential with a decreased likelihood of firing rather than depolarizing and firing more readily.

Correlation of Function with Neurotransmitters in the Central Nervous System

Recently nerve tracts in the brain have been characterized by their neurotransmitter content. These nerve tracts have cell bodies in different areas of the brain that collect information, but the neurons then converge and form synaptic junctions with neurons in other regions of the brain. Through surgery or chemical destruction of specific nerve tracts, researchers have associated control of mental and motor behavior with some of the nerve tracts and their neurotransmitters. Examples include the role of acetylcholine and dopamine in the central coordination of muscle movement (see Chapter 48), the role of dopamine in psychosis (see Chapter 41), the role of dopamine and serotonin in depression (see Chapter 42), and the role of enkephalins in analgesia (see Chapter 44). A current goal in neuropharmacology is to identify how drugs modify behavior through their modification of neurotransmitter synthesis, storage, release, action, and inactivation.

CHAPTER REVIEW

◆ **KEY TERMS**

autonomic nervous system, p. 119
central nervous system, p. 117
efferent neurons p. 117
neurotransmitter, p. 117
parasympathetic nervous system, p. 121
reuptake, p. 119
sympathetic nervous system, p. 121

◆ **REVIEW QUESTIONS**

1. What are neurotransmitters?
2. Describe the synthesis, storage, release, and termination of action of acetylcholine and norepinephrine.
3. What are the two divisions of the autonomic nervous system? How are they involved in dual antagonistic innervation and in determining autonomic tone?
4. Describe the neurons of the autonomic nervous system and the motor nervous system with respect to anatomy and identity of the neurotransmitter used.
5. Describe the "flight or fight" adaptations of the sympathetic nervous system. What objective data would you expect to find?
6. Thought question: What objective change in heart rate would you expect to see if you administer a drug that blocks the adrenergic stimulation?
7. Thought question: What would be the effect on secretions (glands) of administering a drug that blocks the cholinergic stimulation?

SUGGESTED READING

Any current physiology text will elaborate on the principles discussed in this chapter.

CHAPTER 9

Mechanisms of Cholinergic Control

LEARNING OBJECTIVES

After studying this chapter, you should be able to do the following:

- Differentiate between muscarinic and nicotinic receptors.
- Describe the difference between direct- and indirect-acting cholinomimetic drugs.
- Explain the difference between reversible and irreversible acetylcholinesterase inhibitors.
- List three therapeutic uses of cholinomimetic drugs.
- Describe three kinds of cholinergic antagonists.
- Describe six therapeutic uses of muscarinic receptor antagonists such as atropine.

CHAPTER OVERVIEW

- This chapter is intended to be read twice during a course in pharmacology. The beginner should read the chapter for the mechanisms and therapeutic applications but should not be overly concerned with the drugs given as examples. Later in the course the student can return to this chapter to review the drugs' mechanisms of action. The exception is the drug atropine, which is presented in detail in this chapter but not elsewhere.

- In this chapter the basis of selective action of cholinergic drugs is explained. We emphasize how the therapeutic activities of these drugs arise from their selective action on classes of receptors for acetylcholine. Cholinergic drugs achieve their effects through stimulation and inhibition of receptors. The organ systems most prominently affected include the eye, gastrointestinal system, and muscle.

POPULATIONS OF CHOLINERGIC RECEPTORS AS DEFINED BY DRUG ACTION

In Chapter 8, three distinct populations of receptors for acetylcholine in the peripheral nervous system were presented: receptors on striated muscle at the neuromuscular junction, receptors on postganglionic neurons within the ganglia, and receptors on other innervated tissues.

Muscarinic Receptors

The distinction among acetylcholine receptors is not just anatomic. Chemical differentiation is made with **muscarine,** a chemical found in certain mushrooms, which mimics the effects of acetylcholine by slowing the heart rate or stimulating smooth muscle when applied to those tissues. Muscarine produces no effect when applied to skeletal muscles or to ganglia. Muscarine mimics acetylcholine only at the postganglionic receptors. The parasympathetic postganglionic receptors are therefore called *muscarinic receptors.*

As a cholinergic agonist, muscarine is a laboratory tool. It is encountered clinically only as a toxin responsible for acute mushroom poisoning. (Another kind of mushroom poisoning exists, in which symptoms take several hours to appear.) The symptoms of acute mushroom poisoning appear within approximately 1 hour of ingestion and consist of generalized parasympathetic overstimulation that includes glandular stimulation (sweating, tearing, and salivation), symptoms of an overactive gastrointestinal system (nausea, cramps, and diarrhea), cardiovascular symptoms (flushed skin and slow heart rate), constricted pupils, and excessive urination.

Nicotinic Receptors

Nicotine, found in tobacco, is another cholinergic agonist. Nicotine is the laboratory agent that mimics the effects of acetylcholine at the skeletal muscle and ganglionic receptors. Therefore the nicotinic receptors are the ganglionic and neuromuscular receptors for acetylcholine. Nicotine is not an effective agonist for acetylcholine at the muscarinic receptors.

DIRECT- AND INDIRECT-ACTING CHOLINOMIMETIC DRUGS

Drugs that mimic the action of acetylcholine act directly, by mimicking acetylcholine (these drugs are chemically related to acetylcholine) or indirectly, by inhibiting acetylcholinesterase (these drugs allow acetylcholine to remain intact longer because its degradation is inhibited).

Acetylcholine is not commonly used as a therapeutic agent because it produces too many responses and it rapidly degrades in the blood. Rarely, acetylcholine is used topically in eye surgery. Carbachol (Carbacel) and pilocarpine (Pilocar) are examples of direct-acting cholinomimetic drugs used principally in ophthalmology. Bethanechol (Urecholine) is the only direct-acting cholinomimetic drug used systemically.

Reversible and Irreversible Acetylcholinesterase Inhibitors

The acetylcholinesterase inhibitors can be subdivided into the reversible inhibitors and the irreversible inhibitors. The **reversible inhibitors** bind to the enzyme reversibly. The drug effect wears off as the drug is eliminated from the body, usually in a few hours. Examples of reversible inhibitors of acetylcholinesterase include physostigmine (Eserine), pyridostigmine (Mestinon), and neostigmine (Prostigmin).

The **irreversible inhibitors** form a permanent covalent (or electron-sharing) bond with acetylcholinesterase. The enzyme must be completely replaced before the drug effect wears off, a process requiring days to weeks. The most common examples of irreversible acetylcholinesterase inhibitors are the organophosphate compounds, which include potent drugs for constricting the pupil (miotics) such as demecarium (Humorsol), echothiophate (Phospholine), and isofluorophate (Floropryl); the insecticides parathion and malathion; and several agents developed for chemical warfare. Interestingly, the antidote for poisoning by an irreversible acetylcholinesterase inhibitor is pralidoxime (PAM), which is itself an acetylcholinesterase inhibitor. PAM, however, is able to compete with the enzyme for the phosphate group of the inhibitor, thereby eliminating itself and the inhibitor from the enzyme and reversing the irreversible inhibition.

Therapeutic Uses of Cholinomimetic Drugs

Used clinically, cholinomimetic drugs produce three effects in the peripheral nervous system.

1. They restore muscle tone in patients with myasthenia gravis or in surgical patients treated with tubocurarine. This is a nicotinic effect at the neuromuscular junction. All drugs used to increase muscle strength are acetylcholinester-

Table 9-1 Receptor Selectivity of Cholinomimetic Drugs at Therapeutic Doses

Generic and trade names	Muscarinic receptor*	Nicotinic† (neuromuscular) receptor	Therapeutic uses
DIRECT-ACTING			
Bethanechol (Urecholine)	+	0	To stimulate atonic bladder or intestine
Carbachol (Carbacel and others)	+ [topical]		To cause miotic reaction (constriction of pupil)
Pilocarpine (Pilocar and others)	+ [topical] + [topical]		To cause miotic reaction (constriction of pupil)
INDIRECT-ACTING: REVERSIBLE INHIBITORS OF ACETYLCHOLINESTERASE			
Ambenonium (Mytelase)	(+)	+	To restore muscle strength in myasthenia gravis
Edrophonium (Tensilon)	(+)	+	To diagnose myasthenia gravis; to differentiate myasthenic crisis from cholinergic crisis
Neostigmine (Prostigmin)	+	+	To restore muscle strength in myasthenia gravis To stimulate atonic bladder or intestine
Physostigmine (Eserine)	+ [topical]		To cause miotic reaction (constriction of pupil)
Pyridostigmine (Mestinon)	(+)	+	To restore muscle strength in myasthenia gravis
INDIRECT-ACTING: IRREVERSIBLE INHIBITORS OF ACETYLCHOLINESTERASE			
Demecarium (Humorsol)	+ [topical]	(+) near eye	To cause miotic reaction (constriction of pupil)
Echothiophate (Phospholine)	+ [topical]	(+) near eye	To cause miotic reaction (constriction of pupil)
Isofluorphate (Floropryl)	+ [topical]	(+) near eye	To cause miotic reaction (constriction of pupil)
Pralidoxime (Protopam)	+	+	To reactivate acetylcholinesterase

* +, Stimulation. (+), Stimulation, at high concentrations, of muscles near the eye. 0, No stimulation.
†No drugs are used therapeutically that primarily stimulate nicotinic-ganglionic receptors. Stimulation of nicotinic-ganglionic receptors is a toxic effect of cholinomimetic drugs.

ase inhibitors. Cholinomimetic drugs acting at the neuromuscular junction are discussed in Chapter 11.

2. They constrict the pupil (miosis), a muscarinic effect that is used in ophthalmology. Cholinomimetic drugs administered to act in the eye are described in Chapter 12.

3. They stimulate an atonic bladder or intestine. This is a muscarinic effect. Cholinomimetic drugs affecting the gastrointestinal system are discussed in Chapter 13.

Table 9-1 reviews the receptor selectivity of choinomimetic drugs discussed in detail in Chapters 11 to 13. No clinical use is made of drugs stimulating nicotinic receptors of the ganglia. Ganglia are involved in many responses, making their stimulation by drugs clinically useless.

CHOLINERGIC ANTAGONISTS
Anticholinergic Drugs

As illustrated in Figure 9-1, each group of receptors for acetylcholine is characterized by a drug that blocks the action of acetylcholine at that type of receptor by occupying the receptor and preventing cholinergic action. Since each class of acetylcholine antagonist acts on a discrete receptor population, clinical use of each class of antagonist differs greatly. Table 9-2 reviews receptor selectivity of cholinergic receptor antagonists discussed in detail in other chapters.

Neuromuscular Receptor Antagonists

Tubocurarine primarily blocks the receptors for acetylcholine at the neuromuscular junction and thereby causes muscular relaxation or paralysis. Antagonists of the neuromuscular cholinergic receptor are used

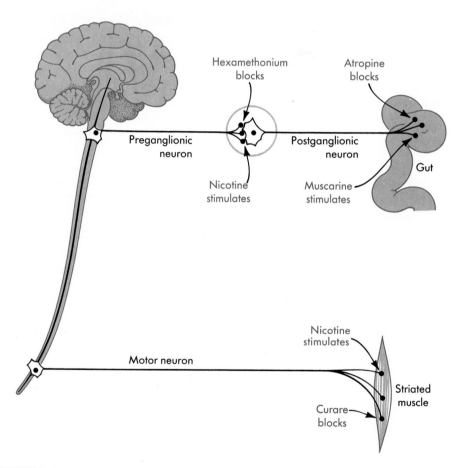

FIGURE 9-1

Acetylcholine is the peripheral neurotransmitter at three receptor populations. Each receptor population is characterized by an agonist and an antagonist. Muscarine is the agonist and atropine is the antagonist of parasympathetic postganglionic (muscarinic) receptors. Nicotine is the agonist and hexamethonium is the antagonist of parasympathetic preganglionic (nicotinic) receptors. Nicotine is the agonist and tubocurarine is the antagonist of neuromuscular junction (nicotinic) receptors.

Table 9-2 Receptor Selectivity of Cholinergic Receptor Antagonists (Anticholinergics) at Therapeutic Doses*

Generic and trade names	Muscarinic receptor	Nicotinic (ganglionic) receptor	Nicotinic (neuromuscular) receptor	Therapeutic uses
Anisotropine	—	0	0	Same as homatropine
Atracurium (Tracrium)	0	0	—	Same as tubocurarine
Atropine	—	0	0	To produce mydriasis (dilated pupil) and cycloplegia (paralysis of accommodation): eye topical; to reduce gastric acid secretion and gastrointestinal motility and tone of the bladder and ureter: systemic use
Cyclopentolate (Cyclogyl)	− [topical]			To produce mydriasis and cycloplegia
Gallamine (Flaxedil)	(—)	0	—	Same as tubocurarine
Glycopyrrolate (Robinul)	—	0	0	Same as homatropine
Homatropine methylbromide (Homapin)	—	0	0	To reduce gastrointestinal hypermotility and gastric acidity
Ipratropium (Atrovert)	—	0	0	To relax bronchial smooth muscle
Methantheline (Banthine)	—	0	0	Same as homatropine methylbromide
Methscopolamine (Pamine)	—	0	0	Same as homatropine methylbromide
Metocurine (Metubine)	0	0	—	Same as tubocurarine
Oxyphencyclimine (Daricon)	—	0	0	To control gastrointestinal hypermotility, gastric acidity, and hypermotility of the genitourinary and biliary tracts
Pancuronium (Pavulon)	0	0	—	Same as tubocurarine
Propantheline (Pro-Banthine)	—	0	0	Same as oxyphencyclimine
Scopolamine	—	0	0	Same as atropine
Succinylcholine (Anectine)	0	0	—	To depolarize skeletal muscle relaxant
Trimethaphan (Arfonad)	0	—	0	To lower blood pressure in selected cases of hypertensive crisis
Tropicamide (Mydriacyl)	− [topical]			Mydriasis and cycloplegia
Tubocurarine (Tubarine)	0	(−)	—	To relax nondepolarizing skeletal muscle
Vecuronium (Nocuron)	0	0	—	Same as tubocurarine

* −, Inhibition. (−), Inhibition at high concentrations. 0, No inhibition.

chiefly as an adjunct to anesthetics and are discussed in Chapter 11.

Ganglionic Receptor Antagonists
The receptors for acetylcholine in the ganglia are blocked by hexamethonium, thus blocking transmission for parasympathetic and sympathetic impulses. Antagonists such as hexamethonium lack specificity in the response produced. Limited use of drugs an-

tagonizing the action of acetylcholine in the ganglia occurs in treating severe cases of hypertension. One such drug, trimethaphan, will be discussed in Chapter 15 with the other antihypertensive drugs.

Muscarinic Receptor Antagonists
Atropine and scopolamine are the prototypes of drugs that block acetylcholine at the muscarinic receptors. These are the parasympathetic, postgan-

glionic receptors for acetylcholine on the heart, smooth muscle, and exocrine glands.

Atropine is an alkaloid originally derived from the leaves of the deadly nightshade, or Atropa belladonna, which belongs to the potato family. Several other plants also contain atropine and a related drug, scopolamine. These two drugs are often referred to as *belladonna alkaloids*. References to the use of these plants as medicinal agents are found in ancient medical literature. Atropine remains the most useful and widely versatile of the antimuscarinic drugs.

THERAPEUTIC USES OF MUSCARINIC RECEPTOR ANTAGONISTS

1. They block secretions. Salivation is readily blocked by atropine. One classic side effect of atropine is a dry mouth (xerostomia). Secretions in the respiratory tract also are inhibited by atropine. This inhibition of bronchial and salivary secretions is the desired effect when atropine is administered as a preanesthetic agent before surgery. The drying effect of atropine reduces secretions that may be involuntarily aspirated when the patient is drowsy or unconscious. Atropine and related drugs are moderately effective in depressing gastric acid secretion in patients with peptic ulcers. The role of cholinergic antagonists in treating gastrointestinal disorders is discussed in Chapter 13. Large doses of atropine and scopolamine dilate the blood vessels in the skin, especially around the face and particularly in children, thus producing a pronounced blushing. The mechanism for this vasodilation is not clear, but since sweating is inhibited by atropine, this flush may represent a mechanism to dissipate heat and a fever may be noted.

2. They depress an overactive gastrointestinal tract. A prominent antimuscarinic effect of atropine is to inhibit the tone and motility of smooth muscle. The gastrointestinal smooth muscle is very sensitive to atropine. Drugs affecting gastrointestinal motility are discussed in Chapter 13.

3. They dilate the eye (mydriasis) and paralyze accommodation (cycloplegia). Atropine is applied by eyedrops to block the actions of acetylcholine. Dilation of the pupil results, since the circular muscles of the iris are relaxed. Blurred vision also occurs, since there is paralysis of accommodation. Mydriasis and cycloplegia allow measurements of lens refraction and examination of the retina and aid in the healing of some infections. Drugs affecting the

eye are discussed further in Chapter 12. Atropine taken orally also reaches the eye. Photophobia (sensitivity to light) as a result of the dilation and blurring of vision (caused by the cycloplegia) are frequent side effects of oral administration of atropine.

4. They increase the heart rate. Atropine is administered to increase the heart rate by antagonizing the acetylcholine released by the vagus nerve at the atrioventricular node of the heart (see Chapter 19).

5. They relax bronchial smooth muscle. Ipratropium alleviates bronchospasm, which is common in many pulmonary diseases.

6. They treat toxicity of cholinergic agents. The most frequent cause of cholinergic toxicity is overexposure to insecticides such as malathion and parathion, which are organic phosphate acetylcholinesterase inhibitors. Atropine reverses the muscarinic effects (i.e., salivation, tearing, diarrhea, and bradycardia) but does not reverse the neuromuscular paralysis. Pralidoxime (PAM), which regenerates acetylcholinesterase at all sites, is therefore the drug of choice.

Side effects may occur in addition to therapeutic effects. The side effects of atropine are extensions of the actions just described. The expected cardiovascular effect is an increase in the heart rate (tachycardia), although a slowing of the heart rate (bradycardia) may be noted with low doses administered intravenously. Dilated pupils and blurred vision are accompanied by an intolerance of the eye to light (photophobia) and sometimes eye pain. In addition to a dry mouth and constipation, patients may experience nausea and vomiting; urinary hesitancy or retention is common. The skin is dry and flushed, and some patients may develop a fever from the inability to dissipate heat through sweating.

Other Uses of Drugs Blocking Muscarinic Receptors

Drugs that are muscarinic receptor antagonists have other uses unrelated to peripheral muscarinic receptors. Many anticholinergic drugs also affect the central nervous system. Some drugs have antitremor activity and are used to relieve certain tremors called **extrapyramidal motor effects** caused by Parkinson's disease, other diseases, and some drugs. Anticholinergic drugs used in the treatment of parkinsonism are discussed in Chapter 48.

Differences in the Central Nervous System Effects of Atropine and Scopolamine

Atropine, particularly in an overdose, produces generalized excitement, which, in the toxic state, may result in hallucinations. Scopolamine can produce hallucinations but also produces sleepiness, sedation, and amnesia. Scopolamine, unlike atropine, is effective in preventing motion sickness.

CHAPTER REVIEW

◆ **KEY TERMS**

extrapyramidal motor effects, p. 128
irreversible inhibitors, p. 125
muscarine, p. 124
reversible inhibitors, p. 125

◆ **REVIEW QUESTIONS**

1. What are muscarine and nicotine? How do they relate to receptors for acetylcholine?

2. Contrast the mechanisms of a direct- and an indirect-acting cholinomimetic drug. How might this knowledge about a drug influence the frequency of patient assessment?

3. What are the three therapeutic uses of cholinomimetic drugs?

4. What are the three prototype antagonists and with which receptor population is each associated?

5. List the five actions of atropine that you would regard as being therapeutically useful.

6. What atropine-like or anticholinergic side effects should you anticipate?

SUGGESTED READING

Bruton-Maree N: Neuromuscular blocking drugs, *J Neurosci Nurs* 21(3):198, 1989.

CHAPTER 10

Mechanisms of Adrenergic Control

LEARNING OBJECTIVES

After studying this chapter, you should be able to do the following:

◆ Define *catecholamines*.

◆ Discuss alpha-1, alpha-2, beta-1, and beta-2 adrenergic receptors, and the effect of stimulation of these receptors.

◆ Relate the activity of the beta-adrenergic receptors to the "fight or flight" concept mentioned in Chapter 8.

◆ Describe the role of cyclic adenosine monophosphate (cyclic AMP) in stimulation of the beta receptors.

◆ Define direct- and indirect-acting adrenergic drugs.

◆ Explain the four mechanisms by which drugs interfere with adrenergic activity.

CHAPTER OVERVIEW

◆ Like Chapter 9, this chapter is intended to be read once at the beginning of a course in pharmacology as an introduction and again at a later time as a review. When reading this chapter as an introduction, pay attention to the mechanisms and their associated effects. The drugs given as examples and their classification by mechanism will be of interest when the chapter is reviewed.

◆ In this chapter, we explain the basis of selective action of adrenergic drugs. Emphasis is given to showing how the therapeutic activities of these drugs arise from their selective action on classes of receptors for norepinephrine and epinephrine. These drugs achieve their effects through stimulation or inhibition of receptors. The organ systems most prominently affected include the eye, bronchial smooth muscle, blood vessel smooth muscle, and heart.

CATECHOLAMINES AND THEIR RECEPTORS

Naturally Occurring Catecholamines

Dopamine, norepinephrine, and epinephrine are naturally occurring **catecholamines,** which function as neurotransmitters and neurohormones. Dopamine is derived from the amino acid tyrosine and is the chemical precursor of norepinephrine:

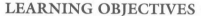

Tyrosine→→Dopamine→
Norepinephrine→Epinephrine

All three catecholamines are important neurotransmitters in the central nervous system. In the autonomic nervous system, norepinephrine is the sympathetic, postganglionic neurotransmitter and epinephrine is the neurohormone released from the adrenal medulla in reaction to stress. Dopamine's role in the autonomic nervous system is not completely understood at present.

Adrenergic Receptors and Responses

Isoproterenol was the first synthetic catecholamine to be studied. The existence of two classes of adrenergic receptors was hypothesized in the late 1940s to explain the different physiologic effects elicited by norepinephrine, epinephrine, and isoproterenol. **Alpha receptors** are receptors for which norepinephrine and epinephrine are equally potent, but isoproterenol is less potent. **Beta receptors** are receptors for which isoproterenol is more potent than or as potent as epinephrine or norepinephrine. Subsequent studies have expanded this classification to include two subtypes in each class, alpha-1, alpha-2, beta-1, and beta-2.

Alpha-1 adrenergic receptors

Alpha-1 receptors account for the primary responses elicited by norepinephrine released from sympathetic postganglionic neurons. Epinephrine is as potent as norepinephrine in stimulating alpha-1 receptors.

Physiologic effects resulting from stimulation of alpha-1 receptors include the following:

1. Contraction of the radial muscles of the iris. The radial muscles are arranged like the spokes of a wheel so that contraction causes dilation of the pupil (mydriasis). Adrenergic drugs used therapeutically for this effect are discussed in Chapter 12.
2. Constriction of arterioles and veins, which causes an increase in blood pressure. Adrenergic drugs that are used to raise the blood pressure are discussed in Chapter 14.
3. Contraction of smooth muscle sphincters in the stomach, intestine, and bladder.
4. Contraction of the uterus (female) and stimulation of ejaculation (male).
5. Reduction of secretions from the pancreas.
6. Breakdown of glycogen in the liver (glycogenolysis) and synthesis of glucose (gluconeogenesis).

Drugs mimicking adrenergic effects listed in items 3 through 6 are not used therapeutically.

Systemic effect of alpha-1 receptor activation

The role of the alpha-1 receptor is to stimulate contraction of smooth muscle. The most prominent effect systemically is an increase in blood pressure resulting from the constriction of blood vessels, mainly arterioles. The blood vessels controlled by alpha-1 receptors service the internal organs, mucosal surfaces, and skin. Blood pressure reflects in part the degree of constriction of these blood vessels, since it is determined by the cardiac output and the peripheral resistance to blood flow in blood vessels.

Local vasoconstriction

Therapeutic use is made of local vasoconstriction by epinephrine and other alpha-1 adrenergic receptor agonists (stimulants). Nasal decongestion is achieved by local application of a vasoconstrictive drug (see Chapter 26). Drug absorption from parenteral sites is slowed when a drug is injected with a vasoconstricting agent. Local anesthetics in particular have a longer duration of action when injected with epinephrine to slow systemic absorption.

Alpha-2 adrenergic receptors

The existence of a second class of alpha receptors, the alpha-2 receptors, was experimentally proved in the 1970s. Alpha-2 receptors originally were found presynaptically on sympathetic neuronal terminals. These presynaptic **alpha-2 receptors** inhibit the further release of norepinephrine when they are stimulated. Therefore presynaptic alpha-2 receptors function as a negative feedback system to limit the amount of norepinephrine released from the neuron. Alpha-2 receptors are found on platelets, where their activation results in platelet aggregation.

Alpha-2 receptors have also been found on the smooth muscle or the blood vessels that determine blood pressure—the resistance vessels. Like alpha-1 receptors, alpha-2 receptors mediate vasoconstriction to increase resistance and thereby increase blood pressure. Current speculation is that the alpha-1 receptors are located primarily where sympathetic neurons innervate the blood vessel. Norepinephrine released from the sympathetic postganglionic nerve terminal activates alpha-1 receptors on the tissue (usually to elicit smooth muscle contraction) and activates alpha-2 receptors on the nerve terminal, which inhibits further release of norepinephrine. Alpha-2 receptors on the blood vessel are believed to mediate vasoconstriction to blood-borne dopamine and catecholamines. The therapeutic potential of drugs acting at alpha-2 receptors remains to be developed. The antihypertensive drugs clonidine and methyldopa stimulate the alpha-2 receptor. This action does not account for their antihypertensive effect, which is a result of their activity in the central nervous system.

Beta-1 adrenergic receptor

The **beta-1 receptor** is stimulated by norepinephrine and epinephrine, but isoproterenol is a more potent stimulant than either. Physiologic responses to activation of beta-1 receptors include the following:

1. Stimulation of the heart. Activation of the beta-1 receptor in the conducting tissue of the heart speeds the repolarization of the cells. Increased heart rate (positive chronotropic effect) and impulse conduction speed (positive dromotropic effect) result. Stimulation of the beta-1 receptors in the ventricular muscle increases the force of contraction (positive inotropic response). In Chapter 14, we discuss drugs that act on beta-1 receptors used for stimulating the heart under certain restricted conditions.
2. Stimulation of the beta-1 receptor of fat tissue. This results in lipolysis, the breakdown of stored fat. Fatty acids released can then be used as energy sources by the heart and liver. Drugs mimicking this adrenergic effect are not used therapeutically.

Beta-2 adrenergic receptor

Epinephrine and isoproterenol are equipotent in stimulating **beta-2 receptors,** whereas norepinephrine is a weak stimulant. Physiologic responses to activation of beta-2 receptors include the following:

1. Dilation of the bronchioles. The relaxation of bronchial smooth muscle decreases airway re-

sistance and makes breathing easier. Drugs acting through activation of beta-2 receptors are used to treat patients with restricted airways, primarily caused by asthma or chronic obstructive lung disease. We will discuss these drugs in Chapter 25.

2. Relaxation of uterine smooth muscle. Drugs acting through activation of the beta-2 receptors ritodrine and terbutaline are used to stop premature labor by relaxing the pregnant uterus (see Chapter 53).

3. Dilation of the blood vessels in the skeletal muscle, brain, and heart. Activation of these beta-2 receptors causes vasodilation and shunts blood to the skeletal muscle, brain, and heart. The drug nylidrin (Arlidin) is used to increase blood flow to these organs (see Chapter 14).

4. Breakdown of glycogen in the liver (glycogenolysis) and synthesis of glucose (gluconeogenesis). Note that this is also an alpha-1 adrenergic effect. This action is not used therapeutically.

Systemic effects of beta-adrenergic receptor activation

The value of the responses to two classes of beta receptors can be appreciated by recalling the "fight or flight" nature of the sympathetic nervous system discussed in Chapter 8. The heart rate and cardiac output increase because epinephrine reinforces the action of norepinephrine on the beta-1 receptors. Blood is shunted to the muscles, brain, and heart, where stimulation of beta-2 receptors results in vasodilation, and from the skin and abdominal organs, where stimulation of alpha-1 receptors causes vasoconstriction. Epinephrine also stimulates the liver to break down glycogen to glucose and stimulates the fat cells to break down lipids to fatty acids to provide readily available energy sources for the body.

Table 10-1 reviews the receptor selectivity of these sympathomimetic drugs, which are discussed in detail in other chapters.

Second Messenger Concept and the Beta Receptor

In the 1950s, Earl Sutherland began the work of elucidating epinephrine caused glycogenolysis (breakdown of glycogen to glucose) in the dog liver. Sutherland and colleagues showed that epinephrine acts by binding to the beta-2 receptor on the liver cell membrane. When the beta-2 receptor is occupied, there is a structural change that activates the membrane-bound enzyme, adenylate cyclase.

As illustrated in Figure 10-1, this structural change is complex. When occupied, the beta receptor activates a transducer protein called G_s (s, stimulatory

protein). G_s then activates adenylate cyclase. The active portion of adenylate cyclase is inside the cell. The enzyme catalyzes the conversion of adenosine triphosphate (ATP) to pyrophosphate (PP) and cyclic adenosine 3′,5′-monophosphate (cyclic AMP). **Cyclic AMP** is the key to the intracellular action of epinephrine. Epinephrine is the hormone released to signal the cell to act. Cyclic AMP is the second messenger that translates the presence of epinephrine at the cell surface to the internal machinery of the cell. Many cyclic AMP molecules are formed as a result of each receptor occupation, amplifying the epinephrine signal.

Cyclic AMP produces cellular effects by stimulating other enzymes. The enzymes present in the cell that can be stimulated by cyclic AMP determine the cellular response. In the liver, the breakdown of glycogen results. In the heart, increases in heart rate, force of contraction, and conduction speed result. In smooth muscle, relaxation results.

Recently it has been shown that the alpha-2 receptor is also linked to the adenylate cyclase. When occupied, the alpha-2 receptor activates a transducer protein called G_i (i, inhibitory protein). G_i then inhibits adenylate cyclase activity. Therefore the beta receptors (beta-1 and beta-2) and the alpha-2 receptor have opposite effects.

The alpha-1 receptor is activated by a different mechanism. Activation of the alpha-1 receptor stimulates the entry of calcium into the cell. The increased cytosolic concentration of calcium changes the activity of certain enzymes. The changes in enzymatic activities account for the actions produced by the activation of the alpha-1 receptor.

We need to point out two more features of the cyclic AMP system. Epinephrine is not the only hormone that stimulates the formation of cyclic AMP. Most polypeptide hormones, discussed in Chapter 36, work through cyclic AMP. The exceptions are insulin, growth hormone, and prolactin. Each hormone has its specific receptor on its target tissues. This is why each hormone can have tissue-specific actions while using the same second messenger system. Second, cyclic AMP is rapidly degraded by the enzyme phosphodiesterase to 5′-adenosine monophosphate (AMP). Drugs that inhibit phosphodiesterase and thereby produce elevated cyclic AMP concentrations include theophylline and its dimer, aminophylline. These drugs produce vasodilation in cerebral ischemia and, more important, treat asthma by promoting bronchial dilation (see Chapter 25).

Therapeutic Uses and Features of Adrenergics

Therapeutic use of **adrenergic drugs** depends on whether they act on alpha-1, beta-1, or beta-2 recep-

Table 10-1   Receptor Selectivity of Adrenergic Drugs*

Generic and trade names	Alpha receptor	Beta-1 receptor	Beta-2 receptor	CNS	Main therapeutic uses
CATECHOLAMINES					
Dobutamine (Dobutrex)	0	+D	0	0	Increases cardiac contractility with little increase in heart rate or conductivity
Dopamine (Intropin)	(+)I	(+)I	0	0	Dilates renal arteries at low doses by activating dopamine receptors and preventing kidney shutdown in shock
Epinephrine	+D	+D	+	(+)	Treats anaphylactic shock Treats acute asthma attacks Limits systemic absorption of drugs applied for local action
Isoproterenol (Isuprel)	0	+D	+	(+)	Improves bronchodilation for asthma
Norepinephrine, levar-terenol (Levophed)	+D	+D	0	(+)	Counteracts hypotension of spinal anesthesia
NONCATECHOLAMINES					
Albuterol (Ventolin, Proventil)	0	0	+	0	Improves bronchodilation
Amphetamine	+I	+I	0	+	Depresses appetite Stimulates respiration Counteracts narcolepsy
Bitolterol (Tornalate)	0	0	+	0	Improves bronchodilation
Ephedrine	+I,D	+I,D	+	+	Improves bronchodilation for asthma Reduces congestion (nasal decongestant) Dilates pupil (mydriasis)
Fenoterol (Berotec)	0	0	+	0	Improves bronchodilation
Hydroxyamphetamine (Paredrine)	+I	+I	0	0	Dilates pupil (mydriasis)
Isoetharine (Bronkosol)	0	0	+	0	Improves bronchodilation
Mephentermine (Wyamine)	+I,D	+I,D	0	+	Counteracts hypotension of spinal anesthesia Depresses appetite
Metaproterenol (Alupent, Metaprel)	0	(+)	+	0	Improves bronchodilation
Metaraminol (Aramine)	+I,D	+I,D	0	0	Counteracts hypotension of spinal anesthesia
Methoxamine (Vasoxyl)	+D	0	0	0	Counteracts hypotension of spinal anesthesia Terminates paroxysmal atrial tachycardia
Naphazoline (Privine)	+	0	0	0	Reduces congestion (nasal decongestant)
Nylidrin (Arlidin)	0	0	+	0	Stimulates blood flow to heart, brain, and muscles
Oxymetazoline (Afrin)	+	0	0	0	Reduces congestion (nasal decongestant)
Phenylephrine	+D	0	0	0	Reduces congestion (nasal decongestant) Terminates paroxysmal atrial tachycardia
Phenylpropanolamine	+I,D	+I,D	+	(+)	Reduces congestion (nasal decongestant)
Pirbuterol (Maxair)	0	0	+	0	Improves bronchodilation

* +I, Indirectly acting (releases norepinephrine). +D, Directly acts on the receptor. (+), Effect is modest except at high concentration. 0, No effect.

Continued.

Table 10-1   Receptor Selectivity of Adrenergic Drugs—cont'd

Generic and trade names	Alpha receptor	Beta-1 receptor	Beta-2 receptor	CNS	Main therapeutic uses
NONCATECHOLAMINES—cont'd					
Procaterol (Pro-Air)	0	0	+	0	Improves bronchodilation
Propylhexedrine Benzedrex)	+	0	0	0	Reduces congestion (nasal decongestant)
Pseudoephedrine	+I,D	+I,D	+	(+)	Reduces congestion (nasal decongestant)
Ritodrine (Yutopar)	0	0	+	0	Stops premature labor
Terbutaline (Brethine, Bricanyl)	0	0	+	0	Improves bronchodilation
Tetrahydrozoline Tyzine)	+	0	0	0	Reduces congestion (nasal decongestant)
Xylometazoline (Otrivin)	+	0	0	0	Reduces congestion (nasal decongestant)

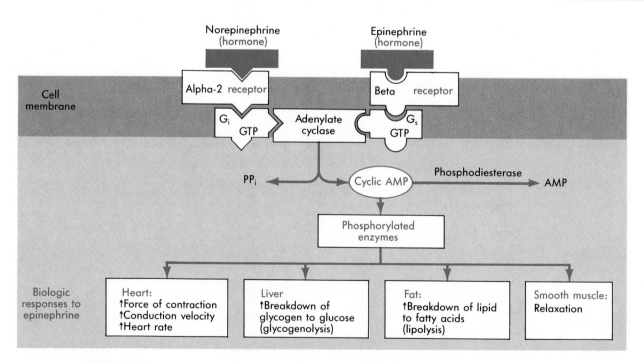

FIGURE 10-1

Second-messenger concept. Binding of hormone at cell surface initiates series of reactions that modify activity through phosphorylation of key enzymes which in turn modify cellular responses. Cyclic AMP is second messenger because it carries message that hormone is at cell surface. It translates this message into action by stimulating phosphorylating enzyme (cyclic AMP dependent protein kinase). Cellular responses to epinephrine characteristic for given organs are given as examples of biologic responses mediated through cyclic AMP.

tors. A variety of drugs have been synthesized that are relatively specific for activating a given receptor type and thereby directly mimic some portion of norepinephrine or epinephrine action. These are called *direct-acting adrenergic drugs*. Other adrenergic drugs act by a second mechanism of action. These are called *indirect-acting adrenergic drugs,* which act by causing the sympathetic, postganglionic neurons to release norepinephrine. This increased amount of norepinephrine activates alpha-1, alpha-2, and beta-1 receptors. Drugs such as amphetamine, ephedrine, and mephentermine also act in the central nervous system, which determines and limits their use. The catecholamines are relatively or completely ineffective when taken orally because they are rapidly destroyed in the gastrointestinal tract or by the liver, whereas many noncatecholamines can be taken orally.

DRUGS INHIBITING ADRENERGIC ACTIVITY

Table 10-2 lists the drugs that interfere with peripheral adrenergic activity and their therapeutic uses. Drug mechanisms that interfere with adrenergic activity include the following:

1. Blockade of alpha-adrenergic receptors
2. Blockade of beta-adrenergic receptors
3. Depletion of peripheral neuronal stores of norepinephrine
4. Inhibition of peripheral sympathetic activity through an action in the central nervous system

We will discuss further the spectrum of physiologic effects produced by each of these mechanisms.

Table 10-2   Drugs Inhibiting Adrenergic Receptor Activity*

Generic and trade names	Alpha receptor	Beta-1 receptor	Beta-2 receptor	CNS	Main therapeutic uses
ALPHA-ADRENERGIC RECEPTOR ANTAGONISTS					
Phenoxybenzamine (Dibenzyline)	—	0	0	0	Treats hypertension secondary to pheochromocytoma / Treats vasospastic disorders of the digits (Raynaud's syndrome)
Phentolamine (Regitine)	—	0	0	0	Treats hypertension secondary to pheochromocytoma
Prazosin (Minipress)	—	0	0	0	Treats chronic hypertension
Terazosin (Hytrin)	—	0	0	0	Treats chronic hypertension
BETA-ADRENERGIC RECEPTOR ANTAGONISTS					
Acebutolol (Sectral)	0	—	0	0	Treats chronic hypertension
Atenolol (Tenormin)	0	—	0	0	Treats chronic hypertension / Treats angina prophylactically
Betaxolol (Betoptic)	0	—	0	0	Treats glaucoma (ophthalmic use)
Carteolol (Cartrol)	0	—	—	0	Treats chronic hypertension
Esmolol (Brevibloc)	0	—	0	0	Controls supraventricular tachycardia
Labetolol (Trandate, Vescal)	—	—	—	0	Treats chronic hypertension / Treats angina prophylactically
Levobunolol (Betagan)	0	—	—	0	Treats glaucoma (ophthalmic use)
Metoprolol (Lopressor)	0	—	0	—	Treats chronic hypertension / Treats angina prophylactically
Nadolol (Corgard)	0	—	—	—	Treats chronic hypertension / Treats angina prophylactically
Oxprenolol (Trasicor)	0	—	—	0	Treats chronic hypertension

*— denotes inhibition, *0* denotes no effect, *I* denotes indirect inhibition resulting from depletion of norepinephrine stores, *−CNS* denotes a decrease in peripheral sympathetic tone through an action in the central nervous system (CNS).

Continued.

Table 10-2   Drugs Inhibiting Adrenergic Receptor Activity*—cont'd

Generic and trade names	Alpha receptor	Beta-1 receptor	Beta-2 receptor	CNS	Main therapeutic uses
BETA-ADRENERGIC RECEPTOR ANTAGONISTS—cont'd					
Penbutolol (Levatol)	0	—	—	0	Treats chronic hypertension Treats angina prophylactically
Pindolol (Visken)	0	—	—	—	Treats chronic hypertension Treats angina prophylactically
Propranolol (Inderal)	0	—	—	—	Treats chronic hypertension Treats angina prophylactically Treats cardiac arrhythmias Treats migraine prophylactically
Sotalol (Sotacor)	0	—	—	0	Treats chronic hypertension
Timolol (Blocadren, Timoptic)	0	—	—	0	Treats chronic hypertension Treats glaucoma (ophthalmic use)
DRUGS DEPLETING NEURONAL STORES OF NOREPINEPHRINE					
Guanadrel (Hylorel)	I	I	I	0	Treats severe chronic hypertension
Guanethidine (Ismelin)	I	I	I	0	Treats severe chronic hypertension
Reserpine (Serpasil)	I	I	I	—	Treats chronic hypertension
DRUGS INHIBITING SYMPATHETIC ACTIVITY THROUGH CNS ACTION					
Methyldopa (Aldomet)	−CNS	0	0	—	Treats chronic hypertension
Clonidine (Catapres)	−CNS	0	0	—	Treats chronic hypertension
Guanabenz (Wytensin)	−CNS	0	0	—	Treats chronic hypertension
Guanfacine (Tenex)	−CNS	0	0	—	Treats chronic hypertension

Blockade of Alpha-Adrenergic Receptors

Phenoxybenzamine, phentolamine, and prazosin each act selectively to antagonize norepinephrine at the alpha-1 receptors. Infusion of one of these drugs into a person with normal blood pressure produces little change in blood pressure as long as the person is lying down. However, any sudden shift to the upright position causes orthostatic (postural) hypotension because the blockade of the alpha-1 receptors prevents the vasoconstriction necessary to redistribute blood flow. Therefore in orthostatic hypotension the blood pools in the legs and drains from the head, causing the person to faint.

Other effects characteristic of blockade of the alpha-1 receptors include pinpoint pupil (miosis), nasal stuffiness, or, in males, inhibition of ejaculation. The uses and pharmacokinetics of the alpha-1 receptor antagonists in the treatment of hypertension are discussed in Chapter 15.

Blockade of Beta-Adrenergic Receptors
Nonselective antagonists

The physiologic effects of beta-receptor antagonists can be anticipated by considering the functions of the beta receptors. Blockade of the beta-1 receptors in the heart causes little change in the normal person at rest but limits the increase in cardiac functions normally elicited by exercise and hypertension. Conditions improved by beta-1 receptor blockade include angina and some cardiac arrhythmias. Recently, propranolol, metoprolol, and timolol have been used effectively to treat patients with angina to prevent recurrent heart attacks.

Beta-receptor antagonists are also effective in treating hypertension. However, when a beta-receptor antagonist is given with a vasodilator drug, the beta-receptor antagonist inhibits the reflex activation of the heart caused by the drop in blood pressure. For this reason, a beta-receptor antagonist combined with a vasodilator drug is especially effective in treating hypertension. The use of beta-receptor antagonists in the therapy of hypertension is discussed in Chapter 15.

Blockade of beta-2 receptors limits bronchiole dilation and therefore can severely compromise pulmonary function in patients with asthma. This has led to development of beta-1 selective antagonists (cardioselective antagonists) such as atenolol (Tenormin) and metoprolol (Lopressor).

Propranolol (Inderal) was the first beta-receptor antagonist approved for clinical use in the United States. Propranolol blocks both beta-1 and beta-2 receptors and is used to treat hypertension, angina, and cardiac arrhythmias. In addition, propranolol is an effective prophylactic in the treatment of migraine headaches, although the mechanisms involved are not clear.

Nadolol (Corgard) was introduced in 1980 as a nonselective beta-receptor antagonist for use in treating angina and hypertension. Additional nonselective beta-receptor antagonists that have been released for clinical use in the United States include labetolol (Trandate, Vescal), penbutolol (Levatol), and pindolol (Visken). Labetolol has alpha- and beta-antagonist action.

Timolol (Trimoptic), betaxolol (Betoptic), levobunolol (Betagan), and metipranolol (OptiPranolol) are beta-receptor antagonists that are effective in treating glaucoma, reducing the production of aqueous humor in the eye. They are discussed with other ophthalmic drugs in Chapter 12. Timolol is also used as an antianginal agent.

Depletion of Peripheral Neuronal Stores of Norepinephrine

Guanethidine (Ismelin) and reserpine (Serpasil) are antihypertensive drugs that deplete norepinephrine from peripheral neurons.

Guanethidine is taken up into the postganglionic sympathetic nerve terminals, where it then prevents the release of norepinephrine. After several days the neuronal content of norepinephrine is depleted. Guanadrel is a more recent drug that has the same mechanism.

Reserpine also causes a depletion of norepinephrine stores not only in the periphery but also in the brain. The central action of reserpine is believed to significantly contribute to the depression of sympathetic tone with this agent.

Reserpine and guanethidine are useful in treating chronic hypertension (see Chapter 15) and Raynaud's disease (see Chapter 14).

Inhibition of Peripheral Sympathetic Activity through an Action in the Central Nervous System

The central nervous system controls sympathetic activity, although the mechanism of this control is not understood. The preceding section indicated that part of the effect of reserpine is believed to be mediated through an action in the central nervous system. It is now recognized that two other antihypertensive drugs, clonidine (Catapres) and methyldopa (Aldomet), decrease sympathetic tone mainly through an action in the central nervous system. Guanabenz (Wytensin) and guanfacine are more recent antihypertensive drugs with the same mechanism. The role of these drugs in the treatment of hypertension is described in Chapter 15.

CHAPTER REVIEW

◆ KEY TERMS.

adrenergic drugs, p. 132
alpha receptors, p. 130
alpha-1 receptors, p. 130
alpha-2 receptors, p. 131
beta receptors, p. 130
beta-1 receptor, p. 131
beta-2 receptors, p. 131
catecholamines, p. 130
cyclic AMP, p. 132

◆ REVIEW QUESTIONS

1. What are the three naturally occurring catecholamines and where are they found?
2. What physiologic actions are associated with stimulation of the alpha-1 adrenergic receptor? With the stimulation of the alpha-2 adrenergic receptor? With the stimulation of the beta-1 adrenergic receptor? With the stimulation of the beta-2 adrenergic receptor? What changes in objective data would you expect to see with each of these?
3. What does the second messenger (cyclic AMP) do?
4. Contrast the mechanism of action of direct- and indirect-acting sympathomimetic drugs.
5. What are the four major drug mechanisms that inhibit adrenergic activity? What therapeutic use is made of each of these actions?

SUGGESTED READING

Andersson DE: Adrenoreceptors—classification, activation and blockade by drugs, *Postgrad Med J* 56(suppl 2):7, 1980.

Dickerson M: Anaphylaxis and anaphylactic shock, *Crit Care Nurse Q* 11(1):68, 1988.

Hancock BG, Eberhard NK: The pharmacologic management of shock, *Crit Care Nurs Q* 11(1):19, 1988.

Hirsch AM: Type A behavior pattern and catecholamine excretion during cardiac catheterization, *West J Nurs Res* 10(3):307, 1988.

Jeffries PR, Shelan SK: Cardiogenic shock: current management, *Crit Care Nurs Q* 11(1):48, 1988.

Johnson GP, Johanson BC: Beta blockers *Am J Nurs* 83(7):1034, 1983.

Mitulsky HJ, Insel PA: Adrenergic receptors in man, *N Engl J Med* 307(1):18, 1982.

Vlietstra RE: Beta-adrenergic blockers—choosing among them, *Postgrad Med J* 76(3):71, 1984.

Wilkins MR, Kendall MH: Clinical and pharmacological considerations in the use of beta blockers in the geriatric patient, *Geriat Med Today* 2(9):99, 1983.

Yacone LA: The nurse's guide to cardiovascular drugs. I. *RN* 51(8):36, 1988.

Yacone LA: The nurse's guide to cardiovascular drugs. II. *RN* 51(9):40, 1988.

SECTION IV

DRUGS AFFECTING SYSTEMS UNDER CHOLINERGIC CONTROL

In this section the cholinergic drug classes are presented within the framework of their major therapeutic targets, the skeletal muscle, the eye, and the gastrointestinal system. This section aims to present the traditional cholinergic drug classes within a systems setting to allow assessment of the therapeutic role of drugs affecting cholinergic mechanisms relative to drugs acting by other mechanisms.

The drug classes in Chapter 11, Drugs to Control Muscle Tone, are the acetylcholinesterase inhibitors and the neuromuscular blocking drugs, so only cholinergic mechanisms are discussed. The drug classes in Chapter 12, Drugs Affecting the Eye, are more diverse, including not only anticholinergic drugs of the atropine type but also adrenergic drugs for pupillary dilation. The discussion of cholinomimetic drugs in treating glaucoma is supplemented by reference to the role of adrenergics, carbonic anhydrase inhibitors, and osmotic diuretics.

In Chapter 13, Drugs Affecting the Gastrointestinal Tract, the role of the cholinergic system is emphasized initially by discussing cholinomimetics to increase and anticholinergics to decrease small intestinal motility. The role of anticholinergic drugs to inhibit stomach acid secretion is discussed, along with the more important roles of antacids to neutralize stomach acid and H_2-receptor antagonists to inhibit stomach acid secretion. Central mechanisms rather than cholinergic mechanisms are cited as the target for drug therapy of nausea and vomiting, which can be considered hyperactivity of the upper gastrointestinal tract. The different roles of antihistamines and the dopamine antagonists are briefly reviewed here but discussed fully in Chapters 24 and 41. Finally, we discuss laxatives and antidiarrheals, the two major drug classes affecting the large intestine. Cholinergic mechanisms play no role in these drug classes. Antidiarrheals rely chiefly on opiate mechanisms to halt hyperactivity, whereas laxatives provide bulk to stimulate activity.

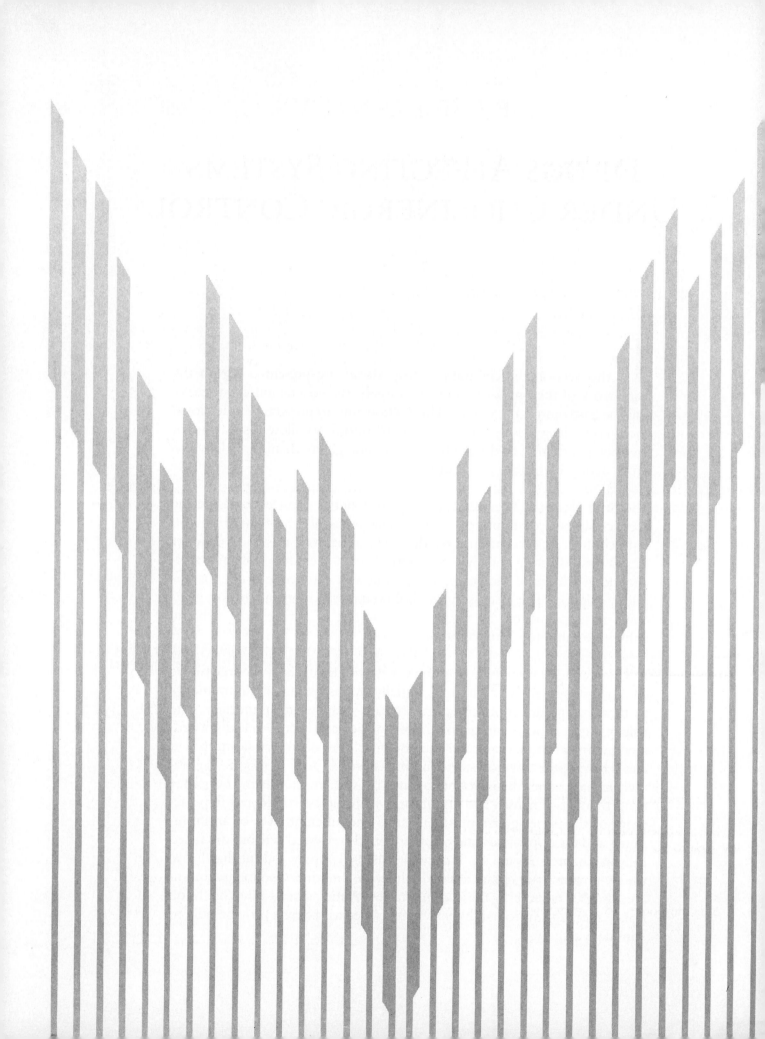

CHAPTER 11

Drugs to Control Muscle Tone

LEARNING OBJECTIVES

After studying this chapter, you should be able to do the following:

◆ Describe the action of acetylcholinesterase inhibitors.

◆ Develop a nursing care plan for patients receiving drug treatment for myasthenia gravis.

◆ Discuss the action of neuromuscular blocking drugs.

◆ Differentiate between nondepolarizing and depolarizing neuromuscular blocking drugs.

◆ Develop a nursing care plan for patients receiving neuromuscular blocking drugs.

CHAPTER OVERVIEW

◆ Motor neurons are single neurons originating in the spinal cord and terminating on the muscle. In this chapter, we discuss two classes of drugs affecting skeletal muscle that act at the neuromuscular junction to affect the neurotransmitter acetylcholine or its receptor. The first class of drugs consists of **acetylcholinesterase inhibitors,** which are indirect-acting cholinomimetic drugs. These drugs are used to diagnose and to treat myasthenia gravis, a disease of muscular weakness, by increasing the quantity of acetylcholine at the neuromuscular junction to restore muscle contraction. The second class of drugs comprises **neuromuscular blocking drugs** that occupy the receptors for acetylcholine on muscles, thus preventing muscle contraction. These drugs produce muscular relaxation for intubation and surgical procedures.

MYASTHENIA GRAVIS

Myasthenia gravis is a disease in which the skeletal muscles quickly show weakness and become fatigued. Muscles controlling facial movements are most commonly involved. One early sign of myasthenia gravis is drooping eyelids (ptosis) (Figure 11-1). As the disease progresses, chewing and swallowing become increasingly difficult, and the voice becomes less distinct. Death can result if the intercostal muscles and the diaphragm, muscles essential for breathing, become affected.

The basic defect in myasthenia gravis is a reduction by 70% to 90% in the available receptors for acetylcholine at the neuromuscular junction. This reduction results from an autoimmune disease. An autoimmune disease is caused by the immune system producing antibodies to a component of the body. Myasthenia gravis is caused by antibodies produced against the neuromuscular receptors for acetylcho-

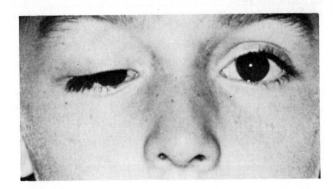

FIGURE 11-1

Myasthenia gravis is often first indicated by drooping eyelid (paresis of levator palpebrae superioris muscle). Only one upper eyelid may be affected. Disease may stay limited to this muscle group.

From Newell FW: Ophthalmology: principles and concepts, ed 7, St Louis, 1992, Mosby–Year Book.

DRUGS THAT MAY WEAKEN A PATIENT WITH MYASTHENIA GRAVIS

Adrenocorticotropic hormone (ACTH) and glucocorticoids
Anesthetics
   Diethyl ether
   Halothane (Fluothane)
   Lidocaine IV (Xylocaine)
Antiarrhythmics
   Procainamide (Pronestyl)
   Propranolol (Inderal)
   Quinidine
Antibiotics
   Bacitracin (Bacitracin)
   Colistimethate (Coly-Mycin M)
   Colistin (Coly-Mycin S)
   Gentamicin (Garamycin)
   Kanamycin (Kantrex)
   Lincomycin (Lincocin)
   Neomycin (Mycifradin, Neobiotic)
   Netilmicin (Nebcin)
   Paromomycin (Humatin)
   Polymyxin B (Aerosporin, Polymyxin B)
   Streptomycin (Streptomycin)
   Viomycin (Viocin)
Anticonvulsants
   Magnesium sulfate
Antimalarials
   Quinine
Diuretics and other drugs or circumstances promoting hypokalemia (low blood potassium concentration)
Muscle relaxants
   Gallamine (Flaxedil)
   Metocurine (Metubine)
   Pancuronium (Pavulon)
   Succinylcholine (Anectine)
   Tubocurarine
Sedatives, especially those with respiratory depressant effects, such as barbiturates, narcotics, and tranquilizers
Thyroid compounds

---

line. These antibodies block the active site for acetylcholine of the neuromuscular (nicotinic) receptor and also increase the rate the receptors are degraded by the cell. A number of drugs are contraindicated for the patient with myasthenia gravis and are listed in the box. These drugs can dangerously weaken the patient with myasthenia gravis but do not noticeably block the neuromuscular receptor of a healthy person.

Nursing Process Overview

DRUGS USED IN MYASTHENIA GRAVIS

Assessment

Patients who have or who are suspected of having myasthenia gravis require acetylcholinesterase inhib-

itors. Symptoms range from mild ptosis and easy fatigue to acute muscular weakness. Assess the temperature, pulse, respiration, blood pressure, vital capacity, ability to swallow, muscle strength, and degree of ptosis. Also assess the patient for additional medical problems that may influence treatment.

Nursing Diagnoses

High risk for ineffective airway clearance related to medication dosage adjustments
High risk for impaired swallowing related to inadequate doses of acetylcholinesterase inhibitors
Anxiety related to frequent swings between myasthenic and cholinergic crises, and apparent inability to obtain adequate drug control of myasthenia gravis

Management

Monitor signs of myasthenia gravis such as ptosis, ability to swallow, vital capacity, muscle strength, and vital signs. Administer medications on time. Keep a suction machine at the bedside if the patient displays any inability to swallow secretions adequately. Keep edrophonium, pyridostigmine, atropine, neostigmine, and syringes at the bedside. Have equipment for intubation readily available. Teach the patient and family about myasthenia gravis management in the home. Refer the patient to other members of the health care team for physical therapy, home nursing care, or social services.

Evaluation

Successful drug therapy helps the patient maintain as normal a lifestyle as possible but does not cure the disease. Patient compliance and understanding are essential to good control of the symptoms. Before discharge the patient should be able to explain how and why the medication should be taken, signs and symptoms of medication overdose and underdose, symptoms that require physician notification, other measures to assist in managing the disease (such as using a nonelectric alarm clock to awaken the patient for nighttime doses of medication), and medications to avoid.

ACETYLCHOLINESTERASE INHIBITORS FOR MYASTHENIA GRAVIS

Mechanism of Action

Drugs that inhibit the degradation of acetylcholine, acetylcholinesterase inhibitors (anticholinesterases), are the first line of treatment for myasthenia gravis. These drugs are listed in Table 11-1. As seen in Figure 11-2, the enzyme acetylcholinesterase is present throughout the neuromuscular junction, where it

Table 11-1 Cholinomimetic Drugs for Myasthenia Gravis

Generic name	Trade name*	Administration/dosage	Comments
Ambenonium chloride	Mytelase	ORAL: *Adults*—5 mg 3 or 4 times daily increased every 1-2 days as required. *Children*—0.3 mg/kg body weight daily in divided doses, increased gradually if necessary to a maximum of 1.5 mg/kg daily.	Mytelase is acetylcholinesterase inhibitor that is rapidly absorbed.
Edrophonium chloride	Tensilon Enlon	For diagnosis of myasthenia gravis: INTRAVENOUS: *Adults*—2 mg injected over 15-30 sec. If no response, 8 mg is given. May repeat test after 1 hr. *Children:* 2 mg initially as above followed by 5 mg (under 75 lb) or up to 10 mg (over 75 lb).	Tensilon is very short-acting acetylcholinesterase inhibitor. Diagnosis is positive if muscle strength increases within 3 min (duration 5 to 10 min).
		To differentiate a myasthenic from a cholinergic crisis: 1 to 2 mg.	Cholinergic crisis if muscle strength decreases (lower medication dose). Patient in cholinergic crisis may require ventilatory assistance after injection.
Neostigmine bromide	Prostigmin bromide	ORAL: *Adults*—15 mg every 3 to 4 hr initially, then adjust upward as required. *Children*—begin with 2 mg/kg body weight daily in divided doses.	Prostigmin bromide is acetylcholinesterase inhibitor with high incidence of side effects.
Neostigmine methylsulfate	Prostigmin methylsulfate	INTRAMUSCULAR: *Adults*—0.022 mg/kg body weight (atropine, intramuscularly, 0.011 mg/kg may be given to control muscarinic side effects). *Children*—0.01 to 0.04 mg/kg body weight (with 0.01 mg/kg atropine, IM).	Prostigmin methylsulfate is injectable form for diagnosis of myasthenia gravis.
Pyridostigmine bromide	Mestinon	ORAL: *Adults*—60 to 120 mg every 3 or 4 hr initially, increased as necessary. *Children*—7 mg/kg in divided doses as required.	Mestinon is acetylcholinesterase inhibitor; it is drug of choice for controlling muscular weakness of myasthenia gravis.
	Regonol	INTRAMUSCULAR, INTRAVENOUS: *Adults*—1/30 of oral dose. *Newborn infants of myasthenic mothers*—0.05 to 0.15 mg/kg body weight.	

*These drugs are available in Canada and United States.

rapidly degrades acetylcholine after release. Acetylcholinesterase inhibitors allow acetylcholine to accumulate at the neuromuscular junction, ensuring that available receptors are activated. Acetylcholinesterase inhibitors used to treat myasthenia gravis are also used to reverse the effects of competitive neuromuscular blocking drugs used in surgery.

Absorption, Distribution, Metabolism, and Excretion

The anticholinesterase drugs used to treat myasthenia gravis are positively charged compounds that are not lipid soluble. These drugs are therefore not readily absorbed orally; the oral dose is 30 times the parenteral dose. The most widely used anticholinesterases are pyridostigmine and neostigmine. The anticholinesterases are metabolized by plasma esterases and by hepatic enzymes to inactive compounds. The drugs and their metabolites are excreted in the urine.

Side Effects

The effective dose must be individualized for each patient. Stress and infection can increase the requirement. Women in the premenstrual part of their cycle may require higher doses. Very ill patients may become unresponsive to their medication, but temporary reduction or withdrawal of the dose over a 3-day period may restore their responsiveness. Parenteral administration may be required.

Side effects arising from overstimulation of neuromuscular (nicotinic) receptors include muscle cramps, rapid small contractions (fasciculations), and

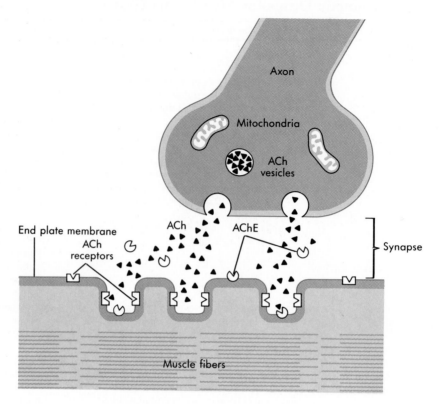

FIGURE 11-2

Acetylcholine is the neurotransmitter released by the nerve to occupy nicotinic receptors on the muscle and thereby initiates biochemical events causing the muscle to contract. Acetylcholine is rapidly degraded by acetylcholinesterase, present throughout the synapse. In myasthenia gravis, the number of receptors is greatly decreased. Acetylcholinesterase inhibitors prevent rapid breakdown of acetylcholine. With more acetylcholine present, fewer receptors are needed, and loss of receptors is partially compensated.

weakness. Acetylcholinesterase inhibitors can also act at sites other than neuromuscular sites. At muscarinic sites, they produce side effects classic for parasympathetic stimulation such as excessive salivation, perspiration, abdominal distress, and nausea and vomiting. Patients frequently develop a tolerance to the muscarinic effects of the anticholinesterases.

Anticholinesterase drugs are contraindicated for patients with intestinal or urinary tract obstruction. These drugs should be used cautiously in patients with bronchial asthma. Individuals sensitive to bromide should be given neostigmine methylsulfate or ambenonium chloride instead of more commonly used bromide-containing anticholinesterases.

Specific Drugs

Ambenonium

Ambenonium (Mytelase) is slightly longer acting than pyridostigmine or neostigmine. Patients may experience side effects not seen with pyridostigmine or neostigmine, such as jitteriness, headaches, confusion, and dizziness. Ambenonium is not a bromide salt, unlike pyridostigmine and neostigmine. It is therefore the drug of choice for patients allergic to bromides.

Edrophonium

Edrophonium (Tensilon) is a short-acting acetylcholinesterase inhibitor used as a diagnostic agent. When a new patient with suspected myasthenia gravis is given 2 mg of edrophonium intravenously, an increase in muscle strength should be seen in 1 to 3 min. If no response occurs, another 4 to 10 mg of edrophonium is given over the next 2 min, and muscle strength is again tested. If no increase in muscle strength occurs with this higher dose, the muscle weakness is not caused by myasthenia gravis. Patients receiving injections of edrophonium commonly show a drop in blood pressure and feel faint, dizzy, and flushed.

A second diagnostic use for edrophonium is to help physicians determine treatment when a patient being treated for myasthenia gravis becomes weaker. The problem is to identify whether the patient is suffering from an overdose of medication (cholinergic crisis) or increasing severity of the disease (myasthenic crisis). An edrophonium injection makes the patient in cholinergic crisis temporarily worse (negative Tensilon test) but temporarily improves the condition when the patient is in myasthenic crisis (positive Tensilon test).

Neostigmine

Neostigmine (Prostigmin) can be used to diagnose and treat myasthenia gravis. As a diagnostic tool, an intramuscular injection of neostigmine should improve the patient's muscular strength in 10 min, and this improvement should last 3 to 4 hr. Neostigmine is also prescribed to relieve the symptoms of myasthenia gravis. Because neostigmine is irregularly absorbed from the gastrointestinal tract, it can be difficult to establish effective drug levels with oral administration. Muscarinic side effects, particularly salivation, cramps, and diarrhea, are common enough to limit the long-term use of neostigmine. If neostigmine is used, atropine may also be prescribed to block the muscarinic effects.

Pyridostigmine

Pyridostigmine (Mestinon) is the drug of choice for the treatment of myasthenia gravis. Compared with neostigmine, pyridostigmine is better absorbed from the gastrointestinal tract and is longer acting. Adverse effects such as miosis, sweating, salivation, gastrointestinal distress, and slow heart rate are less common with pyridostigmine than with neostigmine.

Nursing Process Overview
NEUROMUSCULAR BLOCKING DRUGS
Assessment

As seen in Figure 11-3, neuromuscular blocking drugs produce complete muscle relaxation by preventing muscular contraction. Patients receive neuromuscular blocking drugs when undergoing anesthesia, undergoing diagnostic studies that necessitate brief muscle relaxation, "bucking" ventilators, and undergoing electroconvulsive therapy. Monitor the patient's pulse, respiratory rate, and blood pressure. Assess the patient, focusing on the major problems being treated and the diagnostic or therapeutic procedure to be carried out.

Nursing Diagnoses

Ineffective airway clearance related to drug effect
Anxiety related to inability to swallow, ineffective airway clearance, and weakness

Management

Observe the rate, quality, and depth of respirations and ventilate the patient's airway as needed. Have equipment for intubation and suctioning at the bedside. Use an infusion monitoring device for intravenous administration. Neuromuscular blockade agents alone do not produce anesthesia; medicate the patient for pain if necessary. Position the patient carefully and check to see that instruments and bed linens are not causing unnecessary pressure on the patient's body. After the drug has been administered, it may take minutes to hours for the effect of the neuromuscular blocking agents to wear off. Continue to assess the patient's ability to breathe unassisted, to cough, and to handle secretions. Position the patient on his or her side, and keep the side rails up. Do not leave the patient unattended until he or she can adequately cough, handle secretions, and call for help.

Evaluation

These agents are successful if they produce sufficient muscle relaxation to allow the procedure or activity to proceed. These are all short-acting drugs and are not prescribed for use outside a hospital setting.

NEUROMUSCULAR BLOCKING DRUGS: OVERVIEW
Mechanism of Action

Neuromuscular blocking drugs produce complete muscle relaxation by binding to the receptor for acetylcholine at the neuromuscular junction. The nondepolarizing or competitive blockers bind to the receptor without initiating depolarization of the muscle membrane. The depolarizing drug also binds to the receptor for acetylcholine but does cause depolarization of the muscle membrane. Since the depolarizing drug does not readily dissociate from the receptor, depolarization persists. Larger doses of the depolarizing drug also desensitize the receptor to restimulation. Both types of blockade, nondepolarizing and depolarizing, result in muscle paralysis. The neuromuscular blocking drugs can be differentiated by the response to an injection of a drug such as edrophonium, which inhibits the degradation of acetylcholine by acetylcholinesterase. As concentration of acetylcholine rises in the neuromuscular junction, a nondepolarizing drug is displaced and muscle tone is regained. The depolarizing drug is not displaced. Table 11-2 summarizes neuromuscular blocking drugs and their administration.

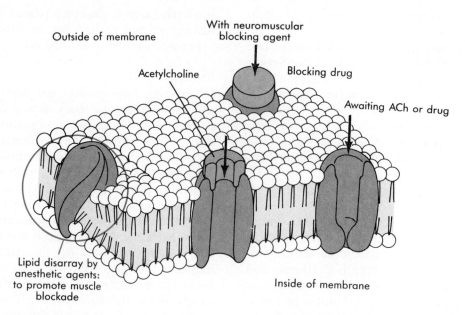

Outside of membrane

With neuromuscular blocking agent

Acetylcholine

Blocking drug

Awaiting ACh or drug

Lipid disarray by anesthetic agents: to promote muscle blockade

Inside of membrane

FIGURE 11-3

Neuromuscular blocking drugs block receptor, preventing acetylcholine from binding to receptor and opening channel. Anesthesia caused by neuromuscular blocking drugs differs from lipid disarray caused by general anesthetic drugs.

Therapeutic Uses

Since neuromuscular blockers can produce complete paralysis, they are administered only to anesthetized patients. Assisted ventilation should be available for short-acting succinylcholine and is mandatory when administering longer-acting neuromuscular blockers. Skeletal muscle relaxants do not inhibit pain. Neuromuscular blocking drugs provide muscle relaxation during surgery, particularly relaxation of the abdominal muscles, without using deep general anesthesia, which would relax abdominal muscles by depressing the spinal cord. Neuromuscular blockers are also used with light anesthesia to allow a tube to be passed down easily to the trachea (endotracheal intubation), to relieve spasm of the larynx, to prevent convulsive muscle spasms during electroconvulsive therapy for depression, and to allow breathing to be controlled totally by a respirator (controlled ventilation) during surgery.

Nondepolarizing Drugs

Tubocurarine

Tubocurarine (curare) was originally isolated as the active principle of the South American arrow poison. An animal hit with an arrow containing curare falls paralyzed a short time later.

Uses. Tubocurarine produces muscle relaxation during surgery or electroconvulsive shock therapy,

reduces muscle spasm in tetanus, and allows controlled ventilation. Administer by slow (60 to 90 sec) intravenous injection. Maximal paralysis occurs within 5 min and persists for 60 min (range: 25 to 90 min). The progression of paralysis begins with the eyelids, then the face, the extremities, and finally the diaphragm, resulting in the cessation of spontaneous breathing. Recovery from neuromuscular blockade can be assisted by injecting edrophonium, neostigmine, or pyridostigmine to increase the amount of acetylcholine at the neuromuscular junction.

Excretion. About 40% of tubocurarine is excreted unchanged in the urine. Patients with renal failure or acidosis excrete tubocurarine less rapidly and require a smaller dose.

Side effects. Tubocurarine can cause release of histamine, which causes hypotension or bronchospasm (see Chapter 24). Hypotension can arise from ganglionic blockade by tubocurarine. Tubocurarine does not cross the placenta or blood-brain barrier.

Drug interactions. Many anesthetics potentiate the action of tubocurarine, including halothane, ether, methoxyflurane, and enflurane. Antibiotics potentiating the action of tubocurarine include the aminoglycosides and the polymyxins (see Chapter 33), bacitracin, lincomycin, and clindamycin. Other drugs that potentiate the action of tubocurarine are the antiarrhythmic drugs, quinidine, the ganglionic blocker

Table 11-2 Neuromuscular Blocking Drugs

Generic name	Trade name	Administration/dosage	Comments
NONDEPOLARIZING (COMPETITIVE) DRUGS			
Atracurium	Tracrium*	INTRAVENOUS: *Adults*—0.3 to 0.6 mg/kg body weight; subsequent doses, 0.05 to 0.1 mg/kg.	Drug is not affected by renal or hepatic impairment and is relatively free of cardiovascular side effects. Doses given are for use with nitrous oxide. Other inhalation anesthetics may require smaller doses.
Doxacurium chloride	Nuromax	INTRAVENOUS: *Adults*—For endotracheal intubation, 0.05 mg/kg body weight will provide 100 min relaxation; after succinylcholine-assisted endotracheal intubation, 0.025 mg/kg body weight to provide 60 min relaxation; maintenance requires 0.005 mg/kg body weight for relaxation. *Children*—0.03 mg/kg body weight initially for halothane anesthesia to provide 30 min relaxation.	Drug does not increase heart rate. Adult doses must be decreased by third if used with enflurane, halothane, or isoflurane anesthesia. Doses for geriatric patients or patients with hepatic or renal disease may need to be reduced. Ideal body weight should be used for obese patients.
Gallamine triethiodide	Flaxedil* triethiodide	INTRAVENOUS: *Adults*—1 to 1.15 mg/kg body weight. Supplemental doses, 0.3 to 1.2 mg/kg. *Children*—2.5 mg/kg initially with 0.3 to 1.2 mg/kg supplemental doses. *Newborns*—up to 1 month of age, 0.25 to 0.75 mg/kg initially, with 0.1 to 0.5 mg/kg supplemental doses.	Drug may cause increased heart rate. Drug is not used for patients in renal failure. Doses given are for use with nitrous oxide. Other inhalation anesthetics may require smaller doses.
Metocurine iodide	Metubine*	INTRAVENOUS: *Adults*—0.1 to 0.3 mg/kg body weight. Supplemental doses, 0.02 to 0.03 mg/kg.	See tubocurarine chloride. Doses given are for use with nitrous oxide. Other inhalation anesthetics may require smaller doses. Drug is not for use in patients with renal failure.
Pancuronium bromide	Pavulon*	INTRAVENOUS: *Adults and children*—0.04 to 0.1 mg/kg body weight initially with 0.01 to 0.02 mg/kg supplemental doses. Newborns may be very sensitive; use a test dose of 0.02 mg.	Drug does not cause hypotension. Drug may stimulate heart rate and cardiac output. Doses given are for use with nitrous oxide. Other inhalation anesthetics may require smaller doses.
Tubocurarine chloride (curare)	Tubarine† Tubocurarine chloride*	INTRAVENOUS: *Adults and children*—0.2 to 0.4 mg/kg body weight initially. Supplemental doses, 0.04 to 0.2 mg/kg. Diagnosis of myasthenia gravis: 1/15 to 1/5 of above dose.	Intravenous injection should be slow (1 to 1½ min). Do not combine with alkaline intravenous barbiturate solutions. Doses given are for use with nitrous oxide. Other inhalation anesthetics may require smaller doses.
Vecuronium	Norcuron*	INTRAVENOUS: *Adults*—0.07 to 0.14 mg/kg body weight for intubation; 0.04 to 0.1 mg/kg initially, followed by 0.015 to 0.02 mg/kg as needed for surgery.	Drug related to pancuronium but shorter (by third to half) in duration. Drug is relatively free of cardiovascular side effects. Doses given are for use with nitrous oxide. Other inhalation anesthetics may require smaller doses.
DEPOLARIZING DRUGS			
Succinylcholine chloride	Anectine* Quelicin* Sucostrin	INTRAVENOUS: *Adults*—0.6 to 1.1 mg/kg body weight initially. Continuous infusion, 0.1% or 0.2% solution at a rate of 0.5 to 10 mg/min. *Children*—1.1 mg/kg body weight initially with 0.3 to 0.6 mg/kg supplemental doses. *Newborns*—2 mg/kg. Continuous infusion is not recommended for children and newborns.	Duration is only 5 min because of hydrolysis by plasma cholinesterase. This enzyme is missing genetically in some patients, and prolonged action is seen. Drug may cause cardiac arrhythmias. Doses given are for use with nitrous oxide. Other inhalation anesthetics require smaller doses.

*Available in Canada and United States.
†Available in Canada only.

drugs, trimethaphan, and magnesium sulfate. Since patients with myasthenia gravis have an exaggerated response to tubocurarine, very small doses of tubocurarine can be used to diagnose myasthenia gravis if tests with edrophonium or neostigmine are inconclusive.

Atracurium

Atracurium (Tracrium) is a nondepolarizing muscle relaxant. It is shorter in duration than tubocurarine, producing adequate relaxation for 15 to 20 min. Atracurium is inactived by hydrolysis. At usual doses, atracurium does not produce cardiovascular side effects.

Doxacurium

Doxacurium (Nuromax) is a new long-acting drug with minimal cardiovascular effects, desirable features for use in patients with coronary disease.

Gallamine triethiodide

Gallamine triethiodide (Flaxedil) is a synthetic drug similar in action to tubocurarine but with a shorter duration of action. Gallamine does not cause histamine release or ganglionic blockade. The major side effect of gallamine is an increase in heart rate (tachycardia), which is seen a few minutes after injection and then declines. Gallamine is excreted unchanged in the urine; do not use it in patients with renal failure.

Metocurine (dimethyl tubocurarine) iodide

Metocurine iodide (Metubine), a semisynthetic derivative of tubocurarine, is two to three times as potent as tubocurarine but otherwise similar. Metocurine is excreted unchanged in the urine and should not be used in patients with renal failure.

Mivacurium

Mivacurium, an investigational drug, has a fast onset of action and is short acting. It does not accumulate since it is rapidly broken down by cholinesterases in the plasma.

Pancuronium bromide

Pancuronium bromide (Pavulon) has a faster onset of action than tubocurarine, although the duration of action is similar. Pancuronium does not cause the histamine release or ganglionic blockade characteristic of tubocurarine. Heart rate, cardiac output, and atrial pressure are increased by pancuronium, effects that may be desired in cardiac surgery. Pancuronium is excreted in the urine, and doses must be decreased for patients with renal failure.

Pipecuronium bromide

Pipecuronium (Ardvan) has a long duration of action and is used for procedures lasting 90 min or longer. Pipecuronium has no vagal blocking action to cause tachycardia, so it can be used in the presence of coronary artery disease in which tachycardia can be dangerous.

Vecuronium

Vecuronium (Norcuron) is a nondepolarizing muscle relaxant chemically related to pancuronium. Vecuronium is shorter acting than pancuronium, and its effects are not cumulative with repeated administration. Unlike tubocurarine, the cardiovascular side effects arising from ganglionic or vagal blockade, interference with norepinephrine reuptake, or release of histamine are minimal with vecuronium. Vecuronium's intensity and duration of action are affected significantly by liver damage and modestly by renal failure.

Depolarizing Neuromuscular Blocking Drug

Succinylcholine chloride

Succinylcholine chloride (Anectine and others) has the briefest duration of action (5 min) of the neuromuscular blocking drugs, since plasma cholinesterases readily degrade succinylcholine. Longer action requires continuous infusion of succinylcholine, but then care must be taken to avoid desensitizing the muscle. The duration of action is increased by drugs that inhibit cholinesterases. Some patients have abnormal plasma cholinesterases that do not readily degrade succinylcholine. In these patients, the action of succinylcholine is prolonged. Conditions that elevate plasma potassium concentration, such as burns, tetanus, massive trauma, or brain or spinal cord injury prolong the action of succinylcholine.

Uses. Succinylcholine's short duration of action makes it a drug of choice for endoscopy, terminating laryngospasm, endotracheal intubation, orthopedic procedures, and electroconvulsive shock therapy.

Side effects. Children are not as sensitive to succinylcholine on a weight basis as adults and require higher doses. Children are more apt to show side effects of succinylcholine resulting from parasympathetic stimulation such as slow heart rate (bradycardia) and cardiac arrhythmias. Succinylcholine does not cross the blood-brain barrier or the placenta.

Succinylcholine initially causes fasciculations before the muscles are paralyzed. This is believed to cause the stiffness and soreness many patients experience 12 to 24 hr after they have received succinylcholine. Succinylcholine also transiently raises intraocular pressure and must be administered before eye surgery.

NURSING IMPLICATIONS SUMMARY

Drugs for Diagnosis and Treatment of Myasthenia Gravis

Drug administration

◆ Assess patients for signs of myasthenic crisis (inadequately treated myasthenia gravis) such as positive Tensilon test; increased blood pressure and pulse; difficulty chewing, swallowing, and coughing; bladder and bowel incontinence; increasing ptosis; difficulty breathing; and cyanosis. Differentiate symptoms of myasthenic crisis from those of cholinergic crisis (overtreated myasthenia gravis) such as negative Tensilon test; abdominal cramps, diarrhea; fasciculations; nausea, vomiting; and blurred vision. The following may be seen in myasthenic or cholinergic crisis: generalized weakness; increased salivation, tearing, and bronchial secretions; general feeling of apprehension; restlessness; and difficulty breathing. Have a suction machine at the bedside.

◆ Keep edrophonium, pyridostigmine, atropine, neostigmine, and syringes and have a tourniquet at the patient's bedside or in a convenient place on the patient care unit for rapid treatment of a myasthenic or cholinergic crisis.

◆ Assess the patient's ability to swallow before preparing an ordered oral dose of acetylcholinesterase inhibitor. If the ability to swallow is deteriorating, it may be necessary to administer a parenteral dose of medication. Ideally, written orders should be obtained for oral and parenteral doses of acetylcholinesterase inhibitors so that time is not lost if the patient can no longer safely swallow.

◆ Schedule off-unit diagnostic studies and therapies for the patient with myasthenia gravis so that medication administration is not delayed while the nurse waits for the patient to return. If the patient is not present when a medication is due, take the dose of the medication to the patient.

◆ Regularly assess blood pressure, pulse, vital capacity, presence and degree of ptosis, muscle strength, and ability to swallow as indicators of adequate drug control.

◆ When neostigmine is used as an antidote for tubocurarine, administer via slow intravenous push. Continue appropriate ventilatory support until the patient is breathing well unassisted. If the pulse is less than 80 beats/min, administer atropine before the neostigmine. For constant infusion of acetylcholinesterase inhibitors, use a volume control device and microdrip tubing. Monitor respiratory and cardiovascular status.

Patient and family education

◆ Teach patients and families about the signs and symptoms of myasthenia gravis, myasthenic crisis, and overdose with acetylcholinesterase inhibitors.

◆ The patient and family should also be taught that medications must be taken exactly as ordered. Forgetting, omitting, or doubling a dose of medication may cause the patient's condition to deteriorate.

◆ No medication, whether prescription or over-the-counter, should ever be taken without the approval of the physician. In addition, give the patient a list of drugs known to be contraindicated for patients with myasthenia gravis (see p. 142). Suggest that patients plan a medication schedule that includes taking doses of acetylcholinesterase inhibitors 30 to 60 min before meals to increase strength for chewing and swallowing. Take acetylcholinesterase inhibitors with milk or a snack to reduce gastric irritation. Use a reliable, nonelectric alarm clock to wake the patient for early morning or nighttime doses of medication.

◆ Keep careful watch on supplies of drugs on hand, and refill prescriptions before they run out. Reinforce to patients and families the need to seek medical assistance immediately if the patient's condition seems to be deteriorating. Encourage patients to wear a medical identification tag or bracelet and to carry a list of the names and doses of medication being taken. Refer patients and families to local, state, or national myasthenia gravis support groups.

Continued.

NURSING IMPLICATIONS SUMMARY—cont'd

Neuromuscular Blocking Agents

Drug administration

◆ Monitor blood pressure, pulse, and respirations and auscultate lungs. Monitor arterial blood gases and electrocardiogram. Use these drugs only in settings where personnel and equipment are available to provide immediate intubation. Have a suction machine, oxygen, mechanical ventilator or resuscitation bag, and resuscitation equipment and drugs handy.

◆ Remember that these drugs cause paralysis but not anesthesia. Unless patients are also anesthetized, they can still hear, feel, and see, if the eyelids are opened. Remember to remain professional in discussions within the patient's hearing, to talk about sounds in the environment and anticipated nursing care activities, and to use television or radio judiciously. Arrange for uninterrupted periods so that the patient can sleep.

◆ If the patient is not anesthetized, avoid rough handling, position the patient in a comfortable position, offer backrubs if possible, and medicate for pain if appropriate. Keep the reversing agent or antagonist readily available. When administering these drugs via constant infusion, a microdrip tubing set and an infusion controlling device should be used.

◆ Consult the manufacturer's literature for specific guidelines regarding calculation of dosage. In many institutions, induction with a neuromuscular blocking agent must be done by the anesthesiologist or nurse anesthetist; follow agency guidelines.

◆ When discontinuing therapy, do not leave the patient unattended until sufficient muscle tone has returned so that the patient can breathe, handle secretions, and call for assistance if needed. In infants, assess for the ability to hold the eyelids open or to hold up the legs. Keep the side rails up and the call bell within reach.

◆ These drugs are not used for home management. Keep the patient and family informed of the patient's condition.

CHAPTER REVIEW

◆ **KEY TERMS**

acetylcholinesterase inhibitors, p. 141

myasthenia gravis, p. 141

neuromuscular blocking drugs, p. 141

◆ **REVIEW QUESTIONS**

1. Contrast the mechanisms by which acetylcholinesterase inhibitors increase activation of the neuromuscular junction and neuromuscular blockers inhibit activation at the neuromuscular junction.

2. What muscarinic side effects of neostigmine and pyridostigmine would you observe? Which drug would you administer as an antidote for neostigmine?

3. Describe two diagnostic uses of edrophonium you might administer.

4. Develop a teaching plan for the patient taking anticholinesterases.

5. Contrast the mechanism of the depolarizing and the nondepolarizing neuromuscular blocking drugs. How could you differentiate between these actions after administering edrophonium?

6. List the nondepolarizing neuromuscular blocking drugs.

7. List the depolarizing neuromuscular blocking drugs.

8. Describe the uses of tubocurarine you would encounter.

9. What genetic alteration do some patients have that prolongs the action of succinylcholine? What supportive actions would you take?

10. How would you assess the patient's ability to handle secretions?

SUGGESTED READING

Bevan DR: Residual neuromuscular blockade, *Curr Rev Nurse Anesth* 12(25):203, 1990.

Bevan DR: Residual neuromuscular blockade, *Post Anesth Care Nurses* 12(7):51, 1990.

Booij LHD: Neuromuscular blockade, *Curr Rev Nurse Anesth* 10(1):3, 1987.

Bruton-Maree N: Neuromuscular blocking drugs, *J Neurosci Nurs* 21(3):198, 1989.

Cronnelly R: Why, when, and how to reverse muscle relaxants, *Curr Rev Nurse Anesth* 13(7):50, 1990.

Hagen NA: Action stat! Myasthenic crisis, *Nurs 91* 21(6):33, 1991.

O'Brien DD: Review and update of neuromuscular blocking agents, *Crit Care Nurse* 9(10):76, 1989.

Van Sickel AD, Spadaccia KI: Muscle relaxants and reversal agents, *Crit Care Nurse Clin North Am* 3(1):151, 1991.

CHAPTER 12

Drugs Affecting the Eye

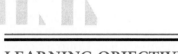

After studying this chapter, you should be able to do the following:

- Define *miosis, mydriasis,* and *cycloplegia,* and give examples of when they are therapeutically produced.
- Discuss the use of anticholinergic drugs for the eye.
- Differentiate between chronic and acute glaucoma.
- Discuss categories of drugs to treat glaucoma, including cholinomimetic drugs, adrenergic drugs, beta blockers, carbonic anhydrase inhibitors, and osmotic agents.

- From a list of drugs used in the treatment of glaucoma, develop a teaching plan to prepare patients for discharge.

- The key functions of the eye are controlled by the autonomic nervous system. Selected drugs with autonomic actions are used in eye examinations, eye surgery, and glaucoma treatment. These ophthalmic drugs are presented in this chapter.

Nursing Process Overview
DRUGS TO TREAT EYE CONDITIONS
Assessment

Patients requiring treatment of eye conditions may have no visible signs of their condition. Assess the patient, focusing on symptoms related to the eye. Check peripheral vision and test visual acuity using a Snellen chart. Question patients about recent difficulties driving or ambulating at home; such difficulties might include tripping or bumping into objects. Examine the eyes for signs of infection, exudate, excessive tearing or dryness, or other deviations.

Nursing Diagnoses

High risk for injury related to impaired vision secondary to the specific eye problem

Altered home maintenance management related to insufficient knowledge about eye medications, their use, or their instillation

Management

The drugs discussed in this chapter are used to assist evaluation of eye problems or to treat glaucoma (elevated intraocular pressure). Other eye medications include antibiotics, glucocorticoids, and lubricants. Caution patients about side effects, particularly those related to vision. Blurred vision, photophobia, and other symptoms can be frightening when they occur without warning. Teach patients about possible systemic side effects.

Evaluation

Drugs used to assist in diagnostic evaluation of the eye are successful if they aid in the examination without producing serious side effects. Drugs used to treat glaucoma are successful if the intraocular pressure is lowered to within safe limits. Before discharge, check that the patient can explain why the drug is being used, demonstrate how to administer the drug correctly, explain potential local and systemic side effects, list the signs and symptoms requiring medical evaluation, and explain the need for continuing therapy as ordered.

AUTONOMIC NERVOUS SYSTEM

The **autonomic nervous system** plays a major role in controlling the amount of light entering the eye and in focusing images. The amount of light penetrating the eye is controlled by the size of the pigmented iris, which contains two sets of muscles, the sphincter and dilator muscles. The sphincter muscles are circular muscles with muscarinic receptors innervated by the parasympathetic nervous system. As shown in Figure 12-1, the pupil is constricted when the sphincter muscles contract so that only a small surface on the eye transmits light. The dilator muscles contain alpha receptors innervated by the sympathetic nervous system. *Miosis* refers to a constricted pupil and is achieved primarily by stimulating the musca-

rinic receptors of the sphincter muscles. *Mydriasis* refers to a dilated pupil and is achieved by blocking the muscarinic receptors of the sphincter muscles or by stimulating the alpha receptors of the dilator muscles.

The cornea and the lens determine the focus of images onto the retina. The cornea accomplishes the coarse focusing, but the fine focusing for sharp images and near vision is accomplished by the lens. The shape of the lens is controlled by muscarinic receptors of the parasympathetic nervous system. As diagrammed in Figure 12-1, the accommodation for near vision requires the contraction of ciliary muscles to change the shape of the lens. Ligaments normally pull the lens to keep it relatively flat. Contraction of the ciliary muscles relaxes the ligaments so that the lens becomes rounder as required for near vision. *Cycloplegia* refers to the paralysis of the ciliary muscles by drugs that block muscarinic receptors. Cyclo-

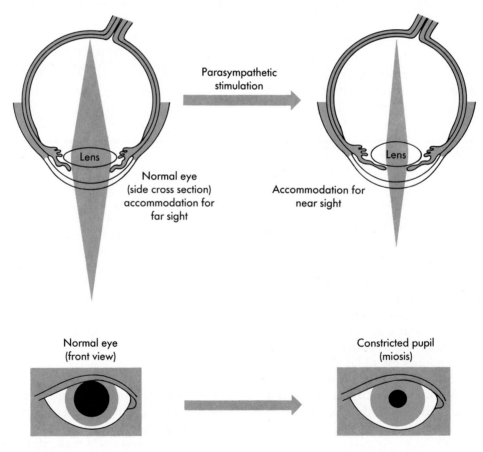

Parasympathetic stimulation

Lens

Normal eye (side cross section) accommodation for far sight

Lens

Accommodation for near sight

Normal eye (front view)

Constricted pupil (miosis)

FIGURE 12-1

Effects of parasympathetic nervous system on eye are mediated through muscarinic receptors. **A,** Pupil is made smaller because circular muscles contract. **B,** Accommodation is made by contracting muscles to thicken lens.

plegia causes blurred vision, since the shape of the lens can no longer be adjusted to near vision.

ANTICHOLINERGIC DRUGS
Actions

Classic anticholinergic actions include dilated pupils (mydriasis) and blurred vision (cycloplegia). Accurate measurement of lens refraction requires both actions. The relaxation of sphincter and ciliary muscles when anticholinergic drugs are instilled into the eye hastens healing of inflammatory conditions, especially after eye surgery. Atropine, scopolamine, and homatropine are used for treatment (Table 12-1).

Side Effects

Anticholinergic drugs used ophthalmically are applied directly to the eye. Systemic reactions may nevertheless occur when the drug is absorbed into the body, particularly with atropine. Systemic reactions are associated with anticholinergic effects such as dry mouth and dry skin, fever, thirst, confusion, and hyperactivity. Children are the most prone to systemic toxicity from ophthalmic drugs.

Specific Drugs
Atropine

Atropine (Atropair and others) is the drug of choice for use in children because it is potent and long acting and children have an active accommodation. Mydriasis may last 12 days, although accommodation usually returns in 6 days. Since atropine is applied for 3 days, watch children for systemic reactions and discontinue application if any reactions appear. Atropine is also used before surgery, often with phenylephrine, to produce mydriasis, and for other conditions requiring prolonged mydriasis. Atropine may cause contact dermatitis of the eyelids.

Cyclopentolate

Cyclopentolate (Cyclogyl) is a rapidly acting mydriatic and cycloplegic drug. It is effective in 25 to 75 min, and accommodation returns in 6 to 24 hr. Cyclopentolate is used as for aiding refraction, for ophthalmoscopy, and for preoperative mydriasis. Systemic reactions have been reported. A combination of cyclopentolate and phenylephrine (Cyclomydril) is used and is the combination of choice for use with premature infants.

Homatropine

Homatropine (AK-Homatropine) is applied 2 or 3 times at 10-min intervals to produce mydriasis and cycloplegia, which are achieved in 60 min. Recovery may take 2 days.

Scopolamine

Scopolamine (Isopto Hyoscine) is a potent mydriatic and is used like atropine, but cycloplegia lasts for only 3 instead of 6 days. Scopolamine can be used in patients who are allergic to atropine.

Tropicamide

Tropicamide (Mydriacyl) acts rapidly, taking effect in 20 to 35 min. Accommodation returns in 2 to 6 hr. Systemic side effects are rare.

ADRENERGIC DRUGS

The adrenergic drugs phenylephrine and hydroxyamphetamine are used as mydriatics when only the interior structures of the eye are examined and cycloplegia is not required (see Table 12-1).

Phenylephrine

Phenylephrine (Neo-Synephrine) acts on the alpha receptors of the dilator muscles to produce mydriasis. Dilation is maximal in 60 to 90 min, and recovery occurs in 6 hr. Cyclomydril is a combination of cyclopentolate and phenylephrine used when maximal dilation is required.

Hydroxyamphetamine

Hydroxyamphetamine (Panedrine) is an indirect-acting alpha-adrenergic drug that acts by releasing neuronal stores of norepinephrine. Dilation is maximal in 45 to 60 min, and recovery occurs in 6 hr.

PROSTAGLANDIN INHIBITORS

Flurbiprofen (Ocufen) and Suprofen (Profenal) are nonsteroidal antiinflammatory drugs specifically for ophthalmic use (see Table 12-1). Ophthalmic surgery may stimulate the synthesis of prostaglandins in the eye. **Prostaglandins** are chemical transmitters synthesized in response to stimulation, locally in tissues. In the eye, newly synthesized prostaglandins cause a miosis that resists the mydriatic action of atropine. The locally applied nonsteroidal antiinflammatory drugs prevent miosis during surgery.

GLAUCOMA
Characteristics

Glaucoma is the increase in intraocular pressure as a result of fluid accumulation between the lens and the cornea. The space between the lens and cornea is filled with aqueous humor. Aqueous humor is a protein-poor fluid formed by the ciliary body. As illustrated in Figure 12-2, this fluid is normally reabsorbed through the trabecular spaces into Schlemm's canal in a region of the cornea called the *anterior chamber*. If the aqueous humor cannot be reabsorbed through the anterior chamber, the fluid accumulates

Table 12-1 Drugs for Mydriasis and Cycloplegia

Drug	Trade name	Administration/dosage	Comments
ANTICHOLINERGIC DRUGS FOR MYDRIASIS AND CYCLOPLEGIA			
Atropine sulfate	Atropine Sulfate* Atropisol* Isopto Atropine* Minims Atropine† Others	Topical solutions, 0.5% to 3% *Adults*—1 drop of 1% to 3% solution to each eye. Frequency of administration depends on condition being treated. *Children*—1 drop of 0.125 to 0.5% solution (under 8 yr) or 0.25 to 1% solution (over 8 yr) 3 times daily for 3 days before and once on morning of day refraction is measured. Duration: 6 days	For children, for refraction measurements For adults, to relax eye muscles during surgery or treatment of eye inflammation, to aid in eye surgery or treatment of eye inflammation
Cyclopentolate hydrochloride	AK-Pentolate* Cyclogyl* I-Pentolate Minims Cyclopentolate† Pentolair Others	Topical solutions, 0.5%, 1%, and 2% *Adults*—1 drop of solution in each eye, repeated after 5 min. Darker irises or children require the stronger solutions. *Children*—1 drop of solution in eye, repeated after 10 min. Onset: 25–75 min Duration: 6–24 hr	To aid in measuring refraction
Homatropine hydrobromide	AK-Homatropine Isopto Homatropine* I-Homatropine† Spectro-Homatropine	Topical solutions, 2% and 5% *Adults*—for refraction 1 drop of 5% solution every 10 min 2 or 3 times Duration: 2 days	To aid in refraction measurements in adults; to aid in treating mild eye inflammation
Scopolamine hydrobromide	Isopto Hyoscine Hydrobromide	Topical solutions, 0.2% to 0.3% *Adults*—1 drop of solution or ointment to each eye, 1 or more times daily depending on condition being treated. *Children*—1 drop of 0.2% to 0.25% solution or ointment twice daily for 2 days before refraction measurement Duration: 3 days	For children, to measure refraction For adults, to treat eye inflammation
Tropicamide	I-Picamide Mydriacyl* Minims Tropicamide† Tropicadyl Others	Topical solutions, 0.5% and 1%. 1 drop in each eye, repeated in 5 min Onset: 20 to 35 min Duration: 2 to 6 hr	To aid in measuring refraction
ADRENERGIC DRUGS FOR MYDRIASIS ONLY			
Hydroxyamphetamine hydrobromide	Paredrine	Topical use, 1 drop of 1% solution	To obtain maximum mydriasis in 45 to 60 min To obtain recovery in 6 hr
Phenylephrine hydrochloride	Minims Phenylephrine† Mydfrin Neo-Synephrine Hydrochloride* Others	Topical use, 1 drop of 2.5% solution	To obtain maximum mydriasis in 60 to 90 min To obtain recovery in 6 hr
Prostaglandin inhibitors			
Flurbiprofen sodium	Ocufen	TOPICAL: 1 drop instilled every 30 min beginning 2 hr before surgery; total dose, 4 drops	To prevent miosis during surgery (Nonsteroidal antiinflammatory drug is applied topically.)
Suprofen	Profenal	TOPICAL: 2 drops are applied 3, 2, and 1 hr before surgery. 2 drops may be applied every 4 hr during waking hours day before surgery	To prevent miosis during surgery (Nonsteroidal antiinflammatory drug is applied topically.)

*Available in Canada and United States.
†Available in Canada only.

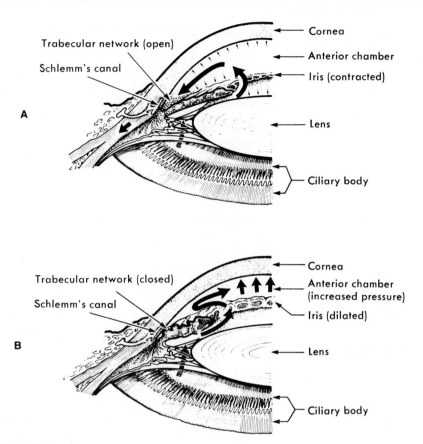

FIGURE 12-2

A, Normal eye or eye with chronic glaucoma. Flow of aqueous humor is shown from ciliary body and around iris. Aqueous humor is normally absorbed into body through trabecular network into Schlemm's canal. In chronic glaucoma, aqueous humor accumulates because trabecular network degenerates. **B,** Eye in acute glaucoma. Flow of aqueous humor is stopped because iris has blocked trabecular network and Schlemm's canal. Aqueous humor can accumulate quickly to cause marked rise in ocular pressure that may damage optic nerve.

and intraocular pressure increases. If the intraocular pressure is not relieved, the optic nerve becomes damaged, resulting in blindness.

Chronic (open-angle) glaucoma is the more common form of glaucoma and is very gradual in its onset. The defect is a slow degeneration of the anterior chamber that impairs the uptake of aqueous humor (see Figure 12-2). Traditionally, drug therapy, applied as eyedrops, has been used to improve the uptake of aqueous humor and thereby lower intraocular pressure. Argon laser treatment is an effective method for treating the drainage area to improve fluid outflow. Recent studies indicate that laser treatment may be the preferred first treatment for glaucoma. Laser treatment appears safe and although it may not eliminate the need for drugs, the amount of medication needed is greatly reduced.

Table 12-2 lists drugs to treat glaucoma. The initial drug therapy for chronic glaucoma is the application of a weak cholinomimetic drug to cause miosis. Therapeutic effectiveness results from the spread of the trabecular spaces of the anterior chamber when the sphincter muscles contract. The larger area allows improved uptake of the aqueous humor, which relieves intraocular pressure.

The adrenergic drug epinephrine is the alternative drug to initiate therapy or the next drug added when the miotic drug alone is inadequate. Epinephrine stimulates alpha and beta receptors. In the eye, stimulation of alpha receptors reduces resistance to the outflow of aqueous humor, whereas stimulation of the beta receptors decreases production of aqueous humor.

The adrenergic beta-blocking drug timolol may

Table 12-2   Drugs to Treat Glaucoma

Generic name	Trade name	Administration/dosage	Comments
CHOLINOMIMETIC DRUGS (WEAK MIOTICS)			
Carbachol	Isopto Carbachol* Miostat*	TOPICAL: 1 drop 0.75% to 3% solution every 8 hr Onset: 15 to 30 min	Carbachol is direct-acting cholinomimetic and miotic for treating chronic glaucoma.
Physostigmine salicylate Physostigmine sulfate	Isopto Eserine Eserine Sulfate	TOPICAL: 1 drop of 0.25% to 1% every 4 to 6 hr Ointment for night use primarily Onset: 30 min	Physostigmine salicylate and sulfate are acetylcholinesterase inhibitors and miotics for chronic glaucoma; conjunctivitis and allergic reactions are common if use is prolonged.
Pilocarpine hydrochloride	Isopto Carpine* Pilocar Various others	TOPICAL: 1 drop, 1% to 2% every 6 to 8 hr Onset: 15 to 30 min Ocular insert: 1 system inserted every 7 days	Pilocarpine hydrochloride is direct-acting cholinomimetic and miotic; it is drug of choice for acute and chronic glaucoma.
Pilocarpine nitrate	P.V. Carpine† Liquifilm Pilagan	TOPICAL: 1 drop, 1% to 2% every 6 to 8 hr Onset: 15 to 30 min	Pilocarpine nitrate is direct-acting cholinomimetic and miotic; it is drug of choice for acute and chronic glaucoma.
CHOLINOMIMETIC DRUGS (STRONG MIOTICS)			
Demecarium bromide	Humorsol	TOPICAL: 1 drop 0.125% to 0.25% solution every 12 to 48 hr Onset: 12 hr	Demecarium bromide is irreversible acetylcholinesterase inhibitor; it is potent miotic for resistant chronic glaucoma. Cataracts can develop with long-term administration.
Echothiophate iodide	Phospholine Iodide*	TOPICAL: 1 drop 0.03% to 0.06% every 12 to 48 hr Onset: 12 hr	Same as for demecarium.
Isofluorphate	Floropryl	TOPICAL: ¼ in strip of 0.025% ointment every 12 to 72 hr Onset: 12 hr	Same as for demecarium.
ADRENERGIC DRUGS			
Apraclonidine hydrochloride	Iopidine	Instillation of 1 drop in affected eye 1 hour before laser surgery; repeated immediately before surgery	Apraclonidine hydrochloride controls or prevents acute, transient spikes in intraocular pressure after laser surgery for glaucoma.
Dipivefrin	Propine*	TOPICAL: 1 drop into conjunctival sac every 12 hr for glaucoma	Dipivefrin is converted to epinephrine by esterases in cornea and anterior chamber.
Epinephrine bitartrate	Epitrate*	TOPICAL: 1 drop of a 0.25% to 2.0% solution 1 or 2 times daily	Persons with darkly pigmented irises may require higher concentration of solution.
Epinephrine borate	Epinal* Eppy	Same as epinephrine bitartrate	
Epinephrine hydrochloride	Epifrin* Glaucon*	Same as epinephrine bitartrate	

*Available in Canada and United States.
†Available in Canada only.

Table 12-2   Drugs to Treat Glaucoma—cont'd

Generic name	Trade name	Administration/dosage	Comments
BETA BLOCKERS			
Betaxolol hydrochloride	Betoptic*	TOPICAL: 1 drop of a 0.5% solution twice daily	This cardioselective (beta-1) beta-adrenergic antagonist has been developed for use in glaucoma.
Levobunolol	Betagan*	TOPICAL: 1 drop of a 0.5% solution once or twice daily	Levobunolol is nonselective beta-adrenergic antagonist.
Metipranolol	Opti-Pranolol	TOPICAL: 1 drop 2 times a day	New beta-adrenergic antagonist to treat glaucoma.
Timolol maleate	Timoptic* Apo-Timop†	TOPICAL: 1 drop of 0.25% solution twice daily; if not sufficient, 0.5% solution is used	Timolol maleate is nonselective beta-adrenergic antagonist.
CARBONIC ANHYDRASE INHIBITORS			
Acetazolamide	Acetazolam† AK-Zol Apo-Acetazol-amide† Diamox* Others	ORAL: *Adults*—250 mg every 6 hr. *Children*—10 to 15 mg/kg body weight daily in divided doses; timed-release capsules taken every 12 to 24 hr but may not be as effective	Acetazolamide is weak diuretic.
Acetazolamide sodium	Diamox, Parenteral*	INTRAVENOUS, INTRAMUSCULAR: *Adults*—500 mg repeated in 2 to 4 hr if necessary. *Children:* 5 to 10 mg/kg body weight every 6 hr	
Dichlorphenamide	Daranide	ORAL: *Adults*—50 to 200 mg every 6 to 8 hr	
Methazolamide	Neptazane*	ORAL: *Adults*—25 to 100 mg every 8 hr	
OSMOTIC AGENTS			
Glycerin	Glyrol Osmoglyn	ORAL: *Adults and children*—1 to 1.5 gm/kg body weight as 50% or 75% solution once or twice daily	Nurse may flavor glycerin with instant coffee or lemon juice to increase palatability. Nurse may chill it with chipped ice. Glycerin may cause hyperglycemia in diabetic patients.
Isosorbide dinitrate	Iso-Bid Isordil* Others	ORAL: *Adults*—1.5 gm/kg body weight up to 4 times daily	Nurse may chill it with chipped ice.
Mannitol	Osmitrol*	INTRAVENOUS: *Adults and children*—0.5 to 2 gm/kg body weight as a 20% solution infused over 30 to 60 min	Nurse may discontinue it when intraocular pressure is decreased, even though full dose has not been given.
Urea	Ureaphil	INTRAVENOUS: *Adults*—0.5 to 2 gm/kg body weight as a 30% solution infused at 60 drops/min. *Children*—0.5 to 1.5 gm/kg body weight of a 30% solution infused over 30 min.	Urea should be infused carefully. Patients with hereditary fructose intolerance should not be given urea made up in invert sugar.

*Available in Canada and United States.
†Available in Canada only.

also be used initially to treat chronic glaucoma or may be applied in addition to the miotic and epinephrine. The mechanism by which blockade of the beta receptors of the eye decreases intraocular pressure is not clear, particularly since stimulation of the beta receptor also causes reduction of intraocular pressure.

The drugs discussed previously are all applied directly to the eye. In resistant cases of glaucoma, systemic drugs are added. A carbonic anhydrase inhibitor is the next drug added because, aside from being weak diuretics, carbonic anhydrase inhibitors are also effective in decreasing the production of aqueous humor.

Osmotic agents such as glycerin, isosorbide, urea, or mannitol provide an immediate but short-term reduction in intraocular pressure by drawing fluid from the eyeball to the hyperosmotic blood.

Acute (closed-angle) glaucoma is characterized by the iris bulging up to shut off access of the aqueous humor to the anterior chamber (see Figure 12-2). This creates an emergency because the buildup of intraocular pressure may rapidly become severe, damaging the optic nerve and causing blindness. Emergency treatment consists of a cholinomimetic drug, a carbonic anhydrase inhibitor, epinephrine, and an osmotic diuretic. This drug regimen provides transient treatment while the patient is being prepared for eye surgery in which the iris is cut to allow fluid access to the anterior chamber once again.

Cholinomimetic (Miotic) Drugs to Treat Glaucoma

Pilocarpine

Pilocarpine (P.V. Carpine, Ocusert Pilo-20/Pilo-40 Systems, Pilopine HS Gel) is the drug of choice for chronic and acute glaucoma. It is a direct-acting cholinomimetic that is active 15 to 30 min after application and lasts 4 to 8 hr. Since pilocarpine is the weakest of the cholinomimetic drugs used, it is the

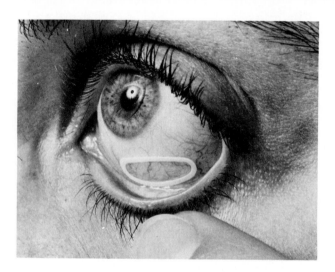

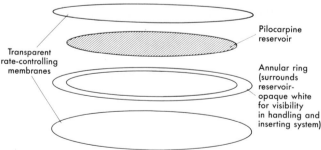

FIGURE 12-3

Ocusert ocular therapeutic system for delivery of pilocarpine for treatment of glaucoma. Flexible wafer is placed under eyelid and provides drug for week. Eyelid is shown displaced to expose device. Expanded view denotes purpose of each component.

Courtesy ALZA Corp.

least likely to produce side effects, although it must be applied more frequently.

The Ocusert system has been devised to overcome the need for frequent application of pilocarpine. The system is placed in the upper or lower cul-de-sac of the eye (Figure 12-3). Pilocarpine is contained in a reservoir between two membranes and is released over 1 week. Drawbacks include occasional sudden leakage of pilocarpine, migration of the system over the cornea, and unnoticed loss of the system. An aqueous gel of pilocarpine provides another long-acting preparation. One application is effective in reducing intraocular pressure for 18 to 24 hr. A persistent superficial corneal haze may develop in about 30% of patients.

Carbachol

Carbachol (Carbacel) is also a direct-acting cholinomimetic agent. It is more potent and slightly longer acting than pilocarpine.

Physostigmine

Physostigmine (Eserine) is a short-acting acetylcholinesterase inhibitor now only rarely used to treat chronic glaucoma. Physostigmine is poorly tolerated with prolonged treatment, since it commonly causes conjunctivitis and allergic reactions. The ointment may cause depigmentation of the eyelids in blacks.

Demecarium, echothiophate, and isoflurophate

The potent acetylcholinesterase inhibitors, Demecarium (Humorsol), echothiophate (Phospholine), and isoflurophate (Floropryl), are used to treat chronic glaucoma that does not respond to the combination of a weak miotic, epinephrine, and timolol. The effect of these acetylcholinesterase inhibitors is not seen for about 24 hr, but a single application is effective for 12 to 72 hr. Unfortunately, side effects are frequent with these miotics. They can cause congestion in the blood vessels of the ciliary body, resulting in a rise in intraocular pressure. For this reason, they are seldom used to treat acute glaucoma. Spasms may be produced in the muscles of the eyelid and the eye itself, resulting in twitching of the eyelids or eyebrows, ocular pain, and headaches.

Additional Drugs to Treat Glaucoma

Epinephrine

Epinephrine (Glaucon) stimulates alpha- and beta-adrenergic receptors to increase uptake of aqueous humor and to decrease production of aqueous humor, respectively. When applied directly to the eye in the treatment of chronic glaucoma, epinephrine produces a fall in intraocular pressure that lasts 12 to 24 hr. Mydriasis is transient. Epinephrine may be used as the initial therapy for glaucoma in young patients, who may suffer spasms of the ciliary muscles controlling accommodation if a miotic is used, and in elderly patients with cataracts, whose vision is compromised by small pupils. Highly pigmented eyes are more resistant to epinephrine than lightly pigmented eyes.

Side effects. Epinephrine can cause browache and eye irritation. With prolonged use, epinephrine can cause swelling of the eyelids and bloodshot eyes. Symptoms of systemic absorption of epinephrine include fast heart rate (tachycardia), high blood pressure, headache, sweating, and tremors.

Dipivefrin hydrochloride

Dipivefrin (dipivalyl epinephrine) (Propine) is a prodrug that is inactive but is converted to epinephrine by esterases in the cornea and anterior chamber of the eye. Dipivefrin is more lipid soluble than epinephrine and therefore concentrates in the eye more readily than epinephrine.

Apraclonidine

Apraclonidine (Iopidine) is an alpha-adrenergic agonist that acts by reducing intraocular aqueous formation. Apraclonidine prevents acute, transient spikes in intraocular pressure after laser surgery for glaucoma. The drug is administered 1 hr before surgery and again just before surgery. Side effects can include upper lid elevation, conjunctival blanching, and mydriasis.

Beta blockers

Beta-adrenergic receptor blockers are effective in lowering intraocular pressure. In many patients, however, drug effectiveness decreases with time. Although there are many beta blockers, only four have proved suitable for ophthalmic use, betaxolol (Betoptic), levobunol (Betagan), metipranolol (Opti-Pranolol), and timolol (Timoptic). Most beta blockers produce corneal anesthesia, which leads to corneal damage. The major advantage of beta blockers is that pupil size nor reactivity to light is altered. Some irritation and blurred vision may occur at the start of therapy, but these effects usually disappear.

Side effects. Betaxolol, levobunol, and timolol may produce systemic effects after absorption into the circulation. The most common effects are a decrease in heart rate (bradycardia) and a fall in blood pressure, effects expected with a drug that blocks beta-1 adrenergic receptors. Bronchospasm resulting from blockade of the beta-2 adrenergic receptors has also been reported. Since betaxolol is selective for beta-1 receptors, it is preferred for patients with pulmonary problems. Betaxolol is also associated with less severe systemic cardiac effects.

Carbonic anhydrase inhibitors. Carbonic anhydrase inhibitors used to treat glaucoma include acetazolamide (Diamox), dichlorphenamide (Daranide), and methazolamide (Neptazane). Although carbonic anhydrase inhibitors are weak diuretics, their effective action in treating glaucoma is to decrease the formation of aqueous humor. A fall in intraocular pressure is seen only in individuals with glaucoma. The fall in intraocular pressure is negligible in individuals with normal ocular pressure.

Carbonic anhydrase inhibitors are taken orally and are maximally effective in 2 hr. The duration of action is 6 to 12 hr. Carbonic anhydrase inhibitors may be added to glaucoma therapy when the combination of a weak miotic, epinephrine, and timolol does not adequately lower the intraocular pressure of chronic glaucoma. Carbonic anhydrase inhibitors are also used with a miotic and epinephrine to lower intraocular pressure in acute (closed-angle) glaucoma.

Side effects. Carbonic anhydrase inhibitors have unpleasant side effects, including appetite loss, gastrointestinal upset, and lethargy and depression. A tingling sensation (paresthesia) in the fingers, toes, and face is common. Carbonic anhydrase inhibitors commonly produce slight hypokalemia early in treatment; thus caution should be used in treating patients who are receiving digitalis.

Osmotic agents

The osmotic agents are used as short-term treatment only to lower the intraocular pressure of glaucoma before surgery or as an emergency treatment of acute (closed-angle) glaucoma. Glycerin and isosorbide are administered orally, whereas mannitol and urea are administered intravenously.

Glycerin. Glycerin (Glyrol, Osmoglyn) lowers intraocular pressure 1 hr after ingestion, and the effect lasts 5 hr. Since glycerin is metabolized, it does not cause diuresis; however, glycerin can cause hyperglycemia in patients who have diabetes. Headache, nausea, and vomiting are additional side effects of glycerin.

Isosorbide

Isosorbide (Ismotic) is used sometimes in the emergency treatment of acute (closed-angle) glaucoma. Isosorbide does produce diuresis but otherwise has few side effects.

Mannitol. Mannitol (Osmitrol) is effective in lowering intraocular pressure in 30 to 60 min, with the effect lasting 6 to 8 hr. Mannitol produces a pronounced diuresis and often causes headache, nausea and vomiting, and dehydration.

Urea. Urea (Ureaphil, Urevert) is less satisfactory than mannitol because it can penetrate the eye and cause a rebound increase in intraocular pressure when the systemic osmotic effect is over, 8 to 12 hr after administration. Urea is also highly irritating on injection.

NURSING IMPLICATIONS SUMMARY

General Guidelines for Use of Eye Medications

Drug administration

◆ Wash hands carefully before administering eye medications to avoid contaminating the eye or applicator. Wash hands after administering eye medications to rinse off any residue that might accidentally be rubbed into your eye. Use a separate bottle or tube of medication for each patient to avoid accidental cross-contamination; wash hands between patients.

◆ Place ordered dose of eye medication in the lower conjunctival sac, never directly onto the cornea. Avoid touching any part of the eye with the dropper or applicator. For additional information on administration, see Chapter 6.

◆ To prevent overflow of medication into nasal and pharyngeal passages, thus reducing systemic absorption, occlude or teach the patient to occlude the nasolacrimal duct with one finger for 1 to 2 min after instilling the medication.

◆ When two or more eye medications are administered, wait at least 3 minutes between drugs. Administer drops or liquid preparations before ointments. Administer glucocorticoid preparations before other drugs. If in doubt, consult the physician. Use atropine and the belladonna alkaloids cautiously in elderly patients, since these drugs may precipitate an acute glaucoma attack.

◆ Monitor the pulse of patients receiving beta blockers and teach patients to do the same.

NURSING IMPLICATIONS SUMMARY—cont'd

If the pulse is below 50 to 60 beats/min in an adult, withhold the next dose of medication and notify the physician. Reassess whether the patient is occluding the nasolacrimal duct correctly after administration of each dose. Use 1 drop of a 1% or 2% epinephrine solution to reverse the redness caused by potent acetylcholinesterase inhibitors; consult the physician.

◆ Use pralidoxime (PAM), 0.1 to 0.2 ml of a 5% solution, to reverse the action of the irreversible acetylcholinesterase inhibitors. PAM must be injected subconjunctivally to be effective in the eye (see Chapter 9).

◆ Glycerin may cause hyperglycemia. Monitor blood glucose levels, especially in diabetic persons.

◆ See Chapter 16 for additional information about carbonic anhydrase inhibitors.

Patient and family education

◆ Teach the patient how to instill medication correctly and supervise instillation until the patient can do it safely (see section on drug administration and Chapter 6). Teach the patient to read labels carefully to ensure administration of correct drug and correct strength. Remind the patient to keep these drugs out of the reach of children.

◆ Warn patient to avoid driving or operating hazardous equipment if vision is blurred. Tell adults that they may be unable to drive home after eye examinations in which medications to dilate the pupil (mydriatics) or drugs to paralyze the ciliary muscle (cycloplegics) were used; a friend or family member should drive until the effects of the medication wear off.

◆ If photophobia occurs, instruct patients to wear sunglasses and avoid bright lights. Tell patients not to wear sunglasses after dusk.

◆ Instruct patients to administer missed doses as soon as they are remembered, unless within 1 to 2 hr of the next dose. Tell patients not to double up for missed doses.

◆ Patients should lie down if headache occurs after doses of glycerin. To make doses of glycerin or isosorbide more palatable, chill them over crushed ice. Flavor glycerin with instant coffee or lemon juice.

◆ Teach patients with glaucoma that it cannot be cured, only controlled. Reinforce the importance of using medications to treat glaucoma as prescribed and not to discontinue these medications without consulting the physician. Drugs used to treat glaucoma may cause pain and blurred vision, especially when therapy is begun. Tell patients that this may diminish with time. Tell patients to try cold compresses to relieve painful eye spasm.

◆ In infants, atropine eye drops may contribute to abdominal distension. Teach caregivers to keep a record of bowel movements of infants. In the health care setting, auscultate bowel sounds of infants and children receiving atropine eye drops.

◆ Instruct patients to report the development of any eye irritation. Teach patients using eye gel to store the gel at room temperature or in the refrigerator but not to freeze it. Discard unused gel kept at room temperature after 8 weeks. After each use, wipe the tip of the tube with tissue and replace the cap tightly.

◆ Soft contact lenses may absorb certain eye medications, and preservatives in eye medications may discolor the contact lenses. Tell patients wearing contact lenses to question the physician carefully about special precautions to observe.

SUSTAINED-RELEASE FORMS

Teach patients to review carefully the instruction sheet provided by the manufacturer. The eye system is inserted into the upper or lower cul-de-sac of the eye, and the drug is released slowly; it should be replaced weekly. Tell patients to check each morning and evening to make sure the system is still in place. If the unit does not seem to be working, is damaged, or is releasing too much medication, remove it and insert a new one. Since vision may change in the first few hours after the eye system is inserted, teach patients to replace it at bedtime. Teach patients to store the eye system in the refrigerator but to avoid freezing it.

CHAPTER REVIEW

◆ KEY TERMS

acute (closed-angle) glaucoma, p. 158

autonomic nervous system, p. 152

chronic (open-angle) glaucoma, p. 155

cycloplegia, p. 152

glaucoma, p. 153

miosis, p. 152

mydriasis, p. 152

prostaglandins, p. 153

◆ REVIEW QUESTIONS

1. Explain what you would observe in a patient given a drug to produce miosis, mydriasis, or cycloplegia.

2. What would you observe when anticholinergic drugs are applied to the eye? How are these actions medically useful?

3. Which anticholinergic drugs might you administer in the eye?

4. What action is mediated by the alpha-adrenergic receptor in the eye? Which drugs might you administer for this effect?

5. Describe glaucoma and the role of aqueous humor.

6. Differentiate between chronic and acute glaucoma.

7. How are cholinomimetic drugs used to treat glaucoma? Which drugs might you administer in the treatment of glaucoma?

8. What role do drugs acting at adrenergic receptors play in the treatment of glaucoma? Describe the actions of epinephrine and timolol.

9. How are carbonic anhydrase inhibitors and osmotic agents used to treat glaucoma?

10. How would you determine whether a patient is administering ordered eye medications correctly?

11. When two or more eye medications are ordered to be given at the same time, what are the guidelines for the sequence of administrations?

12. What are the abbreviations for left eye, right eye, and both eyes that may be used when eye medications are ordered? (See Chapter 7.)

SUGGESTED READING

Everitt DE, Avorn J: Systemic effects of medications used to treat glaucoma, *Ann Intern Med* 112(2):120, 1990.

CHAPTER 13

Drugs Affecting the Gastrointestinal Tract

LEARNING OBJECTIVES

After studying this chapter, you should be able to do the following:

- Discuss the use of drugs in the five categories covered in this chapter, including drugs to alter gastrointestinal tone and motility, treat ulcers, control vomiting, control diarrhea, and relieve constipation.

- Develop a care plan for patients receiving the following drugs or drug groups: bethanechol, metoclopramide, antacids, anticholinergic drugs, histamine H₂-receptor antagonists, sucralfate, misoprostol, scopolamine, antihistamines, antidopaminergic drugs, cannabinoids; paregoric, codeine and other opioids, loperamide, and bismuth salts for diarrhea; and bulk-forming agents, stimulants, saline cathartics, wetting agents, and lubricants for constipation; and lactulose.

- Develop a teaching plan for patients who have xerostomia, constipation, or diarrhea.

CHAPTER OVERVIEW

♦ The gastrointestinal (GI) system processes food and water and eliminates undigestible material. The parasympathetic (cholinergic) nervous system stimulates the digestive processes by increasing digestive secretions and the tone and motility of the smooth muscle of the stomach and intestines. The sympathetic (adrenergic) nervous system plays a minor role in the digestive processes. The autonomic controls are illustrated in Figure 13-1. Although the parasympathetic nervous system acts on all parts of the digestive tract, current research is uncovering a complex system in which activities in each segment of the digestive tract are further regulated by a variety of peptide hormones, prostaglandins, and the biogenic amines histamine and serotonin. The roles of only a few of these factors are well characterized.

♦ This chapter focuses on specific conditions affecting the GI tract for which there are pharmacologic interventions. The five sections of this chapter cover drugs that alter GI tone and motility, treat ulcers, control vomiting and diarrhea, and relieve constipation.

SECTION I: DRUGS ALTERING GASTROINTESTINAL MOTILITY

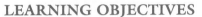

Nursing Process Overview
DRUGS TO INCREASE GASTROINTESTINAL TONE AND MOTILITY
Assessment

Drugs to increase tone and motility are used after trauma or surgery to treat atonic intestines or bladder, and after barium has been used for radiologic examination. They are also used to treat diabetic gastroparesis. Assess the patient to rule out any obstruction of the bladder or intestine. Also assess vital signs, check for the presence of bowel sounds, check intake and output, palpate the bladder for distension, and check patency of urinary catheters.

Nursing Diagnoses

Altered comfort related to abdominal cramps or diarrhea

Diarrhea related to drug action or side effect

Management

After administering bethanechol or neostigmine, remain at the patient's bedside for 15 min to observe for side effects. Side effects often occur with subcutaneous bethanechol. Have the antidote atropine readily available before bethanechol is administered. After the drug is administered, monitor vital signs and measure output. If side effects become serious,

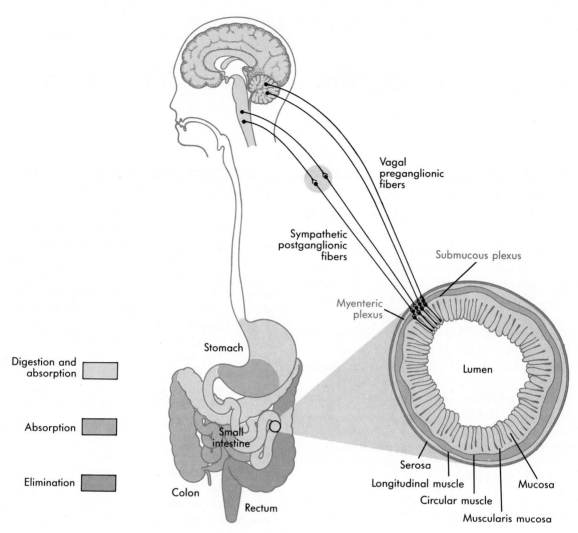

FIGURE 13-1

Overall functions of gastrointestinal tract. Autonomic nervous system modulates longitudinal musculature of small intestine. Small intestine also has complex intrinsic autonomic system controlling circular musculature and secretion.

notify the physician or consider administering atropine (0.6 mg). If administering metoclopramide intravenously, remain at the bedside; oral administration produces much slower effects.

Evaluation

These drugs are effective if they enhance the patient's ability to defecate or urinate. Some patients require only one or two doses, whereas other patients require continued use of these drugs. Before discharging a patient, assess the patient's knowledge of how to take the drug correctly, anticipated effects, possible side effects and what to do about them, and symptoms requiring medical attention.

Specific Drugs to Increase Gastrointestinal Motility

The cholinomimetic drugs listed in Table 13-1 play a minor role in the treatment of GI disorders. Occasionally, bethanechol or neostigmine is administered to stimulate an atonic intestine or bladder. Metoclopramide is a newer drug that stimulates the GI tract, but it is not a cholinomimetic drug.

Table 13-1   Drugs Increasing Gastrointestinal Tone and Motility

Generic name	Trade name	Administration/dosage	Comments
Bethanechol chloride	Urecholine* Duvoid* Urabeth	ORAL: *Adults*—10 to 30 mg every 6 to 8 hr SUBCUTANEOUS: *Adults*—2.5 to 5 mg every 6 to 8 hr; maximum, 10 mg/day. Never give intravenously or intramuscularly Onset: 30 min	Direct-acting cholinomimetic that stimulates atonic bladder and GI tract
Metoclopramide	Reglan* Clopra Emext Others	INTRAVENOUS: *Adults*—10 mg injected over 1 to 2 min. *Children under 6 yr*—0.1 mg/kg body weight. *Children 6 to 14 yr*—2.5 to 5.0 mg/kg ORAL: *Adults*—10 mg 4 times daily, 30 min before bedtime. *Children under 6 yr*—0.1 mg/kg as single dose. *Children 6 to 16 yr*—0.5 mg/kg daily in 3 divided doses	Dopamine antagonist that hastens gastric emptying in diabetic gastroparesis and after barium administration
Neostigmine methylsulfate	Prostigmin methylsulfate*	SUBCUTANEOUS, INTRAMUSCULAR: *Adults*—0.25 to 0.5 mg every 3 to 4 hr to stimulate bladder or GI tract Onset: 10 to 20 min	Acetylcholinesterase inhibitor that stimulates atonic bladder and GI tract

*Available in Canada and United States.

Bethanechol

Bethanechol (Urecholine) is the only direct-acting cholinomimetic drug with sufficient tissue specificity to be administered systemically. At therapeutic doses, bethanechol is relatively specific for the urinary and GI tracts. This stimulation is useful for situations in which the bladder or intestine has lost its tone, such as after childbirth, surgery, or other abdominal trauma. Side effects of bethanechol are expected from muscarinic stimulation such as salivation, flushing of the skin, sweating, diarrhea, nausea and belching, and abdominal cramps.

Bethanechol should never be administered if there is any mechanical obstruction of the GI or urinary tract, such as stones or adhesions, because the hypermotility caused by the drug could lead to rupture of the tissue in the presence of an obstruction. Also, bethanechol is never administered intravenously or intramuscularly because the rate of absorption is so fast that toxic plasma concentrations of the drug are reached, resulting in possible heart block or a severe drop in blood pressure. Bethanechol may be administered subcutaneously if the oral route is not effective.

Metoclopramide

Metoclopramide (Reglan) is a dopamine antagonist, not a cholinomimetic drug. However, it sensitizes the GI tissues to the action of acetylcholine, and this action is abolished by anticholinergic drugs. Metoclopramide stimulates motility of the upper GI tract without stimulating gastric, biliary, or pancreatic secretions. The tone and amplitude of gastric contractions are increased, as is peristalsis of the small intestine, so that gastric emptying and intestinal transit times are increased. These actions are useful in treating diabetic gastroparesis, a condition in which stomach tone is lost and contents are not emptied readily into the intestine. Metoclopramide also facilitates intubation of the small intestine for biopsy and stimulates gastric emptying and intestinal transit of barium in radiologic examinations.

About 10% of patients experience side effects of metoclopramide, including restlessness, drowsiness, fatigue, and lassitude. Sedation is intensified with the concurrent use of alcohol, tranquilizers, sleeping medications, or narcotic analgesics. Metoclopramide is contraindicated in patients with mechanical obstruction, perforation, or possible hemorrhage of the GI tract. An increase in GI motility poses danger for such patients. Anticholinergic drugs and narcotic analgesics inhibit GI tone and thereby antagonize the action of metoclopramide.

Neostigmine

Neostigmine (Prostigmin) is a reversible acetylcholinesterase inhibitor prescribed for its muscarinic and neuromuscular effects (see Chapter 11). Neostigmine may be given subcutaneously or intramuscularly in place of bethanechol to restore bladder or intestinal tone. If urination does not occur within 1 hr, a catheter should be inserted.

Nursing Process Overview
DRUGS TO DECREASE GASTROINTESTINAL TONE AND MOTILITY
Assessment
Assess the patient with attention to vital signs, any subjective complaints, frequency and character of stools, and presence of occult blood in the stool.

Nursing Diagnoses
Colonic constipation related to drug side effects
Altered oral mucous membranes related to dry mouth produced as a drug side effect

Management
These drugs are used with dietary management and other therapies. Continue to monitor the patient's subjective complaints and vital signs and to assess the patient for side effects. Anticholinergic drugs and related compounds produce side effects if administered in effective dosages. Assist patients in dealing with unpleasant side effects (e.g., sucking on hard candy for treatment of dry mouth). Monitor intake and output and assess for constipation. Watch for central nervous system (CNS) effects such as restlessness, tremor, or irritability, which may indicate a need to reduce the drug dose.

Evaluation
These drugs are effective if the patient complains of fewer symptoms or the signs of ulcer disease disappear. Before discharge, patients should be able to explain why and how to take the medications, which side effects will probably occur, how to treat these side effects, which symptoms warrant medical attention, and how to carry out related therapies such as dietary modification for treatment of ulcer disease.

ANTICHOLINERGIC AND ANTISPASMODIC DRUGS TO DECREASE GASTROINTESTINAL TONE AND MOTILITY

A number of anticholinergic and antispasmodic drugs have been developed to decrease GI tone and motility. **Anticholinergic drugs** (drugs that block muscarinic receptors) inhibit gastric acid secretion and depress GI motility. These drugs, listed in Table 13-2, are useful in treating a peptic ulcer or hyperactive bowel disorders.

Table 13-2 lists atropine and its derivatives and the synthetic anticholinergic drugs used to depress gastric acid secretion in treating peptic ulcers. Homatropine and the synthetic drugs are charged compounds that do not cross the blood-brain barrier to act in the CNS. Oxyphencyclimine, an uncharged synthetic compound, is the exception.

Common side effects of anticholinergic drugs include dry mouth (see box), photophobia from dilated pupils (mydriasis), blurred vision (cycloplegia), fast heart rate (tachycardia), constipation, and acute urinary retention. If patients do not have a dry mouth, they are not getting a dose large enough to suppress acid secretion.

Toxic doses of the uncharged anticholinergic drugs atropine (and its L-isomer, hyoscyamine) and oxyphencyclimine reach the CNS and produce CNS stimulation such as restlessness, tremor, irritability, delirium, or hallucinations. Toxic doses of the charged anticholinergic drugs that do not reach the CNS cause ganglionic blockade (usually seen as orthostatic hypotension) or neuromuscular blockade. Death can result from respiratory arrest secondary to neuromuscular blockade.

Table 13-2 also lists drugs that have antispasmodic but not anticholinergic effects. These drugs relax the smooth muscle of the GI tract and are used to treat hyperactivity or spasm of the intestine. Their side effects are not as prominent as those reported for the anticholinergic drugs. Side effects reported include constipation or diarrhea, rash, euphoria, dizziness, drowsiness, headache, nausea, and weakness.

PATIENT PROBLEM: DRY MOUTH

THE PROBLEM

Some drugs produce an excessively dry mouth, or **xerostomia.** This may cause discomfort, trauma to the mouth, bad breath, and potential for injury to the oral mucosa.

SIGNS AND SYMPTOMS

Dry oral mucous membranes, bad breath, mouth feels dry and sticky.

MEASURES TO DECREASE PATIENT DISCOMFORT

Perform thorough, regular oral hygiene, with teeth brushing

Rinse mouth with a pleasant tasting rinse or normal saline (dissolve 1 tsp of salt in 1 pt water)

Sip water frequently

Suck on sugarless hard candy or chew sugarless gum

Avoid drying mouthwashes (those containing alcohol)

Avoid lemon-glycerin swabs for oral hygiene

Keep lips moist with lip moisturizer

Keep environmental air moist with a humidifier

Consider using a commercially available saliva substitute

Table 13-2 Drugs to Decrease Tone and Motility

Generic name	Trade name	Administration/dosage	Comments
BELLADONNA ALKALOIDS (uncharged)			
Atropine sulfate		ORAL, SUBCUTANEOUS: *Adults*—0.3 to 1.2 mg every 4 to 6 hr. SUBCUTANEOUS: *Children*—0.01 mg/kg every 4 to 6 hr.	Atropine sulfate reduces GI motility and gastric acid secretion and reduces tone of the bladder and ureter.
Belladonna extract		ORAL: *Adults*—15 mg every 8 hr.	As above. Atropine is active ingredient.
Belladonna fluid extract		ORAL: *Adults*—0.06 ml every 8 hr.	As above. Atropine is active ingredient.
Belladonna leaf		ORAL: *Adults*—30 to 200 mg.	As above. Atropine is active ingredient.
Belladonna tincture		ORAL: *Adults*—0.6 to 1 ml every 6 to 8 hr. *Children*—0.03 ml/kg in 3 or 4 divided doses.	As above. Atropine is active ingredient.
Hyoscyamine hydrobromide (L-isomer of atropine)		ORAL, INTRAMUSCULAR, SUBCUTANEOUS, INTRAVENOUS: *Adults*—0.25 mg every 6 to 8 hr.	As above. Atropine is active ingredient.
Hyoscyamine sulfate	Anaspaz Levsin Cytospaz	ORAL: *Adults*—0.125 to 0.25 mg every 4 to 6 hr. *Children*—2 to 10 yr, ½ adult dosage; under 2 yr, ¼ adult dosage. INTRAMUSCULAR, SUBCUTANEOUS, INTRAVENOUS: *Adults*—0.25 to 0.5 mg every 4 to 6 hr.	As above. Atropine is active ingredient.
Scopolamine butylbromide	Buscopan†	ORAL: *Adults*—10 to 20 mg 3 or 4 times daily. INTRAMUSCULAR, INTRAVENOUS, SUBCUTANEOUS: *Adults*—10 to 20 mg 3 or 4 times daily.	Elderly patients are more sensitive to scopolamine.
Scopolamine hydrobromide		INTRAMUSCULAR, INTRAVENOUS, SUBCUTANEOUS: *Adults*—0.3 to 0.6 mg as a single dose.	Elderly are more sensitive to scopolamine.
CHARGED DERIVATIVES OF ATROPINE			
Homatropine methylbromide	Homapin	ORAL: *Adults*—2.5 to 10 mg every 6 hr. *Children*—3 to 6 mg every 6 hr. *Infants*—0.3 mg dissolved in water every 4 hr.	Homatropine methylbromide reduces GI hypermotility and gastric acidity
Methscopolamine bromide	Pamine	ORAL: *Adults*—2.5 to 5 mg every 6 hr. *Children*—0.2 mg/kg every 6 hr. INTRAMUSCULAR, SUBCUTANEOUS: *Adults*—0.25 to 1 mg every 6 to 8 hr. Onset: 1 hr.	Methscopolamine bromide reduces GI hypermotility and gastric acidity.
SYNTHETIC SUBSTITUTES FOR ATROPINE			
Anisotropine methylbromide	Valpin	ORAL: *Adults*—50 mg 3 times daily. Onset: 1 hr.	Anisotropine methylbromide treats GI spasms and controls gastric acid secretion.
Clidinium bromide	Quarzan	ORAL: *Adults*—2.5 to 5 mg 3 or 4 times daily before meals and at bedtime. Reduce dosage to 2.5 mg 3 times daily before meals for elderly patients.	Clidinium bromide controls gastric acidity and hypermotility.

*Available in Canada and United States.
†Available in Canada only.

Continued.

Table 13-2 Drugs to Decrease Tone and Motility—cont'd

Generic name	Trade name	Administration/dosage	Comments
Glycopyrrolate	Robinul*	ORAL: *Adults*—1 to 2 mg 3 times daily initially, then 1 to 2 mg 2 times daily for maintenance. Onset: 1 hr. INTRAMUSCULAR, SUBCUTANEOUS, INTRAVENOUS: *Adults*—0.1 to 0.2 mg every 4 hr. Onset: 10 min.	Glycopyrrolate treats gastrointestinal hypermotility and controls gastric acidity.
Hexocyclium methylsulfate	Tral Filmtabs	ORAL: *Adults*—25 mg 4 times daily before meals and at bedtime. May be taken twice daily in combined release capsules.	Hexocyclium methylsulfate controls gastric acidity and hypermotility.
Isopropamide iodide	Darbid*	ORAL: *Adults and children over 12 yr*—5 mg every 12 hr, may increase to 10 mg every 12 hr for severe symptoms.	Mepenzolate bromide controls gastric acidity and hypermotility.
Mepenzolate bromide	Cantil	ORAL: *Adults*—25 mg 4 times daily. Increase to 50 mg if necessary.	
Methantheline bromide	Banthine	ORAL: *Adults*—50 to 100 mg every 6 hr initially; reduce by ½ for maintenance. *Children*—6 mg/kg daily in 4 doses. Onset: 30 min. INTRAMUSCULAR: *Adults*—50 mg every 6 hr. *Children*—6 mg/kg daily in 4 doses. Onset: 30 min.	Methantheline bromide is used like atropine.
Oxyphencyclimine hydrochloride	Daricon	ORAL: 10 mg 2 times daily; can be increased to 50 mg if tolerated.	Oryphencyclimine hydrochloride treats gastric acidity or hypermotility of the GI, genitourinary, or biliary tract.
Oxyphenonium bromide	Antrenyl	ORAL: *Adults*—10 mg 4 times daily; use 5 mg for elderly patients.	Oxyphenonium bromide controls gastric acidity and hypermotility.
Propantheline bromide	Norpanth Pro-Banthine* Propanthel†	ORAL: *Adults*—15 mg 3 times daily plus 30 mg at bedtime or 30 mg timed-release every 8 to 12 hr. *Children*—1.5 mg/kg daily every 6 hr. INTRAMUSCULAR, INTRAVENOUS: *Adults*—30 mg every 6 hr.	Propantheline bromide controls gastric acidity and hypermotility of GI, genitourinary, and biliary tracts.
Tridihexethyl chloride	Pathilon	ORAL: 25 mg 3 times daily before meals and 50 mg at bedtime; timed-release, 75 mg every 6 to 12 hr. INTRAMUSCULAR, SUBCUTANEOUS, INTRAVENOUS: *Adults*—10 to 20 mg every 6 hr.	Tridihexethyl chloride controls gastric acidity and hypermotility of the GI tract.

ANTISPASMODIC DRUGS

Generic name	Trade name	Administration/dosage	Comments
Dicyclomine hydrochloride	Antispas Bentyl Bentylol† Others	ORAL, INTRAMUSCULAR: *Adults*—10 to 20 mg 3 or 4 times daily. *Children*—10 mg 3 or 4 times daily. *Infants*—5 mg 3 or 4 times daily.	Dicyclomine hydrochloride controls hypermotility of colon.
Pirenzepine	Gastrozepin†	ORAL: *Adults*—50 mg 2 times daily. May be increased to 3 times daily if needed.	This new antimuscarinic is relatively specific for GI tract.

*Available in Canada and United States.
†Available in Canada only.

SECTION II: DRUGS TO TREAT AN ULCER

Nursing Process Overview
DRUGS IN THE TREATMENT OF ULCER DISEASE

Assessment

Patients with suspected ulcer disease may have a variety of symptoms. Obtain a baseline patient assessment, focusing on the vital signs, level of consciousness, and character or quality of any emesis or stool, including the presence of occult blood. Monitor patients' intake and output. Question patients about relevant history, such as recent alcohol intake or previous ulcer disease. Monitor the hematocrit and hemoglobin levels.

Nursing Diagnoses

Altered thought processes related to drug side effect (H_2-antagonists)

Altered health maintenance related to complicated dosing regimens when patient is taking several drugs

Management

The goal of treating an ulcer is to stop blood loss and to promote the healing of the ulcerated area. Monitor the patient's vital signs, intake and output, level of consciousness, and character of any emesis or stool. Monitor hematocrit, hemoglobin, and serum electrolyte levels. Prepare the patient for ordered diagnostic studies. Teach the patient about any ordered dietary restrictions.

Evaluation

Before discharge, patients should be able to explain why the drugs have been ordered, how to take them correctly, how to treat side effects, which side effects require medical attention, and how to implement dietary or other restrictions prescribed by the physician.

ULCERS AND STOMACH ACID

An **ulcer** is the loss of the skin or mucosal tissue that provides the protective layer of cells normally surrounding an organ. A **peptic ulcer** occurs in the esophagus, stomach, or duodenum after the mucosal barrier is destroyed, exposing the underlying tissue to stomach acid; as a result the anatomic structure of the stomach and the regulation of stomach secretions are affected. The goal in treating an ulcer is to depress or neutralize stomach acid, thereby allowing the ulcer to heal and preventing the recurrence of the ulcer.

An **esophageal ulcer** results when there is reflux of stomach acid into the esophagus due to a defective esophageal sphincter. An ulcer in the duodenum results from overactive secretion of acid in the stomach so that stomach contents cannot be neutralized in the duodenum. The acidic contents then damage the duodenal mucosa. Stomach ulcers are most frequently caused by a tumor, but a nonmalignant cause of stomach ulcers is the reflux of duodenal contents back into the stomach because of a faulty pyloric sphincter. The duodenal contents contain bile acids that disrupt the mucosal barrier normally protecting the stomach from acid and pepsin.

Factors controlling the secretion of hydrochloric acid by the parietal cells of the stomach are diagrammed in Figure 13-2. The neurotransmitter acetylcholine (released from a branch of the vagus nerve), the hormone gastrin, and histamine all stimulate the secretion of acid. **Hydrochloric acid** aids in breakdown of connective tissue in food, activates pepsinogen to pepsin (which degrades protein), and kills any bacteria ingested in food. The acidic digest leaves the stomach to enter the duodenum. This movement of digested food lessens stomach distension and thereby removes a stimulus for the release of gastrin and for vagal activity. In response to acidity, the duodenum releases **secretin,** a hormone that stimulates the release of bicarbonate and digestive enzymes from the pancreas. Secretin also depresses the release of hydrochloric acid by the parietal cells and depresses the motility of the stomach. The bicarbonate released by the pancreas neutralizes the acidity of the partially digested food entering the duodenum. This neutralization is also necessary for the digestive enzymes in the intestine to be active.

Research has pointed to a bacterial cause of ulcers. The bacterium, *Helicobacter pylori,* may account for 80% of all stomach ulcers and all duodenal ulcers. This bacterium may burrow through and digest the layer of mucus that protects the lining of the stomach and duodenum from acid. A regimen of bismuth and an antibiotic, metronidazole or amoxicillin, effectively destroys *H. pylori.* The bacteria spreads in a family and can cause chronic gastritis or even stomach cancer.

Drug Treatment of Ulcers

Drugs to treat an ulcer are listed in Table 13-3. Ulcers were once treated with antacids and anticholinergic drugs; today, these drugs play a secondary role. The introduction of H_2-receptor antagonists and mucosal protective agents has dramatically improved the treatment of ulcers.

Antacids

Antacids are weak bases that can be ingested to neutralize the hydrochloric acid secreted by the stomach (see Table 13-3).

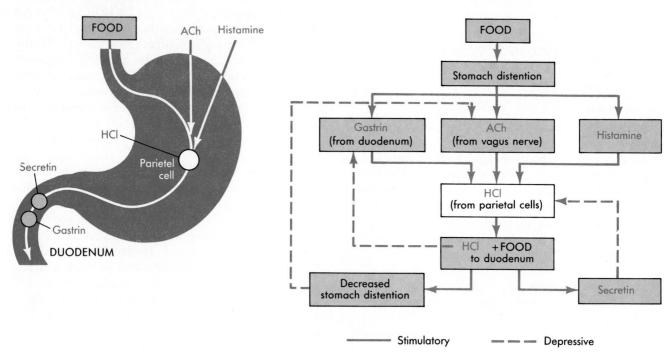

— Stimulatory   --- Depressive

FIGURE 13-2

Secretion of acid parietal cells of stomach is controlled by duodenally released hormone, gastrin; parasympathetic nervous system, via neurotransmitter acetylcholine; and histamine. Histamine is most effective stimulant of gastric acid secretion. Acid secretion is discontinued when food reaches duodenum, where hydrochloric acid (HCl) inhibits gastrin release and stimulates secretin release, and distention of the stomach is lessened, decreasing vagal stimulation.

Table 13-3   Drugs to Treat an Ulcer*

Generic name	Trade name	Administration/dosage	Comments
ANTACIDS			
Aluminum hydroxide gel	Alterna GEL Amphojel†	ORAL: *Adults*—5 to 30 ml up to 40 ml every 30 min if pain is severe	Aluminum hydroxide gel is constipating. Long-term use may cause hypophosphatemia. Complexes with tetracycline and can interfere with absorption of warfarin, digoxin, quinine, and quinidine.
Aluminum carbonate gel	Basaljel	ORAL: *Adults*—5 to 20 ml or 2 capsules every 2 hr up to 12 times daily	See above.
Dihydroxyaluminum aminoacetate	Robalate‡	ORAL: *Adults*—0.5 to 2 gm 4 times daily	Robalate is constipating.
Dihydroxyaluminum sodium carbonate	Rolaids	ORAL: *Adults*—1 to 2 tablets 4 times daily	Rolaids is constipating in large doses.
Calcium carbonate	Dicarbosil Titralac Tums	ORAL: *Adults*—1 to 4 gm 1 and 3 hr after meals and at bedtime (Tablets should be chewed before swallowing.)	Calcium carbonate is constipating. It can be used hourly to keep acid neutralized, but some patients will become hypercalcemic.

*See also Table 13-2, drugs to decrease tone and mobility.
†Available in Canada and United States.
‡Available in Canada only.

Table 13-3   Drugs to Treat an Ulcer—cont'd

Generic name	Trade name	Administration/dosage	Comments
Magnesium carbonate Magnesium hydroxide Magnesium oxide Magnesium phosphate Magnesium trisilicate	Milk of Magnesia		These magnesium salts are laxatives and must be taken with aluminum or calcium antacid to maintain normal stool consistency.
H₂-RECEPTOR ANTAGONISTS			
Cimetidine	Tagamet† Apo-Cimetidine‡ Novocimetidine‡	ORAL: *Adults*—300 mg with meals and at bedtime until ulcer is healed (3 to 6 wk), then 300 mg at bedtime to inhibit nocturnal secretion	Nurse should administer with meals because food slows absorption and prolongs action of cimetidine. Nurse should administer at least 1 hr after antacids or metoclopramide, which reduce absorption of cimetidine if taken concurrently.
Cimetidine hydrochloride	Tagamet Hydrochloride†	INTRAVENOUS: *Adults*—1 to 4 mg/kg/hr or 300 mg diluted and infused over 15 to 20 min INTRAMUSCULAR: *Adults*—300 mg every 6 hr ORAL, INTRAVENOUS: *Children*—20 to 40 mg/kg in divided doses	Nurse should switch to oral doses when ulcer bleeding has stopped.
Famotidine	Pepcid†	ORAL: *Adults*—40 mg daily at bedtime, or in 2 divided doses INTRAVENOUS: *Adults*—20 mg every 12 hr	Famotidine acts longer than cimetidine.
Nizatidine	Axid†	ORAL: *Adults*—300 mg daily at bedtime to heal ulcer, then 150 mg daily to prevent recurrence	Nizatidine acts longer than cimetidine.
Ranitidine hydrochloride	Zantac† Apo-Ranitidine‡	ORAL: *Adults*—150 mg every 12 hr. INTRAMUSCULAR/SLOW INTRAVENOUS: *Adults*—50 mg every 6 to 8 hr. Maximum daily dose is 400 mg.	Ranitidine hydrochloride acts longer than cimetidine.
MUCOSAL PROTECTIVE AGENTS			
Misoprostol	Cytotec	ORAL: *Adults*—100 to 200 μg 4 times daily at meals and bedtime	Misoprostol protects against ulcers from nonsteroidal antiinflammatory drugs used for arthritis. It is also effective for healing peptic ulcer.
Omeprazole	Losec‡ Prilosec	ORAL: *Adults*—20 mg once a day for 4 to 8 weeks	Omeprazole is used for gastroesophageal reflex.
Sucralfate	Carafate Sulcrate‡	ORAL: *Adults*—1 gm 4 times daily taken 1 hr before meals and 1 hr before bedtime	If antacids are prescribed for the pain relief, they should not be taken 30 min before or after sucralfate.

‡Available in Canada only.

Sodium bicarbonate (baking soda) reacts with hydrochloric acid to yield water and carbon dioxide. Carbon dioxide is a gas that causes the frequent belching associated with the ingestion of sodium bicarbonate. Sodium bicarbonate is the only common antacid that is readily absorbed from the GI tract. Taken in excess, sodium bicarbonate also makes the blood slightly alkaline, thus making urine alkaline. Excess bicarbonate stimulates the stomach to secrete more acid (rebound hypersecretion). This hypersecretion can persist after the bicarbonate has been absorbed. For these reasons, sodium bicarbonate is not an antacid of choice when prolonged therapy is required.

Nonsystemic antacids include alkaline salts of aluminum, magnesium, and calcium, which neutralize acid but are not readily absorbed into the bloodstream. Aluminum and calcium salts tend to cause constipation, whereas magnesium salts tend to loosen the bowels. Therefore, most antacids combine a magnesium salt or hydroxide and an aluminum or calcium salt or hydroxide. Nonsystemic antacids are most effective when taken hourly. This regimen neutralizes acid without causing the rebound secretion of acid.

Nonsystemic antacids are available as liquids or chewable tablets. The most common side effect is diarrhea or constipation, even with a combination antacid. The patient must then add more aluminum or calcium antacid to correct diarrhea or more magnesium antacid to correct constipation. Antacids can impede the absorption of drugs, notably tetracyclines (antibiotics), digoxin (a cardiac glycoside), and quinidine (a cardiac antiarrhythmic drug).

Anticholinergic drugs

Anticholinergic drugs used to treat an ulcer were discussed with antispasmodic drugs (see Table 13-2). Anticholinergic drugs are taken before meals so that they can depress the secretion of acid that occurs while eating. Anticholinergic drugs should not be taken with antacids, since antacids slow their absorption. Moreover, the acid would already have been released in response to the meal and neutralized by the antacid, making the anticholinergic drugs useless.

Pirenzepine (Gastrozepin) is a selective anticholinergic drug that inhibits gastric acid secretion without blocking smooth muscle action or causing an increased heart rate. Pirenzepine is available in Canada but not in the United States.

Histamine H$_2$-receptor antagonists

Cimetidine (Tagamet) released in 1977, was the first of a new class of drugs, the H$_2$-histamine receptor antagonists, listed in Table 13-3. These **H$_2$ antagonists** act specifically to block the H$_2$-histamine receptors that control the basal and stimulated secretion of hydrochloric acid by the parietal cells (see Figure 13-2). (H$_1$ receptors are blocked by the antihistamines discussed in Chapter 24.) Gastrin and acetylcholine are believed to act through histamine to cause the release of hydrochloric acid because H$_2$ antagonists are so effective in decreasing acid secretion stimulated by pentagastrin (an active analog of gastrin) or bethanechol (an agonist of acetylcholine), as well as by food, insulin, and caffeine. Because H$_2$ antagonists dramatically decrease stomach acid, they alleviate many conditions in which stomach acid impedes therapy, including the following:

1. Duodenal ulcer. A duodenal ulcer usually heals within 8 weeks of therapy with H$_2$ antagonists,

but maintenance therapy is necessary to prevent recurrence.
2. Gastric ulcer. H$_2$ antagonists increase the healing rate of gastric ulcers. Long-term therapy is moderately effective in preventing recurrences.
3. Reflux esophagitis. H$_2$ antagonists tend to reduce the frequency of symptoms. Long-term therapy may yield sustained improvement.
4. Zollinger-Ellison syndrome. A tumor secretes excessive gastrin that stimulates excessive acid production. H$_2$ antagonists depress this acid production.
5. Gastrointestinal hemorrhage. Stomach acid intensifies inflammation of the stomach, worsening the hemorrhaging.
6. Pancreatic insufficiency. Digestive enzymes must be administered orally. Without H$_2$ antagonists, stomach acid inactivates most of the administered enzymes.

Side effects. H$_2$ antagonists are remarkably free of general side effects. CNS effects include mental confusion, agitation, and hallucinations; these symptoms are reversible when the drug is discontinued. CNS effects are more frequent in patients with liver or renal disease.

Cimetidine (Tagamet) is well absorbed and has a duration of action of about 4 hr. The standard dosage schedule has been 4 times daily, but recent studies indicate that higher doses can be given less frequently and still be effective. Cimetidine is metabolized by the liver and excreted through the kidneys. The dosage must be reduced for patients with impaired kidney function. Cimetidine can cause gynecomastia (breast enlargement) in men and breast tenderness in women resulting from a weak antiandrogenic effect.

Famotidine (Pepcid), nizadepine (Axid), and ranitidine (Zantac) are administered once a day. These drugs are partially metabolized by the liver and excreted by the kidneys. The dosage must be reduced for patients with impaired kidney function. Antacids reduce their absorption. Famotidine, nizadepine, or ranitidine do not have the antiandrogenic activity characteristic of cimetidine. None of these drugs interfere with drug metabolism by the liver.

Mucosal protective agents

Sucralfate (Carafate) is a complex of sulfated sucrose and aluminum hydroxide that is changed by stomach acid into viscous material that binds to proteins in ulcerated tissue. This protects the ulcer from the destructive action of the digestive enzyme pepsin. Sucralfate is used in the initial treatment (first 1 to 2 months) of a duodenal ulcer (see Table 13-3). Sucralfate does not neutralize stomach acid or inhibit acid secretion. Give sucralfate alone 30 to 60 min before mealtime so that it can be activated by stomach acid and coat the ulcer. Sucralfate binds digoxin and tetracycline; thus these drugs should be taken at different times.

Misoprostol (Cytotec) is an ester of prostaglandin E_1 and represents a new drug class for treating ulcers (see Table 13-3). Prostaglandin E_1 is normally synthesized in the stomach, where it blocks gastric acid secretion. The nonsteroidal antiinflammatory drugs (NSAIDs), including aspirin, inhibit the synthesis of naturally occurring prostaglandin E_1 when they dissolve in the stomach. For this reason, bleeding from gastric ulcers is a significant problem with long-term use of NSAIDs. Patients with arthritis who must take NSAIDs to relieve inflammation and pain are a major market for misoprostol. Misoprostol replaces the prostaglandin E_1 that is not produced in the stomach when NSAIDs are present. With the protection of misoprostol, excess acid secretion is blocked, and therefore stomach mucosa is protected. Misoprostol is also used to treat duodenal and peptic ulcers.

Side effects. Minor effects such as diarrhea, mild nausea, abdominal discomfort, and dizziness are occasionally reported. Serious side effects are bleeding and abortion in pregnant women, an action expected of a prostaglandin E_1 analog. In one study there was bleeding in 50% of pregnant women and a 7% incidence of abortion. Therefore misoprostol is contraindicated for pregnant women and should be used cautiously by women of childbearing age.

Omeprazole (Losec) is another new drug with a different mechanism (see Table 13-3). Omeprazole directly inhibits the hydrogen ion pump in the parietal cells of the stomach. Gastric acid secretion can be completely blocked. It has not caused toxicity with long-term use. Omeprazole is a powerful antiulcer agent and is effective in healing peptic ulcer or reflux esophagitis unresponsive to H_2-receptor antagonists.

SECTION III: DRUGS TO CONTROL VOMITING

Nursing Process Overview
DRUGS TO TREAT NAUSEA AND VOMITING
Assessment

Patients develop nausea with associated vomiting from a variety of causes. Assess the patient, focusing on the vital signs, character and quantity of any emesis, presence of bowel sounds, and intake and output. Perform a brief neurologic examination. Obtain a history of precipitating factors, exposure to recent infectious processes, and recent changes in diet or recent medications.

Nursing Diagnoses

Altered thought processes related to drowsiness produced as a drug side effect

High risk for injury related to impaired vision related to drug side effect (e.g., scopolamine)

Management

Antiemetics are used to relieve symptoms. Continue to monitor the vital signs and intake and output, and assess the subjective complaints of nausea and vomiting. Observe the patient for side effects, although these are usually not severe. CNS depression, hypotension, and dry mouth are seen frequently. Limit odors in the patient's environment, limit intake to clear liquids, and provide backrubs or cool washcloths to the forehead to aid comfort.

Evaluation

Success is measured by a reduction in the subjective complaint of nausea and by less vomiting. Before discharge ascertain that patients can explain why and how to take the drug, the frequency of drug administration, the anticipated side effects of the medication, and what to do if nausea and vomiting are unrelieved by the medication.

BACKGROUND

Antiemetics are drugs to control vomiting. **Vomiting** (emesis) is an involuntary act of regurgitating the contents of the stomach and is coordinated by an area in the medulla called the *vomiting center* (Figure 13-3). **Nausea** is the unpleasant sensation that usually precedes vomiting. Input from three major neural sites can stimulate the vomiting center. The first input is controlled by the higher CNS functions, with vomiting being secondary to emotion, pain, or disequilibrium (motion sickness). The second pathway arises from peripheral stimuli, with vomiting secondary to injury or disease of a body tissue or organ. In particular, irritation of the mucosa of the GI tract or bowel or biliary distention stimulates the vomiting center by way of the autonomic neurons carrying information to the CNS (afferent neurons). A third pathway is from the chemoreceptor trigger zone, a medullary center sensitive to stimulation by circulating drugs and toxins.

NONMEDICINAL TREATMENTS OF NAUSEA AND VOMITING

Nausea and vomiting are not necessarily treated with drugs. For instance, the nausea and vomiting of pregnancy is best treated by having patients sip water or tea and eat small meals because antiemetic drugs cause fetal abnormalities in experimental animals. Many

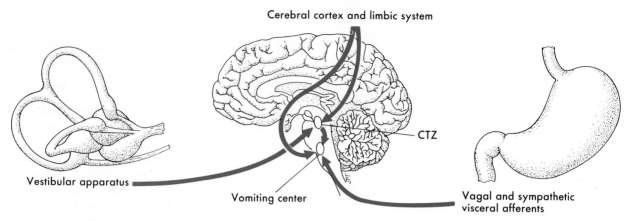

Cerebral cortex and limbic system

CTZ

Vestibular apparatus

Vomiting center

Vagal and sympathetic
visceral afferents

FIGURE 13-3

Vomiting action. Once stimulated, vomiting center acts on cranial nerves, spinal nerves to diaphragm, and abdominal muscles, which results in autonomic response of vomiting.

From Beare PG, Myers JL: *Principles and practice of adult health nursing,* St Louis, 1990, Mosby–Year Book.

drugs cause nausea and vomiting because they act directly on the chemoreceptor trigger zone. Examples of such drugs include levodopa, digitalis, opiates (narcotic analgesics), and aminophylline. The effective treatment is to lower the dose of the offending drug or to increase the dose slowly.

Drugs may also irritate the gastric mucosa, thus causing a reflex stimulation of nausea and vomiting. Aspirin is an example of an irritant drug. To dilute the drug, patients should take it with a large volume of liquid or with a meal.

DRUG THERAPY FOR NAUSEA AND VOMITING

Drugs used to prevent nausea and vomiting are listed by drug class in Table 13-4. These drugs include antagonists of histamine, acetylcholine, and dopamine, as well as drugs whose actions are not yet determined. The choice of an antiemetic is determined by the cause of the nausea and vomiting. Drugs for treating nausea and vomiting are most effective when administered before nausea and vomiting have begun rather than after. For instance, drugs effective in treating motion sickness or vertigo are effective when taken about 30 min before traveling is begun but are relatively ineffective if taken after motion sickness has started. The drugs for treating nausea and vomiting with chemotherapy or radiation therapy are most effective when taken 30 to 60 min before the therapy begins.

Scopolamine and antihistamines are the drugs of choice for treating motion sickness and vertigo. A drug is most effective when given prophylactically, a half hour before travel. These drugs presumably reduce the stimulation of receptors in the labyrinth from which signals governing the sense of equilibrium arise.

Antidopaminergic drugs are effective in reducing vomiting from chemotherapy and radiation therapy of cancer. These drugs act at the chemoreceptor trigger zone and are antagonists of dopamine, the major neurotransmitter of the chemoreceptor trigger zone. Most of these dopamine antagonists are drugs that are used as antipsychotic drugs (see Chapter 41). They include chlorpromazine (Thorazine), droperidol (Inapsine), fluphenazine (Prolixin), haloperidol (Haldol), perphenazine (Trilafon), prochlorperazine (Compazine), promazine (Sparine), thiethylperazine (Torecan), and triflupromazine (Vesprin). They also control postoperative vomiting, although they do not prevent motion sickness.

Cannabinoids are new additions to antiemetic therapy for cancer chemotherapy. Patients who smoked marijuana before receiving cancer chemotherapy reported a decreased incidence of nausea and vomiting. Research revealed that the active ingredients, cannabinoids, appeared to depress the chemoreceptor trigger zone. Dronabinol (Marinol) is the major active substance in marijuana and appears to be an especially effective antiemetic when combined with a phenothiazine. Nabilone (Cesamet) is another active cannabinoid that appears to be especially effective for relieving the nausea from low-dose cisplatin therapy (see box on p. 179).

Text continued on p. 179.

Table 13-4 Drugs to Control Vomiting

Generic name	Trade name	Administration/dosage	Comments
ANTICHOLINERGIC DRUGS			
Scopolamine	Transderm Scop Transderm-V†	TOPICAL: *Adults*—1 adhesive unit is placed behind ear several hours before travel. Duration is 72 hr.	Sustained release protects most patients from motion sickness while greatly reducing anticholinergic side effects (blurred vision, sensitivity to light, dry mouth, and drowsiness).
Scopolamine hydrobromide		ORAL, SUBCUTANEOUS: *Adults*—0.6 to 1.0 mg. *Children*—0.006 mg/kg body weight.	This is one of most effective drugs in preventing motion sickness, but side effects (dry mouth, drowsiness) limit its use.
ANTIHISTAMINIC DRUGS			
Buclizine hydrochloride	Bucladin-S	ORAL: *Adults*—50 mg 30 min before traveling and 4 to 6 hr later. For vertigo, 50 mg 2 times daily.	Drug is effective for preventing motion sickness.
Cyclizine hydrochloride; cyclizine lactate	Marezine Marzin†	ORAL: *Adults*—50 mg 30 min before traveling and 4 to 6 hr later; maximum, 300 mg daily. *Children*—6 to 10 yr, 3 mg/kg body weight divided into 3 doses daily.	Drug is effective for preventing motion sickness and vertigo
Dimenhydrinate	Dramamine* Gravol† Others	INTRAMUSCULAR: *Adults*—50 mg as needed. *Children*—5 mg/kg body weight divided into 4 doses daily; maximum, 300 mg daily. INTRAVENOUS: *Adults*—50 mg diluted in 10-mg saline solution, injected over 2 min. ORAL: *Adults*—50 to 100 mg every 4 hr. *Children*—5 mg/kg body weight divided into 4 doses; maximum, 150 mg daily. RECTAL: *Adults*—100 mg 1 to 2 times daily.	Drug is effective for preventing vertigo, motion sickness, and nausea and vomiting of pregnancy. It also causes drowsiness.
Diphenhydramine hydrochloride	Benadryl Hydrochloride*	DEEP INTRAMUSCULAR: *Adults*—10 mg, increased to 20 to 50 mg every 2 to 3 hr if needed; maximum, 400 mg daily. *Children*—5 mg/kg body weight divided into 4 doses; maximum, 300 mg daily. INTRAVENOUS: *Adults*—same as deep intramuscular. ORAL: *Adults*—50 mg 30 min before traveling, then 50 mg before each meal. *Children*—5 mg/kg body weight divided into 4 doses; maximum, 300 mg daily.	Drug causes sedation. It is effective for preventing vertigo, motion sickness, and nausea and vomiting of pregnancy.
Hydroxyzine hydrochloride	Isaject Vistaril	INTRAMUSCULAR: *Adults*—25 to 100 mg. *Children*—1 mg/kg body weight.	Antianxiety drug is effective for preventing motion sickness and postoperative nausea and vomiting.
Hydroxyzine pamoate	Vistaril	ORAL: *Adults*—25 to 100 mg 3 to 4 times daily. *Children*—over 6 yr, 50 to 100 mg daily divided into 4 doses; under 6 yr, 50 mg daily divided into 4 doses.	

*Available in Canada and United States.
†Available in Canada only.

Continued.

Table 13-4   Drugs to Control Vomiting—cont'd

Generic name	Trade name	Administration/dosage	Comments
Meclizine hydrochloride	Antivert* Bonine† Others	ORAL: *Adults*—25 to 50 mg once daily, taken 60 min or longer before traveling; 25 to 100 mg daily in divided doses for vertigo or radiation sickness.	Drug is effective for preventing motion sickness, vertigo, and nausea and vomiting of radiation therapy. It is longer acting than most antihistamines.
Promethazine hydrochloride	Phenergan* Remsed	INTRAMUSCULAR, RECTAL: *Adults*—25 mg, then 12.5 to 25 mg as needed every 4 to 6 hr. *Children*—under 12 yr, no more than half the adult dose. ORAL: *Adults*—25 mg 2 times daily. *Children*—12.5 to 25 mg twice daily.	Drug is effective for preventing motion sickness and vertigo and postoperative nausea and vomiting.

ANTIDOPAMINERGIC DRUGS

Generic name	Trade name	Administration/dosage	Comments
Chlorpromazine hydrochloride	Thorazine	RECTAL: *Adults*—50 to 100 mg every 6 to 8 hr. *Children*—1 mg/kg body weight every 6 to 8 hr. INTRAMUSCULAR: *Adults*—25 mg, then 25 to 50 mg every 3 to 4 hr to stop vomiting. *Children*—0.5 mg/kg body weight every 6 to 8 hr; maximum, 40 mg (up to 5 yr or 50 lb), 75 mg (5 to 12 yr or 50 to 100 lb) daily. ORAL: *Adults*—10 to 25 mg every 4 to 6 hr. *Children*—0.5 mg/kg body weight every 4 to 6 hr.	Nurse watches for hypotension with initial injection. Drug is effective for postoperative nausea and vomiting and that caused by toxins, radiation therapy, or chemotherapy. It may cause considerable drowsiness.
Droperidol	Inapsine	To prevent postoperative nausea: INTRAVENOUS: *Adults*—1.25 to 2.5 mg. *Children*—0.05 mg/kg. Administer 5 min before termination of anesthesia. To control nausea of cancer chemotherapy, administer 30 to 60 min before treatment. Same or half dose may be given intramuscularly after therapy on request but not more than once every hour. INTRAVENOUS: *Adults*—2.5 to 5 mg. *Children*—1.25 mg/20 kg. For nausea of cisplatin or other potent emetic agents: INTRAVENOUS: *Adults*—15 mg loading dose followed by 7.5 mg every 2 hr for 7 doses.	Drug is effective for postoperative nausea and vomiting and that caused by toxins, radiation therapy, or chemotherapy. With large doses, incidence of dystonic reactions may be high.
Fluphenazine hydrochloride	Prolixin	INTRAMUSCULAR: *Adults*—1.25 mg every 6 to 8 hr as needed.	Drug is effective for postoperative nausea and vomiting and that caused by toxins, radiation therapy, or chemotherapy.
Haloperidol	Haldol*	INTRAMUSCULAR, ORAL: *Adults*—1, 2, or 5 mg every 12 hr as needed.	Drug is effective for postoperative nausea and vomiting and that caused by toxins, radiation therapy, or chemotherapy.

*Available in Canada and United States.
†Available in Canada only.

Table 13-4   Drugs to Control Vomiting—cont'd

Generic name	Trade name	Administration/dosage	Comments
Perphenazine	Trilafon*	ORAL: *Adults*—8 to 24 mg daily in 2 or more divided doses. INTRAMUSCULAR: *Adults*—5 mg daily.	Drug is effective for post-operative nausea and vomiting and that caused by toxins, radiation therapy, or chemotherapy.
Prochlorperazine	Compazine	RECTAL: *Adults*—25 mg 2 times daily. *Children*—over 10 kg, 0.4 mg/kg body weight daily divided into 3 to 4 doses.	Drug is effective for post-operative nausea and vomiting and that caused by toxins, radiation therapy, or chemotherapy.
Prochlorperazine edisylate	Compazine	DEEP INTRAMUSCULAR: *Adults*—5 to 10 mg every 3 to 4 hr; maximum, 40 mg daily. *Children*—over 10 kg, 0.2 mg/body weight daily.	
Prochlorperazine maleate	Compazine	ORAL: *Adults*—5 to 10 mg every 3 to 4 hr; maximum, 40 mg daily. *Children*—over 10 kg, 0.2 mg/body weight daily.	
Promazine hydrochloride	Sparine*	ORAL: *Adults*—25 to 50 mg every 4 to 6 hr as needed. INTRAMUSCULAR: *Adults*—50 mg.	Drug is effective for post-operative nausea and vomiting and that caused by toxins, radiation therapy, or chemotherapy. Nurse watches for hypotension after intramuscular injection. Sedation and anticholinergic effects are common.
Thiethylperazine malate (injection) maleate (oral)	Torecan	INTRAMUSCULAR: *Adults*—10 mg 1 to 3 times daily. ORAL, RECTAL: *Adults*—10 mg 1 to 3 times daily.	Drug is effective for post-operative nausea and vomiting and that caused by toxins, radiation therapy, or chemotherapy.
Triflupromazine hydrochloride	Vesprin	ORAL: *Adults*—20 to 30 mg daily. *Children*—0.2 mg/kg body weight divided into 3 doses; maximum daily dose, 10 mg. INTRAMUSCULAR: *Adults*—5 to 15 mg every 4 hr as needed; maximum daily dose, 60 mg. *Elderly*—2.5 to 15 mg daily. *Children*—0.2 to 0.25 mg/kg body weight; maximum daily dose, 10 mg.	Drug is effective for post-operative nausea and vomiting and that caused by toxins, radiation therapy, or chemotherapy.
CANNABINOIDS			
Dronabinol	Marinol	ORAL: *Adults*—5 to 7.5 mg/M^2 every 3 to 4 hr. Begin 4 to 12 hr before chemotherapy and continue 8 to 24 hr after. Dose may be increased by 2.5 mg/M^2 if necessary.	Dronabinol is delta-9-tetrahydrocannabinol, major active ingredient in marijuana. It is particularly effective antiemetic when combined with phenothiazine. It is Schedule II drug.
Nabilone	Cesamet	ORAL: *Adults*—1 mg twice daily, increasing to 2 mg twice daily if necessary.	Drug is especially effective antiemetic for cisplatin chemotherapy.

*Available in Canada and United States.

Continued.

Table 13-4 Drugs to Control Vomiting—cont'd

Generic name	Trade name	Administration/dosage	Comments
MISCELLANEOUS DRUGS			
Benzquinamide hydrochloride	Emete-Con	INTRAMUSCULAR: *Adults*—0.5 to 1 mg/kg body weight at least 15 min before chemotherapy or emergence from anesthesia. Repeat in 1 hr, then every 3 to 4 hr as required. INTRAVENOUS: *Adults*—0.2 to 0.4 mg/kg body weight diluted in 5% dextrose, sodium chloride injection, or lactated Ringer's injection and administered over 1 to 3 min. Additional doses are given IM.	This rapidly acting antiemetic with a short duration of action is effective in controlling postoperative nausea and vomiting. It acts by inhibiting the chemoreceptor trigger zone.
Diphenidol hydrochloride	Vontrol*	ORAL: *Adults*—25 to 50 mg 4 times daily. *Children over 6 mo and 12 kg*—5 mg/kg body weight daily divided into 4 doses.	Drug acts on vestibular apparatus to prevent vertigo after surgery on middle ear. It is effective for postoperative nausea and vomiting and that caused by toxins, radiation therapy, or chemotherapy.
Domperidone	Motilium†	ORAL: *Adults*—10 mg 4 times/day 15 to 30 min before meals and at bedtime. *Children*—1 drop (0.3 mg)/kg of 1% solution 3 times daily 15 to 30 min before meals and at bedtime if necessary. Oral doses may be doubled if no improvement in 2 weeks.	Drug acts peripherally to enhance stomach peristalsis and to prevent loss of tone associated with vomiting. It is effective in preventing nausea and vomiting that occur after eating in patients with gastroenteritis.
Metoclopramide	Emex† Reglan* Maloxon Maxeran† Reclomide Reglan*	INTRAVENOUS: *Adults*—10 to 20 mg, administered over 2 min. *Children*—up to 6 yr, 0.1 mg/kg body weight; 6 to 14 yr, 2.5 to 5 mg. ORAL: *Adults*—5 to 10 mg 3 times daily 15 to 30 min before meals.	Drug acts centrally to block stimulation of chemoreceptor trigger zone and peripherally to enhance GI tone. High-dose therapy is effective in reducing nausea and vomiting due to cisplatin therapy.
Ondansetron	Zofran*	INTRAVENOUS: *Adults*—150 µg/kg 30 min before chemotherapy, administered over 15 min.	This new drug controls nausea and vomiting with chemotherapy.
Trimethobenzamide hydrochloride	Tigan*	INTRAMUSCULAR: *Adults*—200 mg 3 to 4 times daily. For preventing postoperative nausea and vomiting, give 1 dose before or during surgery and another 3 hr after surgery. ORAL: *Adults*—250 mg 3 to 4 times daily. *Children*—15 mg/kg body weight divided into 3 to 4 doses or 100 to 200 mg divided into 3 or 4 doses.	Drug relieves nausea and vomiting of radiation therapy, in immediate postoperative period, and in gastroenteritis.

*Available in Canada and United States.
†Available in Canada only.

DRUG ABUSE ALERT: MARIJUANA

BACKGROUND

Tetrahydrocannabinols are the active ingredients found in the marijuana plant. The leaves and tops of the marijuana plant are smoked or eaten. Users seek relaxation and feeling of heightened perception. The only medical use of cannabinols, however, is for their antiemetic effect during cancer chemotherapy.

PHARMACOLOGY

Cannabinols impair memory and judgment and raise blood pressure. Characteristically, the user's eyes are bloodshot. When cannabinols are smoked, effects are felt after a few inhalations and reach a maximum about 20 min after the last inhalation. Intoxication includes euphoria, depersonalization, and uncontrollable laughter. Acute effects last about 3 hr.

HEALTH HAZARDS

Acute intoxication may impair judgment; thus the intoxicated individual should not drive or perform potentially dangerous tasks. Anxiety, paranoia, loss of concentration, slower movements, and time distortion are effects of overdose. Long-term health effects have not been clearly shown. Addiction is psychologic. There is no major withdrawal syndrome, although insomnia, hyperactivity, and decreased appetite have been reported.

Additional drugs have antiemetic action. Diphenidol (Vontrol) acts on the aural vestibular apparatus to prevent nausea. Benzquinamide (Emete-con) and trimethobenzamide (Tigan) inhibit stimulation of the chemoreceptor trigger zone and prevent vomiting. Domperidone (Motilium) acts peripherally to prevent the loss of GI tone, which is an early step in vomiting. Metoclopramide (Reglan) also stimulates the GI system, which counteracts the loss of tone in vomiting. In addition, metoclopramide acts at the chemoreceptor trigger zone to prevent vomiting. Ondansetron (Zofran) is a new drug effective against nausea-inducing anticancer drugs. Some anticancer drugs, such as cisplatin, trigger the release from the gut of the transmitter serotonin that stimulates the vagal nerve, resulting in nausea. Ondansetron is a selective blocker of the serotonin (5-HT$_3$) receptor.

Side Effects and Drug Interactions

The side effects of antiemetic drugs are those characteristic of the anticholinergics. All antiemetics cause drowsiness. Scopolamine also causes the usual anticholinergic side effects of blurred vision, dilated pupils, and dry mouth. Because of these anticholinergic effects, antihistamines are more frequently prescribed to prevent motion sickness than scopolamine in spite of the superior effectiveness of scopolamine.

Occasionally, extrapyramidal symptoms are seen with the antidopaminergics. Extrapyramidal symptoms are disorders of motor control associated with too little dopamine in a certain area of the brain. The side effects of the antidopaminergics are more fully discussed in Chapter 41.

The major drug interaction of antiemetics is a synergistic depression with drugs depressing the CNS, particularly when respiratory depression is involved. For instance, vomiting secondary to alcohol intoxication or ingestion of narcotic analgesics can be relieved with an antidopaminergic, but the resultant respiratory depression makes this treatment undesirable.

SECTION IV: DRUGS TO CONTROL DIARRHEA

Nursing Process Overview

DRUGS TO CONTROL DIARRHEA

Assessment

Assess patients, focusing on vital signs, intake and output of solids and liquids, presence and character of bowel sounds, and the character of diarrhea. Question patients about recent exposure to new water or dietary sources, infectious agents, and any medications taken recently. Appropriate laboratory studies include culturing a stool specimen and testing stools for ova, parasites, and occult blood.

Nursing Diagnoses

Altered thought processes related to drowsiness produced as a drug side effect
Colonic constipation related to drug side effects

Management

Diarrhea treatment aims to provide symptomatic relief and identify and treat the cause. Monitor vital signs and intake and output, and observe the frequency and character of bowel movements. Limit the diet to clear liquids. If the diarrhea results from milk intolerance or other dietary cause, refer the patient to a dietitian for instruction. Observe the patient for drug side effects, especially constipation and sedation. If diarrhea is severe, monitor serum electrolyte levels and provide replacement fluids as ordered (see box on p. 180).

Evaluation

Drugs to control diarrhea are effective if the frequency of bowel movements is decreased to the patient's normal range. Before discharge patients should be able to explain when and how to take the medication prescribed, symptoms that may indicate too high a dose, and what to do if drugs do not relieve the symptoms.

DIETARY CONSIDERATION: FIBER

Adequate amounts of dietary fiber may help prevent constipation and colon diseases, maintain blood glucose levels, and lower blood cholesterol levels. Good sources of dietary fiber include fruits and vegetables, especially raw, unpeeled, or with edible seeds; and whole grains and whole-grain products, including bread, cereals, pastas, bran, oats, peas, beans, and lentils.

BACKGROUND

About 8 L of fluid travel through the intestines of the average adult in 24 hr. Water ingested in food or drink accounts for about 2 L, and secretions (salivary, gastric, biliary, and pancreatic) account for about 6 L. Since only 100 to 200 ml of water is normally excreted daily in feces, the intestines are highly efficient in reabsorbing water and electrolytes.

Diarrhea has no precise definition but refers to bowel movements that are frequent (more than three per day), fluid (unformed stools), or large (greater than 200 gm/day). Acute diarrhea lasts for hours or days, whereas chronic diarrhea lasts for more than 3 to 4 weeks. A patient with chronic diarrhea must be thoroughly examined to establish a cause, which can then be specifically treated. Acute diarrhea rarely requires treatment beyond avoidance of food and adequate liquid intake.

REPLACEMENT THERAPY FOR DIARRHEA

The primary treatment of diarrhea is replacement of lost fluids and electrolytes. Glucose is required for the intestinal absorption of water and electrolytes. Mild dehydration can be treated with carbonated drinks, which add glucose and bicarbonate, and broths or clear soups, which add sodium and chloride. Infants and elderly patients can become seriously dehydrated if adequate intake of glucose and salts is not maintained to replace the fluid and electrolytes lost. Commercially available drinks for replacement of glucose and electrolytes include Gatorade and Lytren. A similar drink can be made at home with ½ tsp of corn syrup or honey and a pinch of table salt added to 1 cup (8 oz) of fruit juice (to provide potassium), alternating with a drink made by adding ¼ tsp of baking soda (sodium bicarbonate to 1 cup [8 oz] of water). A simpler drink is made with the following recipe: 1 tsp table salt, 1 tsp baking soda, and 4 tsp of sugar in a quart of boiled water. Since this latter recipe does not provide needed potassium, ½ tsp of potassium chloride should be added to a quart of the solution if possible.

DRUG THERAPY FOR DIARRHEA

Table 13-5 lists the drugs used to treat diarrhea. The most effective nonspecific antidiarrheal agents are the opioids, which decrease the tone of the small and large intestines in a manner that slows the transit of material. The longitudinal contractions propelling the contents (peristalsis) are inhibited by the opioids, but the circular contractions, which cause the segmental activity that mixes the intestinal contents, are stimulated by the opioids. The treatment of diarrhea with opioids is nonspecific, and when diarrhea is caused by poisons, infections, or bacterial toxins, opioids can make the condition worse by delaying the elimination of these agents. Opioids that are used to control diarrhea include opium tincture, paregoric, codeine, difenoxin, and diphenoxylate (Lomotil). The effective antidiarrheal dose is lower than that which can cause euphoria or analgesia. Toxic doses produce respiratory depression, which can be reversed with a narcotic antagonist.

Opium tincture

Opium tincture is a 10% solution of opium containing 10 mg/ml morphine. The antidiarrheal dose of opium tincture is measured in drops (usually 6 to 20 drops), and such a dose does not usually produce euphoria or analgesia.

Paregoric

Paregoric (camphorated opium tincture) contains only 0.4 mg/ml morphine and is administered by the teaspoonful. Paregoric has an unpleasant taste.

Codeine

Codeine can be given orally or administered intramuscularly.

Diphenoxylate and difenoxin

Diphenoxylate (Lomotil) is an opioid that has a lower potential than codeine or opium tincture for causing drug dependence. Difenoxin (Motofen), an active metabolite of diphenoxylate, has about 5 times greater activity than diphenoxylate. These drugs are combined with atropine to diminish abdominal cramping while reducing the loss of water and electrolytes.

Loperamide

Loperamide (Imodium) is a relatively new antidiarrheal drug that depresses longitudinal and circular contractions of the intestinal smooth muscles and decreases the release of acetylcholine. Loperamide has

Table 13-5 Drugs to Control Diarrhea

Generic name	Trade name	Administration/dosage	Comments
OPIOIDS AND RELATED DRUGS			
Codeine phosphate; codeine sulfate		ORAL: *Adults and children over 12 yr*—15 to 60 mg every 4 to 8 hr as needed. INTRAMUSCULAR: *Adults and children over 12 yr*—15 to 30 mg every 2 to 4 hr.	Codeine phosphate and sulfate are Schedule II drugs.
Diphenoxylate hydrochloride with atropine	Lomotil* Lofene Others	ORAL: *Adults*—5 mg 3 to 4 times daily. *Children*—8 to 12 yr, 10 mg daily in 5 divided doses; 5 to 8 yr, 8 mg daily in 4 divided doses; 2 to 5 yr, 6 mg daily in 3 divided doses.	Diphenoxylate hydrochloride with atropine is Schedule V drug.
Difenoxin with atropine	Motofen	ORAL: *Adults*—2 mg initially, then 1 mg after each loose stool or every 3 to 4 hr as needed.	Difenoxin with atropine is Schedule IV drug.
Loperamide	Imodium	ORAL: *Adults*—4 mg initially, then 2 mg with each diarrheal episode, up to 16 mg daily.	Drug is also available as nonprescription drug. It is in FDA Pregnancy Category B.
Opium tincture		ORAL: 0.6 ml 4 times daily. Maximum single dose is 1 ml. Maximum daily dose is 6 ml.	Opium tincture is Schedule II drug.
Paregoric		ORAL: *Adults*—5 to 10 ml 1 to 4 times daily. *Children*—0.25 to 0.5 ml/kg 1 to 4 times daily.	Paregoric is Schedule III drug.
BISMUTH SALTS			
Bismuth subsalicylate	Pepto-Bismol	ORAL: *Adults*—30 ml. *Children*—10 to 14 yr, 20 ml; 6 to 10 yr, 10 ml; 3 to 6 yr, 5 ml.	This nonprescription drug is effective for "traveler's" diarrhea. It may turn stools gray-black.

*Available in Canada and United States.

a broader spectrum of actions on the intestine than the opioids. Loperamide is structurally related to diphenoxylate but has no effects on the CNS and does not appear to produce physical dependence. Originally available as a Schedule V drug, loperamide is now available over the counter. Loperamide is concentrated by the liver and excreted into the bile. Its use is contraindicated in liver disease.

Bismuth salts

In addition to opioids that depress intestinal motility, many agents have been used as antidiarrheal drugs in the belief that they absorb toxins and thus remove the cause of diarrhea. Of these, only bismuth salts have been proved effective.

Bismuth subsalicylate (Pepto-Bismol) is effective in controlling traveler's diarrhea, apparently by binding the bacterial toxins. Bismuth causes the feces to become black, which does not indicate the presence of blood. Use in infants or the elderly may produce feces that cannot be expelled (impacted feces).

SECTION V: DRUGS TO RELIEVE CONSTIPATION

Nursing Process Overview

DRUGS TO RELIEVE CONSTIPATION

Assessment

Assess vital signs, fluid intake and output, and presence of bowel sounds. Perform a digital rectal examination to determine the presence of impacted stools. Obtain a history of previous constipation and its treatment, the patient's perception of constipation, and any recent change in lifestyle, diet, or medications.

Nursing Diagnoses

Diarrhea related to drug side effects
Impaired perianal skin integrity related to diarrhea

Management

The treatment of uncomplicated constipation is usually simple. If constipation is persistent, the physician must rule out serious causes such as cancer. Administer ordered medications, and teach the patient about other factors that influence the frequency of stools such as diet, fluid intake, and exercise.

Evaluation

Drugs to relieve constipation are effective if they produce a bowel movement. Before a patient is discharged, verify that the patient can explain how to take the ordered medications and what the desired effects of the medications are.

BACKGROUND

The major muscular activity of the large intestine is a contraction of circular smooth muscle, which decreases the diameter to segment and knead the fecal mass without moving it along. About 2 L of water are removed from the fecal mass in the large intestine. Bulk in the large intestine stimulates stretch receptors to cause a reflex peristalsis, which moves the fecal mass forward.

Usually 3 to 4 times daily strong propulsive contractions occur spontaneously to move the fecal mass through the large intestine. The strongest movements usually occur after the first meal of the day, and the perception of the need to defecate follows the filling of the rectum. The relaxation of the external anal sphincter is a voluntary act, as are the straining movements to expel the feces. The pattern of defecation described implies that defecation is a regular morning event, but the timing of defecation is highly individual and may occur more or less frequently. A *normal bowel movement* refers to whatever pattern of defecation results in readily passed feces for a given individual. **Constipation** arises when the frequency of bowel movements decreases and defecation yields hard stools that are difficult to pass (see box).

LAXATIVES

Laxative, cathartic, and *purgative* describe agents that act on the large intestine (colon, bowel) to promote defecation, but these terms have evolved to represent different degrees of action. A **laxative** produces soft stools with a minimal incidence of abdominal cramping. A cathartic produces a soft to fluid stool and may also cause abdominal cramping. A purgative produces a watery stool and violent cramping to such an extent

---

PATIENT PROBLEM: CONSTIPATION

THE PROBLEM

The patient is not having bowel movements as often as necessary.

SIGNS AND SYMPTOMS

Abdominal discomfort; feeling a need to defecate but inability to do so; dry, firm, hard stools when bowel movements do occur; infrequent defecation (The meaning of *infrequent* may vary with each patient.)

ASSOCIATED OR CONTRIBUTING FACTORS

Dehydration or inadequate fluid intake; constipating medications; misuse or overuse of antidiarrhea medications or improper use of cathartics, causing the patient to move from constipation to diarrhea; and immobility.

MEASURES TO HELP ELIMINATE CONSTIPATION

Keep a record of bowel movements to help verify the problem, and note any associated factors.

Increase daily fluid intake to 2500 to 3000 ml.

Increase dietary intake of fruit and fruit juices.

Increase dietary intake of fiber (see box on p. 180).

Increase level of exercise.

Examine use of drugs causing diarrhea or constipation.

ADDITIONAL NURSING CARE MEASURES

Keep a record of bowel movements for all hospitalized, immobilized, or institutionalized patients, since constipation is easier to prevent than treat.

Auscultate bowel sounds in patients complaining of constipation.

---

that shock and hemorrhaging may result. Purgatives are no longer used in medical practice, and only some cathartics, also called *stimulant cathartics,* are commonly used.

Table 13-6 lists the drugs used as laxatives. Traditionally, laxatives are classified as bulk-forming, stimulant (irritant) cathartic, saline (osmotic) cathartic, wetting agent (softener), and lubricant. Laxatives are indicated for patients with true constipation. Causes of constipation include poor bowel habits, narcotic analgesics, drugs with anticholinergic side effects, and the intestinal muscle tone loss because of surgery, bed rest, or age. Laxatives are also indicated when straining is painful or risky, such as in women with episiotomies and patients with hemorrhoids, hernias, or aneurysms. Laxatives are also used to clean out the large intestine before surgery or examination. With the exception of mineral oil, laxatives act by providing a greater bulk to the fecal mass, primarily by keeping water in the large intestine. The large,

Table 13-6 Drugs to Relieve Constipation

Generic name	Trade name	Administration/dosage	Comments
BULK-FORMING AGENTS			
Karaya gum		ORAL: 5 to 10 gm daily, taken with water.	Drug is nonprescription.
Methylcellulose; carboxymethyl cellulose	Cologel Citrucel	ORAL: *Adults*—4 to 6 gm daily. *Children*—over 6 yr, 1 to 1.5 gm daily.	Drug is nonprescription.
Plantago (psyllium) seed		ORAL: *Adults*—2.5 to 30 gm daily. *Children*—over 6 yr, 1.25 to 1.5 gm daily. Add to water and drink rapidly.	Drug is nonprescription.
Polycarbophil	Mitrolan† Fibercon	ORAL: *Adults*—4 to 6 gm daily. *Children*—6 to 12 yr, 1.5 to 3 gm daily; 2 to 5 yr, 1 to 1.5 gm daily; to 2 yr, 0.5 to 1 gm daily.	Drug is nonprescription.
Psyllium hydrocolloid Psyllium hydrophilic mucilloid	Fiberall Konsyl Metamucil* Modane Bulk Serutan	ORAL: *Adults*—1 round tsp (7 gm) or 1 packet. Add to glass of water and drink rapidly and then follow with second glass of water. Repeat 1 to 2 times daily if necessary.	Drug is nonprescription.
STIMULANT (IRRITANT) CATHARTICS			
Bisacodyl	Biscolax† Dulcolax* Others	ORAL: *Adults*—10 mg. Up to 30 mg may be given to clear gastrointestinal tract. *Children*—over 6 yr, 5 mg. RECTAL: *Adults and children over 2 yr*—10 mg. *Children under 2 yr*—5 mg.	Drug is nonprescription. Initial response occurs in 6 to 12 hr. Patient should not take it within 60 min of milk or antacids. Rectal administration is effective in 15 min.
Cascara sagrada		ORAL: *Adults*—200 to 400 mg of extract, 0.5 to 1.5 ml of fluid extract, or 5 ml of aromatic extract.	Drug is nonprescription. It is one of mildest of stimulant cathartics.
Castor oil		ORAL: *Adults*—15 to 60 ml. *Children*—over 2 yr, 5 to 15 ml; under 2 yr, 1 to 5 ml.	Drug is nonprescription. Castor oil is degraded to ricinoleic acid, which is active drug.
Castor oil, emulsified	Neoloid	ORAL: *Adults*—30 to 60 ml. *Children*—over 2 yr, 7.5 to 30 ml; under 2 yr, 2.5 to 7.5 ml.	Drug is nonprescription. This emulsion is mint flavored. It turns alkaline urine pink.
Glycerin suppositories		RECTAL: *Adults*—3 gm. *Children*—under 6 yr, 1 to 1.5 gm.	Drug is nonprescription. It is effective in 15 to 30 min.
Phenolphthalein	Ex-lax* Feen-A-Mint Phenolax Others	ORAL: *Adults*—30 to 270 mg daily. *Children*—over 6 yr, 30 to 60 mg daily; 2 to 6 yr, 15 to 20 mg daily.	Drug is nonprescription. It turns alkaline urine pink.
Senna concentrate	Senokot suppositories	RECTAL: *Adults*—1 suppository. *Children*—over 60 lb, ½ suppository.	
Senna pod	Senokot Others	ORAL: *Adults*—twice daily give 1 to 2 tsp (granules), 2 to 3 tsp (syrup), or 2 to 4 tablets. *Children, pregnant or postpartum women, or geriatric patients*—½ adult dose. *Children*—1 mo to 1 yr, 1.25 to 2.5 ml (syrup).	Drug is nonprescription. Not all preparations are recommended for children.

*Available in Canada and United States.
†Available in Canada only.

Table 13-6 Drugs to Relieve Constipation—cont'd

Generic name	Trade name	Administration/dosage	Comments
Senna, whole leaf		ORAL: *Adults*—0.5 to 2 gm or 2 ml of senna fluid extract. *Children*—6 to 12 yr, ½ adult dose; 2 to 5 yr, ¼ adult dose; under 2 yr, ⅓ adult dose.	Drug is nonprescription.
Sennosides A and B	Glysennid† Gentle Nature	ORAL: *Adults*—12 to 24 mg at bedtime. *Children*—over 10 yr same as adult; 6 to 10 yr, 12 mg at bedtime.	Drug is nonprescription.
SALINE CATHARTICS			
Magnesium citrate	Citroma Citro-Mag†	ORAL: *Adults*—1 glassful (about 240 ml). *Children*—0.5 ml/kg body weight.	Drug is nonprescription.
Magnesium hydroxide	Phillips' Milk of Magnesia	ORAL: *Adults*—10 to 15 ml (concentrated) or 15 to 30 ml (regular). *Children*—0.5 ml (regular)/kg body weight.	Drug is nonprescription.
Magnesium sulfate	Epsom salt	ORAL: *Adults*—15 gm in a glass of water. *Children*—0.25 gm/kg.	Drug is nonprescription.
Monosodium phosphate	Sal Hepatica	ORAL: *Adults*—5 to 20 ml with water.	Drug is nonprescription.
Sodium phosphate		ORAL: *Adults*—4 gm in a glass of warm water. *Children*—0.25 gm/kg.	Drug is nonprescription.
Sodium phosphate with biphosphate	Phospho-Soda	ORAL: *Adults*—20 to 40 ml in a glass of cold water. *Children*—5 to 15 ml.	Drug is nonprescription.
LUBRICANTS			
Mineral oil	Agoral, Plain Kondremul Plain* Neo-Cultol Petrogalar Plain	ORAL: *Adults*—15 to 30 ml at bedtime.	Drug is nonprescription. It eases strain of passing hard stools. It should not be used regularly because fat-soluble vitamins (A, D, E, and K) are not absorbed. Response occurs in 1 to 3 days.
FECAL SOFTENERS			
Docusate calcium	Surfak	ORAL: *Adults*—50 to 360 mg daily. *Children*—50 to 150 mg daily.	Drug is nonprescription.
Docusate sodium	Colace D-S-S Others	ORAL: *Adults*—50 to 360 mg. *Children*—6 to 12 yr, 40 to 120 mg; 3 to 6 yr, 20 to 60 mg; under 3 yr, 10 to 40 mg.	Drug is nonprescription.
MISCELLANEOUS			
Lactulose	Chronulac* Constilac Others	ORAL: *Adults*—15 to 30 ml, increased to 60 ml/day if necessary (15 ml = 10 gm).	Drug is nonprescription. It works by osmotic effect in 1 to 3 days.

*Available in Canada and United States.
†Available in Canada only.

hydrated fecal mass can fill the rectum to stimulate defecation, which is then accomplished with minimal irritation or strain.

Bulk-Forming Laxatives

This class of laxatives includes bran, methylcellulose, polycarbophil, and psyllium hydrophilic mucilloid. They act by retaining water so that the stool remains large and soft. Bulk-forming laxatives provide what should be a part of good nutrition. It is generally believed that people in developed countries eat a diet containing too little fiber that favors the formation of small, hard stools. Including bran, whole grain products, and fibrous fruits and vegetables in the diet promotes the formation of large, soft stools that readily stimulate the large intestine and the rectum.

In a patient who does not regularly use laxatives, bulk-forming laxatives are effective in 12 to 24 hr. Bulk-forming laxatives can also relieve a mild water diarrhea by absorbing water to produce a soft stool.

Stimulant Cathartics

Stimulant (irritant) cathartics include cascara, danthron, senna, phenolphthalein, bisacodyl, castor oil, and glycerin. These drugs usually form a soft to fluid stool in 6 to 12 hr (see box). Stimulant cathartics were believed to act only by directly stimulating the motility of the large intestine; however, newer research indicates that these drugs also inhibit the reabsorption of water in the large intestine.

Stimulant cathartics are the most abused laxatives. When a stimulant cathartic is used for more than 1 week, the large intestine loses its tone and becomes less responsive to any stimulation. Continued use of a stimulant cathartic can produce diarrhea severe enough to cause dehydration and to lower blood concentrations of sodium and potassium.

Cascara and senna are extracted from plants. Cascara is the milder and senna the more potent. They should not be used by breast-feeding mothers, since these laxatives are excreted in the milk. Senna and cascara turn acid urine yellow-brown and alkaline urine red.

Phenolphthalein is found in many over-the-counter laxative preparations. Phenolphthalein enters the enterohepatic circulation and may be effective for several days. In alkaline urine, phenolphthalein is pink.

Bisacodyl is a synthetic compound available in suppositories and tablets. As a suppository, bisacodyl is effective in 15 min and as a tablet, in 6 hr. Since bisacodyl irritates the stomach, the tablet is coated to dissolve only in the intestine. This enteric-coated tablet should not be taken within 1 hr of ingestion of milk products or antacids, which neutralize stomach acid. Bisacodyl is often used to clear the large intestine for proctoscopic or colonoscopic examination.

Castor oil is an old remedy for constipation and is still used medically. Castor oil is the most potent of the stimulant cathartics, producing a watery stool in 2 to 6 hr, which thoroughly removes gas and feces from the intestine. Castor oil has an unpleasant taste and is best disguised by chilling and administering with fruit juice.

Glycerin is used only as a suppository. It acts by stimulating the rectum and attracting water to increase bulk. It is effective in 15 to 30 min.

Saline Cathartics

Saline (osmotic) cathartics are poorly absorbed salts of magnesium or sodium such as magnesium carbonate, oxide, citrate, hydroxide, or sulfate; sodium phosphate or sulfate; and potassium and sodium tartrate. Concentrated solutions of these salts attract water osmotically into the lumen of the large intestine, and the resulting bulk stimulates peristalsis. Saline cathartics empty the bowel in 2 to 6 hr.

Patients with poor kidney function should not use saline cathartics, since they cannot excrete the small fraction of the salt that is absorbed systemically.

Wetting Agents

Wetting agents, or stool softeners, are detergents that inhibit the absorption of water so that the fecal mass remains large and soft. This class of laxatives is indicated when the objective is to avoid straining to pass the stools. Such laxatives include dioctyl sodium sulfosuccinate (docusate sodium) and dioctyl calcium sulfosuccinate (docusate calcium).

DRUG ABUSE ALERT: CATHARTICS

BACKGROUND

Cathartics are subject to two types of abuse. Individuals may fixate on being regular. Individuals with eating disorders may use cathartic laxatives in excess to get rid of ingested food.

PHARMACOLOGY

Cathartics are laxatives that produce a soft to fluid stool in 6 to 12 hr. They directly stimulate the colon.

HEALTH HAZARDS

The colon becomes unresponsive when cathartics are used for more than 1 week. Persistent diarrhea may result that in its most severe form causes dehydration and produces electrolyte imbalances. Therapy is supportive as the cathartic is discontinued.

Lubricant

The only lubricant laxative still used is mineral oil, which is indigestible and acts to soften the feces, thus easing the strain of passing stools and lessening irritation to hemorrhoids. Long-term use of mineral oil interferes with the absorption of fat-soluble vitamins A, D, E, and K. Mineral oil can cause a lipid pneumonia if accidentally aspirated. Wetting agents are regarded as superior to mineral oil in softening the stools for easy passage.

Miscellaneous Agent

Lactulose is a synthetic disaccharide that is not hydrolyzed by intestinal enzymes and is not absorbed. Instead, lactulose is degraded by bacteria in the colon to short-chain organic acids that are not absorbed and act as osmotic agents. The net effect is a moderate fluid accumulation in the colon and the formation of a soft stool. Lactulose may initially produce gas and cramps. Lactulose has reduced the incidence of fecal impaction in the elderly. However, elderly patients should have serum electrolyte levels monitored after treatment for more than 6 months.

NURSING IMPLICATIONS SUMMARY

Cholinomimetics: Bethanechol and Neostigmine

Drug administration

◆ Have atropine sulfate (0.5 to 1.0 mg for adults; 10 μg/kg for infants and children) on hand to counteract excessive cholinergic side effects when administering cholinomimetics subcutaneously.

◆ Check doses carefully. The oral dose of bethanechol may be as high as 50 mg, whereas the subcutaneous dose should not exceed 5 mg.

◆ Remain at the bedside of patients for the first 10 min after administering subcutaneous bethanechol to assess for side effects.

◆ The physician may order a test dose of half or less of the usual dose to check for patient response. Monitor vital signs.

◆ Check the pulse before administering neostigmine. Notify the physician if the rate is below 80 beats/min, and withhold the dose pending physician approval. For additional information about neostigmine, see Chapter 11.

Patient and family education

◆ Teach patients to take oral doses of bethanechol on an empty stomach 1 hr before or 2 hr after eating.

◆ If a dose is missed, tell patients to take the missed dose if within 1 to 2 hr of the scheduled time. If close to the next dosing time, omit the missed dose and resume the usual dosing schedule. Do not double up for missed doses.

◆ Remind patients to keep these and all medications out of the reach of children.

Metoclopramide

Drug administration

◆ Administer undiluted intravenous doses over 1 to 2 min. It may be diluted in 50 ml of solution and administered slowly, over at least 15 min. Give doses administered in conjunction with cancer chemotherapy 30 min before chemotherapy is begun. A second dose may be given in 2 hr and a third dose in 3 hr. Doses for this purpose may be as high as 2 mg/kg body weight. Other regimens are also in use.

Patient and family education

◆ Take oral doses 30 min before meals; doses may also be taken at bedtime.

◆ Metoclopramide may produce extrapyramidal reactions (see Table 41-2). Instruct the patient to report any unusual side effects, especially protrusion of the tongue, puffing of the cheeks, chewing movements, and involuntary movements of any body parts. Although rare, these side effects occur more often in children and the elderly.

◆ Caution patients to avoid drinking alcohol or operating hazardous equipment until the effects of the medication can be evaluated.

◆ Caution patients to avoid alcohol while taking this drug, as well as any drug that may depress the CNS such as sleeping medications, tranquilizers, narcotic analgesics, or other drugs that cause drowsiness.

◆ Agranulocytosis occurs rarely. Assess patients for chills, fever, sore throat, and fatigue.

NURSING IMPLICATIONS SUMMARY—cont'd

Anticholinergics and Antispasmodics

Drug administration

◆ Use anticholinergics and antispasmodics cautiously in patients with prostatic hypertrophy, pyloric obstruction, obstruction of the bladder neck, or serious cardiac disease. Assess for preexisting glaucoma, since anticholinergics may precipitate an attack of acute angle-closure glaucoma.

◆ Assess for urinary retention, especially in elderly men with preexisting prostatic hypertrophy. Monitor intake and output. Instruct the patient to report inability to void, increasing difficulty in initiating urination, or a sensation of incomplete bladder emptying. Instruct patients to void before taking each dose.

◆ Monitor the patient's pulse before administering doses. Withhold dose if pulse exceeds 90 to 100 beats/min in an adult. Administer anticholinergics with caution in patients with a history of heart disease characterized by tachycardia. Auscultate bowel sounds. Keep a record of bowel movements. Treat overdose with neostigmine.

◆ Administer intramuscular doses into a large muscle mass such as the dorsogluteal site or rectus femoris muscle in adults or the vastus lateralis muscle in infants and small children. Use careful technique; aspirate before administering dose to avoid inadvertent intravenous administration.

◆ Tincture of belladonna may be prescribed by number of drops. Dilute the dose in 15 to 30 ml of water before administering. If drowsiness or disorientation develops, supervise ambulation, keep side rails up, and use night lights.

Patient and family education

◆ Take doses before meals and at bedtime unless a timed-release form is used. If antacids are also prescribed, take doses 30 min before or 2 hr after antacid doses.

◆ Inform patients that constipation is a common side effect.

◆ Instruct patients to increase the daily fluid intake to at least 3000 ml, to increase dietary intake of fruits and fiber, and to get regular exercise. Tell patients to record bowel movements; if a bowel movement has not occurred in 3 days, consult the physician. Teach patients to avoid cathartics or laxatives unless instructed to use specific ones by the physi-

cian, since they may be contraindicated in certain medical conditions requiring anticholinergics.

◆ Caution patients to avoid driving or operating hazardous equipment until the effects of the medication can be evaluated; drowsiness and blurred vision may occur. Encourage patients to wear sunglasses and avoid bright sunlight if photophobia develops. Keep room lights dim.

◆ Teach patients to suck on sugarless hard candy or to chew sugarless gum to relieve dry mouth. Refer patients to the pharmacist for commercially available saliva substitutes. See Patient Problem: Dry Mouth on p. 166.

◆ Instruct patients to be careful regarding strenuous activities on warm days, since these drugs inhibit the body's ability to perspire. Tell patients to take frequent rest periods to cool off. Inform patients that atropine may produce a fever, especially in children.

◆ Since these drugs often produce side effects when taken in therapeutic doses, patient compliance may be poor. Provide emotional support as needed; teach patients the importance of taking drugs as prescribed. Reinforce the importance of keeping all drugs out of the reach of children. If combination products are prescribed, review side effects of each drug with the patient.

Drugs to Treat Ulcers: Antacids

Patient and family education

◆ Avoid administering antacids with tetracyclines, digoxin, or quinidine. Review with patients their complete list of medications, and schedule home drug administration that prevents the antacids from interfering with absorption of any other drugs. Try to schedule antacids for 30 min before or 1 hr after sucralfate; try to schedule H_2-histamine receptor antagonists 1 hr before or after antacids.

◆ Remind patients to chew antacid tablets, not to swallow them whole.

◆ Tell patients to take a small amount of water after doses of antacid liquid to ensure that the antacid dose is carried to the stomach.

◆ Tell patients to alternate aluminum or calcium salts with magnesium salts to prevent diarrhea or constipation, unless a specific antacid is ordered. Also instruct patients to increase fluid intake to 2500 to 3000 ml/day and increase dietary intake of fruits and fiber to prevent constipation. Patients with renal failure

Continued.

NURSING IMPLICATIONS SUMMARY—cont'd

should not increase fluid intake, and may require concomitant stool softeners.

◆ Teach patients to read labels carefully. Antacids vary in their strength, acid-neutralizing ability, and sodium content, especially if other drugs are included in the formulation. Frequently included drugs are magaldrate, another antacid, and simethicone, an antigas drug.

◆ Teach patients taking aluminum carbonate or aluminum hydroxide products for hyperphosphatemia not to substitute other antacids. Doses of antacids used to bind phosphates are often administered with meals. Refer patients to a dietitian for instruction in following a low-phosphate diet if indicated.

◆ Antacids used to treat ulcers are often administered 1 and 3 hr after meals and at bedtime; review prescription orders with patients. Teach patients taking antacids to prevent kidney stones by increasing daily fluid intake to 3000 ml.

◆ Instruct patients requiring sodium restriction for heart disease or other health problems to avoid antacids high in sodium; consult the physician or pharmacist. Sodium-free products include Advanced Formula Di-Gel, Maalox Plus Extra Strength Oral Suspension, Magaldrate, and Mi-acid; other preparations are very low in sodium. Products relatively high in sodium include Gaviscon-2 chewable tablets (36.8 mg), Gas-is-gon (50.6 mg), and Rolaids (53 mg). Teach patients to use antacids as prescribed and avoid frequent self-medication with over-the-counter products unless advised to do so by a physician.

H₂-Receptor Antagonists: Cimetidine

Drug administration

◆ For direct intravenous injection, dilute 300 mg in at least 20 ml of normal saline. Administer at a rate of 300 mg or less over 2 min. For intermittent intravenous infusion, dilute 300 mg of drug in 100 ml of compatible intravenous solution. Do not add to continuously infusing fluids. Administer over 15 to 20 min. Warn the patient that there may be discomfort associated with intramuscular administration.

◆ Read labels carefully. Prefilled syringes are intended for intramuscular use or for diluting for intermittent infusion. Prefilled syringes are not for direct intravenous injection. This drug is incompatible with many other drugs for infusion. Do not add other drugs to infusions of cimetidine. Usually, administer once-daily doses before bedtime, twice-daily doses in the morning and at bedtime, and more frequent doses with meals and at bedtime. If antacids or metoclopramide are also ordered, they should be administered 1 hr before or after the cimetidine dose.

◆ The action of many drugs, including aminophylline, caffeine, anticoagulants, and some heart medications, may be potentiated when the patient is also receiving cimetidine, since cimetidine is metabolized by the liver and excreted through the kidney. Assess patients carefully for side effects, and monitor appropriate laboratory tests carefully, since dosages of other drugs may need adjustment. Monitor level of consciousness, blood pressure and pulse, intake and output, and complete blood count. Assess patients for skin changes and gynecomastia.

H₂-Receptor Antagonists: Famotidine, Nizatidine, and Ranitidine

Drug administration

◆ Famotidine may be taken with antacids if necessary. For direct intravenous use of famotidine, dilute 20 mg with 5 to 10 ml of compatible solution, and administer over at least 2 min. For intermittent infusion of famotidine, dilute 20 mg in 100 ml of compatible solution, and administer dose over 15 to 30 min. For direct intravenous use of ranitidine, dilute 50 mg with 20 ml of compatible intravenous solution, and administer over at least 5 min. For intermittent infusion of ranitidine, dilute 50 mg in 50 to 100 ml of compatible IV solution, and administer over 15 to 20 min.

◆ Be alert when administering ranitidine intravenously; too rapid administration has been associated with bradycardia, tachycardia, and premature ventricular contractions (PVCs). Monitor pulse and blood pressure. Monitor level of consciousness, blood pressure, and pulse; assess for constipation or diarrhea, and monitor complete blood count. With famotidine, monitor blood urea nitrogen (BUN), serum creatinine level, and urinalysis.

Patient and family education

◆ Review the side effects associated with the prescribed drug, and instruct patients to report the development of these side effects to the physician. Review all prescribed medica-

NURSING IMPLICATIONS SUMMARY—cont'd

tions with the patient, and help the patient develop a dosing schedule that is consistent with the therapy goals and possible drug interactions.

◆ Warn patients to avoid alcohol and smoking while taking these drugs, especially after the final dose of the day. Emphasize the importance of all aspects of therapy, which may include modifying the diet, taking other drugs, and limiting caffeine intake. Warn patients to avoid using over-the-counter preparations while taking antihistamines.

Sucralfate

Drug administration and patient and family education

◆ Instruct patients to take antacids 30 min before or 1 hr after sucralfate. For best effects, instruct patients to take sucralfate with water on an empty stomach 1 hr before meals and at bedtime.

◆ Review all medications prescribed, and develop a dosing schedule that is suitable considering known drug interactions. Patients should take cimetidine, digoxin, phenytoin, tetracyclines, and fat-soluble vitamins at different times than sucralfate.

◆ Instruct patients to keep a record of bowel movements. If constipation develops, teach patients to increase daily intake of fluids to 2500 to 3000 ml, increase level of activity, and increase dietary intake of fruit and fiber. If the patient is taking antacids, changing the brand of antacid may also help; consult the physician.

Misoprostol

Drug administration and patient and family education

◆ Question female patients about possible pregnancy before administering first dose. Make sure that women of childbearing age are informed of the possible side effects of bleeding and abortion before administering first dose.

◆ Instruct patients to report severe or persistent diarrhea. Avoid concurrent use of magnesium-containing antacids; they may aggravate diarrhea. Take misoprostol with or after meals and at bedtime for best effect. Instruct patients to report any new sign or symptom. As more experience is accumulated with this group of drugs, additional information about side effects may be available.

Omeprazole

◆ Take doses before meals. Omeprazole may be taken with antacids if ordered. Tell patients to swallow capsules whole, not to break or chew them.

Antiemetics

Drug administration

◆ Measure emesis as part of fluid intake and output. Intravenous benzquinamide has been associated with an increase in blood pressure and cardiac arrhythmias. The intramuscular route is preferred. Monitor the blood pressure and pulse, and administer intravenous doses slowly. Avoid intramuscular use of trimethobenzamide in children.

◆ Use antiemetics with caution in children who may be suffering from Reye's syndrome. This syndrome is characterized by an abrupt onset of persistent severe vomiting, lethargy, irrational behavior, progressive encephalopathy, convulsions, coma, and death.

◆ Be alert to patient response to the cannabinoids; some patients may hesitate to use drugs derived from marijuana. Inform patients that psychologic or physical dependence is unlikely at therapeutic doses and with short-term use of these drugs.

◆ Since the gelatin capsule form of dronabinol contains sesame seed oil, check for allergy to this oil before administering first dose. The antihistamines are discussed in detail in Chapter 24. The antidopaminergic drugs are discussed in detail in Chapter 41.

Patient and family education

◆ Review the side effects of these drugs with patients. Warn patients to use antiemetics only as prescribed and not to self-medicate with leftover doses. The use of these drugs in pregnant women is contraindicated unless the benefit outweighs the risk. Warn patients to avoid drinking alcohol or operating hazardous equipment when taking antiemetics, since sedation and drowsiness are common side effects. Caution patients to avoid other drugs that may depress the CNS while using antiemetics. These drugs include alcohol, tranquilizers, sleeping medications, and narcotic analgesics.

◆ For treatment of motion sickness, suggest that patients ride in the front seat of the car

Continued.

NURSING IMPLICATIONS SUMMARY—cont'd

if possible, facing forward. Suggest that patients take prophylactic drugs 1 to 2 hr before the trip rather than when nausea develops.

◆ For sustained-release transdermal drugs, emphasize the importance of reading the manufacturer's instructions. Instruct patients to wash hands before applying the device and afterward. The disc is usually applied behind the ear, in front of the hairline. Avoid cut or denuded skin. Replace every 3 days or as directed by the physician. If the disk falls off, apply a new one. Apply the disk 4 hr before a trip.

◆ For dry mouth, suggest the patient chew sugarless gum or suck sugarless hard candy. Provide frequent mouth care, but avoid drying, alcohol-containing mouthwashes or lemon and glycerin swabs. See Patient Problem: Dry Mouth on p. 166. For the person who can have nothing by mouth (NPO) or who has vomited, provide frequent mouth care. Suggest that the patient suck ice chips; consult the physician for the NPO patient.

◆ Keep the environment free of odors. Keep food out of sight of the nauseated person. Try clear liquids in small amounts before progressing to a more complete diet.

◆ If dry eyes are a problem, suggest that the patient use artificial tears on a regular basis; consult the physician. Warn the patient that intramuscular antiemetics often produce burning at the injection site. Remind patients to keep these and all drugs out of the reach of children.

Drugs to Control Diarrhea

Drug administration

◆ Assess patients with diarrhea for a history of recent travel, especially international travel; recent antibiotic use; recent cancer chemotherapy; and recent work with children in day-care centers or other settings where harmful microorganisms are easily spread.

◆ Monitor intake and output, daily weight, skin turgor, level of consciousness, blood pressure, and pulse. Monitor serum electrolyte level. Dilute opium tincture in 15 to 30 ml to ensure that the patient receives the entire dose. Codeine is discussed in greater detail in Chapter 44.

◆ Paregoric tastes unpleasant. Many patients find combination drugs such as Parepectolin more palatable. (Parepectolin 30 ml contains paregoric 2.7 ml, pectin 162 mg, and kaolin 5.5 gm. Note that combination drugs subject the patient to additional ingredients that may or may not be helpful.)

◆ Theoretically, addiction to diphenoxylate or difenoxin is possible. Overdose with this drug resembles an overdose with a narcotic analgesic and is treated in a similar manner (see Chapter 44).

◆ Diphenoxylate and difenoxin preparations contain a small amount of atropine. A single dose of these preparations causes few side effects from the atropine, but the accumulated dose after 1 or 2 days of treatment might cause problems. Review the side effects of and contraindications to atropine use.

Patient and family education

◆ Review side effects with the patients. Note that loperamide is now available over the counter, but patients should be cautioned that side effects may be associated with excessive or long-term use.

◆ Encourage patients to keep a record of bowel movements. After several days of treatment for diarrhea, patients may become constipated.

◆ Teach patients with diarrhea to switch to a clear liquid diet and increase daily intake to 3000 ml but to avoid full-strength fruit juices. If the patient can afford it, commercially available electrolyte solutions or products such as Gatorade may be helpful.

◆ Many cases of diarrhea are self-limiting. Teach patients to consult the physician if diarrhea persists longer than 3 to 5 days; prescribed antidiarrhea medications are not affording relief; stools are especially foul-smelling or contain flecks of blood or large amounts of mucus; or the patient is unable to take in sufficient replacement fluids. Review symptoms of hypokalemia such as muscle weakness, fatigue, anorexia, vomiting, drowsiness, irritability, and eventually coma and death. Review symptoms of hypochloremia, including hypertonic muscles, tetany, and depressed respiration. Caution patients to avoid drinking alcohol and also to avoid driving or operating hazardous equipment if drowsiness develops. This may be dose related.

◆ Remind patients to keep the perianal area clean to avoid anal irritation and to wash hands carefully after defecating to avoid spreading infectious organisms.

NURSING IMPLICATIONS SUMMARY—cont'd

Drugs to Relieve Constipation

Drug administration

◆ Keep a record of bowel movements on all institutionalized, immobilized, or incapacitated patients. Prevention, early detection, and treatment of constipation are much easier and less time-consuming than treatment of severe constipation or impaction. Assess bowel sounds before administering any drug to relieve constipation. If bowel sounds are absent, withhold drug dose and notify the physician.

◆ Read orders and labels carefully. Many of these drugs have similar names. Be alert to the action of each component drug in combination products. For example, Colace contains the stool softener docusate sodium, whereas Peri-Colace contains docusate and casanthranol, a mild stimulant laxative.

◆ Physicians also sometimes prescribe bulk-forming agents to treat diarrhea, especially diarrhea associated with tube feedings. If given through a feeding tube, dilute with sufficient fluid to prevent clogging of the tube, and flush the tube with water after administration. Large-bore tubes are probably better suited to administer these agents.

◆ Castor oil does not mix with a water-based diluent. Add a small amount of baking soda (less than ¼ tsp) immediately before administering to cause the mixture to fizz, and the castor oil will be partially suspended in the juice for 1 or 2 min. Patients may find it easier to drink Castor oil this way. In an institution, the routine use of baking soda for this purpose must be cleared by the pharmacy or physician.

◆ Monitor the serum electrolyte levels of patients receiving lactulose, especially elderly patients. Lactulose is used to treat elevated serum ammonia levels.

Patient and family education

◆ Teach patients that a daily bowel movement is not necessary for normal bowel function. Review with parents the inadvisability of encouraging laxative dependence in small children. To help keep a regular bowel schedule, teach patients to increase daily fluid intake to 2500 to 3000 ml. If necessary, suggest that the patient drink a full (8 oz) glass of water before each meal and a full glass with each meal.

◆ Instruct patients to increase daily dietary intake of bran in cereals and other foods; fruits and vegetables, fruit juices, or foods known by the patient to be stimulating to defecation (e.g., hot chocolate or coffee). Encourage patients to exercise regularly to promote bowel regularity.

◆ Remind patients to use laxatives only as directed. Many laxatives are available without prescription. They may be misused or abused by patients who do not understand that increasing dependence on these drugs can develop with regular use.

◆ Review with patients using laxatives in preparation for GI tract diagnostic procedures the importance of following the prescribed regimen. The major reason that many studies of the GI tract are poor in quality or need to be repeated is that the preparation of the gut or colon was inadequate.

◆ Tell women who are pregnant or lactating that drugs to relieve constipation should be used only under the direction of a physician.

◆ Inform patients that changes in bowel habits should be thoroughly evaluated by a physician.

◆ Special points about bulk-forming laxatives include teaching patients to stir the prescribed dose into an 8-oz glass of fluid and drink the mixture while the drug is still suspended in the liquid. For best results, patients should follow the first glass with a second full glass of water. Patients should never take these drugs dry, since they can cause obstruction. Pills should be swallowed whole and not chewed. Usually, use these agents regularly, 1 to 3 times daily, to promote regular defecation.

◆ Take daily doses of stimulant (irritant) cathartics at bedtime to promote regular defecation in the morning. Swallow enteric-coated preparations, such as bisacodyl, whole and do not chew them. Patients should not take bisacodyl preparations within 1 hr of milk or antacids.

◆ Castor oil has an unpleasant taste; assess whether the patient would like it mixed with fruit juice. Some patients prefer to take castor oil straight and then drink juice as a follow-up so that the taste of the juice is not ruined by the medication.

◆ Teach patients that storing suppositories in the refrigerator will make them firmer and easier to insert.

Continued.

NURSING IMPLICATIONS SUMMARY—cont'd

◆ Note in Table 13-6 that many of these drugs change the color of urine. Warn patients about these changes.

◆ Special points about saline cathartics include chilling magnesium citrate before drinking to make it more palatable. Patients should drink the entire prescribed amount at once for best results. Teach patients on a sodium-restricted diet to avoid saline cathartics. Saline cathartics are often used to eliminate parasites after antihelminthic therapy because the trophozoites are not destroyed and can be examined in the laboratory.

◆ Patients should be warned that when mineral oil is used on a regular basis there may be leakage of the oil or fecal material from the anus. Mineral oil stains clothing. Suggest that patients wear a perianal pad or incontinence shield to protect clothing and sheets. Regular mineral oil use is associated with increased incidence of lipid pneumonia, especially in elderly patients. Encourage patients to always sit upright when taking this medication. For long-term treatment of constipation, drugs other than mineral oil are preferred. Do not use mineral oil or any oil-based substance to lubricate the nose or mouth of immobilized patients, since they may inadvertently aspirate small amounts.

◆ Explain the action of fecal softeners to patients. Many patients misunderstand their function and expect defecation to occur a few hours after taking a single dose. For best results, use fecal softeners on a daily basis as prescribed.

◆ Caution diabetic patients to monitor blood glucose levels carefully when taking lactulose, since the drug contains high concentrations of lactose and galactose. Warn patients taking lactulose that flatulence and abdominal cramps are common initially but subside with continued therapy.

CHAPTER REVIEW

◆ KEY TERMS

anticholinergic drugs, p. 166

antiemetics, p. 173

constipation, p. 182

diarrhea, p. 180

esophageal ulcer, p. 169

H₂-antagonists, p. 172

hydrochloric acid, p. 169

lactulose, p. 186

laxative, p. 182

nausea, p. 173

peptic ulcer, p. 169

secretin, p. 169

ulcer, p. 169

vomiting, p. 173

wetting agents, p. 185

xerostomia, p. 166

◆ REVIEW QUESTIONS

1. How do cholinomimetic drugs act on the GI tract? Name two cholinomimetic drugs that are used for their activity on the GI tract.

2. What is the antidote for bethanechol? Under what circumstances should you consider administering the antidote?

3. What actions do anticholinergic drugs have on the GI tract?

4. The drug atropine is classically given as a preoperative medication. What are the desired effects? For the patient using atropine on a regular (chronic) basis, what are the side effects, and how would you suggest the patient manage them?

5. What three factors stimulate the secretion of stomach acid?

6. How do ulcers arise? What does the location of the ulcer indicate?

7. What do antacids do?

8. Name the major side effects you might expect with the use of sodium bicarbonate, aluminum

and calcium alkaline salts, and magnesium alkaline salts.

9. Patients with renal failure may take antacids to bind phosphate. Give an example of a phosphate-binding antacid. When should you administer it?

10. Why does cimetidine inhibit gastric acid secretion, whereas antihistamines used to treat hay fever do not?

11. What are the three major pathways that stimulate vomiting?

12. What are some nonpharmacologic treatments of nausea and vomiting you might recommend?

13. Describe the major differences in the effectiveness of antihistamines versus the antidopaminergic drugs for types of nausea and vomiting.

14. What is diarrhea? Why do you need to monitor fluid and electrolyte replacement?

15. What drugs might you use for the treatment of diarrhea? What is their mechanism of action?

16. List some teaching points about ways to prevent constipation without using medications.

17. List the five classes of laxatives. How do they differ in the time for a laxative effect to be produced and in the type of stool produced?

18. Why does the continued use of the stimulant (irritant) cathartics not help establish regular bowel habits?

SUGGESTED READING

Brown JK, Everett I: Gentler bowel fitness with fiber, *Geriatr Nurs* 11(1):26, 1990.

Brucker MC: Management of common minor discomforts in pregnancy: managing gastrointestinal problems in pregnancy. III. *J Nurse Midwife* 33(2):67, 1988.

Hockenberry-Eaton J, Benner A: Patterns of nausea and vomiting in children: nursing assessment and intervention, *Oncol Nurs Forum* 17(4):575, 1990.

Hogan CM: Advances in the management of nausea and vomiting, *Nurs Clin North Am* 25(2):475, 1990.

Jordan LN: Effects of fluid manipulation on the incidence of vomiting during outpatient cisplatin infusion, *Oncol Nurs Forum* 16(2):213, 1989.

Karb VB: GI drugs: histamine antagonists, sucralfate and metoclopramide, *J Neurosci Nurs* 20(3):201, 1988.

Lynn MM, Holdcroft C: Preventing NSAID-induced ulcers: the use of misoprostol, *Nurse Pract* 15(10):38, 1990.

Miller TW, Jay LL: Gastrointestinal disorders: diagnosis and treatment, *J Pract Nurs* 39(3):39, 1989.

Rice PS, Phaosawasdi K: Understanding idiopathic chronic constipation: an understated problem, *Gastroenterol Nurs* 12(2):90, 1989.

Ross D: Constipation among hospitalized elders, *Orthop Nurs* 9(3):73, 1990.

Rowland MA: When drug therapy causes diarrhea, *RN* 52(12):32, 1989.

Williams SG, DiPalma JA: Constipation in the long-term care facility, *Gastroenterol Nurs* 12(3):179, 1990.

Yakabowich M: Prescribe with care: the role of laxatives in the treatment of constipation, *J Gerontol Nurs* 16(7):4, 1990.

SECTION V

DRUGS AFFECTING THE CARDIOVASCULAR AND RENAL SYSTEMS

This section is divided into three parts, drugs affecting circulation and blood pressure (Chapters 14 through 17), drugs affecting the heart (Chapters 18 and 19), and drugs affecting the blood (Chapters 20 through 22).

In Chapters 14 and 15, which cover the pharmacologic aspects of circulation and blood pressure, you find drugs with the adrenergic mechanisms discussed in Chapter 10, as well as direct-acting vasodilators. Chapter 14 covers the sympathomimetic amines and their use as short-term agents to maintain circulation or blood pressure. The vasodilators used to treat angina and impaired peripheral vascular circulation are discussed. We also discuss the use of beta-adrenergic blockers and calcium channel blockers as antianginal drugs. Antihypertensive drugs are presented according to their mechanism of action in Chapter 15. The importance of planned drug interaction in the treatment of chronic hypertension is reviewed in the chapter summary.

Chapters 16 through 22 each target a given area of therapeutics for which the pharmacologic factors are distinctly focused on a physiologic process. These chapters focus on diuretics, fluids and electrolytes, cardiac glycosides, antiarrhythmic drugs, drugs affecting blood clotting, drugs to lower blood lipids, and drugs to treat nutritional anemias.

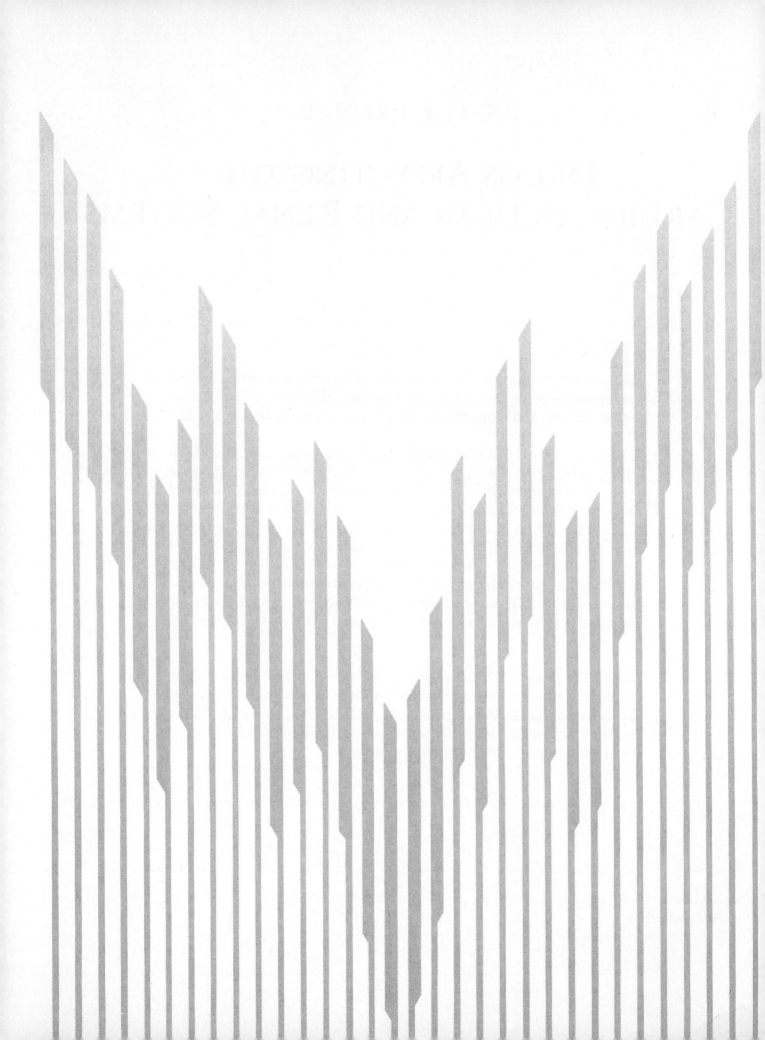

CHAPTER 14

Drugs to Improve Circulation

LEARNING OBJECTIVES

After studying this chapter, you should be able to do the following:

- Discuss the use of sympathomimetic amines in the treatment of shock.
- Describe drug therapy for angina pectoris, including differentiating among the nitrates and nitrites, the beta-adrenergic blocking drugs, and the calcium channel blocking drugs.
- Discuss the rationale for drug treatment of vasospastic disorders.
- Develop nursing care plans for patients receiving sympathomimetic amines, nitrates and nitrites, beta-adrenergic blocking drugs, calcium channel blocking drugs, vasodilating drugs for vascular disease, and pentoxifylline.

CHAPTER OVERVIEW

- This chapter covers sympathomimetic drugs and selected vasodilators used primarily to improve circulation. Beta blockers and calcium channel blockers, also discussed, have gained widespread use in the treatment of angina.
- **Sympathomimetic drugs** restore functions mediated through adrenergic receptors. These drugs are used primarily to treat shock, a condition of poor tissue perfusion in which selective adjustment of cardiac or vascular function may prevent shock from becoming irreversible and progressing to death.
- **Vasodilators** improve blood flow by increasing blood vessel size. Vasodilation is used to treat angina and peripheral vascular disease. Although some of the activity of vasodilators may be related to alpha- or beta-adrenergic receptors, most vasodilators work by a mechanism that was not understood until recently. As understanding of these diseases progresses, the role of vasodilators is being reevaluated. Vasodilators used primarily as antihypertensive agents are discussed in Chapter 15.

Nursing Process Overview
SYMPATHOMIMETIC DRUGS
Assessment

Sympathomimetics treat shock, which can be caused by trauma, blood loss, burns, sepsis, cardiac failure (cardiogenic shock), anaphylaxis, and extreme reactions to some drugs. The patient in shock appears pale and has clammy skin. The blood pressure is usually low or may be absent; the pulse rate may be increased and thready. If alert, the patient may fear death and may be anxious. The respiratory rate may be increased. Perform a rapid assessment, including pulse, respirations, blood pressure, and level of consciousness. Examine for obvious causes of the shock. Monitor appropriate laboratory work, including arterial blood gas concentrations, serum electrolyte concentrations, hematocrit and hemoglobin values, additional blood counts, and blood sugar concentrations.

Nursing Diagnoses

Decreased cardiac output (This may result in several collaborative problems, such as cardiac arrhythmias and hypoxia.)
Altered tissue perfusion
Collaborative problems including fluid overload, metabolic acidosis, hypertension, and fluid and electrolyte imbalance

Management

Administer ordered vasopressors to increase and maintain the blood pressure; use an infusion control device and a microdrip infusion set. Monitor the vital signs frequently, as often as every 5 min. Administer ordered replacement fluids and blood. Monitor intake and output; a Foley catheter may be inserted. Monitor the level of consciousness. Attach the patient to a cardiac monitor. Have available emergency care equipment such as a suction machine and resuscitation equipment. Remain with the patient, and stay calm. Continue to assess for changes in patient, status and drug side effects. Inform the patient and family of what is being done.

Evaluation

Drugs to treat shock are successful if the blood pressure is maintained to provide adequate tissue perfusion. Few vasopressors are used in self-management situations; most are used only in the acute-care setting for the patient in shock. Epinephrine may be prescribed for patients with a history of previous serious allergic response. Before discharge, the patient should be able to explain when epinephrine should be used and how to use it, demonstrate the correct administration technique, and explain the side effects that result from the medication; the patient also should know when to seek emergency assistance.

DIRECT-ACTING SYMPATHOMIMETIC DRUGS
Cardiovascular Actions

The rate of blood flow through a tissue is determined by the size of the blood vessels and the arteriovenous blood pressure differential across the tissue. The systolic blood pressure reflects the cardiac output, and the diastolic blood pressure reflects the resistance of the tissue vessels to flow. As discussed in Chapter 10, the sympathetic nervous system plays a major role in controlling cardiovascular function. Stimulation of the alpha-adrenergic receptors of blood vessels causes vasoconstriction. On a systemic level, this vasoconstriction shows up as a higher blood pressure. Stimulation of the cardiac beta-1 receptors increases heart rate and force of contraction, resulting in an increased cardiac output. Stimulation of the beta-2 receptors, found primarily in the blood vessels of the skeletal muscle, causes vasodilation. Only in unusual circumstances does systemic stimulation of the beta-2 receptors decrease blood pressure. The net change in cardiovascular function produced by direct-acting sympathomimetic drugs depends on the degree of activity at the three adrenergic receptor subtypes.

Uses in Shock

Shock is a disruption of circulation. Frequently, the blood pressure is too low to force blood through vital tissues. Poor perfusion of the brain results in confusion or coma; poor perfusion of the kidney results in low urine output (less than 30 ml/hr); and poor perfusion of the skin results in cold and clammy skin. In shock, the body has already activated the sympathetic nervous system to increase blood pressure. Fluid replacement or addition is often the first choice in treating shock to overcome the decrease in the circulating volume caused by the constriction of the peripheral blood vessels. Direct-acting sympathomimetic amines treat certain types of shock, raise blood pressure by increasing peripheral resistance (activation of alpha-1 adrenergic receptors) or increase cardiac output (activation of beta-1 adrenergic receptors).

Specific Drugs

Specific sympathomimetic drugs are listed in Table 14-1.

Dopamine

Mechanism of action. Dopamine (Dopastat and Intropin) is a naturally occurring catecholamine capable of acting at alpha- and beta-adrenergic receptors, as well as at its own specific dopaminergic receptors. Appropriate doses of dopamine can be selected so that cardiac output is increased while heart rate and mean blood pressure remain unchanged. An unusual and highly desirable property of dopamine is that renal blood flow is directly stimulated at these same doses. Renal function may therefore be maintained in patients being treated for shock as long as supportive therapy maintains adequate blood volume.

Administration and fate. Dopamine must be administered by constant intravenous (IV) infusion. Dopamine is rapidly taken up and stored or destroyed by tissues. The infusion rate must be meticulously adjusted to achieve the desired therapeutic results.

Side effects. Dopamine can cause **tachycardia** (fast heart rate), palpitation, nausea and vomiting, angina, headache, hypertension, and vasoconstriction. A reduction or discontinuance of dopamine infusion is usually sufficient to reverse side effects because dopamine has such a short plasma half-life. Leakage of dopamine around the infusion site must be avoided, but if extravasation occurs, the alpha-adrenergic receptor antagonist phentolamine should be infused into the area to reverse vasoconstriction. Untreated extravasation can cause tissue death and sloughing.

Uses. Dopamine is the most widely used sympathomimetic amine for treating shock. Its action may be controlled by the rate of infusion. Dopamine is used primarily as a renal vasodilator to prevent renal failure in shock and secondarily to increase cardiac output. At low doses (0.5 to 2 μg/kg/min), dopamine acts exclusively on dopamine receptors in the

Table 14-1   Sympathomimetic Drugs Used to Treat Hypotension and Shock

Generic name	Trade name	Administration/dosage	Comments
Dobutamine hydrochloride	Dobutrex*	INTRAVENOUS: *Adults*—2.5 to 10μg/kg/min. A 12.5 to 25 mg/ml solution is made and used.	To stimulate cardiac contractility in cardiogenic shock.
Dopamine hydrochloride	Intropin* Revimine†	INTRAVENOUS: *Adults*—1 ampule (40 mg of chloride salt in 5 ml) is diluted in 250 ml (800 μg/ml) or 500 ml (400 μg/ml) of solution. Initial intravenous infusion is 2 to 5 μg/kg/min. Onset: 5 min. Duration: 10 min.	To maintain renal blood flow in shock with mild cardiac stimulation.
Epinephrine hydrochloride	Adrenalin chloride* EpiPenn Sus-Phrine	INTRAMUSCULAR, SUBCUTANEOUS, INTRAVENOUS: *Adults*—0.5 ml of 1:1000 solution IM or SC followed by 0.25 to 0.5 ml of 1:10,000 solution intravenously every 5 to 15 min. *Children*—0.3 ml of 1:1000 solution intramuscularly. May be repeated every 15 min for 1 hr if necessary. Onset: minutes. Duration: 1 to 4 hr.	To treat anaphylactic shock.
Isoproterenol hydrochloride	Isuprel hydrochloride*	INTRAVENOUS: *Adults*—1 to 2 mg (5 to 10 ml) diluted in 5% dextrose and infused at rate of 1 to 10 μg/min. Onset: minutes. Duration: 1 to 2 hr.	To stimulate cardiac contractility.
Levarterenol (norepinephrine) bitartrate	Levophed bitartrate*	INTRAVENOUS: *Adults*—2 to 8 ml of 0.2% solution in 500 ml 5% dextrose and given by continuous infusion for desired response. Onset: immediate. Duration: minutes.	To maintain blood pressure in life-threatening situations.
Mephentermine sulfate	Wyamine sulfate	INTRAVENOUS: *Adults*—600 mg 1 gm is diluted in 1 L 5% dextrose and given by continuous infusion to maintain pressure. Onset: immediate. Duration: 30 to 45 min.	To maintain arterial blood pressure during spinal, epidural, or general anesthesia.

*Available in Canada and United States.
†Available in Canada only.

Continued.

Table 14-1 Sympathomimetic Drugs Used to Treat Hypotension and Shock—cont'd

Generic name	Trade name	Administration/dosage	Comments
Metaraminol bitartrate	Aramine	INTRAMUSCULAR, INTRAVENOUS: *Adults*—2 to 5 mg as a single intravenous injection or 200 to 500 mg diluted in 1 L 5% dextrose given by continuous infusion to maintain pressure. Alternatively, 5 to 10 mg given intramuscularly. Onset: 1 to 2 min. Duration: 20 to 60 min.	To maintain blood pressure during spinal, epidural, or general anesthesia.
Methoxamine hydrochloride	Vasoxyl*	INTRAMUSCULAR, INTRAVENOUS: *Adults*—5 to 20 mg in a single intramuscular dose or 2 to 5 mg given slowly IV. Onset: immediate Duration: 60 min.	To maintain blood pressure during spinal and general anesthesia To control hypotension after ganglionic blockade.
Phenylephrine hydrochloride	Neo-Synephrine hydrochloride*	ORAL, INTRAMUSCULAR, SUBCUTANEOUS, INTRAVENOUS: *Adults*—1 to 10 mg intramuscularly or subcutaneously,; 0.25 to 0.5 mg given intravenously or 10 mg in 500 ml 5% dextrose infused slowly; 20 mg 3 times per day orally for orthostatic hypotension. Onset: minutes. Duration: 1 to 2 hr	To maintain blood pressure during general and spinal anesthesia. To treat orthostatic hypotension and paroxysmal atrial tachycardia.

*Available in Canada and United States.

renal arterioles to cause vasodilation. At higher doses (1 to 10 µg/kg/min), dopamine acts at cardiac beta-1 receptors to stimulate cardiac contractility. The beta-1 receptors controlling heart rate and the alpha receptors affecting blood pressure are not activated. At doses above these, dopamine causes the release of norepinephrine, thereby increasing heart rate and blood pressure.

Contraindications and drug interactions. Like the other sympathomimetic amines, dopamine is contraindicated for patients predisposed to cardiac arrhythmias. Dopamine is not stable in alkaline solutions and should not be placed in a sodium bicarbonate solution. Patients medicated with a monoamine oxidase inhibitor require only 10% of the usual dose of dopamine. Tricyclic antidepressants potentiate the hypertensive action of dopamine. Dopamine should not be administered to women in labor receiving an oxytocic drug because a severe persistent hypertension may be produced. Patients receiving a general anesthetic that sensitizes the heart to catecholamines may develop arrhythmias if dopamine is administered. Since dopamine dilates renal arteries, the action of diuretic drugs is potentiated.

Dobutamine

Mechanism of action. At low doses dobutamine (Dobutrex), like dopamine, selectively increases the contractility of the heart without increasing the heart rate. Dobutamine neither stimulates the dopamine receptors of the kidney blood vessels nor releases norepinephrine. At high doses, dobutamine increases heart rate and conduction velocity (beta-1 adrenergic receptor) and stimulates beta-2 adrenergic receptors.

Administration and fate. Dobutamine has a plasma half-life of about 2 min and must be administered by continuous IV infusion. Dobutamine is rapidly metabolized to inactive compounds in the liver.

Side effects. Increased heart rate and blood pressure are the most frequent side effects that can be reversed by lowering the infusion rate. Palpitations, shortness of breath, angina, nausea, and headache are infrequent side effects of dobutamine.

Uses. Dobutamine improves cardiac output in patients with congestive heart failure, with little effect on heart rate or systolic blood pressure.

Contraindications and drug interactions. Dobutamine is contraindicated for patients in whom the increased force of contraction would be dangerous, as in idiopathic hypertrophic subaortic stenosis. Drugs that may sensitize the heart to the inotropic effects of dobutamine include hydrocarbon inhalation anesthetics and the reserpine antihypertensives. Dobutamine may reduce the effectiveness of the beta blockers and other antihypertensive agents, including guanadrel, guanethidine, and nitroprusside.

Epinephrine

Mechanism of action. Epinephrine is a potent agonist of the beta-1 receptors of the heart, increasing heart rate and force of contraction. This cardiac stimulation is achieved with an increase in the oxygen demand of the heart, which may not be tolerable in cardiac disease. Epinephrine also stimulates alpha receptors to cause vasoconstriction, particularly of the vessels in the skin, mucosa, kidney, and visceral organs. Epinephrine also stimulates beta-2 receptors, which alter blood flow because beta-2 receptors mediate vasodilation in the blood vessels in skeletal muscle. The overall response to IV administration of epinephrine is a marked increase in heart rate and force of contraction with little or no increase in blood pressure.

Administration and fate. Epinephrine is not active when given orally because it is rapidly inactivated by the gastric mucosa. Epinephrine is administered intramuscularly or subcutaneously. Epinephrine may be inhaled from a nebulizer for relief of bronchospasm. IV administration of epinephrine must be done very slowly and cannot be done using one of the epinephrine suspensions. Intracardiac injection of epinephrine is a last step in attempting cardiac resuscitation when other measures have failed.

Epinephrine is rapidly degraded by the monoamine oxidase and catechol-*O*-methyltransferase of the liver and kidney. Epinephrine is unstable in alkaline solutions and when exposed to light or air. Pink or brown solutions should not be used.

Side effects. Fear and anxiety are side effects of epinephrine, arising from stimulation of the central nervous system (CNS). Other side effects include throbbing headache, dizziness, and pallor caused by vasoconstriction. Stimulation of skeletal muscle causes tremor and weakness, and stimulation of the heart causes palpitation. These effects are usually transient. Hyperthyroid and hypertensive patients are prone to an exaggerated hypertensive response to epinephrine. Cerebral hemorrhage and cardiac arrhythmias are serious reactions to epinephrine.

Uses and contraindications. Epinephrine, administered as soon as possible, is the drug of choice for treating anaphylactic shock. Anaphylactic shock is the result of massive histamine release caused by an allergic reaction and must be promptly treated. Histamine causes profound vasodilation and bronchial constriction. Epinephrine opposes the actions of histamine by producing vasoconstriction, raising blood pressure, and relaxing bronchioles, which restores breathing. Epinephrine quickly reverses the edema of the larynx and the bronchospasm of anaphylactic shock.

Epinephrine may be administered systemically or by inhalation to relieve bronchospasm resulting from asthma or allergic reactions. Because epinephrine causes vasoconstriction, it is applied topically as a hemostatic agent. Epinephrine injection prolongs the action of local anesthetics by slowing their systemic absorption.

Epinephrine is contraindicated for patients under a general anesthetic that sensitizes the heart to catecholamines. Neither patients with narrow-angle glaucoma nor women in labor should receive epinephrine. Epinephrine must be used with extreme care in patients with cardiac arrhythmias, cardiovascular disease, hypertension, or hyperthyroidism. The hyperglycemic, hypoinsulinemic effects of epinephrine interrupt control of diabetes mellitus.

Drug interactions. Epinephrine should not be administered simultaneously with isoproterenol because the combination can cause cardiac arrhythmias. Cardiac effects of epinephrine are also potentiated by tricyclic antidepressants, antihistamines, thyroxine, digitalis, and mercurial diuretics. Patients receiving a monoamine oxidase inhibitor or oxytocin may have a hypertensive response to epinephrine.

Isoproterenol

Mechanism of action. Isoproterenol (Isuprel) is a synthetic catecholamine that stimulates beta-1 and beta-2 adrenergic receptors but has little activity on alpha-adrenergic receptors. Isoproterenol therefore stimulates heart rate and cardiac output. At sufficient doses of isoproterenol, blood pressure falls because activation of the beta-2 receptors of the blood vessels in skeletal muscle shunts blood to the muscles and lowers peripheral resistance. Smooth muscle, particularly bronchial and gastrointestinal smooth muscle, is relaxed by isoproterenol. Isoproterenol can treat bronchospasm when administered by inhalation.

Administration and fate. Isoproterenol is not effective orally. Absorption from a sublingual site is unreliable. Isoproterenol may be given effectively subcutaneously, intramuscularly, or intravenously. The catechol-*o*-methyltransferase of the liver and other tissues is the major enzyme for degrading isoproterenol.

Side effects. Side effects of isoproterenol include palpitation, tachycardia, headache, and flushing of the face. The patient may experience sweating and mild tremors, nervousness, dizziness, and nausea.

Uses. Isoproterenol is used primarily as a bronchodilator (see Chapter 25). Isoproterenol is infrequently used as a cardiac stimulant in heart block and in cardiogenic shock secondary to a myocardial infarction or septicemia.

Contraindications and drug interactions. Patients taking digitalis or otherwise disposed toward cardiac arrhythmias should not receive isoproterenol. Isoproterenol should not be administered with epinephrine because together they can induce severe cardiac arrhythmias.

Levarterenol

Mechanism of action. Norepinephrine, the neurotransmitter of the sympathetic nervous system, is a potent agonist of the alpha-1 and beta-1 adrenergic receptors when administered as the drug levarterenol. Levarterenol does not significantly affect the beta-2 adrenergic receptors.

Levarterenol produces a potent peripheral vasoconstriction and inotropic response. Blood flow shifts from the skin and visceral and renal vessels (where blood vessels are constricted) to the heart and brain (where blood vessels do not have alpha receptors). On administration, levarterenol initially raises blood pressure dramatically. The increase is great enough to stimulate the baroreceptors in the aorta, thereby triggering reflex stimulation of the vagus nerve, a physiologic process called *reflex bradycardia* (slow heart rate). This results because stimulation of the vagus nerve releases acetylcholine. Since acetylcholine slows the heart, this vagal stimulation counteracts the direct stimulation of the heart by levarterenol. The net result of administering levarterenol is therefore an increase in blood pressure with a modest and variable change in heart rate but very strong contractions of the heart.

Administration and fate. Levarterenol is ineffective when taken orally, since it is rapidly degraded in the stomach. It is administered intravenously, and if it does infiltrate the infusion site, the alpha-adrenergic receptor antagonist phentolamine must be infiltrated in the area to counteract the profound vasoconstriction that may lead to tissue ischemia.

Levarterenol is rapidly inactivated by the liver. Like norepinephrine, levarterenol is stored in sympathetic neurons.

Side effects. Anxiety and a slow, forceful heartbeat are common side effects of levarterenol. Some patients develop transient hypertension, evidenced by a severe headache.

Uses and contraindications. Levarterenol is used to restore blood pressure in acute hypotensive states after blood volume has been restored. In the absence of adequate blood volume, tissue perfusion is inadequate after vasoconstriction by levarterenol despite increased blood pressure. Kidney perfusion in particular is poor. Levarterenol provides a temporary treatment when the brain or heart is compromised in shock. Levarterenol may be used immediately after cardiac arrest has been terminated to restore and maintain blood pressure.

Levarterenol is contraindicated for patients who have vascular thrombosis because the resulting vasoconstriction could cause tissue death. Levarterenol should not be used to raise blood pressure in patients anesthetized with a drug that sensitizes the heart to catecholamine-induced arrhythmias (see Chapter 45).

Drug interactions. Administration of levarterenol to a patient taking an antidepressant drug (either a monoamine oxidase inhibitor or a tricyclic antidepressant) may cause a severe hypertensive response, since these drugs interfere with the degradation and reuptake, respectively, of norepinephrine. A persistent hypertensive response may be elicited if levarterenol is administered after an oxytocic drug during labor.

Methoxamine

Methoxamine (Vasoxyl) acts selectively to stimulate alpha-adrenergic receptors. Methoxamine, which is administered intravenously or intramuscularly, increases blood pressure for 60 to 90 min. This vasopressor action treats the hypotension of anesthesia during surgery, primarily for spinal anesthesia when the patient is conscious and aware of the unpleasant effects of hypotension. Increased blood pressure in a patient with normal blood pressure causes reflex bradycardia, which terminates episodes of paroxysmal supraventricular tachycardia. Side effects of methoxamine include sustained hypertension with a severe headache. Goosebumps (pilomotor erection), desire to urinate, and vomiting are occasional side effects.

Like the other sympathomimetic vasopressors, methoxamine should be used with caution in patients with heart disease or hypertension. It potentiates oxytocic drugs, monoamine oxidase inhibitors, tricyclic antidepressants, and general anesthesia that sensitizes the heart to catecholamines.

Phenylephrine

Phenylephrine (Isophrin and Neo-Synephrine) acts selectively to stimulate alpha-adrenergic receptors. Phenylephrine is shorter in duration (20 to 50 min) than methoxamine, but otherwise the description of methoxamine and its uses, side effects, and drug interactions can be applied to phenylephrine. Phenylephrine is used mainly as a nasal decongestant (see Chapter 26); it is also used to dilate the pupil (see Chapter 12). These actions result from stimulation of alpha-adrenergic receptors.

INDIRECT-ACTING SYMPATHOMIMETIC AMINES

Mechanism and Uses

Indirect-acting sympathomimetic drugs cause norepinephrine to be released from sympathetic neurons. Like methoxamine, the indirect-acting sympathomimetic amines are used primarily in treating the hypotension of spinal anesthesia. During spinal anesthesia, the sympathetic ganglia lying near the spinal cord may be affected, thereby disrupting sympathetic control of blood pressure. This is usually not life-threatening, but the sensation is unpleasant to the conscious patient. Indirect-acting sympathomimetic amines act directly on the postganglionic nerve terminals to release norepinephrine, which restores blood pressure.

Specific Drugs

Specific indirect-acting sympathomimetic drugs are listed in Table 14-1.

Ephedrine

Mechanism of action. Ephedrine is the prototype of the indirect-acting sympathomimetic amines, although it can be shown to have direct sympathomimetic actions at alpha- and beta-adrenergic receptors. Ephedrine, which has been isolated from several plants, has been used in Chinese medicine for 2000 years. Ephedrine is primarily used as a bronchodilator (see Chapter 25) and seldom is used as a vasopressor. The vasopressor response to ephedrine is primarily a result of cardiac stimulation, increasing blood pressure through an increase in cardiac output.

Administration. Ephedrine is active administered orally, subcutaneously, intramuscularly, or intravenously for 4 to 6 hr.

Side effects. Ephedrine is a potent stimulant of the CNS. Insomnia, agitation, euphoria, and confusion may be noted. Delirium and hallucinations can occur at high doses. As with other sympathomimetic drugs, headache, palpitation, nausea and vomiting, and difficulty in voiding may be side effects. Repeated administration of ephedrine decreases the effectiveness of the drug. This rapidly developing tolerance (tachyphylaxis) results from the depletion of stored norepinephrine.

Contraindications and drug interactions. Ephedrine should be used cautiously in patients with hypertension, hyperthyroidism, diabetes mellitus, or prostate obstruction. The vasopressor response to ephedrine is potentiated by monoamine oxidase inhibitors, tricyclic antidepressants, and oxytocic drugs. Cardiac arrhythmias may be precipitated by ephedrine in the presence of digitalis or one of the general anesthetics that sensitize the heart to catecholamines.

Metaraminol

Metaraminol (Aramine) has direct alpha-adrenergic agonist activity and indirect sympathomimetic activity. Metaraminol can deplete norepinephrine stores on repeated administration to cause tachyphylaxis.

Metaraminol is administered intravenously, intramuscularly, or subcutaneously, and the onset of action is 1 to 2 min, 10 min, and 15 to 20 min, respectively. Its effects persist for 20 to 60 min. Larger doses are administered by IV infusion, and care must be taken to avoid leakage of the drug at the infusion site. Metaraminol increases diastolic and systolic blood pressure, but heart rate usually decreases as a result of reflex bradycardia. The force of contraction of the heart is increased. Metaraminol is used clinically only to treat certain acute hypotensive states, as in spinal anesthesia.

Metaraminol does not have any pronounced CNS effects. Otherwise, side effects, contraindications, and drug interactions are identical to those described for ephedrine.

Mephentermine

Mephentermine (Wyamine) is an indirect-acting sympathomimetic drug. The major effect of mephentermine is an increased blood pressure resulting from increased cardiac output and peripheral vasoconstriction. The effects of mephentermine persist for 30 to 60 min after subcutaneous administration and continue for up to 4 hr after IM administration. Mephentermine can also be administered as a single IV dose. Mephentermine does not cause the tissue irritation characteristic of most vasopressor drugs.

Side effects of mephentermine are minimal and include drowsiness, weeping, incoherence, and occasionally, convulsions. Contraindications and drug interactions are the same as for other vasopressor drugs.

ANTIANGINAL DRUGS

Blood Circulation to the Heart

The heart has a high requirement for oxygen and nutrients. These needs are met by coronary circulation (Figure 14-1) because the heart muscle cannot use the blood pumped through its chambers. The right and left coronary arteries originate at the aorta as it leaves the heart. The left coronary artery divides into the circumflex branch and the anterior descending branch. The three major vessels of the heart are thus the right coronary artery, the circumflex coronary branch of the left coronary artery, and the anterior descending branch of the left coronary artery. These vessels divide and subdivide to the capillaries that finally service the individual cardiac cells. Normally, the heart receives an adequate supply of blood through these coronary vessels.

Angina Pectoris

Angina pectoris, which means a choking of the chest, results from a temporary insufficient supply of oxygen to the heart. The heart has a large requirement for oxygen and normally extracts maximum amounts of oxygen from the coronary circulation. The increased oxygen demands of the heart associated with increased work are normally met by increased coronary blood flow.

In about 1 of 50 American adults the coronary arteries become narrowed by fatty deposits that develop just underneath the inner lining of the vessel. This condition is called ***coronary atherosclerosis.*** The flow of blood in affected vessels is reduced, and the dependent heart muscle no longer receives an adequate blood supply. As the atherosclerosis worsens, the vascular system in the heart compensates by developing additional blood vessels (collateral circulation) to bypass the affected vessel. If a large enough area of the heart muscle does not receive sufficient oxygen, pain results.

Anginal pain is a sudden, severe, and pressing pain that begins behind the breast bone and radiates up to the left shoulder and arm. Often this pain initially may be a feeling of acute chest discomfort; it also may be felt in the neck, jaw, teeth, arms, or elbows, areas to which cardiac pain is physiologically referred. The pain gradually lessens when the person stops and rests. Drugs that increase the heart rate, decrease blood flow to the heart, or cause fluid retention may precipitate anginal episodes. Drugs shown to increase anginal attacks include bromocriptine, diazoxide, digitalis, dobutamine, dopamine, ergotamine, fluorouracil, hydralazine, indomethacin, minoxidil, nifedipine, prazosin, propranolol, thyroid hormone, and tolazoline.

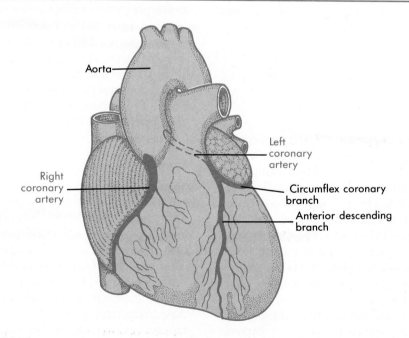

FIGURE 14-1

Coronary arteries. Three major coronary arteries are right coronary artery and two branches of left coronary artery, circumflex coronary branch and anterior descending branch. These arteries supply blood for heart muscle. Occlusion of one or more of these arteries can cause angina.

Classic angina is often called *stable angina* or *exertional angina*. In classic angina the large coronary arteries are obstructed by atherosclerosis so that blood flow cannot increase to supply more oxygen required by increased work. Coronary atherosclerosis is the most common cause of angina.

Variant angina (Prinzmetal's angina) is caused by spasms of the large coronary arteries that result in obstruction of blood flow. These coronary spasms have no relationship to exercise and may occur at rest. Variant angina frequently has a daily rhythm, and episodes are more common in the morning. Most patients with variant angina also have coronary atherosclerosis; in these patients anginal pain may also occur with exertion.

Unstable angina refers to angina that has a changing intensity. Pain comes at decreasing levels of exertion and often at rest. Patients who progress to unstable angina are the most likely to have heart attacks and should be medically reviewed immediately.

Nursing Process Overview
ANTIANGINAL DRUGS
Assessment

Patients with angina pectoris have a primary single complaint, chest pain. Obtain a thorough patient assessment, focusing on the subjective and objective signs. Determine the patient's pulse, respiration, blood pressure, and level of consciousness. Question the patient about the onset and duration of the pain, and ask about previous similar episodes and treatments. Obtain an electrocardiogram and appropriate laboratory work, including serum enzyme concentrations. When the cause of chest pain is uncertain, the usual practice is to treat the patient as if a myocardial infarction has occurred.

Nursing Diagnoses

High risk for altered health maintenance related to insufficient knowledge about prescribed antianginal drugs

High risk for injury related to orthostatic hypotension secondary to vasodilator therapy

Management

Administer drugs as ordered. Assess for further chest pain, monitor for drug side effects, and teach about the drugs in anticipation of discharge. Work with the patient and family to identify and reduce stresses that may precipitate angina attacks. Teach patients about other prescribed therapies such as losing weight, stopping smoking, controlling blood pressure, and exercising regularly. Refer patients as needed to the dietitian, the local heart association, or the visiting nurse association.

Evaluation

The drugs used to treat angina are successful if the pain is relieved and the patient experiences no side effects resulting from drug therapy. These drugs do not halt the progression of disease. Before discharge, make sure that the patient can explain when and how to take the medications prescribed, what side effects might occur and how to treat them, what to do if drug therapy does not relieve the symptoms, how to correctly store the medication, and how to test for its continued effectiveness.

THERAPEUTIC OPTIONS FOR ANGINA

The treatment of angina depends on the recognition that the supply of oxygen to the heart does not meet the demand. Chronically, the demand for oxygen can be decreased by altering secondary factors that affect the heart adversely. These factors include smoking, excess weight, hypertension, arrhythmias, anxiety, anemia, and lack of regular exercise. The major risk factors for the progression of atherosclerosis are cigarette smoking, hypertension, and high serum cholesterol levels. Evidence affirms that alteration of these risk factors in patients with angina secondary to coronary atherosclerosis does prolong life.

Coronary artery bypass surgery may be indicated when angina is severe because of coronary atherosclerosis. In this type of surgery, one or more of the main coronary vessels is bypassed with a graft from the aorta to the lower end of the vessel. Replacement of vessels severely narrowed by atherosclerosis greatly improves coronary blood flow. About 70% of patients have no further angina, and another 20% have markedly reduced angina.

Percutaneous transluminal coronary angioplasty (PTCA) is a nonsurgical procedure for opening a coronary artery narrowed by atherosclerosis. A balloon catheter is inserted into the narrowed area. The balloon is inflated and the vessel is widened. PTCA is most effective in patients with severe angina in whom only one coronary artery is severely narrowed. This is usually the left coronary artery servicing the more worked left ventricle.

Drug therapy for angina pectoris rests with three classes of drugs. The nitrates and nitrites primarily offer acute relief of angina. The beta blockers offer long-term relief in classic angina. The calcium channel blockers are especially effective in relieving the coronary spasms of variant angina.

Nitrates and Nitrites

Mechanism of action. Nitric oxide (NO) is now recognized to be the endothelium-derived relaxing factor (EDRF) responsible for relaxation of vascular smooth muscle resulting in vasodilation (Figure 14-2). Nitrates and nitrites are broken down to nitric oxide. However, within cells, the endogenous source of nitric oxide is the amino acid arginine.

The nitrates and nitrites were originally believed to dilate the coronary blood vessels, thereby increasing blood flow in the heart. Most patients with angina have atherosclerosis of the coronary vessels, and atherosclerotic vessels cannot dilate. Furthermore, insufficient oxygen (ischemia) is itself a potent vasodilator; thus the coronary vessels are already dilated during an anginal attack. The nitrates and nitrites dilate arterioles and veins in the periphery, thereby lowering blood pressure. The reduced blood pressure greatly reduces the work of the heart. This reduced workload lowers the oxygen demand of the heart. The nitrates and nitrites, particularly nitroglycerin, are the mainstay of antianginal medication. The nitrates and nitrites are most effectively used as needed to relieve an acute anginal attack. Patients who understand the factors that precipitate their own anginal attacks can take these medications prophylactically just before those activities.

Administration and fate. The organic nitrates rapidly relieve anginal attacks when administered sublingually. These organic nitrates include nitroglycerin, isosorbide dinitrate, and erythrityl tetranitrate. These drugs produce a general vasodilation by acting directly on blood vessels. The side effects of sublingual nitrates also result from the generalized vasodilation. These side effects include flushing, headache, and dizziness. Flushing results from vasodilation in the "blush" area of the neck and face. The headache results from pressure imposed by dilated blood vessels in the brain. The incidence of headaches decreases 2 to 3 weeks after initial therapy. Dizziness results from generalized hypotension. The patient should sit or lie down to avoid fainting after taking one of these drugs. If the hypotension is severe enough, reflex tachycardia may occur. This increases the cardiac work and makes the pain worse.

The organic nitrates are frequently administered orally in large doses to provide prophylactic treatment for angina. Large doses are required because

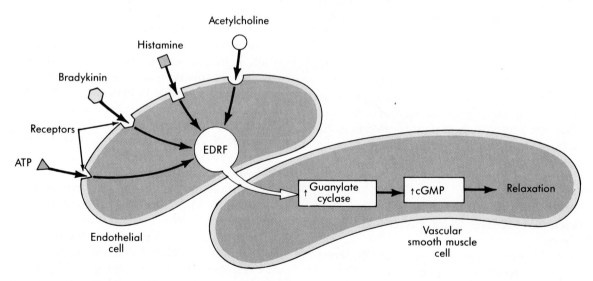

FIGURE 14-2

Endothelium-dependent relaxation factor (EDRF) is nitric oxide (NO). NO is potent vasodilator. Endothelial cell produces NO from arginine, an amino acid, in response to substances such as acetylcholine, histamine, bradykinin, and adenosine triphosphate (ATP). However, nitrates and nitrites are also broken down to nitric oxide. Nitric oxide diffuses into vascular smooth muscle cells and stimulates the enzyme, guanylate cyclase, which produces the second messenger cyclic guanosine monophosphate (GMP). Cyclic GMP activates intracellular events that result in vasodilation.

organic nitrates are rapidly degraded by the liver. However, when large doses of nitrates are given frequently, tolerance rapidly develops, reducing the duration of relief. Studies are underway to determine whether intermittent or pulsed therapy might be best for prophylaxis. The degree of tolerance that is developed to nitrates seems to decrease with intermittent therapy.

Specific Nitrates and Nitrites

Specific nitrates and nitrites are listed in Table 14-2.

Nitroglycerin

Nitroglycerin is considered the drug of choice for angina. When nitroglycerin is taken sublingually, its effect begins in 30 sec, is maximal in 3 min, and lasts for about 10 min. A drawback to nitroglycerin is that it decomposes when exposed to light or heat. Nitroglycerin can also volatilize from the tablets, which therefore must be kept in airtight containers. Nitroglycerin stings when placed under the tongue, which indicates that the drug is still present.

Several dosage forms for nitroglycerin are avail-

Table 14-2   Drugs Prescribed for Relief of Angina Pectoris

Generic name	Trade name	Administration/dosage	Comments
NITRATES AND NITRITES			
Amyl Nitrite	Amyl Nitrite	INHALATION: 0.18 to 0.3 ml. Onset: immediate. Duration: 5 min.	Drug relieves acute angina attacks. Glass pearls are crushed and volatile liquid inhaled. Odor is unpleasant. headache, orthostatic hypotension, and reflex stimulation of heart usually occur.
Erythrityl tetranitrate	Cardilate*	SUBLINGUAL: 5 mg 3 times daily. ORAL, CHEWABLE: 10 mg 3 times daily. If required, dose may be increased every 2 to 3 days up to 30 mg 3 times daily. Onset: 5 min for sublingual or chewable; 30 min for oral. Duration: 4 hr.	Prophylactic treatment prevents anginal attacks. Hypotension, headaches, and tolerance to nitrates are possible side effects.
Isosorbide dinitrate	Iso-Bid Isordil* Isotrate Sorbitrate Others	SUBLINGUAL: 2.5 to 5 mg. CHEWABLE: 5 to 10 mg. Onset: 2 to 5 min. Duration: 1 to 2 hr. ORAL: 5 to 30 mg 4 times daily. Timed-released forms, 40 mg 2 to 4 times daily. Onset: 15 to 30 min. Duration: 4 to 6 hr.	Drug relieves acute angina attacks. It is possibly effective prophylactically, especially if taken in anticipation of stressful situation. Hypotension is side effect limiting dose. It is possibly effective as prophylactic treatment to prevent anginal attacks. Headache can be severe. Tolerance to nitrates may develop.
Nitroglycerin	Nitroglycerin Nitrostat	SUBLINGUAL: Tablets of 0.15 to 0.3 mg initially, up to 0.6 mg as required in individual. Individual dosages may be repeated at 5-min intervals, up to 3 tablets in 15 min. Peak action: 3 min. Duration: 10 min.	Drug is direct-acting vasodilator. It is drug of choice for angina pectoris. Patient takes at onset of acute anginal episodes or in anticipation of an episode, as before exercise or sex. Stoage containers should be kept cool to prevent disintegration and airtight to prevent volatilization.
	Nitrolingual*	SUBLINGUAL: *Adults*—1 or 2 metered doses (400 µg/dose) on or under tongue. Repeat at 5-min interval for relief of anginal attack.	Sublingual spray should afford relief after total of 3 doses in 15 min.
	Niong Nitrong* Nitronet Klavikordal	ORAL, SUSTAINED-RELEASE: 2.5 to 6.5 mg every 8 to 12 hr. Onset: slow variable. Duration: 8 to 12 hr.	Drug provides prophylactic administration of nitroglycerin. Effectiveness of this mode of therapy is not established. Tolerance to nitrates may develop.

*Available in Canada and United States.
†Available in Canada only.

Continued.

Table 14-2 Drugs Prescribed for Relief of Angina Pectoris—cont'd

Generic name	Trade name	Administration/dosage	Comments
NITRATES AND NITRITES			
Nitroglycerin—cont'd	Nitrogard* Nitrogard SR*	BUCCAL: 1 mg 3 times daily. May increase to 2 mg. Kept in mouth for several hours. May increase to 4 times daily or add extra for acute prophylaxis, but no more than every 2 hr.	Nitroglycerin is released from polymer base over several hours to achieve long duration of action.
Nitroglycerin ointment, 2%	Nitro-Bid* Nitrol* Nitrong*	TOPICAL: Initally 1 in is spread over area of skin. This is increased by ½ in increments as required. Absorption is improved by covering area with plastic. Onset: 30 to 60 min. Duration: up to 3 hr.	Drug provides prophylactic administration of nitroglycerin. Effectiveness of this mode of therapy is not established. Excessive dose may cause violent headache. Area of administration will be irritated and should be rotated. On termination of treatment, area and frequency of administration should be reduced gradually over 4 to 6 weeks to prevent withdrawal reactions.
	Nitrodisc Nitro-Dur Transderm-Nitro	TOPICAL: Apply to site free of hair. Do not apply to hands or feet. Change daily to new site.	Nitroglycerin is impregnated into polymer bound to adhesive bandages. Drug is absorbed through skin over 24 hr.
Pentaerythritol tetranitrate	Peritrate* Pentylan Naptrate	ORAL: Initally 10 to 20 mg 4 times daily. If required, dosage may be adjusted up to 40 mg 4 times daily. Onset: 30 min. Duration: 4 to 5 hr.	Drug is possibly effective as prophylactic treatment for angina pectoris. Hypotension, headaches, and tolerance to nitrates are possible side effects. Tablets are taken 30 min before or 1 hr after meals and at bedtime. Drug is taken on empty stomach.
	Duotrate Pentritol Peritrate SA*	SUBSTAINED RELEASE: 30 to 80 mg twice day. Onset: 30 to 60 min. Duration: 12 hr.	Drug is possibly effective as prophylactic treatment for angina pectoris. Hypotension, headaches, and tolerance to nitrates are possible side effects. Tablets are taken 30 min before or 1 hr after meals and at bedtime. Drug is taken on empty stomach.
BETA ADRENERGIC BLOCKING FOR ANGINA			
Acebutolol	Monitan† Sectral*	ORAL: 200 mg 2 times a day initially, then adjusted according to response.	Drug is cardioselective. Dosage should be reduced for patients with reduced liver or kidney function.
Atenolol	Apo-Atenolol† Tenormin*	ORAL: 50 to 200 mg once daily.	Drug is cardioselective. Dose is given every other day to patients with severely impaired renal function.
Carteolol	Cartrol	ORAL: Up to 10 mg daily.	Drug is nonselective. Dosage interval is increased for patients with severely impaired renal function.
Labetalol	Normodyne Trandate*	ORAL: 150 to 300 mg 2 times a day.	Drug is nonselective. It also has alpha-1 adrenergic blocking effects.
Metoprolol	Apo-Metoprolol† Betaloc† Lopressor* Novometoprol†	ORAL: 50 mg 3 or 4 times daily. For prophylaxis after myocardial infarction: 100 mg twice daily.	Drug is cardioselective. It is readily metabolized by liver. Bioavailability is increased by food.
Nadolol	Corgard	ORAL: 40 to 80 mg daily.	Drug is nonselective. It is excreted unchanged in urine. Dosage interval is increased in patients with renal impairment.

*Available in Canada and United States.
†Available in Canada only.

Table 14-2 Drugs Prescribed for Relief of Angina Pectoris—cont'd

Generic name	Trade name	Administration/dosage	Comments
Penbutolol	Levatol	ORAL: 20 to 40 mg once daily.	Drug is nonselective. It is excreted unchanged in urine.
Pindolol	Syn-Pindolol† Visken*	ORAL: 10 mg 4 times daily.	Drug is nonselective. It is well metabolized.
Propranolol	Inderal*	ORAL: 10 to 20 mg 3 or 4 times daily. Increase as required. Maintenance dose is usually 160 to 240 mg daily, in 4 doses.	Drug is nonselective. It is well absorbed and extensively metabolized by liver.
Timolol	Apo-Timolol† Blocadren*	ORAL: 10 to 30 mg twice daily. Prophylaxis for myocardial infarction is 10 mg twice daily.	Drug is nonselective. It is well absorbed and extensively metabolized by liver.
CALCIUM CHANNEL BLOCKING DRUGS			
Bepridil	Vascor	ORAL: Initially, 200 mg once a day, increased after 10 days, if necessary, to 300 mg once a day. Maximum dose is 400 mg/day.	Bepridil is new calcium channel blocker for treating angina.
Diltiazem	Cardizem	ORAL: 60 mg every 6 hr.	Drug is well absorbed. Nitrate therapy is continued.
Nicardipine	Cardene	ORAL: *Adults*—20 mg 3 times daily, adjusted for need and tolerance.	Drug is effective for treating angina and hypertension.
Nifedipine	Procardia Adalat* Apo-Nifed†	ORAL: Initially 10 mg 3 times daily. If required, increase dose every 3 to 7 days. Maximum dosage is 180 mg daily.	Drug is well absorbed and completely metabolized. Nitrate therapy is continued. It is more selective for smooth muscle than for cardiac muscle.
Verapamil	Calan Isoptin*	ORAL: 240 to 480 mg daily in 3 or 4 divided doses.	Drug is well absorbed. It has extensive first-pass metabolism. In patients with cirrhosis, half-life is increased, and dose should be lowered by 70%. Nitrate therapy is continued.

*Available in Canada and United States.
†Available in Canada only.

able. A variation of the sublingual form is nitroglycerin lingual aerosol, which can be sprayed, in a metered form, on or under the tongue. The aerosol substitutes for the sublingual tablets in the acute relief of an anginal attack. Extended-release buccal forms are intended for prophylactic use. Extended-release capsules and tablets have up to 10 times the sublingual dose. These are swallowed and are effective for 8 to 12 hr. Nitroglycerin is very lipid soluble and probably enters the body from the gastrointestinal (GI) tract through the lymphatic system rather than the portal blood.

Nitroglycerin may also be administered through the skin. A measured amount of nitroglycerin oint-ment is spread on a hairless part of the body and held in place with plastic wrap taped over the area. This route of administration is said to produce relief for up to 3 hr. Nitroglycerin is also available impregnated in a polymer bonded to an adhesive bandage. This disk is applied to the skin, and nitroglycerin is absorbed through the skin (transdermally) over 24 hr. The unit should be applied to a site free of hair, and the bandage should be placed at a new site each time to avoid irritation (Figure 14-3).

Nitroglycerin is administered intravenously in acute heart failure. Nitroglycerin can reduce the myocardial ischemia that results when the left side of the heart is failing. Because blood is not being pumped

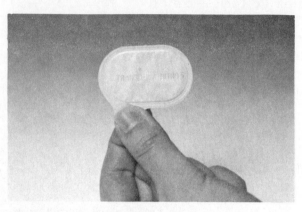

FIGURE 14-3
Transderm-Nitro delivery system for controlled release of nitroglycerin for prevention of angina.
Courtesy Summit Pharmaceuticals, Division of Ciba-Geigy.

---

out effectively, pressure builds in the left ventricle. Pulmonary edema results, since that is where the blood backs up. Nitroglycerin is an effective dilator of the coronary arteries and therefore allows more oxygenated blood to reach the troubled heart muscle. The heart performs better, and the symptoms of acute heart failure are relieved.

Amyl nitrite

Amyl nitrite is the only nitrite used to treat angina. It is a volatile liquid packaged in an easily crushed vial with a woven cover and is self-administered by inhalation. Amyl nitrite is effective 30 sec after inhalation and lasts for 3 to 5 min. Amyl nitrite has an unpleasant odor, is expensive, and is conspicuous to use. The side effects of headache, orthostatic hypotension, and reflex tachycardia can be pronounced. For these reasons amyl nitrite is seldom used. The rush felt when amyl nitrite is inhaled has caused this drug to be abused (see box).

Erythrityl tetranitrate

Erythrityl tetranitrate (Cardilate) is the longest-acting of the sublingual or chewable organic nitrates. This drug becomes effective in 5 min, and its effects last for 4 hr. This is a long duration compared with nitroglycerin or even isosorbide dinitrate, and therefore erythrityl tetranitrate is better for prophylactic use than for relief of acute attacks. Erythrityl tetranitrate is also available for oral administration.

Isosorbide dinitrate

Isosorbide dinitrate (Iso-Bid and Isordil) is another organic nitrate that can be taken sublingually or chewed. It is effective in 2 to 5 min and can act for 1 to 2 hr.

Pentaerythritol tetranitrate

Pentaerythritol tetranitrate (Peritrate) has not been proved effective for the prophylactic treatment of angina.

Beta Blockers for Angina

Mechanism of action. Beta blockers decrease the oxygen requirements of the heart by reducing its workload. Blocking the beta-1 adrenergic receptors of the heart decreases the heart rate and the force of contraction, and a decrease in blood pressure follows. These actions also benefit coronary circulation by decreasing the resistance in the coronary circulation. However, beta blockers are not vasodilators.

There are two subclasses of beta receptors, beta-1 and beta-2. (For further discussion of beta receptors, see Chapter 10.) The cardiac selective beta blockers are relatively selective for the beta-1 receptors. However, this selectivity is diminished at higher doses. There is no evidence that any particular beta blocker is better than another in the management of angina. Patients with asthma, diabetes, or peripheral vascular disease are better able to tolerate the selective beta-1 blockers. The development of new beta blockers has been explosive. Beta-1 selective drugs include acebutolol, atenolol, and metoprolol. Nonselective drugs include oxprenolol, pindolol, propranolol, nadolol, sotalol, and timolol.

Administration. Beta blockers have become widely used in the management of classic angina. A beta blocker is commonly prescribed as prophylactic therapy, and nitroglycerin is prescribed for anginal attacks. Long-term therapy reduces the frequency of anginal pain and decreases the requirements for nitroglycerin. The effective dose is highly individual for each patient. One index of dosage is the decrease in resting heart rate. In patients with severe angina, enough medication may be given to lower the resting pulse to 50 to 60 beats/min. If GI side effects such as nausea, cramping, or diarrhea occur, taking the drug with meals may lessen these symptoms.

Side effects and contraindications. The most common side effects of beta blockers are fatigue and mental lassitude. Depression, nightmares, and psychosis are the more severe CNS side effects sometimes seen. Peripheral vasoconstriction may cause cold hands or feet. Sexual dysfunction, including impotence, is a side effect, especially in patients taking propranolol or timolol. Beta blockers are contraindicated for patients with severely impaired heart or circulatory function (e.g., congestive heart failure, heart block, severe sinus bradycardia, and Raynaud's phenomenon). Withdrawal of beta blockers should be gradual. Sudden withdrawal can lead to unstable angina, myocardial infarction, or sudden death.

Adverse effects of beta blockers include bronchospasm, hypoglycemia, and impairment of peripheral circulation. The bronchospasm arises from blockade of the beta-2 receptors of the bronchi. Hypoglycemia results from the inhibition of glycogen breakdown, a process normally stimulated by epinephrine and norepinephrine. Dilation of peripheral blood vessels is mediated by beta-2 receptors. These adverse effects are less common with the beta-1 selective blockers.

Beta Blockers After Acute Myocardial Infarction

Studies have shown that administration of a beta blocker after a heart attack reduces the incidence of sudden death by as much as 40%. Beta blockers reduce the workload of the heart and have antiarrhythmic and antiplatelet functions that may be important.

Specific Beta Blockers

Beta blockers that have been specifically approved for use as antianginal agents in the United States are atenolol, metoprolol, nadolol, propranolol, and sotalol. Acebutolol, carteolol, labetolol, penbutolol, pindolol, and timolol are beta blockers accepted as antianginal drugs. Atenolol, metoprolol, propranolol, and timolol have been approved for prophylaxis

against myocardial reinfarction. Specific beta blockers are listed in Table 14-2.

Acebutolol

Acebutolol (Monitan and Sectral) is an intermediate-acting, cardioselective beta blocker. The drug is metabolized by the liver and excreted both through the kidney and feces. Dosage should be reduced for patients with reduced liver or kidney function.

Atenolol

Atenolol (Tenormin) is a long-acting, cardioselective beta blocker. It is poorly absorbed from the GI tract and excreted unchanged in the urine. The time between doses must be increased in patients with impaired renal function.

Carteolol

Carteolol (Cartrol) is a long-acting, nonselective beta blocker. It is well absorbed and excreted largely unchanged in the urine. The dosage interval is increased for patients with impaired renal function.

Labetolol

Labetolol (Normodyne and Trandate) is a long-acting, nonspecific beta blocker that also has selective alpha-1-adrenergic blocking effects. It is well absorbed from the GI tract, metabolized by the liver, and excreted in the urine.

Metoprolol

Metoprolol (Lopressor and Betaloc) is a short-acting, cardioselective beta blocker. It is well absorbed from the GI tract and readily metabolized by the liver.

Nadolol

Nadolol (Corgard) is a long-acting, nonselective beta blocker. It is not well absorbed from the GI tract, and up to a fourth of the dose may be excreted in the feces. Absorbed drug is excreted unchanged in the urine. Patients with renal failure should be given the drug less frequently.

Penbutolol

Penbutolol (Levatol) is a short-acting, nonselective beta blocker. It is well absorbed and highly protein bound. The drug is excreted unchanged in the urine.

Pindolol

Pindolol (Visken) is a short-acting, nonselective beta blocker. It is well absorbed and metabolized by the liver.

Propranolol

Propranolol (Inderal), a nonselective beta blocker, is the oldest of the clinically used beta-blocking drugs.

It is well absorbed orally, but it is readily metabolized by the liver.

Timolol

Timolol (Blocadren and Apo-Timol) is a short-acting nonselective beta blocker. It is well absorbed from the GI tract and metabolized by the liver.

Calcium Channel Blockers for Angina

Mechanism of action. Calcium channel blockers, also called *calcium antagonists* or *calcium entry blockers,* are currently used in the treatment of angina, certain arrhythmias (see Chapter 19), and hypertension (Chapter 15). Skeletal muscle has extensive stores of calcium in the sarcoplasmic reticulum, but cardiac muscle and vascular smooth muscle lack these stores and depend on the influx of extracellular calcium for the maintenance of contraction, or tone. Calcium channel blockers interfere with the initial influx of calcium through specific calcium channels on the cell surface.

Calcium channel blockers decrease the oxygen requirements of the heart through several actions. They reduce peripheral vascular resistance by systemic vasodilation. This means that the workload of the heart is decreased. Calcium channel blockers dilate the coronary vessels by inhibiting contractility of coronary smooth muscle. This relieves variant angina, in which coronary spasm prevents blood flow. However, a varying degree of coronary spasm occurs even in classic angina. Patients with asthma, diabetes, and peripheral vascular disease, who cannot tolerate beta blockers, can benefit from calcium channel blockers.

The calcium channel blockers also reduce cardiac contractility (negative inotropy), which decreases the oxygen requirement of the heart. These agents increase coronary blood flow through coronary vasodilation more selectively than they inhibit cardiac contractility. Without this selective preference, calcium channel blockers would not be clinically useful because they would overly compromise cardiac function. These drugs differ in the degree of selectivity in coronary vasodilation versus decreased cardiac contractility.

Side effects. In general, the side effects of calcium channel blockers are mild. Headaches and constipation are the most common. Since the calcium channel blockers were recently introduced, their medical use is still being investigated.

Drug interactions. There are several important interactions of calcium channel blockers with other drugs. Beta blockers and calcium channel blockers, if given concurrently, may cause cardiac problems. These problems include a conduction block or arrhythmias and hypotension. Diltiazem and verapamil may inhibit the liver metabolism of several drugs,

including carbamazepine, cyclosporine, quinidine, theophylline, and valproate. This may allow these drugs to reach toxic levels in the body. Digitalis glycosides may also accumulate in the presence of calcium channel blockers, resulting in excessive slowing of the heart or a heart block. Disopyramide causes negative inotropic effect and should not be administered within 48 hr of a calcium channel blocker.

Specific Calcium Channel Blockers

Calcium channel blockers approved for use in the treatment of angina are bepridil (Vascor), diltiazem (Cardizem), nicardipine (Cardene), nifedipine (Aldalat, Procardia), and verapamil (Calan, Isoptin) (see Table 14-2). Other calcium channel blockers are used in the treatment of hypertension and are covered in Chapter 15.

Bepridil

Bepridil (Vasocor) is a new calcium channel blocker for the therapeutic treatment of angina. It is taken once a day.

Diltiazem

Diltiazem (Cardizem) produces cardiac effects similar to those of verapamil. The incidence of dizziness, headache, and hypotension is less with diltiazem than with nifedipine and verapamil. Diltiazem is well absorbed orally and well metabolized. Only 35% of metabolites are excreted in the urine. The remainder are excreted in the feces.

Nicardipine and Nifedipine

Calcium channel blockers, nicardipine (Cardene) and nifedipine (Adalat and Procardia), are potent coronary and peripheral vasodilators. The cardiodepressant effect is minor because they do not depress the sinoatrial or atrioventricular nodes and because reflex sympathetic activity caused by hypotension counteracts the negative inotropic effect. However, if either drug is combined with a beta blocker, there is risk of severe hypotension and heart failure.

Both drugs are well absorbed orally. The side effects most frequently reported are secondary to peripheral vasodilation and include headaches, hypotension, flushing, tingling in the extremities, and edema.

Verapamil

Verapamil (Calan and Isoptin) depresses the atrioventricular node (negative chronotropy and negative dromotropy), making it a useful antiarrhythmic drug (see Chapter 19). Bradycardia is common. Verapamil does not cause a pronounced decrease in blood pressure, and therefore reflex sympathetic activity to stimulate the heart is minimal. The slowing of the heart rate and the decrease in blood pressure reduce the oxygen requirements of the heart. Verapamil increases coronary blood flow, which increases the oxygen available to the heart.

Although verapamil is readily absorbed, it is rapidly metabolized by the liver. It must be taken 3 or 4 times a day. In the blood, verapamil is 90% bound to albumin. Verapamil is generally well tolerated; constipation is the most common side effect. Verapamil is contraindicated for patients with atrioventricular conduction disturbances or congestive heart failure.

PERIPHERAL VASCULAR DISEASE AND VASODILATOR DRUGS

Vasodilator drugs are prescribed for a variety of circulatory disorders. The effectiveness of drug therapy is not clear, however.

Nursing Process Overview
VASODILATOR THERAPY IN PERIPHERAL VASCULAR DISEASE
Assessment
Assess the patient, and obtain a history about onset and course of vascular disease. Assess the patient's blood pressure and pulses, including peripheral pulses. Assess the patient for altered sensation, poor healing of injuries on the feet, cool extremities, or symptoms of altered cerebral blood flow. Perform a mental status examination.

Nursing Diagnoses
High risk for injury related to orthostatic hypotension secondary to drug therapy
Pain (headache) secondary to vasodilator therapy
Nausea secondary to drug therapy

Management
Monitor the presenting signs and symptoms, especially blood pressure and pulses, and look for drug side effects. Instruct the patient about prescribed medications, and teach the patient about prevention of trauma to areas with decreased perfusion. Teach about exercise programs, weight loss, and restriction of certain activities.

Evaluation
It is difficult to measure the effectiveness of these drugs. Before discharge, determine that the patient can explain when and how to take the ordered medications, what the possible side effects are, and what situations would require notification of the physician.

VASODILATOR DRUGS USED FOR PERIPHERAL VASCULAR DISEASE
Vasospastic Disorders
Blood flow to the arms and legs, particularly the hands and feet, can be limited by peripheral vascular disease. The blood vessels may be narrowed by arteriosclerosis or by spasm of the vessels (vasospasm). If the vessel narrowing is a result of arteriosclerosis, vasodilator drugs will be of little value. Vasodilator drugs may worsen the condition because vessels narrowed by arteriosclerosis will not dilate; adjacent vessels will dilate and shunt the blood away from the occluded area. The occluded vessel therefore has its blood flow reduced, not increased, by vasodilator drugs. On the other hand, if the narrowing of the vessel is a result of vasospasm, drugs will be of benefit.

Raynaud's disease affects primarily the fingers and toes. In Raynaud's disease the blood vessels of the digits are readily thrown into spasm by cold or emotion and turn blue or white. Warming restores blood flow. Currently, the most successful drug treatment of Raynaud's disease is reported with reserpine and guanethidine, drugs that have been used to treat hypertension. These drugs interfere with sympathetic innervation. Reserpine depresses sympathetic tone by depleting stored norepinephrine in the neurons. Guanethidine acts at the sympathetic neuron by blocking the release of norepinephrine and depleting norepinephrine stores. These drugs and their side effects are discussed fully in Chapter 15.

Unfortunately, a large number of vasodilator drugs advertised for treating peripheral vascular spasm are of doubtful clinical value. These drugs include cyclandelate, isoxsuprine, niacin, nylidrin, papaverine, and tolazoline.

Impaired Cerebral Blood Flow
Vasodilator drugs are sometimes prescribed to improve blood flow in the brain, particularly in elderly patients with arteriosclerosis of cerebral vessels who have suffered strokes or show signs of mental impairment. The problem is cerebral ischemia (insufficient oxygen to areas of the brain). Controlled medical trials show that this drug therapy is of little value. Vasodilator drugs may make the situation worse by shunting blood away from the unreactive, damaged vessels to areas with adequate blood flow already, as described for peripheral vascular insufficiency resulting from arteriosclerosis. Cyclandelate, ergot mesylates, and papaverine are sometimes prescribed to improve cerebral blood flow. These drugs do not alter

the progression of cerebral arteriosclerosis. They may improve some symptoms on a short-term basis.

Specific Drugs

Specific vasodilators are listed in Table 14-3.

Cyclandelate

Cyclandelate (Cyclospasmol) acts directly on vascular smooth muscle to cause relaxation. In the laboratory, cyclandelate is a more effective vasodilator than papaverine, but the clinical effectiveness of cyclandelate is considered doubtful. Side effects include belching and heartburn, flushing, headache, weakness, and increased heart rate.

Ergot mesylates

Ergot mesylates (Hydergine) produce vasodilation in contrast to the ergot alkaloids, which produce vasoconstriction (see Chapter 53). Ergot mesylates are of definite value in treating brain disease secondary to hypertension, but the benefit is related to the fall in blood pressure. These alkaloids act centrally to reduce vascular tone and slow heart rate. They act peripherally to block alpha-adrenergic receptors. These alkaloids are available in a sublingual dosage form. Sublingual irritation, nausea, and gastrointestinal upset are the side effects. The dihydrogenated ergot alkaloids can markedly reduce heart rate through their central effect of lowering sympathetic tone.

Table 14-3   Vasodilator Drugs

Generic name	Trade name	Administration/dosage	Comments
Cyclandelate	Cyclospasmol*	ORAL: 300 to 400 mg 4 times daily. Can be decreased gradually to 100 to 200 mg 4 times daily.	Direct vasodilator for use in vasospastic disorders may cause GI disturbances.
Ergot mesylates	Hydergine*	SUBLINGUAL, ORAL: 1 mg 3 times daily.	Drug can cause marked bradycardia. It relieves symptoms in hypertensive brain disease by lowering blood pressure.
Isoxsuprine	Vasodilan* Vasoprine	ORAL: 10 to 20 mg 3 to 4 times daily. INTRAMUSCULAR: 5 to 10 mg 2 to 3 times daily.	Drug is a direct-acting vasodilator with no proven use.
Nicotinyl alcohol	Roniacol† Ronigen Rycotin	ORAL: 50 to 100 mg 3 times daily. TIMED-RELEASE: 300 to 400 mg every 12 hr.	Drug is a direct vasodilator that causes pronounced blushing. GI disturbances, tingling sensation, and rashes are side effects. Use has not been proved effective for any vasospastic disorders.
Nimodipine	Nimotop	ORAL: *Adults*—60 mg every 4 hr, beginning within 4 days after subarachnoid hemorrhage and continuing for 21 days.	Calcium channel blocker treats cerebral vasospasm after subarachnoid hemorrhage.
Nylidrin hydrochloride	Arlidin* PMS Nylidrin†	ORAL: 3 to 12 mg 3 to 4 times daily.	Drug stimulates beta-adrenergic receptors and directly dilates vessels. It may cause dizziness, tachycardia, and hypotension.
Papaverine hydrochloride	Many trade names	ORAL: 100 to 300 mg, 3 to 5 times daily TIMED-RELEASE: 150 mg every 12 hr. Can give up to 150 mg every 8 hr or 300 mg every 12 hr. INTRAVENOUS: 30 to 120 mg, over 1 to 2 min. INTRAMUSCULAR: 30 to 120 mg.	Drug depresses heart. It directly relaxes smooth muscle, particularly of large blood vessels. Use is to relieve smooth muscle spasm in vascular disease or colic. Its effectiveness has not been proved.
Pentoxifylline	Trental*	ORAL: 400 mg 3 times daily, with meals.	Drug is not vasodilator. It reduces blood viscosity and improves red blood cell flexibility to improve blood flow.
Tolazoline hydrochloride	Priscoline*	TIMED-RELEASE: 80 mg every 12 hr. INTRAMUSCULAR, SUBCUTANEOUS, INTRAVENOUS: 10 to 50 mg 4 times daily.	Direct-acting vasodilator may relieve vasospastic disorders.

*Available in Canada and United States.
†Available in Canada only.

Flunarizine

Flunarizine (Sibelium) is a calcium channel blocker available in Canada to treat cerebral vascular disorders. It relieves symptoms of dizziness, vertigo, and tinnitus.

Isoxsuprine

Isoxsuprine (Vasodilan and Vasoprine) was originally thought to stimulate beta receptors, but its vasodilating action is not blocked by drugs that are antagonists of the beta receptors. Clinical tests have not demonstrated any usefulness for isoxsuprine. Side effects include flushing, hypotension, dizziness, an increased heart rate, and occasionally a rash.

Nicotinyl alcohol

Nicotinyl alcohol (Ronigen and Rycotin) has been used as a vasodilator but without good evidence of clinical effectiveness. This drug causes pronounced flushing, postural (orthostatic) hypotension, and GI upset. It can also cause a rash.

Nimodipine

Nimodipine (Nimotop) is a calcium channel blocker approved to treat cerebral vasospasm after subarachnoid hemorrhage. This action alleviates the cerebral ischemia that can follow a stroke, and, by maintaining blood flow, protects the brain from deterioration. Because of these actions, calcium channel blockers are being used to treat various neurologic disorders. Calcium channel blockers for neurologic use cross the blood-brain barrier.

Nylidrin

Nylidrin (Arlidin) stimulates blood flow in muscle. Stimulating the beta receptors of the blood vessels produces vasodilation. However, muscle blood vessels, not the blood vessels of the skin, have beta receptors, so the approach is of little value in vasospastic disorders of the digits. The beta blocker propranolol does not entirely reverse this stimulation, so nylidrin is believed to also act directly on smooth muscle. Side effects attributed to nylidrin include trembling, nervousness, weakness, dizziness, palpitations, and nausea and vomiting.

Papaverine

Papaverine relaxes smooth muscle. In large doses, it also depresses cardiac muscle, slowing conduction and prolonging the refractory period. Papaverine has long been used as a smooth muscle relaxant for ischemia of the brain, periphery, or heart. As with the other vasodilator drugs, there is little evidence that papaverine improves peripheral vascular circulation. Side effects include flushing of the face, malaise, GI upset, and headache. Other side effects include excess perspiration, loss of appetite, increased heart rate, and increased depth of respiration. Rarely, a hypersensitivity reaction involving the liver is seen. Symptoms of liver damage may include jaundice, eosinophilia, and altered results of liver function tests.

Tolazoline

Tolazoline (Priscoline) is an alpha-adrenergic antagonist that has an additional direct vasodilating effect. In theory, a drug that blocks the action of norepinephrine at the alpha receptors of the blood vessels should be helpful, but in practice, alpha-adrenergic antagonists are not very effective in relieving or preventing vasospasm. Tolazoline is not effective by itself but potentiates the action of other drugs. Side effects are frequent with tolazoline therapy and include headache, nausea, chills, flushing, tingling of the skin (especially the scalp), and GI disturbances. Occasionally, irregular heart function is noticed; arrhythmia or a pounding heart is the most common cardiac symptom.

Pentoxifylline

Pentoxifylline (Trental) is a new type of drug for the treatment of peripheral vascular disease. Pentoxifylline increases the flexibility of red blood cells and reduces blood viscosity. These actions improve blood flow through narrowed vessels.

Pentoxifylline is administered as an adjunct to surgery for the treatment of intermittent claudication. Side effects are rare but include dizziness, headache, nausea, or vomiting. Drug interactions include the potentiation of antihypertensive drugs. Smoking may interfere with the therapeutic action of pentoxifylline, since nicotine constricts blood vessels. Toxic symptoms of pentoxifylline include excitement and seizures.

Sympathomimetic Drugs

Drug administration

◆ For safe care of the patient requiring IV sympathomimetic drugs for the treatment of shock or hypotension, use a microdrip IV administration set to regulate the drug dose more accurately. Use an electronic IV monitor or regulator to accurately control the rate of fluid and drug administration. Monitor the blood pressure and pulse every 2 to 5 min until the blood pressure and rate of drug administration are stable, then every 15 min. Do not leave the patient unattended. Monitor the mean arterial pressure, pulmonary capillary wedge pressure (PCWP), central venous pressure (CVP), or other available indicators of hemodynamic response. Monitor the electrocardiogram. Monitor intake and output and urinary output every 30 to 60 min.

◆ Read drug labels carefully, since some drug forms are not indicated for IV administration. Do not administer any drug intravenously if sediment or discoloration is visible. Do not mix two or more drugs in a syringe or in IV solutions. If in doubt, consult the pharmacist. Observe the patient for development of hypertensive crisis. If it occurs, slow or stop vasopressor drugs, notify the physician, and administer specific drug antidotes or phentolamine, an adrenergic blocking drug, as ordered.

◆ Avoid extravasation of these drugs. All sympathomimetic drugs cause vasoconstriction, and levarterenol or dopamine can cause tissue necrosis or sloughing. Administer these drugs through a central venous catheter if possible. In the event of extravasation, the physician may order infiltration of the site of injury with a solution of 5 to 10 mg of phentolamine diluted in 10 to 15 ml of normal saline solution.

◆ Many of these preparations contain bisulfites, which can cause an allergic reaction. Although uncommon in the general population, this reaction may be seen more often in persons with a history of asthma. Symptoms include dizziness; feeling faint; bluish discoloration of the skin; skin rash or hives; swelling of the face, eyelids, or lips; and difficulty breathing. If possible, obtain a history of allergy or previous health problems preceding drug administration. Observe all patients for unexpected drug reactions. Keep patients and families informed of the patient's condition. Provide calm reassurance. Note that shock produces a sense of impending doom and a feeling of anxiety. Administration of adrenergic medication may also produce tachycardia and palpitations, which contribute to a sense of anxiety.

Dopamine

Drug administration

◆ Dilute the concentrate for injection before infusion. Follow dilution guidelines for the agency. One protocol states "Add 5 ml of concentrate containing 40 mg dopamine per ml (total of 200 mg of dopamine) to 500 ml of compatible IV solution to obtain a final concentration of 400 μg/ml."

Dobutamine

Drug administration

◆ Dilute the concentrate for injection to a volume of at least 50 ml with a compatible IV solution before administration. The final concentration should be no greater than 5000 μg/ml. Solutions that are slightly pink in color may still be used. After mixing with IV solution, use within 24 hr.

Epinephrine and Isoproterenol

Drug administration

◆ The usual dose of epinephrine in anaphylactic shock is 0.1 to 1.0 ml (0.1 to 1.0 mg) of 1 : 1000 solution given subcutaneously. Avoid administering epinephrine and isoproterenol simultaneously, since they are both cardiac stimulants. Monitor the blood sugar in patients receiving epinephrine, since this drug causes hyperglycemia.

Levarterenol (Norepinephrine) Bitartrate

◆ Dilute with 5% dextrose injection, with or without sodium chloride before use. In the usual dilution, add 4 mg of drug to 1000 ml of 5% dextrose injection for a concentration of 4 μg/ml.

Phenylephrine

◆ For direct IV administration, dilute 1 mg with 9 ml of sterile water for injection; administer over 20 to 30 sec for paroxysmal supraventricular tachycardia or over at least 1 min for other conditions. For infusion, dilute 10 mg in 500 ml diluent and titrate to patient response.

Ephedrine

◆ Ephedrine may be given undiluted. Administer it at a rate of 10 mg or less over 1 min.

Metaraminol

◆ Dilute metaraminol with 5% dextrose or 0.9% sodium chloride for injection. See manufacturer's directions for further guidelines.

Antianginal Drugs

Drug administration

◆ In patients with chest pain, assess blood pressure and pulse; auscultate lungs and heart; assess intensity, duration, location, and quality of pain; assess response to medication; check for diaphoresis, precipitating factors, electrocardiographic changes, or subjective and objective degree of patient distress, and obtain patient history. Chest pain in the patient with a history of angina pectoris may have other causes.

◆ In the hospital, it is often customary to keep a small supply of nitroglycerin tablets at the bedside of patients with a history of angina pectoris. Instruct patients to use the tablets as needed but to notify the nurse when they are used. Record the frequency of use, as well as a patient assessment, in the nurses' notes. Count and replenish the tablets each shift.

INTRAVENOUS NITROGLYCERIN

◆ Consult manufacturer's literature for specific instructions about dilution, dosage, and administration. Use a microdrip infusion set and a volume control or rate-controlling device to prevent overdosage and to accurately titrate the dose. Nitroglycerin migrates into plastic tubing. Dilutions should be prepared and kept in glass bottles. If standard polyvinyl chloride (PVC) IV tubing must be used, as much as 80% of the drug is lost into the tubing, so adjustments in dose must be made. Use tubing supplied by the manufacturer; do not use filters. Monitor the blood pressure, heart rate, electrocardiogram, and PCWP. Use this drug only in settings where drugs and experienced personnel to treat cardiovascular emergencies are available.

Patient and family education

◆ Encourage patients to make all recommended lifestyle changes, including losing weight to reach desirable body weight, lowering cholesterol levels, ceasing smoking, and engaging in a regular exercise program after approval by the physician. Assist patients and families in identifying activities that trigger anginal attacks such as eating a heavy meal, engaging in strenuous physical activities, lifting heavy ob-jects, being exposed to cold weather, and having sex. Work with the patient to develop ways to decrease the frequency of attacks or to decrease the likelihood that activities will cause anginal pain to develop.

◆ Encourage patients to notify the physician if the frequency, intensity, duration, location, or response to antianginal drugs changes. Instruct patients to avoid the use of alcohol because it potentiates the hypotensive effects of the nitrates and nitrites. Remind patients to keep all health care providers informed of all drugs being used, since diuretics, antihypertensives, CNS depressants, narcotics, and sedatives may potentiate the hypotensive effects of the antianginal drugs. Encourage patients to maintain regular contact with the primary health care provider and not to stop drug therapy without medical consultation.

◆ If headache occurs regularly when antianginal drugs are taken, it may indicate too high a dosage. For some patients it may be necessary to use mild analgesics with antianginal therapy; consult the physician.

Nitrates and Nitrites

Patient and family education

◆ If syncope (fainting), dizziness, or hypotension occurs with nitrate or nitrite use, instruct patients to lie down before taking the prescribed dose of medication. Ascertain that the patient can correctly use sublingual drug forms before discharge. This may be a new dosage form for the patient. In addition, teach the family how to place a dose under the patient's tongue in the event the patient cannot do it. Tell the patient not to eat, drink, chew tobacco, or smoke while the dose is dissolving.

◆ For chewable tablets, have the patient chew the tablet well, then hold it in the mouth for at least 2 min before swallowing. Instruct the patient not to drink, smoke, eat, or chew tobacco while using this form.

◆ For buccal extended-release tablets, place the dose between the cheek and upper gum or between the upper lip and gum, and allow it to dissolve over 5 hr. When eating or drinking, place the dose between the upper lip and gum. If the patient wears dentures, place the tablet between the cheek and gum. Tell the patient not to use chewing tobacco while using this form. Replace the tablet if it is accidentally swallowed. Tell patient not to go to sleep with a tablet still in the mouth.

Continued.

◆ Review the standard instructions with the patient and family for antianginal agents used to relieve an attack of angina. When chest pain develops, sit down, then use one tablet, letting it dissolve under the tongue or in the cheek, or chew a chewable tablet. If relief is not obtained, repeat the dose in 5 min. Repeat again in 5 min if needed, for a total of 3 tablets. If pain persists after 3 tablets, notify the physician or seek medical help. These guidelines may be individualized based on the patient, the patient's condition, and the physician's preference.

◆ Take oral nitrates and nitrites with meals or a snack to reduce gastric irritation. Review the ordered drugs carefully with the patient, as well as exactly how and when to take the prescribed drugs, since there are many dosages and drug forms available for these drugs.

◆ Storage instructions for these drugs include keeping drugs out of the reach of children and not storing them in the bathroom or near the kitchen sink or other damp areas. Check expiration dates, and replace drugs as needed. For sublingual nitroglycerin, follow the previous instructions, and keep tablets in the original glass container. Once the bottle is opened, remove the cotton and do not replace it. Replace the cap tightly and quickly each time the bottle is opened. Do not put other medicines in the same bottle with the nitroglycerin. When pouring a dose (a tablet), pour one or more tablets into the lid of the bottle, take the dose out, and return remaining tablets to the bottle. Avoid replacing tablets from the palm of the hand into the bottle. Instruct the patient to obtain a small glass bottle from the pharmacist for carrying a small number of pills. Do not carry the small bottle too close to the body, since body warmth may cause the pills to lose their strength.

◆ To prevent an angina attack, instruct patients to take the prescribed drug before engaging in the activity expected to produce anginal pain. For sublingual or chewable forms, patients may have to wait 5 to 10 min before engaging in such activities; for extended-release forms, patients may need to take the antianginal drug several hours before the activity. For specific patient needs, consult the physician.

◆ If doses are missed, instruct patients to take the dose as soon as they remember, unless this is within 2 hr of the next dose (extended-release forms or isosorbide dinitrate). Do not double up for missed doses.

LINGUAL AEROSOL FORMS

◆ Review the patient instruction leaflet supplied by the manufacturer. To use, remove the cover. Do not shake the container. Hold the container upright, close to the patient's mouth. Spray once or twice (as prescribed by the physician) under the tongue. Close the mouth. Avoid swallowing for 1 or 2 min. This drug may be used like nitroglycerin tablets; when an attack of angina occurs, administer a dose as prescribed. If no relief is obtained in 5 min, repeat the dose. If there is no relief in another 5 min, repeat the dose. If no relief occurs after a total of 3 doses in 15 min, instruct the patient to seek medical attention or notify the physician. The prescription may be modified for individual patient needs and by physician preference.

TOPICAL TRANSDERMAL FORMS

◆ Review the patient instruction leaflet supplied by the manufacturer. Do not trim or cut the adhesive patch. Remove the previous patch before applying a new patch. Rotate sites to avoid skin irritation. Apply the patch to a clean and dry area, with little or no hair. Avoid scratches, scars, or existing skin irritation. If the patch loosens or falls off, replace it. Side effects are the same as for other antianginal drugs in this group. Transdermal forms should not be used to treat an acute attack of angina. Tolerance to this therapy may be lessened if the patches are not used continuously; some physicians may prescribe a patch-free period each day (e.g., during the night).

TOPICAL OINTMENTS

◆ Review the patient instruction leaflet supplied by the manufacturer. Remove the ointment from a previous dose before applying the ointment. Measure the prescribed amount of ointment, using the measuring paper supplied by the manufacturer. Gently spread the ointment over a small area of about the same size each time with the measuring paper or small applicator (not the fingertips). Do not massage the ointment into the skin. Apply to areas with little or no hair. Avoid scratches and scars. Rotate sites to avoid skin irritation. Cover the area with plastic wrap or other dressing only if ordered by the physician. If a dressing is prescribed, it should be used each time the drug is used. If a dose is missed, apply it as soon as remembered, unless it is within 2 hr of the next dose, in which case

NURSING IMPLICATIONS SUMMARY—cont'd

you follow the usual dosing schedule. Do not use more ointment than ordered, and do not double up for missed doses.

Amyl Nitrate

◆ This drug is rarely used for treatment of angina. Teach the patient and family to wrap the ampule in a cloth or handkerchief, break the glass ampule within its protective covering, then have the patient inhale several deep breaths.

Beta Blockers

◆ See Nursing Implications Summary in Chapter 15.

Calcium Channel Blockers

Drug administration

◆ Assess patients with complaints of chest pain for intensity, duration, location, and quality of pain; response to medications; presence of diaphoresis; vital signs, blood pressure and electrocardiographic changes; precipitating factors; patient history; auscultation of heart and lung sounds; and other subjective complaints. Chest pain in the patient with a history of angina pectoris may be due to other causes.

◆ In patients taking calcium channel blockers, monitor the blood pressure, pulse, intake and output, and weight. Signs of fluid retention are peripheral edema, subjective complaints of tight shoes and rings, signs of congestive heart failure such as dyspnea on exertion, distended jugular veins, orthopnea, or moist rales on pulmonary auscultation.

Patient and family education

◆ See the box on p. 234 for a discussion of orthostatic hypotension and the box on p. 182 for a discussion of constipation.

◆ If appropriate, teach the patient to take and record the pulse daily at home. Instruct the patient to report a change of 10 beats/min in the resting pulse or a pulse rate less than 50 beats/min. Appropriate candidates for such instruction may be those on multiple-drug regimens or those in whom control of side effects has been difficult. If appropriate, teach the patient to monitor and record weight on a regular basis. Instruct patients to report a weight gain of greater than 2 lb/day or 5 lb/week. Instruct patients to report the

development of tight rings, shoes, or clothing, or signs of peripheral edema.

◆ Because of potential drug interactions with other medication, instruct patients to keep all health care providers informed of all drugs being used. Tell patients to avoid the use of any over-the-counter preparations unless first cleared by the physician. In addition to using these drugs as prescribed, patients may find additional relief by losing weight, stopping smoking, limiting caffeine intake, avoiding extremes of temperature, and becoming involved in a regular exercise program; consult the physician.

◆ Emphasize to the patient the importance of taking these drugs as prescribed and not discontinuing them without consulting the physician. If a dose is missed, teach the patient to take the missed dose as soon as remembered but not within 2 hours of the next scheduled dose. Teach patients not to double up for missed doses.

◆ Teach patients to report any signs of liver problems such as right upper quadrant abdominal pain, jaundice, change in color or consistency of stools, and malaise.

◆ Encourage patients to have regular dental examinations. Review oral hygiene practices; encourage regular flossing and brushing.

Nifedipine

◆ To administer nifedipine sublingually or intrabuccally, puncture the fluid-filled capsule and squeeze the drug into the mouth. The patient may chew the capsule to break it and direct the contents to the cheek or under the tongue.

Verapamil

◆ Teach patients to swallow sustained-release formulations whole, without crushing or chewing. The extended-release tablet may be broken along the scored line. Administer IV doses undiluted over at least 2 min in the adult and 3 min in the elderly patient. Monitor the electrocardiogram and blood pressure.

Peripheral Vasodilators

Drug administration

◆ Monitor the blood pressure and pulse when beginning therapy or changing doses. Administer IV doses of papaverine undiluted at a rate

Continued.

NURSING IMPLICATIONS SUMMARY—cont'd

of 30 mg or less over 2 min. IM injection is preferred. Monitor the electrocardiogram, pulse, respiration, and blood pressure during IV administration and for 1 hr afterward. Administer IV doses of tolazoline undiluted at a rate of 10 mg or less over 1 min. It may also be diluted and given as an infusion. IM doses of isoxsuprine may cause hypotension and tachycardia; monitor the blood pressure and pulse. If isoxsuprine is used to prevent labor, monitor intensity, frequency, and duration of uterine contractions. Monitor fetal heart rate at regular intervals.

Patient and family education

◆ Take doses with meals or antacids to diminish GI symptoms. Review box on p. 234 for information about postural hypotension. Hypotension may be potentiated in patients receiving vasodilators who are also receiving other drugs that can cause hypotension, such as diuretics, antihypertensives, CNS depressants, narcotics, and sedatives. Instruct patients to keep all health care providers informed of all medications being taken.

◆ Instruct patients to avoid the use of alcohol, since it potentiates the hypotensive effects of vasodilators. Instruct patients to avoid smoking, since it reduces peripheral blood flow. Inform patients that time-release formulations must be swallowed whole, not crushed or chewed. Encourage patients to maintain desirable body weight to help decrease symptoms from peripheral vascular disease. Warn patients that nicotinyl alcohol, pentoxifylline,

or papaverine may produce pronounced flushing, which is not harmful. Caution patients to avoid driving or operating hazardous equipment if side effects such as dizziness, weakness, drowsiness, or double vision occur.

◆ Encourage patients to take these drugs as prescribed. Regular, long-term use may be necessary for full benefit to occur. Instruct patients to take missed doses as soon as remembered, unless within 2 hr of the next dose. Do not double up for missed doses.

◆ Papaverine may be used to produce erections in some impotent men. The patient should clean off the base of the penis with alcohol, and inject the prescribed dose into the base of the penis as instructed by the physician. After injection, the patient should massage the penis and attempt intercourse within 2 hr. Instruct the patient to consult the physician if the erection lasts more than 4 hr, the erection is painful, there is bleeding at the injection site that does not stop after pressure is applied, a lump develops where the medication was injected, or the penis becomes curved.

◆ Instruct patients taking pentoxifylline to avoid the use of aspirin or aspirin-containing products while taking this drug. Assess patients for hypersensitivity or intolerance to methylxanthines before administering pentoxifylline. Methylxanthines include caffeine, theophylline, and theobromine (the active ingredients in coffee, tea, and chocolate). Pentoxifylline is contraindicated in persons with intolerance to methylxanthines.

CHAPTER REVIEW

◆ **KEY TERMS**

angina pectoris, p. 204
classic angina, p. 205
coronary atherosclerosis, p. 204
percutaneous transluminal coronary angioplasty (PTCA), p. 205

Raynaud's disease, p. 213
reflex bradycardia, p. 202
shock, p. 198
sympathomimetic drugs, p. 197
tachycardia, p. 198
unstable angina, p. 205
variant angina (Prinzmetal's angina), p. 205
vasodilators, p. 197

◆ REVIEW QUESTIONS

1. List the direct-acting sympathomimetic drugs. What is their receptor selectivity and what physiologic actions result?

2. List the indirect-acting sympathomimetic drugs. What is their receptor selectivity and what physiologic actions result?

3. What are symptoms of anaphylactic shock? Which drug would the nurse expect to see used to treat anaphylactic shock? What is the usual dosage range? How is it administered?

4. Develop a teaching plan for the patient discharged to home with a bee-sting kit containing epinephrine.

5. What drug would the nurse expect to see used as a renal vasodilator?

6. What drug is used as a selective stimulant of cardiac contractility?

7. Why are sympathomimetic drugs sometimes administered during spinal anesthesia?

8. What is the origin of angina? Describe the differences between classic, variant, and unstable angina.

9. How do the nitrates and nitrites relieve angina?

10. Outline the main teaching points for patients taking nitrates and nitrites.

11. How do the beta blockers relieve angina? What are their side effects? For which patients are the cardioselective beta blockers especially indicated?

12. What would you include in the teaching plan for a patient taking a beta blocker?

13. How do the calcium channel blockers relieve angina? Why are they especially effective for variant angina?

14. What would you teach a patient about calcium channel blockers?

15. What are two causes of insufficient blood flow to the digits? Which cause is amenable to drug therapy? What role do vasodilators play?

16. List the seven drugs used as vasodilators for improving peripheral circulation. What are some of their common side effects?

SUGGESTED READING

Shock

Adamski DB: Assessment and treatment of allergic response to stinging insects, *J Emerg Nurs* 16(2):77, 1990.

Bochner BS, Lichtenstein LM: Anaphylaxis, *N Engl J Med* 324(25):1785, 1991.

Budny J, Anderson-Drevs K: IV inotropic agents: dopamine, dobutamine, and amrinone, *Crit Care Nurse* 10(2):54, 1990.

Burns KM: Vasoactive drug therapy in shock, *Crit Care Nurs Clin North Am* 2(2):167, 1990.

Cleary JD: Two inotropic agents: dopamine and dobutamine, *Pediatr Nurs* 14(5):414, 1988.

Dickerson M: Anaphylaxis and anaphylactic shock, *Crit Care Nurs Q* 11(1):68, 1988.

Donner C, O'Neill SP: Critical difference: anaphylactic shock, *Am J Nurs* 90(12):40, 1990.

Gawlinski A: Saving the cardiogenic shock patient, *Nurs 89* 19(12):34, 1989.

Hancock BG, Eberhard NK: The pharmacologic management of shock, *Crit Care Nurs Q* 11(1):19, 1988.

Jeffries PR, Whelan SK: Cardiogenic shock: current management, *Crit Care Nurs Q* 11(1):48, 1988.

Jones S, Bagg AM: L-E-A-D drugs for cardiac arrest: lidocaine, epinephrine, atropine, and dopamine, *Nurs 88* 18(1):34, 1988.

Kaliner MA: Calling a halt to anaphylaxis, *Emerg Med* 21(16):51, 1989.

Rimar JM: Shock in infants and children: assessment and treatment, *MCN* 13(2):98, 1988.

Sohl LL, Applefeld MM: A new direction for dobutamine, *Nurs 90* 20(10):41, 1990.

Teplitz L: L-E-A-D drugs for cardiac emergencies: clinical close-up on dopamine, *Nurs 89* 19(12):50, 1989.

Teplitz L: L-E-A-D drugs for cardiac emergencies: clinical close-up on epinephrine, *Nurs 89* 19(10):50, 1989.

Angina

Amsterdam EA, Chatterjee K, Frishman WH: Stable angina: first-line Rx for 1990, *Patient Care* 24(12):42, 1989.

Dix-Sheldon DK: Pharmacologic management of myocardial ischemia, *J Cardiovasc Nurs* 3(4):17, 1989.

Enger EL, Schwertz DW: Mechanisms of myocardial ischemia, *J Cardiovasc Nurs* 3(4):1, 1989.

Gleeson B: Loosening the grip of anginal pain, *Nurs 91* 21(1):33, 1991.

Gleeson B: Teaching your patient about his antianginal drugs, *Nurs 91* 21(2):65, 1991.

Miller CL: Medications in angina, *Focus Crit Care* 15(94):23, 1988.

Shaffer RB, Fritz DL: Preventing nitrate tolerance, *Nurs 91* 21(7):64, 1991.

Calcium channel blockers

Cardin S: Cardiovascular pharmacology: nursing considerations in the administration of verapamil, *J Cardiovasc Nurs* 2(2):73, 1988.

Few BJ: Nifedipine for treatment of premature labor, *MCN* 12(5):309, 1987.

Frohlich ED: Calcium antagonists for initial therapy of hypertension, *Heart Lung* 18(4):370, 1989.

Kedas A, Shively M, Burris J: Nursing delivery of sublingual nifedipine, *J Cardiovasc Nurs* 3(4):31, 1989.

Nagelhout JJ: AANA Journal Course: advanced scientific concepts. Update for nurse anesthetists—cardiac pharmacology: calcium antagonists, *AANA J* 56(4):367, 1988.

Shapiro W: Calcium channel blockers: update on uses in ischemic heart disease, *Consultant* 29(8):132, 1989.

Sosnowski C: Nimodipine: the use of calcium antagonists to prevent vasospasm following subarachnoid hemorrhage, *J Neurosci Nurs* 22(6):382, 1990.

Vidt DG, Borazanian RA: Calcium channel blockers in geriatric hypertension, *Geriatrics* 46(1):28, 1991.

Peripheral vascular disease

Hartshorn JC, Deans KW: Pharmacologic treatment of intermittent claudication with special emphasis on pentoxifylline, *Cardiovasc Nurs* 1(2):65, 1987.

CHAPTER 15

Antihypertensive Drugs

LEARNING OBJECTIVES

After studying this chapter, you should be able to do the following:

- Discuss factors that control blood pressure.
- Outline the stepped-care approach to treating hypertension.
- Develop a nursing care plan for patients receiving drugs altering peripheral sympathetic activity (beta blockers, alpha-adrenergic receptor antagonists, alpha- and beta-adrenergic receptor antagonists); drugs interfering with the storage or release of norepinephrine; centrally-acting antihypertensive drugs; or vasodilators (angiotensin converting enzyme (ACE) inhibitors, calcium channel blockers, and others).
- Develop a nursing care plan for a patient with a hypertensive emergency being treated with diazoxide, sodium nitroprusside, or trimethaphan.
- Develop a teaching plan for a patient who has orthostatic hypotension or needs to reduce sodium intake.

CHAPTER OVERVIEW

◆ *Hypertension* is generally defined as resting systolic blood pressure greater than 140 mm Hg or diastolic blood pressure greater than 90 mm Hg or both in an adult. In the United States, it is estimated that 15% of adults have hypertension. High blood pressure reflects an increased tone of the arteries and arterioles. Renal, endocrine, or neurogenic diseases cause hypertension in 10% of patients with hypertension. Hypertension in these patients is treated by treating its cause. No primary cause can be found in the remaining 90% of patients; this condition of unknown origin is called *essential hypertension*. Patients with hypertension may have no symptoms but do have an increased risk of stroke, blindness, and heart and renal disease after 10 or more years of sustained high blood pressure that produces vascular and organ damage. The incidence of hypertension is higher in men than in women, in blacks than in whites, in older than in younger adults, and in individuals with diabetes mellitus, hyperlipidemia, or a family history of hypertension. This chapter discusses drugs used to control hypertension and the rationale for their use.

Nursing Process Overview
ANTIHYPERTENSIVE DRUGS
Assessment

Assess the blood pressure when the patient is at rest. Check both arms; some physicians order lying, sitting, and standing blood pressure measurements. Monitor weight, serum electrolyte levels, blood urea nitrogen (BUN) levels, and measures of renal and cardiovascular function. Obtain a dietary history, focusing on sodium intake.

Nursing Diagnoses

Sexual dysfunction related to drug's side effect (impotence)
Noncompliance related to intolerable side effects
High risk for orthostatic hypotension

Management

Patients in hypertensive crisis may be admitted to the acute-care setting for cardiac monitoring and intravenous (IV) drug therapy. Otherwise, therapy may be started in the hospitalized or ambulatory patient. Monitor the patient's blood pressure and other vital signs, intake and output, weight, serum electrolyte and blood glucose levels, and other laboratory data specific to side effects of individual drugs. Instruct patients who are to be discharged about prescribed drugs and other prescribed therapies such as sodium restriction, weight loss, and regular exercise.

Evaluation

Ideally, therapy lowers the blood pressure to below 140/90 mm Hg without serious side effects. Make sure patients can explain what the hazards of untreated hypertension are, how to take the prescribed medications safely, why additional drugs such as diuretics or potassium may be needed, what to do about anticipated side effects, how to follow any dietary restrictions, and when to call the physician. If necessary, instruct patients to record weight or blood pressure on a regular basis.

BLOOD PRESSURE REGULATION

The major factors regulating blood pressure are diagrammed in Figure 15-1. These factors influence the circulating volume through adjustments of body salt and water (renal mechanisms) and the activity of the heart and blood vessels (cardiovascular mechanisms).

Renal Mechanisms

The kidney helps maintain blood pressure through control of the salt and water content of the body (see Chapter 16). A decrease in blood pressure stimulates the release of renin from the kidney. Renin release may be partly controlled by beta-adrenergic receptors. Renin is a proteolytic enzyme that acts on protein in the blood to produce the peptide angiotensin I. Angiotensin I is converted to angiotensin II, a small peptide that is a potent vasoconstrictor and therefore

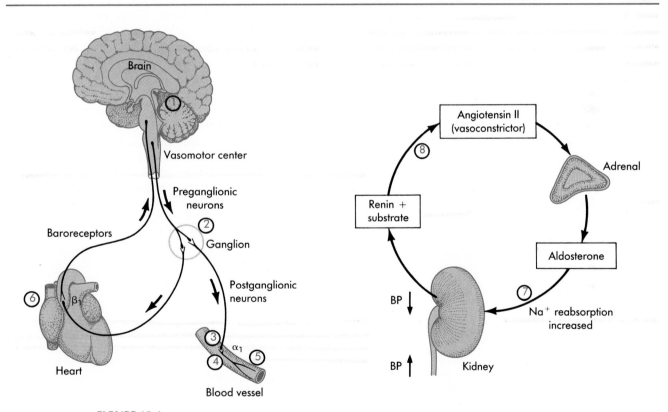

FIGURE 15-1

Numbers in diagram refer to mechanisms by which various antihypertensive drugs act. *1*, Drugs acting centrally to depress sympathetic tone (clonidine, methyldopa, guanabenz, reserpine). *2*, Drug blocking ganglionic receptor for acetylcholine (trimethaphan). *3*, Drugs interfering with norepinephrine synthesis, storage, or release (metyrosine, guanethidine, guanadrel, reserpine, pargyline). *4*, Drugs *A* blocking alpha-adrenergic receptor (prazosin, phenoxybenzamine, phentolamine, labetalol) or *(B)* blocking angiotensin II receptor (saralasin). *5*, Drugs directly dilating smooth muscle (hydralazine, minoxidil, sodium nitroprusside, diazoxide, calcium channel blockers). *6*, Drugs decreasing cardiac output (beta blockers, calcium channel blockers). *7*, Drugs blocking sodium reabsorption (diuretics). *8*, Drugs inhibiting angiotensin II formation (ACE inhibitors).

increases blood pressure. Angiotensin II also acts on the adrenal cortex to stimulate the secretion of aldosterone. Aldosterone is the mineralocorticoid hormone that acts on the kidney to decrease sodium excretion and to increase potassium excretion. The resulting sodium retention expands the plasma and extracellular fluid volumes, which contributes to the elevation of blood pressure.

Cardiovascular Mechanisms

Within the blood vessels, blood pressure depends on the cardiac output and the resistance to blood flow in the blood vessels. As illustrated in Figure 15-1, baroreceptors in the aorta and carotid sinus monitor the blood pressure and send the information to the brain. The brain integrates this information and adjusts the heart rate and resistance of the blood vessels, largely through the sympathetic nervous system, to fine tune the blood pressure. The vasomotor center in the medulla controls blood pressure. As the neurotransmitter of the sympathetic nervous system, norepinephrine raises blood pressure by stimulating the beta-1 receptors of the heart to increase cardiac output and by stimulating the alpha-1 receptors of the blood vessels, which causes constriction and increases the resistance to blood flow. In contrast, in the central nervous system (CNS), norepinephrine is the neurotransmitter for nerve tracts that ultimately decrease blood pressure.

Atrial natriuretic peptide (ANP) is an antihypertensive hormone derived from a peptide released from the heart into the circulation. ANP lowers blood pressure by relaxing the smooth muscle of blood vessels. ANP also causes diuresis and sodium excretion, inhibits the release of renin from the kidney and vasopressin from the hypothalamus, and antagonizes the action of aldosterone to retain sodium. The discovery and characterization of ANP is recent. Future antihypertensive drugs may work by enhancing or mimicking the activity of this hormone.

Antihypertensive Therapy

There has been an explosion of new drugs for the treatment of hypertension. Table 15-1 outlines drugs used to treat hypertension. These drugs can be divided into four categories, including diuretics, sympathetic depressants, vasodilators, and angiotensin antagonists. The sympathetic depressant drugs en-

Table 15-1 Categories of Antihypertensive Drugs

Type	Drugs	Antihypertensive action
DIURETICS		
Thiazide-type	See Table 16-3	Drug reduces body salt and water, which decreases arterial blood pressure. It may reduce plasma volume. It counteracts fluid retention caused by certain antihypertensive drugs (methyldopa, reserpine, guanethidine, guandrel, prazosin, hydralyzine, minoxidil, and diazoxide). It enhances action of most antihypertensive drugs given in long-term therapy.
Loop	Bumetanide Furosemide Ethacrynic acid	
Potassium-sparing	Spironolactone Triamterene Amiloride	
SYMPATHETIC DEPRESSANT DRUGS		
Beta-adrenergic receptor antagonist (beta blockers)	Acebutolol Atenolol Betaxolol Carteolol Metoprolol Nadolol Oxprenolol† Penbutolol Pindolol Propranolol Sotalol† Timolol	Drug reduces cardiac output. It reduces renin release from kidney. It may have central antihypertensive action. Drug preferred for individuals with high renin levels, typically young whites. It decreases incidence of sudden death in patients with recent heart attacks. Cardioselective [beta-1 adrenergic receptors] drugs are acebutolol, atenolol, and metoprolol.
Alpha-adrenergic receptor antagonist	Prazosin Terazosin Phenoxybenzamine Phentolamine	Drug blocks vasoconstrictive action of norepinephrine, thereby decreasing peripheral resistance.

†Available in Canada only.

Table 15-1   Categories of Antihypertensive Drugs—cont'd

Type	Drugs	Antihypertensive action
Alpha- and beta-adrenergic receptor antagonist	Labetalol	Both alpha- and beta-receptor antagonistic actions apply. Alpha receptor antagonist actions predominate. This is new drug class.
Centrally acting drug	Clonidine Methyldopa Guanabenz Guanfacine	Drug inhibits sympathetic outflow from brain by stimulating alpha receptors in vasomotor center of medulla. The result is decrease in peripheral resistance.
Centrally and peripherally acting drug	Reserpine	Drug depletes norepinephrine stores peripherally and centrally, resulting in decreased peripheral resistance.
Ganglionic blocking drug	Trimethaphan Mecamylamine	Drug blocks nicotinic receptors of autonomic ganglia to inhibit sympathetic and parasympathetic functions. Peripheral resistance is decreased.
Drug blocking norepinephrine release	Guanethidine Debrisoquine† Guanadrel	Loss of peripheral sympathetic tone decreases peripheral resistance by reducing cardiac output and peripheral resistance. Drug is used for severe hypertension.
Drug blocking norepinephrine synthesis	Metyrosine	Drug decreases peripheral resistance, particularly with norepinephrine-producing tumor (pheochromocytoma). It is rarely used.
Monoamine oxidase inhibitor	Pargyline	Drug decreases peripheral resistance. It is rarely used because of serious drug-food interactions.
VASODILATORS		
Arterial vasodilator	Hydralazine Minoxidil Diazoxide	Drug relaxes arterial smooth muscle to lower peripheral resistance. When used alone, it causes rebound tachycardia (increased heart rate) and edema.
Arterial and venous vasodilator	Nitroprusside	Drug dilates blood vessels. It is useful in hypertensive emergencies.
Calcium channel blocker	Diltiazem Felodipine Isradipine Nicardipine Nifedipine Verapamil	Drug reduces tone of blood vessels by reducing intracellular calcium, thereby causing arteriolar dilation and decreased total peripheral resistance.
Angiotensin converting enzyme (ACE) inhibitor	Benazepril Captopril Enalapril Fosinopril Lisinopril Quinapril Ramipril	Drug reduces peripheral resistance in individuals with high plasma renin levels.

†Available in Canada only.

compass several adrenergic mechanisms, since adrenergic drugs can lower blood pressure by decreasing the activity of the sympathetic nervous system peripherally or centrally. (Drug mechanisms that modify the activity of the sympathetic nervous system are reviewed in Chapter 9.) Figure 15-1 shows the sites of action of antihypertensive drugs.

Hypertension is commonly treated when the diastolic pressure is greater than 105 mm Hg, which indicates moderate to severe hypertension. If untreated, moderate to severe hypertension is associated with the development of congestive heart failure, renal failure, aneurysms, and strokes. Diastolic pressures of 90 to 105 mm Hg indicates mild hypertension, which is associated with increased morbidity when atherosclerosis is also a factor. A greater incidence of sudden death, usually caused by electrical dysfunction of the heart secondary to poor coronary circulation or of myocardial infarction, is seen among patients having mild hypertension and atherosclerosis. Many physicians reserve treatment of mild hypertension for patients with significant risk factors for atherosclerosis such as smoking, high cholesterol values (above 185 mg/dl), high lipid levels, abnormal glucose tolerance tests, electrocardiographic abnormalities, and family histories of atherosclerosis.

In general, drug therapy for hypertension is standard. However, therapy is changing as more is being learned about hypertension and as new drugs become available. Current therapy is based on a modified **stepped-care approach** in which drugs are added by class until blood pressure is controlled. The Joint National Committee on Detection, Evaluation, and Treatment of High Blood Pressure updated and published its recommendations in 1988.

Step 1 is the administration of a single drug from one of four drug classes (diuretics, beta blockers, calcium channel blockers, or ACE inhibitors). The most common choice is an oral diuretic, usually a thiazide or thiazide-like diuretic. Diuretics are especially effective as single agents for black hypertensive patients. Diuretics inhibit renal tubular reabsorption, causing diuresis that leads to reduction of body salt and water (extracellular fluid). The loss of extracellular fluid is associated with reduction of arterial blood pressure, but the mechanism of this hypotensive action remains obscure. This hypotensive effect is not seen in normotensive patients. Volume depletion also produces a reduction in plasma volume, although it is not clear that this reduction persists after the first month of therapy. In addition, many antihypertensive drugs cause fluid retention, which limits their antihypertensive effect. Diuretics are therefore commonly given with other antihypertensive drugs. Diuretics are discussed in Chapter 16.

Instead of a diuretic, a beta blocker may be given as the first drug. Hypertensive individuals with high plasma renin levels are especially responsive to beta blockers and rather unresponsive to diuretics. This is because beta blockers inhibit the release of renin from the kidney. Unfortunately, renin levels cannot be reliably or readily determined at present. In general, white hypertensive patients in the younger age groups have high renin levels, whereas black hypertensive patients in the older age groups have low renin levels. A beta blocker is also indicated for patients who have coronary artery disease. Beta blockers protect against sudden death in individuals who have had heart attacks, whereas diuretics may, through a lowering of potassium levels, increase the vulnerability of compromised hearts to sudden failure.

Calcium channel blockers have been added as step 1 drugs. They prevent the entry of calcium into the smooth muscle layer of blood vessels. This diminishes the contraction of the blood vessels and results in vasodilation. Calcium channel blockers decrease hypertension without causing reflex sympathetic stimulation or fluid retention. These drugs are especially effective as single agents for older patients and for those with low plasma renin activity.

ACE inhibitors treat most forms of hypertension and congestive heart failure. The ACE inhibitors are now step 1 drugs. They block the formation of angiotensin II. The antihypertensive response is not associated with an increase in heart rate or cardiac output. ACE inhibitors are effective as single agents for many hypertensive patients.

In Step 2 therapy step 1 therapy is evaluated after 1 to 3 months. If the antihypertensive response is not adequate, one of four actions is taken. First, the patient is evaluated for compliance. Second, the dose of the drug may be increased. Third, the first drug may be discontinued and a new drug started. Fourth, a second drug may be added to the therapeutic regimen. The most common second drug added to diuretic therapy is a sympathetic depressant drug. The sympathetic drug is commonly a beta-receptor blocker. However, methyldopa, clonidine, or occasionally prazosin or reserpine is an alternative drug used in step 2. The newer drugs guanabenz and guanadrel are also used in step 2.

Step 3 therapy is a further evaluation of step 2 therapy. If the antihypertensive response is still not adequate, a new second drug may be substituted or a third drug may be added. The most common three-drug regimen involves a vasodilator being added to the antihypertensive therapy. Hydralazine, minoxidil, and prazosin are the vasodilators most frequently used.

Step 4 therapy begins with a careful assessment of the factors limiting the antihypertensive response. A third or fourth drug may be added.

Patients with essential hypertension may have to take drugs for the rest of their lives to control the condition. Drug therapy can rarely be discontinued after the blood pressure is brought into a normal range. Frequently the drug dosage can be reduced with time. This is important, since antihypertensive drugs can produce uncomfortable side effects, whereas the hypertension itself may not produce uncomfortable symptoms, a situation that can make patient compliance with drug therapy difficult. Obesity and high salt intake are factors that aggravate hypertension. If a patient reduces weight and salt intake, drug requirements frequently are also reduced.

Antihypertensive therapy for special patient populations

Black patients. Hypertension is more prevalent in black Americans than in white Americans. In general, black hypertensive patients respond best to diuretics as monotherapy. ACE inhibitors and beta blockers are generally less effective as single agents for black patients than for white patients. However, in combination with diuretics, ACE inhibitors and beta blockers are equally effective in white and black hypertensive patients. Other antihypertensive drug classes are equally effective in both racial groups.

Elderly patients. Approximately two thirds of the U.S. population over 65 years of age has hypertension. A recent study examined the effect of treating elderly patients who have an elevated systolic pressure but normal diastolic pressure. The incidence of strokes and heart attacks was reduced. Older patients are more sensitive to diuretics, beta blockers, and the orthostatic hypotensive effects of other antihypertensive drugs. Thiazides and calcium channel blockers are generally well tolerated.

Pregnant patients. Hypertension as a complication of pregnancy is called *preeclampsia* and entails risk for the mother and fetus. Diet and bed rest are the first line of treatment, but if high blood pressure persists, methyldopa, hydralazine, and beta blockers have proved effective in controlling blood pressure and improving fetal survival. ACE inhibitors and calcium blockers have not yet been proved safe for use in pregnant patients.

DRUGS ALTERING PERIPHERAL SYMPATHETIC ACTIVITY

Antihypertensive drug classes include drugs that block the alpha- and beta-adrenergic receptors and drugs that interfere with the storage or release of norepinephrine, the adrenergic neurotransmitter. Each of these drug classes is discussed separately, and they are summarized in Table 15-2.

Text continued on p. 232.

Table 15-2 Drugs for Treatment of Chronic Hypertension

Generic name	Trade name	Administration/dosage	Comments
BETA-ADRENERGIC RECEPTOR ANTAGONISTS			
Acebutolol hydrochloride	Sectral* Monitan†	ORAL: *Adults*—400 mg once a day initially. Maintenance dose range: 200 to 1200 mg daily to control hypertension. Do not exceed 800 mg daily in elderly. Reduce dose 50% to 75% for patients with renal failure. FDA Pregnancy Category B.	Drug is cardioselective. It is also used as antiarrhythmic.
Atenolol	Apo-Atenolol† Tenormin*	ORAL: *Adults*—50 mg daily; increase to 100 mg if needed. Reduce dose to 50 mg on alternate days for renal failure. FDA Pregnancy Category C.	Drug is cardioselective. It is also used as antianginal.
Betaxolol	Kerlone	ORAL: *Adults*—10 mg once a day initially, dosage being doubled, if necessary, after 7 to 14 days.	Cardioselective. Also used for the treatment of glaucoma.
Carteolol	Cartrol	ORAL: *Adults*—2.5 or 5 mg. FDA Pregnancy Category C.	Drug is nonselective beta blocker.
Metoprolol tartrate	Apo-metoprolol† Betaloc† Lopresor† Lopressor	ORAL: *Adults*—50 mg 2 times daily. Dosage may be increased to 200 mg daily to control hypertension, maximum 450 mg. FDA Pregnancy Category B.	Drug is cardioselective. It is also used as antianginal and as prophylaxis against myocardial reinfarction.
Nadolol	Corgard* Syn-Nadolol†	ORAL: *Adults*—40 mg once daily to start. Dosages are increased by 40 to 80 mg every 3 to 7 days until optimum blood pressure control is achieved. The dosage range for maintenance is 80 to 120 mg daily. FDA Pregnancy Category C.	Drug is nonselective beta blocker. It is also used as antianginal.
Oxprenolol hydrochloride†	Trasicor†	ORAL: *Adults*—20 mg 3 times daily initially. Daily dosage may be increased every 2 to 3 weeks by 60 mg to achieve desired response.	Drug is nonselective beta blocker.

*Available in Canada and United States.
†Available in Canada only.

Continued.

Table 15-2 Drugs for Treatment of Chronic Hypertension—cont'd

Generic name	Trade name	Administration/dosage	Comments
Penbutolol sulfate	Levatol	ORAL: *Adults*—20 mg once daily.	Drug is nonselective beta blocker.
Pindolol	Visken* Syn-Pindolol†	ORAL: *Adults*—10 mg twice daily or 5 mg 3 times daily. Dose may be increased in increments of 10 mg/day every 2 to 3 weeks to achieve satisfactory response. Maximum dose, 60 mg daily. FDA Pregnancy Category B.	Drug is nonselective beta blocker.
Propranolol hydrochloride	Inderal* Apo-Propranolol† Detensol† Novopranol†	For hypertension: ORAL: *Adults*—20 mg 3 times daily with a diuretic. Dosage may be increased to 480 mg daily to control hypertension. FDA Pregnancy Category C. *Children*—0.5 to 1 mg/kg daily in 2 to 4 divided doses.	Drug is nonselective beta blocker. It is also used as antianginal, antiarrhythmic, prophylaxic against myocardial reinfarction, as prophylaxic in treatment of vascular headaches. It is also used in treatment of tremors and for symptomatic treatment of thyrotoxicosis.
Propranolol hydrochloride—cont'd		For pheochromocytoma: ORAL: *Adults*—30 mg 3 times daily with alpha-adrenergic blocking drug to control symptoms from pheochromocytoma. Dosage is increased to 60 mg 3 times daily for 3 days before surgery to remove pheochromocytoma.	Drug is nonselective beta blocker. Propranolol blocks beta action on heart from excess epinephrine produced by tumor of the adrenal medulla called *pheochromocytoma* Alpha receptor blocking drug must also be used to control hypertension.
Sotalol hydrochloride†	Sotacor†	ORAL: *Adults*—80 mg 2 times daily. Daily dosage may be increased by 80 mg every 2 to 3 weeks to achieve desired results.	Drug is nonselective beta blocker.
Timolol maleate	Apo-Timolol† Blocadren*	ORAL: *Adults*—10 mg daily initially. Maintenance is 20 to 40 mg daily. Maximum, 60 mg daily in 2 doses. FDA Pregnancy Category B.	Drug is nonselective beta blocker. It is also used as prophylaxic for myocardial reinfarction and for treatment of glaucoma.

ALPHA-ADRENERGIC RECEPTOR ANTAGONISTS

Generic name	Trade name	Administration/dosage	Comments
Phentolamine hydrochloride; phentolamine mesylate	Regitine Rogitine†	ORAL: *Adults*—50 mg every 4 to 6 hr. *Children*—25 mg every 4 to 6 hr. INTRAMUSCULAR, INTRAVENOUS: *Adults*—5 mg. *Children*—1 mg.	Drug is alpha-adrenergic blocker. It is used to diagnose hypertension resulting from pheochromocytoma. It treats hypertensive crisis secondary to pheochromocytoma, clonidine withdrawal, or tyramine ingestion during monoamine oxidase therapy. It reverses ischemia of levarterenol infiltration.
Phenoxybenzamine hydrochloride	Dibenzyline	ORAL: *Adults*—10 mg daily. May be increased by 10 mg/day to maximum dose of 60 mg daily. *Children*—0.2 mg/kg body weight up to 10 mg, once a day.	Drug is irreversible alpha-adrenergic blocker. Drug treats hypertension secondary to pheochromocytoma. Drug improves peripheral circulation in Raynaud's disease, ulceration, frostbite, and diabetic gangrene.
Prazosin hydrochloride	Minipress*	ORAL: *Adults*—initial dosage 2 to 3 mg in divided doses. Dosage may be increased gradually to 20 to 30 mg/day	Drug is alpha-adrenergic blocker. It is usually added to diuretic and sympathetic depressant, usually beta blocker.

*Available in Canada and United States.
†Available in Canada only.

Table 15-2   Drugs for Treatment of Chronic Hypertension—cont'd

Generic name	Trade name	Administration/dosage	Comments
Terazosin hydro-chloride	Hytrin*	ORAL: *Adults*—initially, 1 mg daily at bedtime; may increase to 5 mg daily if necessary, in increments. FDA Pregnancy Category C.	Drug is alpha-adrenergic blocker. It is usually added to diuretic and sympathetic depressant, usually beta blocker.
ALPHA- AND BETA-ADRENERGIC RECEPTOR ANTAGONIST			
Labetalol hydro-chloride	Trandate* Normodyne	ORAL: *Adults*—100 mg twice daily, initially. Maintenance doses are 200 to 800 mg daily for mild to moderate hypertension; 600 to 1200 mg daily for moderately severe hypertension; 1200 to 2400 mg daily for severe hypertension. FDA Pregnancy Category C.	Drug is taken with diuretic as step 2 drug. It has greater effect on standing blood pressure than pure beta-adrenergic antagonists. It also has effective vasodilator activity. Injectable preparation is available for hypertensive emergencies. See Table 15-3.
DRUGS INTERFERING WITH STORAGE AND/OR RELEASE OF NOREPINEPHRINE			
Alseroxylon	Rauwiloid	ORAL: *Adults*—initial dosage 2 to 4 mg daily; maintenance dosage 2 mg daily.	Active ingredient is reserpine.
Deserpidine	Harmonyl	ORAL: *Adults*—initial dosage 0.75 to 1 mg daily; maintenance dosage 0.25 mg daily.	Drug is chemically related to reserpine.
Guanadrel	Hylorel	ORAL: *Adults*—10 mg daily initially, increased daily or less often until desired response is obtained. Maintenance dose is usually 25 to 75 mg daily. May divide daily dosage. FDA Pregnancy Category B.	Drug is taken with a diuretic. It acts more rapidly and lasts a shorter time than guanethidine. It is being tested as step 2 drug for moderate hypertension. Side effects are similar to those of guanethidine but are milder.
Guanethidine sulfate	Apo-Guanethidine† Ismelin*	ORAL: *Adults*—initial dosage 12.5 mg daily. Dosage may be increased every 7 days by increments of 12.5 mg to maximum daily dosage of 100 mg. Further increments of 25 mg to daily dosage may then be added every week to maximum of 300 mg daily. *Children*—initial dosage 0.2 mg/kg of body weight daily. Increments of 0.2 mg/kg may then be added to daily dosage every 7 to 10 days.	Drug is used with diuretic to control severe hypertension. It inhibits release of norepinephrine and eventually depletes neuronal stores of norepinephrine. Guanethidine does not enter CNS to cause depression. Common side effects include orthostatic hypotension and diarrhea.
Rauwolfia serpentina	Raudixin Rauval Rauverid Wolfina	ORAL: *Adults*—initial dosage 200 to 400 mg daily in 1 or 2 doses; maintenance dosage 50 to 300 mg daily in 1 or 2 doses.	Active ingredient is reserpine.
Reserpine	Serpasil* Novoreserpine† Reserfia† Serpalan	ORAL: *Adults*—initial dosage 0.25 to 0.5 mg daily; maintenance dosage 0.1 to 0.25 mg daily. *Children*—0.25 to 0.5 mg daily.	Drug depletes norepinephrine stores. It is used with diuretic for control of essential hypertension. Reserpine is also used to treat vasospasm of Raynaud's disease (see Chapter 14).

*Available in Canada and United States.
†Available in Canada only.

Continued.

Table 15-2   Drugs for Treatment of Chronic Hypertension—cont'd

Generic name	Trade name	Administration/dosage	Comments
CENTRALLY ACTING ANTIHYPERTENSIVE DRUGS THAT INHIBIT ACTIVITY OF SYMPATHETIC NERVOUS SYSTEM			
Clonidine hydro-chloride	Catapres* Dixarit†	ORAL: *Adults*—0.1 mg 2 or 3 times daily. Dosage may be increased daily in increments of 0.1 to 0.2 mg. Maintenance doses are commonly 0.2 to 0.8 mg daily and are seldom larger than 2.4 mg daily. Withdrawal symptoms occur when doses are larger than 1.2 mg daily unless doses are reduced gradually. FDA Pregnancy Category C.	Centrally acting drug reduces sympathetic output. It is used with diuretic for control of essential hypertension. It is also being tested to treat nicotine and opioid withdrawal.
	Catapres-TTS	TRANSDERMAL: *Adults*—1 system applied once a week. Systems deliver 100, 200, or 300 µg/day.	Drug is used as transdermal patch, changed weekly.
Guanabenz acetate	Wytensin	ORAL: *Adults*—4 mg twice daily. May increase gradually to 32 mg twice daily or 64 mg once a day. FDA Pregnancy Category C.	Drug is taken with diuretic as step 2 drug. It reduces blood pressure and heart rate. Withdrawal reaction with rebound hypertension may be seen after discontinuing large doses.
Guanfacine	Tenex	ORAL: *Adults*—0.5 mg twice a day, increased gradually. Maintenance dose is 1 to 3 mg as single or divided dose. FDA Pregnancy Category B.	Drug is used alone or with diuretic. It reduces blood pressure and may reduce heart rate. Withdrawal reaction with rebound hypertension may be seen after discontinuing large doses.
Methyldopa	Aldomet*	ORAL: *Adults*—initial dose 250 mg in morning. After 1 week, dose may be doubled, with second 250 mg given at bedtime. Dosage may then be increased to maximum of 2 gm daily. *Children*—initial dosage 10 mg/kg body weight divided into 2 to 4 doses. Dosage may be increased gradually after 2 days in increments to maximum dosage of 65 mg/kg daily.	Drug acts centrally to depress sympathetic tone. It is used with thiazide diuretic for control of essential hypertension. Injectable preparation is available for hypertensive emergencies. See Table 15-3.
VASODILATORS **Direct acting**			
Hydralazine hydro-chloride	Apresoline* Novo-Hylazin†	ORAL: *Adults*—initial dosage 20 mg 2 or 3 times daily. Dosage may be increased by 10 to 25 mg daily. Maximum dosage, 400 mg in 4 divided doses. *Children*—initial dosage 0.75 mg/kg body weight in 4 divided doses. Dosage may be increased over 3 to 4 weeks to a maximum dosage of 7.5 mg/kg daily.	Drug is usually addded to diuretic and sympathetic depressant (particularly beta-adrenergic antagonists) for control of essential hypertension.

*Available in Canada and United States.
†Available in Canada only.

Table 15-2 Drugs for Treatment of Chronic Hypertension—cont'd

Generic name	Trade name	Administration/dosage	Comments
Minoxidil	Loniten Minodyl	ORAL: *Adults*—initial dosage 2.5 mg twice daily, increased to 5 mg twice daily after 1 week if needed. Up to 40 mg daily may be given. FDA Pregnancy Category C. *Children*—initial dosage 0.1 to 0.2 mg/kg body weight daily in 2 doses. Increase gradually to 1.4 mg/kg of body weight daily if required.	Drug is usually added to therapy with diuretic and beta-adrenergic antagonist.
Calcium channel blockers			
Diltiazem hydrochloride	Cardizem	ORAL: *Adults*—initially, 30 mg 3 or 4 times daily, increasing at 1- or 2-day intervals as needed, up to 360 mg daily. FDA Pregnancy Category C.	Drug is good vasodilator. It is also used as antianginal agent.
Felodipine	Plendil	ORAL: *Adults*—initially, 5 mg once a day. Adjust dosage as needed but no more often than at 2-week intervals. MAINTENANCE: 5 to 10 mg once a day. Maximum 20 mg daily.	New drug.
Isradipine	DynaCirc	ORAL: *Adults*—initially, 2.5 mg twice a day. Increase if necessary, in increments of 5 mg/day every 2 to 4 weeks, up to 20 mg daily.	New drug.
Nicardipine	Cardene	ORAL: *Adults*—initially, 20 mg 3 times a day.	A good vasodilator. Also used as an antianginal agent.
Nifedipine	Adalat* Apo-Nifed* Novo-Nifedin* Procardia	ORAL: *Adults*—initially, 10 mg 3 times daily, increasing gradually as needed, to maximum dose of 180 mg daily. FDA Pregnancy Category C.	Drug is good vasodilator. It does not depress sinoatrial (SA) or atrioventricular (AV) nodes. It is also used as antianginal agent.
Verapamil hydrochloride	Calan Isoptin*	ORAL: *Adults*—initially, 80 mg 3 or 4 times daily. Increase gradually as needed, up to 480 mg daily. FDA Pregnancy Category C.	Drug depresses SA and AV nodes. It is also used as antianginal and antiarrhythmic agents. It also treats hypertrophic cardiomyopathy.
Angiotensin converting enzyme inhibitors			
Benazepril	Lotensin	ORAL: *Adults*—initially, 10 mg once a day, reduced to 5 mg a day if diuretic is also taken.	New drug.
Captopril	Apo-Capto† Capoten*	ORAL: *Adults*—12.5 mg 3 times daily. May increase up to 25 mg 3 times daily in 1 to 2 weeks. FDA Pregnancy Category C.	Drug may be used alone but is often combined with diuretic. It also treats congestive heart failure.
Enalapril maleate	Vasotec*	ORAL: *Adults*—initially, 5 mg once a day. Increase gradually to maximum of 40 mg daily if needed. FDA Pregnancy Category C.	Drug may be used alone but is often combined with diuretic. This drug is converted to its active form by liver.

*Available in Canada and United States.
†Available in Canada only.

Continued.

Table 15-2   Drugs for Treatment of Chronic Hypertension—cont'd

Generic name	Trade name	Administration/dosage	Comments
Fosinopril	Monopril	ORAL: *Adults*—initially, 10 mg daily. Maintenance range is 20 to 40 mg daily.	New drug.
Lisinopril	Prinivil Zestril	ORAL: *Adults*—initially, 10 mg once a day; increased gradually to maximum of 40 mg if needed.	Drug may be used alone but is often combined with diuretic.
Quinapril hydrochloride	Accupril	ORAL: *Adults*—initially, 10 mg once a day or 5 mg if patient is taking a diuretic. MAINTENANCE: 20 to 80 mg daily as a single dose or divided into 2 doses.	New drug.
Ramipril	Altace	ORAL: *Adults*—initially, 2.5 mg daily, adjusted if necessary. Maintenance range is 2.5 to 20 mg daily as single or 2 divided doses.	New drug.

Beta Blockers

Mechanism of action. **Beta blockers** are more precisely the beta-adrenergic receptor antagonists. They are effective as antihypertensive drugs. Beta-1 adrenergic receptors are found principally in heart and fat tissue and stimulate heart function and lipolysis, respectively. Beta-2 adrenergic receptors mediate bronchodilation and peripheral vasodilation. The antihypertensive action of beta blockers is not entirely clear but appears to result from the decreased cardiac output and from the inhibition of renin production by the kidney. The decreased cardiac output is a result of the inhibition of the beta-1 adrenergic receptors to decrease heart rate, contractility, and automaticity.

One goal in the development of new beta blockers has been to develop cardioselective agents (drugs specific for the beta-1 receptor). The adverse side effects associated with blockade of beta-2 receptors include bronchospasm, prolongation of insulin-induced hypoglycemia, and aggravation of peripheral vascular insufficiency. However, the superiority of the cardioselective beta blockers for avoiding these complications is not clear.

Another goal in the development of new beta blockers has been to find drugs with some intrinsic beta-adrenergic activity (partial agonists), as seen in acebutolol, carteolol, oxprenolol, and pindolol. These drugs should produce less cardiac depression and should be safer for patients with compromised cardiac function. The improved safety remains to be proved.

Comparison of beta blockers. Beta blockers do not differ in their antihypertensive effects. However, they differ in their physiologic distribution and metabolism. Dosages must be individualized for the patient. Some drugs must be given 2 or more times a day, whereas others require only one daily dose.

Use as antihypertensive drugs. Beta blockers are used as step 2 drugs, added to a diuretic in long-term antihypertensive therapy. However, growing evidence shows beta blockers are most effective when given as a sole drug to hypertensive patients with high plasma renin levels. These patients are usually young and white. Older black hypertensive patients tend to have low plasma renin concentrations and respond better to a diuretic alone or to a diuretic with another type of sympathetic depressant.

Beta blockers are especially effective when a step 3 direct-acting vasodilator, such as hydralazine or minoxidil, is added to therapy. These vasodilators alone cause a reflex increase in cardiac output because of their marked hypotensive effect. This reflex cardiac stimulation is blocked by the beta blockers.

Side effects and contraindications. Adverse effects of beta blockers are usually mild. The most common side effects are dizziness, fatigue, cool extremities, reduced exercise tolerance, tingling in the fingers or toes, gastrointestinal (GI) upset, bronchospasm, depression, and sexual dysfunction (impotence in men). Patients with abnormal cardiovascular function are likely to encounter more serious side effects such as pulmonary edema, hypotension, cardiac failure, and an AV nodal block.

Beta blockers should not be discontinued abruptly because such an action may exacerbate angina, myocardial infarction, or ventricular arrhythmias. Instead, the dosage should be reduced gradually over 1 to 2

DIETARY CONSIDERATION: SODIUM AND HYPERTENSION

Excessive intake of sodium is associated with fluid retention and hypertension in some individuals. The first step in decreasing sodium intake is to stop adding salt to food while cooking or to cooked food during meals. The next step is to eliminate processed foods that contain a large amount of added sodium, including

- Relishes and pickles
- Salted popcorn, nuts
- Sauerkraut
- Bouillon cubes
- Salted crackers
- Potato chips, pretzels
- Canned, frozen, or dehydrated soup
- Bread, rolls, bran, bran flakes
- Processed cheese, cheese spreads
- Canned meat such as tuna and Vienna sausages
- Salt-cured meat such as bacon, ham, corned beef, salt pork, luncheon meats, frankfurters, and sausage
- Seasonings such as garlic, onion salts, or prepared mustard; meat extracts and tenderizers such as monosodium glutamate, soy sauce, and Worcestershire sauce; catsup; steak sauce; and cooking with salt pork or bacon grease

Instruct patients to read food ingredient lists and to limit or avoid foods containing salt, baking soda, monosodium glutamate, baking powder, and sodium compounds such as sodium benzoate, sodium citrate, sodium propionate, sodium alginate, sodium sulfite, sodium hydroxide, disodium phosphate, and sodium saccharin. Finally, instruct patients to limit or avoid foods naturally high in sodium such as milk, eggs, meat (including fish and poultry), cheese, beets and greens, carrots, celery, chard, spinach, kale, and white turnip roots.

weeks with careful monitoring of the patient for these possible complications.

Beta blockers are used with caution in patients whose health status could be worsened by this class of drugs; specific conditions include poor cardiac function, asthma, peripheral vascular disease, and diabetes. Blockade of beta receptors can compromise cardiac function, induce bronchospasm, and inhibit peripheral vasodilation. Hypoglycemia normally elicits the discharge of epinephrine. The effects of this released epinephrine will not be noticed easily in a patient taking a beta-receptor blocking drug. This is an important point for patients with diabetes mellitus who are taking insulin or an oral hypoglycemic drug.

Other uses. Beta blockers are also used to treat angina (see Chapter 14) and certain arrhythmias (see Chapter 17) and after myocardial infarction. These drugs are used after myocardial infarction to prevent sudden death resulting from electrical abnormalities

in the recovering heart. Recent studies have specifically shown timolol, propranolol, and metoprolol to be effective in reducing the incidence of sudden death after a heart attack.

Specific Beta Blockers

Acebutolol

Acebutolol (Monitan and Sectral) is an intermediate-acting, cardioselective beta blocker. It is moderately well absorbed when taken orally. Acebutolol is metabolized by the liver but is excreted mostly unchanged, both in the urine and in the feces, through enterohepatic circulation.

Atenolol

Atenolol (Tenormin) is a long-acting, cardioselective beta blocker. Poorly absorbed from the GI tract, the drug is not metabolized but is excreted unchanged in the urine. Time between doses must be increased in patients with impaired renal function.

Betaxolol

Betaxolol (Kerlone) is a long-acting, cardioselective beta blocker structurally related to metoprolol. It is well absorbed after oral administration and metabolized by the liver. Doses should be decreased for patients with renal impairment and for elderly patients. Betaxolol is also available for ophthalmic administration to treat glaucoma.

Carteolol

Carteolol (Cartrol) is a long-acting, nonselective beta blocker. Doses should be decreased in patients with renal impairment.

Esmolol

Esmolol (Brevibloc) is an ultra-short-acting, cardioselective beta blocker. It is administered intravenously for rapid, short-term control of ventricular rate in patients with atrial fibrillation or atrial flutter during surgery or medical emergencies. (See Chapter 19 for discussion of drugs to control cardiac arrhythmias.)

Metoprolol

Metoprolol (Lopressor and Betaloc) is a short-acting, cardioselective beta blocker. It is well absorbed from the GI tract and readily metabolized by the liver.

Nadolol

Nadolol (Corgard) is a long-acting, nonselective beta blocker. It is not well absorbed from the GI tract, and up to a fourth of the dose may be excreted in the feces. The absorbed drug is excreted unchanged in the urine. Patients with renal failure should be given the drug less frequently.

Oxprenolol

Oxprenolol (Trasicor) is a short-acting, nonselective beta blocker. It is well absorbed from the GI tract and metabolized by the liver. Oxprenolol is available in Canada but not in the United States.

Penbutolol

Penbutolol (Levatol) is a long-acting, nonselective beta blocker.

Pindolol

Pindolol (Visken) is a short-acting, nonselective beta blocker. It is well absorbed when taken orally. Pindolol is metabolized by the liver, but about half the dose is excreted unchanged in the urine.

Propranolol

Propranolol (Inderal), a nonselective beta blocker, is the oldest of the clinically used beta-blocking drugs. It is well absorbed orally and readily metabolized by the liver. Propranolol is short acting, but is available in extended-release forms.

Sotalol

Sotalol (Sotacor) is a long-acting, nonselective beta blocker. It is moderately well absorbed from the GI tract and poorly metabolized by the liver. Most of the drug is excreted unchanged in the urine. Patients with renal failure should be given the drug less frequently. Sotalol is available in Canada but not in the United States.

Timolol

Timolol (Blocadren and Apo-Timol) is a short-acting, nonselective beta blocker. It is well absorbed from the GI tract and metabolized by the liver.

Alpha-Adrenergic Receptor Antagonists

Prazosin and Terazosin

Mechanism of action. Prazosin (Minipress) and terazosin (Hytrin) are *vasodilators.* They lower blood pressure by blocking alpha-1 adrenergic receptors. Both arterioles and veins dilate, reducing the total peripheral resistance. Prazosin and terazosin are largely used as second or third drugs in the treatment of hypertension. A diuretic is usually necessary because the alpha-1 adrenergic blockers may cause fluid retention. Prazosin must be taken 2 or 3 times daily. Terazosin is taken once daily.

Side effects. The most common side effects are dizziness, lightheadedness, palpitations, and fainting attributable to orthostatic hypotension. Other complaints may include weakness, fatigue, drowsiness, blurred vision, nasal congestion, nausea, edema, and weight gain.

Drug interactions. Because blood pressure is lowered to a degree that can interfere with the perfusion of blood in the heart, attacks of angina may be precipitated by alpha-1 adrenergic blockers. They can also interact with nitroglycerin to relieve an anginal attack. However, the blood pressure may be lowered so much that the patient faints. Antiinflammatory drugs tend to cause fluid retention, which may worsen with alpha-1 adrenergic blockers.

Phentolamine

Phentolamine (Regitine) is a short-acting and reversible alpha-adrenergic receptor antagonist. The major effects of phentolamine are vasodilation resulting from blockade of alpha-1-adrenergic receptors

---

PATIENT PROBLEM: ORTHOSTATIC HYPOTENSION

THE PROBLEM

The blood pressure drops markedly as the individual moves from lying to sitting or sitting to standing positions.

SIGNS AND SYMPTOMS

Dizziness, lightheadedness, weakness, and syncope (fainting)

ASSOCIATED OR CONTRIBUTING FACTORS

Long periods of standing; hot weather; hot showers or baths; ingestion of alcohol; exercise, especially when followed by immobility; and dehydration

PATIENT AND FAMILY EDUCATION

◆ Tighten calf muscles regularly while standing, or take a break to walk around frequently.

◆ If possible, sit instead of standing at work.

◆ Reduce the temperature of baths and showers.

◆ Wear support stockings. In severe cases, tailor-made waist-high stockings may be needed.

◆ Avoid the use of alcohol.

◆ Move slowly from lying to sitting positions. Hold on to something to provide support while moving from lying to sitting or standing positions.

◆ Maintain adequate fluid intake to avoid dehydration, especially in the summer or if perspiring profusely.

◆ If the problem is severe, consult the physician. A change in drug or dose may be needed.

ADDITIONAL NURSING CARE MEASURES

◆ Monitor the blood pressure with patient lying, sitting, and standing. To document hypotension, check both arms.

◆ Supervise ambulation. Instruct patients with marked hypotension to call for assistance when moving from a reclining to a standing position.

and cardiac stimulation believed to be secondary to blockade of the presynaptic alpha-2-adrenergic receptors. (Presynaptic alpha-2 adrenergic receptors are associated with uptake of norepinephrine; see Chapter 10.) This drug is not well absorbed orally, and IV or intramuscular (IM) administration is more common.

Phentolamine has specific clinical uses as a vasodilator. It lowers blood pressure in patients with a tumor (pheochromocytoma) of the adrenal medulla, which secretes large amounts of epinephrine. Phentolamine also lowers blood pressure in patients who are being treated with a monoamine oxidase (MAO) inhibitor and are suffering from the "cheese reaction," a hypertensive crisis that can be reversed with phentolamine. (See Chapter 29 for a discussion of the cheese reaction.) It also treats patients being withdrawn from the antihypertensive drug clonidine, who may suffer a temporary hypertensive crisis.

A major use of phentolamine is to infiltrate a site where levarterenol (norepinephrine) or metaraminol has leaked into the tissue surrounding the infusion site. Phentolamine reverses the profound vasoconstriction that can otherwise cause tissue death. Side effects of the systemic use of phentolamine include hypotension, a fast heart rate (tachycardia) as a reflex response of the body to the hypotension, nasal congestion secondary to the vasodilation, and general GI upset.

Phenoxybenzamine

Phenoxybenzamine (Dibenzyline) is an irreversible alpha-receptor antagonist with a duration of action lasting several days. The prominent side effect of phenoxybenzamine is postural hypotension, which refers to a fall in blood pressure when a patient rises from a recumbent to a standing position. In a healthy person, postural hypotension is not seen because compensatory vasoconstriction redirects blood flow so that blood does not drain from the head to the legs on standing, which would cause fainting. In a person treated with phenoxybenzamine or other drugs that deplete peripheral norepinephrine, the compensatory vasoconstriction is lost. Reflex tachycardia, nasal congestion, and GI upset are other common side effects of phenoxybenzamine resulting from its alpha-adrenergic antagonist activity.

Phenoxybenzamine controls the high blood pressure caused by the elevated plasma levels of epinephrine in patients with pheochromocytoma when they are not yet ready for surgical removal of the tumor. Phenoxybenzamine is also used to dilate blood vessels in the skin, as in the treatment of Raynaud's phenomenon, in which there is a prominent neurogenic vasoconstriction of the blood vessels of the skin, par-

ticularly in the hands and feet (see Chapter 14).

A major source of drug interactions with phenoxybenzamine is overstimulation of beta-adrenergic receptors by drugs such as epinephrine that have alpha- and beta-adrenergic receptor agonist activity. The blockade of alpha receptors allows beta-receptor activation to go unopposed. Tachycardia is exaggerated. The vasodilator activity of drugs (such as the opioids) is exaggerated by phenoxybenzamine.

Investigational drugs

Indoramin (Baratrol) and trimazosin (Cardovar) are alpha blockers currently under study as antihypertensive agents for use in treating chronic hypertension.

Alpha- and Beta-Adrenergic Receptor Antagonist

Labetalol

Labetalol (Normodyne and Trandate) has alpha- and beta-receptor antagonist activities. It reduces the heart rate and myocardial contractility, slows AV conduction, and lowers blood pressure. The decrease in heart rate is not as pronounced with labetalol as with other beta antagonists. Alpha-antagonist effects are more prominent with labetalol than beta-antagonist effects, and a decrease in peripheral resistance is probably the major therapeutic effect. Labetalol is especially useful for treating hypertensive patients who also have angina.

Labetalol is effective orally and is metabolized by the liver and excreted in the urine. The drug is normally administered twice daily and is best taken with a meal, since food increases its bioavailability. Orthostatic hypotension may be experienced early in therapy. Other adverse effects noted include GI upset, fatigue, nervousness, dry mouth, and tingling of the scalp. Side effects characteristic of other beta blockers are also seen.

Drugs Interfering with the Storage or Release of Norepinephrine

Guanadrel

Guanadrel (Hylorel) has actions similar to those of guanethidine but with more rapid onset of action and shorter duration of action. The side effects of guanadrel are similar to those of guanethidine but are less severe.

Guanethidine

Mechanism of action. Guanethidine (Ismelin) is a potent antihypertensive drug that is restricted for use in controlling severe hypertension. It enters peripheral sympathetic neurons, being taken into the cell by the same mechanism as for the reuptake of norepinephrine. Inside the neuron, guanethidine blocks norepinephrine release. Guanethidine does not cross the blood-brain barrier and therefore produces no central effects. Because norepinephrine is not available for release from peripheral sympathetic neurons, the peripheral vascular resistance and cardiac output are decreased.

Administration and duration. The effects of guanethidine may take 1 to 2 weeks to reach the maximum therapeutic response to a given dosage regimen. Moreover, effects persist for 7 to 10 days after therapy is discontinued.

Side effects. A number of uncomfortable side effects arise from the depletion of peripheral norepinephrine stores. Postural hypotension makes guanethidine therapy difficult. The tone of blood vessels is diminished by guanethidine, and if the patient moves suddenly from a reclining to a standing position, the appropriate vascular changes cannot take place quickly enough for proper blood redistribution. The blood stays in the periphery and drains from the head when the patient stands, resulting in fainting. Instruct patients taking guanethidine to change body positions slowly. Other side effects resulting from the depletion of norepinephrine include slow heart rate (bradycardia) and diarrhea. Diarrhea can be severe after meals. In men, failure of erection or ejaculation may occur secondary to the loss of vascular tone. Guanethidine also causes sodium retention; therefore a diuretic is administered concurrently.

Contraindications. Contraindications for guanethidine therapy include angina, cerebral insufficiency, or coronary artery disease, conditions that are further compromised by the loss of vascular tone.

Drug interactions. A number of drug interactions have been noted for guanethidine. Patients taking guanethidine are supersensitive to administered catecholamines. Patients become less responsive to guanethidine when an indirect-acting adrenergic drug such as amphetamine or ephedrine or a tricyclic-antidepressant drug is taken. These indirect-acting adrenergic drugs release stored norepinephrine from neurons, thus overcoming the effect of guanethidine in blocking release of norepinephrine. Tricyclic antidepressants block the uptake of guanethidine into the neuron so that guanethidine cannot reach its site of action.

Reserpine

Reserpine (Serpasil) and related drugs are often called *rauwolfia alkaloids* because reserpine was originally isolated from the *Rauwolfia serpentina* bush of India. Reserpine was originally used as an antipsychotic drug but has been replaced by the phenothiazine tranquilizers. Reserpine effectively lowers blood pressure because it depletes stores of norepinephrine from neurons in both the central and peripheral nervous systems. Reserpine's central action produces sedation and tranquilization. The reported incidence of depression with reserpine varies from 27% to 40%. Occasionally, patients taking reserpine become suicidal. More commonly, patients complain of a lethargic feeling, an increased appetite, and increased dreaming. Patients sometimes complain of nightmares.

Vasodilation and nasal congestion, other side effects of reserpine, are related to the decreased sympathetic tone. Salivation, stomach cramps, and diarrhea are related to the predominant parasympathetic tone when sympathetic tone is depressed. Since reserpine augments gastric acid secretion through the increased parasympathetic tone, it should not be used in patients with a peptic ulcer.

CENTRALLY ACTING ANTIHYPERTENSIVE DRUGS THAT INHIBIT THE ACTIVITY OF THE SYMPATHETIC NERVOUS SYSTEM

Clonidine, guanabenz, guanfacine, and methyldopa exert their antihypertensive activity through actions in the CNS.

Specific Drugs

Clonidine

Clonidine (Catapres) has an antihypertensive effect resulting from its action in the CNS. It activates alpha receptors in the vasomotor center of the medulla, which inhibits activity of the sympathetic nervous system. Heart rate and cardiac output are decreased and account for the reduction in blood pressure.

Clonidine is commonly used with a diuretic in antihypertensive therapy. New therapeutic uses for clonidine have developed. Clonidine is used to prevent vascular headaches and to treat the vasomotor symptoms of menopause. The symptoms of opioid and nicotine withdrawal can often be controlled by clonidine. Tourette's syndrome, a condition marked by severe and multiple tics, is alleviated by clonidine therapy.

Common side effects of clonidine therapy include drowsiness, dry mouth, and constipation. Sudden discontinuance can be dangerous. After therapeutic doses are discontinued for 12 to 48 hr, many patients experience symptoms of a sympathetic rebound, including restlessness, insomnia, tremors, increased salivation, and tachycardia. If clonidine is not reinstated, further symptoms, such as headaches, abdominal pain, and nausea, follow. The most severe reaction is a hypertensive crisis that is best treated in the hospital with a combination of alpha- and beta-blocking drugs such as phentolamine and propranolol. To avoid these withdrawal problems, clonidine doses are gradually reduced over 1 week or more.

Guanabenz (Wytensin)

Guanabenz (Wytensin) has a mechanism of action similar to that of clonidine, inhibiting sympathetic activity by activating alpha receptors in the CNS. Guanabenz has a long duration of action, 12 to 24 hrs, and may require only one daily dose. It is metabolized in the liver and excreted in the urine. The most common side effects are drowsiness, dry mouth, dizziness, weakness, and headache. Withdrawal rebound hypertension can occur if guanabenz is discontinued abruptly.

Guanfacine

Guanfacine (Tenex), like clonidine and guanabenz, appears to act in the CNS. By stimulating central alpha-adrenergic receptors, it decreases sympathetic outflow and blood pressure lowers. Guanfacine has a long duration of action, about 24 hr, and can be taken once a day. It is well absorbed and is metabolized in the liver. The most common side effects are drowsiness, dry mouth, depression, and confusion.

Methyldopa

Methyldopa (Aldomet) is taken into sympathetic neurons and metabolized to methylnorepinephrine. Methylnorepinephrine is stored in granules and released on stimulation of the neuron. Methylnorepinephrine is called a *false transmitter,* since it takes the place of norepinephrine. Until recently the antihypertensive effect of methylnorepinephrine was believed to result from the ineffectiveness of methylnorepinephrine as a vasoconstrictor. Recently, it has been shown that methylnorepinephrine is a potent vasoconstrictor, so the action of methylnorepinephrine as a false transmitter for peripheral sympathetic neurons does not account for the antihypertensive effects of methyldopa. The action of methyldopa in the CNS to decrease the activity of the sympathetic nervous system is now believed to account for the antihypertensive effect of the drug. Methyldopa decreases sympathetic tone and has a tranquilizing effect on behavior.

Side effects common to methyldopa are related largely to the decrease in central sympathetic activity. Drowsiness is common at the beginning of treatment. Unpleasant sedation, depressed mood, and nightmares are occasional complaints. Tiredness and fatigue may be noted. Peripheral effects include bradycardia, diarrhea, dry mouth, and occasional ejaculatory failure in males.

Occasionally, methyldopa causes a false positive Coombs' test. A positive Coombs' test indicates hemolytic anemia, but it is rare for the patient taking methyldopa to have hemolytic anemia despite the positive test. Methyldopa may also cause a mild alteration of liver function tests. Methyldopa should not be used for patients who already have impaired liver function, since it will interfere with evaluating the course of the disease. This alteration of liver tests ordinarily occurs during the first 6 weeks of therapy, and it is reversed by discontinuing methyldopa.

VASODILATORS FOR TREATING CHRONIC HYPERTENSION

Angiotensin Converting Enzyme (ACE) Inhibitors

The **angiotensin converting enzyme (ACE) inhibitors** have rapidly found a role in the treatment of chronic hypertension. These drugs are used alone or with a diuretic or other drug in the treatment of mild to severe hypertension. ACE inhibitors are also useful in treating renovascular hypertension by altering renal blood flow in patients with diabetic nephropathy or renal scleroderma. Patients with severe congestive heart failure may also be helped by treatment with ACE inhibitors.

Mechanism of action. Angiotensin II is a potent vasoconstrictor. As seen in Figure 15-1, angiotensin II is formed from angiotensin I by ACE. When this enzyme is inhibited, the amount of angiotensin II formed decreases. ACE inhibitors therefore decrease the amount of angiotensin II. ACE inhibitors also block the degradation of bradykinin and therefore increase the amounts of this important vasodilator peptide. In effect, ACE inhibitors decrease peripheral vascular resistance. This action makes the ACE inhibitors useful in treating congestive heart failure and hypertension.

Side effects and drug interactions. ACE inhibitors are well tolerated and have little, if any, adverse effects on CNS function or on carbohydrate or lipid metabolism. Dizziness, a skin rash, swelling, and an increase in serum potassium levels (hyperkalemia) have been reported. Drug interactions have been reported for the ACE inhibitors. Foods or drugs high in potassium may contribute to hyperkalemia. The hypotensive effect of ACE inhibitors is enhanced by diuretics, alcohol, and beta blockers. Nonsteroidal antiinflammatory drugs (NSAIDS), especially indomethacin, may antagonize the antihypertensive effect of the ACE inhibitors and cause sodium retention leading to edema.

Specific ACE Inhibitors

Benazepril

Benazepril (Lotensin) is a newly introduced ACE inhibitor to treat hypertension.

Captopril

Captopril (Capoten) is rapidly absorbed after oral administration and is effective within 1 hr. About half of the drug is excreted unchanged in the urine.

Enalapril

Enalapril (Vasotec) is a prodrug, designed to be absorbed orally. During absorption, enalapril is deesterified to the active drug, enalaprilat, which is an ACE inhibitor like captopril. However, patients with liver disease may be unable to activate enalapril. Enalaprilat injection (Vasotec injection) is the active form of enalapril in a dosage form to treat a hypertensive emergency.

Fosinopril

Fosinopril (Monopril) is a newly introduced ACE inhibitor used to treat hypertension.

Lisinopril

Lisinopril (Prinivil and Zestril) has a longer duration of action than captopril or enalapril. Most patients require just one daily dose.

Quinapril

Quinapril (Accupril) is a newly introduced ACE inhibitor to treat hypertension.

Ramipril

Ramipril (Altace) is metabolized in part to ramiprilat, which has about 6 times the activity of ramipril itself. Metabolites are excreted in the urine and feces. Ramipril may be taken alone or with a diuretic. The most common side effects include headache, dizziness, and numbness.

Calcium Channel Blockers

Calcium channel blockers have rapidly become important in the treatment of various cardiovascular diseases. These drugs treat angina, arrhythmias, and hypertension. In the treatment of hypertension, calcium channel blockers may be used alone or with one or more other drugs, most commonly a diuretic.

Mechanism of action. Calcium channel blockers decrease the entry of calcium into smooth muscle and thereby lower vascular tone, an action that reduces peripheral resistance and blood pressure. This reduction in blood pressure can produce a reflex increase in heart rate. Cardiac function is also depressed because of reduced intracellular calcium. The various calcium channel blockers each differ in their relative effect on vascular and cardiac tissue. In general, calcium channel blockers are useful for patients with coexisting angina (see Chapter 14).

Side effects. Calcium channel blockers are well tolerated by various age and ethnic groups, and side effects are generally mild. Headaches, dizziness, and edema are complaints in 20% or less of patients. The depression of AV nodal conduction may lead to heart block. Beta-adrenergic blockers act synergistically with calcium channel blockers to depress AV conduction and depress cardiac contractility. The digitalis glycosides act additively with the calcium channel blockers to depress AV conduction. These drugs should be used with caution in patients with congestive heart failure.

Specific Calcium Channel Blockers

Diltiazem

Diltiazem (Cardizem) depresses the SA and AV nodes but produces little negative inotropic effect (decrease in the strength of the heartbeat). Diltiazem is effective in dilating coronary vessels, making it a good antianginal agent. It is well absorbed orally and extensively metabolized.

Felodipine

Felodipine (Plendil) is a new calcium channel blocker.

Isradipine

Isradipine (DynaCirc) is a new calcium channel blocker structurally related to verapamil.

Nicardipine

Nicardipine (Cardene) is more selective for vascular smooth muscle than for cardiac muscle. Nicardipine is a potent vasodilator and also dilates the coronary vessels with little or no depression of conductivity.

Nifedipine

Nifedipine (Procardia and Adalat) is similar to nicardipine in being more selective for smooth muscle than for cardiac muscle. It has no real effect on the AV node and thus does not directly depress the heart rate.

Verapamil

Verapamil (Calan and Isoptin) depresses the SA and AV nodes, making it a useful antiarrhythmic drug (see Chapter 19). Bradycardia is a common side effect.

Investigational drugs

Calcium channel blockers currently under clinical investigation include anipamil, gallopamil, lidoflazine, nisoldipine, nilvadipine, nitrendipine (Baypress), and ronipamil.

Other Vasodilators

Hydralazine

Hydralazine (Apresoline) acts directly on arteriolar smooth muscle to cause relaxation. The mechanism is not known. The drop in arterial blood pressure is great enough to activate the baroreceptors of the aorta. This activation causes a reflex stimulation of the heart, which increases cardiac output and partially compensates for the fall in blood pressure (reflex tachycardia). Hydralazine also causes sodium retention. Because hydralazine causes reflex stimulation of the heart and increases sodium retention, it is most effective in reducing hypertension when added to a diuretic to counteract the sodium retention and a beta blocker (propranolol, nadolol, or metoprolol) to block the reflex stimulation of the heart.

Side effects of hydralazine include headache, palpitation, loss of appetite, nausea, vomiting, and diarrhea. In the absence of a beta antagonist, hydralazine can cause angina in susceptible individuals as a result of the reflex stimulation of the heart. Hydralazine should not be used for a patient with angina, coronary artery disease, or congestive heart failure because of the indirect cardiac effects.

The main problem that has been documented after long-term therapy at high doses of hydralazine is the appearance of a lupuslike syndrome. Lupus erythematosus (LE) is an autoimmune disease wth symptoms of fever, joint pain, chest pain, edema, and appearance of circulating anti-DNA antibodies. The syndrome induced by hydralazine is similar, but it is reversed when the drug is discontinued. The appearance of lupuslike symptoms is infrequent when smaller doses of hydralazine are used with diuretic and sympathetic blocking drugs. Patients on hydralazine therapy are monitored for anti-DNA antibodies and LE cells.

Minoxidil

Minoxidil (Loniten) is a direct-acting vasodilator like hydralazine but is more potent. It must be given with a diuretic to control fluid retention and a beta-receptor blocker to prevent reflex tachycardia. A side effect of minoxidil is excessive hairiness, which may develop after a few weeks of treatment. Some patients experience transient nausea, headaches, or fatigue when treatment is started.

DRUGS USED IN HYPERTENSIVE EMERGENCIES

A **hypertensive emergency** cannot be simply defined. The blood pressure may be severely or only moderately elevated. The important feature is that there is impending end-organ damage, usually of the brain, heart, or eyes. Unstable neurologic symptoms suggesting damage to the brain include headache, restlessness, confusion, and even convulsions. Hemorrhaging may be apparent in the eye. Drugs used to treat hypertensive emergencies by rapidly lowering blood pressure are listed in Table 15-3.

Vasodilators

Diazoxide

Diazoxide (Hyperstat) acts directly to relax arteriolar smooth muscle. This action lowers blood pressure but does not affect the venous side of circulation. Diazoxide is therefore not useful for conditions requiring the decreased venous return produced by trimethaphan.

The advantage of diazoxide treatment is that a bolus of the drug can be given intravenously over 30 sec, is usually effective in 5 min, and remains effective for 2 to 12 hr. Blood pressure does not need to be continuously monitored as with trimethaphan treatment. The patient rarely becomes excessively hypotensive. Diazoxide causes retention of sodium and water, which must be treated with a diuretic. Diazoxide also causes hyperglycemia.

Sodium nitroprusside

Sodium nitroprusside (Nipride) acts directly on the smooth muscle of arterioles and venous vessels. Blood pressure decreases immediately, with no increase in venous return. There are no notable side effects with short-term use of nitroprusside. Blood pressure must be constantly monitored, and the drug is administered by IV drip. Nitroprusside is unstable in light; therefore it should not be used more than 4 hr after it is dissolved. Side effects arise from the use of nitroprusside for several days. Some of it is metabolized to thiocyanate, which can produce ringing in the ears (tinnitus), blurred vision, and hypothyroidism.

Ganglionic Blocking Drug

Trimethaphan

Trimethaphan (Arfonad) is a ganglionic blocking drug that blocks the receptors for acetylcholine in the ganglia. Ganglionic blocking drugs inhibit sympathetic and parasympathetic activity and therefore have limited clinical uses. Trimethaphan is used in treating some hypertensive emergencies. Because trimethaphan has a short duration of action, it is administered by continuous IV drip, during which blood pressure must be constantly monitored. Side effects result from the inhibition of sympathetic and parasympathetic tone. Severe hypotension can result from the inhibition of sympathetic tone. IV drip is then discontinued until the blood pressure begins to rise again. Side effects from loss of parasympathetic tone include pupillary dilation, loss of accommodation, drying of mucous surfaces, constipation, and urinary retention.

The disadvantages of trimethaphan therapy are that blood pressure must be carefully monitored and that the loss of pupillary reflexes makes it difficult to monitor ongoing neurologic damage to the brain, if neurologic damage was the presenting symptom. Tri-

Table 15-3 Drugs Used in Hypertensive Emergencies

Generic name	Trade name	Administration/dosage	Comments
Diazoxide	Hyperstat*	INTRAVENOUS: *Adults*—150 mg or 5 mg/kg body weight. *Children*—5 mg/kg body weight. Administered over 30 sec. May be repeated after 30 min.	Drug is direct-acting vasodilator. It acts rapidly (2 to 5 min) and lasts 2 to 12 hr. It increases venous return and cardiac output. Blood pressure fall is rarely excessive, so blood pressure monitoring is not critical.
Enalaprilat	Vasotec	INTRAVENOUS: *Adults*—1.25 mg administered over 5 min every 6 hr. Use 0.625 mg for patients on diuretic therapy or in renal failure.	An ACE inhibitor, it is in its active form for IV administration. Clinical response should be seen in 1 hr.
Labetalol	Normodyne Trandate*	INTRAVENOUS: *Adults*—20 mg or 0.25 mg/kg injected over 2 min. Additional injections of 40 to 80 mg may be given in 10-min intervals until blood pressure control is achieved or total dose of 300 mg has been given. Alternatively, may be infused at rate of 2 mg/min.	Drug is mixed alpha and beta blocker. Clinical response is seen in about 5 min.
Methyldopate hydrochloride	Aldomet*	INTRAVENOUS: *Adults*—250 to 500 mg in 100 ml 5% dextrose, administered slowly over 30 to 60 min. Maximum dose is 1 gm in 6 hr. INTRAVENOUS: *Children*—5 to 10 mg/kg in 5% dextrose, administered over 30 to 60 min. Maximum dose is 65 mg/kg body weight or 3 gm daily.	Drug is centrally acting antihypertensive. Clinical response may take several hours. Duration of action is 10 to 16 hr.
Nitroglycerin	Nitro-Bid* Nitrol Nitrostat* Tridil*	INTRAVENOUS: *Adults*—initially 5 μg/min; increase in 5-μg increments every 3 to 5 min until clinical response or 20 μg/min is reached.	Drug is direct-acting vasodilator. Doses are stated for non-PVC infusion sets. PVC may absorb nitroglycerin. IV nitroglycerin is also used to reduce cardiac load or as antianginal agent in emergency situation. Effective immediately.
Sodium nitroprusside	Nipride* Nitropress	INTRAVENOUS: *Adults*—dissolve 50 mg in 500 to 1000 ml of 5% dextrose. Infuse 0.5 to 10 μg/kg/min. Solution must be protected from light and discarded after 4 hr. *Children*—1.4 μg/kg/min.	Drug is direct-acting vasodilator. It acts rapidly (1 to 2 min). Continuous infusion is necessary to maintain hypotensive effect. Decreased venous return occurs with no change in heart rate. Blood pressure must be carefully monitored and infusion rate adjusted to maintain desired level.
Trimethaphan camsylate	Arfonad*	INTRAVENOUS: *Adults*—0.1% (1 mg/ml) infusion in 5% dextrose. Rate of infusion is begun at 0.5 to 1 mg/min and increased gradually until blood pressure falls by 20 mm Hg. After several minutes, rate is again increased until blood pressure reaches desired level.	Rapidly acting drug blocks acetylcholine receptors in ganglia. It inhibits sympathetic and parasympathetic nervous systems and decreases venous return and cardiac output. Blood pressure must be carefully monitored, since hypotensive effect is variable and unpredictable.

*Available in Canada and United States.

methaphan can also be unpredictable in its effects. Patients already on antihypertensive medication or with a reduced blood volume may be unusually sensitive to trimethaphan. Some patients do not respond readily to trimethaphan; others are initially responsive but become unresponsive.

Trimethaphan decreases venous return of blood and lowers cardiac output. These actions are helpful in patients with dissecting aortic aneurysm, hypertensive encephalopathy, acute left ventricular failure, or cerebral hemorrhage, since the pressure is removed from the weakened tissue.

NURSING IMPLICATIONS SUMMARY

Antihypertensives

Drug administration and patient education

◆ Encourage the patient to reach desirable body weight and to restrict dietary intake of sodium, since these may reduce the need for antihypertensive drug therapy.

◆ Assess patients thoroughly and thoughtfully on a regular basis. Poor compliance with drug therapy may result from patients possibly feeling worse, not better, while on antihypertensives. Patients may be reluctant to discuss side effects such as impotence and may discontinue a drug if this or other side effects occur. In addition, the cost of drug therapy, especially when two or more drugs are required, may be prohibitive.

◆ Reinforce the need to take these medications as directed and not to discontinue therapy abruptly or without consulting the physician.

◆ Work with patients to develop a system for remembering to take their medication. Activities such as marking off a calendar when doses are taken or preparing a week's doses at one time may keep patients more involved and serve as a reminder.

◆ Instruct patients about orthostatic hypotension, a common side effect of antihypertensive therapy (see box on p. 234).

◆ Monitor blood pressure and pulse at least every 4 hr when patients begin antihypertensive therapy, during periods of dosage adjustment, or when orthostatic hypotension is a problem. Assess the blood pressure with the patient lying, then sitting, and then standing; check both arms. For selected patients, it may be necessary to instruct a family member how to measure and record the blood pressure in the home.

◆ Supervise the ambulation of the hospitalized patient on antihypertensive therapy to guard against injury in case the patient becomes dizzy or faint. Be especially alert with elderly patients, who are more sensitive to drug effects.

◆ Teach patients to keep all health care providers informed of all drugs being used and to avoid over-the-counter medications unless approved by the physician. The incidence of hypotensive episodes is increased if patients taking antihypertensives take other drugs that also cause hypotension, including diuretics, CNS depressants, barbiturates, or alcohol.

◆ Monitor daily weight of the hospitalized patient. Weigh patients under standard conditions (same time, same scales, same amount of clothing). Observe for signs of fluid retention such as pitting edema (edema characterized by indentations that remain in the skin for seconds to minutes after pressure has been applied by the examiner's finger), dependent edema, tight rings, shoes, and clothing. Auscultate the lungs to detect pulmonary rales. If possible, instruct patients to monitor and record their weight at home. Report to the physician a weight gain in excess of 2 lb/day or 5 lb/week. Record intake and output in the hospitalized patient. Refer the patient to a dietitian or teach the patient about dietary sodium (see box on p. 233).

◆ When patients are taking combination products containing two or more drugs, teach them about each drug in the product, and assess for side effects for each drug. For example, Apresoline contains hydralazine and hydrochlorothiazide; Ser-Ap-Es contains hydralazine, hydrochlorothiazide, and reserpine. If a dose is missed, instruct patients to take the dose as soon as remembered, unless within 2 hr of the next dose, then resume the usual dosing schedule. Do not double up for missed doses.

◆ Caution patients to avoid driving or operating hazardous equipment if sedation or sleepiness occurs. Review the box on p. 166 for measures to help patients with dry mouth.

INTRAVENOUS ANTIHYPERTENSIVE THERAPY

◆ Monitor blood pressure and pulse every 3 to 5 min until stable, then every 15 to 30 min. Use an electronic infusion monitor and a microdrip infusion set to titrate drug dose more accurately. Monitor the electrocardiogram. Ensure that patients remain in bed for up to 3 hr after drug administration. Keep call bell within reach and siderails up.

Beta Blockers

Drug administration

◆ See general guidelines for antihypertensive drugs. Take the apical pulse for a full minute before administering the dose. If the pulse is less than 60 beats/min in an adult or 90 to 100 beats/min in a child, withhold the dose and notify the physician. Specific guidelines

Continued.

may vary with an individual patient or by physician preference. Be especially alert to bradycardia if the patient is also taking a cardiac glycoside. Monitor the blood pressure. Review the general guidelines. Monitor general parameters of cardiovascular function, including intake, output, daily weight, and serum electrolyte levels. Because these drugs accumulate in the presence of renal failure, monitor the BUN levels. Treatment of overdose with beta blockers is symptomatic. Bronchospasm occasionally occurs. Assess for signs of respiratory distress, auscultate lung sounds, and monitor respiratory rate. Assess patients for signs of depression, including withdrawal, insomnia, anorexia, and lack of interest in personal appearance.

INTRAVENOUS ESMOLOL

◆ Dilute according to manufacturer's directions to a concentration of 10 mg/ml. Dosage is individualized, but one regimen specifies a loading dose of 500 μg/kg/min for 1 min, followed by a maintenance infusion of 50 μg/kg/min for 4 min. These dosages may be repeated at regular intervals. Monitor blood pressure, pulse, and electrocardiogram.

INTRAVENOUS METOPROLOL

◆ Metoprolol may be given by direct IV push. Administer the dose over at least 1 min. Monitor blood pressure, pulse, and electrocardiogram.

INTRAVENOUS PROPRANOLOL

◆ Check the dose carefully: IV dose is much smaller than oral dose. Propranolol may be given undiluted or diluted in 5% dextrose solution. Administer at a rate of 1 mg/min or more slowly. Monitor blood pressure, pulse, and electrocardiogram.

Patient and family education

◆ Emphasize the importance of taking these drugs as prescribed for optimal benefit. Caution patients not to discontinue these drugs without consulting the physician and not to let prescriptions run out. Stress to patients that several weeks of therapy may be needed to gain maximum effects. Orthostatic hypotension may be a problem; review the box on p. 234.

◆ Instruct patients to take oral doses with meals or a snack to reduce gastric irritation. Many side effects can occur with beta blockers. Tell patients to report any unexpected sign or symptom to the physician. Instruct patients to report signs of thrombocytopenia (unexplained bruising or bleeding) or signs of agranulocytosis (unexplained fever or sore throat). Teach diabetic patients that beta blockers may mask the symptoms of hypoglycemia; patients should monitor blood glucose levels carefully during periods of dosage adjustment or when starting or stopping the drug. Tell patients that if drowsiness occurs, they should avoid driving or operating hazardous equipment until it wears off. If drowsiness is severe or persistent, notify the physician.

Alpha-Adrenergic Receptor Antagonists
Drug administration and patient and family education

◆ See general guidelines for antihypertensives. Nasal congestion may be a problem. Inform patients that this side effect may decrease with continued use of the prescribed drug. Caution patients to avoid the use of over-the-counter medications to self-treat this annoying side effect.

◆ Sexual dysfunction is common. Question patients tactfully about sexual problems; many patients are reluctant to discuss sexual difficulties. Sexual problems may prompt patients to discontinue medications. Provide emotional support as needed. Remind patients not to discontinue medications without notifying physician.

◆ Caution patients to avoid driving or operating hazardous equipment until the effects of these medications are known. Dizziness and lethargy may be common. Before discharge, teach patients how to monitor for fluid retention. If diuretics are also prescribed, teach patients the importance of taking all drugs as ordered for maximum effects.

◆ For overdose with phenoxybenzamine, place patient supine with head lowered and feet elevated if possible. An abdominal binder and leg bandages may also be used. Epinephrine is contraindicated, but IV norepinephrine (levarterenol) may be helpful.

INTRAVENOUS PHENTOLAMINE

- Dilute 5 mg with 1 ml of sterile water; you may dilute drug further. Administer the drug at a rate of 5 mg or less over 1 min. Monitor blood pressure and pulse every 30 sec, and obtain an electrocardiogram. Do not leave patient unattended until he or she is stable. Treat overdose with dopamine; do not use epinephrine.
- Prazosin and terazosin are especially prone to cause orthostatic hypotension, particularly when therapy is started and during periods of increasing dosage. See box on p. 234 for a discussion of orthostatic hypotension. Instruct patients to take the first dose and any increased dosages at bedtime and to be especially careful when getting up at night during the first few days of therapy. Warn families about this side effect so that they will not be frightened and will know that they should lie the patient down until the patient is no longer dizzy.

Alpha- and Beta-Adrenergic Receptor Antagonist
Labetalol

- See general guidelines for antihypertensive therapy and information about beta blockers.

INTRAVENOUS LABETALOL

- Labetalol may be given undiluted or diluted in most common IV solutions. Administer at a rate of 20 mg over at least 2 min. Monitor patient's blood pressure and pulse every 5 to 10 min until he or she is stable. Monitor electrocardiogram. Keep patients supine for several hours after injection and supervise ambulation.

Drugs Interfering with Storage or Release of Norepinephrine
Guanethidine and Guanadrel
Drug administration and patient and family education

- See general guidelines for antihypertensives. Diarrhea may be severe; see p. 180. These drugs may cause hypoglycemia. Instruct diabetic patients to monitor blood glucose levels closely during the start of therapy and periods of dosage adjustment. Dry mouth may occur; see box on p. 166. Nasal congestion may be a problem. Caution patients to avoid treatment with over-the-counter products without consulting the physician.

Reserpine and Related Drugs
Drug administration and patient and family education

- See general guidelines for antihypertensives. Serious mental depression is a side effect. Monitor patients carefully for changes in mood or affect; assess for anorexia, insomnia, impotence, withdrawal, and mood swings. Instruct families to report the development of any change in the patient's personality.
- Take doses with meals or a snack to reduce gastric irritation. Monitor the patient's pulse. Tell the patient to notify the physician if noticeable changes in heart rate occur. Instruct patients that several weeks of therapy may be necessary to see full drug benefit.

Centrally Acting Antihypertensive Drugs
Clonidine, Guanabenz, and Guanfacine
Drug administration and patient and family education

- See general guidelines for antihypertensives. Dry mouth may occur; see box on p. 166. Constipation may occur; see box on p. 182. Caution patients to avoid driving or operating hazardous equipment if drowsiness occurs.
- Emphasize to patients the importance of not discontinuing these drugs abruptly. Instruct patients to have prescriptions refilled before the supply on hand runs out. Patients who may not comply with dosage schedules should not take these drugs. See discussion of withdrawal symptoms. If an oral dose is missed, instruct patients to take it as soon as they remember, unless within 2 hr of the next dose. Teach patients not to double up for missed doses. If two or more doses are missed, patients should notify the physician.
- Clonidine is available in a transdermal form. Review instruction leaflet provided by manufacturer with patients. Patients should not cut or trim patch. Remove old patch, Apply it to clean, heirless area, but avoid areas of skin irritation or scars. Rotate sites. If patch becomes loose or falls off, replace it with a fresh one; if it is only slightly loose, cover with adhesive tape. Replace it weekly. If a patch is overdue for replacement by 3 days or more, notify physician; do not apply 2 patches at once.

Continued.

NURSING IMPLICATIONS SUMMARY—cont'd

Methyldopa

Drug administration and patient and family education

◆ See general guidelines for antihypertensives. Dry mouth may occur; see box on p. 166. Depression is a side effect. Assess patients carefully for changes in mood or affect; assess for anorexia, insomnia, impotence, withdrawal, and mood swings. Instruct families to report the development of any change in the patient's personality. Diarrhea may occur; see p. 180. Nasal congestion may be a problem. Caution patients to avoid treatment with over-the-counter products without consulting the physician.

◆ Methyldopa may alter liver function tests. Teach patients to report the development of malaise, fever, right upper quadrant abdominal pain, or change in the color or consistency of stools. Monitor liver function tests. Tell patients that urine may darken if exposed to the air. The IV form of methyldopa is methyldopate hydrochloride. Dilute dose in 100 to 200 ml of 5% dextrose in water. Administer dose as an infusion over 30 to 60 min. Avoid IM or subcutaneous administration.

Vasodilators for Chronic Hypertension
ACE inhibitors

Drug administration

◆ Monitor serum potassium levels.

INTRAVENOUS ENALAPRIL

◆ Check dose; a single IV dose is much smaller than an oral dose. It may be given undiluted, or dilute with up to 50 ml of a compatible IV solution (see manufacturer's guidelines). Administer dose over at least 5 min. Monitor blood pressure and pulse. Keep patients supine until blood pressure is stable.

Patient and family education

◆ See general guidelines for antihypertensives. Caution patients to avoid excessive amounts of foods high in potassium (see box on p. 252). Instruct patients to avoid salt substitutes, unless approved by the physician, since these products often contain large amounts of potassium.

◆ Tell patients to take captopril on an empty stomach, 1 hr before meals, unless instructed otherwise by the physician. If a dose is missed, take it as soon as remembered, unless close to the time for the next dose. Do not double up for missed doses. Instruct patients to report the development of fever, sore throat, or signs of infection. Caution patients to avoid driving or operating hazardous equipment if dizziness develops; if dizziness is severe, consult the physician.

Calcium Channel Blockers

◆ See Chapter 14.

Hydralazine

Patient and family education

◆ See general guidelines for antihypertensives. Diarrhea may occur; see p. 180. Teach patients to monitor weight and to assess themselves for fluid retention. Tell patients to notify the physician if lupuslike symptoms develop; see p. 239. Instruct patients to report the development of tingling of fingers or numbness, since this sensation may signal peripheral neuropathy; pyridoxine may be prescribed. Instruct patients to take oral doses with food or a snack to reduce gastric irritation.

Minoxidil

Patient and family education

See general guidelines for antihypertensives. Minoxidil may cause hypertrichosis (excessive hairiness) after several weeks of therapy. Instruct patients to report this side effect. The hair can be shaved, bleached, or removed depending on the location and severity. Caution patients not to discontinue the medication without contacting the physician. The excessive hair growth may slowly disappear after several months of therapy.

◆ The side effect of hypertrichosis led to the development of topical minoxidil (Rogaine), used to stimulate hair growth in balding men. Instruct patients to follow instructions supplied by the manufacturer. Patients should wash hair daily before applying solution, and dry scalp and hair thoroughly. Instruct pa-

NURSING IMPLICATIONS SUMMARY—cont'd

tients to apply the prescribed amount, using the applicator supplied. Patients should wash hands to remove any solution left on the hands. They should not use a hair dryer to dry the scalp after drug application. If patients use topical minoxidil at night, instruct them to wait at least 30 min after applying solution before going to bed. If a dose is missed, it should be applied as soon as the patient remembers, unless it is close to the time for the next dose; patients should not double up for missed doses. Tell patients to report local side effects (e.g., itching, scalp burning, skin irritation) or systemic effects such as dizziness, flushing, headache, tingling of hands or feet, and weight gain. Instruct patients to report the development of shortness of breath, increased heart rate, or changes in heart rhythm. Assess patients for distended jugular veins and pulmonary rales.

Drugs Used in Hypertensive Emergencies

Drug administration

◆ Drug dose may be titrated to patient blood pressure. Do not leave patients unattended until they are stable. Keep siderails up. Ideally, the patient should be in an intensive care unit. Monitor electrocardiogram, blood pressure, pulse, respirations, level of consciousness, and intake and output; insertion of a Foley catheter may be necessary. These drugs should not be mixed with other drugs in an infusion or a syringe.

INTRAVENOUS DIAZOXIDE

◆ IV diazoxide should be administered quickly, undiluted (e.g., 150 mg over 10 to 30 sec). Because it is highly alkaline, avoid IM or subcutaneous injection. Make certain that the IV line is patent before administration, and inspect the insertion site for irritation or redness. If extravasation occurs, apply ice packs. Treat drug overdose or severe hypotension with dopamine. Monitor the blood glucose level because diazoxide may cause hyperglycemia; insulin may be necessary.

INTRAVENOUS SODIUM NITROPRUSSIDE

◆ Dilute as directed by manufacturer. Do not use an IV filter. Do not use drug if it is highly discolored; it may be used if faintly brownish in color. Cover the prepared infusion with aluminum foil to protect it from light. Titrate dose based on physician guidelines and patient response; a typical dose is 3 μg/kg of body weight/min (adults) or 1.4 μg/kg/min (small children). Use microdrip tubing and an infusion-control device.

◆ To treat overdose, discontinue nitroprusside and administer amyl nitrate (see Chapter 14) for 15 to 30 sec every minute until a sodium nitrite solution for IV administration can be prepared. Administer a 3% sodium nitrite solution at a rate of 2.5 to 5 ml/min up to a total dose of 10 to 15 ml. After this, inject sodium thiosulfate intravenously, 12.5 gm in 50 ml of 5% dextrose in water over 10 min. Monitor patients carefully. Signs of overdose can reappear for up to several hours, and sodium nitrite and sodium thiosulfate can be repeated at half the dose listed. Monitor thiocyanate levels if the drug is used longer than 72 hr. Use dopamine to correct hypotension.

INTRAVENOUS TRIMETHAPHAN

◆ Dilute as directed by the manufacturer. Titrate dose based on physician guidelines and patient response; a typical dose is 0.5 to 1.0 mg/min. Use microdrip tubing and an infusion-control device. Monitor patient response closely. If blood pressure does not drop with patient in supine position, lower the head of the bed. Monitor patients closely for signs of cerebral anoxia; the drug produces pupillary dilation, so this sign may be of little significance. To treat severe hypotension, use phenylephrine or dopamine.

CHAPTER REVIEW

◆ **KEY TERMS**

angiotension converting enzyme (ACE) inhibitors,
p. 237
beta blockers, p. 232
calcium channel blockers, p. 238
essential hypertension, p. 222
hypertensive emergency, p. 239
stepped-care approach, p. 226
vasodilators, p. 234

◆ **REVIEW QUESTIONS**

1. Describe the renal mechanisms controlling blood pressure.

2. Describe the cardiovascular mechanisms controlling blood pressure.

3. Name the beta blockers you might use as antihypertensive drugs. How does blockade of the beta receptors lower blood pressure? What are the side effects of these drugs? What are cardioselective beta blockers? List three cardioselective beta blockers.

4. For what situations might you use phentolamine as an antihypertensive drug? What is its mechanism of action?

5. How does the action of phenoxybenzamine differ from that of phentolamine?

6. How does the use of prazosin differ from that of phentolamine?

7. List which antihypertensives act by interfering with storage or release of norepinephrine.

8. List which antihypertensives act centrally to inhibit sympathetic activity.

9. How do ACE inhibitors work? What are their limiting side effects? Develop a teaching plan for a patient taking an ACE inhibitor.

10. How do calcium channel blockers decrease hypertension? Develop a teaching plan for a patient taking a calcium channel blocker.

11. List antihypertensives used in the chronic treatment of hypertension that are direct-acting vasodilators.

12. Which drug is both an alpha- and a beta-adrenergic antagonist?

13. List three drugs used to control a hypertensive emergency and their mechanisms of action.

14. What is a limiting side effect of reserpine? How should you assess the patient?

15. What is orthostatic hypotension? Which antihypertensive drugs are commonly associated with orthostatic hypotension as a side effect? What information can you provide to the patient?

16. Which antihypertensive is associated with the synthesis of a false transmitter?

17. What reaction may occur with the sudden discontinuance of clonidine? What information can you provide to the patient?

18. Describe reflex tachycardia. Which antihypertensive drugs would you expect to cause it?

19. Why is patient compliance with antihypertensive therapy frequently poor? What actions can you take?

20. Hypertension is a major health problem that requires chronic drug therapy. The drugs required may be costly and may cause annoying or embarrassing side effects. Treatment of hypertension may also necessitate changes in patients' lifestyle (e.g., sodium restriction and weight loss). If time permits, try some role playing activities in which one student practices asking another student (the patient) about how well the patient is complying with drug therapy. Develop questions that are nonjudgmental and do not put the patient on the defensive.

SUGGESTED READING

Allinger RL: Folk beliefs about high blood pressure in Hispanic immigrants, *West J Nurs Res* 10(5):629, 1988.

Blake GJ: Metoprolol for myocardial infarction, *Nurs 91* 21(1):91, 1991.

Christlieb AR: Treating hypertension in diabetics: achieving therapeutic success without dangerous side effects, *Consultant* 29(12):24, 1989.

Cunningham SG: Nonpharmacologic management of high blood pressure, *Cardiovasc Nurs* 23(4):18, 1987.

Evans MJ: Tips for taking a child's blood pressure quickly, *Nurs 83* 13(3):61, 1983.

Fontana SA: Update on high blood pressure: highlights from the 1988 national report, *Nurse Pract* 13(2):8, 1988.

Manzo M: Sodium nitroprusside for hypertensive crisis, *Nurs 87* 11:98, 1987.

Maree SM: Esmolol: a unique beta adrenergic antagonist, *J Neurosci Nurs* 22(2):121, 1990.

Nakagawa-Kogan H and others: Self-management of hypertension: predictors of success in diastolic blood pressure reduction, *Res Nurs Health* 1192):105, 1988.

National High Blood Pressure Education Program: The 1988 report of the Joint National Committee on Detection, Evaluation, and Treatment of High Blood Pressure, *Arch Intern Med* 148:1023, 1988.

Plawecki HM and others: Compliance and health beliefs in the Black female hypertensive client, *J Natl Black Nurses Assoc* 2(1):38, 1987.

Powers MJ, Jalowiec A: Profile of the well-controlled, well-adjusted hypertensive patient, *Nurs Res* 36(2):106, 1987.

Rodman MJ: Hypertension: step-care management, *RN* 54(2):24, 1991.

Rodman MJ: Hypertension: first-line drug therapy, *RN* 54(1):32, 1991.

Sabo CE, Michael SR: Drug therapy for the hypertensive diabetic patient: implications for the diabetes educator, *Diabetes Educ* 15(4):377, 1989.

Stuart EM and others: Nonpharmacologic treatment of hypertension: a multiple-risk-factor approach, *J Cardiovasc Nurs* 1(4):1, 1987.

Teplitz L: Action stat! Hypertensive crisis, *Nurs 90* 20(4):33, 1990.

Winer N: Hypertensive crisis: *Crit Care Nurs Q* 13(3):23, 1990.

CHAPTER 16

Diuretics

LEARNING OBJECTIVES

After studying this chapter, you should be able to do the following:

- Explain why increasing sodium excretion is a desirable action of diuretics.
- Name the loop diuretics.
- Identify the class of diuretics with the highest potency.
- Name conditions for which loop diuretics or thiazide diuretics must be used.
- Develop a nursing care plan for a patient receiving a loop, thiazide, potassium-sparing, carbonic anhydrase inhibitor, or osmotic diuretic, or combination of two diuretics.

CHAPTER OVERVIEW

- **Diuretics** are drugs that increase urine flow. There are several mechanisms by which drugs can produce this effect, but the clinically important drugs of this class act on the kidney. This chapter reviews pertinent renal physiology and discusses the mechanism of action and clinical properties of diuretic drugs.

Nursing Process Overview

DIURETICS

Assessment

Perform a total patient assessment, focusing on the presenting signs and symptoms and appropriate laboratory and other objective data that would help further define the nature of the patient's problems. Assess the patient's intake, output, weight, and blood pressure, and observe for signs of electrolyte imbalance, fluid retention, or dehydration.

Nursing Diagnoses

Fluid volume deficit related to furosemide therapy as manifested by excessive urine output, decreased skin turgor, and orthostatic hypotension
High risk for hypokalemia
High risk for sleep pattern disturbance related to nocturia secondary to diuretic therapy

Management

Determine what actions are required to aid drug therapy. For example, dietary and fluid restrictions may be required to speed fluid removal and to prevent reaccumulation. Monitor fluid intake and output, serum electrolyte levels, blood urea nitrogen (BUN) level, uric acid level, body weight, and blood pressure, and observe for the appearance of new signs or symptoms. Watch for side effects, such as ototoxicity with ethacrynic acid.

Evaluation

Diuretic therapy is effective if excess fluid is lost and blood pressure is maintained and if abnormalities in electrolyte status or side effects do not result. For some patients, it is necessary to tolerate minor side effects to achieve required diuresis. Potassium depletion may be treated with potassium supplements. Teach the patient why the medication is necessary, what the major possible side effects are, and what symptoms should be reported to the physician. Discuss why additional medications such as potassium supplements may be needed. Teach selected patients to record daily weight, fluid intake and output, and blood pressure. If the physician has prescribed a restricted diet, verify that the patient can choose menus within the limits of the diet plan. Be aware of the potential for abuse with these compounds (see box).

FUNCTION OF THE NEPHRON

The functional unit of the kidney is the **nephron** (Figure 16-1). Glomerular filtration is the first step in the production of urine. Blood contacts a filtering surface in the glomerulus, where water and small molecules pass into the tubule, leaving behind most proteins and protein-bound small molecules. The remainder of the nephron adjusts the salt and water content of the tubular fluid to achieve **homeostasis**, a balanced condition in which the body retains the salt and water required for proper function and eliminates the excess. For the purpose of understanding diuretic drugs, this discussion is limited to six ions or molecules: sodium (Na^+), chloride (Cl^-), potassium (K^+), water (H_2O), bicarbonate (HCO_3^-), and organic ions.

Sodium Ion Sites

Sodium ion freely enters the tubular fluid from the glomerulus so that the fluid entering the proximal convoluted tubule has the same sodium ion content as blood. The proximal convoluted tubule actively removes sodium ion from the tubule. No further sodium ion is removed in the descending limb of Henle's loop, but in the ascending limb, sodium ion passively follows chloride ion out of the tubule. In the distal convoluted tubule, sodium ion is removed by an active pump like that in the proximal convoluted tubule or by a pump that exchanges sodium ion for potassium ion. With the latter pump, sodium ion is reabsorbed, while potassium ion is excreted.

Chloride Ion Sites

Chloride ion is primarily removed from tubular fluid in the ascending limb of Henle's loop. This active removal of chloride ion draws sodium ion along with it and effectively dilutes the tubular fluid.

Potassium Ion Sites

Potassium ion is not the primary ion involved in the action of any diuretic drug; these drugs are designed to alter sodium ion excretion patterns. Nevertheless, potassium excretion is altered by some of these agents, and the effects on some patients may be detrimental. Potassium ion may be reabsorbed in the ascending limb of Henle's loop. Secretion of potassium occurs in the distal convoluted tubule, where the ion is exchanged for sodium ion (see Figure 16-1).

Water Sites

The kidney is the primary site for maintenance of water balance. Water may be recovered from the tubule by diffusion in the proximal convoluted tubule and in the descending limb of Henle's loop. The ascending limb of Henle's loop and the distal convoluted tubule are relatively impermeable to water. Final urine concentration is achieved in the collecting duct. Removal of water at this site is regulated by antidiuretic hormone (ADH), which increases permeability of the tissue to water and thereby increases water retention.

Bicarbonate Sites

Bicarbonate, which is the main buffer for the blood, freely enters tubular fluid from the glomerulus and must be recovered for the body to maintain proper acid-base balance. Reabsorption of bicarbonate occurs in the proximal convoluted tubule. Reabsorption of bicarbonate, which is indirect, involves the action of the enzyme carbonic anhydrase. Carbonic anhydrase converts hydrogen ion and bicarbonate ion in the tubular fluid to carbon dioxide and water. Carbon dioxide can freely pass into the tubular epithelial cell and is reabsorbed, whereas bicarbonate ion stays in the tubule. The reabsorbed carbon dioxide is quickly reconverted to bicarbonate within the kidney cell and may reenter the bloodstream.

$$H^+ + HCO_3^- \rightleftharpoons CO_2 + H_2O$$

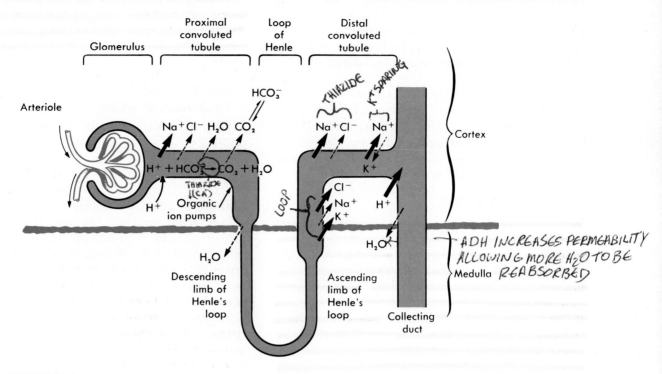

FIGURE 16-1

Sites of secretion and reabsorption of salt and water in nephron. Active (energy-requiring) processes are designated by bold arrows; passive diffusion is designated by broken arrows.

Table 16-1 Diuretic Effects on Tubular Transport

Drug	Excretion increased					Excretion blocked		
Loop diuretics	Na^+	H_2O	K^+	Cl^-	—	Uric acid	Li^+	—
Thiazides and related drugs	Na^+	H_2O	K^+	Cl^-	HCO_3^-	Uric acid	Li^+	—
Potassium-sparing diuretics	Na^+	H_2O	—	—	HCO_3^-	—	—	K^+, H^+
Carbonic anhydrase inhibitors	Na^+	H_2O	K^+	—	HCO_3^-	Uric acid	—	—
Osmotic diuretics	(Na^+)†	H_2O	(K^+)†	(Cl^-)†	—	—	—	—

*Li^+, Lithium ion; H^+, hydrogen ion.
†Large doses.
NOTE: The effects on ion transport shown are those commonly observed in humans during chronic therapy with normal clinical doses. With prolonged therapy, those ions whose excretion is increased may become depleted from the body, whereas those whose excretion is blocked may accumulate. Lithium ion accumulation is clinically important only for those patients receiving lithium carbonate therapy for mania. Uric acid accumulation is usually important only for those patients predisposed to gout.

Organic Ion Pumps

The kidney can rapidly secrete complex ions such as amino acids and other natural compounds. This secretion occurs near the proximal convoluted tubule in the cortical portion of the descending limb of Henle's loop. Many drugs, including several diuretics, enter tubular fluid by this mechanism, which is referred to as an *organic ion pump*. Since some di-uretics work only from within the tubule, the action of the drug depends at least in part on the proper function of the organic ion pump.

Mechanism of Diuretic Action

The diuretics considered in this chapter achieve their effects by increasing sodium ion excretion. Since water tends to follow sodium ion in the kidney, it is excreted when sodium ion is excreted. Several distinct mechanisms for increasing sodium ion excretion exist, and all may be understood in terms of the renal physiology just discussed. Specific mechanisms with the individual drugs are summarized in Table 16-1.

Clinical Uses of Diuretics

Diuretics are widely used, not only for their effects on kidneys but also for other actions in the body. For example, these drugs are used to treat hypertension (see Chapter 15). The range of clinical uses of diuretics is summarized in Table 16-2.

LOOP DIURETICS

Ethacrynic acid, furosemide, and bumetanide are called **loop diuretics** because the primary site of their diuretic action is in Henle's loop. These drugs (Table 16-3) inhibit the active reabsorption of chloride ion in the ascending limb of Henle's loop. Since chloride ion reabsorption is prevented, the passive reabsorption of sodium ion is also blocked. Therefore sodium chloride is retained in the tubule and excreted in the urine, carrying body water with it. Although ordinarily 99.4% of the sodium ion entering the tubule is reabsorbed, under the influence of loop diuretics only 70% to 80% of the sodium ion is reabsorbed, along with an equivalent amount of chloride ion. Potassium ion is also excreted in higher than normal amounts in response to these drugs (see Table 16-1). The loop diuretics are the most potent diuretics known. Their rapid, powerful action must be carefully monitored to avoid profound dehydration and salt depletion. Since loop diuretics promote the loss of excess salt and body water, they can control

edematous states, such as those occurring in congestive heart failure, renal disease, cirrhosis of the liver, lymphedema, nephrotic syndrome, and ascites associated with cirrhosis or malignancies (see Table 16-2).

Ethacrynic Acid
Mechanism of action

Ethacrynic acid has all the actions of the loop diuretics.

Absorption, distribution, and excretion

Ethacrynic acid is well absorbed from the gastrointestinal (GI) tract, producing a diuretic effect within 1 hr of administration. The drug is also appropriate for intravenous (IV) administration, producing diuresis within 2 to 10 min of administration. Ethacrynic acid should not be given by intramuscular (IM) or subcutaneous injection, since the drug can cause severe pain and irritation at the injection site.

Ethacrynic acid is bound to proteins in the bloodstream and in the protein-bound form is not available for glomerular filtration. The drug is secreted into the tubule by the organic anion pump in the descending limb of Henle's loop (cortical portion). The effectiveness of ethacrynic acid depends on its ability to enter the tubule, since diuresis is produced from within the tubule. About two thirds of the normal dose of ethacrynic acid is excreted by the kidney, the remainder being eliminated by the liver. In the kidney, ethacrynic acid exists primarily as the free drug and as a complex with cysteine. The cysteine-ethacrynic acid complex is much more effective than the free drug.

Table 16-2   Clinical Uses of Diuretics

Conditions responding to diuretics	Loop diuretics	Thiazides and related compounds	Potassium-sparing diuretics	Carbonic anhydrase inhibitors	Osmotic diuretics
Essential hypertension	+	+	+		
Edema caused by congestive heart failure, renal disease, or cirrhosis of liver	+	+	+		
Pulmonary edema	+				
Diabetes insipidus		+			
Acute mountain sickness				+	
Open-angle glaucoma				+	
Excessive intraocular pressure				+	+
Brain edema					+

Table 16-3 Loop Diuretics

Generic name	Trade name	Administration/dosage	Diuretic effect		
			Onset	Peak	Duration
Bumetanide	Bumex	ORAL: *Adults*—1 mg each morning; if needed, a second dose may be given 6 to 8 hr later. Usual daily doses are less than 4 mg, except in severe renal failure, when doses may reach 15 mg daily. FDA Pregnancy Category C.	30 min	1 to 2 hr	4 to 6 hr
		INTRAVENOUS: *Adults*—initially 0.5 to 1 mg to relieve pulmonary edema; repeat dose in 20 min if necessary.	5 to 10 min	15 to 20 min	3 to 4 hr
Ethacrynic acid	Edecrin*	ORAL: *Adults*—50 to 100 mg initially; thereafter 50 to 200 mg daily. FDA Pregnancy Category B. *Children*—25 mg initially, increasing by 25 mg to maintain.	30 min	1 to 2 hr	6 to 8 hr
		INTRAVENOUS: *Adults*—50 mg. Not recommended for children by this route.	5 to 10 min	15 to 20 min	1 to 3 hr
Furosemide	Lasix* Myrosemide Novosemide† Uritol†	ORAL: *Adults*—20 to 80 mg once or twice daily. FDA Pregnancy Category C. *Children*—2 mg/kg initially, increasing by 1 or 2 mg/kg after 6 to 8 hr; maximum dose, 6 mg/kg.	30 to 60 min	1 to 2 hr	6 to 8 hr
		INTRAVENOUS: *Adults*—20 to 40 mg once or twice daily. *Children*—1 mg/kg initially, increasing by 1 mg/kg after 2 hr; maximum dose 6 mg/kg.	5 to 10 min	15 to 20 min	1 to 3 hr

*Available in Canada and United States.
†Available in Canada only.

Toxicity

The most likely toxic reaction to ethacrynic acid is an excess of the action for which the drug is prescribed. Ethacrynic acid is so potent that excessive salt and water loss can occur quickly. Dehydration with reduction in blood volume can precipitate circulatory collapse. Vascular thromboses and emboli may be generated, especially in elderly patients (see box). Electrolyte depletion, marked by weakness or lethargy, dizziness, leg cramps, anorexia, vomiting, and possibly mental confusion, may occur gradually.

Orthostatic hypotension may occur. Patients who tend to rise quickly from a sitting or lying position need to learn to move slowly to allow accommodation of blood pressure (see box on p. 234). The most serious danger is risk of injury from falls.

Ethacrynic acid increases the loss of potassium and calcium ions, as well as sodium and chloride ions. Excessive potassium loss impairs proper functioning

---

GERIATRIC CONSIDERATION: DIURETICS

THE PROBLEM

Elderly patients are often more sensitive to the effects of diuretic drugs than are other adult patients. For example, loop diuretics and thiazides can cause excessive hypotension and severe electrolyte imbalances. Potassium sparing diuretics more often cause hyperkalemia in the elderly than in others.

SOLUTIONS

◆ Dosages of these drugs for the elderly may be lower than for other adults.
◆ Blood pressure should be carefully monitored.
◆ Precautions should be taken against orthostatic hypotension.
◆ Electrolyte balance should be carefully monitored.
◆ Dietary counseling may be required to maintain potassium balance.

DIETARY CONSIDERATION: POTASSIUM SOURCES

Some drugs, especially the loop and thiazide diuretics, steroids, and amphotericin B, cause excessive loss of potassium, resulting in hypokalemia (low blood potassium levels). In mild cases, hypokalemia may go unnoticed but in severe cases may contribute to toxicity from other drugs, as well as cardiac toxicity. Good dietary sources of potassium include:

◆ Citrus fruits and juices
◆ Bananas
◆ Grape, cranberry, apple, pear, and apricot juices
◆ Cereals
◆ Leafy vegetables
◆ Meat, fish, and fowl
◆ Salt substitutes (read label)
◆ Coffee, tea, and cola beverages
◆ Nuts and peanut butter

Some sources of potassium may be contraindicated in persons who must also limit sodium intake. Licorice can cause potassium excretion and should be avoided by patients experiencing hypokalemia.

---

of the heart, skeletal muscle, kidneys, and other organs. Many physicians routinely prescribe a potassium replacement for their patients receiving ethacrynic acid for prolonged periods (see box). Loss of calcium may rarely be sufficient to produce tetany. Most patients do not require calcium replacement, but serum calcium levels should be observed periodically.

Uric acid excretion is partially blocked by ethacrynic acid (see Table 16-1). Therefore in susceptible patients gout may develop. For most patients the increase in serum uric acid produces no symptoms.

Ethacrynic acid has caused GI disturbances in a few patients, especially those receiving the drug continually for several months. A sudden severe, watery diarrhea indicates the drug should be withdrawn. The physician may discontinue the drug permanently if these symptoms arise.

Ethacrynic acid affects ion transport in several body organs other than the kidneys. Altered sodium and potassium transport may be associated with toxicity to certain cells in the inner ear. Transient or permanent deafness has been observed in patients receiving ethacrynic acid, especially those who receive high doses or those who have reduced renal function in whom the drug accumulates.

Drug interactions

The potassium-depleting effect of ethacrynic acid makes this drug dangerous for patients receiving digitalis. Lowered potassium content in the tissue predisposes the heart to toxicity from the cardiac glycosides, which may include fatal arrhythmias. Corticosteroids are also potassium-depleting agents and may add to the danger of electrolyte imbalance when given with ethacrynic acid.

Ethacrynic acid lowers the renal clearance of lithium, a drug used to control manic cycles in manic-depressive psychosis (see Table 16-1). Under these conditions, lithium may accumulate and severe toxicity may occur. These drugs are ordinarily not given together.

Ethacrynic acid has an antihypertensive action that may be additive with that of other antihypertensive agents. Care is required to prevent excessive hypotension when these drugs are used together.

The ototoxic effect of ethacrynic acid may be potentiated by aminoglycoside antibiotics (see Chapter 33), which are also ototoxic. This combination should be avoided, since permanent deafness may result. Ethacrynic acid is strongly bound to serum proteins and may therefore displace other drugs from protein-binding sites. This action increases the concentration of the free, active form of the displaced drug. The anticoagulant warfarin is displaced in this manner by ethacrynic acid. Higher concentrations of unbound warfarin produce greater anticoagulant effects and may produce toxicity.

Furosemide

Mechanism of action

Furosemide has all the actions of the loop diuretics. At high doses, furosemide may occasionally increase bicarbonate excretion, whereas other loop diuretics have little direct effect on such excretion. Furosemide is the loop diuretic most likely to be included in therapy to control hypertension; it is used alone or with other antihypertensive agents.

Absorption, distribution, and excretion

Furosemide is well absorbed from the GI tract, producing diuresis within 1 hr. Diuresis occurs within minutes of an IV dose. Furosemide can also be administered intramuscularly.

A significant portion of furosemide in the bloodstream is bound to protein. Free drug is filtered in the glomerulus; furosemide also enters the tubular fluid by the organic anion pump. As with ethacrynic acid, it is only the drug within the tubule that is active in producing diuresis. About two thirds of an ingested dose of furosemide passes through the kidney, with most of the remainder excreted in the feces. A small amount is metabolized.

Toxicity

Furosemide can produce the same acute dehydration, orthostatic hypotension, salt depletion, and potassium depletion as ethacrynic acid. Calcium loss and uric acid accumulation also occur with furosemide.

Various types of dermatitis and occasional blood dyscrasias have been reported. The brisk diuresis produced by furosemide may be associated with urinary bladder spasm, thirst, perspiration, muscle cramps, weakness, or dizziness. It also impairs glucose tolerance in some patients, and rarely the drug has precipitated diabetes mellitus. GI effects and ototoxicity are less common with furosemide than with ethacrynic acid. Furosemide may produce allergic interstitial nephritis that can result in reversible renal failure. Lupus erythematosus may be activated by furosemide.

Drug interactions

Furosemide causes potassium depletion to the same extent as ethacrynic acid, so it should be used with great care in patients receiving digitalis or potassium-depleting steroids. Furosemide, like ethacrynic acid, blocks lithium excretion and may lead to toxic lithium accumulation. Its potential for ototoxicity may be increased by aminoglycoside antibiotics or other ototoxic drugs.

Furosemide may potentiate tubocurarine, which can lead to muscular and respiratory paralysis. The drug is usually discontinued a few days before surgery, if possible.

Furosemide and salicylates are secreted by the organic anion pump. Since this pump system has limited capacity, furosemide may block salicylate excretion. If patients receiving high doses of salicylates for rheumatoid diseases are also given furosemide, salicylates may accumulate and cause salicylate toxicity.

Bumetanide

Mechanism of action

Bumetanide is similar to furosemide in inhibiting the active reabsorption of chloride ions in the ascending limb of Henle's loop. Bumetanide is much more potent than other loop diruetics. For example, 1 mg of bumetanide given orally is as effective as approximately 40 mg of furosemide. Like the other loop diuretics, bumetanide controls edematous states caused by various medical conditions (see Table 16-2).

Absorption, distribution, and excretion

Bumetanide is completely absorbed after oral administration. The pharmacokinetics of bumetanide and furosemide are similar (see Table 16-3). In the bloodstream, bumetanide is almost completely bound to plasma protein. The drug is eliminated by renal mechanisms and by other routes. In renal failure the half-life of bumetanide is unchanged, which suggests that these alternative routes of elimination may be highly effective.

Toxicity

Because of its potent diuretic action, bumetanide can cause acute dehydration, orthostatic hypotension, salt depletion, and potassium depletion like the other loop diuretics. Azotemia, high uric acid concentration in the blood, and impaired glucose tolerance can also occur.

Ototoxicity, blood dyscrasia, GI distress, and rashes are all possible reactions to bumetanide. Large doses may cause severe muscle pain (myalgia) in patients in renal failure.

Drug interactions

Bumetanide can interact similarly to furosemide. In addition, indomethacin reduces the diuretic action of bumetanide. Since bumetanide is a relatively new drug, more interactions may become evident as additional clinical experience is gained.

Thiazide Diuretics
Mechanism of action

Thiazide diuretics have multiple effects on the nephron. These diuretics block sodium and chloride ion reabsorption in the distal convoluted tubule. This action leads to increased excretion of sodium chloride and body water and establishes a new state of salt and water balance in which there is a lower level of body sodium than before the drug was given. Thiazide diuretics also inhibit carbonic anhydrase in the proximal convoluted tubule, thereby elevating the excretion of bicarbonate ion and an additional increment of sodium ion. This effect is lost after a few days. Potassium excretion is also enhanced by the thiazide diuretics, but this effect is not required for diuresis and is usually considered a toxic side effect.

Thiazide diuretics are less potent than ethacrynic acid or furosemide and are more suitable for use in outpatients. The drugs can control edema associated with heart or kidney disease, as well as that caused by corticosteroid or estrogen therapy. The use of thiazide diuretics in controlling hypertension is discussed in Chapter 15.

Absorption, distribution, and excretion

Thiazide diuretics are well absorbed from the GI tract and may take action in the kidney within 1 hr of ingestion. Peak diuretic action can occur from 2 to 6 hr or more after the oral dose, depending on which thiazide preparation is used. Various preparations differ in timing and duration of diuretic effects (Table 16-4). In general, the longer-acting thiazide diuretics

Table 16-4 Thiazide Diuretics and Agents with Similar Mechanisms

Generic name	Trade name	Administration/dosage	Diuretic effect		
			Onset	Peak	Duration
THIAZIDE DIURETICS					
Bendroflumethiazide	Naturetin*	ORAL: *Adults*—initially, 5 mg once daily; maintenance, 2.5 to 15 mg once daily or less frequently. *Children*—maximum dosage 0.4 mg/kg daily in 2 doses; reduce dose for maintenance.	1 to 2 hr	6 to 12 hr	18 to 24 hr
Benzthiazide	Exna Hydrex	ORAL: *Adults*—50 to 200 mg; once daily for low doses, divide doses over 100 mg daily. FDA Pregnancy Category B. *Children*—1 to 4 mg/kg daily in 3 doses initially; dose reduced for maintenance.	2 hr	4 to 6 hr	12 to 18 hr
Chlorothiazide	Diuril	ORAL: *Adults*—0.5 to 1 gm once or twice daily. FDA Pregnancy Category B. *Children*—22 mg/kg daily in 2 doses. *Infants*—under 6 months, 10 to 20 mg/kg daily in 2 divided doses.	2 hr	4 hr	6 to 12 hr
Chlorothiazide sodium	Diuril (sodium)	INTRAVENOUS: *Adults*—500 mg twice daily	15 min	30 min	6 to 12 hr
Cyclothiazide	Anhydron	ORAL: *Adults*—1 to 2 mg once daily; maintenance 1 mg 2 to 4 times weekly. FDA Pregnancy Category C. *Children*—initially, 0.02 to 0.04 mg/kg daily, reduce dose for maintenance.	6 hr	7 to 12 hr	18 to 24 hr
Hydrochlorothiazide	Diuchlor-H† Esidrix HydroDIURIL* Novohydrazide† Oretic Urozide†	ORAL: *Adults*—initially, 25 to 200 mg once or twice daily; maintenance, 25 to 100 mg daily or less frequently. FDA Pregnancy Category B. *Children*—1 to 2 mg/kg daily in 2 doses. *Infants*—under 6 months, up to 3 mg/kg daily.	2 hr	4 hr	6 to 12 hr
Hydroflumethiazide	Diucardin Saluron	ORAL: *Adults*—50 to 200 mg; once daily for low doses; divided doses over 100 mg daily. FDA Pregnancy Category D. *Children*—1 mg/kg daily; adjust as needed for maintenance	1 to 2 hr	3 to 4 hr	18 to 24 hr
Methyclothiazide	Aquatensen Duretic† Enduron	ORAL: *Adults*—2.5 to 10 mg once daily. FDA Pregnancy Category C. *Children*—0.05 to 0.2 mg/kg daily.	2 hr	6 hr	24 hr
Polythiazide	Renese	ORAL: *Adults*—1 to 4 mg once daily; maintenance, 0.5 to 8 mg daily, according to response. *Children*—0.02 to 0.08 mg/kg daily.	2 hr	6 hr	36 hr

*Available in Canada and United States.
†Available in Canada only.

Table 16-4   Thiazide Diuretics and Agents with Similar Mechanisms—cont'd

Generic name	Trade name	Administration/dosage	Diuretic effect		
			Onset	Peak	Duration
Trichlormethiazide	Metahydrin Naqua Trichlorex	ORAL: *Adults*—1 to 4 mg once daily. FDA Pregnancy Category B. *Children*—0.07 mg/kg daily in single or divided dose.	2 hr	6 hr	24 hr
NONTHIAZIDE DIURETICS WITH THIAZIDE-LIKE MECHANISMS					
Chlorthalidone	Hygroton* Novothalidone† Thalitone	ORAL: *Adults*—25 to 100 mg after breakfast daily or less frequently. FDA Pregnancy Category B. *Children*—2 mg/kg once daily for 3 days per week.	2 hr	2 hr	24 to 72 hr
Indapamide	Lozide† Lozol	ORAL: *Adults*—2.5 mg/day taken in the morning; may be increased after few days to 5 mg/day. FDA Pregnancy Category B.	1 to 2 hr	2.3 to 3.5 hr	24 to 72 hr
Metolazone	Diulo Mykrox Zaroxolyn*	ORAL: *Adults*—5 to 20 mg once daily for extended tablets. For Prompt Metolazone tablets, dose is 0.5 mg once daily. FDA Pregnancy Category B.	1 hr	2 hr	12 to 24 hr
Quinethazone	Hydromox	ORAL: *Adults*—50 to 100 mg once daily, or 150 to 200 mg alternate days or 3 times weekly.	2 hr	6 hr	18 to 24 hr

*Available in Canada and United States.
†Available in Canada only.

are highly bound to serum proteins. Their long duration of action is related to their slow elimination from these protein-binding sites.

Thiazide diuretics remain primarily in the extracellular water in the body except for the drug concentrated in the kidneys. Thiazides are secreted into the renal tubule by the organic anion pump. Most of the dose leaves the body by this route. Some drug is eliminated by the liver, which secretes these drugs into the bile.

Chlorothiazide may be administered intravenously. The onset of action is somewhat more rapid by this route, but the duration of effect is not greatly altered from that of oral doses. This preparation must never be administered intramuscularly or subcutaneously. Great care should be taken to prevent leakage of the drug into the tissues when it is given intravenously.

Toxicity

Long-term administration of thiazide diuretics can lead to fluid and electrolyte imbalance, which may produce thirst, weakness, lethargy, restlessness, muscle cramps, and fatigue. The electrolyte imbalance most likely to occur is excessive potassium and chloride ion loss. The loss of these ions leads to metabolic alkalosis. Potassium supplements may be required to remedy this situation. Chloride loss alone is usually mild and does not need to be treated.

Calcium excretion is blocked by thiazide diuretics, and increased serum calcium levels may result. The parathyroid glands may also be affected by long-term therapy with these diuretics. Uric acid excretion is also blocked, and the increased blood levels may precipitate an attack of gout in susceptible individuals.

Thiazide diuretics irritate the GI tract and may cause side effects ranging from simple nausea and vomiting to constipation, jaundice, and pancreatitis.

Thiazides affect the central nervous system (CNS). Mild symptoms include dizziness, headache, and paresthesia. At high concentrations such as those found in drug overdose, mental lethargy may progress to coma, although heart function and respiration are not markedly depressed.

Blood dyscrasias and allergic reactions have been observed. Although urticaria or other mild forms of allergy are more common, severe serum sickness and anaphylactic reactions have been noted.

Thiazides cause hypotension by a mechanism apparently unrelated to their action as diuretics. Some patients suffer orthostatic hypotension when receiving these drugs. Thiazides occasionally lower glomerular filtration rate when given intravenously. This does not affect most patients, although a patient with already reduced renal function may be adversely affected.

Drug interactions

Since thiazide diuretics have intrinsic hypotensive activity, they may potentiate the action of other antihypertensive agents, especially those that act at ganglionic or peripheral adrenergic sites (see Chapter 15). Thiazide diuretics are commonly included in fixed combinations that are marketed primarily for use as antihypertensives. Examples of some of these fixed combinations are listed in Table 16-5.

Potassium loss is enhanced when thiazide diuretics are given with corticosteroids or adrenocorticotropic hormone (ACTH). Hypokalemia may render the patient more sensitive to digitalis toxicity.

Thiazides may increase the response to tubocurarine, a muscle relaxant commonly used in surgery. Carefully observe patients receiving both of these drugs for signs of excessive tubocurarine activity.

Thiazide diuretics frequently alter the requirement for insulin or other hypoglycemic agents. A diabetic patient who must receive one of the thiazides should be carefully observed during the first few days of thiazide therapy to prevent loss of diabetes control.

Lithium excretion is blocked by thiazides and other diuretics. The increased danger of lithium toxicity prevents the safe concurrent use of these drugs.

Potassium-Sparing Diuretics

Mechanism of action

Potassium-sparing diuretics (Table 16-6) inhibit the pump mechanism that normally exchanges potassium for sodium in the distal convoluted tubule (Figure 16-1). This pump is controlled by mineralocorticoid hormones, such as aldosterone, which increase sodium retention and promote potassium loss. Aldosterone is present in greater than normal amounts in edematous states resulting from congestive heart failure, nephrotic syndrome, and hepatic cirrhosis.

Spironolactone competitively blocks the action of aldosterone in the sodium-potassium exchange pump, thereby causing sodium to remain in the tubule and to be excreted. Potassium is not pumped into the tubule, so it is not excreted.

Triamterene produces the same effects as spironolactone but by a direct mechanism that does not depend on aldosterone. Spironolactone is most effective when the aldosterone level is elevated, whereas the more rapidly and directly acting triamterene is effective at any level of aldosterone.

Amiloride, the newest of the potassium-sparing diuretics, acts in the same way as triamterene.

Since the sodium-potassium pump in the distal convoluted tubule is ordinarily responsible for reabsorbing only a small fraction of the sodium from the tubule, blockage of this pump increases sodium excretion only slightly. This limits the effectiveness of the potassium-sparing diuretics.

Spironolactone controls edema in congestive heart failure, cirrhosis of the liver, and nephrotic syndrome. Spironolactone may ameliorate the effects of excessive aldosterone levels in patients suffering from the endocrine disorder hyperaldosteronism. It may also be useful in treating hypertension and reversing potassium loss. Triamterene is used in many of the same situations as spironolactone. Amiloride has uses similar to those of the other potassium-sparing diuretics. If amiloride is used in long-term therapy, less sodium excretion and less potassium retention are observed than with other drugs of this class. Amiloride also corrects metabolic alkalosis more effectively than spironolactone or triamterene.

Absorption, distribution, and excretion

Spironolactone is a steroid derivative related in structure to natural mineralocorticoids (see Chapter 51). Spironolactone is not highly water soluble but is formulated using very fine particles to improve absorption from the GI tract. Peak therapeutic effects with spironolactone are observed several days after treatment begins (Table 16-6). This delay is related to the mechanism of action of the drug and is not a result of delay in absorption or other pharmacokinetic properties of the drug.

Spironolactone is extensively metabolized much the same as the natural steroids it chemically resembles. Metabolites of spironolactone appear in urine and in lesser quantities in bile.

Triamterene, although not a steroid like spironolactone, is also relatively insoluble in water. Intestinal absorption is somewhat variable but usually satisfactory. Most of the orally administered dose appears in the urine within 24 hr. The drug enters the renal tubule by glomerular filtration and tubular secretion. Unlike spironolactone, the peak effect of this drug is observed within hours of an oral dose.

Amiloride is excreted primarily by the kidneys. About 60% of an oral dose is recovered unchanged in the urine within 48 hr of administration. Absorption of the drug is impaired if it is taken with food.

Table 16-5   Fixed Combinations That Include a Thiazide

Components	Trade names
THIAZIDE WITH POTASSIUM-SPARING DIURETICS	
Hydrochlorothiazide + amiloride	Moduretic
Hydrochlorothiazide + spironolactone	Aldactazide, Spirozide
Hydrochlorothiazide + triamterene	Dyazide, Maxzide
THIAZIDE WITH ACE INHIBITOR	
Hydrochlorothiazide + captopril	Capozide
Hydrochlorothiazide + enalapril	Vaseretic
Hydrochlorothiazide + lisinopril	Prinzide, Zestoretic
THIAZIDE WITH ALPHA BLOCKER	
Polythiazide + prazosin	Minizide
THIAZIDE WITH BETA BLOCKER	
Bendroflumethiazide + nadolol	Corzide
Chlorthalidone + atenolol	Tenoretic
Hydrochlorothiazide + labetalol	Normozide, Trandate HCT
Hydrochlorothiazide + metoprolol	Lopressor HCT
Hydrochlorothiazide + pindolol	Viskazide
Hydrochlorothiazide + propranolol	Inderide
Hydrochlorothiazide + timolol	Timolide
THIAZIDE WITH CENTRALLY ACTING ANTIHYPERTENSIVE	
Chlorthalidone + clonidine	Combipres
Chlorothiazide + methyldopa	Aldoclor
Hydrochlorothiazide + methyldopa	Aldoril
THIAZIDE WITH RAUWOLFIA	
Hydrochlorothiazide + reserpine	Hydropres, Mallopres
Polythiazide + reserpine	Renese-R
Trichlormethiazide + reserpine	Metatensin, Naquival
THIAZIDE WITH VASODILATOR	
Hydrochlorothiazide + hydralazine	Apresazide, Aprozide
THIAZIDE WITH RAUWOLFIA AND VASODILATOR	
Hydrochlorothiazide + reserpine + hydralazine	Ser-Ap-Ex, Unipres

Includes many commonly used fixed combinations but does not include every available combination.

Table 16-6 Potassium-Sparing Diuretics

Generic name	Trade name	Administration/dosage	Diuretic effect		
			Onset	Peak	Duration
Amiloride	Midamor*	ORAL: *Adults*—5 to 10 mg daily as a single dose. FDA Pregnancy Category B.	Effects similar to triamterene		
Spironolactone	Aldactone* Novospiroton†	ORAL: *Adults*—25 to 200 mg daily in divided doses. *Children*—3.3 mg/kg daily in divided doses.	Effects build over period of days		
Triamterene	Dyrenium*	ORAL: *Adults*—25 to 100 mg daily with meals; do not exceed 300 mg daily. FDA Pregnancy Category B. *Children*—2 to 4 mg/kg daily in divided doses.	2 to 4 hr (maximal effect not seen for several days)	6 hr	7 to 9 hr

*Available in Canada and United States.
†Available in Canada only.

Toxicity

Spironolactone, triamterene, and amiloride may cause serum potassium levels to increase dangerously. Patients with impaired renal function or excessively high potassium intake are especially at risk. Fatal cardiac arrhythmias may result.

Spironolactone can cause various endocrine alterations, since the drug chemically resembles not only mineralocorticoids but also androgens and progestins. Women may observe menstrual irregularities, hirsutism, and deepening of the voice. Men may observe gynecomastia (breast development) and have difficulty in achieving or maintaining erection. Symptoms in both sexes are usually reversed when the drug is discontinued.

Spironolactone produces tumors in rats exposed to the drug for long periods. It should be restricted to cases in which the benefit clearly outweighs this risk. Spironolactone should not be used to control edema in pregnancy. If the drug is used in lactating women, breast-feeding should be discontinued, since metabolites appear in breast milk.

Triamterene and amiloride may produce a reversible azotemia revealed by an increased BUN level. Skin rashes, GI disturbances and fever have been observed in patients receiving spironolactone, triamterene, or amiloride.

Drug interactions

Two potassium-sparing diuretics should not be administered concurrently, nor should these drugs be administered to a patient receiving potassium supplements or ingesting a diet high in potassium.

Use of the potassium-sparing diuretics with anti-

hypertensive agents may require reduction in doses of the latter drugs, since spironolactone, triamterene, and amiloride may have additive antihypertensive effects with these agents.

When spironolactone is combined with other diuretics, dosages may have to be reduced. It can prevent distal tubular reabsorption of sodium, making diuretics that act upstream of this site in the nephron even more effective. Amiloride given in fixed combination with hydrochlorothiazide is not as effective in preventing hypokalemia as are spironolactone and triamterene.

Spironolactone reduces vascular responsiveness to norepinephrine. This effect may impair maintenance of normal blood pressure in patients under local or general anesthesia.

Carbonic Anhydrase Inhibitors

Mechanism of action

Diuretics that inhibit carbonic anhydrase in the kidney prevent the secretion of hydrogen ion into the renal tubule and the reabsorption of carbon dioxide from the renal tubule (Table 16-7). As a result, the excretion of bicarbonate is rapidly increased and the urine becomes alkaline. **Carbonic anhydrase inhibitors** have diuretic action because sodium ion accompanies the excreted bicarbonate. However, bicarbonate excretion is much greater than sodium ion excretion, and these drugs are classified as weak diuretics. Moderate amounts of potassium, phosphate, and chloride ion are also lost in the urine. When carbonic anhydrase inhibitors are given over long periods, metabolic acidosis may occur. Since metabolic acidosis prevents the action of these diuretics, they are not suitable for long-term continuous administration as diuretics.

Table 16-7   Carbonic Anhydrase Inhibitors

Generic name	Trade name	Administration/dosage	Clinical effect		
			Onset	Peak	Duration
Acetazolamide	Acetazolam† Diamox*	ORAL, INTRAVENOUS: *Adults*—250 to 375 mg once daily; alternate day therapy may be used	About 1 hr (oral) IV: 2 min	2 to 4 hr (oral) IV: 15 min	6 to 12 hr (oral) IV: 4 to 5 hr
Dichlorphen-amide	Daranide	ORAL: *Adults*—initially 100 to 200 mg, then 100 mg every 12 hr until desired effect achieved; maintenance, 25 to 50 mg 1 to 3 times daily.	0.5 to 1 hr	2 to 4 hr	6 to 12 hr
Methazolamide	Neptazane*	ORAL: *Adults*—25 to 100 mg 2 or 3 times daily.	2 to 4 hr	6 to 8 hr	10 to 18 hr

*Available in Canada and United States.
†Available in Canada only.

Carbonic anhydrase inhibitors are primarily used to treat glaucoma, congestive heart failure, and convulsive disorders.

Absorption, distribution, and excretion

Many carbonic anhydrase inhibitors are chemically related to the sulfonamide antibiotics. These drugs are well absorbed from the GI tract. The most widely used drug of this class, acetazolamide, has a plasma half-life of about 2 hr and is concentrated in the kidneys. Tissue levels in the kidneys may be 2 to 3 times the plasma concentration within 30 min to 2 hr of an oral dose. Acetazolamide enters the tubule by the organic anion pump. The drug also inhibits carbonic anhydrase in other tissues.

Acetazolamide and other carbonic anhydrase inhibitors are sometimes given on alternate days rather than continuously (see Table 16-6). This therapy is designed to prevent the kidney from becoming resistant to the action of the drug (e.g., to prevent metabolic acidosis). During the day without the drug, the carbonic anhydrase inhibitors are cleared from the body and kidney function returns to its predrug condition. When the drug is readministered on the following day, it is as effective as when first given.

Toxicity

Reactions to these drugs are not very common, especially when they are used in intermittent or short-term therapy. These sulfonamide derivatives are capable of causing blood dyscrasias, fever, and rash. Drug precipitation in the urine has occurred, causing the formation of stones.

These drugs have direct actions on the CNS. Paresthesia, nervousness, sedation, lassitude, depression, headaches, vertigo, and other symptoms have been reported. The conditions of patients already suffering from respiratory acidosis may worsen from these drugs, which tend to produce metabolic acidosis.

Drug interactions

Acetazolamide and other carbonic anhydrase inhibitors produce more marked potassium excretion than sodium excretion. Potassium depletion is therefore likely to occur. This possibility is made even more likely by corticosteroids or ACTH given concomitantly. Digitalis toxicity is increased in the presence of low serum potassium levels.

Osmotic Diuretics

Osmotic diuretics are nonelectrolytes that are filtered by the glomerulus but not significantly reabsorbed or metabolized. Therefore osmotic diuretics enter the renal tubule and are highly concentrated in renal tubular fluid. The high osmolality in the tubule reduces reabsorption of water, which increases urine production. At high doses, some increase in sodium excretion is produced, but this is not observed in most clinical circumstances. These drugs are therefore exceptions to the generalization that sodium excretion precedes water excretion during diuretic therapy.

Osmotic diuresis may be used clinically to prevent permanent damage during acute renal failure. The usefulness of osmotic diuresis in these cases frequently depends on maintaining adequate urine volume without altering electrolyte balance. Osmotic diuretics also increase the osmolality of the plasma, which allows reduction of osmotic pressure inside the eye and in the cerebrospinal fluid.

The agents currently used as osmotic diuretics, mannitol and urea, are usually administered intravenously. Mannitol is the preferred agent.

Toxicity produced by these agents depends on how much drug is administered and how much the drug affects fluid balance. These drugs are retained within the extracellular space and can cause an acute expansion of extracellular fluid volume during IV administration. This volume expansion may be hazardous to a patient with reduced cardiac reserve.

Fluid and electrolyte imbalances may develop, especially if a degree of renal impairment exists. Under these circumstances the diuretics tend to accumulate in the blood and may cause dangerous shifts in salt and water balance. Pulmonary congestion, acidosis, thirst, blurred vision, convulsion, nausea and vomiting, diarrhea, tachycardia, fever, and anginalike pain may be noted occasionally. Local irritation with thrombophlebitis can also occur. Urea should not be used in a patient with liver failure, since the high levels of urea may place additional demands on liver function.

NURSING IMPLICATIONS SUMMARY

General Guidelines

◆ Carefully measure and record fluid intake and output. Report unexpected findings to the physician. For example, oliguria (scanty urine output) or anuria (no urine output) are unexpected after an increase in a diuretic dose. Patients at home are not usually required to measure intake and output, except in the case of severe kidney or heart disease, but encourage such patients to report abnormal output.

◆ Weigh patients in the acute care setting at least daily. Weigh patients under standard conditions (e.g., at the same time [usually in the morning], after patients have voided or catheter bags are emptied, but before breakfast). Use the same scale each day, and have patients wear the same amount of clothing. If appropriate to their ability and resources, teach patients at home how to keep daily or weekly weight records. Instruct patients to report to the physician weight gains or losses greater than 2 lb/day, or 5 lb/week, unless otherwise instructed by the physician.

◆ Monitor the blood pressure regularly. Although all patients receiving diuretic therapy would be expected to experience an initial drop in blood pressure, the elderly, those receiving IV diuretics, and those also taking antihypertensives may experience a precipitous fall in blood pressure and in rare instances may go into shock. Other drugs that can cause hypotension, and can thus potentiate hypotension in patients receiving diuretics, include CNS depressants, barbiturates, narcotics, and antihypertensives. Initially, monitor the blood pressure with the patient in the sitting and lying positions, and compare the measurements from each arm.

Review with the patient the symptoms of orthostatic hypotension (see box on p. 234).

◆ Caution patients to avoid the use of alcohol because it enhances hypotension.

◆ To monitor for fluid retention, measure abdominal girth or circumference of one or both legs. To ensure accurate measurement, mark the patient's skin with small ink marks to indicate the correct placement of the tape measure from day to day.

◆ Check dependent areas daily for the presence of or change in the amount of pitting edema. In pitting edema, an indentation or depressed area made by the examiner's finger remains visible in the skin for seconds to minutes after the pressure has been released. Dependent areas where this is more likely to occur include the sacral area and the feet and legs.

◆ Observe patients for symptoms of dehydration, including thirst, decreased skin turgor, nausea, lightheadedness, weakness, increased pulse, oliguria, decreased blood pressure, and elevated hemoglobin, hematocrit, and BUN levels.

◆ Assess patients for electrolyte abnormalities, and monitor the serum levels of potassium, sodium, calcium, magnesium, and bicarbonate. The signs and symptoms of common electrolyte abnormalities are summarized in Table 17-1.

◆ Teach patients the importance of taking potassium supplements, if prescribed, and work with them to find a preparation they are willing to take (see Chapter 17). Many effervescent preparations are unpalatable. Enteric-coated tablets have been implicated in small bowel ulceration. Oral solutions are the preferred form of therapy, but they are often unpleasant tasting. Dilute these solutions in

NURSING IMPLICATIONS SUMMARY—cont'd

juice or milk to reduce the risk of gastric irritation and to make the taste tolerable. Instruct patients to take potassium with meals to reduce gastric irritation. Encourage hypokalemic patients to increase dietary intake of potassium-rich foods (see box on p. 252).

◆ Caution patients taking diuretics not to switch to salt substitutes without first consulting the physician. Salt substitutes contain a variety of electrolyte salts, and the exact proportions vary from product to product. A patient may inadvertently contribute to electrolyte abnormalities by using a salt substitute. For example, a patient taking a potassium-sparing diuretic may develop hyperkalemia if a salt substitute containing a high portion of potassium salts is used.

◆ Refer patients as needed to the dietitian for instruction about special dietary restrictions, which may include sodium, calories, cholesterol, and other factors.

◆ Teach patients about their need for diuretic therapy, and review the anticipated side effects of the prescribed drugs. Poor compliance may stem from patient annoyance caused by frequent and excessive urination. Instruct patients to take diuretics ordered once a day in the morning and twice-daily diuretics in the morning and afternoon to avoid interrupting sleep to urinate.

◆ Dehydration and hypovolemia can contribute to thromboembolic disorders. Assess the patient for pain in the chest, calves, and pelvis that might indicate thromboembolism.

◆ For some patients, intermittent therapy will achieve the desired effects with fewer side effects.

◆ Teach patients to take diuretics as ordered. If a dose is missed, it should be taken as soon as remembered, unless within a few hours of the next dose (this varies with the frequency of the dosing schedule), in which case it should be omitted and the regular dosing schedule resumed. Tell patients not to double up for missed doses.

◆ Thirst is often a frequent side effect. Review Patient Problem: Dry Mouth on p. 166.

Loop Diuretics

Drug administration

◆ Review general guidelines for patients receiving diuretics. Assess patients for development of hyponatremia, hypocalcemia, hypokalemia, and hypochloremic alkalosis (see Table 17-1).

Monitor serum electrolyte levels. Monitor blood glucose levels because these drugs may cause hyperglycemia.

◆ Review drug interactions and counsel patients as appropriate.

◆ Assess patients receiving warfarin and loop diuretics for signs of excessive anticoagulation (see Chapter 20).

◆ Monitor serum uric acid levels and assess patients for signs of gout.

◆ Assess patients for signs of ototoxicity, which include tinnitus (ringing in the ears), reduced hearing acuity, and vertigo.

◆ Question patients about allergy to sulfonamides before administering first doses. Observe for allergic response, including development of rashes.

INTRAVENOUS BUMETANIDE

◆ Bumetanide is usually given undiluted but may be mixed with 5% dextrose in water, 0.9% sodium chloride, and lactated Ringer's solution.

◆ Administer dose over 1 to 2 min. After IV administration, monitor blood pressure every 15 to 30 min until stable, keep siderails up, and supervise ambulation.

INTRAVENOUS ETHACRYNIC ACID

◆ Ethacrynic acid may be given undiluted, or 50 mg may be diluted in 50 ml of 5% dextrose in water or 0.9% sodium chloride. Do not mix with other drugs. Do not administer if solution is discolored or contains particulate matter. Administer at a rate of 10 mg or less over 1 min, or infuse total dose over 30 min. Check infusion site carefully; thrombophlebitis is common, and extravasation causes pain and tissue irritation. After IV administration, monitor blood pressure every 15 to 30 min until stable, keep siderails up, and supervise ambulation.

FUROSEMIDE

◆ Furosemide may be given undiluted or added to 5% dextrose in water or normal saline. Inspect the solution before administering, and do not use it if it is yellow. Do not mix furosemide with other drugs.

◆ Administer at a rate of 20 mg 1 to 2 min. After IV administration, monitor blood pressure every 15 to 30 min until stable, keep siderails up, and supervise ambulation.

Continued.

NURSING IMPLICATIONS SUMMARY—cont'd

INTRAMUSCULAR FUROSEMIDE

◆ IM injection of furosemide may cause transient pain at the injection site.

Patient and family education

◆ See general guidelines for patients receiving diuretics.

◆ Potassium supplements are often prescribed concomitantly. As noted in the general guidelines, emphasize the importance of taking these as prescribed, refer to the dietitian as needed, and review good dietary sources of potassium. Teach patients that diarrhea, vomiting, and anorexia (loss of appetite), if prolonged or severe, may also cause hypokalemia and should be reported to the physician. Caution patients also taking a cardiac glycoside to be especially careful to avoid hypokalemia. Review other drug interactions with the patient, as appropriate.

◆ Caution diabetic patients to monitor blood glucose levels carefully, since hyperglycemia may occur, requiring an adjustment in diet or dose of insulin.

◆ Instruct patients to report signs of agranulocytosis (depressed production of white blood cells), including unexplained fever, chills, sore throat, or enlarged lymph nodes. This is a rare but serious side effect of drug therapy. See Patient Problem: Depressed White Blood Cell Production on p. 560.

◆ Instruct patients to take oral preparations with meals or just after eating to reduce gastric irritation. Warn patients in renal failure that bumetanide may cause myalgia. Tell patients to report skin changes, rashes, photosensitivity, nausea, vomiting, or any unexpected sign or symptom. See Patient Problem: Photosensitivity on p. 629.

Thiazide Diuretics

Drug administration

◆ See the general guidelines for diuretics therapy. Thiazides may cause hypokalemia, hypochloremia, alkalosis, hyponatremia, and hypomagnesemia. Monitor patients for these electrolyte abnormalities, and monitor serum electrolyte levels (see Table 17-1).

◆ Monitor patient's blood glucose levels because these drugs may cause hyperglycemia.

Review drug interactions and counsel patients as appropriate.

◆ Monitor serum uric acid levels and assess for signs of gout.

◆ Monitor the serum BUN levels and lipid levels.

PARENTERAL CHLOROTHIAZIDE

◆ Dilute each vial (0.5 gm) with at least 18 ml of sterile water. Dilute further if desired with 5% dextrose in water or sodium chloride injection. Do not mix with other drugs or blood products. Administer at a rate of 0.5 gm or less over 5 min.

◆ Check insertion site and avoid extravasation as the drug is extremely alkaline. Do not administer intramuscularly or subcutaneously. Thiazides can cause a paradoxical antidiuretic effect in patients who have diabetes insipidus (see Chapter 50).

Patient and family education

◆ See general guidelines for diuretic therapy. Potassium supplements may be prescribed, but patients may be able to prevent hypokalemia by increasing their daily dietary intake of potassium-rich foods (see box on p. 252). If potassium supplements are prescribed, emphasize the importance of taking these as prescribed. Instruct patients that diarrhea, vomiting, and anorexia, if prolonged or severe, can also cause hypokalemia and should be reported to the physician. Concomitant administration of adrenal corticosteroids may also predispose the patient to hypokalemia.

◆ Caution diabetic patients to monitor blood glucose levels carefully, as hyperglycemia may occur, requiring an adjustment in diet or insulin dosage. Instruct patients to take oral doses with meals to reduce gastric irritation.

Potassium-Sparing Diuretics

Drug administration

◆ See general guidelines for diuretic therapy. Potassium-sparing diuretics may cause hyperkalemia or hyponatremia. Assess patients for these electrolyte imbalances and monitor serum electrolyte levels (see Table 17-1).

◆ Many combination products are available containing both a potassium-depleting diuretic and a potassium-sparing diuretic. The combination is designed to promote diuresis while maintaining normal serum potassium levels. Patients receiving combination drugs are potentially at risk for side effects due to any of the component drugs (see Table 16-5). Instruct patients to report the development of any unexpected sign or symptom.

◆ Monitor blood glucose and BUN levels.

Patient and family education

◆ Instruct diabetic patients to monitor blood glucose levels, since these drugs may produce hyperglycemia.

◆ Patients should take doses with meals or a snack to reduce gastric irritation. Spironolactone tablets may be crushed and mixed in syrup or fluid of the patient's choice. The triamterene capsule may be opened and the contents mixed with food or fluid for patients who have difficulty swallowing.

◆ If patients have been switched to a potassium-sparing diuretic or if a potassium-sparing diuretic is prescribed in addition to a potassium-depleting diuretic, impress on patients the need to omit previous potassium supplements that may have been ordered; consult the physician. In addition, the patient should limit intake of potassium-rich foods (see box on p. 252).

◆ Instruct patients to avoid salt substitutes that contain potassium while taking potassium-sparing diuretics.

◆ Caution patients taking triamterene that photosensitivity may develop; (see box on p. 629).

Carbonic Anhydrase Inhibitors

Drug administration

◆ Review general guidelines for diuretic therapy.

◆ Monitor serum electrolyte levels and assess patients for electrolyte abnormalities, especially metabolic acidosis (see Table 17-1). Intermittent therapy may be used to limit the development of acidosis.

◆ Read physician's orders carefully; tablets and extended-release capsules are available. Review drug interactions and counsel patients as appropriate.

◆ Monitor serum uric acid and blood glucose levels.

◆ Monitor patients for signs of kidney stone formation such as renal colic (severe flank pain), hematuria (blood in the urine), and oliguria.

INTRAVENOUS ACETAZOLAMIDE

◆ Dilute each 500 mg of acetazolamide with at least 5 ml of sterile water for injection, and administer at a rate of 500 mg over at least 1 min. The drug may be further diluted with standard IV fluids and administered over 4 to 8 hr. Avoid IM injection, since it is very painful.

Patient and family education

◆ Review guidelines for diuretic therapy.

◆ Instruct diabetic patients to monitor blood glucose levels; a change in diet or insulin dose may be needed. Review expected effects and possible side effects. Instruct patients to report any unexpected sign or symptom. Instruct patients to avoid driving or operating hazardous equipment if drowsiness, dizziness, lightheadedness, or visual changes occur; notify the physician.

◆ A metallic taste in the mouth may occur. Sucking sugarless hard candy, chewing sugarless gum, brushing the teeth or rinsing the mouth frequently may help.

◆ Photosensitivity may occur (see box on p. 629)

Osmotic Diuretics

Drug administration and patient and family education

◆ See general guidelines for diuretic therapy.

◆ Monitor serum electrolyte levels and assess for electrolyte abnormalities (see Table 17-1). Assess patients for signs of circulatory overload. Monitor vital signs for blood pressure, intake and output, and daily weight. Assess breath and heart sounds. Monitor patients for signs of pulmonary congestion or congestive heart failure, including dyspnea, labored respiration, tachypnea, tachycardia, distended neck veins, rales, agitation, fluid retention, and weight gain.

◆ These drugs are often administered to patients with increased intracranial pressure. Assess level of consciousness and monitor indicators of cerebral function, including blood

NURSING IMPLICATIONS SUMMARY—cont'd

pressure, pulse, intracranial pressure, and Glasgow coma scale or institutional equivalent.

◆ Determine with physician the desired daily fluid balance. Infusion rate may be titrated to output. Diuresis may be copious, especially intitially; a urinary catheter may be needed. If the urine output falls below 30 to 50 ml/hr, notify the physician.

◆ Oral fluids may not be permitted. Occasional ice chips may be permitted to help relieve thirst.

◆ If extravasation occurs, osmotic diuretics cause local skin and tissue damage. Before instituting infusion, ascertain that the IV line is secure and patent, with no signs of redness or infiltration, and that the rate of flow is not sluggish. Inspect infusion site regularly. If infiltration is suspected, discontinue infusion and restart in another site.

INTRAVENOUS MANNITOL

◆ Read physician's order carefully. Mannitol is available in several concentrations. Do not confuse mannitol with mannitol hexanitrate, an antianginal drug. It is not necessary to dilute mannitol. Check ampule or bottle for crystallization, a common problem. If crystals are present, warm the container under running water until crystals dissolve. Let cool to body temperature before administering. Use an in-line IV filter for 15%, 20%, and 25% solutions. Do not add to other IV solutions, medications, or blood products. The rate of administration is usually 1 to 2 gm/kg over 30 to 90 min but is variable.

INTRAVENOUS UREA

◆ Urea must be diluted to make a 30% solution (30% solution equals 30 gm of urea/100 ml or 300 mg/ml). Dilute with 5% or 10% dextrose in water or with 10% invert sugar in water; some manufacturers supply the diluent. Patients with hereditary fructose intolerance (aldolase deficiency) may have a severe reaction to the invert sugar solution if it is used as a diluent. Symptoms include hypoglycemia, nausea, vomiting, tremors, coma, and convulsions. Infuse at a rate of 4 ml/min (1200 mg/min) or slower. Use only fresh solutions, and discard any unused portions. Do not mix with blood or other drugs in the same syringe.

◆ These drugs are rarely used outside of the acute-care setting; keep patient and family informed of the patient's condition.

CHAPTER REVIEW

◆ KEY TERMS

◆ REVIEW QUESTIONS

1. What is the nephron?
2. What is the function of the glomerulus?
3. Where is sodium reabsorbed from the renal tubule?
4. What is the mechanism by which bicarbonate ion is recovered from the tubular fluid? Where does this occur?
5. What is the general mechanism by which all diuretics act?
6. What is the specific mechanism of action of loop diuretics?

7. What toxicity is characteristic of ethacrynic acid?

8. What toxicity is characteristic of furosemide?

9. How does bumetanide differ from the other loop diuretics?

10. What is the specific mechanism of action of thiazide diuretics?

11. What toxicity is characteristic of thiazide diuretics?

12. What is the specific mechanism of action of the potassium-sparing diuretics?

13. What toxicity is associated with the potassium-sparing diuretics?

14. How are carbonic anhydrase inhibitors used clinically?

15. What toxicity is characteristic of carbonic anhydrase inhibitors?

16. What reactions occur with the osmotic diuretics?

17. Develop a nursing care plan for a patient receiving one of the diuretics discussed in this chapter. How can you assess the drug's effectiveness? About what drug interactions should you instruct the patient?

SUGGESTED READING

Gahart BL: *Intravenous medications,* St Louis, 1992, Mosby–Year Book.

Horne MM, Swearingen PL: *Pocket guide to fluids and electrolytes,* St Louis, 1989, Mosby–Year Book.

Karb VB: Electrolyte abnormalities and drugs which commonly cause them, *J Neurosci Nurs* 21(2):125, 1989.

Moser M: Controversies in the management of hypertension: diuretic use in the 1990s, *Physician Assist* 14(5):81, 1990.

Stanley R: Drug therapy of heart failure, *J Cardiovasc Nurs* 4(3):17, 1990.

Todd B: Diuretics danger, *Geriatr Nurs* 10(4):212, 1989.

Weinberger MH: Diuretics and their side effects. II. Dilemma in treatment of hypertension, *Hypertension* 2(2):16, 1988.

CHAPTER 17

Fluids and Electrolytes

LEARNING OBJECTIVES

After studying this chapter, you should be able to do the following:

- Explain what forces control the movement of water between body compartments.
- Describe causes and signs of dehydration, and suggest fluids to reverse dehydration.
- Describe causes and signs of fluid excess, and suggest ways to control it.
- Describe appropriate nursing actions in response to common problems encountered with IV fluids.

CHAPTER OVERVIEW

- Fluids and electrolyte solutions are used to re-establish proper salt and water balance. Since these solutions are used to return the body to homeostasis, they may be thought of as drugs. This chapter reviews the general classes of fluids and solutions that are commonly used in clinical practice. Although a full discussion of the clinical indications for these solutions is outside the scope of a pharmacology text, the most important physiologic and clinical factors in the use of these solutions are covered.

Nursing Process Overview

FLUIDS AND ELECTROLYTES

Assessment

Observe patients for edema, especially in dependent areas; check skin turgor; auscultate breath and heart sounds; and monitor the vital signs, weight, and fluid intake and output. Observe patients for specific electrolyte level imbalances. Observe for signs of nutritional deficiency, remembering that weight and intake measures alone are poor indicators. Monitor appropriate laboratory values, including serum electrolyte, blood urea nitrogen (BUN), and blood gas levels. If the patient is receiving IV fluids or nutrition, observe the administration setup, starting at the level of the patient. Check the insertion site; observe for signs of infiltration or infection; and check the placement and patency of the tubing, the rate of flow, and the amount of fluid remaining.

Nursing Diagnoses

Fluid volume excess related to malnutrition as manifested by edema and low protein levels

High risk for hypervolemia

High risk for infection related to long-term total parenteral nutrition (TPN)

Management

The decision to initiate, terminate, or change the fluid and electrolyte therapy depends on the ongoing and cumulative data base gathered during assessment. Keep the patient informed about the goals of therapy. Enlist the help of the patient and family in monitoring the IV line, and encourage them to report any unexpected subjective or objective finding. Continue to monitor the parameters identified above. Observe patients for the desired and undesired effects of therapy. Label all IV fluids and medications carefully, monitor their rate of flow and their effects, and record carefully.

Evaluation

Therapy with fluids and electrolytes is effective if desired goals have been achieved without harmful consequences to the patient. If the patient is being switched to an oral electrolyte replacement, review with the patient and family how the medication is administered, work with the patient to find an acceptable dosage form, review the need to continue the medication as desired, review side effects, and discuss situations that should cause the patient to call the physician or nurse (e.g., signs of electrolyte overload). Teach the patient to measure fluid intake and output or weight at home. If the patient is to continue hyperalimentation at home, instruct the patient and family about the desired goals of therapy, and review the technical tasks associated with the therapy (how to care for the insertion site, how to change the bottle, and what to do if the infusion line fails to function). Refer patients to social service and a visiting nurse agency as needed.

REGULATION OF SALT AND WATER BALANCE

Fluid Compartments

Water comprises 60% of the weight of an average person. Although water passes easily through most tissues, certain physical and permeability barriers allow the body to be divided into compartments in which water content may be independently regulated. For example, a 70-kg person would contain 42 L of water, of which 28 L are inside cells (Figure 17-1). This water, along with its dissolved solutes, is called *intracellular fluid.* The *interstitial fluid* bathes the outside of the cell and allows it to excrete waste products and receive nutrients. Plasma constitutes an important separate fluid compartment similar to interstitial fluid, but it is more accessible to manipulation and testing. Extracellular fluid primarily includes interstitial fluid and plasma but also other fluids such as lymph and cerebrospinal fluid.

Composition of Body Fluids

The fluid compartments in the body differ in the concentration of important ions and other solutes. In plasma the major solute is sodium chloride (Figure 17-2). The primary buffers maintaining the pH of blood at 7.4 are bicarbonate (HCO_3^-, 27 mEq/L) and protein (16 mEq/L). Interstitial fluid is similar to plasma except that the protein content is much reduced.

Inside the cell, high concentrations of protein and potassium are found, but the sodium ion concentration is much lower. The major buffer for the intracellular fluid is phosphate, shown in Figure 17-2 as PO_4^{-3} but actually present as a mixture of HPO_3^{-2} and $H_2PO_3^{-1}$. Magnesium ion, an important component of critical enzyme systems, is also a significant constituent of intracellular fluid.

Movement of Fluid and Electrolytes between Compartments

Water moves freely through the vascular walls separating plasma from interstitial fluid and through the cell membranes separating intracellular fluid from interstitial fluid. Movement of ions and other solutes is rigidly controlled so that optimum concentration differences are maintained between the compartments. The concentrations of these solutes influence the disposition of water among the compartments. To understand the distribution of water and the var-

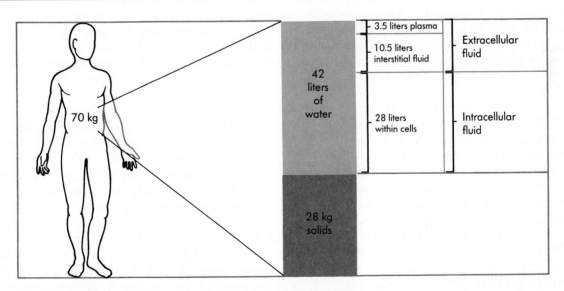

FIGURE 17-1

Distribution of water in males. In females, about 50% of body weight is found as water, but proportion of intracellular to extracellular fluid is the same as for males.

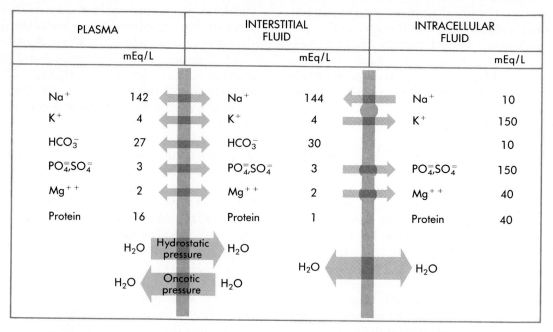

	PLASMA			INTERSTITIAL FLUID			INTRACELLULAR FLUID	
	mEq/L			mEq/L			mEq/L	
Na^+	142		Na^+	144		Na^+	10	
K^+	4		K^+	4		K^+	150	
HCO_3^-	27		HCO_3^-	30			10	
$PO_4^=,SO_4^=$	3		$PO_4^=,SO_4^=$	3		$PO_4^=,SO_4^=$	150	
Mg^{++}	2		Mg^{++}	2		Mg^{++}	40	
Protein	16		Protein	1		Protein	40	

FIGURE 17-2

Movement of water and solutes between body compartments. Double-headed arrows represent simple diffusion; straight arrows represent pressure-regulated processes. Arrows passing through or in contact with circles represent active transport of solutes.

ious solutes, certain concepts from chemistry and physiology must be recalled.

Osmosis describes the movement of water across a semipermeable membrane (a membrane that selectively limits the passage of some chemicals). For example a cell membrane is semipermeable. The direction of movement is determined by the concentration of solutes in the water on either side of the membrane. Water moves toward the solution having the higher concentration. Osmosis reduces the difference in concentration of the solutions on either side of a semipermeable membrane.

The movement of water by osmosis across semipermeable membranes creates osmotic pressure. For example, if a sugar solution is enclosed in a synthetic membrane that allows water but not sugar to pass through the membrane and the sealed sac is submerged in pure water, two things will happen. Water will enter the sac at a greater rate than it leaves the sac. As water enters the solution-filled sac, pressure inside the sac increases and opposes the entry of more water. The pressure required to completely prevent the net movement of water into the sac is a measure of the osmotic pressure of the solution.

The osmotic properties of a solution relate to the concentration of solute, but the number of particles (ions, atoms, or molecules) is important, not the mass of the solute. For example, a 0.5 molar solution of

glucose contains 90 gm/L of glucose and has a potential osmotic pressure of 9650 mm Hg. In contrast, a 0.5 molar solution of sodium chloride contains 29 gm/L of sodium chloride and has a potential osmotic pressure of 19,300 mm Hg. The greater potential osmotic pressure of the sodium chloride solution results from the ionization of sodium chloride to release two particles for every molecule of salt, a sodium ion and a chloride ion. Glucose does not ionize, and each molecule of the sugar remains a single particle.

Osmolarity of the extracellular fluid is determined mainly by the concentration of sodium chloride. Solutions that have the same osmolarity as plasma are called *isotonic*. Isotonic solutions include 5% dextrose and 0.9% sodium chloride solutions. Hypertonic solutions have an osmolarity above that of plasma (>310 milliosmoles/L); hypotonic solutions have lower osmolarity than plasma.

Oncotic pressure regulates the movement of water between the plasma and the interstitial fluid. This pressure is generated by the difference in protein concentration between plasma and interstitial fluid. Although most solutes in plasma pass freely through the pores of the vascular walls that separate plasma from interstitial fluid, proteins cannot leave plasma by that route. Since proteins act like any other solute to cause the movement of water, movement of water from interstitial fluid toward plasma is promoted.

Without a balancing force, oncotic pressure tends to dilute the protein in plasma and increase pressure in the plasma compartment. Oncotic pressure is balanced by **hydrostatic pressure** generated by the force of contraction of the heart. In the arteriolar vasculature where blood pressure is highest, hydrostatic pressure predominates over oncotic pressure. In the arteriolar side of the capillaries, water, along with dissolved nutrients and other solutes, moves from the plasma into the interstitial fluid, where it is available to the cells. Pressure on the venous side of the capillaries is lower. This lower venous pressure is not sufficient to fully block the movement of water. Therefore oncotic pressure is the predominant regulator on the venous side of the capillaries and allows water and solutes, including waste products, to move back into the plasma compartment.

Diffusion describes the movement of solutes across semipermeable membranes. The direction of movement is toward the less concentrated solution. As with osmosis the process lowers the difference in concentration between the two solutions. Free diffusion of most ions and solutes takes place between plasma and interstitial fluid, but the cell membrane is not normally permeable to most solutes found in extracellular fluid. Sensitive control of uptake and release of solutes is maintained by active transport systems on the cell membrane. For example, the high intracellular concentration of potassium is maintained by the action of Na^+, K^+-ATPase, an active transport system that hydrolyzes a molecule of ATP to exchange three sodium ions for two potassium ions. Other active transport systems maintain the high intracellular concentrations of phosphate and magnesium ion.

CLINICAL INDICATIONS FOR FLUID THERAPY
Loss of Extracellular Fluid Volume

Several clinical conditions can cause water and solutes to be lost from the extracellular fluid compartment. For example, sudden hemorrhage, prolonged vomiting, excessive diarrhea, or plasma loss through large areas of burned skin may cause fluid and salt loss, but the fluid remaining in the extracellular compartment may for a time stay essentially normal in composition. If the fluid loss is excessive and uncompensated, the patient may enter hypovolemic shock, in which the blood volume becomes so depleted that organ perfusion is compromised. The symptoms of this condition include lowered blood pressure, increased heart rate, rapid respiration, restlessness, pale and clammy skin, and decreased urine output. Without adequate perfusion, the kidneys may fail completely. Hypovolemic shock is potentially life threatening and requires rapid replacement of fluid and electrolytes to restore the proper distribution of volume throughout the body.

In certain conditions, extracellular fluid volume may be decreased primarily by water loss. For example, patients who fail to take in adequate water may suffer dehydration. This condition is common in elderly persons who may have inefficient thirst centers in the brain. Unconscious patients lose between 1000 and 1700 ml of water in insensible perspiration, breath, and urine each day; this water must be replaced daily to avoid dehydration. In certain circumstances, violent, watery diarrhea and high-volume renal failure may cause loss of water in excess of salt loss (see box). All these circumstances may require replacement of lost volume and restoration of the proper proportion of solutes in the extracellular fluid.

PEDIATRIC CONSIDERATION: DIARRHEA IN INFANTS

THE PROBLEM

In most cases, diarrhea is mild and self-limiting, but infants and young children may be thrown into dangerous states of dehydration and electrolyte imbalance if diarrhea is severe or prolonged. Hypotension and coma can arise when fluid losses equal 5% of body weight; losses of 10% can cause shock, and death ensues at higher losses.

ASSOCIATED OR CONTRIBUTING FACTORS

In underdeveloped nations, diarrhea is a significant cause of mortality in infants and children, with death resulting from dehydration and electrolyte imbalance. Poor sanitation may expose children and adults to infectious agents that cause diarrhea. Even if the diarrhea is caused by bacterial contamination of food or water, treatment is often successful if salt and water balance are maintained. IV replacement of fluids is expensive, unavailable to many people, and unnecessary in the majority of cases. Aggressive oral replacement with properly balanced solutions is first-line treatment.

SOLUTIONS

◆ Oral rehydration therapy (ORT) should begin early in the course of the disease
◆ In the United States, preparations are available under the trade names Lytren, Pedialyte, Rehydralyte, and Resol
◆ In Canada, Lytren and Pedialyte are available
◆ In other countries, the World Health Organization (WHO) Diarrheal Disease Control Program supplies ORS-bicarbonate or ORS-citrate in premeasured packets that are mixed with 1L of potable water before use

Fluid deficiency requiring therapy is associated with weight loss in excess of 5% of normal body weight, dry lips and eyes, decreased blood pressure, and depressed central nervous system (CNS) activity. Skin turgor is also diminished.

Fluid Excess

In certain conditions, extracellular fluid volume is expanded to a degree that may impair cardiovascular functioning, in part by increasing venous pressure. Fluid excess may arise from conditions impairing the body's ability to eliminate fluid such as heart failure or renal impairment. Alternatively, fluid excess can arise from the improper administration of IV fluids. The main route for elimination of excess fluid is through the kidneys. Treatment aims to prevent further overload and, if necessary, to assist the kidney by pharmacologic means. For example, digitalis given to strengthen the contraction of the heart in heart failure improves perfusion of the kidneys and assists in mobilizing and eliminating excess fluid. Diuretics also enhance urine production.

Signs of fluid excess include swelling and edema, bounding pulse, distension of the jugular vein, difficult or noisy breathing, and warm, moist skin.

Electrolyte Imbalances

The proper concentrations of ions and solutes in the extracellular compartment can be disrupted by diseases or medical interventions. (Table 17-1).

Sodium ion

Sodium is the major ion determining the osmolarity of the plasma and interstitial fluid. **Hypernatremia** (excessive sodium ion concentration in the plasma) can arise when a patient loses water but retains salt. Alternatively, hypernatremia may arise when excessive sodium has been administered with fluids or medications. In hypernatremia, water moves from the cells into the extracellular fluid in an attempt to reduce the sodium ion concentration and restore equal osmolarity between the fluid compartments. **Hyponatremia** (plasma sodium concentrations less than 130 mEq/L) arises most commonly in patients who are losing water and electrolytes but are receiving water without adequate electrolyte replacement. In an extreme case, this condition is called *water intoxication*. The low sodium ion concentration of the extracellular fluid causes water to move into the cells in an attempt to restore equal osmolarity between the two compartments.

Potassium ion

Hyperkalemia (excessive potassium ion concentration in the plasma) causes less osmotic disturbance than a sodium ion imbalance, but potassium ion imbalances can be life threatening because cardiac function may be impaired. Potassium-induced cardiac dysfunction appears in the electrocardiogram (ECG) as depressed ST segments, widened QRS complexes, and peaked T waves. Hyperkalemia may result from massive tissue injury when large numbers of cells die, releasing their high intracellular concentrations of potassium into the extracellular fluid. Renal failure may also cause retention of potassium, as may the potassium-sparing diuretics discussed in Chapter 16. **Hypokalemia** (low potassium ion concentration in the plasma) can result from the use of diuretics such as

Table 17-1 Common Electrolyte Imbalances

Solute	Normal concentration in plasma	Signs of deficiency	Signs of excess
Sodium ion	136 to 145 mEq/L	Anorexia, nausea, vomiting; increased intracranial pressure; oliguria leading to anuria	Dry, sticky membranes; fever; weakness and disorientation; oliguria
Potassium ion	3.5 to 5.0 mEq/L	Muscle weakness; diminished tendon reflexes; paralytic ileus; cardiac arrhythmia	Nausea and vomiting; muscle weakness; changes in ECG
Bicarbonate ion	24 to 31 mEq/L (pH 7.35 to 7.45)	Metabolic acidosis (pH <7.35); weakness; deep, rapid breathing (Kussmaul); stupor or unconsciousness	Metabolic alkalosis (pH >7.45); hypertonicity of muscles; depressed respirations; tetany
Calcium ion	4.7 to 5.6 mEq/L	Tetany; prolonged QT interval on electrocardiogram (ECG)	Weakness, fatigue, thirst; nausea, anorexia; muscle cramping
Magnesium ion	1.3 to 2.3 mEq/L	Flushing, hypertension; neuromuscular irritability	Nausea, vomiting; diarrhea, colic

furosemide, ethacrynic acid, or the thiazides. Poor nutrition or poor gastrointestinal (GI) absorption may also result in hypokalemia. Vomiting depletes the body of potassium, along with fluid and other salts. Replacement of potassium is necessary to restore normal function, but the replacement should be spread out over several days to avoid excessive cardiac stress.

Hydrogen ion and bicarbonate ion

The balance of these ions regulates the pH of the plasma and interstitial fluid. An increase of hydrogen ion over bicarbonate ion lowers the pH of extracellular fluid, causing acidosis. An increase of bicarbonate ion over hydrogen ion causes a rise in pH of the extracellular fluid, or alkalosis. Acid-base imbalances arise from respiratory or metabolic causes. **Respiratory acidosis** arises when pulmonary ventilation is impaired. Without adequate ventilation, the carbon dioxide concentration in the blood rises. In the blood, carbon dioxide becomes carbonic acid, which lowers blood pH. Pneumonia, pulmonary obstructive disease, and depressed respiration can produce respiratory acidosis. Therapy is aimed at the underlying disease. **Metabolic acidosis** arises when excess acid is produced, as in diabetic acidosis, lactic acidosis, starvation, or certain types of poisoning.

Respiratory alkalosis can be induced by hyperventilation, through which excessive amounts of carbon dioxide are lost. **Metabolic alkalosis** arises when excess hydrogen ion is lost, as in prolonged vomiting or nasogastric suctioning. Respiratory alkalosis seldom requires IV therapy, but metabolic alkalosis may often be treated with isotonic saline. During metabolic alkalosis, bicarbonate excretion becomes limited by the progressive depletion of sodium. Administering isotonic saline allows the kidney to sacrifice the sodium required to accompany excreted bicarbonate. With this assistance the kidney usually reestablishes acid-base balance.

FLUID AND ELECTROLYTE SOLUTIONS

Hydrating Solutions

Conditions such as hemorrhage or shock, in which plasma volume is acutely reduced, require replacement of fluid as initial therapy. Replacement of lost fluid volume allows maintenance of kidney function, preventing further development of dangerous electrolyte imbalances. Perfusion of other vital organs is also maintained by this strategy.

Sodium chloride in water

Isotonic saline (Table 17-2) replaces extracellular fluid volume and treats sodium depletion and metabolic alkalosis. Dangers associated with its use include circulatory overload and hypernatremia. Metabolic acidosis may arise when excess chloride ion promotes bicarbonate ion loss in the kidney. Hypokalemia may arise as excess sodium ion forces potassium ion excretion by the kidney. Hypertonic saline solutions should be used in small volumes and administered carefully for the correction of severe hyponatremia (see also box on p. 273).

Ringer's solution and lactated Ringer's solution

These solutions are used to replace fluid, sodium, and other electrolytes (see Table 17-2). Often called *balanced* or *maintenance solutions,* these preparations are appropriate to replace volume if renal function is not seriously compromised. The potassium found in these solutions cannot be eliminated by the body and may accumulate to dangerous levels unless the kidney is functioning. For this reason, renal function must be established before these fluids are administered.

Ringer's solution is appropriate replacement therapy for patients who have lost fluid and electrolytes through the alimentary tract, for burn patients, for postoperative patients, and for patients with dehydration or sodium depletion. Lactated Ringer's solution is most appropriate for patients who, along with other electrolyte imbalances, have acidosis. The lactate in this solution, converted to bicarbonate by the liver, provides stronger basic cations in the blood than the simple inorganic salt solutions.

Dextrose in water

Dextrose, or glucose, in an isotonic solution (5%) is appropriate for most situations in which rehydration is needed. In addition to the fluid, the solution supplies about 170 cal/L or 560 KJ/L. Electrolytes are not supplied in this solution. Hypertonic glucose solutions are given slowly to avoid tissue damage. These hypertonic solutions may be used to shift fluid from the interstitial space into the plasma. Isotonic dextrose solutions may be infused through peripheral veins, but hypertonic dextrose solutions should be infused through a central vein to avoid excessive irritation.

Dextrose solutions may have other components added for infusion, but not all additives are compatible. For example, dextrose solutions are never used in the same IV line with whole blood because the sugar causes hemolysis (rupture of red blood cells). The pharmacist can provide information about compatibilities of IV fluids.

Solutions to Correct Specific Electrolyte Imbalances

Dextrose in saline may be used to hydrate patients and to replace sodium loss. Five percent dextrose in

Table 17-2 Parenteral Therapy Solutions

Solution	IV dosage	Comments
Calcium gluceptate (22%, or 0.9 mEq Ca^{++}/ml) or Calcium gluconate (10%, or 0.45 mEq Ca^{++}/ml)	Doses are individualized.	Calcium solutions may be used to resuscitate the heart, to treat hyperkalemia, to treat magnesium intoxication, or to replace calcium in patients receiving large volumes of citrated blood.
Dextrose in water (2.5%, 5%, 10%, 20%, 25%, 38%, 40%, 50%, 60%, 70%)	Isotonic (5%) 90 to 125 ml/hr is usual but may range much higher; doses of hypertonic solutions are individualized for specific purposes.	Isotonic dextrose (D5W) maintains or replaces fluid without altering electrolytes. Hypertonic dextrose is used to prevent brain damage caused by hypoglycemic shock or to supply extra calories (see Table 17-4).
Dextrose in saline (2.5%, 5%, or 10% dextrose in various combinations with 0.11%, 0.2%, 0.225%, 0.3%, 0.45%, or 0.9% NaCl)	Doses are adjusted as needed for specific fluid and electrolyte needs of patient.	Hypotonic solution (2.5% dextrose, 0.45% NaCl) drives fluid from plasma into interstitial space. Isotonic solutions supply calories and replenish salt and water.
Dextrose in saline with (5% dextrose with 0.2%, 0.225%, 0.33%, 0.45% or 0.9% NaCl and 0.075%, 0.15%, 0.224%, or 0.3% KCl)	Doses are adjusted as needed for specific fluid and electrolyte needs of patient.	Mixture replenishes salt and water when potassium replacement is also required. Dosage must be carefully monitored to avoid potassium overload, especially when renal function is compromised.
Dextrose with electrolytes (5% with Elecrolyte No. 48, No. 75, Ionosol, Isolyte, Normosol, Plasmalyte; 50% with Electrolytes pattern A, B, 1 or 2)	Refer to specific information supplied with each individual preparation.	Complex mixtures are used in special circumstances to correct massive electrolyte imbalances.
KCl in water (0.2, 0.3, 0.4, 1.5, 2, or 3 mEq/ml)	Solution must be diluted before use and administered at rates less than 10 to 15 mEq/hr for minimally depleted patients or up to 40 mEq/hr for severely depleted patients.	These solutions are strongly hypertonic (15% = 2000 mEq/L) as supplied and must be diluted before administration. Concentrations are commonly 40 to 60 mEq/L.
Lactated Ringer's solution (0.6% NaCl, 0.03% KCl, 0.02% $CaCl_2$, 0.31% Na lactate)	90 to 125 ml/hr is commonly used.	Balanced salt solution supplies, in mEq/L, these ions: Na^+ 130, K^+ 4, Ca^{++} 3.0, Cl^- 109. It is used to maintain or restore fluid and electrolyte balance, especially when mild acidosis is also present. A portion of the lactate present is converted to bicarbonate, which elevates blood pH.
Magnesium sulfate (10%, 12.5%, 50%)	10% solution should be infused at rates less than 1.5 ml/min. More concentrated solution is for IM administration.	Nearly isotonic solution (10%) is used to reverse severe magnesium deficiencies such as maintenance during TPN and to control convulsions of eclampsia.
NaCl in water (0.45%, 0.9%, 3.0%, 5.0%)	Isotonic (0.9%) and hypotonic (0.45%) solutions are infused at 90 to 125 ml/hr but may range much higher for initial therapy; 3% solution is infused up to 80 ml/hr and 5% solution up to 50 ml/hr.	Isotonic saline supplies 154 mEq/L of Na^+ and 154 mEqL of Cl^-. Used to replace sodium and water loss.
Ringer's solution (0.86% NaCl, 0.03% KCl, and 0.033% $CaCl_2$)	90 to 125 ml/hr is commonly used.	Balanced salt solution supplies, in mEqL, these ions: Na^+ 147, K^+ 4, Ca^{++} 4.5, Cl^- 156. It is used to maintain or restore fluid and electrolyte balance. Additional K^+ is required to correct severe potassium depletion.
Sodium bicarbonate in water (4.2%, 5%, 7.5%, 8.4%)	Doses are calculated to reverse acidosis (individualized for each patient)	Commercially available solutions are hypertonic and must be diluted before use. One liter of 1.4% $NaHCO_3$ contains 167 mEq/L of Na^+. This essentially isotonic solution is used to reverse metabolic acidosis.

PEDIATRIC CONSIDERATION: BENZYL ALCOHOL

THE PROBLEM
Benzyl alcohol is a bacteriostatic agent commonly used in solutions of sodium chloride and other drugs. Neonates are especially sensitive to this agent, and deaths have occurred when solutions containing benzyl alcohol were used in this age group.

SOLUTIONS
◆ Avoid administration of bacteriostatic saline (with benzyl alcohol) to newborns
◆ Do not dilute drug with bacteriostatic saline if the drug is to be used in newborns
◆ Do not flush newborns' IV lines with bacteriostatic saline

0.9% saline has about the same properties as normal saline.

Five percent dextrose in 0.45% saline may be used to shift fluid from plasma into the interstitial space, which may cause difficulty for patients with cardiac,

renal, or liver disease already suffering from edema and poor venous return.

Potassium chloride is often added to IV fluids to replace potassium lost from the GI tract or through the kidney. Replacement must be undertaken carefully to avoid causing hyperkalemia and its dangerous side effects. Dosage is calculated from a knowledge of approximate loss for the individual patient.

Magnesium sulfate is used to correct severe magnesium deficiencies. The 10% solution is nearly isotonic and may be used intravenously, but the 50% solution is strongly hypertonic and is used intramuscularly.

Plasma Expanders

In hemorrhage or hypovolemic shock, rapid filling of the plasma compartment may be a lifesaving measure. This volume replacement may be accomplished in several ways (Table 17-3), depending on the needs of the patient.

Whole blood can be used in patients who have lost more than 20% of their blood volume. Cross-matching to test for blood-group compatibility is required, although O-negative blood can be used until cross-

Table 17-3 Blood, Blood Components, and Blood Substitutes

Preparation	Dosage/administration	Comments
Whole blood	One unit = 450 ± 45 ml blood + 63 ml CPD (citrate-phosphate-dextrose) or CPDA-1 (citrate-phosphate-dextrose-adenine), administered intravenously through a 170 μm filter.	Whole blood is used to treat patients who have lost more than 20% of their blood volume. Whole blood acts as a volume expander and maintains oxygen transport.
Plasma	Monitored by clinical response to IV infusion.	Plasma is used as volume expander when oxygen transport is not seriously impaired.
Albumin, human (5%, 25%) (Albuminar, Buminate, Plasbumin)	Adjusted according to patient's need, but should be less than 250 gm/48 hr.	Albumin is used to expand plasma volume. Normal human serum albumin preparations contain significant amounts of Na^+, which may be dangerous for patients on sodium-restricted diets.
Plasma protein fraction (5%) (Plasmanate, Plasma Plex, Plasmatein, Protenate)	*Adults*—1 to 1.5 L of 5% solution infused at 5 to 8 ml/min, adjusted as necessary. *Children*—33 ml/kg infused at 5 to 10 ml/min to correct dehydration.	Plasma protein fraction is used to correct hypovolemic shock in adults, to correct dehydration in children, and to supply protein to patients with deficiencies. Human plasma protein fraction is 83% albumin, <17% globulin, and <1% gamma globulin.
Dextrans (Dextran 40, Dextran 70, Dextran 75)	Infusion rates may be rapid initially, but total daily dose should not exceed 20 ml/kg.	Dextran 40 (molecular weight 40,000) has effects that last 2 to 4 hr. Dextran 70 (molecular weight 70,000) and Dextran 75 (molecular weight 75,000) are cleared by kidney more slowly than Dextran 40; duration of action of these preparations is about 12 hr. They are used for shock.
Hetastarch (6% in 0.9% NaCl) (Hespan)	Rates of infusion for acute hemorrhagic shock are 20 ml/kg/hr or less.	Hetastarch is used as plasma volume expander in shock or hypovolemia.

matched blood is available. Whole blood replaces fluid, electrolytes, and oxygen-carrying capacity lost through hemorrhage. Before use, whole blood must be tested for evidence of viruses, including hepatitis and human immunodeficiency virus (HIV).

Plasma is a natural cell-free fluid that performs all the functions of whole blood except for oxygen transport. Cross-matching is not required.

Human albumin and plasma protein fractions expand plasma volume by increasing the plasma protein concentration. The resulting increase in plasma oncotic pressure causes water to move from the interstitial space into the plasma compartment. The albumin preparation contains appreciable amounts of sodium that may cause problems for certain patients with cardiovascular disease.

Dextran and hetastarch are complex carbohydrate molecules too large to pass out of the capillaries or vascular walls. Therefore these compounds are restricted to the vascular space. They generate osmotic forces that cause water to enter the blood vessels, thereby expanding plasma volume.

IV Hyperalimentation

Patients unable to take oral foods and fluids require maintenance with IV nutrients. Dextrose solutions supply some calories, but since only about 3 L of fluid can be administered daily without overloading the circulatory system, only about 500 calories can be supplied each day from isotonic dextrose solutions. For longer-term therapy, more calories from different sources are required. Total parenteral nutrition (TPN) is now possible using synthetic amino acids, dextrose, and fat emulsions (Table 17-4).

Hypertonic dextrose is required for TPN. Solutions for administration are prepared from 50% or 60% dextrose stock solutions, but as they are administered the concentration of dextrose is only 25% to 30%. This hypertonic solution must be administered via a large central vein, in which blood flow is sufficient to dilute the strong sugar solution and prevent tissue damage. A 10% dextrose solution is hypertonic but can be given peripherally without damage to veins.

Amino acids are used in TPN to prevent negative

Table 17-4   Fluids Used for Total Parenteral Nutrition

Solution	IV dosage	Comments
Hypertonic dextrose (50% or 70%)	This solution is diluted with water or amino acid solutions to about 12.5% before use. Longer term therapy may require 25% to 30% solutions. Minimum adult requirement for dextrose is about 150 gm daily. Initial infusion of 1000 to 1200 ml of 12.5% dextrose approximates that requirement; dosage can be gradually increased as needed to meet caloric requirements.	Solutions must be administered into central vein with sufficient blood flow to dilute sugar. Special care is taken to maintain aseptic conditions, since these catheters remain in use for prolonged periods. Infusion should be terminated gradually to avoid rebound hypoglycemia.
Crystalline amino acids (Aminosyn, BranchAmin, FreAmine, HepatAmine, NephrAmine, Novamine, ProcalAmine, RenAmin, Travasol, TrophAmine)	Solution may be given at about 1 gm/kg body weight per day, as needed to prevent protein breakdown and negative nitrogen balance. Solutions contain mixtures of essential and nonessential amino acids. TrophAmine and Aminosyn contain taurine, amino acid required by neonates.	3.5% solution is nearly isotonic, supplies 140 cal/L, and may be administered via peripheral vein. Various commercial amino acid solutions include appreciable amounts of sodium and other electrolytes.
Intralipid, Liposyn, Nutrilipid (10% or 20%)	Solution may be given by peripheral vein 1 ml/min for 10% or 0.5 ml/min for 20% over 30 min initially as needed to supply calories (20% contains 2000 cal/L) or to replace essential fatty acids. Children and infants require lower infusion rates. Lipids should supply no more than 60% of total calories. Dosage should not exceed 2.5 gm fat/kg body weight daily.	Soybean oil 10% or 20% is stabilized with egg yolk phospholipids with glycerol to adjust to isotonicity. Major fatty acids contained in these preparations are linoleic and oleic.
Liposyn (10% or 20%)	Same as Intralipid.	Safflower oil 10% or 20% is stabilized with egg phospholipids. This preparation contains more linoleic acid but much less linolenic acid than Intralipid.

nitrogen balance and breakdown of protein in the body. Pure amino acid solutions, rather than protein hydrolysates, are preferred. At 3.5% concentrations the amino acid solutions offer about 140 cal/L, and a variety of electrolytes. Extra potassium is often required by patients receiving amino acid solutions, since that element is depleted by amino acid metabolism.

Fat emulsions may be administered intravenously during TPN to prevent essential fatty acid deficiency. Since fats have a high caloric content, these preparations may supply a significant proportion (up to 60%) of the daily caloric requirement.

Vitamin and mineral supplements may need to be added to the TPN fluids. A variety of these preparations exist, allowing individual design of the nutrition program (see box).

DIETARY CONSIDERATION: VITAMINS

Vitamins are among the essential nutrients. If the patient's diet is varied and plentiful, vitamin deficiencies are rare. Digestive disorders and certain drugs can interfere with vitamin absorption. Good sources of major vitamins are listed in the following examples.

Vitamin A (retinol)

Liver, kidney, fish liver oils, cream, butter, whole milk, whole-milk cheese, fortified margarine, skin milk, skim-milk products, and dark green and deep yellow fruits and vegetables (all contain a precursor of vitamin A).

Vitamin D

Exposure to sunlight, fortified milk, liver, egg yolk, butter, cream, fish, and liver oils

Vitamin E

Widely distributed in foods, especially wheat germ and vegetable oils

Vitamin K

Fruits and leafy vegetables, cereals, dairy products, meat, and tomatoes

Vitamin C (ascorbic acid)

Citrus fruits, other fruits, and vegetables

B-COMPLEX VITAMINS

Thiamine

Organ meats, legumes, nuts, whole or enriched grain products, wheat germ, and brewer's yeast

Riboflavin

Milk and milk products, organ meats, eggs, leafy green vegetables, and whole or enriched grain products

Niacin

Meats, legumes, nuts, peanut butter, and whole-grain and enriched-grain products. Tryptophan, a niacin precursor, is also found in protein foods of animal origin.

Pantothenic acid

Liver, kidney, salmon, eggs, legumes and peanuts, whole grains, milk, fruits, vegetables, molasses, and yeast

Biotin

Organ meats, egg yolk, legumes, nuts, and mushrooms

Folic acid

Leafy green vegetables, orange juice, liver, peanuts, legumes, whole-grain products, and wheat germ

Vitamin B$_{12}$

Animal protein products only (meat, milk, fish and shellfish, eggs, and cheeses)

Pyridoxine

Meat, fish, egg yolks, legumes and nuts, potatoes, whole grains, wheat germ, yeast, prunes and raisins, and bananas

Table 17-5　Intravenous Infusion: Problems, Signs and Symptoms, and Suggested Nursing Actions

Problem	Signs and symptoms	Nursing actions
Pain during infusion	Patient discomfort	Slow rate of infusion because some drugs are irritating to veins. Warm IV fluids to room temperature before hanging. Rule out phlebitis (below).
Occluded infusion	Decreased rate of infusion or no infusion Backup of blood into tubing Possible discomfort	Check to see that clamp is open or electronic device is turned on. Inspect tubing for kinks. Remove dressing over insertion site (using aseptic technique); check for kinks, remove old dressing, and retape insertion site. If fluid level in bag or bottle is low, raise level of bag or bottle, or replace it with full bag or bottle. With some infusion devices (e.g., Port-A-Cath) or with multilumen central catheters, use thrombolytics such as urokinase to dissolve clots occluding IV flow; follow agency policies. If all else fails, restart IV.
Extravasation (leaking of fluid or drug into tissue surrounding vein, caused by tear in vein)	Decreased rate of infusion or no infusion Patient discomfort Puffiness, edema of extremity or insertion site Coolness distal to insertion site No blood return when bag or bottle is lowered below level of insertion site	Discontinue IV and restart line at another site. Apply warm soaks (follow agency procedure). If drug is known to be caustic (e.g., mechlorethamine), carry out any specific measures, including infiltration of area with steroids or drug antidote; consult physician or agency policies.
Phlebitis (irritation or inflammation of the vein)	Patient discomfort Red streak coursing arm Site is warm to touch Possible edema	Slow rate of infusion, while doing further assessment. If phlebitis is confirmed, discontinue IV and restart line at another site. Apply warm soaks (follow agency procedure).
Septicemia	Fever, chills, symptoms of shock, malaise, hypotension Normal appearance of IV insertion site Headache, nausea, vomiting	Notify physician. Rule out other causes (respiratory tract infection, urinary tract infection, wound infection). Discontinue IV line, culture catheter tip and fluid (or as agency procedure directs), and restart IV line at another site.
Fluid overload	Noisy, rapid respiration, rales Distended neck veins Increased pulse rate or blood pressure Distress Puffiness, edema of dependent areas Weight gain	Slow infusion to keep open rate. Notify physician.
Embolism	Shortness of breath Chest and shoulder pain Cyanosis Hypotension, weak pulse Loss of consciousness	Place patient on left side, in Trendelenburg position. Notify physician. Remain with patient, taking vital signs.

General Guidelines

◆ Maintain vigilance whenever working with IV fluids or drugs because the administration of any substance directly into the vascular system can cause serious and rapid consequences.

◆ Inspect the patient receiving IV fluids at least hourly. Assess for correct infusion rate; and inspect the bag or bottle, tubing, monitoring devices, and area surrounding insertion site. Assess for signs of fluid overload, and observe for any of the common problems associated with IV fluid therapy. See Table 17-5 for a summary of common IV problems and suggested nursing actions.

◆ Monitor skin turgor, intake and output, and weight; inspect dependent areas for edema; monitor vital signs; auscultate heart and lung sounds; and monitor central venous pressure and pulmonary capillary wedge pressure if available.

◆ Be familiar with agency or institutional policies and procedures regarding IV administration. Policies may specify who may start IV administrations, who may add electrolyte solutions or drugs to infusions, and what the procedures are for routinely changing the tubing or insertion site or for redressing central line insertion sites.

◆ Use measures to prevent complications of IV administration, in addition to assessing for their development and subsequent treatment. For example, cleanse insertion sites thoroughly before initiating IV therapy, and wear sterile gloves when starting IV line. Cleanse injection ports well with an alcohol or povidone-iodine solution before puncturing them. Use Luer-Lok connections to prevent accidental pulling apart of IV tubing. Choose insertion sites where catheters are less likely to be dislodged by patient movement, and tape catheters securaly. Wear gloves when discontinuing IV catheterization.

◆ Become familiar with the IV equipment used in the agency. Read the package inserts, and attend in-service programs about new equipment.

◆ Check infusion rates carefully. If you have difficulty calculating IV drip rates, check calculations with another nurse. If a drip rate seems excessively fast or slow, discuss this with another nurse. Some agencies require that two nurses check the infusion rate for infants and small children. See Chapter 7 for information about calculating IV rates of infusion.

◆ Inspect IV solutions carefully before using. Do not use solutions that are discolored, are leaking, or that contain particulate matter.

◆ Choose a needle or catheter, administration set, and tubing length appropriate for the patient and the drug. For example, the larger the diameter of the needle or catheter, the faster the fluid will infuse, but the larger the diameter, the more difficult it is to insert the needle or catheter into the chosen vein. The higher the fluid reservoir (bag or bottle) is above the patient, the faster the rate of infusion; generally, the reservoir should be about 36 in above the insertion site. The viscosity of the fluid influences the rate of flow; for example, blood infuses more slowly than normal saline or 5% dextrose solutions. The greater the length of tubing from the fluid reservoir to the patient, the slower the rate of flow. Choose a tubing long enough to allow safe movement by the patient but short enough to ensure that the tubing will not get tangled in the siderails or significantly restrict flow. Finally, choose an administration set appropriate to the ordered rate of flow. For example, if the rate of flow is 150 ml/hr, the drip rate on a minidrip set that delivers 60 gtt/ml would be 150 gtt/min, almost too fast to count. That same rate of administration with a set that delivers 10 gtt/ml would be 25, an easy rate to count. Use a minidrip set for infants or small children, when a patient is on a keep-open or slow rate, or when drug dose is measured according to patient response such as when an IV drug (e.g., dopamine) is adjusted based on the patient's blood pressure.

◆ Use volume-control devices to limit the volume a patient could receive in a specified time period; an example is Buretrol, a volume-control device attached to the IV tubing between the fluid reservoir and the patient. The nurse fills the volume control device with a specified volume of fluid and adjusts the flow rate. The patient can receive only the volume contained in the device, until it is refilled. For example, consider an infant requiring IV fluids. Even if a 500-ml reservoir bag were hung instead of a 1000-ml bag, the danger of fluid overload would be significant if all 500 ml were to infuse rapidly. The nurse could fill the volume-control device with the amount ordered for 1 hr (e.g., 30 ml for this patient) and adjust the flow rate. Even if all of the fluid in the device would infuse rapidly, the danger of fluid overload would be much less than with 500 ml. Volume control devices permit the addition of medications to the fluid in the chamber.

Continued.

NURSING IMPLICATIONS SUMMARY—cont'd

◆ IV pumps and controllers are widely available today. These electronic devices help maintain a constant rate of flow. Because they contain alarms, they warn the nurse when a problem has occurred. The IV pump delivers the IV fluid with pressure, whereas the IV controller adjusts the rate of fluids infusing via gravity. Become familiar with devices used in the agency. Electronic devices do not replace careful patient assessment and nursing care but can assist in managing IV therapy.

◆ The use of in-line IV filters for all medications and solutions is not universally accepted. Nevertheless, many agencies require them. Familiarize yourself with the advantages of the filters in use in your agency. For example, some filters remove only particulate matter, and some do not have air-eliminating capability. The 0.22-µm filter can remove particulate matter, fungi, bacteria, and air but cannot filter TPN solutions because it is too small. Tubing for blood administration is equipped with a filter. Fat emulsions cannot be filtered.

◆ Label all fluid reservoirs as directed by agency procedure. A common way is to place a length of adhesive tape along the side of the bag or bottle next to the volume markers on the container. The correct fluid level per hour is marked on the tape. For example, if 1000 ml of fluid is started at 8 AM, there should be 900 ml remaining at 9 AM and 800 ml at 10 AM. Thus any nurse on duty can determine at a glance whether the infusion is running properly. If the infusion is not correctly timed, do not try to catch up by doubling or increasing the rate for the next hour or two. Assess the situation and, if necessary, restart the infusion at another site. If the solution is infusing too rapidly, slow the rate and assess the patient for signs of fluid overload (see Table 17-5). If the extra volume infused was minimal and the patient's condition is satisfactory, resume the prescribed rate. If the volume is excessive or signs of fluid overload are present, maintain the IV at the keep-open rate, and notify the physician.

◆ Label all IV solutions carefully, especially when additives, such as potassium, vitamins, heparin, insulin, and other drugs, have been included. Record the administration of all IV solutions carefully. See Chapter 6 for additional information about IV administration.

Oral and IV Potassium
Drug administration

◆ Potassium chloride (KCl) is the most frequently administered electrolyte added to IV fluids. (Most sodium chloride administered is supplied by manufacturers in commonly used concentrations; potassium chloride is more often added by the nurse or pharmacy). Ascertain that the patient has adequate kidney function before administering IV potassium. Always dilute potassium chloride before administering it intravenously. Carefully check the dose before adding it. Carefully label containers to which potassium has been added.

◆ Monitor the patient's ECG and serum potassium level. See Table 17-1 for signs of common electrolyte imbalances. The classic ECG changes seen with potassium imbalances are hypokalemia (with ST-segment depression, flattened T waves, presence of U waves, and ventricular dysrhythmias) and hyperkalemia (with tall, thin T waves, prolonged PR interval, ST depression, widened QRS, and loss of P waves.)

◆ Carefully check the rate of administration of IV potassium. The usual dose is 20 to 60 mEq/24, but if needed, it may be given at a rate of 10 to 15 mEq/hr of a solution containing 40 mEq/L, unless the patient is severely potassium depleted.

◆ To treat hyperkalemia, discontinue potassium replacements (IV or oral), and limit potassium-rich foods (see box on p. 252). Emergency treatment includes IV sodium bicarbonate, calcium gluconate (if not contraindicated by existing cardiac conditions), and IV glucose and insulin (which helps shift potassium into the cell). Dialysis may also be used.

◆ Subacute hyperkalemia is treated with cation exchange resins such as Kayexalate, which exchanges sodium for potassium in the intestine. The effect is not evident for several hours to 1 day after administration. The resin is given orally, via nasogastric tube, or as a retention enema. Adverse effects include hypokalemia, hypocalcemia, anorexia, nausea, vomiting, and constipation. Monitor electrolyte levels. When the resin is given orally or via nasogastric tube, constipation is common, so a mild laxative may be administered concurrently. For oral administration, dilute the drug in water, syrup, fruit juice, or soft drink.

NURSING IMPLICATIONS SUMMARY—cont'd

◆ Monitor potassium levels carefully in patients with cardiac conditions, since hypokalemia potentiates the effects of cardiac glycosides. Do not administer potassium to patients receiving potassium-sparing diuretics (see Chapter 16).

Patient and family education

◆ Review with patients the importance of taking potassium preparations as ordered. Some patients will be able to maintain potassium levels through dietary intake of potassium-rich foods; (see box on p. 252).

◆ Work with patients to find an acceptable form of potassium. Oral preparations are often unpalatable or difficult to swallow. Enteric-coated tablets have been implicated in small bowel ulceration. Effervescent preparations are often unpalatable, and patients soon stop taking them. Oral solutions work well but often have a bitter, salty taste.

◆ Dilute oral solutions in juice or milk if acceptable to the patient. Avoid tomato juice if the patient is on a low-sodium diet.

◆ Dissolve the soluble powders, granules, or tablets in at least 4 oz of juice or water; avoid tomato juice if the patient is on a low-sodium diet.

◆ Extended-release tablets and capsules should be swallowed whole without being chewed or crushed. (A few tablets may be crushed or broken and a few capsules may be opened, but most should not be; check with the pharmacist.) Instruct patients to take potassium with meals to reduce gastric irritation.

Magnesium Sulfate

Drug administration and patient and family education

◆ Magnesium sulfate is useful orally to promote defecation (see Chapter 13) and parenterally to treat or prevent hypomagnesemia. It is also available as an anticonvulsant, especially in pregnancy-induced hypertension (PIH).

◆ See Table 17-1 for signs of magnesium imbalances. If magnesium imbalance is suspected, monitor the serum magnesium level.

◆ IM administration of magnesium is painful. Use large muscle masses and rotate sites. Inject the drug slowly.

◆ The goal in treating PIH is to obtain a serum level that will inhibit seizures but will not cause respiratory or cardiac paralysis. Several dosage regimens are followed for this purpose; most are initiated with a loading dose, followed by a maintenance dose. Assess the deep tendon reflexes, respiratory rate, and urinary output. If reflexes diminish or cease, if the respiratory rate decreases, or if the urinary output falls below 30 to 100 ml/hr, the dose of magnesium sulfate may need to be reduced. Monitor vital signs, intake and output, and serum magnesium levels. Monitor fetal heart sounds. In severe cases, monitor maternal ECG and attach a fetal monitor to assess infant status. Monitor newborns of mothers who received magnesium sulfate for several hours after delivery for signs of hypermagnesemia (see Table 17-1).

◆ Administer the 10% solution at a rate of 1.5 ml/min.

◆ Have available equipment for resuscitation in settings where parenteral magnesium sulfate is administered. Have available calcium gluconate and calcium gluceptate as specific antidotes for magnesium overdose.

Sodium Bicarbonate

Drug administration and patient and family education

◆ Sodium bicarbonate is given orally to neutralize gastric acid (see Chapter 13), and to alkalinize the urine. During resuscitation efforts, administer sodium bicarbonate via direct IV push to help correct metabolic acidosis. It is usually included in the emergency drug box or on the resuscitation cart, packaged in labeled, filled syringes. For IV administration the drug is diluted and administered at a rate of 2 to 5 mEq/kg over 4 to 8 hr. Signs of overdose are metabolic alkalosis and hypernatremia (see Table 17-1). Monitor serum electrolyte and arterial blood gas levels.

Calcium

Drug administration and patient and family education

◆ Calcium compounds are antacids (see Chapter 13). Read physician's orders carefully. IV calcium compounds include calcium gluco-

Continued.

nate, calcium chloride, and calcium gluceptate. When possible, warm drug to body temperature before administering. The IV route is preferred in infants, but avoid scalp veins because extravasation may cause tissue necrosis. Monitor ECG during IV administration. Keep patient recumbent for 30 min after IV administration; monitor blood pressure and serum calcium levels.

◆ If IV administration is not possible, calcium gluceptate, calcium gluconate, or a combintaion of calcium glycerophosphate and calcium lactate may be administered intramuscularly. (Do not give calcium chloride IM.) Use large muscle masses and rotate injection sites. If greater than 5 ml is to be administered intramuscularly to an adult, divide the dose in half and administer via two injections. With children, determine whether the dose should be divided.

◆ Severe hypocalcemia may manifest as tetany. Chvostek's sign and Trousseau's sign may be positive (see a text on physical assessment). Pad the siderails. Have resuscitation equipment readily available. Review with patients taking oral calcium supplements foods that are rich in calcium. (See box on p. 768). Hypercalcemia is discussed in Chapter 52.

Blood, Plasma, Albumin, and Plasma Protein Fraction

Drug administration

◆ Review the general guidelines for care of patients receiving IV fluids and other replacement solutions.

◆ Whole blood is administered via a blood infusion tubing set, which usually contains an in-line filter. The infusion is established, usually with normal saline in the primary line (solutions with dextrose may hemolyze the blood, and solutions containing calcium, as in lactated Ringer's solution, may clot the blood). The blood is then piggybacked to the primary solution via the second port in the set. This method helps prevent the blood from clotting toward the end of the infusion; it also helps maintain a patent IV access line, even if infusion of the blood must be stopped, as might happen with an allergic reaction.

Monitor hematocrit and hemoglobin levels, intake and output, and vital signs.

◆ Before beginning the transfusion, carefully check the patient's identification bracelet and the label on the container of blood. Blood-type incompatibility is potentially fatal; death can occur after infusion of as little as 50 to 100 ml of an incorrect blood type. Most institutions provide specific, detailed procedures to ensure that blood is carefully checked beforehand. Signs and symptoms of a transfusion reaction include flushing, nausea, hypotension, increased pulse rate, difficulty breathing, tightness in the chest, chills, fever, headache, substernal chest pain, vomiting, and sense of impending doom. In addition, hematologic changes may occur, including disseminated intravascular coagulation (DIC), thrombocytopenia, and spontaneous bleeding. If the patient is anesthetized or unconscious, it may be difficult to recognize this reaction.

◆ After initiating the transfusion, remain with the patient for 10 to 15 min, monitoring and recording the vital signs. Thoroughly investigate any unanticipated occurrence; stop the infusion (but maintain a patent IV access line by restarting the priming solution), and notify the physician. Hypersensitivity reactions include rashes, itching, and the symptoms noted above. Minor reactions can frequently be treated with antihistamines or corticosteroids, but occasionally emergency life support measures, including epinephrine, are needed. Know beforehand where emergency drugs and equipment are kept.

◆ Febrile reactions usually begin within the first 15 min of infusion but may not begin until 1 to 2 hr later. They are characterized by fever (39.4° to 40° C [103° to 104° F]), chills, headache, and malaise. Stop the infusion, notify the physician, and investigate the cause.

◆ Circulatory overload is more common when whole blood is administered, when the patient is elderly or an infant, or when the patient has cardiac disease. Monitor vital signs and cardiac and lung sounds, and observe for respiratory difficulty and cough.

◆ Do not mix any medications with blood. If it is necessary to administer an IV medication via the same IV access line, stop the blood infusion, flush the line with saline, inject the medication, flush the line again with saline, and resume the blood infusion. Blood cells are large, so a large-diameter needle or catheter should be used.

◆ When fluid overload is a concern or large volumes must be transfused, whole-blood components may be prescribed, such as packed red cells, platelets, cryoprecipitated factor VIII (for patients with hemophilia), and fibrinogen. These products are smaller in volume than whole blood but are generally administered the same way.

◆ Complete administration of whole blood within 2 to 4 hr; after this time, the blood may clot. (In extreme emergencies, pressure applied to the bag will afford delivery within 10 min or less.)

◆ Blood products deteriorate rapidly if not stored properly and used promptly. Do not thaw frozen products until they are to be used. Do not procure blood from the blood bank until the patient is ready for the infusion. Do not leave blood products in the patient care unit. Check and observe expiration dates of all blood products. Plasma, albumin, and plasma protein fraction are derived from blood, and the same general guidelines apply.

Dextran
Drug administration

◆ Monitor weight, blood pressure, pulse, and intake and output. Assess for signs of fluid overload (see p. 276). Monitor hematocrit, hemoglobin, serum protein, and serum protein electrophoresis levels. Assess patients for bleeding.

◆ Notify physician if urine output falls below 30 to 5 ml/hr.

◆ Monitor patients for signs of allergic reaction.

◆ If blood must also be administered, flush tubing thoroughly between blood and dextran infusion because dextran causes blood to coagulate in tubing.

◆ Use only clear solutions. If crystallization has occurred, heat bottle in warm water until crystals dissolve before administering. If you are drawing blood for laboratory tests, note on the requisition that dextran is being administered, as it may cause false high serum glucose levels and alterations in other blood tests.

Hetastarch
Drug administration

◆ Monitor for allergic reactions. Monitor vital signs. Monitor hematocrit, hemoglobin, plasma proteins, and platelet levels. Assess patients for signs of bleeding.

TPN
Drug administration and patient and family education

◆ Review the general guidelines for care of patients receiving IV fluids.

◆ TPN, or hyperalimentation, must be administered via a central infusion line for solutions more concentrated than 10% dextrose. The central line is placed by the physician under aseptic technique, as described in Chapter 6.

◆ Follow aseptic technique when manipulating the TPN infusion. These fluids provide favorable conditions for harmful bacteria—It is essential to prevent infection. Follow agency procedures for maintenance of TPN. They will usually specify how often to dress the insertion site, what method to use for dressing, what agent to use to clean injection sites (e.g., povidone-iodine or alcohol), and how often to change tubing.

◆ Monitor vital signs, and assess for fluid overload (see p. 276). Monitor patient's temperature every 4 hr in the hospital. Instruct the patient at home to notify the physician if fever develops.

◆ Hypertonic dextrose, amino acids, and fat emulsions are the mainstay of TPN therapy. The rate of flow, additives (vitamins, minerals, and electrolytes), and their concentrations must be ordered specifically by the physician. Most agencies have devised a protocol for monitoring the patient, including the frequency of blood work such as serum electrolyte levels, albumin levels, BUN levels, liver function studies, and blood glucose levels; the frequency of vitamin and mineral infusions; the procedures for culturing the catheter tip and fluid if infection develops; and the frequency of weighing the patient.

◆ Do not add medications to the solution or administer medications via the TPN line unless specifically permitted by agency protocol. Usually, if other IV medications are needed, a separate peripheral IV line must be started and maintained.

Continued.

NURSING IMPLICATIONS SUMMARY—cont'd

◆ Maintain the infusion at a steady rate; usually an electronic monitoring device is used. Erratic infusion rates may cause fluctuations in blood glucose levels, which will induce hyperglycemia and hypoglycemia. If the infusion stops or must be discontinued abruptly, standing orders are (at most facilities) to begin a peripheral infusion of dextrose 10% to prevent hypoglycemia. When the need for TPN therapy has resolved, gradually slow the rate of infusion to prevent hypoglycemia.

◆ Assess the patient for appearance of dry, flaky skin; hair loss; and rashes. These signs may indicate essential fatty acid or zinc deficiency.

◆ Prepare TPN solutions in a laminar flow hood, where risk of contamination is low.

◆ Some patients are suitable candidates for TPN administration at home. Assess learning needs with patient and family. Provide reassurance. Ascertain that they are able to manipulate the equipment. Refer the patient to social services agency and to a community-based nursing care service.

Amino Acid Infusions
Drug administration

◆ Review the general guidelines for TPN. Assess for common side effects (nausea, vomiting, flushing, and a sensation of warmth). Less common are chills, headache, abdominal pain, dizziness, rashes, hyperglycemia, and glycosuria.

◆ Monitor intake and output; serum electrolyte, magnesium, blood ammonia, phosphate, serum protein, cholesterol, and BUN levels; liver function studies; and blood glucose levels. Observe for signs of essential fatty acid deficiency (hair loss and dry, flaky skin).

◆ Vitamins, electrolytes, trace elements, heparin, and insulin can be administered via the same IV line, but other medications should not be. Do not premix these drugs with amino acid infusions; administer via a Y-connector.

◆ Use an IV filter. Infuse at a rate not exceeding 4 mg/kg/hr of nitrogen.

◆ Infuse at a steady rate; use an electronic infusion monitor if available.

Fat Emulsions
Drug administration and patient and family education

◆ See the general guidelines for IV therapy. Administer fat emulsions via central or peripheral IV line. Read the manufacturer's information supplied with the bottle of fat emulsion. Fat emulsion should comprise no more than 60% of the total daily caloric intake. Inspect before using. If the emulsion has cracked (the oil separated from the other products), it should not be used. Do not shake the emulsion.

◆ Assess for side effects including thrombophlebitis, vomiting, chest pain, back pain, and allergic reactions. Begin the infusion slowly (e.g., 1 ml/min) and observe the patient. If no untoward effect has occurred after 15 to 30 min, increase the rate of infusion to the desired rate. Monitor serum triglyceride levels. Fat emulsions can cause hyperlipidemia, which should clear between infusions; if not, withhold the next dose and notify the physician.

◆ Do not filter a fat emulsion. If it is piggybacked into a line incorporating a filter, the fat emulsion must be inserted below the level of the filter (closer to the patient).

Vitamins

◆ Water-soluble vitamins may be administered intravenously, whereas fat-soluble vitamins are administered via IM injection. Vitamins should be administered parenterally when oral intake and digestion are compromised. Patients with vitamin deficiencies who are able to eat and digest food should be counseled to increase their dietary intake of vitamin-rich foods (see box on p. 275).

CHAPTER REVIEW

◆ KEY TERMS

diffusion, p. 269

hydrostatic pressure, p. 269

hyperkalemia, p. 270

hypernatremia, p. 270

hypokalemia, p. 270

hyponatremia, p. 270

interstitial fluid, p. 267

intracellular fluid, p. 267

metabolic acidosis, p. 271

metabolic alkalosis, p. 271

oncotic pressure, p. 268

osmosis, p. 268

respiratory acidosis, p. 271

respiratory alkalosis, p. 271

◆ REVIEW QUESTIONS

1. What are the three main fluid compartments of the body?

2. What are the major buffers of plasma?

3. What is the major difference in composition between plasma and interstitial fluid?

4. What is osmosis?

5. What solute primarily determines the osmotic strength of plasma?

6. What is oncotic pressure?

7. Does the protein content of plasma cause water to move into or out of blood vessels?

8. What is hydrostatic pressure?

9. Does hydrostatic pressure cause water to move into or out of blood vessels?

10. How are cells able to maintain high intracellular concentrations of potassium, phosphate, and magnesium?

11. What are signs of dehydration or fluid deficit? Give examples of patients who might manifest dehydration.

12. What can cause fluid excess or overload? Give examples of patients who might manifest fluid overload.

13. What are signs of fluid overload?

14. What is hypernatremia? Hyponatremia? How would you assess for these?

15. What is hyperkalemia? Hypokalemia? How would you assess for these?

16. What is respiratory acidosis? How does it differ from metabolic acidosis? How would you assess for these?

17. What is respiratory alkalosis? How does it differ from metabolic alkalosis? How would you assess for these?

18. What are the uses of isotonic saline?

19. What are the dangers associated with saline administration?

20. How do isotonic saline, Ringer's solution, and lactated Ringer's solution differ?

21. What is the primary use for isotonic dextrose?

22. Why must you never mix dextrose solutions with whole blood for administration?

23. What organ system must be functioning before potassium replacement is begun?

24. Why are solutions of large-molecular-weight proteins or carbohydrates able to expand plasma volume?

25. What special precautions for administration are necessary with hypertonic dextrose for parenteral nutrition?

26. What additional supplement may be required by patients receiving amino acid solution for parenteral nutrition?

27. What is the primary advantage of fat emulsions in parenteral nutrition? What are some nursing care precautions in administering fat emulsions?

SUGGESTED READING

American Association of Blood Banks: Blood transfusions outside the hospital, *Am J Nurs* 89(4):486, 1989.

Anthony CP, Thibodeau GA: Fluid and electrolyte balance. In *Textbook of anatomy and physiology,* ed 13, St Louis, 1990, Mosby–Year Book.

Fluid, electrolyte, and acid-base therapy. In *Drug Evaluations Subscription,* Chicago, 1990, American Medical Association.

Fuller AK: Platelet transfusion therapy for thrombocytopenia, *Semin Oncol Nurs* 6(2):123, 1990.

Gahart BL: *Intravenous medications: a handbook for nurses and other allied health personnel,* St Louis, 1992, Mosby–Year Book.

Gasparis L, Murray EB, Ursomanno P: IV solutions: which one's right for your patient? *Nurs 89* 19(4):62, 1989.

Graves L III: Disorders of calcium, phosphorus and magnesium, *Crit Care Nurs Q* 13(3):3, 1990.

Horne MM, Swearingen PL: *Pocket guide to fluids and electrolytes,* St Louis, 1989, Mosby–Year Book.

Janusek LW: Metabolic alkalosis: pathophysiology—and the resulting signs and symptoms, *Nurs 90* 20(6):52, 1990.

Janusek LW: Metabolic acidosis: pathophysiology, signs, and symptoms, *Nurs 90* 20(7):52, 1990.

Karb VB: Electrolyte abnormalities and drugs which commonly cause them, *J Neurosci Nurs* 21(2):125, 1989.

Kresevic DM, Kralik K: Understanding therapeutic plasma exchange, *Nurs 90* 20(4):68, 1990.

La Rocca JC, Otto SE: *Pocket guide to intravenous therapy,* St Louis, 1989, Mosby–Year Book.

McCormac M: Managing hemorrhagic shock, *Am J Nurs* 90(8):22, 1990.

Metheny NM: Why worry about IV fluids? *Am J Nurs* 90(6):50, 1990.

Nacker JG, Brubakken KM: Accuracy of infusing IV fluids: a Q.A. approach, *J Intravenous Nurs* 13(1):23, 1990.

Nursing Education Working Group of the National Blood Resource Education Program: Transfusion nursing: trends and practices for the '90s. I. Autologous transfusion, *Am J Nurs* 91(6):47, 1991.

Nursing Education Working Group of the National Blood Resource Education Program: Transfusion nursing: trends and practices for the '90s. II. Choosing blood components and equipment, *Am J Nurs* 91(6):42, 1991.

Nursing Education Working Group of the National Blood Resource Education Program: Transfusion nursing: trends and practices for the '90s. III. Preventing and managing transfusion reactions, *Am J Nurs* 91(6):482, 1991.

Parenteral and enteral nutrition. In *Drug evaluations subscription,* Chicago, 1990, American Medical Association.

Querin, JJ, Stahl LD: 12 simple sensible steps for successful blood transfusions, *Nurs 90* 20(10):68, 1990.

Sherman JE, Sherman RH: I.V. therapy that clicks, *Nurs 89* 19(5):50, 1989.

Sommers M: Rapid fluid resuscitation: how to correct dangerous deficits, *Nurs 90* 20(1):52, 1990.

Taylor DL Respiratory acidosis: pathophysiology, signs, and symptoms, *Nurs 90* 20(9):52, 1990.

Taylor N and others: Comparison of normal versus heparinized saline for flushing infusion devices, *J Nurs Qual Assur* 3(4):49, 1989.

Thomason SS: Using a Groshong central venous catheter, *Nurs 91* 21(10):58, 1991.

Walpert N: An orderly look at calcium metabolism disorders, *Nurs 90* 20(7):60, 1990.

Weber BB: Timely tips on adhesive tape, *Nurs 91* 21(10):52, 1991.

Yarnell RP, Craig MP: Detecting hypomagnesemia: the most overlooked electrolyte imbalance, *Nurs 91* 21(7):55, 1991.

CHAPTER 18

Cardiac Glycosides and Other Drugs for Congestive Heart Failure

---

LEARNING OBJECTIVES

After studying this chapter, you should be able to do the following:

- Explain where the signal to beat originates in the heart and how it is transmitted throughout the heart.
- Explain what the mechanism of action of cardiac glycosides is and why they are used in congestive heart failure.
- Discuss other classes of drugs used in congestive heart failure.
- Discuss the toxicity expected with cardiac glycosides.
- Develop a nursing care plan for a patient receiving a cardiac glycoside.

CHAPTER OVERVIEW

◆ Congestive heart failure leads to symptoms that may all be traced back to the failure of the heart muscle to adequately pump the blood delivered to it. Although the condition cannot be cured, many medications can improve the situation by acting directly on the heart or by acting at other sites to relieve symptoms and indirectly aid the heart.

◆ To understand the actions of cardiotonic drugs covered in this chapter and the antiarrhythmic agents covered in the next chapter, a review of certain features of the anatomy and physiology of the heart is necessary.

Nursing Process Overview

CARDIOTONIC THERAPY

Assessment

Obtain baseline assessment data, including the vital signs and blood pressure, weight, fluid intake and output, serum electrolyte and blood urea nitrogen (BUN) levels, electrocardiogram (ECG), and other laboratory data. Auscultate heart and lungs, and assess for the presence and location of edema. Obtain any subjective history of recent dysfunction such as dyspnea on exertion, shortness of breath, and orthopnea (needing to sleep with the head supported or elevated on several pillows).

Nursing Diagnoses

Potential altered health maintenance related to insufficient knowledge of cardiac glycoside therapy
High risk for electrolyte imbalance or hypokalemia

Management

Monitor the weight, fluid intake and output, ECG, serum electrolyte levels, blood pressure, and other parameters of cardiovascular function. Auscultate the heart and lungs.

Evaluation

Before discharge, make sure patients can explain why and how to take all prescribed medication, what interrelations may exist (e.g., the need to take potassium supplements if certain diuretics and cardiac glycosides are prescribed together), how to plan meals within prescribed dietary limitations, what side effects are anticipated, and what situations require consultation with a physician. If appropriate, patients should be able to measure pulse, correctly record weight or pulse, and state what decisions should be made based on assessment of these data.

FUNCTIONS OF THE HEART
Cardiac Function

To understand the action of drugs on the heart, it is important to understand the following terms relating to cardiac physiology.

Automaticity is the ability of certain heart cells to depolarize spontaneously to initiate a beat (contraction of the whole heart). Normally a heartbeat is initiated in the sinoatrial (SA) node, but any of the conductive fibers of the heart are capable of spontaneously depolarizing and initiating beats and do so in certain types of heart disease.

Depolarization is the process by which cells become less negatively charged than extracellular fluid. Depolarization occurs when sodium rushes into the cell as the first event in the generation of the action potential.

Excitability of a cell or fiber in the heart is a measure of the ease with which the cell may be stimulated to depolarize. Certain drugs increase the excitability of cells by reducing the energy necessary to depolarize the cell, and some drugs can decrease cell excitability.

Action potential is a burst of electrical activity in a cell. Frequently described as cell firing, the process is similar to the conduction of impulses along a nerve fiber. The cell undergoes rapid depolarization followed by a slower repolarization phase, and in the process, it stimulates adjacent cells to do likewise. In the heart the generation of an action potential initiates ionic changes inside the cell that cause the myocardial fibers to contract.

Conduction velocity is the rate at which an electrical impulse passes through the atrioventricular (AV) node. There is a delay in transmission of the impulse to beat from the atrium to the ventricle produced by the AV node. This delay regulates the temporal separation in atrial and ventricular contractions. *Dromotropic* refers to factors affecting conduction velocity. A positive dromotropic response is an increase in conduction velocity, whereas a negative dromotropic response is a decrease in that velocity.

Rate is the number of beats or ventricular contractions per minute. In normal hearts, this is the rate of SA node firing. *Bradycardia* means a slow heart rate. *Tachycardia* means a fast heart rate. ***Chronotropic*** refers to changes in heart rate. Positive chronotropic effects are increases in heart rate; negative chronotropic effects are decreases in heart rate.

Contractility is measured as the strength of the muscular contraction of the heart. *Inotropic* refers to factors affecting the strength of cardiac contraction. A positive inotropic response is an increase in cardiac contractility. A negative inotropic response is a decrease in cardiac contractility.

Conductive Tissues of the Heart

The heart is formed of muscle similar in many respects to skeletal muscle but different in that many of the fibers conduct as well as contract. This property facilitates rapid conduction of action potentials. Action potentials do not pass directly between the atria and ventricles because they are insulated from each other by a ring of nonconductive tissue. The independence of the atria and ventricles as contractile units is important in regulating the heartbeat.

Within the heart the impulse to beat normally originates at the **SA node,** a specialized group of automatic cells in the right atrium (Figure 18-1). Another group of specialized fibers, the **AV node,** transmits this impulse to the ventricles after an important delay.

The heart is innervated by the sympathetic and parasympathetic branches of the autonomic nervous system (Figure 18-2). The vagus nerve is part of the parasympathetic nervous system; its action is localized in the nodes. Stimulation of the vagus nerve releases acetylcholine, which decreases the rate of depolarization and makes the cells less excitable. In the SA node, these actions decrease the rate of firing, which reduces heart rate. Stimulation of the vagus nerve also decreases conduction velocity through the AV node. This slowing of conduction velocity increases the temporal separation between contraction of atria and ventricles and therefore slows heart rate.

Sympathetic nerve fibers innervate the atria and ventricles. Stimulation of the sympathetic nerves releases norepinephrine, which activates the beta-1 adrenergic receptors of the heart. Activation of the beta-1 receptors in the conducting tissue of the heart speeds the repolarization of the cells. The results are an increase in heart rate (positive chronotropic effect) and an increase in conduction velocity (positive dromotropic effect). Stimulation of the beta-1 adrenergic receptors in the ventricular muscle increases the force of contraction (positive inotropic response).

Regulation of Myocardial Output
Frank-Starling law

The volume of blood that the heart delivers per second to the arteries varies with stress, exertion, and

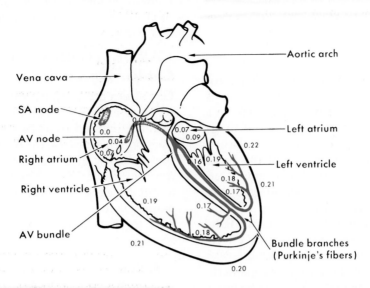

FIGURE 18-1

Transmission of action potentials through heart. Initiation of heartbeat occurs at SA node, and action potential is transmitted throughout atria before passing through AV node to ventricles. Numerals designate seconds it takes for impulse to travel from SA node to anatomic site designated by numeral. All parts of atria have received impulse within 0.09 sec, but transmission to ventricles is delayed during its passage through AV node so that ventricles do not begin to contract until 0.16 sec after SA node firing. Delay allows atria to contract and fill ventricles before ventricles begin to contract to force blood from heart.

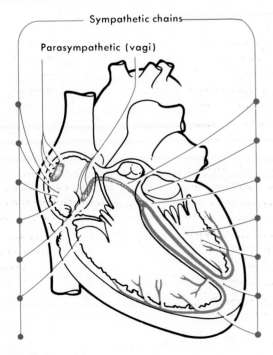

FIGURE 18-2

Autonomic innervation of heart.

other factors. How the heart regulates its output to meet these variable demands is described by the **Frank-Starling law** of the heart. This principle of physiology states that the force of muscular contraction is directly related to the stretch of the muscle; the more a muscle is stretched, within mechanical limits, the stronger is its subsequent contraction. With respect to the heart, this principle means that, when the ventricles are filled with larger than normal volumes of blood, they contract with greater than normal force to deliver their entire contents to the arteries. Normally, blood does not accumulate in the veins, and all the blood coming to the heart is pumped into the arteries.

When the healthy heart responds to acute exercise, the Frank-Starling law applies. The heart increases its force of contraction and hence its output. Sympathetic stimulation also increases the rate of contraction, which is a second mechanism for increasing output. The peak efficiency of the heart under these conditions is reached at about 150 to 175 beats/min. Faster rates result in incomplete filling of the ventricles and reduce the overall efficiency of the pump.

To summarize the Frank-Starling law, up to a certain limit the more a muscle fiber is stretched, the greater its subsequent strength of contraction, but beyond that limit, greater stretching diminishes the strength of contraction.

Cardiac hypertrophy

If the heart is subjected to chronic demands for increased output, it may enlarge. This condition is called **hypertrophy** of the myocardium and may be a normal response to chronic stress. For example, long-distance runners and tennis players may have enlarged hearts. In other cases the enlargement of the heart may signal a pathologic process. For example, in chronic heart failure the myocardial output gradually falls below the required level resulting from the failure of the myocardium as a pump. As the output falls, the normal regulatory mechanisms come into effect. Hypertrophy of the heart may occur as the body seeks to increase the efficiency of the pump. Sympathetic stimulation may also be increased to increase the heart rate and hence the output. In many cases, in the absence of acute demands on the heart, these mechanisms enable a weakened heart to maintain sufficient output. Patients may not complain of symptoms, but on examination may have an enlarged heart and high heart rate.

Congestive heart failure

If the regulatory mechanisms fail and cardiac output falls below venous return, **congestive heart failure** results. The symptoms arise directly from insufficient cardiac output. The blood pooled in the veins produces increased venous pressure. The excessive venous pressure stretches cardiac muscle fibers beyond their limit, and as predicted by the Frank-Starling law, the strength of contraction falls further. The kidneys do not receive sufficient blood flow to maintain salt and water balance. Edema of the lungs and periphery develops as fluid leaks into the tissues from the capillaries. The typical patient in congestive heart failure is therefore short of breath and has a rapid pulse resulting from sympathetic stimulation of the heart, obvious swelling of the hands and feet, and an enlarged heart. All of these acute symptoms may be

relieved by increasing the cardiac output. The drugs discussed in the next section are used primarily for this purpose.

CARDIOTONIC DRUGS
Cardiac Glycosides

Glycosides are complex steroidlike structures linked to sugar molecules. The drugs discussed in this section are referred to as **cardiac glycosides** because of their potent action on the heart. Many of the clinically useful cardiac glycosides come from species of *Digitalis* (see Table 18-3). The term *digitalis* may refer to a specific drug prepared from the leaf of *Digitalis purpurea;* it may also be used as a generic term to refer to all cardiac glycosides derived from *Digitalis* species.

Actions

The cardiac glycosides are used to treat congestive heart failure because they directly improve the strength of the heart muscle, elevating cardiac output. Biochemically, these drugs inhibit Na^+, K^+-ATPase and promote accumulation within the heart cells of the calcium necessary for contraction. These actions cause increased contractility, which increases cardiac output, improves blood flow to the kidneys and periphery, reduces venous pressure, and allows excess fluid to be excreted as edema clears. This diuretic effect of digitalis is secondary to its action on the heart. Cardiac glycosides are also widely used to control cardiac arrhythmias (see Chapter 19).

Administration

Half-lives of the cardiac glycosides may extend to 7 days (Table 18-1). With repeated equal doses of a drug, the plateau of drug concentration in the blood is not achieved for about 4 elimination half-times (see Chapter 1). Therefore these long half-lives for cardiac glycosides mean that the final desired therapeutic concentration of drug in the blood is not achieved for weeks after the start of therapy. For many patients, such a delay is intolerable. To avoid a long delay in achieving therapeutic concentrations, cardiac glyco-

Table 18-1   Pharmacokinetics of Cardiac Glycosides

Drug	Oral absorption	Plasma protein binding	Plasma half-life	Route of excretion
Digoxin	60% to 100%*	23%	32 to 48 hr	Renal
Digitoxin	90% to 100%	97%	5 to 7 days	Hepatic
Deslanoside	Unreliable	25%	33 to 36 hr	Renal

*Absorption is 60% for tablet form and up to 100% for soft gelatin capsule form.

sides are frequently administered first in a loading dose. The loading dose is designed to rapidly raise the concentration in the blood to the therapeutic range. After the loading dose or doses, a smaller dose is administered on a regular schedule. This smaller dose, called the *maintenance dose,* maintains the concentration of drug in the therapeutic range. This dose is continued indefinitely or until some change in the patient's condition requires adjustment.

The available cardiac glycosides are similar in intrinsic potencies, but they differ markedly in pharmacokinetic properties (Tables 18-1 and 18-2). These properties largely determine the dosage and dosing schedule for the individual preparations (Table 18-3) (see box on p. 291).

Digitoxin. Digitoxin is usually given orally in a dose to produce and to maintain the therapeutic level in plasma of 14 to 26 ng/ml. The dose required to produce the maximum therapeutic effect varies considerably from patient to patient and must be individualized. Digitalizing, or loading, doses range from 0.4 to 1.2 mg/day. Since 97% of this drug is reversibly bound to protein in the bloodstream and is inactive, the dose must reflect that only 3% of the dose in the bloodstream is active. Since the half-life of digitoxin is about 6 days, about 10% of the total body store of the drug is excreted each day. The routine daily dose of the drug must compensate for this loss. Maintenance doses should be expected to range from 0.05 to 0.2 mg/day. Consideration of the half-life of the drug is also important when toxicity occurs; toxicity may persist for long periods because the drug is slowly removed from the system.

Digoxin. Digoxin is usually given orally in a dose that produces and maintains the therapeutic plasma level of 0.8 to 1.6 ng/ml. Dosage regimens must be individualized. Digitalizing doses should range from 0.75 to 1.25 mg/day. This drug is less highly bound to plasma protein than digitoxin and has a much shorter half-life. The maintenance dose must replace the 37% of the total body store of the drug that is lost every day. Maintenance doses commonly range from 0.125 to 0.5 mg/day.

Deslanoside. Deslanoside is used only in emergencies when IV administration is required. Deslanoside has no role in long-term therapy of congestive heart failure, its only advantage being rapid action when given intravenously. However, it is usually no more rapid in onset of action than digoxin given intravenously. Morever, adjustment of doses when the patient is switched to oral maintenance therapy is more problematic with deslanoside than with digoxin. For these reasons, deslanoside is not widely used.

Toxicity of the cardiac glycosides

There is such a small difference between the therapeutic dose and doses that cause side effects that most patients taking cardiac glycosides experience drug-related difficulties. The symptoms may be neurologic, visual, cardiac, or even psychiatric. They often tend to be vague and easily confused with those of congestive heart failure.

The neurologic or central nervous system (CNS) effects of cardiac glycosides are now recognized as significant sources of much of the toxicity observed with these drugs. Anorexia, nausea, and vomiting caused by these drugs result from stimulation of the chemoreceptor trigger zone in the CNS. Weakness, fatigue, fainting, and other neurologic symptoms also point to an origin in the CNS. Visual disturbances such as dimness of vision, double vision, blind spots, flashing lights, or altered color vision also occur. Psychiatric disturbances range from mood alterations to psychoses or hallucinations.

The toxic action of cardiac glycosides on the heart may also result partly from CNS effects. Whatever the mechanism, the result may be bradycardia, various arrhythmias that may occasionally induce tachycardia, and ultimately ventricular fibrillation and death (see Chapter 19). Patients receiving cardiac glycosides must be checked frequently for the appearance of extra heartbeats or other arrhythmias. It is routine practice in many hospitals to omit the dose if the heart rate is less than 60 beats/min. Although bradycardia is the most common sign of digitalis-induced arrhythmias, other changes in heart rate are

Table 18-2 Time Course of Action of Cardiac Glycosides

Drug	Route	Onset	Peak	Duration
Digoxin	Oral	1 to 2 hr	2 to 6 hr	2 to 6 days
	IV	5 to 30 min	1 to 4 hr	2 to 6 days
Digitoxin	Oral	1 to 4 hr	8 to 14 hr	14 days
Deslanoside	IV	10 to 30 min	1 to 3 hr	2 to 5 days

Table 18-3   Summary of Inotropic Agents

Generic name	Trade name	Administration/dosage	Comments
Digitoxin	Crystodigin	ORAL: *Adults*—loading doses may be 0.6 mg then 0.4 mg in 4 to 6 hr, followed by 0.2 mg 4 to 6 hr later (for rapid loading) or 0.2 mg twice daily for 4 days (for slow loading). Maintenance doses range from 0.05 to 0.3 mg daily. FDA Pregnancy Category C. *Children*—Dosage forms are inconvenient for children. Digoxin is more conveniently administered.	Digitoxin is purified form of primary active glycoside from *Digitalis purpurea* (purple foxglove). Most patients can be safely started on oral loading doses.
Digoxin	Lanoxin* Novodigoxin†	ORAL (tablets): *Adults*—loading dose initially 0.75 to 1.25 mg divided into 2 or more doses given at 6 to 8 hr intervals (for rapid loading). Maintenance dose, also used for slow loading, is 0.125 to 0.5 mg daily. FDA Pregnancy Category C. *Children* (elixir)—loading doses that follow should be divided and administered every 6 hr. Premature infants: 0.02 to 0.035 mg/kg. Newborns: 0.025 to 0.035 mg/kg. Infants to 2 yr: 0.035 to 0.06 mg/kg. 2 to 5 yr: 0.03 to 0.04 mg/kg. 5 to 10 yr: 0.02 to 0.035 mg/kg. Over 10 yr: usual adult dose (tablets). Maintenance dose for premature infants is 20% to 30% of loading dose; for all other children, 25% to 35% of loading dose.	Digoxin is purified form of active glycoside from *Digitalis lanata* (white foxglove). Patients started on therapy with maintenance dose given orally will achieve stable blood concentrations of drug within 7 days. Bioavailability of digoxin from tablet is variable and may be as low as 60%. Oral absorption from solution in soft gelatin capsule is nearly 100%. Since digoxin is eliminated primarily by kidneys, dosage may need to be lowered in patients with diminished renal function.
		ORAL (capsule) and INTRAVENOUS: *Adults*—loading dose of 0.4 to 0.6 mg followed by 0.1 to 0.3 mg 2 or 3 more times at 4- to 6-hr intervals. Maintenance dose ranges from 0.05 to 0.35 mg daily. *Children*—loading doses that follow are divided and administered every 6 hr. Premature infants: 0.015 to 0.025 mg/kg. Newborns: 0.02 to 0.03 mg/kg. Infants to 2 yr: 0.03 to 0.05 mg/kg. 2 to 5 yr: 0.025 to 0.035 mg/kg. 5 to 10 yr: 0.015 to 0.03 mg/kg. Over 10 yr: 0.008 to 0.012 mg/kg. Maintenance dose for premature infants is 20% to 30% of oral loading dose; for all other children, 25% to 30% of oral loading dose.	
Deslanoside	Cedilanid-D Cedilanid†	INTRAVENOUS: *Adults*—initially 0.8 mg, then repeated at 4 hr intervals. FDA Pregnancy Category C. *Children*—divide doses into 2 or 3 portions and administer at 3- or 4-hr intervals. Newborns, 0.022 mg/kg. Infants to 3 yr: 0.025 mg/kg. Over 3 yr: 0.0225 mg/kg. INTRAMUSCULAR: *Adults*—IV usually preferred. *Children*—same as for IV.	Deslanoside is desacetyl form of lanatoside C, a glycoside found in *Digitalis lanata* (white foxglove). It is used only for emergencies; oral glycosides must be used for maintenance.
Amrinone	Inocor	INTRAVENOUS: *Adults*—initially, 0.75 mg/kg body weight given slowly over 2 or 3 min. Repeat after 30 min if needed. Maintenance, 0.005 to 0.01 mg/kg/min, according to clinical response. FDA Pregnancy Category C.	Patients with atrial flutter may need pretreatment with digitalis to prevent ventricular arrhythmia. Patients need adequate fluid intake to maintain adequate cardiac fluid filling so that response to amrinone is optimal.

*Available in Canada and United States.
†Available in Canada only.

Table 18-4 Treatment of Cardiac Glycoside Overdose

Generic name	Trade name	Administration/dosing
Digoxin immune FAB	Digibind	INTRADERMAL: *Adult*—0.1 ml of 0.1 mg/ml solution. Inspect for redness and wheal 20 min later. Do not administer full dose if reaction is positive. FDA Pregnancy Category C. INTRAVENOUS: *Adult*—give amount equimolar to total amount of digoxin or digitoxin in body. Digoxin immune FAB in a dose of 40 mg binds approximately 0.6 mg of drug. Consult package insert for aid in calculating dosage.

possible. For this reason, any change in heart rate or rhythm should be noted and reported.

Because the toxic reactions caused by cardiac glycosides are dose related, they are somewhat predictable (see Chapter 2). Many hospitals have developed an assay to measure active cardiac glycosides to aid in establishing safe doses and in diagnosing drug toxicity. Toxicity of the cardiac glycosides may be increased by the presence of other drugs. For example, potassium-depleting diuretics such as thiazides or loop diuretics (see Chapter 16) may predispose a patient to cardiac toxicity, because a low intracellular potassium level increases the likelihood of arrhythmias.

Accidental poisoning of children with preparations of cardiac glycosides is not uncommon. Patients who are around small children should be warned of the potential danger their medicine poses to curious toddlers.

Interest in deriving new inotropic agents that may be administered orally for chronic congestive heart failure has been sparked by the realization that the cardiac glycosides are severely limited in usefulness by their low therapeutic index (see Chapter 2).

Treatment of digitalis toxicity

With digoxin or digitoxin overdose, patients may continue to be at risk during the lengthy period required to eliminate these long-acting agents. If arrhythmias or hyperkalemia become life-threatening, digoxin immune FAB (Table 18-4) can be administered to rapidly neutralize free drug. Arrhythmias and electrolyte imbalance can be reversed within 30 min. The inotropic effect of the cardiac glycosides persists for several hours longer.

Adrenergic Agents

Stimulation of the beta-1 class of adrenergic receptors in the heart directly increases cardiac contractility by increasing cyclic adenosine monophosphate (cAMP) in heart muscle. An increase in cAMP can also be achieved by blocking phosphodiesterase, the enzyme that degrades cAMP. Drugs with these actions may be of value in treating symptoms of acute or chronic congestive heart failure.

Dobutamine. Dobutamine directly stimulates myocardial beta-1 receptors, but it has little effect on beta-2 receptors and alpha receptors, which predominate in blood vessels. Dobutamine does not activate dopamine receptors in the renal vasculature. The drug has little tendency to increase heart rate or to elevate blood pressure. These properties make it an attractive agent for increasing cardiac output in severely ill patients. A disadvantage of dobutamine is that it must be given intravenously and has a short duration of action. This drug is therefore appropriate only for acute cardiac decompensation. See Chapter 14 for a more detailed discussion of this drug.

Dopamine. Dopamine directly stimulates myocardial beta-1 receptors but also causes indirect stimulation at this site by releasing norepinephrine from the nerve terminals in the heart. Dopamine also stimulates alpha receptors in blood vessels and dopamine receptors in the renal vasculature. Low doses increase renal blood flow, thus promoting diuresis. Higher doses directly stimulate the heart. Vasoconstriction caused by alpha-receptor stimulation appears with the highest doses. Since dopamine can limit cardiac output by these actions in peripheral vessels, it is usually selected only for patients in congestive heart failure complicated by hypotension. Like dobutamine, dopamine must be administered intravenously and has a very short duration of action. See Chapter 14 for a more detailed discussion of this drug.

Amrinone. Amrinone is intended for short-term IV use in congestive heart failure when response to other agents has been poor. The drug rapidly increases cardiac output and is additive in its effects with digitalis. The exact mechanism of action of amrinone is not yet completely understood, although the drug inhibits phosphodiesterase. In addition, it has some activity as a vasodilator in the periphery.

OTHER CLASSES OF DRUGS USED IN CONGESTIVE HEART FAILURE
Diuretics

Diuretics control the pulmonary edema that accompanies severe congestive heart failure. The agent most commonly selected is furosemide, although other diuretics may also be effective (see Chapter 16).

In addition to relieving pulmonary edema, a side effect of congestive failure, diuretics may directly improve cardiac function in some patients. In end-stage congestive heart failure, venous pressure is elevated sufficiently to cause heart muscle fibers to excessively stretch during filling of the chambers. Diuretics reduce preload by lowering the pressure forcing blood into the heart chambers. As a result, the muscle fibers are not so abnormally stretched; they are then able to contract with greater power. Therefore contractility of the heart muscle is improved.

The major consideration limiting the use of diuretics in congestive heart failure is the risk of causing electrolyte or fluid imbalances, which may be especially dangerous to the patient in heart failure. Volume depletion or excessive dehydration must be avoided. Patients receiving digitalis should be carefully observed to prevent complications, because diuretics tend to alter potassium concentration in the blood (see Chapter 14).

Vasodilators

Vasodilators reverse the persistent vasoconstriction in late chronic congestive heart failure resulting from long-term compensatory sympathetic nervous system stimulation. Sympathetic nervous system stimulation may drive the failing heart, but in the vasculature, it constricts vessels, thereby reducing cardiac output and increasing the workload of the heart. Vasodilators reduce the resistance against which the left ventricle must force blood. Cardiac output is therefore increased, and workload is reduced.

Several classes of vasodilators are available for use in congestive heart failure. For outpatient therapy, nitroglycerin or isosorbide dinitrate (see Chapter 14) can be employed. Nitroglycerin injection can be used as therapy for acute congestive heart failure. Alternatively, the related drug nitroprusside (see Chapter 15) can be used for short-term IV therapy in severely ill patients. This agent is often given with an adrenergic agent such as dobutamine or dopamine.

Angiotensin-converting enzyme (ACE) inhibitors captopril and enalapril (see Chapter 15) may also produce vasodilation that is useful in controlling congestive heart failure. These oral agents are used with diuretics and cardiac glycosides for therapy for chronic congestive heart failure.

NURSING IMPLICATIONS SUMMARY

Cardiac Glycosides
Drug administration
◆ Observe patients carefully. Desired effects of therapy include a decrease in pulse rate; slower, less labored respirations; diuresis with accompanying weight reduction; less coughing; less distended neck veins; and better tolerance of exertion. At the same time, observe for signs of toxicity. Many of the symptoms are seen in older or chronically ill persons and may not be recognized as drug toxicity. Symptoms include abdominal discomfort, fatigue, confusion, restlessness, anorexia, nausea, and vomiting, among others.

◆ Take the apical pulse for a full minute before administering a cardiac glycoside. Withhold the dose if the pulse is below 60 beats/min in an adult or below 90 to 110 beats/min in an infant or small child; notify the physician. Guidelines may vary according to institution or physician.
◆ Monitor the serum potassium and other electrolyte levels. Digitalis toxicity is aggravated in hypokalemia. If the potassium level is below normal range, notify the physician. Signs of hypokalemia are noted in Table 17-1. Recall that vomiting, chronic diarrhea, nasogastric suctioning, and alkalosis contribute to hy-

NURSING IMPLICATIONS SUMMARY—cont'd

pokalemia, as can administration of potassium-depleting diuretics, chronic steroids, amphotericin B, and chronic glucose.

◆ Monitor serum drug levels when available. Withhold the drug and notify the physician if the serum drug level is higher than the therapeutic range.

◆ Monitor intake and output, daily weight, vital signs, and heart and lung sounds. Assess for dependent edema in the sacral area and feet and ankles. Assess for jugular venous distention. Use data from central venous or arterial lines if available. Monitor the ECG; the cardiac glycosides can cause PR interval prolongation, ST segment sagging, AV blockage, and other arrhythmias.

◆ Read orders and drug labels carefully; do not confuse digoxin with digitoxin.

INTRAVENOUS DIGOXIN

◆ Monitor the apical pulse, and check serum electrolyte and drug levels before administering. It may be administered undiluted or diluted in 4 ml of sterile water, normal saline, or 5% dextrose for injection; use diluted solution as soon as prepared. Administer each dose over at least 5 min. If possible, monitor ECG during IV administration.

INTRAVENOUS DESLANOSIDE

◆ Monitor the apical pulse, and check serum electrolyte and drug levels before administering. It may be administered undiluted or diluted in 10 ml sodium chloride injection. Administer at a rate of 0.2 mg or less over 1 min. If possible, monitor the ECG during IV administration.

Patient and family education

◆ Review with patients the expected benefits and possible side effects of drug therapy. Review in detail the signs of drug toxicity, especially if the patient is elderly, since the elderly are more sensitive to the effects of the cardiac glycosides.

◆ Discuss the importance of maintaining an adequate potassium level. Review sources of dietary potassium (see box on p. 252). Patients with heart disease may need instruction about sodium-restricted, weight-reduction, and low-cholesterol diets; refer patients to a dietitian as needed.

◆ Review all medications the patient is taking, and emphasize the importance of taking them as prescribed. These may include diuretics, potassium replacements, and antihypertensives.

◆ If appropriate for their abilities, resources, and medical conditions, teach patients to monitor and record the apical pulse on a regular basis. It may also be appropriate to instruct patients to measure and record weight on a regular basis. Instruct patients to report weight gain greater than 2 lb/day (1 kg/day) or 5 lb/week (2 kg/week) to the physician.

◆ Instruct patients to take cardiac glycosides with meals or snacks to lessen gastric irritation.

◆ For maintenance therapy, cardiac glycosides are usually taken once a day. For missed doses, instruct patients to take the dose as soon as remembered on the day it was missed if within 12 hr of the usual time the dose is taken. Instruct patients not to double up for missed doses; take only one dose a day unless otherwise directed by the physician. Refer patients as needed to community-based nursing care services.

◆ Remind patients to keep these drugs out of the reach of children, to keep all health care providers informed of all drugs being taken, and not to self-medicate with over-the-counter drugs without consulting the physician.

◆ Suggest that patients wear medical identification tags or bracelets indicating that they are taking cardiac glycosides.

Amrinone

Drug administration

◆ Review the information about cardiac glycosides.

◆ Monitor the platelet count and other parameters noted above.

◆ Follow the dosage charts supplied by the manufacturer. It may be given as a bolus; administer dose over 2 to 3 min. If given as an infusion use microdrip tubing and an electronic infusion monitor. Monitor the ECG and other data available from central venous or arterial lines.

◆ Amrinone is used only in the acute-care setting. Keep the patient and family informed of the patient's condition.

Continued.

NURSING IMPLICATIONS SUMMARY—cont'd

Digoxin Immune FAB
Drug administration
♦ Review the manufacturer's insert for the latest guidelines.
♦ Skin testing may be prescribed before the full dose is given (see manufacturer's guidelines). Be prepared to treat an anaphylactic reaction. Patients who are allergic to digoxin immune FAB should not be given the full dose unless absolutely necessary. Have personnel, equipment, and drugs for resuscitation available.

♦ Prepare ordered dose, and administer over 30 min, using IV tubing with a 0.22 µg filter, unless cardiac arrest is imminent. It may be given as a bolus in that situation. Monitor the ECG and data from central venous and arterial lines as available.
♦ Monitor serum level of cardiac glycosides and serum electrolyte levels.
♦ Keep patient and family informed of the patient's condition.

CHAPTER REVIEW

♦ KEY TERMS
action potential, p. 286
automaticity, p. 286
AV node, p. 286
cardiac glycosides, p. 288
chronotropic, p. 286
conduction velocity, p. 286
congestive heart failure, p. 288
contractility, p. 286
depolarization, p. 286
dromotropic, p. 286
excitability, p. 286
Frank-Starling law, p. 287
hypertrophy, p. 288
rate, p. 286
SA node, p. 286

♦ REVIEW QUESTIONS
1. How does heart muscle differ from skeletal muscle?
2. What is the purpose of the ring of nonconductive tissue that separates the atria from the ventricles?
3. Where does the impulse to beat originate in the healthy heart?
4. What structure transmits the impulse to beat from the atria to the ventricles?
5. What is the effect of parasympathetic stimulation on the heart?
6. What is the effect of sympathetic stimulation on the heart?
7. What is the Frank-Starling law of the heart?
8. What symptoms are typical of congestive heart failure? How would you assess for these?
9. What is digitalis?
10. What is the physiologic effect of digitalis on the heart?
11. What is the mechanism of action of digitalis?
12. What is the mechanism by which digitalis produces diuresis in a patient with congestive heart failure?
13. How do digitoxin and digoxin differ in plasma protein binding and route of excretion?
14. Which digitalis preparation has the longest elimination half-time?
15. What is the purpose of the loading dose at the beginning of digitalis therapy?
16. What is the purpose of the maintenance dose in digitalis therapy?
17. Does digitalis have a high or a low therapeutic index?
18. What toxicity is common with digitalis therapy? What should you assess while monitoring for this toxicity?
19. Why are pulse rates measured before administering each prescribed dose of digitalis? What parameters should you use in assessing pulse rate data?
20. What drugs increase the likelihood of digitalis toxicity?

21. What inotropic drugs other than cardiac glycosides are used in congestive heart failure? What is the basis for their action in congestive heart failure?

22. How do diuretics relieve pulmonary congestion in congestive heart failure? How should you assess for this?

23. How may diuretics improve function in a failing heart?

24. How do vasodilators relieve symptoms of congestive heart failure?

SUGGESTED READING

Bachman J, Bolton ED, Cooke DH: The failing heart, *Patient Care* 23(1):132, 1989.

Gever MP: Top 25 discharge drugs, *Nurs 91* 21(6):53, 1991.

Porterfield L, Porterfield JG: How digoxin interacts with other drugs: a practical guide, *Nurs 90* 20(1):50, 1990.

Purcell JA, Holder CK: Cardiomyopathy: understanding the problem . . . supporting cardiac function, *Am J Nurs* 89(1):57, 1989.

Schwertz DW, Piano MR: New inotropic drugs for treatment of congestive heart failure, *Cardiovasc Nurs* 26(2):7, 1990.

Yacone LA: The nurses' guide to cardiovascular drugs. I. *RN,* 51(8):36, 1988.

Yacone LA: The nurses' guide to cardiovascular drugs. II. *RN* 51(9):40, 1988.

CHAPTER 19

Drugs to Control Cardiac Arrhythmias

LEARNING OBJECTIVES

After studying this chapter, you should be able to do the following:

◆ Explain how normal heart rhythm is maintained.

◆ Describe the four classes of antiarrhythmic agents.

◆ Explain how each class of antiarrhythmics suppresses arrhythmias.

◆ Discuss the cardiotoxicity of antiarrhythmic drugs.

◆ Develop a nursing care plan for a patient receiving an antiarrhythmic.

CHAPTER OVERVIEW

◆ **Cardiac arrhythmias** are defined as any deviation from the normal rate or pattern of heartbeat. Heart rates that are too slow (**bradycardia**), too fast (**tachycardia**), or irregular are all included in this classification. Arrhythmias are also referred to as *dysrhythmias*.

◆ To understand the pharmacologic control of arrhythmias, recall the physiologic control mechanisms of the heart. The impulse to beat originates in the sinoatrial (SA) node; it spreads through the atria, causing them to contract then passes through the artioventricular (AV) node and enters the ventricles, causing contraction of that tissue (see Chapter 18). The electrical activity that allows this communication is discussed first in this chapter, followed by a description of classes of antiarrhythmic agents and individual drugs.

Nursing Process Overview

ANTIARRHYTHMIC THERAPY

Assessment

Antiarrhythmic therapy is used in patients with cardiac arrhythmias. An arrhythmia is diagnosed by use of the electrocardiogram (ECG), although patients may complain of missed beats, fluttering in the chest, pounding in the chest, or irregular heart rates or patterns. Perform a thorough cardiovascular assessment, and question the patient about previous cardiac problems.

Nursing Diagnoses

High risk for cardiac arrhythmias
Possible activity intolerance related to fatigue and weakness secondary to drug side effects

Management

Treatment may take place in the coronary care unit or in the nonacute care setting if the arrhythmia is less serious. Perform periodic or continuous ECG monitoring as needed. Monitor vital signs and blood pressure, weight, fluid intake and output, serum electrolyte levels, and laboratory work appropriate for the drug prescribed. Observe the general physical condition of the patient, and watch for the appearance of side effects (see box).

Evaluation

Before discharge, determine that the patient can explain interactions among prescribed drugs, plan meals within prescribed dietary restriction, state how to manage persistent side effects, describe side effects and the signs and symptoms of toxicity, and understand when to notify the physician.

ELECTROPHYSIOLOGY OF THE HEART
Normal Action Potential

Typical action potentials for three types of cardiac tissue are illustrated in Figure 19-1. Atrial and ventricular patterns are quite similar. Both begin with a rapid depolarization, marked by 0 on the curves, which is caused by a rapid rush of sodium ion (Na^+) into the cells. The inside of the cell therefore becomes more positive as the electrical potential shifts from about -90 mV to about $+20$ mV. Shortly thereafter, chloride ion (Cl^-) enters the cardiac cell, so the electrical potential becomes more negative. This phase is marked by 1 on the curve. During the relatively long plateau period, marked phase 2 on the curve, sodium ion and calcium ion (Ca^{++}) slowly enter the cell, while potassium ion leaves. As time progresses, the sodium and calcium ions stop flowing in but potassium ion continues to flow out (phase 3). During this phase the electrical potential continues to become more negative. In the final phase of the action potential, sodium ion flows out of the cell in exchange for potassium ion, which enters the cell. At the end of this cycle, the cell has returned to the resting potential of about -90 mV and has regained the ability to generate another normal action poten-

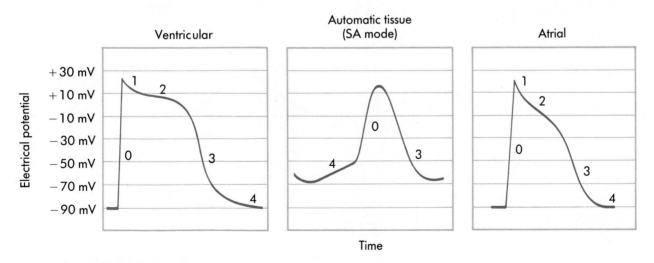

FIGURE 19-1

Typical action potential for three types of cardiac tissues. Action potentials are determined in the laboratory in tissues from experimental animals.

tial. From the beginning of phase 0 until sometime during the middle of phase 3, atrial or ventricular cells cannot be stimulated to beat again. This span of time is referred to as the ***refractory period.*** In nodal tissue the refractory period lasts well beyond phase 3 of the action potential.

Automaticity of Normal SA Nodal Cells

The action potential for the SA nodal tissue differs from that of atrial and ventricular cells. Most important in terms of cardiac physiology is the gradual depolarization that occurs during phase 4 (see Figure 19-1). This ability to gradually shift from a potential of about -70 mV to -50 or -40 mV triggers the start of the action potential (phase 0) in SA nodal cells. This process is called ***automaticity:*** the cells need no externally applied stimulus to initiate an action potential.

Electrocardiogram (ECG)

In the clinical setting, information about the function of a patient's heart must be gained from ECG tracings (Figure 19-2). These ECG tracings may be related to action potentials in various parts of the heart. The change in potential marked in Figure 19-2 as P (the P wave) is produced by the initial depolarization of atrial cells (phase 0 on the action potential). Very

shortly after this wave of depolarization, the atrium contracts to complete filling of the ventricles. The waves marked Q, R, and S (QRS complex) result from depolarization of the ventricles. Repolarization of the atria occurs at this time but is masked by large changes produced by the ventricles. Ventricular contraction occurs between the QRS complex and the midpoint of the T wave. The T wave is generated by repolarization (phase 1 through 3 of the action potential) of the ventricles.

MECHANISMS PRODUCING ARRHYTHMIAS

Arrhythmias occur because of disorders in the pacing of the heartbeat and/or disorders in conducting the impulse to beat through the heart tissues. Disorders in heart pacing are frequently related to changes in the automaticity of the heart. For example, the normal pacemaker of the heart, the SA node, may become overstimulated by the sympathetic nervous system. The catecholamine neurotransmitters for this branch of the nervous system increase the automaticity of the SA node. As a result, phase 4 on the action potential curve is steepened and shortened, phase 0 is triggered more frequently, and the heart beats more rapidly. In contrast, if the vagus nerve is predominant and sympathetic stimulation is re-

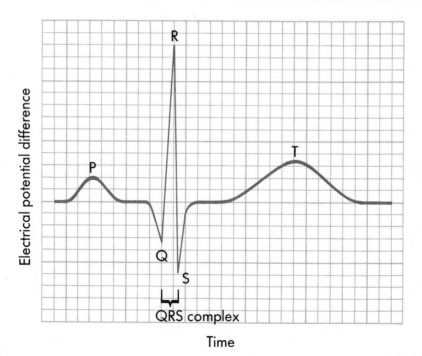

FIGURE 19-2

ECG tracing showing pattern typical of normal heart function.

moved, the heart rate decreases. This action occurs because acetylcholine from the vagus nerve decreases the automaticity of the SA node.

In addition to these disorders in automaticity at the SA node, the heart may suffer altered rates resulting from **ectopic foci** of automatic cells. These ectopic foci are groups of cells in the atria or the ventricles that spontaneously beat independently of the SA node. These groups of automatic cells may replace the SA node as the primary pacer for the heart, work in combination with the SA node so that the heart responds to both pacemakers, or interfere with SA nodal pacing so that neither pacing system is effective.

Conduction disorders are primarily of two types. One involves an alteration in the conduction time across the AV node. The AV node prevents the ventricles from receiving the impulse to beat until the atria have contracted and filled the ventricles (see Chapter 18). If the ventricles contract prematurely, ineffective pumping action occurs, because the chambers will be only partially filled. If the delay in transmission through the AV node becomes too long, skipped heartbeats may occur, since the AV node may still be in the refractory period from the last beat when the next impulse arrives from the SA node.

The second type of conduction disorder involves conduction through the contracting tissue. If an area of heart muscle becomes oxygen starved (ischemic)

or damaged, it may not only fail to contract, but it may also fail to properly conduct an action potential. Ordinarily the action potential spreads across the tissue in a pattern that allows all parts of the tissue to contract at the proper time so that the heart pumps efficiently. This damaged region alters the pattern of stimulation, and the subsequent contraction may not be rhythmic or effective. Occasionally the damaged area may alter conduction so that a phenomenon called *reentry* occurs. In reentry, the action potential from a single impulse to beat passes more than once through the same group of cells. In the extreme case, reentry may produce a continuous cycle or loop of electrical activity through part of the tissue that prevents the heart from contracting properly.

ANTIARRHYTHMIC DRUGS

The classification system described in Table 19-1 is based on the effects of the drugs on the action potential (see Figure 19-1). The classification system demonstrates the mechanistic relatedness of drugs that might otherwise seem unrelated. Even within groups, however, effects of the drugs may differ somewhat. Table 19-2 lists the specific actions and reactions generated by each drug.

Antiarrhythmics may have other applications. For example, propranolol, esmolol, and acebutolol block beta-adrenergic receptors (see Chapters 10 and 15);

Table 19-1   Classification of Antiarrhythmics with Indications for Use

Class	Drugs	Effect on action potential	Indications
I	Moricizine	Properties of all three subclasses	Ventricular arrhythmias
I-A	Disopyramide Procainamide Quinidine	Depress phase 0; prolong action potential duration	Ventricular and some supraventricular arrhythmias
I-B	Lidocaine Mexiletine Phenytoin Tocainide	Depress phase 0 slightly; may shorten action potential duration	Ventricular arrhythmias
I-C	Encainide Flecainide Propafenone	Depress phase 0 markedly; profound slowing of conduction	Ventricular arrhythmias
II	Acebutolol Esmolol Propranolol	Depress phase 4 depolarization	Supraventricular and other tachyarrhythmias; acebutolol for premature ventricular contractions
III	Amiodarone Bretylium	Prolong phase 3 repolarization	Ventricular tachycardia, ventricular fibrillation
IV	Verapamil	Depress phase 4 depolarization; lengthen phase 1 and 2	Supraventricular tachyarrhythmias

Table 19-2   Mechanism of Action of Antiarrhythmics

Drug	Predominant mechanism of antiarrhythmic action	Summary of cardiac actions			Adverse reactions
		Conduction velocity	Automaticity	Contractility	
Acebutolol	Selective blockade of beta-1 receptors in heart increases AV nodal refractory period.	Slowed	Decreased	Decreased	Bradycardia, lowered cardiac output; congestive heart failure; bronchospasm in asthmatics. FDA Pregnancy Category B.
Adenosine	Slows conduction through AV and SA nodes	Slowed	Decreased	Decreased	Transient depression of left ventricular function; new arrhythmias possibly including heart block. FDA Pregnancy Category C.
Amiodarone	Prolongs action potential duration and refractory period throughout heart.	Slowed	Decreased	Decreased	Bradycardia; pulmonary toxicity; neurotoxicity; hypothyroidism. FDA Pregnancy Category C.
Atropine	Blocks effects of vagus nerve stimulation.	Hastened	Increased	No change	Dry mouth, mydriasis, fever, urinary retention, confusion.
Bretylium	Prolongs effective refractory period.	No change	No change or slight increase	No change or slight increase	Bradycardia, hypotension, and precipitation of anginal attacks.
Digoxin	Slows conduction through AV node.	Slowed	Increased at high doses	Increased	Bradycardia, premature ventricular beats, AV nodal tachycardia, anorexia, nausea.
Disopyramide	Suppresses automaticity, especially in ectopic foci, by membrane-stabilizing and anticholinergic effects.	No change or slightly slowed	Decreased	Decreased	Anticholinergic effects: dry mouth, constipation, urinary retention, blurred vision; hypoglycemia. FDA Pregnancy Category C.
Encainide	Prolongs refractory period in conductive fibers; markedly slows conduction in atria.	Slowed	Decreased	No change	New ventricular arrhythmias; bradycardia; AV block; congestive heart failure. FDA Pregnancy Category B.
Esmolol	Cardioselective beta adrenergic receptor blockade; increases AV nodal refractory period.	Slowed	Decreased	Decreased	Bradycardia; confusion; impaired peripheral circulation. FDA Pregnancy Category C.
Flecainide	Prolongs refractory period in conductive fibers; markedly slows conduction in atria.	Slowed	Decreased	Slightly decreased	New ventricular arrhythmias; AV block; bradycardia; congestive heart failure. FDA Pregnancy Category C.
Lidocaine	Increases electrical threshold for ventricular stimulation.	No change	Decreased	No change	Confusion, drowsiness, convulsions. FDA Pregnancy Category B.
Mexiletine	Prolongs refractory period in conductive fibers.	No change	Decreased	No change	Ventricular arrhythmias; shortness of breath; hepatic necrosis. FDA Pregnancy Category C.
Moricizine	Decreases excitability, conduction velocity, automaticity in nodal tissue; also potent local anesthetic and membrane stabilizing effects.	Slowed	Decreased	Decreased	Congestive heart failure, new ventricular arrhythmias, neurotoxicity, dizziness. FDA Pregnancy Category B.

Table 19-2   Mechanism of Action of Antiarrhythmics—cont'd

Drug	Predominant mechanism of antiarrhythmic action	Summary of cardiac actions			Adverse reactions
		Conduction velocity	Automaticity	Contractility	
Phenytoin	Depresses spontaneous depolarization in ventricular and atrial but not nodal tissue.	No change or slightly hastened	Decreased	No change	Severe myocardial toxicity caused by rapid intravenous injection; cerebellar side effects caused by chronic use.
Procainamide	Suppresses automaticity, especially in ectopic foci, by membrane-stabilizing and anticholinergic effects.	Slowed	Decreased	Decreased	Hypotension, decreased cardiac output, ventricular tachycardia, allergy, gastrointestinal (GI) distress; lupuslike syndrome caused by chronic use. FDA Pregnancy Category C.
Propafenone	Slows conduction in AV node and ventricular tissue.	Slowed	Decreased	Decreased	Congestive heart failure, new ventricular arrhythmias, AV blockade, sinus arrest, convulsions, dizziness. FDA Pregnancy Category B.
Propranolol	Increases AV nodal refractory period by beta-adrenergic blockade and membrane-stabilizing effects.	Slowed	Decreased	Decreased	Bradycardia, lowered cardiac output; congestive heart failure; bronchospasm in persons with asthma.
Quinidine	Suppresses automaticity, especially in ectopic foci, by membrane-stabilizing and anticholinergic effects.	Slowed	Decreased	Decreased	Peripheral vasodilation, hypotension, paradoxical ventricular tachycardia, decreased cardiac output, cinchonism, allergy, fever, GI distress. FDA Pregnancy Category C.
Tocainide	Increases threshold of excitability in conductive fibers.	No change	Decreased	No change	Pulmonary toxicity, allergic reactions, blood dyscrasias. FDA Pregnancy Category C.
Verapamil	Blocks calcium channels and slows conduction through AV node.	Slowed	No change or slightly decreased	Decreased	IV: Hypotension, bradycardia, asystole; ORAL: GI disturbances, lightheadedness, headache, nervousness. FDA Pregnancy Category C.

in the heart this action slows the rate at the SA node and slows conduction through the AV node. The effect at both sites is to slow heart rate. Anticholinergic drugs, such as atropine, may produce the opposite effect by blocking the muscarinic receptors by which the heart responds to vagal nerve stimulation. Calcium channel blocking drugs such as verapamil primarily change the responses of cells highly dependent on the so-called slow calcium current (e.g., AV nodal cells or cells in ischemic regions of muscle). Local anesthetics, such as lidocaine and related drugs, alter cardiac cell membranes, and thus change the sodium ion influx that causes phase 0 of the action potential. Table 19-3 describes drugs for controlling arrhythmias.

Class I Antiarrhythmic Drugs

Class I antiarrhythmic drugs block sodium channels that are required for phase 0 of the action potential. This class of agents has been subdivided based on additional properties of the drugs. Moricizine does not clearly fit into any one of these subclasses but has properties of all.

Moricizine

In addition to blocking sodium channels, moricizine also has potent local anesthetic activity and membrane-stabilizing activity. It may also have anticholinergic effects. The AV node and the His-Purkinje system are most sensitive to moricizine. Conduction through these tissues is slowed considerably, but there is little effect on the SA node.

Table 19-3 Drugs Used to Control Cardiac Arrhythmias

Generic name	Trade name	Administration/dosage	Comments
Acebutolol	Monitan† Sectral*	ORAL: *Adults*—200 mg twice daily; adjust according to response.	Mild intrinsic sympathomimetic effect and cardioselectivity should reduce risk of bronchospasm, hypoglycemia, and impaired peripheral circulation.
Adenosine	Adenocard	INTRAVENOUS: *Adults*—6 mg given rapidly over 1 to 2 sec. If not effective, 12 mg may be given 1 to 2 min later.	Extremely short half-life, thus side effects are usually self-limiting.
Amiodarone	Cordarone*	ORAL: *Adults*—800 mg to 1.6 gm daily in divided doses; reduce dose when control is adequate or side effects occur, 600 to 800 mg daily for 1 month; maintain with lowest effective dose. *Children*—10 mg/kg body weight or 800 mg/1.72 M² daily until control is adequate or side effects occur; reduce to 5 mg/kg or 400 mg/1.72 M² for several weeks; maintain with lowest effective dose.	Very long duration of action (weeks or months) and very slow onset (2 days to 2 months). Persists in the body for months after the drug is discontinued.
Atropine		INTRAVENOUS: *Adults*—0.4 to 1 mg every 1 to 2 hr as needed, up to a maximum of 2 mg. *Children*—0.01 to 0.03 mg/kg body weight.	Rapidly effective; excreted by the kidney within 12 hr of administration.
Bretylium tosylate	Bretylol Bretylate†	INTRAMUSCULAR: *Adults*—5 to 10 mg/kg repeated in 1 to 2 hr, then every 6 to 8 hr. INTRAVENOUS: *Adults*—5 to 10 mg/kg repeated every 15 to 30 min to a maximum dose of 30 mg/kg.	Excreted unchanged by the kidneys. One intramuscular site should receive no more than 5 ml of undiluted drug.
Digoxin	Lanoxin*	ORAL: *Adults*—tablets or elixir, load with 0.5 to 0.75 mg, followed by 0.25 to 0.5 mg every 6 to 8 hr to a total dose of 1 to 1.5 mg; maintain with 0.125 to 0.5 mg daily. *Children*—doses are individualized for age and body weight.	Effective serum level 1 to 2 ng/ml and toxic at 3 ng/ml; elimination half-time is about 36 hr. Bioavailability with capsules is higher so that 0.1-mg dose is equivalent to 0.125 mg in tablets.
Disopyramide	Norpace* Rythmodan†	ORAL: *Adults*—100 to 140 mg every 6 hr. Maintenance may use extended-release forms 300 mg every 12 hr. *Children*—6 to 30 mg/kg body weight daily divided into 4 doses.	Effective serum level 2 to 4 μg/ml; serum half-life 4 hr, kidneys eliminate 80% of the active drug and metabolites.
Encainide	Enkaid	ORAL: *Adults*—25 mg every 8 hr; after 3 to 5 days may be increased to 35 mg every 8 hr, then 50 mg every 8 hr. Individual dose should not exceed 75 mg.	Rapidly metabolized to active metabolites in liver.
Esmolol	Brevibloc	INTRAVENOUS: *Adults*—0.5 mg/kg body weight in 1 min, then 0.05 mg/kg/min for 4 min. Increase maintenance dose as necessary up to 0.2 mg/kg.	This very short-acting drug must be given by continuous infusion. May be used up to 48 hr.
Flecainide	Tambocor*	ORAL: *Adults*—100 mg every 12 hr, increasing in increments of 50 mg twice daily every 4 days as needed. Maximum daily dose 400 to 600 mg.	Toxicity increases at plasma concentrations above 0.7 to 1 μg/ml.
Lidocaine	Xylocaine HCl* (for cardiac arrhythmias) Xylocard†	INTRAMUSCULAR: *Adults*—emergency use, 4.3 mg/kg, or 3 ml of 10% solution (300 mg). INTRAVENOUS: *Adults*—up to 300 mg in any 1-hr period. *Children*—continuous infusion, 20 to 50 μg/kg body weight/min.	Effective serum level 1 to 5 μg/ml; serum half-life 15 to 20 min; metabolized in liver; toxicity increased by reduced liver blood flow or function.

*Available in Canada and United States.
†Available in Canada only.

Table 19-3   Drugs Used to Control Cardiac Arrhythmias—cont'd

Generic name	Trade name	Administration/dosage	Comments
Mexiletine	Mexitil*	ORAL: *Adults*—200 mg every 8 hr; adjust up or down by 50 to 100 mg per dose every 2 to 3 days. Doses not to exceed 1200 mg daily.	Effective plasma concentrations are 0.5 to 2 μg/ml, but toxicity may be observed even at these levels.
Moricizine	Ethmozine	ORAL: *Adults*—200 to 300 mg every 8 hr, not to exceed 900 mg daily.	Adverse cardiac effects occur in many patients. Careful monitoring is essential.
Phenytoin	Dilantin*	INTRAVENOUS: *Adults*—50 to 100 mg given over 10 min. Repeat if necessary at 5- to 15-min intervals. Dose held under 1 gm, or 15 mg/kg body weight.	Arrhythmias are not official indications for phenytoin, but it has been used for digitalis-induced arrhythmias.
Procainamide	Promine Pronestyl*	ORAL: *Adults*—500 mg to 1 gm every 4 to 6 hr. *Children*—50 mg/kg daily in 4 to 6 divided doses. INTRAMUSCULAR: *Adults*—250 to 1000 mg every 4 to 8 hr. INTRAVENOUS: *Adults*—100 mg over 5 min as needed.	Effective serum level 4 to 8 μg/ml; serum half-life about 3 hr.
Procainamide sustained release	Procan-SR* Pronestyl-SR*	ORAL: *Adults*—50 mg/kg/day divided into 4 doses.	Absorption is variable and may be extremely low.
Propafenone	Rythmol*	ORAL: *Adults*—initially 150 mg every 8 hr, increasing gradually to a maximum of 300 mg every 8 hr.	Adverse cardiac effects occur in many patients. Careful monitoring is essential.
Propranolol	Inderal* Detensol†	ORAL: *Adults*—10 to 30 mg 3 or 4 times daily. *Children*—0.5 to 4 mg/kg daily in 2 to 4 doses. INTRAVENOUS: *Adults*—1 mg/min for 1 to 3 min; repeat after 2 min and 4 hr. *Children*—0.01 to 0.10 mg/kg over 3 to 5 min up to 1 mg.	Effective serum level is highly variable; serum half-life 2½ to 4 hr; metabolized in the liver.
Quinidine gluconate	Duraquin Quinaglute* Quinalan Quinate†	ORAL: *Adults*—325 to 650 mg every 6 hr. INTRAMUSCULAR: *Adults*—initially 600 mg; 200 to 400 mg every 2 to 6 hr. INTRAVENOUS: *Adults*—20 mg each min with ECG and blood pressure monitoring.	More slowly absorbed than quinidine sulfate.
Quinidine polygalacturonate	Cardioquin	ORAL: *Adults*—as for quinidine sulfate (1 tablet of 275 mg is equivalent to 200 mg of quinidine sulfate).	Less irritating to gastrointestinal tract than other forms of quinidine.
Quinidine sulfate	Cin-Quin Quinidex Extentabs* Quinora	ORAL: *Adults*—200 to 400 mg 4 times daily. *Children*—6 mg/kg every 4 to 6 hr.	Effective serum level 3 to 6 μg/ml.
Tocainide	Tonocard*	ORAL: *Adults*—400 mg every 8 hr, adjusted as necessary; maintenance 1200 to 1800 mg daily divided into 3 doses.	Bioavailability is high and is unaffected by food.
Verapamil	Calan Isoptin*	ORAL: *Adults*—240 to 480 mg daily divided into 3 or 4 doses. *Children*—4 to 8 mg/kg daily in divided doses. INTRAVENOUS: *Adults*—initially 5 to 10 mg over 2 to 5 min, repeated if necessary at 30 min. *Infants to 1 yr*—0.1 to 0.3 mg/kg over 2 min, repeated if necessary at 30 min.	Therapeutic serum levels are 0.08 to 0.3 μg/ml.

*Available in Canada and United States.
†Available in Canada only.

Absorption, distribution, and excretion. Moricizine is extensively biotransformed by the liver and has a half-life of about 2 hr. The drug is well absorbed orally but is subject to first-pass effects (see Chapter 1) that lower the absolute bioavailability to about 38%. The onset of action is usually within 2 hr. Elimination is by the biliary/fecal route and by the kidneys, but little unchanged drug is eliminated.

Side effects. Moricizine, like other antiarrhythmics, can induce new arrhythmias in some patients. About 4% of patients receiving the drug in controlled trials suffered new or exacerbated ventricular arrhythmias. Other patients developed signs of congestive heart failure, AV block, or sinus arrest. Dizziness and other central nervous system (CNS) effects may also be observed with chronic administration.

Toxicity. Overdoses of moricizine have been fatal, producing cardiotoxicity, coma, and respiratory failure. Most of the side effects are dose-related and become more pronounced as doses exceed the normal therapeutic range.

Class I-A Antiarrhythmic Drugs

Class I-A antiarrhythmic drugs depress phase 0 of the action potential (see Figure 19-1) and prolong the action potential duration. The effective refractory period is therefore prolonged in atria and ventricles, making the tissue less electrically responsive. Class I-A antiarrhythmics are indicated for prophylaxis and treatment of ventricular arrhythmias (premature contractions and tachycardia); quinidine and procainamide may also be used for atrial tachycardia or fibrillation.

Quinidine and procainamide

Quinidine and procainamide have virtually identical mechanisms of action. They alter calcium distribution within the cardiac cell, thereby decreasing contractility of the heart muscle. Quinidine and procainamide have atropine-like effects that block the effect of the vagus nerve on the heart. Finally, both drugs alter the membranes of cardiac cells, resulting in a prolonged refractory period. The ability of these drugs to prolong the refractory period of cardiac tissues may explain their ability to suppress ectopic foci. Quinidine and procainamide have equipotent membrane effects; however, quinidine has more potent anticholinergic effects.

Absorption, distribution, and excretion. Quinidine sulfate is relatively rapidly absorbed by oral routes. The half-life of quinidine in serum is about 6 hr. Quinidine gluconate is more slowly absorbed orally and hence slightly longer acting. Quinidine polygalacturonate is less irritative to the gastrointestinal (GI) tract than other forms of quinidine. Quinidine

is partially metabolized in liver; up to 50% of a dose may be excreted unchanged in the urine, and the drug may accumulate in patients in renal failure.

Procainamide reaches effective concentrations in the serum (4 to 8 μg/ml) within 1 to 3 hr of an oral dose or within 30 min of an IM dose. The half-life of the drug in serum is 3 hr and about half the drug dose is eliminated unchanged in the kidney.

Side effects. The anticholinergic effects of quinidine and procainamide in some ways oppose the direct action of the drugs. The dual effects of quinidine have caused serious complications in the treatment of atrial fibrillation. Although the direct effects of quinidine might be expected to slow the atrial rate, the first observed effect may be an anticholinergic action producing increased conduction through the AV node, with the result that ventricular rates soar dangerously high before quinidine can slow atrial rates.

Toxicity. The primary difference between quinidine and procainamide is in the toxic effects produced. Quinidine is commonly associated with GI reactions, but the most serious reactions include allergic responses and cardiovascular toxicity. When the drug is given intravenously, hypotension may result. Quinidine is an arteriolar and venous dilator. This action may account for the reduction in cardiac output in some patients taking quinidine. At higher doses, usually resulting in blood levels above 8 μg/ml, quinidine may produce ventricular arrhythmias, including ectopic beats, tachycardia, and fibrillation. Quinidine causes a dose-dependent widening of the QRS complex. This effect can monitor its therapeutic activity.

Like quinidine, procainamide may cause GI discomfort to patients receiving the medication orally. Procainamide is less completely bound to plasma proteins than quinidine and therefore less subject to unexpected drug interactions resulting from displacement from plasma protein binding sites (see Chapter 2). Allergic and immunologic reactions are among the most striking adverse effects of procainamide. With long-term use the drug may produce a syndrome that resembles lupus erythematosus, including symptoms such as arthritis and arthralgia, myalgia, fever, and pericarditis. Direct toxic effects on the heart usually relate to changes in conduction within the heart, especially at the AV nodal tissue and the conducting fibers of the ventricles. These direct toxic effects on the heart are usually produced when blood levels exceed 12 μg/ml. Since normal therapeutic concentrations range from about 4 to 8 μg/ml, this drug, like the other antiarrhythmic drugs, has a very narrow safety margin. Like quinidine, procainamide widens the QRS complex on the ECG and lengthens the refractory period.

Disopyramide phosphate

Disopyramide phosphate is similar in action to procainamide and quinidine.

Absorption, distribution, and excretion. Disopyramide is rapidly and almost completely absorbed following oral administration. Biotransformation by the liver produces metabolites with antimuscarinic, as well as antiarrhythmic, activities. About half of each dose is eliminated unchanged by the kidneys.

Side effects. Difficulty in urination, which is an antimuscarinic effect, may be experienced by 10% to 20% of treated patients. Up to 10% of patients suffer hypotension (dizziness or fainting), altered heart function (change in rhythm or heart failure), or fluid retention (congestive heart failure). Dry mouth, another antimuscarinic effect, is very common but not dangerous.

Toxicity. Overdose causes pronounced widening of the QRS complex and the QT interval of the ECG. Cardiac arrhythmias may ensue. Apnea, loss of spontaneous respirations, and unconsciousness precede death by cardiovascular collapse.

Class I-B Antiarrhythmic Drugs

Class I-B antiarrhythmic drugs slightly depress phase 0 of the action potential (Figure 19-1) and may shorten the action potential duration. As a group, these drugs have much less effect on atria than the class I-A drugs. Class I-B antiarrhythmic agents are indicated for ventricular arrhythmias, including those arising from myocardial infarction (MI), cardiac surgery, cardiac catheterization, or digitalis toxicity.

Lidocaine

Lidocaine is a local anesthetic (see Chapter 46) that alters sodium ion conduction in heart cells. Its antiarrhythmic action affects ventricular tissue more than atrial or nodal tissues.

Absorption, distribution, and excretion. Lidocaine is eliminated primarily by the liver, and over 90% of a dose is rapidly destroyed in that tissue. For this reason the drug is useful primarily when administered as a continuous infusion.

Side effects and toxicity. Lidocaine causes a variety of CNS reactions, ranging from muscle twitching and drowsiness to paresthesia, respiratory depression, convulsions, and coma. These reactions may be dose-dependent; CNS reactions are expected when serum concentrations exceed 8 μg/ml. Toxic reactions to lidocaine are more common in patients with reduced hepatic function, because the drug may accumulate in these patients.

When administering lidocaine, recall that the drug has two separate clinical uses and is packaged differently for each. When intended for use as a local anesthetic, lidocaine is frequently packaged in solution with epinephrine (e.g., Xylocaine or other trade names with epinephrine). When used with the local anesthetic, epinephrine acts as a vasoconstrictor to reduce local blood flow and prolong the action of the anesthetic. If lidocaine with epinephrine were inadvertently administered to treat a cardiac arrhythmia, the epinephrine might trigger a severe arrhythmia by stimulating automaticity of the heart. Lidocaine intended for use in cardiac emergencies is labeled "lidocaine preservative-free" or "Xylocaine for ventricular arrhythmias or continuous infusion."

Mexiletine

Mexiletine is an oral antiarrhythmic drug with a mechanism of action similar to parenteral lidocaine. Both drugs have local anesthetic properties. Mexiletine also has anticonvulsant actions.

Absorption, distribution, and excretion. Mexiletine is well absorbed from the GI tract, making oral administration practical and effective. The onset of effect is within ½ to 2 hr. Elimination is primarily by hepatic metabolism; the half-life of the drug in the blood may be doubled in severe hepatic disease but only slightly increased in renal impairment.

Side effects and toxicity. Side effects of mexiletine are generally dose-related, with the incidence increasing when plasma concentrations exceed 2 μg/ml. New ventricular arrhythmias may arise, including premature ventricular contractions and torsades de pointes. Heartburn, nausea, and vomiting usually occur within 2 hr of administration. Agranulocytosis, leukopenia, and thrombocytopenia may cause fever, chills, and unusual bruising or bleeding. CNS effects include dizziness, trembling, nervousness, and unsteady gait. Overdose can cause death due to respiratory failure and asystole.

Phenytoin

Phenytoin, a drug also used as an anticonvulsant (see Chapter 34), may alter cardiac function by CNS effects. In heart cells, phenytoin changes membrane responsiveness, reducing the possibility for reentry, a process that contributes to severe arrhythmias. The major use of phenytoin is for digitalis-induced arrhythmias. Phenytoin is less effective for arrhythmias of other types.

Therapeutic, nontoxic levels of phenytoin do not cause significant depression of myocardial contractility. However, the drug can produce dangerous myocardial depression if intravenous (IV) administration is too rapid. Bradycardia, hypotension, AV blockade, and cardiac arrest have been observed with venous injection faster than 50 mg/min. The patient is observed for nausea, dizziness, or drowsiness, which are signs of excessive blood levels of the drug. Chronic use of phenytoin for its antiarrhythmic action is not recommended.

Tocainide

Tocainide, like lidocaine, is an amide-type of local anesthetic. Its action in the heart is similar to that of lidocaine.

Absorption, distribution, and excretion. Tocainide is completely absorbed orally, whether taken with or without food. The onset of action is within ½ to 2 hr, and the half-life is about 15 hr. Elimination is nearly equally divided between hepatic metabolism and renal excretion.

Side effects and toxicity. Shaking and trembling signal that maximal doses have been approached. Blisters, peeling skin, or skin rashes may signal a dangerous allergic reaction that can culminate in Stevens-Johnson syndrome. After several weeks of therapy, pulmonary damage can occur, with coughing and shortness of breath. Allergic reactions or pulmonary damage can be fatal.

Class I-C Antiarrhythmic Drugs

Class I-C antiarrhythmics drugs markedly depress phase 0 of the action potential (see Figure 19-1) and profoundly slow conduction, especially in conductive fibers. Class I-C antiarrhythmic agents are indicated only for control of life-threatening ventricular arrhythmias.

Encainide

Encainide may have greater effect in ischemic than in normal heart tissue. The drug has little effect on cardiac contractility.

Absorption, distribution, and excretion. Oral absorption is nearly total, with onset of action within 1 to 3 hr. Encainide is eliminated by hepatic metabolism to active metabolites. About 90% of the population rapidly form these metabolites while the remaining 10% metabolize encainide slowly and accumulate few of these metabolites.

Side effects and toxicity. Encainide has been associated with development of new and potentially fatal arrhythmias, especially when daily doses exceed 200 mg. Congestive heart failure, AV blockade, sinus bradycardia, sinus pause, or sinus arrest may occur. Overdose produces widening of the QRS complex, prolongation of the QT interval, AV dissociation, hypotension, bradycardia, asystole, and seizures and finally can cause death.

Flecainide

Flecainide is very similar to encainide but has local anesthetic action and may decrease contractility of the heart more than encainide.

Absorption, distribution, and excretion. Flecainide is nearly completely absorbed following oral administration with or without food. The major route of elimination is by hepatic metabolism, and the drug has a long half-life of approximately 20 hr.

Side effects and toxicity. Flecainide has been associated with development of new and potentially fatal arrhythmias, especially when plasma concentrations exceed 1 μg/ml. Ventricular arrhythmias, congestive heart failure, and AV block are most common.

Propafenone

Propafenone primarily affects the AV node, slowing conduction markedly. The drug also has a weak beta-adrenergic blocking effect (¹⁄₄₀ as effective as propanolol) and a strong local anesthetic action. Propafenone has a negative inotropic effect that increases the risk for congestive heart failure.

Absorption, distribution, and excretion. Propafenone is well absorbed orally, but a first-pass effect (see Chapter 1) reduces the absolute bioavailability to 10% or less. The liver converts propafenone to several products, some of which are also active as antiarrhythmics. Elimination is primarily by renal mechanisms. The half-life of the drug is 2 to 10 hr in most patients, but up to 10% of the population metabolize the drug much more slowly. For slow metabolizers, the half life is 10 to 32 hr. Steady-state concentrations of the drug are achieved after 4 or 5 days, but the steady-state plasma concentrations vary widely as a result of variations in metabolism.

Propafenone interferes with metabolism or elimination of digoxin and can significantly increase the serum concentrations of digoxin. Doses of digoxin may have to be reduced and serum concentrations monitored when propafenone is also being given.

Side effects and toxicity. Propafenone, like other antiarrhythmics, can induce new arrhythmias in some patients. About 5% of patients receiving the drug in controlled trials suffered new or exacerbated ventricular arrhythmias. Other patients developed signs of congestive heart failure, AV block, or sinus bradycardia. Dizziness and other CNS effects may also be observed with chronic administration. Many patients also report a change in their sense of taste.

The side effects of propafenone are dose related, and at high doses the cardiotoxic effects can become severe, with dangerous new arrhythmias, heart block, and severe congestive heart failure.

Class II Antiarrhythmic Drugs

Class II antiarrhythmic drugs are beta-adrenergic receptor blockers that depress phase 4 depolarization of the action potential (see Figure 19-1). Acebutolol and esmolol primarily block beta-1 receptors in the heart, but propranolol blocks beta receptors in many tissues.

Acebutolol

Acebutolol differs from the other antiarrhythmic drugs of this class by having mild-to-moderate intrinsic sympathomimetic activity. In theory, blockade with this type of agent would never be complete, which would minimize risk of certain side effects. Acebutolol primarily controls premature ventricular contractions.

Absorption, distribution, and excretion. About 70% of an oral dose of acebutolol is absorbed. Metabolism by the liver produces an active metabolite with a longer half-life than that of the parent drug. The peak effect is obtained within 2 ½ hr and persists for several hours. Elimination also involves renal excretion.

Side effects and toxicity. Like all beta-adrenergic blockers, acebutolol may cause hypoglycemia, peripheral vasoconstriction, and bronchospasm, but because the blockade is relatively selective for cardiac beta receptors, these effects may in theory be less likely. Overdose may cause slow or irregular heartbeat, dizziness, fainting, difficulty breathing, blue fingernail beds, or seizures.

Esmolol

Esmolol is intended for rapid, short-term control of ventricular rates in atrial flutter or fibrillation. It is primarily an emergency medication for perioperative or postoperative use.

Absorption, distribution, and excretion. Esmolol is administered by IV, is distributed to tissues within 2 min, and achieves therapeutic effect within 5 min. The duration of effect lasts only 10 to 20 min after the infusion is stopped. The drug is rapidly destroyed by esterases in red blood cells.

Side effects and toxicity. Hypotension is very common in patients receiving esmolol and may be symptomatic in up to 12% of patients. Reduced peripheral circulation and difficulty breathing may also occur. Overdose may cause slow or irregular heartbeat, dizziness, fainting, difficulty breathing, blue fingernail beds, or seizures.

Propranolol

Propranolol is a beta-adrenergic blocking drug (see Chapter 10) that decreases contractility in the heart. It may decrease cardiac automaticity by blocking the effects of the sympathetic nervous system. The most important antiarrhythmic action of propranolol is to increase the refractory period of the AV node. In addition, the drug has a quinidine-like membrane effect that slows phase 0 of the action potential. Propranolol is used for supraventricular arrhythmias,

ventricular tachycardias, and drug-induced tachyarrhythmias.

Absorption, distribution, and excretion. Propranolol is well absorbed orally, but blood levels are diminished by a substantial first-pass effect (see Chapter 2). Elimination is primarily by hepatic mechanisms.

Side effects and toxicity. The most significant dangers of propranolol used as an antiarrhythmic agent result from the beta-adrenergic blockade. This effect is especially dangerous in patients with a significant degree of heart failure that has been compensated by increased sympathetic stimulation of the heart. Blockade of these sympathetic influences may produce bradycardia or heart arrest, especially if partial AV block already exists. In addition, propranolol may precipitate severe bronchospasm, because it also blocks the beta receptors in the lung (see Chapter 25). This reaction is more common in patients with a history of asthma or allergies.

Of the beta-adrenergic drugs commonly used as antiarrhythmics, propranolol is most likely to cause CNS side effects, such as mental depression, dizziness, drowsiness, insomnia, or weakness.

Class III Antiarrhythmic Drugs

Class III antiarrhythmics primarily prolong phase 3, the repolarization phase, of the action potential (see Figure 19-1).

Amiodarone

Amiodarone has many actions on cardiac tissues, which result in prolonging the refractory period and reducing automaticity. Amiodarone also may depress contractility and may cause vasodilation. The drug produces noncompetitive beta-adrenergic blockade and blocks calcium channels. It is used for prophylaxis or therapy for life-threatening ventricular arrhythmias.

Absorption, distribution, and excretion. Oral absorption is variable, and most patients absorb much less than half the administered dose. Amiodarone is highly lipid soluble and is sequestered in adipose tissue, as well as other sites. As a result the onset of action is measured in days or even months. The duration of action is also greatly prolonged. The drug may be detectable in plasma up to 9 months after it has been discontinued.

Side effects and toxicity. Sinus bradycardia is common, and arrest or heart block may occur. New arrhythmias may be generated in up to 5% of patients. Up to 15% of patients suffer significant pulmonary toxicity, which may be fatal. Neurotoxicity, signaled by weakness, numbness, or ataxia, may occur in up to 40% of patients. Sensitivity to sun, ocular toxicity, and hypothyroidism are also expected effects. Reversal of side effects may take months after cessation of therapy.

Bretylium

Bretylium has a mechanism of action different from that of other antiarrhythmic drugs. The drug increases the action potential duration and hence prolongs the refractory period. It does not directly suppress automaticity or conduction velocity. Bretylium accumulates in sympathetic neurons and causes an initial release of norepinephrine that may stimulate contractility, heart rate, and automaticity, but ultimately the drug produces an adrenergic blockade by preventing norepinephrine release. Bretylium is used primarily for life-threatening ventricular tachycardia, especially episodes refractory to lidocaine or cardioversion, and for ventricular fibrillation.

Absorption, distribution, and excretion. Bretylium is administered by IV or intramuscularly (IM). The duration of action is 6 to 8 hr and most of the drug is excreted by the kidneys.

Side effects and toxicity. The major reactions to this drug are precipitation of anginal attacks, bradycardia, and hypotention. Bretylium does not alter the ECG.

Class IV Antiarrhythmic Drugs

Class IV antiarrhythmic drugs primarily depress phase 4 depolarization and lengthen phase 1 and 2 repolarization. The heart rate may slow significantly.

Verapamil

Verapamil is a calcium channel blocking drug used not only as an antiarrhythmic agent but also as an antianginal agent (see Chapter 14). The slow calcium ion current blocked by verapamil is more important for the activity of the AV node than for many other tissues in the heart. By interfering with this current, the calcium channel blockers achieve some selectivity of action. The major antiarrhythmic effect of verapamil is a delay in conduction through the AV node.

The drug is well absorbed by the oral route, but is rapidly metabolized by the liver. This first-pass phenomenon significantly reduces its bioavailability (see Chapter 1). Some of its metabolites may be active. Cirrhosis of the liver significantly diminishes drug elimination. Verapamil may be administered intravenously when the oral route is inappropriate.

Miscellaneous Antiarrhythmic Drugs

Adenosine

Adenosine is a naturally occurring metabolite that is recognized as an autocoid. Receptors for adenosine exist on the outer surface of many cells in the body, including cells in blood vessels and organs such as the brain, heart, and kidneys. Large doses of adenosine given by rapid IV injection are effective in terminating supraventricular tachycardia and returning the heart to normal sinus rhythm. Adenosine slows conduction in the SA and AV nodes and can interrupt reentry. In addition, adenosine may impair ventricular function, but because the drug has a half-life of about 10 sec, this undesired action is considered minor and transient for most patients. The antiarrhythmic effect persists after the drug has been metabolized and removed.

Atropine

Atropine, previously discussed as a blocker of muscarinic cholinergic receptors (see Chapter 9), may also be used to treat certain arrhythmias. Its action as an antiarrhythmic drug depends on its ability to reduce the effects of vagal nerve stimulation, primarily on the SA node. Since stimulation of the vagus nerve slows heart rate, atropine increases heart rate by blocking that effect. Because it also speeds conduction through the AV node, it may lessen heart block in certain cases.

Digitalis

Digitalis is primarily a cardiotonic agent (see Chapter 18). However, in addition to its ability to strengthen contraction of the heart muscle, digitalis also increases vagal tone at the AV node. Through this action and the direct effects on nodal tissue, digitalis slows conduction through the AV node. This action is sought when digitalis is used as an antiarrhythmic agent.

As with the other antiarrhythmic drugs, higher concentrations of digitalis may also cause arrhythmias of various types, most characteristically bradycardia and premature ventricular contractions (PVCs). Bradycardia may be a sign of impending heart block (no impulse passes through the AV node to the ventricles). PVCs arise because digitalis increases the spontaneous rate of ventricular depolarization (phase 4 of the action potential). It increases the automaticity of Purkinje fibers in the ventricles. Any digitalis preparation can be used as an antiarrhythmic agent. However, in practice digoxin is commonly given IV in an emergency and then continued orally for maintenance or prophylaxis (see Table 19-3). Deslanoside (Cedilanid-D) may sometimes be used in emergencies.

PHARMACOLOGIC THERAPY OF ARRHYTHMIAS

Atrial flutter and **fibrillation** are usually serious arrhythmias that demand treatment. Several useful drugs are available. The digitalis glycoside, digoxin, is frequently selected. The rationale for this therapy is that by lowering the conduction of impulses through the AV node, digoxin protects the ventricles from overstimulation. The short-term therapeutic goal is not to slow the atrial rate, but to produce a partial heart block that allows fewer of the impulses from the atria to stimulate the ventricles to beat. The patient may therefore be maintained with rapid atrial rates but with ventricular rates from 60 to 80 beats/min. Many patients spontaneously convert to normal sinus rhythm after a few days of treatment.

Beta-adrenergic blockers such as esmolol or propranolol can also slow ventricular rates in atrial flutter, fibrillation, or tachycardia. These agents prolong AV conduction times and block beta-adrenergic receptors, which may also reduce catecholamine stimulation of the heart. Both effects slow heart rate.

Occasionally, quinidine may be selected to control atrial flutter or fibrillation. Since its anticholinergic action may speed conduction through the AV node, the first result of this therapy may be a dramatic increase in the ventricular rate. Digoxin or a related drug should always be used before quinidine in this case to prevent a dangerous overstimulation of the ventricles during the initial phases of treatment. Once atrial rates have been sufficiently reduced, this action of quinidine on the AV nodes poses no particular problem to the patient.

Verapamil may also effectively slow AV conduction and protect the ventricles when atrial flutter or fibrillation is present.

Sinus tachycardia, a rapid atrial rate, may not be harmful unless the ventricular rate is also abnormally increased. Many physicians do not administer antiarrhythmic drugs to patients with rapid atrial rates and no other symptoms. Sinus tachycardia may be produced in normal persons by anxiety; ingestion of coffee, tea, or alcoholic beverages; or smoking. Nitrites, sympathomimetics, anticholinergics, or phenothiazines may also induce transient sinus tachycardia.

Paroxysmal supraventricular tachycardia, a rapid heart rate produced by sudden overactivity in the atria, is often treated with adenosine. Given by rapid IV injection, this drug can convert the heart back to normal sinus rhythm.

Sinus bradycardia is usually of minor importance and not treated. If bradycardia is associated with reduced cardiac output, atropine or isoproterenol may be prescribed. Atropine increases the heart rate by blocking the effects of vagal nerve stimulation, whereas isoproterenol directly stimulates the heart through the beta-adrenergic receptors.

Premature ventricular contractions (PVCs) occur when the ventricles beat in response to both the SA node and an abnormal pacemaker. The ECG pattern shows a normal QRS complex following a P wave (see Figure 19-2), plus an abnormal QRS complex that is isolated from a P wave. These arrhythmias are found even among normal persons. If these PVCs are rare, they are ordinarily not treated, unless the patient is recuperating from a myocardial infarction (MI). If the patient complains of palpitations with the PVCs, mild sedatives may be prescribed. Abstaining from coffee, tea, and cigarettes may also control the condition.

When PVCs occur frequently or in rapid succession or with other signs of cardiac disease, treatment may be instituted with lidocaine, acebutolol, disopyramide, mexiletine, tocainide, quinidine, or procainamide. If these contractions are caused by a previous MI, lidocaine is the drug of choice in the hospital.

Ventricular tachycardia usually relates to ectopic foci that are stimulating PVCs. Lidocaine is the drug of choice and may be used to control or prevent this arrhythmia. Many other drugs are effective against ventricular tachycardia. Mexiletine, procainamide, propranolol, quinidine, and tocainide can treat or prevent ventricular tachycardia. Disopyramide can be used for therapy or prophylaxis of episodic arrhythmias of this type. Amiodarone, bretylium, encainide, and flecainide are reserved for life-threatening arrhythmias.

Digitalis-induced arrhythmias constitute a significant fraction of arrhythmias, usually arising in patients receiving digitalis as a cardiotonic agent. Digitalis may induce any type of arrhythmia, but the most common ones are bradycardia, PVCs, and AV nodal tachycardia. The first step in therapy is to discontinue the digitalis. If the arrhythmia is not severe, no further therapy may be required. However, digitalis preparations routinely used as cardiotonics are relatively long-acting drugs, and it may be necessary to treat the arrhythmia while the digitalis is being eliminated from the system. Potassium levels should be assessed in these patients, because a low potassium level increases the sensitivity of the heart to digitalis and may predispose it to arrhythmias. Potassium supplements may be given if required.

Phenytoin is most often selected to treat digitalis-induced arrhythmias of all types. Empirically, phenytoin seems more effective in most patients than the other drugs, although a mechanistic explanation for this observation is lacking. If phenytoin does not control the arrhythmia satisfactorily, lidocaine or propranolol may be tried.

NURSING IMPLICATIONS SUMMARY

General Guidelines

Drug administration

◆ Monitor the vital signs and blood pressure. Although a change in the heart rate is frequently a desired outcome of therapy, a heart rate less than 60 beats/min or greater than 120 beats/min in an adult should usually be avoided.

◆ Establish specific guidelines for each patient in consultation with the physician.

◆ Monitor the ECG. In the acute care situation, monitor the continuous ECG tracing. Check the tracing on a regular basis on outpatients.

◆ Monitor other indicators of cardiovascular functioning as appropriate, including blood pressure, pulse, intake and output, weight, and heart and lung sounds. Assess for edema, especially in dependent areas, and jugular venous distention. Assess for activity tolerance with daily activities.

◆ Monitor the blood urea nitrogen (BUN) level, liver function studies, and serum drug levels if available.

◆ For IV administration, use microdrip tubing and an electronic infusion monitor. Usually, monitor the ECG during IV administration. Monitor the blood pressure and pulse. Keep patient supine after IV doses until vital signs are stable. Keep siderails up. Have available emergency equipment and drugs to treat toxicity or for resuscitation.

Patient and family education

◆ Teach patients about the desired effects and common side effects of prescribed drugs. Tell patients to report the development of any unexpected sign or symptom. Point out that drugs or doses may need to be changed or adjusted if unusual side effects develop, so patients should not hesitate to contact the physician.

◆ Review with patients the importance of taking medications as ordered. Antiarrhythmic drugs are most effective when taken on a regular basis, as prescribed. If a dose is missed, patients should not double up for it. Refer patients as appropriate to community-based nursing care agencies.

◆ Instruct patients not to discontinue antiarrhythmic medications without first consulting the physician.

◆ Stress the importance of concomitant therapies, if ordered, including modifying diet; losing weight; restricting sodium; using potassium replacements, diuretics, and antihypertensives; limiting caffeine intake; and stopping smoking.

◆ Assess the need for patients to monitor weight, pulse, blood pressure, or other parameters in the home. Consider the patient's medical condition, prescribed medication, ability, and resources when making this decision.

◆ Suggest that the patient carry a medical identification tag or bracelet indicating that antiarrhythmics are being used.

◆ Instruct patients to avoid drinking alcoholic beverages unless approved by the physician.

◆ Keep all health-care providers, including dentists, informed of all medications being used.

◆ Keep all medications out of the reach of children.

◆ Digoxin is discussed in Chapter 18.

◆ Beta-adrenergic receptor blockers are discussed in Chapter 15.

◆ Calcium channel blockers are discussed in Chapter 14.

◆ Phenytoin is discussed in Chapter 47.

Moricizine

◆ See general guidelines for antiarrhythmic therapy.

◆ Caution patients to avoid driving or operating hazardous equipment if dizziness develops; notify the physician.

◆ For missed doses, take as soon as remembered, unless within 2 hr of next dose, in which case the missed dose should not be taken.

Quinidine

Drug administration

◆ See general guidelines for antiarrhythmic therapy.

◆ Read labels carefully; do not confuse quinidine with quinine.

◆ Monitor liver function tests, blood count, platelet count, serum electrolyte levels, and prothrombin time.

◆ A test dose may be ordered before the full dose to test for possible idiosyncrasy to quinidine.

◆ Assess for rash or skin changes.

NURSING IMPLICATIONS SUMMARY—cont'd

INTRAVENOUS ADMINISTRATION

◆ Dilute 800 mg (10 ml) in at least 40 ml of 5% dextrose in water. Do not add to IV solutions or mix with other drugs in a syringe. Administer at a rate of 1 ml (16 mg)/min.

◆ IM injections may be painful and may increase serum creatine phosphokinase (creatine phosphokinase [CPK] or creatine kinase [CK]) levels.

Patient and family education

◆ See general guidelines for antiarrhythmic therapy.

◆ Review symptoms of cinchonism such as ringing in the ears, headache, nausea, or changes in vision with the patient. Tell the patient to notify the physician if these occur.

◆ Review Patient Problem: Photosensitivity on p. 629 with patients.

◆ Warn patients to avoid driving or operating hazardous equipment if visual changes occur; notify the physician.

◆ Doses are best taken on an empty stomach with a full glass (8 oz) of water 1 hr before or 2 hr after meals. If GI symptoms are severe, take doses with meals. Notify the physician if diarrhea develops.

◆ Patients may develop bitter taste in the mouth. There is little that can be done for this, but caution the patient not to discontinue the drug without consulting with the physician.

◆ Teach patients taking extended-release tablets to swallow tablets whole without crushing or breaking.

◆ Review Patient Problems: Bleeding Tendencies on p. 570 and Depressed White Blood Cell Count on p. 560 with patients. Tell patients to report the development of any unexpected sign or symptom.

◆ For missed doses, take as soon as remembered, unless within 2 hr of next dose, in which case the missed dose should not be taken.

Procainamide

Drug administration

◆ See general guidelines for antiarrhythmic therapy.

◆ Monitor antinuclear antibody (ANA) tests.

INTRAVENOUS ADMINISTRATION

◆ For direct IV injection, dilute each 100 mg with 10 ml of 5% dextrose in water or sterile water. Administer at a rate of 20 mg/min. For infusion, add 1 gm to 500 ml 5% dextrose in water for a dilution of 2 mg/ml. Use microdrip tubing, and infuse at a rate of 2 to 6 mg/min.

Patient and family education

◆ See general guidelines for antiarrhythmic therapy.

◆ Doses are best taken on an empty stomach with a full glass (8 oz) of water 1 hr before or 2 hr after meals. If GI symptoms are severe, take doses with meals, but take doses consistently with meals or on an empty stomach.

◆ Teach patients taking extended-release formulations to swallow whole without crushing or breaking.

◆ Instruct patients to report the development of arthritis, polyarthralgia, pleuritic pain, myalgia, skin lesions, fever, or any other new sign or symptom.

◆ Caution patients to avoid driving or operating hazardous equipment if dizziness develops; notify the physician.

◆ For missed doses, take as soon as remembered, unless within 2 hr of next dose (4 hr for sustained–release preparations), in which case the missed dose should not be taken.

◆ Caution patients that they may see the matrix from extended–release tablets in stool and that this is normal.

Disopyramide

Drug administration

◆ See general guidelines for antiarrhythmic therapy.

◆ Assess for urinary retention. Monitor intake and output, question patient about hesitancy or difficulty voiding; palpate bladder.

◆ Monitor blood sugar, since this drug can cause hypoglycemia.

Patient and family education

◆ See general guidelines for antiarrhythmic therapy.

◆ See Patient Problems: Xerostomia on p. 166; Orthostatic Hypotension on p. 234; and Constipation on p. 182. Tell patient to report any difficulty urinating.

Continued.

NURSING IMPLICATIONS SUMMARY—cont'd

◆ Review the signs of hypoglycemia including fast heart rate, cold sweats, headache, hunger, nausea, nervousness, shakiness, unsteady walk, and anxious feeling. Tell patients to eat or drink a food containing sugar if this develops and to notify the physician. Instruct diabetic patients to monitor blood glucose levels.

◆ Caution patients to avoid driving or operating hazardous equipment if dizziness or blurred vision develop; notify the physician.

◆ This drug may cause patients to sweat less. Tell patients to take frequent rest periods if engaging in strenuous activities, and to limit time in hot environments or in direct sunlight.

◆ Teach patients taking extended-release formulations to swallow whole without crushing or breaking.

◆ For missed doses, take as soon as remembered, unless within 4 hr of next dose, in which case the missed dose should not be taken.

Lidocaine

Drug administration and patient and family education

◆ See general guidelines for antiarrhythmic therapy.

◆ This drug is rarely used outside of the acute care setting. Keep patient and family informed of the patient's condition.

◆ Assess for the side effects noted in the text. Instruct patients to report any subjective changes.

INTRAMUSCULAR ADMINISTRATION

◆ Read labels carefully. Lidocaine with epinephrine is not given as an antiarrhythmic. Administer IM doses into the deltoid muscle. IM injection may cause elevations in the CPK or CK levels.

INTRAVENOUS ADMINISTRATION

◆ Read labels carefully. Lidocaine with epinephrine is not used as an antiarrhythmic. Label must state "for IV use." Bolus doses may be given undiluted at a rate of 50 mg/min; too rapid administration may cause seizures. For continuous infusion, dilute per agency protocol or consult manufacturer's literature. Use microdrip tubing and adjust dose to patient response.

Mexiletene

Drug administration

◆ See general guidelines for antiarrhythmic therapy.

◆ Monitor white blood cell count, white blood cell differential, and platelet count.

◆ Assess patients for ataxia, nystagmus, and development of CNS side effects.

Patient and family education

◆ See Patient Problems: Bleeding Tendencies on p. 570 and Depressed White Blood Cell Production on p. 560. Instruct patients to report the development of these rare but serious side effects.

◆ Caution patients to avoid driving or operating hazardous equipment if dizziness or blurred vision develop; notify the physician.

◆ Take doses with meals or a snack to lessen GI irritation.

◆ For missed doses, take as soon as remembered, unless within 4 hr of next dose, in which case the missed dose should not be taken.

Tocainide

Drug administration

◆ See general guidelines for antiarrhythmic therapy.

◆ Assess regularly for skin changes or rashes. Auscultate breath sounds and assess respiratory rate.

Patient and family education

◆ See general guidelines for antiarrhythmic therapy.

◆ Take doses with food or milk to lessen gastric irritation.

◆ Tell patients to notify the physician immediately if rashes, skin changes, peeling or scaling of skin, blisters on skin or mouth, cough, or shortness of breath develop.

◆ Caution patients to avoid driving or operating hazardous equipment if dizziness, lightheadedness, confusion, or visual changes develop; notify the physician.

◆ Instruct patients to take missed dose as soon as remembered, unless within 4 hr of next dose, in which case the missed dose should not be taken.

NURSING IMPLICATIONS SUMMARY—cont'd

Encainide and Flecainide

Drug administration and patient and family education

◆ See general guidelines for antiarrhythmic therapy.

◆ Caution patients to avoid driving or operating hazardous equipment if dizziness or visual changes develop; notify the physician.

◆ Some patients develop a metallic taste in the mouth. Monitor patient's weight. If patients cannot tolerate this side effect, consult the physician. Instruct patients not to discontinue medication without consulting the physician.

◆ For missed doses, take as soon as remembered, unless within 4 hr of next dose (encainide) or within 6 hr of the next dose (flecainide), in which case the missed dose should not be taken.

Propafenone

Drug administration and patient and family education

◆ See general guidelines for antiarrhythmic therapy.

◆ Caution patients to avoid driving or operating hazardous equipment if dizziness, blurred vision, or lightheadedness develop; notify the physician.

◆ Review Patient Problems: Xerostomia on p. 166 and Constipation on p. 182.

◆ Some patients develop a metallic taste in the mouth. Monitor weight. If patient is unable to tolerate this side effect, consult the physician. Remind patients not to discontinue medication without consulting the physician.

◆ For missed doses, take as soon as remembered, unless within 4 hr of next dose, in which case the missed dose should not be taken.

Amiodarone

Drug administration

◆ See general guidelines for antiarrhythmic therapy.

◆ Assess breath sounds and respiratory rate for signs of pulmonary toxicity.

◆ Assess visual acuity at the start of therapy.

Patient and family education

◆ See general guidelines for antiarrhythmic therapy. Review the common side effects. Instruct patients to report the development of respiratory difficulties, weakness, numbness, or ataxia.

◆ Review Patient Problem: Photosensitivity on p. 629. Patients on this drug who develop photosensitivity may be sensitive to sunlight coming through windows.

◆ Instruct the patient to report subjective visual or eye changes. Encourage patients who wear glasses to continue periodic ophthalmic examinations.

◆ Warn patients that the skin may turn a bluish-gray color, but the discoloration should fade when therapy is discontinued. Notify the physician if skin color begins to change.

◆ Review Patient Problem: Constipation on p. 182.

◆ Some patients develop a metallic taste in the mouth. Monitor weight. If patients are unable to tolerate this side effect, consult the physician. Remind patients not to discontinue medication without consulting the physician.

◆ For missed doses, instruct patients not to take missed dose, and do not double the next one; go back to the regular dosing schedule. If two or more doses are missed, contact the physician.

Bretylium

Drug administration

◆ See general guidelines for antiarrhythmic therapy.

INTRAMUSCULAR ADMINISTRATION

◆ Administer in large muscle masses. Record and rotate injection sites. Do not dilute. Do not administer more than 5 ml into a single injection site; if a larger volume is ordered, divide the dose into two equal volumes for injection into two sites.

INTRAVENOUS ADMINISTRATION

◆ May be given undiluted, one dose over 1 min or less.

INTERMITTENT ADMINISTRATION

◆ Dilute drug in at least 50 ml diluent, or use commercially prepared diluted solutions. Administer dose over 10 to 30 min. Too rapid infusion may contribute to nausea and vomiting.

CONTINUOUS INFUSION

◆ Use microdrip tubing and an infusion control device. Monitor continuous ECG recording.

Continued.

NURSING IMPLICATIONS SUMMARY—cont'd

◆ This drug is rarely used outside of the acute care setting. Keep patient and family informed of patient's condition.

Adenosine

Drug administration and patient and family education

◆ See general guidelines for antiarrhythmic therapy.

INTRAVENOUS ADMINISTRATION

◆ Read labels carefully. Do not confuse with adenosine phosphate. May be given undiluted and should be given in an injection site as close to the IV insertion site as possible. Administer as a rapid bolus, over 1 to 2 sec. Follow with a rapid normal saline flush (± 50 ml) if given via IV line.

◆ Monitor ECG and blood pressure.

◆ A variety of side effects have been reported but usually last less than 1 min. These include chest pressure or pain, hyperventilation, hypotension, metallic taste in the mouth, neck or back pain, tight throat, nausea, PACs or

PVCs, and others. Notify the physician of side effects that last longer than 1 min. Because side effects are short-lived, overdose is rarely a problem, but xanthines are competitive antagonists that may be used if necessary.

◆ This drug is rarely used outside of the acute care setting. Keep patient and family informed of the patient's condition.

Atropine

Drug administration and patient and family education

◆ See general guidelines for antiarrhythmic therapy and review the patient care implications for anticholinergic drugs at the end of Chapter 13.

◆ See Patient Problems: Xerostomia on p. 166 and Constipation on p. 182.

INTRAVENOUS ADMINISTRATION

◆ May be given undiluted, or dilute dose in at least 10 ml of sterile water. Do not add to infusing fluids or drugs. Administer at a rate of 1.0 mg or less over 1 min.

CHAPTER REVIEW

◆ **KEY TERMS**

arrhythmias, p. 296
atrial flutter, p. 308
automaticity, p. 298
bradycardia, p. 296
ectopic foci, p. 299
fibrillation, p. 308
premature ventricular contractions, p. 309
refractory period, p. 298
tachycardia, p. 296

◆ **REVIEW QUESTIONS**

1. What is an action potential?
2. What tissues in the heart are normally automatic?
3. Describe how the waves on an ECG are related to electrical activity of different portions of the heart.
4. What is the normal pacemaker of the heart?
5. What is the effect of vagus nerve stimulation on the heart?
6. What is the effect of sympathetic stimulation on the heart?
7. What is the refractory period?
8. What is reentry?
9. What are the classes of antiarrhythmic drugs? On what is the classification based? How would you include this information in teaching plans?
10. What is the mechanism of action of quinidine and procainamide?
11. What secondary action do both quinidine and procainamide share?
12. How do the toxic effects of quinidine and procainamide differ? How would you assess the patient for them?
13. What is the mechanism of action of disopyramide?
14. Lidocaine, mexiletine, moricizine, propafenone, and tocainide are most effective on which tissue in the heart?

15. How does the use of lidocaine differ from that of mexiletine and tocainide?

16. For what type of arrhythmias is phenytoin especially useful?

17. Encainide and flecainide are reserved for what clinical indication? Why?

18. What is the antiarrhythmic effect shared by acebutolol, esmolol, and propranolol?

19. What is the mechanism of action of amiodarone?

20. What are the uses of amiodarone?

21. What are the side effects of amiodarone? How would you assess for them?

22. What is the mechanism of action of bretylium as an antiarrhythmic agent?

23. What is the mechanism of action of verapamil as an antiarrhythmic agent?

SUGGESTED READING

Andrews LK: ECG rhythms made easier with algorithms, *Am J Nurs* 89(3):365, 1989.

Atchison JJ: Arrhythmia or artifact? *Am J Nurs* 89(2):210, 1989.

Dibianco R, Estes NAM III, Horowitz LN: Oral antiarrhythmics in 1990, *Patient Care* 24(15):145, 1990.

Frye SJ, Lounsbury PS: *Cardiac rhythm disorders: a nursing process approach,* St Louis, 1992, Mosby–Year Book.

Guzzetta, CE, Dossey, BM: *Cardiovascular nursing: holistic practice,* St Louis, 1992, Mosby–Year Book.

Lazarus M, Nolasco VM, Luckett C: Cardiac arrhythmias: diagnosis and treatment, *Crit Care Nurse* 8(7):57, 1989.

Porterfield LM: Antiarrhythmic drug therapy, *Adv Clin Care* 4(4):20, 1989.

Porterfield LM: Propafenone (rythmol) for ventricular arrhythmias, *Adv Clin Care* 5(5):41, 1990.

Teplitz L: L-E-A-D drugs for cardiac emergencies: clinical close-up on lidocaine, *Nurs 89* 19(9):44, 1989.

CHAPTER 20

Agents Affecting Blood Coagulation

LEARNING OBJECTIVES

After studying this chapter, you should be able to do the following:

- Discuss the groups of drugs used in anticoagulation.
- Develop a care plan for patients receiving an anticoagulant.
- Identify the antidotes for hemorrhage caused by drug overdose.
- Describe the use of antiplatelet therapy, thrombolytic therapy, and hemostatic therapy.
- Differentate between treatments for hemophilia.
- Develop nursing care plans, including teaching plans, for patients receiving drugs affecting blood coagulation.

CHAPTER OVERVIEW

◆ Blood can quickly produce plugs and clots when blood loss is threatened. This chapter describes blood cogulation and drugs and agents used to control it. Anticoagulants interfere with the process of coagulation. Antiplatelet drugs inhibit the aggregation of blood platelets and play a prophylactic role against heart attacks and strokes. Thrombolytic drugs degrade blood clots and can limit the damage of a heart attack. Hemostatic agents aid in promoting blood coagulation.

Nursing Process Overview

ANTICOAGULANTS AND ANTIPLATELETS

Assessment

Anticoagulation *prevents* clot formation; it does not dissolve existing clots. Obtain a history of problems with clots. Assess the general physical condition of the patient, including bruising or easy bleeding. Monitor blood coagulation studies, including prothrombin time (PT), partial thromboplastin time (PTT), platelet count, and clotting times. Document the presence of any bleeding.

Nursing Diagnoses

High risk for hemorrhage
Potential altered health maintenance related to insufficient knowledge of the implication of anticoagulant therapy

Management

Assess for bleeding from any site, and check stools for occult blood. Evaluate any symptoms signaling possible thrombus formation such as chest or leg pain or any symptom of internal bleeding such as headache. Monitor blood coagulation studies carefully. Use an infusion monitoring device for infusions of heparin, and check dosages carefully. Keep antidotes readily available for the drugs being used.

Evaluation

Before discharge, determine that the patient can explain why the drug is needed, how to take the drug, what signs and symptoms of bleeding should be reported, how to avoid injury and bruising, what side effects may be related to the drug but do not involve bleeding, and which additional side effects require notification of the physician. Finally, verify that the patient can state which other drugs, such as aspirin, to avoid while taking anticoagulants.

ANTICOAGULANT DRUGS

Review of Coagulation Steps

The process of **blood coagulation** is diagrammed in Figure 20-1. The initial step can be in the intrinsic pathway with the activation of the blood component factor XII (the Hageman factor) by contact with exposed collagen, or an event in the extrinsic pathway, (e.g., the release of tissue factor by damaged tissue). Either pathway results in the activation of factor X. Factor Xa (activated factor X) forms a complex with platelet phospholipids, calcium, and factor V. This complex, which is sometimes called *thromboplastin,* catalyzes the conversion of prothrombin (factor II) to thrombin. Thrombin then catalyzes the conversion of fibrinogen to fibrin. After cross-linking of fibrin by factor XIIIa, fibrin becomes insoluble, forming a mesh that is the blood clot, also called a ***thrombus.***

Blood clots in the arterial system are initially composed largely of platelets with a fibrin mesh (white thrombus). Blood clots in the venous system have only a few platelet aggregates and are composed largely of fibrin with trapped red blood cells (red thrombus). A thrombus in the arterial or venous system may dislodge, becoming an **embolus.** Venous emboli often lodge in the small arteries of the pulmonary circulation, thereby markedly blocking the oxygenating capacity of the lungs and increasing the blood pressure in the pulmonary system, a life-threatening situation. Thrombi form in veins in which blood flow is low, favoring the accumulation of activated clotting factors. Patients at risk for experiencing venous thrombosis include those immobilized as a result of trauma or surgery and those with a history of thromboembolism.

Anticoagulant drugs interfere with any of the steps depicted in Figure 20-1, leading to the formation of fibrin. Blood coagulation is often referred to as a *cascade phenomenon,* since the process becomes magnified at every step. Each activated factor is a catalyst leading to the formation of many molecules of the next actvated factor. The earlier in the process that a step can be blocked, the more efficient is the inhibition of blood coagulation.

Anticoagulant drugs prevent clot formation; they do not affect existing clots. They can be classified into three groups: agents that remove calcium, the drug heparin, and oral anticoagulants. Antiplatelet drugs inhibit the aggregation of platelets and inhibit coagulation in the arterial system.

Agents that Remove Calcium

Calcium is a cofactor for each of the steps through the activation of prothrombin. The removal of calcium prevents the coagulation of blood. Citrate and ethylenediaminetetraacetic acid (EDTA) are compounds that complex calcium, making calcium unavailable for blood coagulation. When blood is drawn for testing or storage, citrate or EDTA may be used to keep the blood from clotting in the container. Since calcium is essential for many biochemical events, anticoagulants that complex calcium can be used only in storage containers (**in vitro**), not in a patient (**in vivo**).

Heparin

Heparin is an anticoagulant that can either be administered to the patient (Table 20-1) or added to a storage container.

Mechanism of action

Heparin activates a plasma protein, antithrombin III, which neutralizes thrombin. However, antithrombin III also neutralizes factor Xa, the step before the activation of prothrombin to thrombin. This inhibition of factor Xa, rather than the inhibition of thrombin, appears to be primarily responsible for the effective anticoagulant action of heparin in low doses. Heparin is also an antiplatelet drug. In vitro, heparin stimulates platelet aggregation. In vivo, however, heparin appears to coat the endothelial lining of the vessels. Since heparin is a highly negatively charged polymer, it adds a negative charge to the endothelium that keeps platelets from attaching and forming a thrombus.

Clinical uses

The clinical uses of heparin differ in dose and route of administration. It achieves anticoagulation (in high doses), prevents postoperative thromboembolism (in low doses), and prevents coagulation of laboratory samples and stored blood in vitro.

High-dose administration. Heparin is used in the hospital to prevent the further growth of venous thrombi. Large doses (35 to 100 units/kg) must be administered intravenously to achieve this anticoagulation. Heparin cannot be taken orally, since it is not absorbed and causes a painful hematoma if administered intramuscularly. Heparin may be given as an intravenous (IV) injection, achieving immediate anticoagulation, with the same or lesser dose repeated every 4 to 6 hr. Blood levels of heparin decrease by half every 1½ hr. Intermittent IV administration results in virtual incoagulability after administration and is associated with a higher risk of bleeding than continuous IV infusion. Thus an initial IV injection followed by continuous infusion at approximately 1000 units/hr is commonly given. An IV drip must be carefully monitored if used to deliver heparin, or overdosing may result; an infusion monitor is usually used.

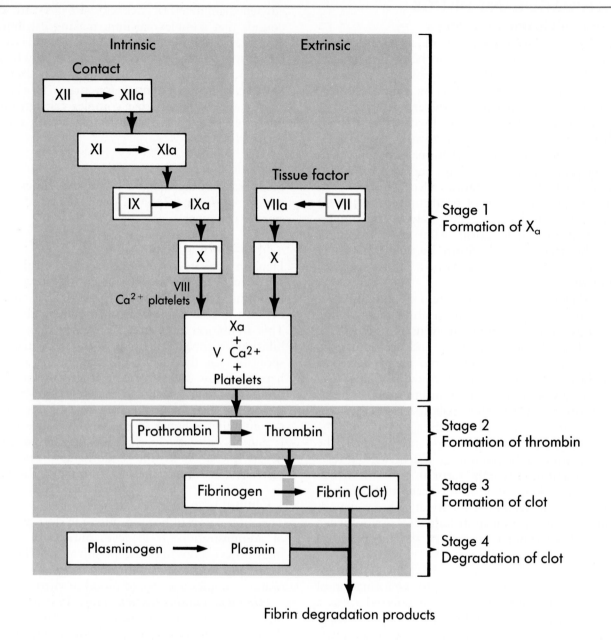

Intrinsic

Contact

XII ⟶ XIIa

XI ⟶ XIa

IX ⟶ IXa

X

VIII
Ca^{2+} platelets

Extrinsic

Tissue factor

VIIa ⟵ VII

X

Xa
+
V, Ca^{2+}
+
Platelets

Stage 1
Formation of X_a

Prothrombin ⟶ Thrombin

Stage 2
Formation of thrombin

Fibrinogen ⟶ Fibrin (Clot)

Stage 3
Formation of clot

Plasminogen ⟶ Plasmin

Stage 4
Degradation of clot

Fibrin degradation products

▨ Indicates the step is blocked by heparin

☐ Indicates a clotting factor that is not synthesized when
oral anticoagulants are present

FIGURE 20-1

Stages of blood coagulation. Actions of drug classes include four stages: *Stage I,* Antiplatelet drugs inhibit platelet aggregation in intrinsic pathway. Citrate and EDTA, which chelate calcium, prevent formation of factor Xa. Heparin, by activating antithrombin III, neutralizes factor Xa and stops coagulation at stage 1. Oral anticoagulants prevent synthesis of factors VII, IX, and X, which are necessary for stage 1. Local hemostatic agents provide contact to activate intrinsic pathway; *Stage II,* Oral anticoagulants prevent synthesis of prothrombin; *Stage III,* Heparin activates antithrombin III to prevent thrombin activity; *Stage IV,* Aminocaproic acid inhibits activation of profibrinolysin and thus inhibits clot degradation. TPA, streptokinase, and urokinase activate profibrinolysin to aid clot digestion.

Table 20-1   Anticoagulant Drugs

Generic name	Trade name	Administration/dosage	Comments
Heparin	Calciparine* Calcilean† Liquaemin Hepalean†	SUBCUTANEOUS: 10,000 to 20,000 units, then 8000 to 10,000 units every 8 hr or 15,000 to 20,000 units every 12 hr. INTRAVENOUS: *Intermittent*—10,000 units, then 5000 to 10,000 units every 4 to 6 hr. *Continuous*—20,000 to 40,000 units daily in 1000 ml. SUBCUTANEOUS: 5000 units 2 hr before surgery, then every 8 to 12 hr until ambulatory. FDA Pregnancy Category C.	High dose is for therapeutic anticoagulation. Low dose is for prophylaxis of postoperative thromboembolism.
ORAL ANTICOAGULANTS			
Anisindione	Miradon*	ORAL: 300 mg day 1; 200 mg day 2; 100 mg day 3, 25 to 250 mg daily for maintenance.	Half-life is 3 to 5 days. Peak effect occurs in 2 to 3 days. Anticoagulant effect persists 1 to 3 days after discontinuance. Dermatitis is a side effect. Drug imparts an orange color to an alkaline urine.
Dicumarol (bishydroxycoumarin)	Generic	ORAL: 200 to 300 mg day 1; 25 to 200 mg daily for maintenance.	The prototype oral anticoagulant. Half-life is 1 to 2 days. Peak effect occurs in 1 to 4 days. Anticoagulant effect persists 2 to 10 days after discontinuance. This coumarin is poorly and erratically absorbed.
Warfarin	Coumadin* Panwarfin Warfilone* Sofarin	ORAL, INTRAMUSCULAR, INTRAVENOUS: 10 to 15 mg daily until prothrombin time is in therapeutic range. 2 to 10 mg daily for maintenance. A loading dose of 40 to 60 mg (20 to 30 mg in elderly patients) may be given initially.	Half-life is 2 days. Peak effect occurs in 1 to 3 days. Anticoagulant effect persists 4 to 5 days after discontinuance.

*Available in Canada and United States.
†Available in Canada only.

Low-dose administration. Heparin may also be given subcutaneously to achieve a slow, continual administration over 8- to 12-hr. Low-dose heparin is used for patients over 40 years of age undergoing thoracoabdominal surgery who are at increased risk. It is not used in brain, spinal cord, or eye surgery, in which even minor hemorrhage could be catastrophic. It is not effective in hip replacement surgery. Heparin is administered subcutaneously (5000 units) 2 hr before surgery, and then 5000 units are administered every 8 to 12 hr until the patient is walking. This regimen can reduce the incidence of deep leg vein thrombosis by 50% in these patients without significantly affecting their bleeding or clotting times. The effectiveness of this therapy results from heparin activating antithrombin III, which in turn rapidly inactivates newly formed factor Xa. After antithrombin III has inactivated factor Xa, the heparin can dissociate from this inactive complex and act again to cause further inactivation.

In vitro use. Heparin prevents the coagulation of blood after it leaves the body. Tubing used to shunt blood can be pretreated with heparin to prevent clotting. The negative charge of the heparin coating on the wall of the tubing that prevents platelet adherence is probably the effective anticoagulant mechanism. Heparin is also added to containers used for blood collection. For transfusions, 4 to 6 units of heparin/ml of blood is used. For laboratory samples, 7 to 15 units of heparin/ml of blood is used.

Side effects

Heparin is a natural compound, extracted from animal lungs or intestines. Some patients become allergic to heparin. The usual symptoms of heparin hypersensitivity are chills, fever, and urticaria, but other allergic reactions such as asthma, rhinitis, lacrimation, or anaphylaxis have been reported. In some patients, heparin has caused thrombocytopenia; thus the platelet count should be measured daily after therapy.

Protamine and hemorrhage. The major side effect of heparin is hemorrhage. Since the half-life of intravenously administered heparin is only 1½ hrs, discontinuing heparin therapy is usually sufficient to reverse a hemorrhagic episode. If hemorrhaging must be stopped immediately, protamine sulfate may be given by slow IV infusion. Protamine is a highly positively charged molecule that complexes the negatively charged heparin. Protamine is an anticoagulant and has a longer half-life than heparin. Protamine may persist and cause bleeding after heparin is eliminated. One milligram of protamine sulfate neutralizes 100 units of heparin. No more than 50 mg of protamine sulfate should be administered in 10 min.

Oral Anticoagulants

Mechanism of action

Clotting factors II (prothrombin), VII, IX, and X are synthesized in the liver, with vitamin K as a necessary cofactor. If vitamin K is deficient, these clotting factors are synthesized in a functionally inactive state, impairing blood coagulation.

The coumarins and the indandiones interfere with the regeneration of active vitamin K in the liver and thereby produce vitamin K deficiency. Since the synthesis of functional clotting factors II, VII, IX, and X is inhibited, the anticoagulant effect does not appear until preexisting factors II, VII, IX, and X are removed by normal degradation. This takes 1 day or longer. Factor II, prothrombin, is the longest lived of these clotting factors, and requires 24 hr to deplete half the existing prothrombin. A one-stage prothrombin test frequently determines if the dose of oral anticoagulants is appropriate. Therapeutic doses of the oral anticoagulants increase the prothrombin time by 1½ to 2½ times the baseline values. Anticoagulant therapy must be individualized for each patient (see Table 20-1).

Clinical use of oral anticoagulants

The major indication for the oral anticoagulants is the prophylaxis or treatment for a deep venous or pulmonary thrombus. However, low-dose heparin administered during surgery has significantly reduced the risk of thrombus formation. The oral coumarins were widely used as prophylaxis against myocardial reinfarction, a use never well substantiated by controlled studies. Recently, the number of available oral anticoagulants has dropped to two coumarins, warfarin and dicumarol; and one indandione, anisindione.

Anticoagulants that are vitamin K antagonists do not prevent coagulation of blood after it is drawn, since the clotting factors are already synthesized and present.

Coumarins

Warfarin is the most widely used coumarin. It is the only coumarin that can be administered intramuscularly or intravenously. Warfarin is well absorbed orally. Its peak effect occurs 36 to 72 hr after administration, and the duration of action is 4 to 5 days.

Dicumarol is longer acting than warfarin. The peak action is 3 to 5 days after administration, and the duration of action is up to 10 days. Dicumarol is not well absorbed and cuases flatulence and diarrhea.

Importance of protein binding to the pharmacokinetics of coumarins. The coumarins stay in the body a long time because they are bound tightly to plasma albumin. This tight binding has several consequences. Only a small amount of the total drug in the body is free to diffuse to the site of action in the liver. The liver also degrades the coumarin to inactive forms that are then excreted in the urine so that only a small amount of the total coumarin is available for degradation. Other drugs can displace coumarins from albumin. This displacement dramatically increases the effective concentration of coumarin. For example, if only 1% of the total coumarin is not bound and displacement causes another 1% to be free, the concentration of free coumarin drug has doubled. The albumin-bound coumarin acts as a reservoir for the drug. After administration is discontinued, several days are required for the drug to dissociate from the albumin and to be degraded by the liver.

Drug interactions. Drug interactions are especially numerous with the coumarins. Many drugs alter their effectiveness. No drug should be added to or deleted from a therapeutic regimen that includes a coumarin without considering drug interactions and appropriately modifying dosages.

The anticoagulant action of both heparin and coumarins is enhanced by drugs that decrease platelet adhesion (e.g., aspirin, clofibrate, dextran, dipyridamole, hydroxychloroquine, ibuprofen, indomethacin, and phenylbutazone). The anticoagulant action of coumarins is enhanced by drugs that inhibit coumarin degradation, such as clofibrate, disulfiram, metronidazole, oxyphenbutazone, phenylbutazone, and trimethoprim; drugs that displace bound anticoagulant, such as chloral hydrate, oxyphenbutazone, and phenylbutazone; and drugs that interact by unknown mechanisms, such as anabolic steroids, cimetidine, D-thyrozine, glucagon, quinidine, and sulfinpyrazone. The anticoagulant action of coumarins is diminished by drugs that accelerate coumarin degradation, such as barbiturates, ethchlorvynol, glutethimide, griseofulvin, and rifampin; drugs that decrease gastrointestinal (GI) absorption of coumarins, such as cholestyramine; and drugs that interact by unknown mechanisms, such as 6-mercaptopurine. Dicumarol enhances the action of phenytoin. This list summarizes the major drug interactions but is not exhaustive.

Side effects. The principal side effect is hemorrhage. Signs of coumarin overdose include blood in the urine or stools, causing them to turn red, orange, smoky, or black. The drug can be discontinued temporarily when minor hemorrhaging occurs. When hemorrhaging is severe, fresh or frozen plasma may be transfused to replace clotting factors immediately. Less severe hemorrhage can be trated by administering 10 mg (up to 50 mg) of vitamin K_1 phytonadione. This adds excess vitamin K to overcome the block caused by the coumarins. Clotting factors are then again synthesized by the liver, returning the PT to normal in about 24 hr. Side effects other than hemorrhaging are rare.

Indandiones

The indandiones more frequently cause side effects, including rashes, depression of the bone marrow, hepatitis, and renal damage, than the coumarins and are not widely used in the United States. Drug interactions are not prominent with the indandiones.

Anisindione (Miradon) is the only indandione in clinical use in the United States and Canada. It is long acting, and the peak effect occurs 48 to 72 hr after the initial dose. The PT returns to normal 24 to 72 hr after the last dose.

ANTIPLATELET DRUGS

Mechanism of action

Platelets (**thrombocytes**) are the small cell fragments in blood derived from giant bone marrow cells called *megakaryocytes*. Ordinarily, platelets do not stick to each other or to the endothelial lining of the blood vessels. When there is a break in the endothelial lining, however, platelets readily attach to the collagen in the exposed tissue. This attachment causes the platelets to aggregate, rapidly forming a plug that stops the bleeding and aids in the formation of a thrombus. This aggregation of platelets in the presence of abnormal surfaces is the initial step in the normal repair system for the blood vessels. Drugs that interfere with this process are termed *antiplatelet* or *antithrombic drugs.*

In the late 1970s, it was discovered that when the platelets adhere to a surface, they synthesize thromboxane A_2, a substance related to the prostaglandins. Thromboxane A_2 is a potent stimulus for the further aggregation of platelets and thereby accelerates the formation of the platelet plug. Therefore drugs blocking the synthesis of thromboxane A_2 inhibit the aggregation of platelets to form a plug. Aspirin and sulfinpyrazone (Anturane) are inhibitors of thromboxane A_2 synthesis. Dipyridamole (Persantine) and sulfinpyrazone prolong the survival of platelets in persons with thromboembolic diseases so that platelets do not initiate thrombus formation as readily. These drugs are listed in Table 20-2.

The role of platelet aggregation as the initial step leading to blood coagulation is well established. In particular, the blood clots forming in the arterial system, as opposed to the venous system, are highly linked to conditions promoting platelet aggregation. Patients at risk for developing arterial clots are those who have already suffered a myocardial infarction (MI) or a stroke. Another established clinical use of antiplatelet drugs is for heart valve prostheses, disorders, and shunts.

Aspirin

Aspirin is the most widely studied antiplatelet drug. It provides effective prophylactic treatment for the following:

Patients who have experienced a **transient ischemic attack (TIA),** (a ministroke) have a decreased incidence of further TIAs, strokes, or death. This is a dramatic effect in men but probably not in women. Sulfinpyrazone and dipyridamole were not effective.

Patients who have had an MI or who have stable or unstable angina, have a decreased incidence of subsequent heart attacks. These results are from studies in men and may not apply to women.

Primary prevention of heart attacks has been demonstrated. Over 22,000 doctors in the United States volunteered to take a buffered aspirin or a placebo every other day. At the end of 5 yr, the aspirin takers had half the heart attacks and a third the deaths from heart attacks experienced by the placebo takers. However, because these doctors were initially screened and found to be in normal health, the applicability of this study to the general population is not yet known. A retrospective study of nurses indicated that those who took six or more aspirins each week had a 32% decrease in the incidence of heart attacks.

The dose of aspirin may be important to its effectiveness in preventing thrombus formation. A low dose of aspirin (80 to 180 mg/day) inhibits the synthesis of thromboxane A_2 by the platelets. A higher dose of aspirin (1000 mg/day) also inhibits the synthesis of prostacyclin (prostaglandin I_2) by the epithelial lining of the blood vessel. Prostacyclin inhibits the aggregation of platelets, an action directly opposite that of thromboxane A_2. Prostacyclin therefore prevents the formation of a platelet plug. For this reason a high dose of aspirin may be less effective

Table 20-2   Antiplatelet Drugs

Generic name	Trade name	Administration/dosage	Comments
Aspirin	Various	ORAL: *Adults*—After TIA: 325 mg with each meal and at bedtime or 650 mg twice a day. Prosthetic heart valve: 325 mg with each meal. Atrioventricular (AV) shunt or fistula: 160 mg with each meal and at bedtime. Graft patency: 325 mg after each meal. Prevention of MI or sudden death in patient with unstable angina: 325 mg with each meal and at bedtime. Prevention of recurrent MI or coronary death post-MI: 325 to 1300 mg/day.	Taken with a coumarin for prosthetic heart valve. Taken with dipyridamole for graft patency.
Dipyridamole	Persantine* Apo-Dypridamole†	ORAL: *Adults*—400 mg daily. FDA Pregnancy Category B.	Taken to prevent thrombi formation with a prosthetic heart valve or to maintain graft patency. Taken with warfarin for prosthetic heart valve. May also be taken with aspirin for a prosthetic heart valve or graft patency.
Sulfinpyrazone	Anturan† Anturane Antazone† Apo-sulfinpyrazone† Novopyrazone†	ORAL: *Adults*—200 mg 4 times a day.	Taken to prevent thrombi formation with a prosthetic heart valve, AV shunt or fistula, mitral stenosis, or to prevent sudden death after MI. Taken with a coumarin for prosthetic heart valve or mitral stenosis.
Ticlopidine†	Ticlid*	ORAL: *Adults*—250 mg 2 times a day with food.	A new drug. Used as a prophylactic for stroke.

*Available in Canada and United States.
†Available in Canada only.

than the low dose in preventing the formation of a thrombus. However, for prophylaxis following a TIA, only high doses have been found effective.

Dipyridamole

Dipyridamole (Persantine) combines with warfarin for patients with artificial heart valves. It has not been shown effective as prophylaxis in preventing heart attacks or strokes.

Sulfinpyrazone

The effectiveness of sulfinpyrazone (Anturane) as prophylaxis in preventing heart attacks or strokes is not clear.

Ticlopidine

Ticlopidine (Ticlid) is a new drug, curently available in Canada. Ticlopidine inhibits platelet aggregation irreversibly. It may be effective in preventing strokes and MI.

Nursing Process Overview
THROMBOLYTIC DRUGS

Thrombolytic drugs have revolutionized the treatment of MI. They promote the digestion of fibrin, thereby dissolving the clot.

Assessment

Anticoagulant therapy prevents clots, and thrombolytic therapy dissolves clots. Both alter the normal coagulation mechanism to cause anticoagulation. Assess the size and location of the clot and the signs and symptoms caused by the clot. A recent patient history of streptococcal infection would influence the choice of agents and should be documented.

Nursing Diagnoses

High risk for hemorrhage

High risk for anaphylaxis or severe allergic reaction to streptokinase

Management

Use thrombolytic drugs only in acute care settings. Monitor patients for signs of clot dissolution and hemorrhage.

Monitor the usual tests for blood coagulation and check the hematocrit level daily because it may drop even when bleeding is not present. Use an infusion monitoring device for infusions. Have available appropriate drugs to control bleeding, such as aminocaproic acid.

Evaluation

If effective, a thrombolytic drug dissolves the existing clot without causing hemorrhage. Patients are not discharged while still on thrombolytic therapy.

Mechanisms and Use of Thrombolytic Drugs

As shown in Figure 20-1, the plasma contains the enzyme plasmin, which degrades the fibrin network of a clot into small, soluble fragments. Plasmin normally exists in an inactive form, plasminogen. Plasminogen is activated to plasmin by various factors in the plasma, primarily tissue-type plasminogen activator (TPA), which originates in the blood vessel wall. Plasminogen and TPA bind to fibrin, and TPA converts plasminogen to plasmin and plasmin digests fibrin. Degradation products of fibrin act as anticoagulants, thereby limiting further clot formation.

Although the steps in coagulation occur very rapidly, the dissolution of a blood clot may take several days. Drugs to speed the clot dissolution process are widely used. The treatment of choice for an acute MI has become the injection of a clot-dissolving drug as quickly as possible, which prevents the myocardial ischemia that leads to tissue death. Patients can leave the hospital after 3 days instead of 10 and may not require prolonged recovery at home. The drugs available are streptokinase, TPA, and anistreplase (Table 20-3). Thrombolytic therapy is also used in acute pulmonary embolism, deep vein thrombosis, or peripheral arterial occlusion. This therapy helps locally to clear AV shunts in patients receiving long-term renal dialysis; however, clotting often recurs.

Table 20-3   Thrombolytic Drugs

Generic name	Trade name	Administration/dosage	Comments
Alteplase, recombinant	Activase Activase rt-PA*	INTRAVENOUS: *Adults*—Initially, a bolus of 6 to 10 mg over 1 to 2 min, followed by infusion of 60 mg for 1 hr and 20 mg for the next 2 hr. For patients weighing less than 65 kg, the total dose is 1.25 mg/kg.	Monitor for arrhythmias, reocclusion. Very expensive, about $2300/dose.
Anistreplase (APSAC)	Eminase	INTRAVENOUS: *Adults*—30 units injected for 2 to 5 min via IV	Monitor for bleeding. Very expensive, about $1700/dose.
Streptokinase	Kabikinase Streptase*	INTRAVENOUS: *Adults*—Loading dose of 250,000 IU in 30 min, then infusion of 100,000 IU/hr. Dosage is continued for 24 to 72 hr for pulmonary embolism and for 72 hr for deep vein embolism. For coronary thrombosis: INTRAVENOUS: *Adults*—1.5 million IU, administered within 1 hr. INTRAARTERIAL (via coronary artery catheter)—20,000 IU initially, followed by 2000 IU/min for 1 hr.	Monitor thrombin times every 12 hr. Allergic reactions are common (15% of patients); usually of the milder variety (itching, flushing, nausea, headache). Treat with antihistamines.
Urokinase	Abbokinase	INTRAVENOUS: *Adults*—Loading dose of 2000 IU/lb in 10 min by infusion, then 2000 IU/lb/hr for 12 hr. FDA Pregnancy Category B.	Isolated from human urine. Not as allergenic as streptokinase but very expensive.

*Available in Canada and United States.

The thrombolytic agents are proteins and must be infused. Except for anistreplase, they are relatively short-acting, 30 min or less.

Specific Drugs

Anistreplase

Anistreplase (Anisoylated Plasminogen-Streptokinase Activator Complex [APSAC] and Eminase) is a complex of streptokinase and human plasminogen. The human plasminogen has been modified with a blocking group so that it is not readily activated. The injected complex binds to the fibrin of a clot, and the plasminogen slowly loses its blocking group and is activated by streptokinase. This happens at a controlled rate and at the fibrin network of the clot. Anistreplase is active for about 6 hr.

Alteplase

Alteplase (Activase; TPA) is produced for pharmacologic use by recombinant DNA technology. Alteplase is infused intravenously following MI and activates fibrin-bound plasminogen.

Streptokinase

Streptokinase (Streptase) is isolated from group C beta-hemolytic streptococci; it acts by forming a complex with plasminogen to activate it. Streptokinase is antigenic and may cause allergic reactions. The cost of streptokinase treatment is about one tenth that of alteplase or anistreplase and appears to be as effective in treating coronary thrombosis.

Urokinase

Urokinase (Abbokinase) is isolated from human urine; it is an enzyme that cleaves plasminogen to plasmin. Bleeding or its complications are potential side effects of all three agents. Urokinase treats thromboembolisms but not coronary thrombosis.

Nursing Process Overview

HEMOSTATICS

Hemostatics are local or systemic agents used to control excessive bleeding.

Assessment

Assess the type, location, and amount of bleeding; the symptoms related to the bleeding, such as pain, swelling, and level of consciousness; appropriate blood coagulation tests such as PTT, PT, clotting time, platelet count, and hematocrit; and general physical condition of the patient.

Nursing Diagnosis

High risk for deep vein thrombosis

Management

Observe the patient for signs that bleeding is stopping and for side effects of the drugs. Overmedication with the systemic hemostatic agents is possible; ensure that the patient receives the correct dose. Monitor the appropriate coagulation studies and the hematocrit.

Evaluation

The goal of therapy with hemostatic agents is to stop bleeding without causing side effects resulting from the drug therapy. These patients will rarely be sent home on hemostatic therapy but should be able to explain what to do if bleeding recurs.

Systemic Hemostatic Drugs

Epsilon aminocaproic acid

Epsilon aminocaproic acid (Amicar) inhibits the activation of profibrinolysin (plasminogen) to the active enzyme fibrinolysin (plasmin). The lack of fibrinolysin inhibits dissolution of blood clots. Aminocaproic acid is used in instances in which it is desirable to protect blood clots, such as surgery on the prostate; after a ruptured cerebral aneurysm; or for patients with hemophilia, after a tooth extraction.

Aminocaproic acid can be given orally or by IV. It is rapidly excreted in the urine. Side effects are transient and minor and include nausea, cramps, dizziness, headache, ringing in the ear, or stuffy nose. When IV therapy is used, aminocaproic acid can irritate the veins and give rise to thrombophlebitis. This effect may be minimized by diluting the drug before use and by carefully placing the needle.

Tranexamic acid

Tranexamic acid (Cyklokapron), like epsilon aminocaproic acid, inhibits the activation of plasminogen to the active enzyme plasmin. Tranexamic acid also directly inhibits plasmin. As an antifibrinolytic agent, it is 5 to 10 times more potent than epsilon aminocaproic acid. The major indication for the drug is in hemophiliac patients undergoing dental surgery.

Patients receiving tranexamic acid should be monitored for signs of thromboembolic complications. If they are to receive the drug for more than a few days, they should also receive an ophthalmologic examination; animal studies have indicated that high doses of the drug can cause focal areas of retinal degeneration. More frequent side effects are GI upsets, including diarrhea, nausea, and vomiting. Tranexamic acid is eliminated largely unchanged in the urine.

Vitamin K

Vitamin K is a fat-soluble vitamin required for the synthesis of clotting factors II, VII, IX, and X in the liver. Vitamin K is contained in many foods. Humans cannot synthesize vitamin K, but bacteria in the GI tract can synthesize vitamin K for absorption by the host. Conditions that can produce vitamin K deficiency include the following:

1. Long-term IV feeding
2. Debilitation resulting from poor diet
3. Prolonged oral antibiotic therapy
4. Malabsorption syndrome
5. Acute diarrhea in infants
6. Biliary disease

In addition, the oral anticoagulant drugs—produce a relative vitamin K-deficiency by inhibiting the reactivation of vitamin K.

Administration and side effects. Vitamin K is available as vitamin K_1 (phytonadione) and vitamin K_3 (menadione) for replacement therapy, but only phytonadione is effective as an antidote for severe bleeding episodes caused by an overdose of one of the oral anticoagulants. They are safest when taken orally. IV injection must be made slowly with a dilute solution and even then may cause a severe reaction. Reactions to IV injection include flushing, a heavy feeling on the chest, sweating, vascular collapse, and an anaphylactic reaction. Intramuscular (IM) and subcutaneous administration may cause pain and bleeding at the injection site.

In infants and anyone with a deficiency of the enzyme, glucose-6-phosphate dehydrogenase, menadione can produce hemolysis but phytonadione does not. These vitamins do not promote clotting in a patient with liver disease or a hereditary deficiency of one of the vitamin K-dependent clotting factors.

Local Absorbable Hemostatics

Local absorbable hemostatics provide a surface that promotes platelet adhesion and thereby promotes blood clotting where the agent is applied (Table 20-4).

Absorbable gelatin sponge

Gelfoam is a sterile absorbable gelatin sponge (Figure 20-2) that is moistened with sterile saline solution and applied to bleeding capillary beds that cannot be readily sutured. It is absorbed in 4 to 6 weeks.

Absorbable gelatin film

Gelfilm is a thin, sterile absorbable gelatin film used in neurologic, thoracic, and ocular surgery to repair membrane surfaces. Reabsorption may take from 1 week to 6 months, depending on the size and site of the film.

Oxidized cellulose

Oxidized cellulose (Oxygel) and oxidized regenerated cellulose (Surgicel) are used much like the absorbable gelatin sponge. They interfere with bone regeneration and therefore cannot be packed around fractures. Oxygel retards formation of new skin and cannot be used as a surface dressing. Small implants are reabsorbed in 1 week, but large ones may require 6 weeks for reabsorption.

Microfibrillar collagen hemostat

Microfibrillar collagen hemostat (Avitene) is a water-insoluble powder that is applied to a bleeding surface to activate natural clotting. The collagen is absorbed in 7 weeks. Microfibrillar collagen is used during surgery to control bleeding in capillary beds, liver, and skin-graft sites. It does not interfere with the healing of skin or bone. Microfibrillar collagen must be kept dry and cannot be resterilized after the container is opened.

Thrombin

Thrombin is an activated clotting factor (see Figure 20-1). Thrombin is applied topically only as a sterile protein powder to bleeding surfaces. It must be kept cold and dry until use or it becomes inactive. Thrombin can be applied topically as a solution; however, it is important to note that it must not be injected.

Replacement Therapy for Hemophilia

Hemophilia is an inherited disorder in which there is a deficiency of one of the factors necessary for coagulation of the blood. Hemophilia A or classic hemophilia is a deficiency of factor VIII, which is important in the activation of factor X. Hemophilia A is inherited as an X-linked recessive disorder and is seen almost exclusively in males. Hemophilia B or Christmas disease is an inherited X-linked recessive disorder characterized by a deficiency of factor IX. Von Willebrand's disease is a nonsex-linked (autosomal) codominant disorder in which von Willebrand factor is decreased or abnormal. Von Willebrand factor is important for the adhesion of platelets to the blood vessels and as a carrier for factor VIII.

Desmopressin

Desmopressin (DDAVP, Stimate) temporarily increases the concentrations of factor VIII and von Willebrand factor. This action controls mild-to-moderate bleeding. Desmopressin is a synthetic analogue of the pituitary hormone, vasopressin.

Adverse reactions to desmopressin may be seen in patients who have certain blood disorders that predispose them to reactions. For this reason, desmopressin should not be used for patients with type IIB of von Willebrand's disease and should be used with caution for patients with coronary artery disease, hypertension, or atherosclerosis, or who are elderly.

Table 20-4 Hemostatic Agents

Generic name	Trade name	Administration/dosage	Comments
REPLACEMENT THERAPY FOR HEMOPHILIA			
Antihemophilic factor—human	Hemofil M Koate HS Factor VII-SD Profilate SD Others	INTRAVENOUS: *Adults and children*—usually a single dose of 15 to 20 units/kg given at a rate of 10 to 15 ml/min maintains activities sufficient for clotting.	There are four different methods of purifying factor VIII from plasma.
Cryoprecipitated antihemophilic factor—human		INTRAVENOUS: *Adults and children*—Usually a single dose of 15 to 20 units/kg given at a rate of 10 to 15 ml/min maintains activities sufficient for clotting.	This product is prepared by the hospital blood bank. Thaw in a water bath at 37° C; keep at room temperature and use within 3 hr.
Antihemophilic factor (AHF)—porcine	Hyate:C	INTRAVENOUS: *Adults and children*—Initially, 100 to 150 units/kg. If this is insufficient, a second larger dose should then be given, followed by a third dose if necessary.	This is a purified freeze-dried concentrate of AHF from pig plasma. This can be used for patients who have developed antibodies to the human product.
Antithrombin III	ATnativ KobiVitrum	INTRAVENOUS: *Adults and children*—Initially, 50 to 100 units/min is administered over 5 to 10 min. The final dosage is determined by the level of deficiency, the response, and the weight of the patient.	This is an orphan drug. It is prepared from human plasma tested to be free of HIV and hepatitis B and is heat treated.
Desmopressin	DDAVP Stimate	INTRAVENOUS: *Adults and children*—0.3 μg/kg is infused slowly over 15 to 30 min. The dosage should not be repeated within 24 hr.	This synthetic analogue of arginine vasopressin is used for short-term hemostatic control in patients with mild or moderate factor VIII deficiency and in those with type I von Willebrand's disease.
Factor IX complex human	Konyne-HT Profilnin, heat treated	INTRAVENOUS: *Adults and children*—For nonlife-threatening bleeding in patients with hemophilia who have factor VIII inhibitors, 75 units/kg is the initial dose, repeated in 8 to 12 hr if necessary.	Factor IX complex treats bleeding associated with Christmas disease or deficiency of one or more of the other factors in this preparation (factors II, VII, and X).
SYSTEMIC HEMOSTATIC AGENTS			
Aminocaproic acid	Amicar*	ORAL, INTRAVENOUS: *Adults*—5 to 6 gm initially orally or by slow IV infusion, then 1 gm hourly or 6 gm every 6 hr. Maximum in 24 hr is 30 Gm. Reduced dosage is used with low renal output or renal disease. *Children*—100 mg/kg body weight every 6 hr for 6 days.	Prevents activation of plasminogen (fibrinolysis) so that blood clots are not broken down. Used in special surgical situations.

*Available in Canada and United States.

Table 20-4 Hemostatic Agents—cont'd

Generic name	Trade name	Administration/dosage	Comments
Phytonadione (vitamin K₁)	AquaMEPHYTON Konakion* Mephyton	ORAL, INTRAMUSCULAR, SUBCUTANEOUS: *Adults and children*—2.5 to 25 mg. INTRAMUSCULAR, SUBCUTANEOUS, INTRAVENOUS: *Newborns*—0.5 to 1 mg immediately after birth. Alternatively the mother is given 1 to 5 mg 12 to 24 hr before delivery.	IV route can be dangerous. Use only in emergencies for oral anticoagulant overdose, and dilute so that no more than 1 mg is given per min. Subcutaneous and IM injection may be painful.
Menadiol sodium diphosphate (vitamin K₄)	Synkayvite*	ORAL, INTRAMUSCULAR, SUBCUTANEOUS, INTRAVENOUS: *Adults*—5 to 15 mg once or twice daily. *Children*—5 to 10 mg once or twice daily.	Used to correct secondary hypoprothrombinemia. Converted to menadione (vitamin K₃) in the body.
Tranexamic acid	Cyklokapron*	ORAL: *Adults and children*—25 mg/kg 3 or 4 times the day before surgery and 2 to 8 days after surgery. INTRAVENOUS: *Adults and children*—10 mg/kg before surgery, administered with factor VIII or IX, and 10 mg/kg 3 or 4 times daily for 2 to 8 days after surgery. FDA Pregnancy Category B.	Indicated use is for hemophiliac patients undergoing dental surgery.

LOCAL HEMOSTATIC AGENTS

Generic name	Trade name	Administration/dosage	Comments
Absorbable gelatin sponge	Gelfoam	Blocks and cones of various sizes. Also a sterile (surgical) and nonsterile (dental) powder.	Used to control bleeding in a wound or at an operative site.
Absorbable gelatin film	Gelfilm	Thin film strips.	Used to repair membranes in neural, thoracic, and ocular surgery.
Oxidized cellulose	Oxycel*	Gauze-type pads or strips. Also as sponges 2 × 1 × 1 inch.	Used to control hemorrhage and absorb blood. May be left in wound. Not for packing around bone fractures or to be left on skin.
Oxidized regenerated cellulose	Surgicel	Knitted fabric strips.	Used like oxidized cellulose, but may be left on skin.
Microfibrillar collagen hemostat	Avitene	Sterile powder. 1 gm should cover 50 × 50 cm (20 × 20 inches) to control light bleeding.	Used to control bleeding in a wound or at an operative site. May be used on skin. Discard unused material, since it cannot be resterilized.
Thrombin	Fibrindex Thrombin, topical	Sterile powder. Packaged by units. May be dissolved in sterile saline solution and applied in absorbable gelatin sponge.	Used to control bleeding in a wound or at an operative site. Discard unused material, since it cannot be resterilized and the solution is unstable.

*Available in Canada and United States.

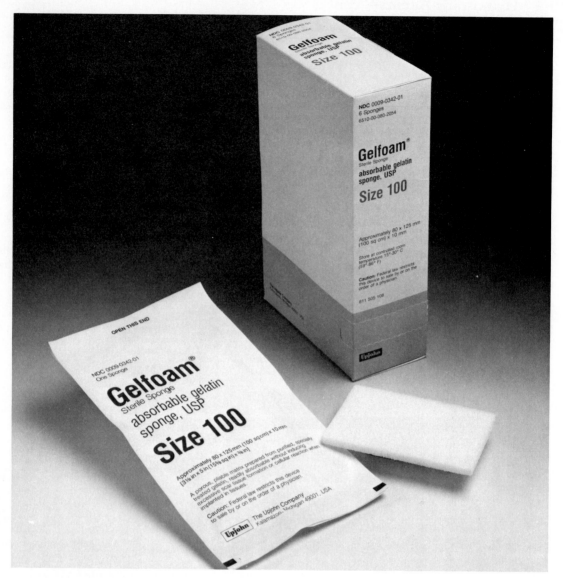

FIGURE 20-2

Absorbable gelatin sponge (Gelfoam) promotes platelet adhesion and promotes blood clotting.
Courtesy Upjohn, Kalamazoo, MI.

Antihemophilic factor

There are several methods of isolating factor VIII from human plasma. A unit of antihemophilic factor may represent a pool from as many as 25,000 donors because of the viral inactivation steps now needed. (It is estimated that 80% of severe hemophiliacs are human immunodeficiency virus (HIV) positive because of contaminated supplies of antihemophilic factor from the early 1980s.) Cryoprecipitated antihemophilic factors are made from the plasma of one unit of whole blood. This product may be kept frozen for about 1 year.

Factor VIII, produced by recombinant DNA technology, is currently being tested clinically. Availability of Factor VIII from a source other than the blood supply would eliminate the risk of blood-transmitted diseases such as HIV and hepatitis.

Antithrombin III, human

A deficiency of antithrombin II is seen in several thousand Americans and results in an increased risk of thromboembolic diseases and venous thrombosis, especially after surgery and obstetric procedures. Antithrombin III (ATnative and KabiVitrum) is now prepared from plasma tested and treated to exclude viruses.

Factor IX complex, human

Factor IX is derived from human plasma and used to treat bleeding episodes in hemophilia B or factor IX deficiency (Christmas disease). Patients receiving factor IX may experience transient fever, chills, itching, nausea, vomiting, headache, flushing, or tingling. Slow administration can reduce these reactions. Patients, particularly those undergoing surgery, may experience thromboembolic complications.

NURSING IMPLICATIONS SUMMARY

General Guidelines for Patients Receiving Anticoagulants

Drug administration

◆ Inspect the patient at least twice daily for the appearance of bruising and petechiae.

◆ Check stool for guaiac/blood at least twice a week.

◆ Monitor vital signs at regular intervals. Be alert to signs of hemorrhage such as hypotension, rapid pulse, pale color, or weakness. In pregnant women, hemorrhage occurs most often in the third trimester or immediate postpartum period.

◆ Avoid the use of restraints. If necessary to use them, pad the extremities well, and remove the restraints frequently to inspect the area.

◆ Handle patients carefully to avoid bruising.

Patient and family education

◆ Teach patients to notify the physician if nosebleeds, bleeding gums, blood in stool or urine, unexplained or severe bruising, severe headache, or stiff neck occurs.

◆ Instruct patients to wear a medical identification tag or bracelet indicating that they are taking anticoagulants.

◆ Keep all health-care providers informed of anticoagulant use, including dentists and oral surgeons.

◆ Avoid using razors with blades; use electric shavers instead.

◆ Do not take any medications except those prescribed without checking with the physician. This applies especially to aspirin or over-the-counter drugs which might contain aspirin.

◆ Brush teeth with a soft-bristle brush if bleeding from gums is prolonged. Avoid flossing. Use water-spray oral care devices on low settings only.

◆ Do not go barefoot.

◆ Avoid rough contact activities or sports while on anticoagulants.

Heparin

Drug administration

◆ Review the general guidelines.

◆ Monitor blood work before administering doses, especially with high-dose heparin (>15,000 units/24 hr). Monitor activated PTT (aPTT); the goal of anticoagulation therapy is 1.5 to 2 times control in seconds. Other tests that may be monitored include the Lee-White whole blood clotting time and the activated clotting time (ACT). There will be little or no change when low-dose heparin is used. Blood specimens for these tests are usually obtained ½ hr before ordered doses for intermittent therapy. If the laboratory work indicates anticoagulation above the desired range, notify the physician before administering dose of heparin.

◆ Monitor platelet counts.

◆ If the patient is receiving heparin and an oral anticoagulant, monitor laboratory work appropriate to both drugs.

◆ For mild heparin overdose, discontinue heparin until the laboratory findings return to the therapeutic range. Keep protamine sulfate handy for treatment of severe overdose (see Protamine).

◆ Read labels carefully, since there are several strengths available. Check calculations carefully; some institutions require that two nurses check doses of heparin before administration.

◆ Place a note above patient's bed (or as is customary in the institution) that the patient is receiving heparin therapy so that laboratory personnel will use care to avoid excessive bleeding after venipuncture.

◆ Avoid IM injections in patients on high-dose heparin.

Continued.

NURSING IMPLICATIONS SUMMARY—cont'd

SUBCUTANEOUS ADMINISTRATION, INTERMITTENT DOSES

◆ Use any subcutaneous injection site (see Chapter 6), but the abdomen is preferred because it contains few muscles, and bruising is less of a cosmetic problem. Avoid the arms.

◆ Keep a record of sites used, and rotate sites, even if only the abdomen is being injected.

◆ Avoid the area 2 inches around the umbilicus and any abdominal scars.

◆ Use careful technique to avoid bruising, but know that bruising may occur with even the best technique. Avoid areas that are already bruised. Do not rub the area after injecting drug.

◆ After drawing up the dose, change needles. Inject at 45- to 90-degree angle with ⅝ to ½ inch, 25- to 28-gauge needle, after careful assessment to avoid injection into a muscle. Do not aspirate before injecting the drug.

◆ There is disagreement about the desirability of pinching the skin, which would be done when administering insulin; pinching may contribute to more bruising.

CONTINUOUS IV INFUSION OF HEPARIN

◆ Use microdrip tubing and an electronic infusion monitoring device.

◆ Many drugs are incompatible with heparin. If other IV drugs must be administered, establish a second IV infusion line for these medications, or flush the tubing containing heparin with normal saline before and after administering other medications. Heparin blood levels will be erratic if the heparin infusion is interrupted frequently or for long periods.

INTERMITTENT IV HEPARIN VIA HEPARIN WELL OR OTHER INFUSION ACCESS DEVICES

◆ Insert heparin well (heparin lock) into vein using accepted venipuncture technique, and secure in place.

◆ Prime the well with a small amount (1 to 2 ml) of heparin of the same strength that will be used for anticoagulation.

◆ Inject each dose of heparin into the heparin well. The injected dose displaces the heparin remaining in the well each time a dose is given, so flushing the well after the dose is administered is not necessary. Follow agency procedures if different from those listed.

OTHER IV MEDICATIONS VIA HEPARIN WELL OR HEPARIN-PRIMED INFUSION ACCESS DEVICES

◆ Insert heparin well into vein using accepted venipuncture technique, and secure in place.

◆ Prime the heparin well with 1 ml of a solution of normal saline containing 10 or 100 units of heparin/ml. Implanted ports may require up to 5 ml; consult manufacturer's literature. These solutions are available in prepackaged syringes, multiple-dose vials, or can be prepared by the nurse or pharmacist. Some institutions use only normal saline for flushing.

◆ Each time a dose of medication is given, flush the heparin well with 1 to 2 ml of saline (unless there is only saline in the heparin well); administer the prescribed medication via IV push or infusion; flush the well again with 1 to 2 ml of normal saline; finally, flush with 1 ml of the dilute heparin solution. Follow agency procedures if different from those listed.

◆ Check for patency and correct location of the heparin well before administering heparin or other medications. Assess for pain, tenderness, swelling, or redness. It should be possible to gently aspirate blood from the heparin well. It should be possible to smoothly but slowly inject drugs via the well with no patient discomfort or resistance. If in doubt that the heparin well is patent and in the vein, it should be removed and another one inserted elsewhere.

Patient and family education

◆ See the general guidelines.

◆ If heparin is prescribed for home management, instruct the patient in the necessary psychomotor tasks involved (subcutaneous injection or injection via implanted ports, heparin wells, or catheters). Provide positive reinforcement and encouragement. Supervise return demonstrations of the necessary techniques. Refer patients to a community-based nursing care agency.

◆ Tell patients that a variety of side effects may occur, including alopecia (hair loss), burning sensation of the feet, myalgia, and bone pain. Encourage the patient to notify the physician of any unusual sign or symptom.

NURSING IMPLICATIONS SUMMARY—cont'd

Protamine Sulfate

Drug administration

◆ The dose of protamine sulfate is based on the amount of heparin administered during the preceding 3 to 4 hr. Dilute to 10 mg/ml. Administer at a rate of 20 mg or less over 1 to 3 min. Do not exceed 50 mg in 10-min. May be further diluted for infusion.

◆ Monitor vital signs; protamine may cause hypotension.

◆ Warn patients that flushing and a feeling of warmth may occur.

◆ Patients receiving protamine zinc insulin may be sensitized to protamine and may experience a severe reaction.

◆ Keep available drugs and equipment to treat anaphylactic shock.

◆ Continue to assess patient and monitor blood work, since the effects of the heparin may persist longer than the protamine, necessitating additional doses of protamine. Monitor the ACT, aPTT, or thrombin time (TT).

◆ Protamine sulfate is rarely used outside of a hospital setting. Keep patient and family informed.

Coumarins and Indandiones

Drug administration

◆ See general guidelines for patients receiving anticoagulants.

◆ Monitor the PT. The goal for anticoagulation is 1.2 to 2 times the control value in seconds. Check the daily laboratory work before administering the dose, and if higher than the therapeutic range, notify the physician before administering the dose. If the patient is receiving an oral anticoagulant and heparin, monitor laboratory studies of both drugs.

◆ Monitor white blood count, white blood cell differential, and platelet count.

◆ For mild overdose, withhold the anticoagulant until the blood chemistry returns to the therapeutic range. Keep phytonadione available to treat severe overdose with the oral anticoagulants.

PARENTERAL ADMINISTRATION OF WARFARIN

◆ Reconstitute with diluent provided. May be given IM, although this route is used infrequently. For IV use, administer via IV push at a rate of 25 mg/min. May be mixed in a syringe with heparin. Do not mix with IV fluids.

◆ Pregnant women requiring anticoagulants are usually treated with heparin, since the oral agents cross the placenta and cause birth defects. Anticoagulation is usually discontinued at about the thirty-seventh week of pregnancy in anticipation of labor and delivery.

Patient and family education

◆ See general guidelines for patients receiving anticoagulants.

◆ Tell patients that anisindione may turn alkaline urine orange, which may be mistaken for blood. If in doubt, consult the physician.

◆ Rare side effects may develop in patients taking oral anticoagulants. Emphasize the importance of notifying the physician if unexpected signs or symptoms develop.

◆ Instruct patients to avoid drinking alcoholic beverages while taking anticoagulants.

◆ Emphasize the importance of returning for follow-up visits to monitor laboratory studies.

◆ If a dose is missed, take it as soon as remembered if it is during the same day. If it is the next day, omit the forgotten dose and resume the original dosing schedule. Do not double up for missed doses.

Aspirin

◆ For a detailed discussion of aspirin, see Chapter 23.

Dipyridamole

Patient and family education:

◆ Take doses with a full glass (8 oz) of water. It is best to take doses on an empty stomach, 1 hr before or 2 hr after meals. However, if gastric irritation is a problem, take doses with meals, milk, or a snack.

◆ Dipyridamole may be prescribed with aspirin or another anticoagulant. Review with the patient the importance of taking both drugs as prescribed.

◆ Remind patients to keep all health care providers informed of all drugs being taken. Instruct patients not to take aspirin or any blood thinner, unless prescribed by the same doctor who prescribed the dipyridamole.

◆ Tell patients to avoid over-the-counter medications, especially aspirin-containing products, unless approved by the physician.

Continued.

NURSING IMPLICATIONS SUMMARY—cont'd

◆ Instruct patients to space doses throughout the day. If a dose is missed, tell the patient to take the dose as soon as remembered, unless within 4 hr of the next dose, in which case the missed dose should be omitted and the usual schedule resumed with the next dose. Instruct patients not to double up for missed doses.

◆ Tell the patient to notify the physician if bruising, bleeding gums, nosebleeds, or bleeding in the stool occurs.

Sulfinpyrazone

◆ For a detailed discussion of sulfinpyrazone, see Chapter 23.

Anistreplase and Alteplase

Drug administration

◆ Monitor vital signs. Be alert to signs of hemorrhage such as hypotension, rapid pulse, or other signs of shock. Monitor pupil size and reactivity and level of consciousness. Assess for nosebleeds, bleeding gums, blood in urine, stool, vomitus, or bleeding at IV sites; notify the physician. Heparin may also be prescribed, which puts the patient at greater risk for hemorrhage.

◆ Assess patients systematically. Many other side effects have been reported, including nausea, vomiting, rash, fever, muscle aches, and dyspnea. Sometimes it is difficult to distinguish drug side effects from symptoms of the underlying medical condition.

◆ Monitor laboratory work, including complete blood count (CBC), TT, aPTT, PT, creatine phosphokinase (CPK), fibrinogen level, and platelet count.

◆ Monitor continuous electrocardiogram (ECG). Reperfusion arrhythmias occur frequently.

◆ Check stools daily for presence of blood.

◆ Use caution in handling and moving patients to avoid excessive bleeding or bruising. Do not restrain patients.

◆ If arterial puncture is necessary, apply pressure to the puncture site for 30 min after the procedure. Check the site regularly for signs of bleeding.

◆ For continuous infusion, use microdrip tubing and an electronic infusion monitoring device.

◆ Do not administer IM injections to patients receiving these drugs.

◆ Avoid venipuncture unless absolutely necessary. Apply pressure to the site for at least 15 min after venipuncture. Label the bed (or as agency custom dictates) so that personnel from the laboratory use appropriate technique to minimize bleeding after venipuncture.

◆ Anaphylaxis has been reported. Keep available drugs and equipment to treat acute allergic reactions.

◆ These drugs are used only in acute care settings. Keep patients and family informed of patient's condition.

INTRAVENOUS ALTEPLASE

◆ Dilute as directed by manufacturer. Administer initial bolus dose over 2 min. Give remaining first dose over 1 hr. Administer each successive dose over 1 hr. Do not use filters.

INTRAVENOUS ANISTREPLASE

◆ Assess for history of allergic response to streptokinase. Anistreplase contains streptokinase.

◆ Dilute as directed by manufacturer. Administer dose over 2 to 5 min (at least 4 min is preferred).

Streptokinase and Urokinase

Drug administration

◆ Monitor the vital signs. Be alert to signs of hemorrhage: including hypotension, rapid pulse, or other signs of shock. Monitor pupil size and reactivity and level of consciousness. Assess for nosebleeds, bleeding gums, blood in urine, stool, or vomitus; notify the physician.

◆ Temporary increases in blood pressure have been reported with streptokinase. If systolic blood pressure increases more than 25 mm Hg, notify the physician.

◆ Monitor laboratory work, including hemoglobin and hematocrit, TT, aPTT, PT, and platelet count. If the patient has been receiving heparin therapy, streptokinase or urokinase is withheld until the TT is less than 2 times normal. If heparin is to be started after thrombolytic therapy, heparin is withheld until the TT is less than 2 times normal control.

◆ Check stools daily for the presence of blood or guaiac.

◆ Use caution in handling and moving patients to avoid excessive bleeding or bruising. Do not restrain patients.

NURSING IMPLICATIONS SUMMARY—cont'd

- If arterial puncture is necessary, use the radial or brachial artery rather than the femoral. Apply pressure to the puncture site for 30 min after the procedure. Check the site regularly for signs of bleeding.
- Monitor the ECG during therapy.
- For continuous infusion, use microdrip tubing and an electronic infusion monitoring device.
- Do not administer IM injections to patients receiving these drugs.
- Avoid venipuncture unless absolutely necessary. Apply pressure to the site for at least 15 min after venipuncture. Label the bed (or as agency custom dictates) so that personnel from the laboratory use appropriate technique to minimize bleeding after venipuncture.
- Streptokinase is highly antigenic. Observe the patient for the signs and symptoms of allergic response, including anaphylaxis, urticaria, itching, flushing, nausea, headache, and musculoskeletal pain. Have available drugs, equipment, and personnel to treat serious allergic response. Use antihistamines and corticosteroids to treat allergic response; do not use aspirin to reduce fever.
- Before using these drugs to clear occluded cannulae, attempt to clear the occluded cannulae with heparinized saline. Follow institutional guidelines. Do not mix either of these drugs with any other drug in a syringe.
- These drugs are used only in acute care settings. Keep patient and family informed of patient's condition.

Aminocaproic Acid

Drug administration

- This drug may be used to treat overdose with fibrinolytic drugs.

INTRAVENOUS AMINOCAPROIC ACID
- Available in a concentration of 250 mg/ml or 1 gm/4 ml. Further dilute with compatible solution, 50 ml of diluent for each 1 gm of drug (4 ml). Administer at a rate of 5 gm/hr for the first hour, then 1 gm/hr after the first hour. Too rapid administration can cause cardiovascular side effects. Monitor the pulse, blood pressure, and if possible ECG during administration.

- Since the drug can cause clot formation, be alert to signs of possible thrombosis such as pain in extremities, one extremity colder than another, loss of pulse in an extremity, shortness of breath, chest pain, and Homan's sign.

Patient and family education

- Review the goals of therapy with the patient. Therapy is usually on a short-term basis, but side effects may develop. Encourage patients to notify the physician if any unexpected sign or symptom develops.
- Tell patients to take any missed doses as soon as remembered, unless close to the time for the next dose, in which case the missed dose should be omitted. Do not double up for missed doses.

Tranexamic Acid

Drug administration

- This drug may be used to treat overdose with fibrinolytic drugs.

INTRAVENOUS TRANEXAMIC ACID
- May be given undiluted or further diluted in IV infusion solutions. Administer undiluted at a rate of 100 mg (1 ml)/min. Too rapid administration can cause cardiovascular side effects. Monitor the pulse, blood pressure, and if possible ECG during IV administration.
- Since the drug can cause clot formation, be alert to signs of possible thrombosis such as pain in extremities, one extremity colder than another, loss of pulse in an extremity, shortness of breath, chest pain, and Homan's sign.

Patient and family education

- Review the goals of therapy with the patient. Therapy with this drug is usually on a short-term basis, but side effects may develop. Encourage patients to notify the physician if any unexpected sign or symptom develops.
- Tell patients to take any missed doses as soon as remembered, unless close to the time for the next dose, in which case the missed dose should be omitted. Do not double up for missed doses.
- The physician may recommend that patients on long-term tranexamic acid therapy receive an ophthalmic examination to detect side effects.

Continued.

NURSING IMPLICATIONS SUMMARY—cont'd

Phytonadione

Drug administration

◆ Assess for history of allergy before administering. Monitor vital signs and blood pressure. Remain with the patient for 5 to 10 min after administration. Have available drugs, equipment, and personnel to treat an acute allergic response.

◆ IM injection is painful, and the injection site may be tender. Use large muscle masses. Record and rotate injection sites.

◆ Monitor the prothrombin time.

◆ Read labels carefully. Konakion is for IM injection only; AquaMEPHYTON may be given IM, IV, or subcutaneously.

INTRAVENOUS PHYTONADIONE

◆ Dilute only with designated fluids (see manufacturer's instructions). Use only preservative-free diluents. Administer diluted solution at a rate of 1 mg/min. The drug is light sensitive. Administer immediately after preparing.

◆ Patients with bile deficiency who are receiving oral preparations need concomitant administration of bile salts.

Patient and family education

◆ Review with patients the expected benefits of therapy.

◆ Dietary deficiency of vitamin K is rare in adults. For dietary sources of vitamin K, see Dietary Consideration: Vitamins on p. 275.

Menadiol Sodium Diphosphate

Drug administration

◆ Assess for glucose-6-phosphate dehydrogenase deficiency before administering; if present, do not administer.

◆ IM injection is painful, and the injection site may be tender. Use large muscle masses. Record and rotate injection sites.

INTRAVENOUS MENADIOL SODIUM DIPHOSPHATE

◆ May be given undiluted or added to most infusion solutions. Administer dose in undiluted form over at least 1 min.

◆ Monitor PT.

◆ Patients with bile deficiency who are receiving oral preparations need concurrent administration of bile salts.

Patient and family education

◆ Review with patients the expected benefits of therapy.

◆ Dietary deficiency of vitamin K is rare in adults. For dietary sources of vitamin K, see Dietary Consideration: Vitamins on p. 275.

◆ Take oral doses with meals to decrease gastric irritation.

Desmopressin

◆ This drug is also discussed in Chapter 50.

◆ For treatment of hemophilia A and von Willebrand's disease, dilute a single dose in 10 ml of normal saline for children under 10 kg and in 50 ml for children over 10 kg and adults. Administer a dose over 15 to 30 min.

◆ Monitor blood pressure and pulse. Other side effects include headache, nausea, flushing, abdominal cramps, and pain at the injection site. Assess patients systematically.

◆ Desmopressin does have an antidiuretic effect. Monitor intake and output. Caution patients to limit fluid intake, unless the desired effect is antidiuresis.

◆ Monitor blood work such as factor VIII coagulant, factor VIII antigen, aPTT, factor VIII ristocetin cofactor, bleeding time, and the von Willebrand factor antigen in von Willebrand's disease (Type I).

Antihemophilic Factor, Cryoprecipitated Antihemophilic Factor, Antithrombin III, and Factor IX Complex

◆ See Chapter 17 for a general discussion of administration of blood products.

◆ Monitor vital signs. If severe allergic reaction is suspected, discontinue blood products, but keep IV line patent. Notify the physician. Have available drugs and equipment to treat acute allergic response.

◆ Consult the physician for questions about dosing, and manufacturer's literature for information about reconstitution (if applicable).

CHAPTER REVIEW

◆ KEY TERMS

anticoagulant drugs, p. 317

antiplatelet drugs, p. 321

antithrombic drugs, p. 321

blood coagulation, p. 317

embolus, p. 317

hemophilia, p. 325

hemostatics, p. 324

in vitro, p. 317

in vivo, p. 317

thrombocytes, p. 321

thrombus, p. 317

transient ischemic attack (TIA), p. 321

◆ REVIEW QUESTIONS

1. Describe the major steps in blood coagulation.

2. What are the groups of anticoagulants you see in clinical practice? What is the mechanism of action of each group?

3. Describe how you would administer heparin in high-dose and low-dose therapy.

4. Which anticoagulants would you expect to see in test tubes when blood is drawn for storage or testing?

5. How do protamine and vitamin K function as antidotes for hemorrhaging induced by drugs?

6. How does protein binding affect the pharmacodynamics of the coumarins?

7. What are the therapeutic limitations of the indandiones?

8. How do platelets initiate clot formation?

9. What drugs might you see prescribed to inhibit platelet aggregation?

10. What roles do thromboxane A_2 and prostacyclin play in platelet aggregation?

11. What is the action of thrombolytic drugs? Name the thrombolytic drugs.

12. Briefly describe hemophilia A, hemophilia B, and von Willebrand's disease.

13. What drugs are used to treat hemophilia? What are the nursing care implications of these drugs?

14. What is the mechanism of action of aminocaproic acid? Of vitamin K? When would these drugs be used?

15. List the agents used as local hemostatics. What is their mechanism of action?

SUGGESTED READING

Fields WS, Goldhaber SZ, Lewis HD Jr: Who should have prophylactic aspirin? *Patient Care* 22(8):28, 1988.

Relman AS: Aspirin for the primary prevention of myocardial infarction, *N Engl J Med* 318(4):245, 1988.

Schwartz L and others: Aspirin and dipyridamole in the prevention of restenosis after percutaneous transluminal coronary angioplasty, *N Engl J Med* 318:1714, 1988.

Steering Committee of the Physicians' Health Study Research Group: Preliminary report: findings from the aspirin component of the ongoing physicians' health study, *N Engl J Med* 318:262, 1988.

Anticoagulant therapy

Baldwin DR: Heparin-induced thrombocytopenia, *J Intravenous Nurs* 12(6), 1989.

Currie DL: Pulmonary embolism: diagnosis and management, *Crit Care Nurs Q* 13(2):41, 1990.

Irvin S: White clot syndrome: a life-threatening complication of heparin therapy, *Focus Crit Care* 17(2):107, 1990.

Kuhar PA, Hilll KM: When heparin goes haywire, *Am J Nurs* 91(3):59, 1991.

Paulsen JT, Kersting GL: A systematic approach to heparin administration for pediatric hemodialysis, *ANNA J* 14(4):265, 1987.

Swithers CM: Tools for teaching about anticoagulants, *RN* 51(1):57, 1988.

Todd B: Use heparin safely, *Geriatr Nurs* 8(1):43, 1987.

Thrombolytic therapy

Bilodeau ML, Capasso VC: Peripheral arterial thrombolytic therapy, *Crit Care Nurs Clin North Am* 2(4):673, 1990.

Blake GJ: Anistreplase for acute MI, *Nurs 90* 20(10):113, 1990.

Dillon J and others: Rapid initiation of thrombolytic therapy for acute MI, *Crit Care Nurs* 9(2):55, 1989.

Emde KL, Searle LD: Current practices with thrombolytic therapy, *J Cardiovasc Nurs* 4(1):11, 1989.

Kline EM: Comparison of thrombolytic agents: mechanisms of action, *Crit Care Nurs Q* 12(2):1, 1989.

Niemyski P, Hellstedt LF: Patient selection and management in thrombolytic therapy: nursing implications, *Crit Care Nurs Q* 12(2):8, 1989.

Reidy SJ, O'Hara PA, O'Brien P: Streptokinase use in children undergoing cardiac catheterization, *J Cardiovasc Nurs* 4(1):46, 1989.

Wilson V: Action stat! Complications of thrombolytic therapy, *Nurs 91* 21(1):41, 1991.

IV and intraarterial lines

Cyganski JM, Donahue JM, Heaton JS: The case for the heparin flush, *Am J Nurs* 87:796, 1987.

Dunn DL, Lenihan SF: The case for the saline flush, *Am J Nurs* 87:798, 1987.

Harper J: Use of heparinized intraarterial lines to obtain coagulation samples, *Focus Crit Care* 15(5):51, 1988.

Taylor N and others: Comparison of normal versus heparinized saline for flushing infusion devices, *J Nurs Qual Assur* 3(4):49, 1989.

CHAPTER 21

Drugs to Lower Blood Lipid Levels

LEARNING OBJECTIVES

After studying this chapter, you should be able to do the following:

◆ Differentiate between the two main types of lipids in the blood and the four major classes of lipoproteins.

◆ Discuss the five types of hyperlipidemias.

◆ Develop a teaching plan for a patient who needs to decrease cholesterol intake.

◆ Develop a nursing care plan for a patient taking one of the drugs discussed in this chapter.

CHAPTER OVERVIEW

◆ **Atherosclerosis** is the gradual blocking of arteries by a buildup of plaque. This clogging of the arteries is the major factor behind heart attacks, strokes, and peripheral vascular disease. Lipids, particularly cholesterol, are a major component of atherosclerotic plaques. The association of high blood levels of cholesterol with atherosclerosis has led to preventive measures to control cholesterol. This chapter reviews the current pharmacologic approaches to controlling blood cholesterol.

Nursing Process Overview

BLOOD LIPID LEVELS

Assessment

Baseline assessment should include a general physical assessment and weight, serum cholesterol and triglyceride levels, blood pressure, and dietary history.

Nursing Diagnoses

Altered bowel elimination: diarrhea secondary to antilipemic therapy.

Management

These drugs have few side effects in usual doses. Evaluate new signs or symptoms. Discharge planning should include instruction by the dietitian, particularly if the type of hyperlipidemia can be better treated by dietary restriction or weight loss.

Evaluation

By discharge, ascertain that the patient can explain why and how to take the prescribed drug, when to take it in relation to meals, what anticipated side effects to expect and what to do about them, which symptoms should be reported immediately to the physician, and how to plan meals within prescribed dietary restrictions.

ORIGIN OF BLOOD LIPIDS AND THEIR ROLE IN ATHEROSCLEROSIS

The **lipids** in the blood are triglyceride and cholesterol. These lipids are bound to special proteins to form soluble **lipoproteins**. The major classes of lipoproteins are chylomicrons, very-low-density lipoproteins (VLDL), low-density lipoproteins (LDL), and high-density lipoproteins (HDL). Chylomicrons and VLDL are largely composed of triglycerides and transport triglycerides to tissues for metabolic use or storage. LDL and HDL transport cholesterol. The role and composition of the lipoproteins are summarized in Figure 21-1.

Chylomicrons

Chylomicrons are very large lipoproteins that contain about 90% triglyceride by weight. After a meal the ingested fat is processed by the intestine into chylomicrons, which are transported through the lymphatic system to the plasma. Chylomicrons are normally found in the blood only during the 8 to 12 hr after a meal. Since chylomicrons represent dietary fat,

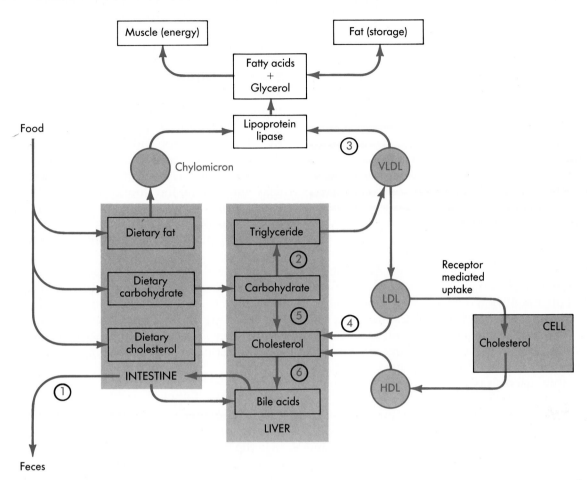

FIGURE 21-1

Diagram of origin and fate of lipids. Sites of action of drugs that can lower excessive plasma concentrations of lipids include (1) drugs that lower cholesterol by increasing the excretion of bile acids (cholestyramine and colestipol); (2) drugs that lower triglycerides by inhibiting hepatic triglyceride synthesis (gemfibrozil and niacin); (3) drug that lowers VLDL, inhibiting its release and activating lipoprotein lipase (clofibrate); (4) drug that lowers cholesterol by stimulating LDL degradation (dextrothyroxine); (5) drug that lowers cholesterol by inhibiting cholesterol synthesis (lovastatin, and probucol); (6) drug that lowers cholesterol by increasing cholesterol excretion into bile (clofibrate).

patients being evaluated for triglyceride abnormalities should not eat for 12 to 16 hr before a blood sample is drawn.

Very-Low-Density Lipoproteins

VLDLs are 60% triglyceride by weight. This triglyceride pool is synthesized by the liver from carbohydrate sources for export as fuel to other tissues. Triglycerides cannot be transported directly into cells for use. Tissues that require triglycerides, particularly muscle and fat tissues, secrete an enzyme called *lipoprotein lipase*, which breaks down the triglycerides to fatty acids and glycerol, compounds that can be taken into the cells.

Low-Density Lipoproteins

LDLs are only 5% triglyceride but are 50% cholesterol by weight. LDLs are the remains of the VLDLs after removal of triglycerides and some protein. When cells need cholesterol, they synthesize receptors for LDL. LDLs bind to these receptors and are taken into the cell by pinocytosis and degraded. Most cells can synthesize cholesterol, but this synthesis is turned off when the cholesterol from LDL is used. When the cell has sufficient cholesterol, it stops making LDL receptors.

Role of LDL in atherosclerosis

Recent studies have examined the role of LDL in atherosclerosis because the concentration of LDL reflects the total cholesterol concentration. Increased total plasma cholesterol concentration is linked to increased incidence of atherosclerosis. When there is an injury to the epithelial cells of arteries or when the amount of circulating LDL becomes high, the receptor mechanism controlling LDL uptake no longer operates properly, and the cell becomes overwhelmed with cholesterol. This is believed to be an origin of atherosclerotic plaques.

Atherosclerotic plaques

Platelets may also initiate atherosclerosis. Aggregated platelets release factors that stimulate smooth muscle growth. This stimulation of growth heals the minute breaks in the normal blood vessel. When the epithelial cells are overloaded with cholesterol and aggregated platelets stimulate an overgrowth of smooth muscle cells, an atherosclerotic plaque is formed. The outcome of atherosclerosis is the narrowing of an artery so that the blood flow is reduced and may not be sufficient to maintain tissue function (Figure 21-2). Reduced blood flow also favors the formation of a clot that may completely obstruct flow. A stroke may result when the cerebral arteries are involved, or a myocardial infarction (MI) may result when the coronary arteries are involved. When the legs are affected, limbs may be lost to gangrene. Renovascular hypertension is associated with atherosclerosis.

High-Density Lipoproteins

HDLs are 50% protein, 20% cholesterol, and 5% triglyceride by weight. Only about 20% of the total plasma cholesterol is found in HDL. Until recently the HDLs were not widely studied. It appears that the HDLs help remove excess cholesterol from peripheral tissues. HDL can remove cholesterol from cells and can inhibit the uptake of LDL by cells. Recent studies indicate that persons with high concentrations of HDL have a lower incidence of atherosclerosis and the related problems of heart disease and strokes.

The liver degrades cholesterol to bile acids, which are excreted into the small intestine. Bile acids emulsify lipids to aid in fat absorption. Some bile acids are absorbed into the portal vein for transport back to the liver. This circulation between the liver and small intestine is called *enterohepatic circulation*.

HYPERLIPIDEMIA
Origin and Types

Hyperlipidemia is an abnormal concentration of one or more of the four lipoproteins. Five major types of hyperlipidemia have been described, depending on which lipoproteins are present in abnormally high

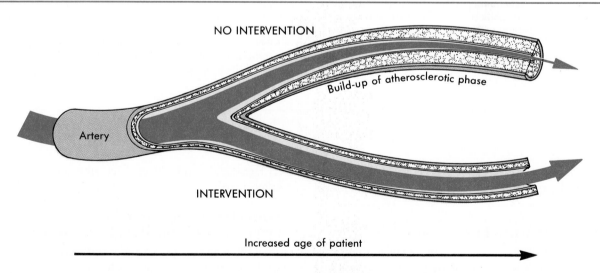

FIGURE 21-2

Diagram of increasing blockage of artery due to atherosclerotic plaque. Buildup of plaque is shown as time-dependent phenomenon. Intervention, through diet, exercise, or drugs, can slow buildup. Recent studies have shown that some interventions can reverse atherosclerosis.

concentrations. Since it is easier to measure cholesterol than LDL and easier to measure triglyceride than VLDL, hyperlipidemias are usually detected by measuring cholesterol and triglyceride. The characteristics of hyperlipidemia are listed in Table 21-1. All hyperlipidemias can be genetically determined but may also be secondary to diabetes, obesity, alcoholism, hypothyroidism, and liver and kidney disease. Only type II and type IV are commonly encountered.

Type II hyperlipidemia is characterized by high concentrations of LDL but normal or modestly increased amounts of VLDL. Persons with elevated LDL are most at risk for atherosclerosis. In genetically determined type II hyperlipidemia, patients homozygous for the type II trait have evidence of severe heart disease by age 20. In addition, type II hyperlipidemia can occur in individuals who are obese or hypothyroid, or who suffer from liver or kidney disease.

Type IV hyperlipidemia is characterized by high concentrations of VLDL with relatively normal levels of LDL. It is the most common lipid abnormality and also carries a high risk of coronary artery disease. Type IV hyperlipidemia is common among obese, alcoholic, or diabetic patients. Oral contraceptives or estrogen can elicit type IV hyperlipidemia.

The common types of hyperlipidemia are associated with a high production of triglycerides (type IV) or cholesterol (type II) by the liver. Type IV hyperlipidemia is often well controlled by calorie restriction with emphasis on losing weight and on reducing carbohydrates from which the liver synthesizes triglycerides. A decrease in foods high in cholesterol such as egg yolk, liver, and shellfish and a decrease in saturated fats are recommended dietary modifications for patients with type II hyperlipidemia (see box on p. 340). When diet alone does not reduce blood lipid levels to acceptable ranges, a few drugs lower the concentration of blood lipids. The type of hyperlipidemia determines which drug may be effective. These drugs have not been in use long enough to evaluate whether they are associated with long-term side effects.

Drug Therapy

The Lipid Research Study, conducted by the National Heart, Lung, and Blood Institute and completed in 1983, found that in a high-risk group whose cholesterol levels were lowered through diet and drug therapy there was as much as a 40% reduction in heart disease risk. The group had blood cholesterol levels above 265 mg/dl. They were treated with diet and up to 24 gm daily of cholestyramine. The better the compliance of the test group, the greater the reduction of heart attacks and deaths from heart disease, the lower the need for bypass surgery, and the lower the incidence of heart disease symptoms. A 4.4% reduction in cholesterol concentration was associated with an 11% decrease in heart disease risk. A 19% reduction in cholesterol concentration was associated with a 40% decrease in heart disease risk.

Table 21-1   Types of Hyperlipidemias

	Type I	Type II	Type III	Type IV	Type V
Lipoprotein content of fasting plasma					
Chylomicrons	Markedly increased	Absent	May be present	Absent	Increased
VLDL	Normal or decreased	Normal or increased	Increased	Increased	Increased
LDL	Normal or decreased	Increased	Increased	Normal	Normal or decreased
Lipids					
Cholesterol	Increased	Increased	Increased	Normal or increased	Increased
Triglyceride	Increased	Normal or increased	Increased	Increased	Increased
Incidence	Rare	Common	Relatively uncommon	Common	Relatively uncommon
Usual age at detection	Early childhood	Early adulthood (can be detected in infancy or childhood)	Early adulthood	Adulthood (middle age)	Early adulthood
Risk of atherosclerosis	Normal	Greatly increased	Greatly increased	Probably increased	Unknown

DIETARY CONSIDERATION: REDUCING CHOLESTEROL

Dietary changes to lower serum cholesterol levels involve decreasing cholesterol intake, lowering the intake of saturated fat, and increasing the intake of polyunsaturated fat. As with all major dietary prescriptions, refer patients to a dietitian for more extensive teaching and explanation if necessary.

FOODS ALLOWED

Meat

Lean, well-trimmed meat. Prefer poultry, fish (not shrimp), veal, with occasional ham, pork, lamb, and beef

Eggs and other alternatives

Egg white only, no-cholesterol egg substitutes, legumes, soy protein, peanut butter, and nuts (such as walnuts, pecans, and almonds)

Milk and cheese

Skim milk and skim milk products, buttermilk; low-fat cheese, cottage cheese, yogurt containing up to 1% milkfat, and sherbet

Vegetables and fruits

Fresh, canned, frozen or dried fruits or vegetables; juices; vegetables prepared without animal fat; and vegetarian baked beans

Fat

Vegetable oils, soft margarine listing an allowed liquid oil as the first ingredient, and mayonnaise and salad dressings not containing sour cream or cheese

Breads and cereals

Cooked and dry cereal; rice; flour; pasta; breads made with a minimum of saturated fat; white, whole wheat, rye, pumpernickel, raisin, Italian, and French bread, English muffins; hard rolls; matzo; pretzels; saltines; and homemade breads made without whole milk, egg yolk, or saturated shortening

Soup

Bouillon, clear broths, fat-free vegetable soup and pot liquor, cream soups made with skim milk and allowed fat; and packaged dehydrated soup

Desserts and sweets

Angel food cake; fruit ices; sherbet (1% to 2% fat), gelatin desserts; meringues and homemade pastries made with allowed fat, skim milk, and egg white; pure sugar candies; jam and jelly; honey and syrup made without fat; molasses; and sugar

Miscellaneous

Coffee, tea, caffeine-free coffee, carbonated beverages, relishes, fat-free barbecue sauce, catsup, chili sauce, spices, herbs, extracts, lemon juice, and vinegar

FOODS TO AVOID OR LIMIT

Fatty meat, regular ground beef, bacon, sausage, luncheon meat, fried meat, meat in gravy, shrimp, organ meats, and fish roe

Egg yolk, canned pork and beans, cashews, and macadamia nuts

Whole milk and milk, malted milk and milkshakes, cream (sweet and sour), ice cream and ice milk, nondairy substitutes for cream, whipped toppings containing coconut or palm oil, and cheese made from cream or whole milk

Buttered, creamed, or fried vegetables; pork and beans; and avocado (use sparingly)

Other margarines (including low-calorie), butter, hydrogenated vegetable shortening, bacon, lard, meat drippings, salt pork, suet, cream, coconut, palm and peanut oils; and gravies (unless made with allowed fat and skim milk)

Egg noodles; egg bread; commercial biscuits, muffins, donuts, pancakes, waffles, and butter rolls; mixes for above; corn chips, potato chips, and other deep-fried snacks; and cheese crackers

All other soups

Commercial pies, cakes, and mixes; desserts and candy containing nonallowed fat, egg yolk, and whole milk; chocolate; and coconut

Earlier studies had not been as conclusive. The Coronary Drug Project trial studied males with coronary atherosclerosis who were treated with clofibrate, dextrothyroxine, or niacin to lower blood lipid concentration. None of the drugs reduced mortality, and dextrothyroxine increased mortality. In patients with established coronary atherosclerosis, reducing lipid levels may be less effective in preventing complications than in patients who have yet to develop clinical signs of heart disease and atherosclerosis.

SPECIFIC DRUGS TO LOWER BLOOD LIPID LEVELS

Drugs that are used to reduce blood lipid concentrations are listed in Table 21-2.

Table 21-2 Drugs That Reduce Blood Lipid Concentrations

Generic name	Trade name	Administration/dosage	Comments
Cholestyramine resin	Questran* Cholybar	ORAL: Adults—4 gm 4 times daily (at meals and bedtime). May be increased to 6 gm 4 times daily. Alternatively, the dosage may be divided into 2 or 3 doses. Material must be mixed with a liquid (1 oz for each gram). Children—over 6 yr, 8 gm twice daily with meals. Total maximum dosage, 24 gm daily.	Type II hyperlipidemia (high LDL). Stays in the intestine removing bile acids and thereby increasing cholesterol degradation by the liver. Available as a chewable bar, 4 gm per bar.
Clofibrate	Atromid-S* Clariplex† Novofibrate†	ORAL: Adults—500 mg 3 to 4 times daily.	Types III, IV, and V hyperlipidemia. Type II hyperlipidemia if VLDL is elevated. Inhibits triglyceride synthesis in the liver and inhibits the breakdown of triglycerides in fat tissue.
Colestipol hydrochloride	Colestid*	ORAL: Adults—15 to 30 gm daily in 2 to 4 doses with meals. Mix 1 oz liquid with each 4 to 6 gm. Children—not established.	Like cholestyramine.
Dextrothyroxine	Choloxin*	ORAL: Adults—with normal thyroid function, initially, 1 to 2 mg daily. May be increased monthly by 1 to 2 mg to a maximum of 8 mg daily (4 mg daily maximum in patients taking digitalis). Children—initially, 0.05 mg/kg body weight. May be increased monthly by 0.05 mg/kg to a maximum daily dose of 4 mg.	Type II hyperlipidemia. Lowers cholesterol by increasing LDL degradation.
Gemfibrozil	Lopid*	ORAL: Adults—600 mg twice daily 30 min before breakfast and dinner. FDA Pregnancy Category B.	Types IV and V hyperlipidemia. Lowers total triglyceride levels. Effects on cholesterol levels are mixed. LDL levels may fall and HDL levels increase.
Lovastatin	Mevacor*	ORAL: Adults—20 mg/day with the evening meal. May adjust at 4-week intervals. Maintenance dose: 20 to 80 mg daily. FDA Pregnancy Category X.	Type II hyperlipidemia. Inhibits cholesterol synthesis in the liver.
Niacin (nicotinic acid)	Nicobid Niac Nicolar Tri-B3†	ORAL: Adults—initially 100 mg 3 times daily, increasing to a total of 2 to 6 gm daily in divided doses with or after meals. FDA Pregnancy Category C.	Types II, III, IV, and V hyperlipidemia. Inhibits the synthesis of VLDL by the liver.
Pravastatin	Pravachol*	ORAL: Adults—10 to 20 mg once a day at bedtime initially. Maintenance dosage is 10 to 40 mg daily.	Type II hyperlipidemia. Inhibits cholesterol synthesis in the liver.
Probucol	Lorelco*	ORAL: Adults—500 mg twice daily (with breakfast and dinner). Children—not established.	Type II hyperlipidemia. Lowers cholesterol probably by inhibiting cholesterol biosynthesis in the liver.
Simvastatin	Zocor*	ORAL: Adults—5 to 10 mg once a day in the evening. Maintenance dosage is 5 to 40 mg daily.	Type II hyperlipidemia. Inhibits cholesterol synthesis in the liver.

*Available in Canada and United States.
†Available in Canada only.

Cholestyramine resin

Cholestyramine (Questran) is a resin with a sandlike texture that stays in the intestine and binds bile acids. Bile acids are the degradation products of cholesterol produced in the liver and excreted into the intestine through the biliary tract. The binding of bile acids by cholestyramine decreases the reabsorption of bile acid through the enterohepatic circulation and therefore increases the amount of fecal bile acid. Cholestyramine increases the excretion of cholesterol, but it must be taken several times a day to achieve this goal. Cholestyramine is effective in treating type II hyperlipidemia only. ∴ no effect on TG

The patient may experience bloating, nausea, and constipation at the beginning of cholestyramine therapy. During therapy, cholestyramine may interfere with the absorption of fat-soluble vitamins (A, D, K), digitalis, thyroxine, and coumarin anticoagulants.

Colestipol hydrochloride

Colestipol (Colestid) is similar to cholestyramine.

Clofibrate

Clofibrate (Atromid-S) reduces the plasma concentration of triglycerides by several mechanisms. It activates the enzyme lipoprotein lipase. This accelerates the breakdown of VLDL. It inhibits the release of VLDL by the liver. Clofibrate also decreases plasma cholesterol concentrations. This action appears to result from increased excretion of cholesterol into bile and subsequently into the feces. Clofibrate treats type IV hyperlipidemia, type II if there is elevated VLDL, and the rare type III and V hyperlipidemias.

Clofibrate produces few side effects. About 10% of patients initially experience some gastrointestinal (GI) upset. Clofibrate may cause impotence in men and muscle cramps and should be used with caution in patients with liver or kidney disease. It is contraindicated during pregnancy or for nursing mothers. Clofibrate displaces several drugs from albumin, including coumarins, phenytoin, and tolbutamide. The higher concentration of displaced drug can cause toxic effects.

Long-term use of clofibrate increases the incidence of gallstones. In studies of men with ischemic heart disease or a history of an MI, clofibrate increased the incidence of gallstones and symptoms of ischemic heart disease while not decreasing, and perhaps increasing, the overall death rate.

Dextrothyroxine

Dextrothyroxine (Choloxin) is the inactive stereoisomer of the hormone thyroxine. It enhances LDL degradation and thereby lowers plasma cholesterol levels. Since it lowers LDL, dextrothyroxine is only useful for type II hyperlipidemia. When plasma cholesterol levels are high, it produces a 20% to 30% decrease in 1 to 2 months. Side effects include dizziness, diarrhea, and an altered sense of taste. Some patients show symptoms of hyperthyroidism, such as weight loss, nervousness, insomnia, sweating, and menstrual irregularities. Others may be hypersensitive to iodine and experience itching or a rash. Angina may be aggravated.

Dextrothyroxine can decrease glucose tolerance in diabetic patients. It enhances the action of coumarin anticoagulants. Contraindications to dextrothyroxine use include pregnancy and hypertension, as well as heart, renal, or liver disease. Since the latter conditions are common among patients with type II hyperlipidemia, the use of dextrothyroxine is limited.

Gemfibrozil

Gemfibrozil (Lopid) is chemically related to clofibrate. Like clofibrate, it lowers VLDL levels to lower total triglyceride levels. Gemfibrozil interferes with the transfer of fatty acids from adipose tissue to the liver and with the hepatic production of VLDL. Gemfibrozil has variable effects on total cholesterol levels. LDL levels appear to fall while HDL levels appear to rise. It is not known whether this is associated with a reversal of atherosclerotic risks.

Gemfibrozil is prescribed for the treatment of severe hypertriglyceridemia, types IV and V. Side effects include GI upset and rashes. Gemfibrozil increases the incidence of gallstones and therefore is contraindicated for patients with gallstones. Blood glucose levels may rise in diabetic patients.

Lovastatin, Pravastatin, and Simvastatin

Lovastatin (Mevacor) is a relatively new antilipemic drug that inhibits an early step in synthesis of cholesterol by the liver. This inhibition leads to an overall reduction in LDL production, making lovastatin effective in the treatment of type II hyperlipoproteinemia. LDL levels decrease after 2 weeks of therapy; if therapy is discontinued, a therapeutic effect may remain for up to 6 weeks. Lovastatin is effective and may become the preferred treatment if long-term safety can be demonstrated.

Patients may complain of GI discomfort, headaches, dizziness, or skin rash. Side effects may include muscle aches or cramps, fever, tiredness or weakness, and blurred vision. Liver function tests may change with therapy. Yearly ophthalmic examinations are recommended. Lovastatin is contraindicated during pregnancy because skeletal abnormalities have been noted in animal studies. Lovastatin is primarily excreted unchanged in the feces through the bile.

Pravastatin (Pravachol) and Simvastatin (Zocor) are newly released drugs that act like lovastatin.

Niacin

Niacin (nicotinic acid) is a B vitamin for which the minimun daily requirement (MDR) is 20 mg. At doses 10 to 20 times higher than the MDR, niacin is a vasodilator (see Chapter 15). At doses 100 to 200 times higher than the MDR, niacin depresses the synthesis of VLDL by the liver and thereby reduces LDL. Niacin treats types II, III, IV and V hyperlipidemias. However, the high doses needed produce troublesome side effects in most patients, and only a few patients can tolerate continued use of niacin. Most patients experience marked flushing because of its vasodilator action. Itching and GI upset are also frequent side effects. Tolerance may develop to these symptoms; thus the dosage is usually low at first and increased gradually to avoid severe reactions. Niacin can cause or aggravate peptic ulcer, glucose intolerance (diabetes), and high plasma uric acid (gout).

Probucol

Probucol (Lorelco) inhibits cholesterol synthesis. It decreases plasma LDL and cholesterol and therefore is potentially useful in type II hyperlipidemia. Its main side effects are those of GI upset, including diarrhea, gas, abdominal pain, nausea, and vomiting. A clinical response to probucol occurs after 1 to 3 months of therapy. Cholesterol, but not triglyceride levels, is decreased. You should carefully monitor patients with a history of cardiac arrhythmias.

Other Lipid-Lowering Agents

Conjugated estrogens

Conjugated estrogens have been used as lipid-lowering agents because premenopausal women have a low incidence of MI. However, recent studies show that estrogen given to males not only causes feminization but also increases the incidence of heart attacks. Post-menopausal women are protected from an MI by conjugated estrogens.

Progestins and androgens

Progestins may decrease hyperlipidemia in women with type V hyperlipidemia. Progestins aggravate other types of hyperlipidemia and cannot be given to males. Anabolic androgens may reduce elevated plasma triglyceride concentrations in males only. Androgens can cause water retention and therefore must be used with care in males with heart, kidney, or liver disease.

Neomycin

Neomycin is an antibiotic that is not well absorbed. Neomycin prevents cholesterol absorption in the intestine, thereby promoting bile acid secretion. These effects may lower elevated LDL levels in some patients with type II hyperlipidemia.

NURSING IMPLICATIONS SUMMARY

Drugs to Lower Blood Lipid Levels

Patient and family education

◆ Most of these drugs cause GI side effects. Forewarn patients about this. Provide emotional support as needed. Instruct patients about the importance of taking the drug as prescribed for best effect.

◆ Review Patient Problem: Constipation on p. 182.

◆ Tell patients to report persistent or severe diarrhea to the physician.

◆ Teach patients about necessary changes in diet to lower fat, carbohydrate, and cholesterol; see Dietary Consideration: Cholesterol on p. 340. Refer patients to the dietitian as appropriate. Teach patients that these drugs must be taken for weeks to months before full benefit can be seen. If the drugs prove to be beneficial, they may then be prescribed on a long-term basis.

◆ Remind patients not to discontinue taking the drugs without consulting the physician. Doses of other medications may be prescribed based on their effect when the patient is taking the prescribed antilipemic. Discontinuing the antilipemic therapy may result in incorrect doses of other drugs being taken. Because these drugs may interfere with absorption of other prescribed drugs, remind patients to keep all health care providers informed of all drugs being taken.

◆ It may be appropriate to screen children for the presence of familial hyperlipidemias and if necessary to place them on therapeutic diets to lower lipid levels.

Cholestyramine and Colestipol

Drug administration

◆ Monitor intake and output, weight, urinalysis, and vital signs. Assess patients for skin changes and rashes.

Continued.

NURSING IMPLICATIONS SUMMARY—cont'd

◆ Schedule drug administration times to allow as much time as possible between cholestyramine or colestipol and other drugs taken orally. At minimum, take other drugs 1 hr before or 4 hr after cholestyramine or colestipol.

Patient and family education

◆ Review the general guidelines.
◆ GI side effects are the most common. Instruct patients to report the development of any unexpected sign or symptom.
◆ Review all of the drugs the patient is taking, and plan a dosing schedule to allow as much time as possible to elapse between the antilipemic and other medications.
◆ For the chewable bar, instruct patients to chew each bite well before swallowing. Instruct patients not to take the powder in dry form. Always mix it with fluid or food or fruit with a high fluid content such as applesauce, crushed pineapple, or thin soups, or with milk in hot or regular breakfast cereals. Fill a glass with 4 to 6 oz of chosen fluid. Put the correct dose of medication on top of the fluid and let it stand, without stirring, for 1 to 2 min. This allows the medicine to absorb moisture and helps prevent formation of lumps. Instruct patients to stir and drink the mixture while the drug is still suspended. The drug will not dissolve in the fluid. Add a little more of the selected beverage to rinse the glass, and drink this also. If a carbonated beverage is chosen, use a large glass to prevent spillover, since the mixture will foam up. To prevent swallowing air, especially if a carbonated beverage is chosen, patients should drink the mixture slowly. Instruct patient to take doses before meals and at bedtime, as ordered.
◆ Since these drugs interfere with absorption of fat-soluble vitamins, supplemental vitamins may be necessary; consult the physician. If these drugs are used to treat the pruritus of biliary stasis, the pruritus may reappear if the drug is discontinued.

Clofibrate
Patient and family education

◆ See the general guidelines.
◆ Nausea is the most common side effect, but others occasionally occur. Tell patients to report the development of any unexpected sign or symptom. Impotence and decreased libido have occurred; patients may be reluctant to mention these. Assess patient carefully for

sexual side effects. Provide emotional support. It may be possible to change dose or drug; consult the physician.
◆ Patients should take doses with meals to lessen gastric irritation. Nausea may diminish with continued use of the drug.

Dextrothyroxine
Patient and family education

◆ Review general guidelines for antilipemic therapy (see Chapter 52). The effects of treatment with dextrothyroxine mimic those of any thyroid replacement hormone. Overdose results in symptoms of hyperthyroidism.

Gemfibrozil
Patient and family education

◆ Review general guidelines for antilipemic therapy.
◆ GI upset is the most common side effect but others occasionally occur. Tell patients to report the development of any unexpected sign or symptom.
◆ Caution diabetic patients to monitor blood glucose levels closely, since this drug may cause an increase in fasting glucose and a decrease in glucose tolerance. Changes in diet or insulin dose may be necessary.

Lovastatin, Pravastatin, and Simvastatin
Patient and family education

◆ Review general guidelines for antilipemic therapy.
◆ GI discomfort may occur, and a variety of other side effects have been reported. Instruct patients to report the development of any unexpected sign or symptom.
◆ Warn patients to avoid driving or operating hazardous equipment if blurred vision or weakness develops; notify the physician.
◆ Patients should take doses with the evening meal.
◆ Encourage patients to have regular eye examinations.

Niacin
Patient and family education

◆ Review general guidelines for antilipemic therapy.
◆ Most patients experience flushing of the face and neck after taking the dose needed for its antilipemic effect. This usually diminishes with continued use of the drug. Starting with low doses and gradually increasing them may

NURSING IMPLICATIONS SUMMARY—cont'd

also help. Flushing may be ameliorated by taking 1 aspirin tablet 30 min before the niacin dose (check with physician). GI discomfort may occur, and a variety of other side effects have been reported. Instruct patients to report the development of any unexpected sign or symptom. Patients should take doses with meals to lessen gastric irritation.

◆ For information about dietary sources of niacin, see Dietary Consideration: Vitamins on p. 275.

◆ Caution diabetic patients to monitor blood glucose levels carefully during periods of dosage adjustment while on niacin.

Probucol
Patient and family education

◆ Review general guidelines for antilipemic therapy.

◆ GI discomfort may occur, and a variety of other side effects have been reported. Instruct patients to report the development of any unexpected sign or symptom. Impotence and decreased libido may occur; patients may be reluctant to mention these. Assess patient carefully for such side effects. Provide emotional support. It may be possible to change dose or drug; consult the physician. Instruct patients to take doses with meals for best effect.

CHAPTER REVIEW

◆ **KEY TERMS**

atherosclerosis, p. 336
hyperlipidemia, p. 338
lipids, p. 336
lipoproteins, p. 336

◆ **REVIEW QUESTIONS**

1. List the four categories of lipoproteins and describe the role of each.

2. What is hyperlipidemia? What causes it? What is the most frequently seen type of hyperlipidemia? The least common form?

3. Name five drugs you might see prescribed for lowering plasma cholesterol and their mechanism of action.

4. Name drugs and their mechanism of action for lowering triglyceride levels.

5. Develop a teaching plan for the patient who needs to decrease dietary intake of cholesterol.

SUGGESTED READING

Becker DM, Larosa JH, Watson JE: Interpreting the new guidelines, *Am J Nurs* 89(12):1622, 1989.

Grundy SM: Cholesterol and coronary heart disease, *JAMA* 264(23):3053, 1990.

Hartshorn JC, Deans K: Treatment of hyperlipidemia with gemfibrozil, *J Cardiovasc Nurs* 1(4):76, 1987.

Schulman KA and others: Reducing high blood cholesterol level with drugs, cost-effectiveness of pharmacologic management, *JAMA* 264(23):3025, 1990.

Schultheis AH: Hypercholesterolemia: prevention, detection, and management, *Nurs Pract* 15(1):40, 1990.

Steinberg D, Witztum JL: Lipoproteins and atherogenesis, current concepts, *JAMA* 264(23):3047, 1990.

Stoy DB: Controlling cholesterol with diet, *Am J Nurs* 89(12):1625, 1989.

Stoy DB: Controlling cholesterol with drugs, *Am J Nurs* 89(12):1628, 1989.

Stoy DB: Diet and drug therapy for hypercholesterolemia: principles and perspectives for the occupational health setting, *AAOHN J*, 38(5):222, 1990.

Stoy DB: Pharmacotherapy for hypercholesterolemia: guidelines and nursing perspectives, *J Cardiovasc Nurs* 5(2):34, 1991.

Todd B: Cholesterol reducers: worth the price? *Geriatr Nurs* 10(1):39, 1989.

CHAPTER 22

Drugs to Treat Anemia

LEARNING OBJECTIVES

After studying this chapter, you should be able to do the following:

◆ Explain the role of iron in normal body functioning.

◆ Develop a care plan for the patient receiving iron therapy.

◆ Describe the treatment of iron toxicity.

◆ Explain the treatment of pernicious anemia, and develop a care plan for patients receiving vitamin B_{12}.

◆ Outline dietary sources of iron, folic acid, and vitamin B_{12}.

◆ Explain the use of Epoetin Alpha, and develop a nursing care plan for patients receiving it.

CHAPTER OVERVIEW

◆ This chapter covers iron, vitamin B_{12}, folic acid, and related agents used to treat anemia. These agents are most commonly associated with anemia of nutritional origin. They play a major role in the production of new red blood cells—the process of *hematopoiesis*.

◆ Erythropoietin, a growth factor produced by the kidney, promotes hematopoiesis. Erythropoietin is a new product available through recombinant DNA technology.

Nursing Process Overview

IRON THERAPY

Assessment

Patients requiring iron therapy may have fatigue, pallor, and lethargy. Folic acid and vitamin B_{12} deficiency are usually diagnosed from blood studies but may be seen in patients with iron deficiency anemia. Assess vital signs, weight, and diet history; blood studies, including hemoglobin level, peripheral blood smear, and reticulocyte count; and any neurologic symptoms such as tingling in the fingers or toes.

Nursing Diagnosis

Altered bowel elimination: constipation secondary to iron therapy

Management

At usual dosages, there are few side effects with these drugs. If the source of anemia is diet related, provide dietary instruction about iron-rich foods.

Evaluation

Determine that patients can explain what kind of anemia is present, what the goals of drug therapy are, how to take the prescribed medications correctly, what anticipated side effects are and what to do about them, and which symptoms can be expected to improve and which will not. (The neurologic damage in pernicious anemia may be permanent.) Verify that patients can identify dietary sources of needed iron or folic acid.

IRON

Functions

Iron is an essential component of several key proteins that carry or use oxygen. Over 70% of body iron is part of hemoglobin, the protein of red blood cells that transports oxygen to tissues and carbon dioxide away from tissues. The red color of blood is caused by the iron-oxygen complex in the heme portion of hemoglobin. Iron is also part of several of the electron transport enzymes of the mitochondria responsible for the oxidation-reduction reactions essential to functioning cells.

Absorption, Storage, and Excretion

Given the importance of iron, it is not surprising that the body uses iron efficiently. The total iron content of a 70-kg male is about 4 gm, yet iron is reused so efficiently that less than 1 mg of iron is lost daily. Not only is the iron of the red blood cell reused after cell degradation, but 10% to 35% of the iron is in a storage form for use when required. Iron is lost only as body cells are lost through shedding of cells from the gastrointestinal (GI) tract, skin, fingernails, and hair and in fluids such as bile, urine, and sweat.

The absorption of iron from food is regulated. Iron is taken up by active transport into the mucosal cells of the duodenum and upper jejunum in the small intestine. These cells contain the protein ferritin, which binds the iron. When ferritin is saturated with iron, further absorption of iron is limited. It remains in the mucosal cells unless transferred to the plasma protein transferrin. Iron not transferred within 5 days is lost in the feces when the mucosal cell is sloughed. Iron bound to transferrin is carried in the plasma and transferred to the proteins ferritin and hemosiderin, which act as storage forms of iron within the liver, spleen, and bone marrow.

Iron as a Therapeutic Agent

Iron deficiency anemia

When the intake of iron is inadequate to meet the demand, iron is first taken from the iron stores in hemosiderin and ferritin. Absorption of iron from the GI tract can increase twofold when the ferritin within the mucosal cells is no longer saturated with iron. When iron stores are exhausted and the intake of iron is still inadequate, the newly made red blood cells are small (microcytic) and do not have much color (hypochromic) because there is not enough iron to make an adequate amount of hemoglobin to fill the cells. **Iron deficiency anemia** is therefore a microcytic, hypochromic anemia.

Requirements for iron

Iron deficiency anemia commonly results from blood loss or rapid growth. This is reflected in the varying requirements for dietary iron. The average American diet contains about 6 mg of iron per 1000 calories, and only 10% of dietary iron is actually absorbed, although up to 20% may be absorbed in iron-deficient individuals. Adult males and postmenopausal females have the lowest daily requirement for dietary iron (5 to 10 mg). Menstruating females have a higher daily requirement, depending on the amount of blood loss during menstruation (7 to 20 mg).

DIETARY CONSIDERATION: IRON

Inadequate iron intake contributes to iron deficiency anemia, the most common nutritional deficiency in the United States. Good dietary sources of iron include the following:
- Red meats
- Legumes and nuts
- Whole grains
- Molasses
- Dried fruits
- Organ meats
- Green leafy vegetables
- Enriched bread and cereal
- Brewer's yeast
- Oysters

Pregnant females have the highest daily requirement because of the added demand of the placenta and developing fetus (20 to 58 mg). Children and adolescents have a higher requirement per unit weight than adults because of their rapid growth (4 to 20 mg total) (see box).

Administration of replacement iron

Iron for replacement therapy is most commonly given orally as a ferrous salt. Iron preparations are listed in Table 22-1. Ferrous sulfate is the standard for these preparations. The usual daily dose in iron deficiency anemia is 50 to 100 mg of iron. The amount of iron per tablet depends on the ferrous salt used. A 300-mg tablet of ferrous sulfate contains 60 mg of iron and 240 mg of sulfate; a 300-mg tablet of ferrous gluconate contains 37 mg of iron and 263 mg of gluconate; and a 300-mg tablet of ferrous fumarate contains 99 mg of iron and 201 mg of fumarate.

Iron in the ferrous form is absorbed most readily in the presence of acid. Therefore optimum absorption occurs when a tablet of ferrous sulfate or other soluble ferrous salt is taken before meals. However, iron is also highly irritating to the GI tract; many patients cannot tolerate iron tablets taken on an empty stomach and have to take iron with meals. Enteric forms are not satisfactory, since they generally dissolve past the duodenum, where there is little capacity for the absorption of iron. Infants and children given iron-supplemented formula or vitamins may develop acute diarrhea from the GI irritation.

Patients with iron deficiency anemia respond to iron therapy in the first 2 days with increased energy and appetite. Since this is too soon to correct the hemoglobin deficiency, the response may be due to restoration of the cellular enzymes containing iron. After 1 week there is an increase in the number of

Table 22-1   Drugs to Treat Nutritional Anemias

Generic name	Trade name	Administration/dosage	Comments
IRON SALTS FOR IRON DEFICIENCY ANEMIA			
Ferrous fumarate (33% elemental iron)	Femiron Fumerin Palafer† Various others	Replacement therapy requires 90 to 300 mg of elemental iron daily in divided doses before meals if tolerated or with meals.	Timed-release or enteric coated forms considered less effective because of poor iron absorption beyond the duodenum.
Ferrous gluconate (11.6% elemental iron)	Fergon Fertinic† Various others	See above.	See above.
Ferrous sulfate (20% elemental iron)	Feosol Fer-In-Sol* Fero-Gradumet Various others	See above.	See above.
Iron-dextran injection	Imferon* Various others	INTRAVENOUS: *Adults and children*—no more than 100 mg daily, no faster than 50 mg (1 ml)/min of the undiluted solution, or dilute in 500 to 1000 ml normal saline solution and administer by drip over 10 hr. (FDA) Pregnancy Category C.	Reserved for use in severe iron deficiency anemia where oral iron is contraindicated (GI disease) or unsuccessful. Serious toxic effects, including anaphylaxis, may accompany parenteral administration and are more common with IM than with IV administration.
Iron-polysaccharide complex	Hytinic Niferex	See above.	Not well absorbed. May be milder to the stomach than other formulations.
ANTIDOTE FOR IRON TOXICITY			
Deferoxamine mesylate	Desferal*	INTRAMUSCULAR: preferred route; 1 gm followed by 0.5 gm at 4 hr and 8 hr. INTRAVENOUS: in face of cardiovascular collapse; as for intramuscular (IM) but infused at 15 mg kg/hr. Not to exceed 6 gm in 24 hr.	A specific chelator for iron. To manage acute iron intoxication. Will turn urine pink to red. Can be administered long-term to manage secondary hemochromatosis.
VITAMIN B₁₂ (CYANOCOBALAMIN) FOR PERNICIOUS ANEMIA			
Hydroxocobalamin	Alphamine Acti-B₁₂† Various others	As for cyanocobalamin.	Like cyanocobalamin. Somewhat longer acting.
Vitamin B₁₂ (cyanocobalamin)	Betalin 12 Redisol Rubramin PC* Various others	INTRAMUSCULAR: 30 to 50 μg daily for 5 to 10 days, then 100 to 200 μg monthly.	For pernicious anemia, only IM injection effective. Oral forms taken for dietary deficiency.
FOLIC ACID FOR ANEMIA			
Folic acid	Apo-Folic† Folvite*	ANY ROUTE: *Adults or children*—1 mg daily.	Solutions of the sodium salt used for parenteral administration.
Leucovorin calcium	Wellcovorin Generic	For megaloblastic anemia, 1 mg daily. To counter folic acid antagonists, give in amounts equal to the weight of antagonist.	The metabolically active form of folic acid. The expense does not justify use for anemia, but protects normal tissue when given with methotrexate (antineoplastic drug) or pyrimethamine (antimalarial drug)
HORMONE FOR ANEMIA			
Epoetin Alpha	Epogen EPO	INTRAVENOUS, SUBCUTANEOUS: *Adults and children*—initially, 50 to 100 units/kg 3 times weekly. The dosage is adjusted to reach a hematocrit of 30% to 33%.	Epoetin is the protein hormone, erythropoietin, produced by recombinant DNA technology. Used to treat the anemia of chronic renal failure.

IM, Intramuscular; *IV,* intravenous.
*Available in Canada and United States.
†Available in Canada only.

reticulocytes (immature red blood cells) and the rate of hemoglobin synthesis. Although the microcytic anemia of iron deficiency is eliminated after a few weeks of therapy, at least 6 months of therapy is necessary to restore iron storage sites.

Iron may also be given parenterally as iron dextran when oral administration is not possible. Slow intravenous (IV) injection is preferred. Deep intramuscular (IM) injection is painful and can discolor the injection site. An anaphylactic response is more common after IM than after IV injection.

Food and drug interactions

Absorption of iron salts is increased with ingestion of large doses of ascorbic acid (vitamin C). Cereal and eggs decrease absorption, as do antacids, particularly magnesium trisilicate, and tetracyclines, since all of these bind to iron and prevent its uptake by the mucosal cells in the small intestine.

Iron Toxicity

Acute toxicity from excess iron

Acute toxicity from iron is uncommon in adults and is primarily seen in young children. The population most likely to take iron tablets are pregnant women who may also have small children. Many iron tablets are brightly colored and look like candy, leading young children to swallow many tablets at once. Commonly the child experiences acute nausea and vomiting 30 to 60 min after ingesting the tablets. Treatment is gastric lavage with sodium phosphate or sodium bicarbonate to remove undissolved tablets, to create an alkaline environment that retards absorption, and to complex the ferrous iron into insoluble salts.

Within a few hours of ingestion, metabolic acidosis is common and cardiovascular collapse can occur. If supportive treatment carries the child through these stages, the next stage originates from tissue injury. The high concentration of iron overloads the uptake capacity of the mucosal cells so that a high concentration of free ferrous iron enters the portal circulation. Signs of extensive damage to the liver and kidney are evident in children who die of iron toxicity after 24 hr.

To avoid damage from high plasma concentrations of iron, a specific antidote, deferoxamine mesylate (Desferal), is given as soon as possible and concurrently with lavage and supportive measures. Deferoxamine is given IM or IV, and combines with iron in the plasma to form a water-soluble complex that is excreted in urine (67%) and in bile (33%). This complex gives a pink to red color to urine, which shows elevated concentrations of iron in the plasma. The free deferoxamine imparts no color to urine.

Chronic toxicity from iron overload

Since the body has no mechanisms to remove excess iron, excess intake can cause iron overload, called **hemosiderosis** (after the storage protein for iron). Chronic iron overload can occur in patients treated with parenteral iron who receive frequent blood transfusions, since each milliliter of blood contains 0.5 mg of iron. Some patients have a genetic tendency to store excess iron; this genetic disorder is called **hemochromatosis.** Iron overload traditionally imparts a bronze color to the skin of the face, neck, upper chest, genitalia, hands, and forearms. The pancreas is especially sensitive to damage, and diabetes mellitus can result. Liver damage is seen on biopsy but is generally not serious unless superimposed on liver disease. Patients with iron overload generally die of heart failure. Treatment for iron overload is weekly bleeding (phlebotomy).

MEGALOBLASTIC MACROCYTIC ANEMIAS

Both vitamin B_{12} and folic acid are required for a key reaction in the synthesis of thymidylate, a component of DNA. Whereas folic acid is the immediate cofactor in this synthesis, vitamin B_{12} regenerates the active form of folic acid. Deficiency of folic acid or vitamin B_{12} results in the release of too few red blood cells. Those red blood cells that are released are large and immature because of the deficiency of DNA synthesis required for cell division and maturation. This is a **megaloblastic macrocytic anemia,** or immature large cell anemia. Other tissue cells that turn over rapidly and require active DNA synthesis include some white and mucosal cells of the GI tract. A deficiency in white cell counts and GI upset can appear in vitamin B_{12} or folic acid deficiency.

Vitamin B_{12} and Pernicious Anemia

Vitamin B_{12} is unique because it requires a special binding protein for transport into the intestinal cells. This binding protein is called **intrinsic factor,** which is produced and released by the parietal cells of the stomach. (Parietal cells also release hydrochloric acid.) **Pernicious anemia** is the relative or complete lack of intrinsic factor so that vitamin B_{12} is no longer absorbed. The body has a large store of vitamin B_{12}, 4 to 5 mg, and a deficiency will not occur for 2 to 5 years after intrinsic factor is no longer released. Stomach atrophy is a normal part of the aging process, and pernicious anemia appears more frequently in patients over 50 years of age than in younger patients. Any condition that damages the stomach can also cause pernicious anemia.

Origin, absorption, and distribution of vitamin B_{12}

A diet including animal protein, eggs, and dairy products contains adequate vitamin B_{12}. The usual American diet contains 5 to 15 μg of vitamin B_{12}, although the minimum daily requirement is only 1 to 2 μg. Only strict vegetarians develop dietary vitamin B_{12} deficiency over a period of several years. Vitamin B_{12} bound to intrinsic factor is absorbed in the distal ileum, the part of the small intestine just ahead of the large intestine, and this absorption requires a slightly alkaline pH. Conditions in which the distal ileum is damaged or removed or in which the pancreas fails to secrete sufficient bicarbonate to keep the intestine at a slightly alkaline pH slow absorption of vitamin B_{12}. After absorption, vitamin B_{12} is carried to storage sites. Some vitamin B_{12} is excreted in the bile but is later reabsorbed.

Vitamin B_{12} deficiency

Neurologic damage may result from deficiency of vitamin B_{12}. This damage arises because vitamin B_{12} is a cofactor for an enzymatic step necessary for producing the myelin sheath of nerves. A frequent initial neurologic symptom of vitamin B_{12} deficiency is a tingling sensation of the extremities (paresthesia) from neurologic damage. Neurologic damage becomes irreversible if vitamin B_{12} deficiency persists.

Administration of replacement vitamin B_{12}

The IM injection of vitamin B_{12} to bypass the intestine for systemic absorption is the treatment for pernicious anemia. Initial therapy is administered daily for about 1 week, then monthly throughout life. Oral vitamin B_{12} is indicated only for the rare dietary deficiency of vitamin B_{12} when there is an adequate amount of intrinsic factor released.

Vitamin B_{12} injections have been given indiscriminately to older patients as a general tonic, which it is not. Vitamin B_{12} injections are also not of therapeutic value for general neurologic disorders, psychiatric disorders, general malnutrition, or loss of appetite. Folic acid taken in large doses will overcome the block in DNA synthesis caused by the deficiency of vitamin B_{12}. Folic acid will thereby cure the anemia, but folic acid cannot affect the vitamin B_{12}–dependent reaction necessary for myelin synthesis. If folic acid is taken indiscriminately, the anemia of vitamin B_{12} deficiency will never appear, but neurologic damage may proceed until it is irreversible.

Vitamin B_{12} injections are virtually free of side effects. Patients receiving vitamin B_{12} injections for pernicious anemia must understand that injections must be continued for the rest of their lives to avoid irreversible neurologic damage.

Folic Acid

Folic acid is found in most meats, fresh vegetables, and fresh fruits but is destroyed when these are cooked for longer than 15 min. Folic acid preparations are listed in Table 22-1. The minimum daily requirement is 50 gm, and the average American diet contains 200 to 300 gm. Unlike vitamin B_{12}, stores of folic acid are not large and can be depleted in a few weeks when the diet is deficient in folic acid. It is readily absorbed in the intestine and administered orally. Individuals with poor diets and chronic alcoholics may be deficient in folic acid. Pregnant women and nursing mothers have increased requirements for folic acid, and it is commonly given as a routine supplement to these women. Studies have shown that folic acid taken during pregnancy reduces the incidence of neurologic defects in newborn infants.

Some drugs interfere with the use of folic acid including phenytoin, oral contraceptives, glucocorticoids, and aspirin. Methotrexate, antineoplastic drugs, and pyrimethamine (an antimalarial drug) are folic acid antagonists. When these drugs are used, folinic acid (leucovorin), the metabolically active form of folic acid, can be given to protect normal tissues from folic acid deficiency. Folic acid is nontoxic. The greatest danger of indiscriminate ingestion of folic acid is that it may correct the anemia of pernicious anemia but leave the neurologic damage untreated.

ANEMIA SECONDARY TO KIDNEY FAILURE

Chronic renal failure is associated with underproduction of red blood cells. This happens because the kidney is the major producer of the growth factor, erythropoietin, which is critical to the production of red blood cells. When the kidneys fail, erythropoietin is not produced in sufficient quantity to maintain adequate red blood cell production in the bone marrow.

Epoetin Alpha

Epoetin Alpha (Epogen and EPO) is the human hormone, erythropoietin, manufactured by recombinant DNA technology. It is a protein and must be administered intravenously or subcutaneously. This hormone stimulates the production of red blood cells. The effect is seen in 1 to 2 weeks.

Epoetin counteracts the anemia associated with chronic renal failure. This avoids the need for transfusion of red blood cells and greatly improves patients' quality of life. Patients should be evaluated to ensure that they have adequate iron stores to support red blood cell production.

Epoetin is being evaluated for treatment of anemia resulting in a number of other conditions, including azathioprine (AZT) treatment, prematurity, rheumatoid arthritis, and cancer.

Side effects of epoetin are minimal. Occasional headaches or joint pain are reported. About one-third of patients have elevated blood pressure that may require drug therapy. However, renal function does not worsen.

Abuse of epoetin has been reported among athletes in high-endurance sports, especially cyclists. The increased production of red blood cells enhances athletic performance by increasing the blood's ability to carry oxygen. The increased number of red blood cells makes the blood more viscous, and this viscosity is enhanced by the dehydration of performance. Death from heart blockage was reported in one young athlete taking epoetin.

NURSING IMPLICATIONS SUMMARY

General Guidelines for Patients Receiving Iron Therapy

Drug administration

◆ Parenteral and oral iron preparations should not be given at the same time, since this increases the incidence of toxic reactions.

◆ Parenteral doses of iron may cause anaphylactic reactions. Before the first dose of IM or IV iron dextran, administer a 25-mg test dose. Monitor vital signs. Wait at least 1 hr before administering the remaining dose. Have available equipment, drugs, and personnel to treat anaphylactic reactions. Other reactions may include fever, arthralgias, myalgia, headache, transitory paresthesia, nausea, shivering, and rash.

INTRAMUSCULAR IRON DEXTRAN

◆ Use large muscle masses, preferably in the buttocks. The drug may stain the skin, which on the thigh is cosmetically unacceptable. Consult the physician when administering to small children and infants. Draw up the prescribed dose. Put a fresh needle on the syringe. Use the Z-track method of administration (see Chapter 6).

INTRAVENOUS IRON DEXTRAN

◆ Read the vial carefully; use preparations labeled "for IV use." May be given undiluted or diluted in 50 to 250 ml normal saline. Administer a test dose over at least 5 min. Administer other doses at a rate of 50 mg/min. Flush the IV line with normal saline before and after administering dose. Keep the patient in a supine position for 30 min after IV doses; monitor vital signs and blood pressure.

Patient and family education

◆ Review dietary sources of iron with patients (see Dietary Consideration: Iron on p. 347). Remind patients to keep all medications out of the reach of children. Tell patients to notify the physician immediately if overdose with iron is suspected.

◆ Instruct patients to take liquid iron preparations through a straw to avoid staining the teeth. Patients should dilute the preparation well with water or fruit juice and should rinse the mouth well after taking the dose.

◆ Ideally, instruct patients to take iron preparations on an empty stomach, although this may cause significant GI upset. Patients should take the drug with meals or a snack to reduce gastric irritation, but note that absorption is significantly reduced in the presence of milk, antacids, tetracycline, many cereals, and eggs. Vitamin C increases the absorption of iron; some patients may take the iron with orange or other citrus juice.

◆ Inform patients that regular use of iron causes the feces to turn dark green or black and to become more tarry in consistency. If there is doubt whether the cause of a change in color or consistency in stools is due to blood or ingestion of iron, the stool should be tested for presence of blood. Some patients experience diarrhea while taking iron preparations, and others experience constipation (see Patient Problem: Constipation on p. 182). If diarrhea is severe or persistent, notify the physician. To decrease gastric irritation, suggest that the patient take smaller but more frequent doses of iron.

Continued.

Deferoxamine Mesylate

Drug administration

◆ Deferoxamine may be administered via IM, IV, or subcutaneous injection, usually by subcutaneous pump. IM or subcutaneous injection may cause swelling, irritation, pain, and itching at the injection site. Deferoxamine has been associated with allergic reactions, including anaphylactic reactions. Monitor vital signs. Have available equipment and drugs to treat acute allergic reactions.

INTRAVENOUS DEFEROXAMINE

◆ Dilute as directed in the manufacturer's literature. Administer at a rate not exceeding 15 mg/kg/hr. Monitor the blood pressure and vital signs. Treatment of acute iron overdose should be performed in the acute care setting.

Vitamin B_{12}

Drug administration

◆ Administer parenteral doses via the IM route only. Allergic reactions have been reported. Monitor vital signs and blood pressure. Have available drugs and equipment to treat acute allergic reactions.

Patient and family education

◆ Teach patients with pernicious anemia about their disease. It may be difficult for patients to understand why the vitamin B_{12} cannot be taken orally and why it must be continued for life. Review dietary sources of vitamin B_{12} (see Dietary Consideration: Vitamins on p. 275) with patients in whom vitamin B_{12} deficiency is due to dietary causes. Teach patients to avoid the use of alcohol while taking vitamin B_{12}.

Folic Acid

Drug administration

◆ In addition to the more common oral administration, folic acid may be given IM, IV, or via the subcutaneous route.

◆ Folic acid may be given undiluted or added to most IV solutions and given as an infusion. For direct IV administration, administer at a rate not to exceed 5 mg/min.

◆ Allergic reactions, although rare, have been reported. Monitor vital signs after parenteral administration. Have available drugs and equipment to treat acute allergic reactions.

Patient and family education

◆ Review dietary sources of folic acid (see Dietary Consideration: Vitamins on p. 275).

◆ Warn patients that self-treatment with large doses of vitamins is unwise and may mask some health problems. Large doses of vitamins should be taken only under the direction of a physician.

Leucovorin

Drug administration and patient and family education

◆ Leucovorin is the calcium salt of folinic acid, a metabolite of folic acid. Read orders carefully. It may be given orally, IM, or IV. Parenteral administration is usually used when the drug is given to counteract some of the toxic effects of the folic acid antagonists, especially some cancer chemotherapy drugs (called *leucovorin rescue*) (see Chapter 39).

PARENTERAL ADMINISTRATION

◆ Reconstitute as directed on the vial. Further dilute in 100 to 500 ml of common IV fluid. Administer dilute volume over 15 min to 1 hr (depending on volume and patient condition). Monitor vital signs.

◆ For leucovorin or folinic acid rescue, several protocols may be used. The dose is based on the dose of methotrexate and the body surface area of the patient. Monitor the creatinine level.

◆ Review with patients and families the reason leucovorin is being used. Instruct them to report the development of any unexpected sign or symptom.

Epoetin Alpha

Drug administration

◆ May be given undiluted as an IV bolus. Read accompanying literature. Do not shake vial. Prepare only 1 dose per vial. Administer dose over at least 1 min. For dialysis patients, it may be administered via the venous line at the end of dialysis. May also be administered IV or subcutaneously in patients not receiving dialysis.

◆ Monitor blood pressure, and report increases to the physician. Dose and length of therapy are based on patient response. Monitor the complete blood count (CBC) with differential; platelet counts; blood urea nitrogen (BUN) levels; and uric acid, creatinine, phosphorus, and potassium levels.

Patient and family education

◆ Review the reasons for epoetin therapy. Instruct the patient to report the development of any new sign or symptom.

CHAPTER REVIEW

◆ KEY TERMS

hemochromatosis, p. 349
hemosiderosis, p. 349
intrinsic factor, p. 349
iron, p. 346
iron deficiency anemia, p. 347
megaloblastic macrocytic anemia, p. 349
pernicious anemia, p. 349

◆ REVIEW QUESTIONS

1. What is the role of iron?
2. Describe factors governing the absorption of iron.
3. What are the symptoms of iron toxicity?
4. How does deferoxamine function as an antidote for iron toxicity?
5. What is pernicious anemia?
6. Why does vitamin B_{12} have to be injected intramuscularly to treat pernicious anemia?
7. What role do vitamin B_{12} and folic acid play in red blood cell maturation?
8. Why is folic acid contraindicated for treatment of pernicious anemia?
9. Why is chronic renal failure associated with underproduction of red blood cells?
10. How would you respond to a student athlete colleague who wants to know about epoetin to increase athletic endurance?

SUGGESTED READING

Beutler E: The common anemias, *JAMA* 259(16):2433, 1988.
Biggers PB: Administering epoetin alfa, *Nurs 91* 21(4):43, 1991.
Erslev AJ: Erythropoietin, *N Engl J Med* 234(19):1339, 1991.
Froberg JH: The anemias: causes and courses of action, parts 1 and 2, *RN* 52(1):24 and 52(3):52, 1989.
Stockman JA III: Iron deficiency anemia: have we come far enough? *JAMA* 258(12):1645, 1987.

SECTION VI

DRUGS TO TREAT MILD PAIN AND FEVER, INFLAMMATION, ALLERGY, AND RESPIRATORY OBSTRUCTION

Many chemicals such as histamine and the prostaglandins are released or synthesized in response to injury. These substances act locally and systemically through receptors to produce a physiologic response. This section covers the pharmacologic basis of mild pain and fever, inflammation, allergy, and respiratory obstruction in which substances like histamine and prostaglandins play a major role.

Chapter 23, Drugs for Pain and Inflammation, relates the various uses of aspirin. Aspirin is an inhibitor of the synthesis of prostaglandins. Certain prostaglandins affect pain, fever, and inflammation. Several categories of antiinflammatory drugs are included in Chapter 23, including those for rheumatoid arthritis and gout. Antihistamines, covered in Chapter 24, are used primarily to treat allergies. Chapter 25, Bronchodilators and Other Drugs to Treat Asthma, deals with the therapeutics of asthma, for which the pharmacology principally involves adrenergic mechanisms. Chapter 26, Drugs to Control Bronchial Secretions, discusses classes of drugs used to treat respiratory problems, including nasal congestion, cough, and thickened mucus, to complete the coverage of respiratory pharmacology.

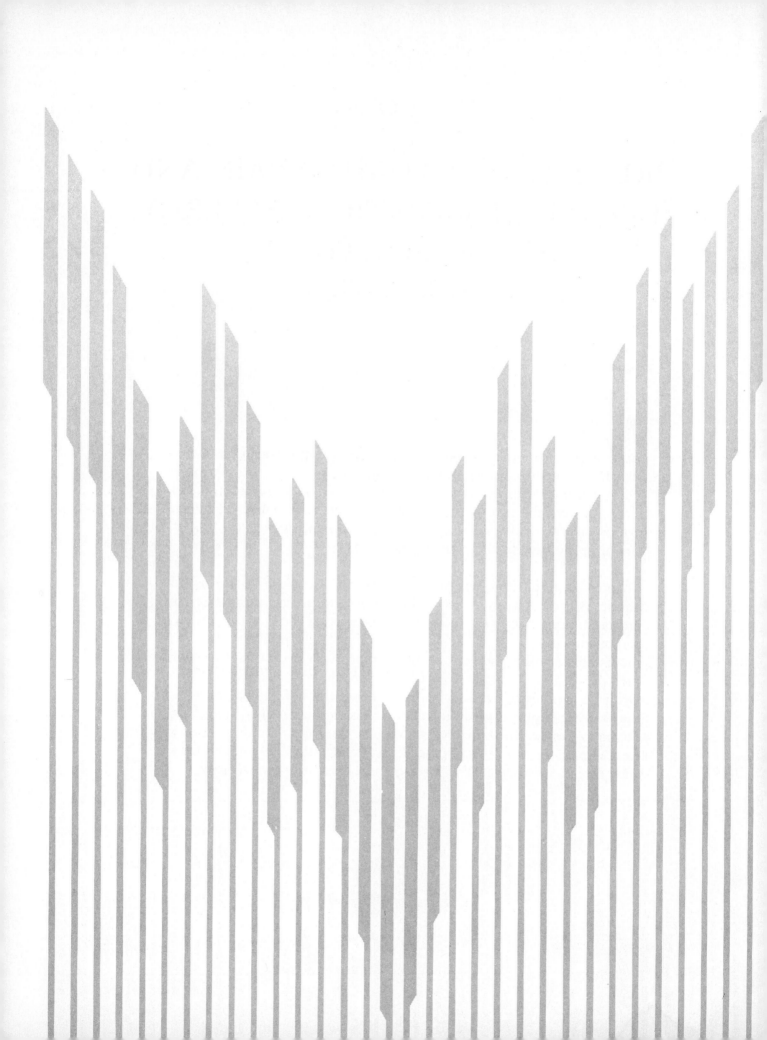

CHAPTER 23

Drugs for Pain and Inflammation

(see Chapter 20)

LEARNING OBJECTIVES

After studying this chapter you should be able to do the following:

◆ Differentiate among the actions, side effects, and uses of aspirin and acetaminophen.

◆ Discuss drug therapy with nonsteroidal antiinflammatory drugs (NSAIDs), and differentiate between individual drugs.

◆ Discuss drug therapy for rheumatoid arthritis and gout.

◆ Develop a nursing care plan for a patient receiving one of the drugs discussed in this chapter.

CHAPTER OVERVIEW

◆ This chapter covers analgesic-antipyretic drugs, NSAIDs, drugs to treat rheumatoid arthritis, and drugs to treat gout. These are all classifications for the actions of aspirin, although aspirin is no longer used to treat gout. Aspirin is used to promote antipyresis (reducing fever), to promote analgesia for mild-to-moderate pain, and to reduce inflammation. Although aspirin inhibits prostaglandin synthesis (see Chapter 20), it is not clear that this explains more than the antiinflammatory action. In addition to aspirin, the sections consider other drugs that are used clinically.

Nursing Process Overview
ANALGESIC-ANTIPYRETIC DRUGS

An analgesic-antipyretic drug relieves pain and reduces fever. Aspirin and acetaminophen are the major analgesic-antipyretic drugs. They are available without a prescription as over-the-counter (OTC) drugs.

Assessment

The patient requiring a drug to reduce fever is one who has a temperature above 38.5° C (101° F) or above the locally accepted limit of normal. Fever is not a disease; it is a symptom. Monitor temperature and other vital signs; note the presence of diaphoresis, chills, or seizures; assess the level of consciousness and the fluid intake and output. Assess the patient for possible causes of fever such as pulmonary infections, wound infection, and urinary tract infection.

Nursing Diagnosis

Potential impaired home maintenance management related to knowledge deficit of safe use of antipyretic agents

Management

The treatment of fever is twofold: to reduce the fever and to determine the cause. Administer antipyretics when the temperature exceeds the ordered upper limit or every 4 hr around the clock, as ordered. Monitor the temperature every 4 hr, ensure adequate fluid intake, monitor fluid intake and output, and monitor blood counts and other vital signs. Maintain patient comfort. Use additional measures if needed such as cool water baths and hypothermia mattresses. If aspirin is used, monitor patients for bruising or bleeding.

Evaluation

Verify that patients know the correct dose and frequency of administration and the possible side effects of antipyretics. They should also know when to seek medical assistance for fever, and what other drugs and substances to avoid during antipyretic therapy.

Mechanism of Action

Analgesia

An **analgesic** drug relieves pain. The analgesics discussed in this chapter, also called the *nonnarcotic analgesics*, inhibit the enzyme cyclooxygenase. This enzyme is key to the synthesis of local mediators, prostaglandin endoperoxides, PGG and PGH, released in damaged tissue to stimulate nerve endings. In the presence of the nonnarcotic analgesics, the nerves are not stimulated. Objective pain, pain arising from stimulation of peripheral nerve endings, is therefore not felt. This mechanism contrasts that of the narcotic analgesics, which interfere with subjective pain at the level of the central nervous system (CNS) (see Chapter 44).

Antipyresis

An **antipyretic** drug reduces fever. The balance between heat production and heat dissipation is regulated by the brain. An area of the preoptic anterior hypothalamus is the thermostat of the body. Fever results from an increase in the set point of this hypothalamic center. An endogenous fever-producing agent (pyrogen) is released by white cells engulfing foreign matter (phagocytic leukocytes). This pyrogen enters the CNS and stimulates the synthesis of prostaglandin E_2. This prostaglandin is the mediator elevating the temperature set point in the hypothalamus. The cyclooxygenase inhibitors prevent the synthesis of prostaglandin E_2.

Analgesic-antipyretic drugs

Acetaminophen (Datril, Tylenol, Panadol, and others) and several salicylates, including aspirin, are so widely used by the public that a patient may not mention them when asked, "What drugs have you taken recently?" Acetaminophen and the salicylates produce analgesia and antipyresis and are safe enough to be available without a prescription. However, they do have side effects and can interact with other drugs. Aspirin and acetaminophen are frequently found in OTC and prescription combination drugs that are marketed for relief of colds and allergies.

In addition to acetaminophen and the salicylates, the NSAIDs are also antipyretics and analgesics. Except for ibuprofen, they are prescription drugs used primarily to treat inflammation and resulting pain.

Specific Drugs

Acetaminophen (Datril, Tylenol, Panadol, and others)

Mechanism of action. Acetaminophen is identical to aspirin in its antipyretic and analgesic properties. However, acetaminophen is not an effective antiinflammatory agent. Acetaminophen therefore does not treat rheumatoid arthritis inflammation, but reduces pain in mild osteoarthritis (Table 23-1).

Administration and use. Acetaminophen provides the same analgesic-antipyretic actions as aspirin and can be combined with aspirin or other analgesics, including codeine. Unlike aspirin, the drug can be formulated as a liquid for infants and young children. Elixirs, solutions, suspensions, chewable tablets, wafers, tablets, caplets, and capsules are available. Acetaminophen is preferred to aspirin in treating the fever and discomfort of flu and chickenpox in childhood and early adulthood. Aspirin is implicated in the development of Reye's syndrome in young people who

experience those viral diseases. Acetaminophen has also become a popular alternative to aspirin for treating simple pain and fever because it does not cause gastric irritation or alter platelet funding and bleeding times, as does aspirin. Furthermore, acetaminophen does not interact with oral anticoagulants or other drugs.

Side effects. Acetaminophen can cause allergic reactions, usually involving skin rashes. Persons with a known glucose 6-phosphate dehydrogenase deficiency can develop hemolytic anemia if they take acetaminophen. Chronic daily ingestion of acetaminophen is reportedly associated with an increased risk of renal disease.

Toxicity. In adults, overdose of acetaminophen causes liver damage. Alcoholics are especially prone to this. Children rarely suffer permanent liver damage from the drug, but adults who take more than 2.6 gm in 24 hr may show mild symptoms of liver damage such as loss of appetite, nausea, vomiting, and slight jaundice. In deliberate overdoses of 10 gm or more, adults are highly susceptible to severe liver damage; death has been reported after ingestion of 15 gm. This toxicity arises because the liver normally conjugates toxic metabolites of acetaminophen with a sulfhydryl compound, glutathione, to produce an inactive, readily excreted compound. The amount of glutathione available for conjugation is exceeded when large amounts of acetaminophen are ingested. The unconjugated metabolites then bind to and destroy liver cells. Acetylcysteine is most effective if administered within 8 hr of an acetaminophen overdose. Cimetidine, which inhibits hepatic metabolism of acetaminophen, is being tested as an additional antidote for overdose.

Acetylcysteine (Mucomyst) prevents liver damage caused by excessive acetaminophen. Acetylcysteine degrades bronchial mucus in respiratory therapy (see Chapter 26). When given to counteract acetaminophen, it provides the sulfhydryl groups needed to conjugate and inactivate the toxic metabolites of acetaminophen. Treatment should begin within 12 hr after overdose. The stomach is first emptied by lavage or induced vomiting. An initial dose of 140 mg/kg is given as a 5% solution; doses of 70 mg/kg are then administered every 4 hr for approximately 17 doses. Since acetylcysteine has the pervasive flavor of rotten eggs, it must be disguised in a flavored iced drink and preferably drunk through a straw to minimize contact with the mouth.

Acetylsalicylic acid (aspirin)

Indications for use. Aspirin in low doses (325 to 650 mg or 1 to 2 adult tablets) reduces fever and relieves mild pain. Two aspirin tablets are the anal-

Table 23-1   Analgesic-Antipyretic Drugs

Generic name	Trade name	Administration/dosage	Comments
Acetaminophen	Tylenol* Datril Panadol* Liquiprin Various others	ORAL: *Adults*—325 to 650 mg every 6 to 8 hr. No more than 2.6 gm in 24 hr. *Children*—7 to 12 years, ½ adult dose; 3 to 6 years, ⅙ adult dose. Available without prescription.	Acts as an analgesic and antipyretic only. It has little antiinflammatory action and no inhibition of platelets. It is contraindicated in patients with glucose 6-phosphate dehydrogenase deficiency. Nonprescription.
Aspirin (acetyl-salicylic acid)	A.S.A. Aspergum Bayer Aspirin Children's Aspirin Ecotrin* Measurin	For analgesia or antipyresis: ORAL, RECTAL: *Adults*—650 mg every 4 hr, or 1.3 gm of timed-release form every 8 hr. *Children*—65 mg/kg over 24 hr in divided doses, every 4 to 6 hr.	Oral doses should be taken with a large glass of water or milk to decrease stomach irritation. Some patients may need to take aspirin after a meal to avoid gastrointestinal (GI) distress. Nonprescription.
Aspirin, buffered	Aluprin Ascriptin Bufferin Alka-Seltzer Various others	Same as for aspirin. There are no smaller dose tablets for children.	Alka-Seltzer contains 1.9 gm sodium bicarbonate and 1 gm citric acid per tablet. To avoid acid-base disturbances, limit ingestion to occasional use only. Remaining products contain magnesium and aluminum antacid salts. These salts are not absorbed systemically to any great extent. Nonprescription.
Sodium salicylate	Dodd's Pills† Uracel	Same as for aspirin. An injectable form is available by prescription.	Less effective than an equal dose of aspirin. May be tolerated by patients who are allergic to aspirin. Does not affect platelet function, but does retain vitamin K antagonist effect, which can increase prothrombin time. Nonprescription.

*Available in Canada and United States.
†Available in Canada only.

gesic equivalent of 60 mg of codeine. Aspirin is an effective analgesic for most common mild-to-moderate headaches and generalized mild muscular aches. Aspirin or aspirin-codeine combinations also treat mild-to-moderate pain of tooth extractions, episiotomies, cancer, and bone fractures. A dose of 1.2 gm/day of aspirin produces the maximum analgesic effect. At much higher doses (3 to 6 gm/day) aspirin treats the inflammation of rheumatoid arthritis. At this concentration, aspirin is the prototype for the NSAIDs (see Table 23-1).

Absorption and distribution. Aspirin is a weak acid and is rapidly absorbed from the stomach and upper small intestine. Buffering agents are present in several aspirin brands to hasten dissolution of the tablet and to reduce gastric irritation from the tablet. Advantages of buffering agents are minimal, and if several doses are taken, the buffering agents may cause loose stools. Alka-Seltzer contains so much sodium and bicarbonate that it should be used only on a short-term basis.

Once aspirin is absorbed, 50% to 90% binds loosely to plasma albumin. Aspirin can displace oral anticoagulants, oral hypoglycemic drugs, phenytoin, and methotrexate. Since the unbound drug is the effective concentration, free drug may reach toxic levels when displaced by aspirin.

Metabolism and excretion. Aspirin is rapidly hydrolyzed in the blood. The acetyl group of aspirin is readily transferred to the enzyme cyclooxygenase of the blood platelets. Cyclooxygenase is the key enzyme for the formation of prostaglandins. Acetylation of cyclooxygenase is irreversible and therefore persists for the 3- to 7-day lifetime of the platelet. Acetylated cyclooxygenase is inactive, and synthesis of the prostaglandin thromboxane A_2 is therefore blocked. Thromboxane A_2, a potent agent promoting platelet aggregation, is normally synthesized by platelets as they begin to aggregate. Even one aspirin tablet inhibits blood clotting by inhibiting platelet aggregation. This observation has led to the examination of aspirin as a prophylactic agent to prevent myocardial infarctions (MI) and strokes, processes associated with an increased tendency toward platelet aggregation (see Chapter 20).

Salicylic acid is the other product of the hydrolysis of aspirin. Salicylate (the basic salt to which salicylic acid dissociates at the pH of blood) is an analgesic-antipyretic and a reversible inhibitor of prostaglandin synthesis. Salicylate does not affect platelet aggregation, and therefore a salicylate salt is sometimes used in place of aspirin.

In acidic urine, salicylic acid is uncharged and therefore diffuses back into the blood. Vitamin C (ascorbic acid) maintains an acidic urine when taken in large doses and can therefore delay the excretion of salicylic acid. This interaction can be dangerous if large doses of aspirin are being taken, such as for arthritis. In alkaline urine, salicylic acid dissociates to salicylate, which is charged, cannot diffuse back into the blood, and is therefore eliminated in the urine. Salicylate is metabolized to inactive salicyluric acid by the liver. However, a 325-mg aspirin tablet saturates this liver inactivation system; thus the liver cannot readily metabolize large doses of aspirin.

Side effects. Approximately 2% to 10% of those taking an occasional aspirin tablet experience GI upset. This may be felt as heartburn or nausea. Aluminum and calcium-urea salts of aspirin have been formulated to be less irritating to the stomach than aspirin. When aspirin is taken regularly in large doses for arthritis, this incidence becomes 30% to 50% and may be the factor limiting the use of aspirin. Sometimes antacids are prescribed to minimize stomach irritation, but antacids also raise the pH of the urine and increase the rate of excretion of salicylic acid. Alternatively, enteric-coated or timed-release preparations may be tried to decrease gastric irritation.

Aspirin is directly irritating and damaging to gastric mucosal cells. Since alcohol also has these gastric effects, aspirin should not be taken when alcohol is in the stomach. The combination of alcohol and aspirin is greater than additive in producing gastric bleeding. Advise patients with active peptic ulcers not to use aspirin.

Long-term aspirin ingestion can cause the loss of 10 to 30 ml of blood daily from GI irritation. This may lead to iron deficiency anemia in women with heavy menses. Rarely, massive GI bleeding occurs in patients taking aspirin on a long-term basis.

Some people develop an allergy to aspirin. The most common form of aspirin intolerance is manifested as a rash. Patients with a skin rash caused by aspirin may tolerate other salicylates. A few people develop nasal polyps and sometimes later develop an asthma that is triggered by aspirin.

Patients sensitive to aspirin may be sensitive to a variety of other compounds. Most commonly, individuals sensitive to aspirin may show cross-sensitivity to the following:

1. Salicylin-containing foods (e.g., apples, oranges, and bananas)
2. Processed foods or drugs containing tartrazine dye or sodium benzoate
3. Iodide-containing substances
4. Various other NSAIDs
5. Tartrazine (see box)

As can be seen from this list, the origin of these cross-sensitivities is not always the classic cross-reactivity due to structural similarities of the agents.

Reye's syndrome. When treated with aspirin, children and teenagers who have an acute febrile illness such as flu or chickenpox seem to be at increased risk for contracting **Reye's syndrome.** Reye's syndrome is rare but serious. It is characterized by vomiting and rapidly progressive encephalopathy. Acetaminophen and other NSAIDs have not been so implicated. Nonprescription aspirin products now contain a warning against administration to children and teenagers who manifest chickenpox or flu symptoms.

Salicylism. Mild intoxication with aspirin is called *salicylism* and is commonly experienced when the daily dosage is more than 4 gm. Tinnitus (ringing in the ears) is the most frequent effect and may be accompanied by a degree of reversible hearing loss. Since salicylate stimulates the respiratory center, hyperventilation (rapid breathing) may occur. Fever

---

PATIENT PROBLEM: TARTRAZINE ALLERGY

THE PROBLEM

Tartrazine (FD & C yellow dye #5) is used by many drug companies in manufacturing drugs. Ingestion of this dye may cause an allergic reaction in susceptible individuals. This rare reaction is seen more often in persons with aspirin hypersensitivity. Example drugs containing tartrazine include Pronestyl procainamide film-coated tablets; Choloxin 2- and 6-mg dextrothyroxine tablets; and Nicolar 500-mg niacin tablets.

SOLUTIONS

◆ Instruct patients with a known allergy to tartrazine to wear a medical identification tag or bracelet.
◆ Assess patients with an allergy to aspirin for associated allergy to tartrazine before giving medications that contain tartrazine.
◆ Instruct patients to warn the pharmacist of tartrazine allergy before prescriptions are filled so that tartrazine-containing products can be avoided. Instruct patients with this allergy not to switch brands of a drug without consulting the pharmacist, to avoid accidental exposure to tartrazine.

Tartrazine is known to be associated with allergic reactions, but many other dyes, fillers, and preservatives are used in the manufacture of drugs. Patients experiencing an unusual reaction to a drug may be manifesting an allergic response to an ingredient used in its manufacture. Read ingredient labels carefully. Take a thorough drug history. Consult the pharmacist.

may result because salicylate interferes with the metabolic pathways coupling oxygen consumption and heat production.

Toxicity. Acute overdose of aspirin causes serious disturbances in the body's acid-base balance. A child is more likely to die from a large overdose of aspirin than an adult. Fatalities among children have been dramatically reduced since 1970 when the Poison Prevention Packaging Act required that orange-flavored baby aspirin (81-mg tablets) be limited to 36 tablets per bottle and that safety caps be used. If a child has ingested more than 150 mg/kg (36 baby tablets [one bottle] or 9 adult tablets for a 45-lb child), vomiting may be induced, or gastric lavage is used to get rid of undissolved tablets. Since charcoal absorbs about half its weight in aspirin, it is given orally to reduce absorption of aspirin.

Children, particularly those under 4 years of age, can rapidly develop metabolic acidosis. This is because of the acidic nature of aspirin and its metabolites and because salicylate inhibits metabolism in a manner that favors the accumulation of organic acids, which would normally have been metabolized to carbon dioxide and water. The hyperthermia that is also produced with this metabolic block must be treated with sponge baths. Profuse sweating can produce dehydration. The supportive treatment of aspirin toxicity therefore consists of careful monitoring of the acid-base and electrolyte levels and appropriate fluid administration. Intravenous (IV) sodium bicarbonate can counter the tendency toward metabolic acidosis and produce an alkaline urine that hastens the excretion of salicylate. Osmotic diuretics or dialysis may be necessary in extreme cases to remove salicylate. Salicylate is a weak vitamin K antagonist and in large doses acts like an oral anticoagulant. A day or two after massive aspirin ingestion, increased bleeding tendency and signs of minor hemorrhaging may be noted (see box).

Drug interactions. The drug interactions characteristic of aspirin are especially important because of its widespread and uncritical use. Drug interactions arise because aspirin enhances the potential for GI bleeding and ulcers with glucocorticoids, alcohol, and phenylbutazone. It also enhances anticoagulation with coumarins. Aspirin antagonizes the uricosuric effect of probenecid and sulfinpyrazone.

Other OTC salicylates

Salicylamide. Salicylamide is a chemically modified form of salicylate and is not hydrolyzed to salicylic acid. It is used only in combination with other drugs.

Sodium salicylate. Sodium salicylate (Uracel and Dodd's Pills) does not alter platelet function as does aspirin. Salicylates bind to plasma albumin and dis-

---

PATIENT PROBLEM: ASPIRIN TOXICITY

TOXIC SALICYLATE PLASMA CONCENTRATIONS

Mild	45 to 65 mg/dl
Moderate	65 to 90 mg/dl
Severe	90+ mg/dl
Usually fatal	>120 mg/dl

TREATMENT STEPS

1. Undissolved tablets are removed through induced vomiting or absorption with charcoal.

2. Plasma salicylate, acid-base, glucose, sodium, and potassium concentrations are determined every 4 to 5 hr.

3. Hyperthermia is treated with sponge baths, and dehydration is treated with fluid replacement.

4. Fluids are administered as required to treat electrolyte imbalances and acidosis.

5. If salicylate concentration is dangerously high or does not fall with supportive treatment, dialysis or exchange transfusions may be used.

---

place other drugs, particularly the oral anticoagulants (see Table 23-1).

Methyl salicylate. Methyl salicylate (oil of wintergreen) is only used topically. It causes vasodilation in the applied areas and thereby creates a warmth that relieves muscle or joint stiffness.

Nursing Process Overview
NONSTEROIDAL ANTIINFLAMMATORY DRUGS

Aspirin is the prototype of the NSAIDs. For many years, aspirin has been the first drug used to control the pain and inflammation of rheumatoid arthritis. Recently several new drugs have been developed, which like aspirin are analgesic, antipyretic, and antiinflammatory. These drugs are all prescription drugs, although ibuprofen is also available OTC. They are prescribed as analgesic antiinflammatory drugs for patients with rheumatoid arthritis who cannot tolerate aspirin. In addition, they are prescribed for patients with painful joint disorders, with or without inflammation, such as osteoarthritis, ankylosing spondylitis, low back pain, and gout.

Assessment

Assess temperature, pulse, respiration, blood pressure, blood counts, and other laboratory data relevant to the possible or probable diagnosis. Perform a brief neurologic examination. Assess patients' ability to perform activities of daily living to assist in planning for discharge.

Nursing Diagnoses

High risk for GI distress or bleeding
Possible complication: hematologic disorders

Management

For individualized care, develop a plan with the patient to reach the goals of drug therapy. Reinforce the importance of other therapies including heat or cold application, immobilization, special exercises, and restricted activity. Monitor vital signs and subjective and objective data related to the specific problem and the laboratory data appropriate to the problem and the drug therapy.

Evaluation

Check that patients can explain why and how to take the prescribed drugs and what other therapies are being used to treat the problem, which other drugs should be avoided while receiving therapy, whether alcohol should be avoided, what are reasonable expectations of the regimen (e.g., will joint pain disappear or only diminish), what are possible side effects and what to do if they occur, how to implement a plan for prophylactic treatment, and when to return for follow-up or assistance.

GENERAL PHARMACOLOGY OF NSAIDS

Mechanism of Action

The primary mechanism of action of the NSAIDs is the inhibition of the enzyme cyclooxygenase so that prostaglandins are not formed. Aspirin is an irreversible inhibitor of cyclooxygenase because cyclooxygenase is acetylated by aspirin. Other salicylates and NSAIDs also inhibit cyclooxygenase but reversibly, since they do not acetylate cyclooxygenase.

How prostaglandins affect pain receptors is not known. The actions of prostaglandin E_2 include vasodilation and increased bone resorption. Large amounts of prostaglandin E_2 have been present in the synovial fluid of affected joints in patients with rheumatoid arthritis, synthesized by cells in the mesenchymal synovial lining. Presumably this production of prostaglandin E_2 contributes to the swelling and eventual bone erosion of rheumatoid arthritis. In addition, inflammation at other sites may involve prostaglandin E_2 synthesis.

Dysmenorrhea (menstrual cramps) appears to be caused by the overproduction of prostaglandins by the uterus at the time of menstruation. The prostaglandins can cause the uterus to contract to the point of cramping, producing dysmenorrhea. Aspirin is not effective for treating dysmenorrhea, but the NSAIDs are effective in averting menstrual cramps, particularly if therapy is begun a few days before the start of menses.

Recent studies have clarified other mechanisms of the NSAIDs that contribute to their action. These include inhibition of various enzymes, inhibition of transmembrane ion fluxes, and inhibition of the chemoattractant binding that affects the inflammatory process.

Side Effects

The major side effect of the NSAIDs is gastric irritation leading to an increase in peptic ulcers. Prostaglandins protect the gastric mucosa by inhibiting gastric acid secretion. GI irritation commonly caused by aspirin and other NSAIDs may arise because this protection is absent when these drugs, which inhibit prostaglandin synthesis, are present in the stomach. These effects can be minimized by taking the drugs with meals. All prescription NSAIDs now carry a warning to reflect concern about the GI side effects seen with their chronic use.

Misoprostol (Cytotec) controls gastric irritation associated with aspirin and other NSAIDs. Misoprostol, and analogue of prostaglandin E_1, is protective by inhibiting excessive gastric acid secretion. Thus it replaces the prostaglandin that is suppressed by the NSAIDs (see Chapter 13 and Table 13-2).

Inhibition of platelet aggregation is another common side effect of the NSAIDs. Although this effect is irreversible with aspirin, it is reversible with the other NSAIDs. The inhibition of prostaglandin synthesis is responsible also for the platelet phenomenon.

Patients who develop a rash or other allergic reactions to one of the NSAIDs may be intolerant of the others. This is especially true of patients who have experienced bronchospasm resulting from aspirin ingestion or who are sensitive to aspirin because they have asthma.

Elderly patients are more likely to develop GI distress, liver toxicity, or renal damage while taking NSAIDs and should be carefully monitored. Also, patients with clinical conditions such as congestive heart failure, cirrhosis, and renal insufficiency are at risk for impaired renal function when taking NSAIDs. These patients require the local synthesis of vasodilating prostaglandins to maintain renal perfusion. NSAIDs, by inhibiting these prostaglandins, can allow unopposed vasoconstriction. This renal ischemia can lead to a deterioration of renal function.

Drug Interactions

In general, the NSAIDs are protein bound and displace other drugs, particularly hydantoins, sulfonamides, sulfonylureas, and calcium channel blockers, leading to exacerbation of side effects because of these drugs. NSAIDs may increase the risk of renal damage if acetaminophen is used concurrently over long periods. The risk of GI complications, especially ulceration or hemorrhage, is increased if NSAIDs are taken concurrently with alcohol, anticoagulants, thrombolytics, or glucocorticoids. NSAIDs may diminish the effectiveness of diuretics and intensify the risk of renal failure. They potentiate drugs that inhibit platelet aggregation. NSAIDs should be discontinued when a gold compound or methotrexate is administered to treat rheumatoid arthritis, because of their potential for renal damage.

SPECIFIC DRUGS
Salicylates

Aspirin

Aspirin, (many trade names) given initially to control the symptoms of arthritis. Doses of 2.6 to 7.8 gm/day are required to produce the plasma concentrations of 20 to 30 mg/dl needed for an effective antiinflammatory response. These doses are associated with considerable gastric irritation with or without bleeding, salicylism, decreased platelet aggregation, and interactions with other drugs. Aspirin must be taken continuously for at least 2 weeks before an improvement may be noted. Timed-release or enteric-coated formulations may improve patient compliance by decreasing the number of times aspirin must be taken each day and by bypassing the stomach, thereby reducing gastric irritation (Table 23-2).

Table 23-2   Nonsteroidal Antiinflammatory Drugs

Generic name	Trade name	Administration/dosage	Comments
ASPIRIN AND SALICYLATES			
Aspirin	Bayer Timed-Release Bufferin, Arthritis Strength Measurin Various others	ORAL: *Adults*—arthritis: 2.6 to 5.2 gm daily in divided doses (every 8 hr for timed-release forms). For acute rheumatic fever, up to 7.8 gm daily in divided doses. *Children*— 65 mg/kg over 24 hr in divided doses every 6 hr. Available without prescription.	Dose needed to achieve blood levels for antiinflammatory activity of 20 to 30 mg% may vary from person to person. Doses given are average ones. Children who have a viral illness and are given aspirin have an increased risk of developing Reye's syndrome.
Choline salicylate	Arthropan	ORAL: *Adults and children over 12 years*—870 mg (1 teaspoon) every 3 to 4 hr, up to 6 times daily. Available without prescription.	A mint-flavored liquid formulated for patients with arthritis.
Diflunisal	Dolobid*	ORAL: *Adults*—500 to 1000 mg daily, taken as 2 doses. Maximum dose is 1.5 gm daily. Prescription drug.	A long-acting salicylic acid derivative. Has a lower incidence of the same side effects as aspirin.
Magnesium salicylate	Doan's* Magan Mobidin	Same as aspirin. No pediatric forms. Prescription drug. FDA Pregnancy Category C.	Contains no sodium; low incidence of GI upset. Contraindicated in renal failure.
Olsalazine	Dipentum	ORAL: *Adults and adolescents*—1 gm daily divided in 2 doses.	Prophylaxis for inflammatory bowel disease for patients intolerant to sulfasalazine.
Salsalate	Amigesic* Disalcid*	ORAL: *Adults only*—1 gm 3 times daily. Prescription drug. FDA Pregnancy Category C.	A dimer of salicylate. Absorption is from the intestine only after hydrolysis to salicylic acid. Delayed onset compared to free salicylic acid.
Sodium salicylate	Dodd's Pills† Uracel	Same as aspirin. Available without prescription. An injectable form is available by prescription.	Less effective than an equal dose of aspirin. May be tolerated by patients with allergic reaction to aspirin. Does not affect platelet function but does retain vitamin K antagonist effect, which can increase prothrombin time.

*Available in Canada and United States.
†Available in Canada only.

Continued.

Table 23-2 Nonsteroidal Antiinflammatory Drugs—cont'd

Generic name	Trade name	Administration/dosage	Comments
ASPIRIN AND SALICYLATES—cont'd			
Sodium thiosalicylate	Asproject Rexolate Tusal	INTRAMUSCULAR: *Adults*—prescription drug. For arthritis, 100 mg daily. For musculoskeletal disorders, 50 to 100 mg daily or every other day. For rheumatic fever, 100 to 150 mg every 4 to 6 hr for 3 days, then 100 mg twice daily.	An injectable, longer-acting form of salicylate that can be given in doses lower than for oral aspirin.
OTHER NONSTEROIDAL ANTIINFLAMMATORY DRUGS			
Diclofenac	Voltaren*	ORAL: *Adults*—150 to 200 mg daily divided into 2 to 4 doses. Also available in extended release form for once-daily administration. Available in Canada in suppository form. FDA Pregnancy Category B.	For rheumatoid arthritis, osteoarthritis, and ankylosing spondylitis.
Etodolac	Lodine	ORAL: *Adults*—800 to 1200 mg daily for osteoarthritis. For pain, 400 mg, then 200 to 400 mg every 6 to 8 hr as needed. Daily dose should not exceed 20 mg/kg of body weight or 1200 mg, whichever is less.	New drug
Fenoprofen	Nalfon*	ORAL: *Adults*—300 to 600 mg 3 or 4 times daily for rheumatoid arthritis. For pain or dysmenorrhea, 200 mg every 4 to 6 hr.	For mild-to-moderate pain, dysmenorrhea, and rheumatoid arthritis.
Floctafenine	Idaract†	ORAL: *Adults*—200 to 400 mg every 6 to 8 hr.	For mild-to-moderate pain and inflammation. Not available in United States.
Flurbiprofen	Ansaid* Froben†	ORAL: *Adults*—for arthritis, 100 to 200 mg daily in 3 or 4 divided doses. For dysmenorrhea, 50 mg 4 times daily. FDA Pregnancy Category B.	For arthritis or dysmenorrhea.
Ibuprofen	Advil Motrin* Nuprin Various others	ORAL: *Adults*—for mild pain, fever, or dysmenorrhea, 200 to 400 mg every 4 to 6 hr. For antiinflammatory response, 1.2 to 3.2 gm daily in 3 or 4 divided doses.	Nonprescription for mild pain, fever, or dysmenorrhea. Higher doses available in prescription form for arthritis.
Indomethacin	Apo-Indomethacin† Indameth Indocid† Indocin Novomethacin†	ORAL: *Adults*—25 mg 2 to 3 times daily. If necessary, total daily dose can be increased by 25 to 50 mg daily at weekly intervals, but the total daily dose should not exceed 200 mg. *Children*—1.5 to 2.5 mg/kg body weight per day, divided into 3 or 4 doses. Maximum dose is 4 mg/kg of body weight daily or 200 mg daily, whichever is less. *Premature infants*—0.3 to 0.6 mg/kg/24 hr to close the ductus arteriosus. Available in capsules, extended-release capsules, oral suspension, and suppositories.	Administer with meals or with antacids to minimize gastric irritation. For acute inflammatory episodes. Also given to premature infants to close the ductus arteriosus.

*Available in Canada and United States.
†Available in Canada only.

Table 23-2 Nonsteroidal Antiinflammatory Drugs—cont'd

Generic name	Trade name	Administration/dosage	Comments
OTHER NONSTEROIDAL ANTIINFLAMMATORY DRUGS—cont'd			
Ketoprofen	Orudis*	ORAL: *Adults*—150 to 300 mg daily divided into 3 or 4 doses. Available in capsules, delayed-release capsules, and suppositories. FDA Pregnancy Category B.	For rheumatoid arthritis and dysmenorrhea.
Ketorolac tromethamine	Toradol	ORAL: *Adults*—10 mg every 4 to 6 hr, up to a maximum of 40 mg/day. INTRAMUSCULAR: *Adults*—60 mg initially, followed by 30 mg every 6 hr. Maximum 150 mg the first day, then 120 mg daily thereafter.	NSAID with analgesia equivalent to morphine. Useful for outpatient surgery.
Meclofenamate	Meclomen	ORAL: *Adults*—200 mg daily divided into 3 or 4 doses. May be increased up to 400 mg daily if necessary.	For rheumatoid arthritis. Not available in Canada.
Mefenamic Acid	Ponstel Ponstan†	ORAL: *Adults*—500 mg initially, then 250 mg every 6 hr as needed. FDA Pregnancy Category C.	For mild-to-moderate pain. Administer after meals to avoid gastric irritation.
Nabumetone	Relafen	ORAL: *Adults*—initially 1000 mg a day, taken as a single dose. May increase dose to 1500 or 2000 mg, taken as a single dose or in 2 divided doses.	New drug for rheumatoid arthritis and osteoarthritis.
Naproxen	Anaprox* Naprosyn* Various others	ORAL: *Adults*—250 to 750 mg 2 times daily for rheumatoid arthritis; 500 mg initially, then 250 mg every 6 to 8 hr for mild-to-moderate pain, including dysmenorrhea; 750 mg initially, then 250 mg every 8 hr for acute gout. FDA Pregnancy Category B.	For dysmenorrhea, mild to moderate pain, acute gout, and rheumatoid arthritis.
Phenylbutazone	Butazolidin* Butazone Novobutazone Various others	ORAL: *Adults*—initially, 300 to 600 mg daily divided into 3 or 4 doses. Maintenance dose is 100 mg 1 to 4 times daily. For acute gout, 400 mg initially, then 100 mg every 4 hr for 4 days or a maximum of 1 week. Available in capsules, tablets, and delayed-release and buffered tablets. FDA Pregnancy Category C.	For rheumatoid arthritis and acute attacks of other arthritic conditions, including gout. Administer after meals to avoid gastric irritation.
Piroxicam	Apo-Piroxicam† Feldene* Novopirocam†	ORAL: *Adults*—20 mg once a day or 10 mg twice a day.	For rheumatoid arthritis and osteoarthritis. Administer after meals to avoid gastric irritation.
Sulindac	Apo-Sulin† Clinoril* Novo-Sundae†	ORAL: *Adults*—150 to 200 mg twice a day.	For rheumatoid arthritis, acute gout, and bursitis.
Tiaprofenic Acid	Surgam†	ORAL: *Adults*—600 mg daily divided into 2 o 3 doses.	For rheumatoid arthritis and osteoarthritis. Not available in U.S.
Tolmetin	Tolectin*	ORAL: *Adults*—initially, 400 mg every 8 hr, then 600 to 1800 mg daily, divided into 3 or 4 doses. FDA Pregnancy Category C.	For rheumatoid arthritis and osteoarthritis.

*Available in Canada and United States.
†Available in Canada only.

Because aspirin is highly irritating to the stomach, salicylate salts have been introduced that replace aspirin and cause less GI upset. These salicylates do not affect platelet aggregation but displace oral anticoagulants from albumin.

Diflunisal

Diflunisal (Dolobid) is a derivative of salicylic acid having a long duration of action. It relieves the symptoms of rheumatoid arthritis and osteoarthritis. Diflunisal has fewer side effects than aspirin, including GI reactions, dizziness, edema, and tinnitus.

Olsalazine

Olsalazine (Dipentum) is an alternative to sulfasalazine in patients with ulcerative colitis. Olsalazine does not have the sulfa component that causes intolerance in some patients. Currently, olsalazine is only indicated for patients in remission from ulcerative colitis.

Salicylate salts

Sodium salicylate, sodium thiosalicylate, magnesium salicylate, and choline salicylate are all salicylate salts that produce less GI upset than aspirin.

Salsalate

Salsalate (Disalcid) is a dimer of salicylic acid. It is slowly hydrolyzed to two molecules of salicylic acid in the small intestine and absorbed into the bloodstream.

Thiosalicylate

Thiosalicylate (Asproject and others) is a chemically modified form of salicylate for (IM) injection.

Nonsalicylate Nonsteroidal Antiinflammatory Drugs (NSAIDs)

Recently many NSAIDs have been introduced into clinical practice; four have been withdrawn because they were excessively toxic to kidneys in elderly patients. NSAIDs are derived from several chemical classes and are discussed on the basis of their chemical group (see Table 23-2).

Diclofenac

Diclofenac (Voltaren) is new to the U.S. market. It treats rheumatoid arthritis, osteoarthritis, and ankylosing spondylitis.

Etodolac

Etodolac (Lodine) is a new drug introduced to control the pain of osteoarthritis.

Ibuprofen and related NSAIDs

About half the NSAIDs are propionic acid derivatives. These include fenoprofen (Nalfon), floctafenine (Idarac), flurbiprofen (Ansaid), ibuprofen (Advil, Mediprin, Motrin, Nuprin, and others), ketoprofen (Orudis), naproxen (Anaprox, Naprosyn), and tiaprofenic acid (Surgam). They provide good analgesic and antiinflammatory action. They often treat dysmenorrhea, rheumatoid arthritis, osteoarthritis, and gout (see Table 23-2).

Ibuprofen is available OTC. It is rapidly absorbed and has a plasma half-life of 2 hr. It appears to be well tolerated. GI irritation and bleeding occur less frequently than with aspirin and may be decreased by taking the drug with meals.

Indomethacin

Indomethacin (Indocin, Indocid, and others) is prescribed for its analgesic and antiinflammatory actions. GI disturbances such as nausea, vomiting, loss of appetite, indigestion, or diarrhea are common, but can be reduced by taking the drug after meals. Occasionally, indomethacin can cause ulceration along the GI tract that may become serious if bleeding or perforation results. Headaches and dizziness are the most common side effects. These can often be minimized if the dose is lowered and then increased gradually. Other CNS disturbances that can limit the use of indomethacin include confusion, light-headedness, fainting, or drowsiness.

Ketorolac tromethamine

Ketorolac tromethamine (Toradol) is a new NSAID. However, it is being used principally as an analgesic, equivalent in potency to morphine. It is given by IM injection for the short-term management of moderate-to-severe pain, particularly in postoperative patients. The lack of mental effects is especially beneficial in outpatient surgery.

Meclofenamate and mefenamic acid

Meclofenamate (Meclomen) and mefenamic acid (Ponstel, Ponstan) are fenamate derivatives. Mefenamic acid is prescribed for mild-to-moderate pain. However, therapy with this drug is limited to 1 week because of the frequent occurrence of toxicity associated with the GI, kidney, and blood-forming systems. Side effects may include GI upset, diarrhea, and rash.

Meclofenamate is prescribed for rheumatoid arthritis and osteoarthritis. Side effects are similar to those of mefenamic acid.

Nabumetone

Nabumetone (Relafen) is a new drug for the treatment of rheumatoid arthritis and osteoarthritis. This is a prodrug that undergoes hepatic biotransformation to the active substance.

Phenylbutazone

Phenylbutazone (Azolid, Butazolidin and Butazone) is a potent antiinflammatory drug with a long plasma half-life of 2 to 3 days. It binds strongly to plasma albumin and can displace other bound drugs, particularly oral anticoagulant and oral hypoglycemic drugs. Phenylbutazone causes fluid retention and gastric irritation and prolongs platelet function, thereby inhibiting blood clotting. Occasionally, phenylbutazone causes liver damage or bone marrow suppression. Because of these problems, it is commonly prescribed for only 1 to 2 weeks to treat an acute inflammatory response.

Piroxicam

Piroxicam (Feldene) is well absorbed and has a long half-life of 45 hr, making once-a-day dosing adequate. Piroxicam is rapidly excreted in the urine as a glucuronide. Piroxicam is prescribed principally for rheumatoid arthritis and osteoarthritis.

Sulindac and tolmetin

Sulindac (Clinoril) and tolmetin (Tolectin) are chemically related to indomethacin. In general, their side effects are similar to those of aspirin, although the incidence is less than with aspirin. Sulindac has a plasma half-life of 8 hr and can be taken less frequently than indomethacin or tolmetin. It is a prodrug, activated after conversion by the liver. The active drug is excreted in the bile and reabsorbed from the intestine. Tolmetin induces fewer side effects in the CNS than does indomethacin. Tolmetin is absorbed rapidly and has a plasma half-life of only 1 hr.

Nursing Process Overview
RHEUMATOID ARTHRITIS

Rheumatoid arthritis is an autoimmune disease. The primary target of this major crippling disorder initially is the synovium, or joint lining. This tissue, which normally is smooth and shiny, becomes inflamed, painful, and swollen. Rheumatoid arthritis occurs in about 1% of the population (over 2 million people in the United States) affecting females about 3 times more often than males. Although the disease can occur at any age, the peak incidence in females is between the ages of 40 to 60 years.

Assessment

Obtain a careful history of the presenting problem in addition to vital signs, weight, and subjective and objective data related to the complaint and the overall condition of the patient. Monitor laboratory work including hematocrit and hemoglobin level, blood counts, tests to confirm the diagnosis or to monitor diseases such as the rheumatoid factor, antinuclear antibody (ANA), complement, erythrocyte sedimentation rate (ESR), and tests to monitor the activity or side effects of drugs the patient is taking. Assess joint function and ability to perform activities of daily living.

Nursing Diagnoses

High risk for stomatitis (with gold compounds)
Possible complication: hematologic disorders
Possible anxiety related to chronic disease, changing medical therapies, and use of drugs with a high potential for causing side effects

Management

No drug can cure rheumatoid arthritis. Goals of drug therapy are to provide analgesia, to reduce inflammation, which decreases pain, and to maintain or increase joint function. Monitor response to the therapeutic regimen including pain, joint function, subjective and objective data related to the patient's complaints, new signs and symptoms possibly because of the therapy, and laboratory work specific for the drugs being used or the patient's problems. Plan goals so that patient management is directed to a mutually satisfactory outcome. Teach patients that maintaining ideal weight is less stressful to joints in cases of arthritis; dietary restriction and instruction may be necessary. Refer to occupational therapy, physical therapy, and visiting nurses.

Evaluation

Ascertain that the patient can explain the disease process and the specific drugs being used, is aware of possible side effects of the drugs and what action to take if they should appear, knows how to take ordered drugs correctly, understands the need for frequent follow-up and data that will be obtained at these visits to monitor for effectiveness and side effects, and recognizes the need to avoid self-medication with OTC drugs unless approved by the physician.

DRUGS FOR RHEUMATOID ARTHRITIS

Rheumatoid Arthritis

Rheumatoid arthritis is a highly variable disease process. It frequently goes into remission for months or years. In early rheumatoid arthritis only the synovial membranes are inflamed, causing painful swelling. In this situation, aspirin and the other NSAIDs may be effective. The antiinflammatory effect added to the analgesic effect eases the pain and increases the mobility of the affected joint. In mild cases, NSAIDs may be sufficient to control symptoms. These drugs do not affect the progression of rheumatoid arthritis, however, which is marked by erosion of the bone at the joint and eventual bone deformation. Drugs that may alter the progression of joint erosion include gold therapy, hydroxychloroquine, penicillamine, and immunosuppressive drugs, in that order. Glucocorticoids have a restricted role in treating rheumatoid arthritis. All these antirheumatic drugs have potentially serious side effects that must be monitored carefully.

Specific Drugs

Disease-modifying drugs for rheumatoid arthritis are presently reserved for patients with severe, difficult-to-manage rheumatoid arthritis (Table 23-3). They are tried with a patient, one at a time, over several months, until an assessment of effectiveness can be made. Although a NSAID may be continued, these drugs are not combined with each other. Many have potentially severe side effects that must be monitored. Some clinicians believe that the disease-modifying drugs should be used much earlier in the course of rheumatoid arthritis, before inflammatory processes have been in place for decades.

Auranofin

Auranofin (Ridaura) is a gold compound that can be taken orally. Clinical trials indicate that auranofin is as effective as the injectable gold drugs in inducing remission in rheumatoid arthritis. Auranofin is taken twice daily. GI reactions, including diarrhea, abdominal pain, nausea, and loss of appetite are common early in therapy but usually subside in the first month. The toxicity of auranofin is similar to that of injectable gold compounds.

Aurothioglucose and gold sodium thiomalate

Aurothioglucose (Solganal) and gold sodium thiomalate (Myochrysine) are injectable gold salts. It is not known how gold affects the synovial tissues to suppress rheumatoid arthritis. Therapy is started with weekly injections into the gluteal muscle until a total of 1 gm has been given. Further therapy depends on the patient's response. Gold requires a long time to come to plateau levels in the tissues, and a response usually requires 2 to 6 months. Only 30% to 60% of patients treated with gold respond over a 2- to 3-year course of treatment. Patients in whom remission is induced usually continue receiving monthly injections.

The most common reason for discontinuing successful gold therapy is the appearance of serious side effects such as skin reactions, mouth ulcers, fever, kidney damage, or abnormalities in the blood count. About 40% of patients develop an adverse reaction. Skin reactions and mouth ulcers are the most common side effects. If these are mild, gold therapy may be halted temporarily and then tried again. Blood counts and a urinalysis to measure protein should be done before each dose early in gold therapy and continued periodically throughout therapy.

Azathioprine

Azathioprine (Imuran) is an immunosuppressive agent used to suppress rejection in organ transplantation. It also manages severe, active rheumatoid arthritis unresponsive to conventional medications. Azathioprine also has a steroid-sparing effect, which allows a reduction in steroid dose when the two are combined in chronic inflammatory diseases. About 28% of patients taking azathioprine have hematologic reactions, including anemia and a decrease in white cell and thrombocyte counts.

Glucocorticoids

Glucocorticoids dramatically relieve inflammation and the accompanying pain of arthritis. They indirectly inhibit prostaglandin E_2 synthesis. However, glucocorticoids do not alter the course of rheumatoid arthritis. Long-term administration suppresses the pituitary-adrenal axis with serious consequences (see Chapter 51). Although oral administration is rarely given for rheumatoid arthritis, injection into the articular space of the joint may relieve acute inflammatory episodes without causing systemic reactions. Glucocorticoids may treat certain nonarticular manifestations of rheumatoid arthritis, such as vasculitis and rheumatoid lung. Small doses may treat joint symptoms. *Hydrocortisone acetate, triamcinolone hexacetonide,* and depot *methylprednisolone* are the preferred glucocorticoids because they have a longer duration of action than other injectable glucocorticoids. If a glucocorticoid is injected, patients should avoid strenuous use of the affected joint. This is because the drug masks the normal signals of stress at the joint, and therefore strenuous use may damage the stressed joint.

Table 23-3   Drugs for Rheumatoid Arthritis

Generic name	Trade name	Administration/dosage	Comments
Auranofin	Ridaura	ORAL: *Adults*—6 mg daily. FDA Pregnancy Category C.	Effective orally. Appears as effective as injected gold drugs in inducing remission of rheumatoid arthritis.
Aurothioglucose Gold sodium thiomalate	Solganal Myochrysine*	INTRAMUSCULAR (GLUTEAL): *Adults*—weekly injections of 10 mg week 1, 25 mg week 2, 25 to 50 mg week 3, 50 mg each week thereafter until a total of 800 mg to 1 gm has been administered. If the patient has improved and there are no toxic signs, 50-mg injections are continued every 2 weeks (4 doses) then every 3 weeks (4 doses), then every 3 to 4 weeks. *Children*—1 mg/kg (up to 25 mg) weekly for 20 weeks, then every 2 to 4 weeks if the therapy is beneficial. FDA Pregnancy Category C.	About 40% of patients develop serious side effects, most commonly an allergy marked by skin reactions or mouth ulcers. Blood counts and urinalysis are done routinely to monitor for suppression of blood cells and kidney damage. Therapy is discontinued if no improvement is seen in 5 months.
Azathioprine	Imuran	ORAL: *Adults*—1 mg/kg body weight per day, the dosage being increased in increments of 0.5 mg/kg body weight per day after 6 or 8 weeks, then every 4 weeks as necessary. Maximum dose: 2.5 mg/kg body weight daily. For maintenance, the dosage should be reduced in 0.5 mg/kg body weight increments every 4 to 8 weeks.	For the management of severe active rheumatoid arthritis unresponsive to rest or conventional medications.
Hydroxychloroquine sulfate	Plaquenil* Sulfate	ORAL: *Adults*—200 mg once or twice daily at meals, not more than 3.5 mg/lb.	Regular ocular examination to detect retinopathy if required.
Methotrexate	Rheumatrex	ORAL: *Adults*—2.5 to 5 mg every 12 hr for 3 doses weekly. FDA Pregnancy Category X.	Low-dose weekly therapy.
Penicillamine	Cuprimine* Depen	ORAL: *Adults*—initially 125 to 250 mg daily as a single dose. May be raised every 2 to 3 months by 250 mg daily to 500 to 750 mg daily.	Patient must be carefully monitored to detect suppression of blood cells and autoimmune responses.
Sulfasalazine	Azulfidine Salazopyrin† Various others	ORAL: *Adults*—500 mg daily initially, gradually increasing to 2 gm daily. Use enteric-coated tablets.	Investigational for rheumatoid arthritis. Primary use is for inflammatory bowel disease.

*Available in Canada and United States.
†Available in Canada only.

Hydroxychloroquine

Hydroxychloroquine (Plaquenil) is an antimalarial drug that is also used as an alternative to gold therapy or after gold therapy has failed. A response may not be seen for 3 to 6 months after the start of therapy, and therapy is discontinued after 1 year if no response is seen. This drug is taken orally, and some remains in the body for months or years. Occasionally, patients develop retinopathy that can progress to blindness even when the drug is discontinued. Therefore regular ophthalmic examination is necessary. Skin rashes, peripheral neuropathy, and depressed white cell count are other complications.

Penicillamine

Penicillamine (Cuprimine and Depen) is a chelating drug that is used to treat rheumatoid arthritis. Side effects are frequent but reversible when dosage is reduced or drug is discontinued. These include taste loss, nausea, depression of platelets and white cells, and proteinuria. Side effects are minimized by starting with a low dose and increasing the dose every 4 to 6 weeks until a response is obtained or a total of 1 gm/day is given.

Methotrexate

Methotrexate (Rheymatrex) is a folic acid antagonist used to treat cancer and psoriasis. Low doses are approved to treat rheumatoid arthritis when other treatments have failed. Side effects include nausea, mucositis, GI discomfort, rash, diarrhea, and headaches. Toxic reactions are possible but most are reversible if detected early; these include liver damage, lung disease, bone marrow depression, severe diarrhea, and ulcerative stomatitis. Baseline studies include blood chemistry, renal function, liver function, and chest x-ray films; these are repeated periodically throughout treatment. Contraindications to the use of methotrexate include pregnancy and nursing, alcoholism, blood dyscrasias, immunodeficiency syndromes, or hypersensitivity to the drug.

Sulfasalazine

Sulfasalazine (Azulfidine, Salzopyrin, and others) is composed of a sulfa compound and a 5-aminosalicylic acid. In the colon, the drug is metabolized by bacteria to the component drugs. Sulfasalazine is particularly effective in the treatment of inflammatory bowel disease. Its effectiveness in treating rheumatoid arthritis and ankylosing spondylitis is being investigated.

Nursing Process Overview

GOUT

Gout is a type of arthritis caused by a specific metabolic disorder. If gout is diagnosed early and therapy begun promptly, the disease can be arrested and complications of the disease prevented.

Assessment

Assess vital signs, weight, history of previous attacks, family history of gout, subjective complaints, and objective data. Monitor blood work, including the serum uric acid level. X-ray films and joint aspiration may be required.

Nursing Diagnoses

Possible impaired home maintenance management related to the need to increase daily fluid intake to 2500 ml
High risk for GI distress

Management

Encourage a high urinary output (2000 to 3000 ml/day) to prevent the formation of kidney stones; this requires a high fluid intake. Monitor fluid intake and output until certain that the high fluid output is being maintained. Monitor vital signs, blood pressure, con-dition of affected joints, subjective complaints, objective signs, and appropriate laboratory work.

Evaluation

Before discharge, check that patients can describe the disease, the medications that have been prescribed and their actions, the administration of the drugs to achieve maximum benefit, and the possible side effects and the ones that should be reported immediately. In addition, verify that patients can demonstrate how to plan meals within any prescribed dietary restrictions and explain how to maintain a fluid intake that will ensure adequate urinary output.

DRUGS FOR GOUT
Gout

Gout is a metabolic disease in which total body pools of uric acid (a product of DNA and RNA degradation) are elevated. The uric acid crystallizes in joints or, less commonly, in tendons or bursae. The joint at the base of the big toe is most commonly affected. During an attack of acute gouty arthritis there is a marked inflammation of the joint accompanied by significant pain. This acute attack is treated with the drug colchicine, which acts (in an unknown manner) to relieve the pain, with one of the NSAIDs already discussed, or in special circumstances with adrenocorticotropic hormone (ACTH) (see Chapter 51). Some patients develop a tophus in a joint (crystals of uric acid with fibrous tissue surrounding them). Patients with tophi or recurrent attacks of gouty arthritis must receive long-term treatment, often for the rest of their lives, with drugs that will reduce uric acid levels in the body.

Aspirin was used in doses over 5 gm to treat gout based on the action of salicylates by increasing excretion of uric acid. However, effects are variable, and aspirin is no longer used. (Lower doses have no effect, and doses of 1 to 2 gm may decrease uric acid excretion).

With the newer drug therapy, tophi, if present, often regress with long-term therapy, restoring the joint to a normal range of function. About 25% of such patients overproduce uric acid. These patients are treated with the drug allopurinol, which prevents the formation of uric acid from xanthine and hypoxanthine, the purine metabolites of DNA and RNA metabolism. Other patients are treated with a uricosuric drug, probenecid or sulfinpyrazone. These drugs increase the renal excretion of uric acid by inhibiting its reabsorption from the proximal kidney tubule.

Specific Drugs

Drugs used to treat gout are listed in Table 23-4.

Table 23-4 Drugs to Treat Gout

Generic name	Trade name	Administration/dosage	Comments
Allopurinol	Lopurin Zyloprim*	ORAL: *Adults*—200 to 300 mg daily as a single dose; maximum, 800 mg daily. Dose is reduced if there is renal insufficiency. FDA Pregnancy Category C.	Inhibits the formation of uric acid from hypoxanthine or xanthine; these are excreted instead.
Colchicine	Generic	ORAL: *Adults*—0.5 to 0.6 mg hourly or 1 to 1.2 mg initially and 0.5 to 0.6 mg every 2 hr. This is regimen for an acute gouty attack and is continued until the pain subsides or GI symptoms appear. Maximum dose, 7 to 8 mg. For prophylaxis, 0.5 to 1 mg daily. INTRAVENOUS: for an acute attack, 1 to 2 mg initially, then 0.5 mg every 3 to 6 hr or 1 dose of 3 mg; maximum dose, 4 mg. FDA Pregnancy Category D.	Terminates an acute gouty attack. Appearance of GI distress usually limits the amount given. Dilutes the drug 10-fold with sterile saline solution before injecting to minimize tissue damage.
Probenecid	Benemid* Benuryl† Various others	ORAL: *Adults*—250 mg 2 or 3 times daily the first week, then 500 mg twice daily thereafter. May increase to 2.0 gm daily if necessary.	Inhibits reabsorption of uric acid by the kidney. A prophylactic drug to reduce existing tophi and to prevent recurrence of a gouty attack.
Sulfinpyrazone	Anturan† Anturane	ORAL: *Adults*—100 to 200 mg 2 times daily with meals or with milk at bedtime. The dosage is raised as needed to control blood urate levels (400 to 800 mg daily). The dose is then reduced to the minimum effective level, usually 300 to 400 mg daily.	Acts like probenecid. May also prevent the recurrence of MI.

*Available in Canada and United States.
†Available in Canada only.

Colchicine

Colchicine provides relief from the pain of an acute attack of gouty arthritis, usually within 24 hr. The earlier in an episode colchicine is taken, the more effective it is. (Antiinflammatory drugs are similarly more effective if taken early in an acute episode). Colchicine taken orally at the doses required to treat an acute gouty attack may cause nausea and vomiting followed by diarrhea. These effects limit the amount of colchicine that can be taken. Alternatively, the drug may be given intravenously to minimize these side effects. Since it causes severe tissue inflammation, it is diluted before IV administration to minimize the effect of any drug leakage.

Colchicine may be continued at reduced dosages once the acute episode is over. Continuance of colchicine is most common if a drug to reduce uric acid is begun. A sudden change in body uric acid concentration often precipitates a new acute attack of gouty arthritis. This can often be avoided with prophylactic colchicine.

Allopurinol

Allopurinol (Zyloprim) inhibits the formation of uric acid from xanthine or hypoxanthine so that xanthine or hypoxanthine is excreted instead. A patient whose morning urine has a ratio of uric acid to creatinine greater than 0.75 or whose 24-hr urine contains more than 600 mg or uric acid is classified as an overproducer of uric acid. These overproducers and patients with renal uric acid crystals or impaired renal function are those for whom allopurinol will be most effective. It is also effective for patients with gout resulting from drug therapy that increases uric acid production, particularly cancer therapy. Side effects are rare; they appear to be allergic reactions (see box).

Probenecid and sulfinpyrazone

Probenecid (Benemid) and sulfinpyrazone (Anturane) inhibit the reabsorption of uric acid by the kidney tubules and thereby promote the excretion of uric acid in the urine. The patient should drink at least eight glasses of water daily to keep the uric acid dilute so that it does not crystallize in kidney tubules or the bladder. Since these drugs flood the kidney tubules with uric acid, they are contraindicated in patients with renal failure or with a history of renal stones.

Probenecid is generally well tolerated but occasionally causes GI upset or an allergic reaction. It interferes with the renal excretion of many compounds.

Sulfinpyrazone is also well tolerated. The incidence of GI upset is higher with sulfinpyrazone than with probenecid. Recent studies show that sulfinpyrazone decreases the incidence of sudden death in the first 8 months after an MI. This effect is believed to be due to decreased platelet aggregation. Since many patients with gout also have conditions such as diabetes, hypertension, or coronary artery disease (high-risk factors for MI), sulfinpyrazone may be more desirable than probenecid despite the higher incidence of GI upset.

Drug Interactions in the Therapy of Gout

Factors that diminish the effectiveness of the uricosuric drugs probenecid and sulfinpyrazone include the following:

1. A diet high in purines produces too much uric acid (see box).
2. Inhibition of uric acid secretion counteracts the block in reabsorption by the uricosuric drugs.
   a. Heavy alcohol consumption produces enough lactic acid to inhibit uric acid secretion.
   b. Aspirin and other salicylates at low doses (300 to 650 mg) inhibit uric acid secretion. Acetaminophen should be substituted for simple pain relief.
   c. Diuretics, particularly the thiazides, furosemide, ethacrynic acid, triamterene, and spironolactone inhibit uric acid secretion. Drugs used to treat gout can potentiate other drugs.

DIETARY CONSIDERATION: PURINE

Uric acid is produced when purine is catabolized. Gout is a problem of elevated uric acid. Formerly, a mainstay of gout therapy was purine restriction in the diet. With better drug therapy, purine restriction is a less significant component of therapy. Patients should probably modify their diets to limit excessive purine intake, unless more severe restriction is indicated on an individual basis. High purine foods to avoid or limit include the following:

◆ organ meats   ◆ mincemeat
◆ roe   ◆ herring
◆ sardines   ◆ shrimp
◆ scallops   ◆ mackerel
◆ anchovies   ◆ gravy
◆ broth and consomme ◆ yeast

The uricosuric drugs inhibit the secretion or degradation of several medications:

1. Probenecid inhibits the renal secretion of penicillin, indomethacin, methotrexate, sulfonylureas (oral hypoglycemics), sulfinpyrazone, salicylates, and rifampin keeping their plasma levels high.
2. Sulfinpyrazone inhibits the degradation of sulfonamides, particularly sulfadiazine and sulfisoxazole, sulfonylureas, and coumarins.
3. Allopurinol inhibits the degradation of azathioprine, 6-mercaptopurine, antipyrine, coumarins, and cyclophosphamide.

NURSING IMPLICATIONS SUMMARY

Acetaminophen

Patient and family education

◆ When used in usual doses, there are few side effects associated with this drug. Instruct patients to report the development of any new sign or symptom to the physician.

◆ Remind patients to keep these and all drugs out of the reach of children. Never encourage children to take medications by telling them that drugs are candy. Tell parents to seek medical help immediately if overdose is suspected.

◆ Tell patients to be alert to signs of acute toxicity such as nausea, vomiting, and abdominal pain. Severe poisoning may result in CNS stimulation, excitement, and delirium; followed by CNS depression; stupor; hypothermia; rapid, shallow breathing; tachycardia; hypotension; and circulatory failure.

◆ Teach patients to read labels of all medications carefully. Many OTC products for pain and sinus problems or colds contain acetaminophen alone or in combination with other drugs. Tell patients to avoid taking several drugs simultaneously unless absolutely necessary.

◆ Review with parents the dosages appropriate for children of various sizes and ages. Assist parents in finding a drug form that is easy to administer. Note that absorption from a rectal suppository is variable, and there may be rectal irritation; this route may be the least desirable.

◆ Pain or fever that persists beyond 3 to 5 days may signal a more serious health problem. Instruct patients to seek medical help rather than to self-medicate indefinitely. Take only the recommended dose; too much may cause liver damage.

◆ Remind patients to inform all health-care providers of all drugs they take.

◆ To take effervescent preparations, pour the granules into a glass. Fill the glass with 4 oz of cool water. Drink all of the contents of the glass, whether still fizzing or not.

◆ Avoid alcoholic beverages while taking acetaminophen.

◆ Instruct patients who are also taking tetracycline to take it at least 1 to 2 hr before or after acetaminophen. Acetylcysteine is discussed in Chapter 26.

Aspirin and Related Drugs

Drug administration

◆ Monitor platelet count and hematocrit level.

◆ Regularly check stools for presence of blood or guaiac.

Patient and family education

◆ Instruct patients about the signs of aspirin toxicity.

◆ Instruct patients to report the development of tinnitus, unexplained bleeding or bruising, severe or persistent gastric irritation, or blood in the stool. Salicylates other than aspirin do not affect platelet aggregation.

◆ Warn parents that aspirin and other salicylates should not be used to treat fever and discomfort of the flu or chickenpox in children, since aspirin is associated with the development of Reye's syndrome. Acetaminophen is preferred over aspirin to treat childhood flu and chickenpox symptoms.

◆ Remind patients to keep these and all drugs out of the reach of children. Never encourage children to take medications by telling them that drugs are candy. Instruct parents to seek medical help immediately if overdose is suspected.

◆ Teach patients to read labels of all medications carefully. Many OTC products for pain and for sinus problems or colds contain salicylates alone or in combination with other drugs. Instruct patients to avoid taking several drugs simultaneously unless necessary.

◆ To reduce gastric irritation, teach patients to take oral doses with a full glass of fluid, or with meals or a snack.

◆ Pain or fever that persists beyond 3 to 5 days may signal a more serious health problem. Instruct patients to seek medical help rather than self-medicate indefinitely. Patients should take only the recommended dose; too much may result in salicylism or other complications.

◆ Remind patients to keep all health-care providers informed of all medications being taken, including aspirin; this includes dentists and oral surgeons. Note the drug interactions on p. 361.

◆ Do not take aspirin products that smell strongly of vinegar, as they may have broken down and may not be effective.

Continued.

NURSING IMPLICATIONS SUMMARY—cont'd

◆ To take effervescent preparations, pour the granules into a glass. Fill the glass with 4 oz of cool water. Drink all of the contents of the glass, whether still fizzing or not.

◆ Enteric-coated preparations should be swallowed whole, without chewing or crushing. Chewable aspirin tablets may be crushed, chewed, or swallowed whole. Patients should chew aspirin chewing gum for several minutes (or as directed on the package label) for best effect Extended-release preparations should be broken along scored lines. Some should not be chewed or crushed; consult the pharmacist about specific brands.

◆ Instruct patients to avoid alcoholic beverages while taking aspirin or salicylates. Buffered aspirin and choline and magnesium salicylates should not be taken at the same time as tetracyclines. Patients taking one of these drugs and tetracycline should allow 1 to 2 hr between doses.

◆ Patients on long-term therapy may find extended-release preparations helpful, particularly at night, since morning blood levels of aspirin may not be so low.

◆ Teach patients taking aspirin for arthritis and other musculoskeletal conditions that the best effect is achieved through regular use of the drug, as prescribed.

◆ Warn diabetics that chronic or excessive use of aspirin-containing products may cause false urine sugar results. Monitor blood glucose levels. Consult the physician or pharmacist.

◆ Low-dose aspirin may be used for its antiplatelet effect. It may be prescribed to decrease the incidence of thromboembolism in immobilized patients and postoperative orthopedic patients. It is also used to prevent other vascular problems; see Chapter 20.

◆ Encourage patients who are allergic to aspirin to wear a medical identification tag or bracelet indicating this.

Nonsteroidal Antiinflammatory Drugs
Drug administration

◆ Monitor vital signs, blood pressure, and weight. Monitor the complete blood cell count, differential, platelet count, blood urea nitrogen level (BUN), serum creatinine level, and liver function tests. Check stools for presence of blood or guaiac. If diarrhea or vomiting is severe or persistent, monitor intake and output.

◆ Question patients about history of allergy to other drugs before administering. If unsure that an allergy to a NSAID exists, consult physician before administering the first dose.

◆ In patients with cardiovascular, renal, or hypertensive disease, assess for possible fluid retention. Auscultate lung sounds. Assess for jugular venous distention. Monitor daily weight.

Patient and family education

◆ Review anticipated benefits and possible side effects of drug therapy. Instruct patients to report the development of bruising, bleeding gums, nosebleeds, blood in stool, fever, rash, sore throat, mouth ulcers or irritation, jaundice, right upper quadrant abdominal pain, and malaise. Instruct patients to notify the physician if unexpected symptoms develop.

◆ Tell patients with long-term musculoskeletal problems that several weeks of therapy may be necessary before full benefit is seen. Best effects are seen if the drugs are taken regularly, as ordered. Tell patients not to discontinue or increase therapy without consulting the physician.

◆ Ensure that patients take doses with meals, a snack, or milk to reduce gastric irritation. Doses are taken with a full glass (8 oz) of fluid. Patients should not lie down for at least 15 to 30 min after an oral dose.

◆ Review the other medications and drug interactions noted in the text; counsel patients as appropriate. Remind patients to keep all health-care providers including dentists and oral surgeons, informed of all drugs they take. Tell patients not to take OTC products without consulting the physician. This applies especially to products containing aspirin or acetaminophen.

◆ Warn patients to avoid driving or operating hazardous equipment if visual changes, dizziness, fatigue, or weakness occur and to notify the physician.

◆ Patients should avoid drinking alcoholic beverages while taking NSAIDs.

◆ NSAIDs may cause photosensitivity. Warn patients to limit time in the sun or under sun lamps until the effects of the drug can be evaluated. (See Patient Problem: Photosensitivity on p. 629.)

◆ NSAIDs may be used to treat fever, even in children.

NURSING IMPLICATIONS SUMMARY—cont'd

- Long-term use of these drugs is associated with visual changes. Encourage patients to get recommended ophthalmic examinations.
- Enteric-coated forms should be swallowed whole, not chewed or crushed. Capsules may be opened and the contents mixed with food. Some tablets may be crushed and mixed with food. Work with patients to find a form the patient can take. Consult the pharmacist for information about crushing, breaking, or mixing an individual product.
- Instruct patients taking nonprescription NSAIDs to review the manufacturer's literature supplied with the package. Emphasize the importance of continuing with other prescribed therapies, which might include a prescribed exercise program, weight reduction, application of heat and cold, and physical therapy.
- Some of these drugs cause fluid retention. Assess patient's ability, resources, and other health problems (e.g., hypertensive, cardiovascular, or renal disease). If appropriate, teach patients to monitor and record weight on a daily basis. Report weight gain in excess of 2 lb/day or 5 lb/week to the physician.
- Remind pregnant or lactating women that no drugs should be used without consulting the physician.

Gold Compounds

Drug administration

- Assess respiratory rate and auscultate lung sounds. Monitor intake and output, and weight. Monitor complete blood count and differential, platelet count, BUN level, serum creatinine level, and liver function tests. Monitor urinalysis to detect proteinuria, and hematuria. Inspect skin and mouth for presence of rashes, ulcers, stomatitis, and irritation.
- For IM injection, use large muscle masses. Record and rotate injection sites. Aspirate before administering dose to prevent inadvertent IV administration. Keep patient supine for at least 15 minutes after dose. Monitor vital signs and blood pressure. Have available drugs, equipment, and personnel to treat an acute allergic reaction when parenteral gold compounds are administered.

INTRAMUSCULAR AUROTHIOGLUCOSE

- This drug form is an oil-based suspension. (See box on p. 87.)

Patient and family education

- Review anticipated benefits and possible side effects of drug therapy with patients. Instruct patients to notify the physician if severe or persistent vomiting or diarrhea, rashes, skin irritation, itching, mouth ulcers, oral irritation, stomatitis, metallic taste, unexplained bruising, bleeding of gums, bleeding in stool, nosebleeds, jaundice, right upper quadrant abdominal pain, malaise, fever, sore throat, eye irritation, or visual changes develop. Reinforce the importance of reporting new signs or symptoms to the physician.
- Instruct patients to take oral compounds with meals or a snack to lessen gastric irritation.
- Review oral hygiene with the patient if stomatitis develops. (See Patient Problem: Stomatitis on p. 561.)
- Review Patient Problem: Photosensitivity on p. 629 with the patient.
- Explain that weeks to months of therapy may be necessary before full benefit of gold therapy can be seen. Emphasize the importance of continuing other prescribed therapies, including prescribed exercise program, weight reduction, application of heat and cold, and physical therapy.
- Women of childbearing age may wish to use some form of birth control while on gold therapy; discuss this before initiating gold therapy.

Azathioprine

- See Chapter 28 for a discussion of this drug.

Glucocorticoids

- See Chapter 51 for a detailed discussion of these drugs.

Hydroxychloroquine

- See Chapter 38 for a detailed discussion of this drug, also used to treat malaria.

Methotrexate

- See Chapter 39 for a detailed discussion of this drug, used in higher doses to treat cancer.

Continued.

NURSING IMPLICATIONS SUMMARY—cont'd

Penicillamine

Drug administration

◆ Penicillamine is a copper chelating agent and is therefore used in the treatment of Wilson's disease, a disorder of copper metabolism. Patients with Wilson's disease should avoid foods higher in copper including chocolate, nuts, shellfish, mushrooms, liver, molasses, broccoli, and copper-enriched cereals.

◆ Monitor weight and blood pressure. Auscultate lung sounds. Inspect for presence of skin rashes and lesions. Monitor complete blood count and differential, platelet count, serum creattinine level, BUN level, and liver function tests. Monitor urinalysis to detect proteinuria.

◆ Assess penicillin allergy before administering. Cross-sensitivity between the two drugs is possible, though rare.

Patient and family education

◆ Review anticipated benefits and possible side effects of drug therapy. Instruct patients to notify the physician if severe or persistent vomiting or diarrhea, skin rashes, lesions, scaling, dermatitis, hair loss, fever, inflamed mouth, mouth lesions, stomatitis, swelling or edema, bruising, bleeding, nosebleeds, blood in stool, malaise, sore throat, jaundice, or abdominal pain develop. Explain that side effects may develop any time during therapy. Report new signs and symptoms to the physician.

◆ Review Patient Problem: Stomatitis on p. 561.

◆ Emphasize the importance of taking drugs as ordered. Sporadic or intermittent use (unless prescribed by the physician) may contribute to further allergic reactions.

◆ Capsules may be opened and contents mixed with 15 to 30 ml of chilled applesauce, other pureed foods, or fruit juice for ease in administering.

◆ For treatment of arthritis, patients should take doses 1 hr before or 2 hr after meals, and 1 hr before or after other medications, food, or milk.

◆ For treatment of Wilson's disease, doses should be taken on an empty stomach, 30 to 60 min before or 2 hr after meals.

◆ For prevention of cystinuria, tell patients to take the bedtime dose with at least two 8-oz glasses of water, and to drink two more 8-oz glasses of water during the night. Take daytime doses with a full glass of water. Patients taking oral iron preparations should allow at least 2 hr to elapse between the two drugs.

◆ Patients with Wilson's disease should avoid multivitamin preparations containing copper.

◆ Penicillamine increases the body's requirement for pyridoxine. If pyridoxine is also prescribed, emphasize the importance of taking this supplement. See Dietary Consideration: Vitamins on p. 275 for dietary sources of pyridoxine.

◆ Women of childbearing age may wish to use some form of birth control while on penicillamine therapy; discuss this before initiating therapy.

◆ Emphasize that weeks to months of therapy may be necessary before full benefit of penicillamine can be seen. Reinforce the importance of continuing other prescribed therapies, which might include a prescribed exercise program, weight reduction, application of heat and cold, and physical therapy.

Sulfasalazine

Patient and family education

◆ Assess patients for allergy to other sulfonamides, furosemide, thiazide diuretics, salicylates, carbonic anhydrase inhibitors, or sulfonylureas. (See Chapter 34).

◆ Take doses with meals or a snack to lessen gastric irritation.

◆ Take enteric-coated tablets whole, without chewing or crushing.

◆ Teach patients to maintain a daily fluid intake of at least 2000 to 2500 ml.

◆ Patients should avoid driving or operating hazardous equipment if dizzy.

◆ See Patient Problems: Photosensitivity on p. 629; Depressed White Blood Cell Production on p. 560; and Bleeding Tendencies on p. 570.

◆ Encourage regular dental care and good dental hygiene (flossing and brushing). Leukopenia and thrombocytopenia may contribute to gum infections and bleeding gums.

◆ Encourage patients to return for regularly scheduled follow-up.

NURSING IMPLICATIONS SUMMARY—cont'd

Allopurinol

Drug administration

◆ Inspect patients to detect rash and skin changes. Assess vision. Monitor serum creatinine level, BUN level, uric acid levels, complete blood count, differential, platelet count, and liver function tests.

Patient and family education

◆ Review anticipated benefits and possible side effects of drug therapy. Instruct patients to report bruising, bleeding, nosebleeds, blood in stool, fever, sore throat, malaise, jaundice, or abdominal pain. GI discomfort is common. Encourage patients to notify the physician of GI discomfort.

◆ Tell patients to maintain daily fluid intake sufficient to ensure a daily urinary output of at least 2 L; this may require an intake of 2500 ml/day (about ten 8-oz glasses of water).

◆ Caution patients to avoid analgesics containing salicylates unless approved by the physician.

◆ Remind patients to inform all health-care providers of all drugs they take. Allopurinol may interfere with the effects of other drugs.

◆ Instruct patients to take oral doses with meal or a snack to reduce gastric irritation.

◆ Review Dietary Consideration: Purine on p. 372.

◆ Patients should limit the intake of alcoholic beverages. They should not take vitamin C concurrently with allopurinol since it may increase urine acidity and promote the formation of kidney stones.

Colchicine

Drug administration

◆ Inspect patients to detect hair loss and skin changes. Assess for GI discomfort. Monitor serum creatinine level, BUN level, complete blood count, differential, platelet count, liver function tests, and uric acid levels.

INTRAVENOUS COLCHICINE

◆ May be given undiluted or dilute with 0.9% sodium chloride without a bacteriostatic agent. Administer 0.5 mg/1 min. Avoid extravasation or IM administration. Check that IV line is patent before administering.

Patient and family education

◆ Review anticipated benefits and possible side effects of drug therapy. Instruct patients to report change in the color of urine (hematuria), bruising, bleeding, nosebleeds, blood in stool, fever, sore throat, malaise, jaundice, or abdominal pain. GI discomfort is common. Encourage patients to notify the physician of any GI discomfort.

◆ Instruct patients to maintain daily fluid intake sufficient to ensure daily urinary output of at least 2 L; this may require an intake of 2500 ml/day (about 10 8-oz glasses of water).

◆ Instruct patients to take oral doses with meals or a snack to reduce gastric irritation.

◆ Caution patients to avoid the use of analgesics containing salicylates without approval of the physician.

◆ Remind patients to inform all health care providers of all drugs they take. Colchicine may interfere with the desired effect of other drugs.

◆ Review Dietary Consideration: Purine on p. 372.

◆ Patients should limit the intake of alcoholic beverages.

Probenecid

Drug administration

◆ Inspect for development of skin changes. Monitor blood pressure. Monitor liver function tests and serum creatinine, BUN, and uric acid levels.

◆ Probenecid is sometimes used concurrently with some antibiotics such as penicillins and cephalosporins; the probenecid helps increase the plasma and tissue antibiotic concentration.

Patient and family education

◆ Review anticipated benefits and possible side effects of drug therapy. Instruct patients to report malaise, jaundice, or abdominal pain. GI discomfort is common. Encourage patients to notify physicians of GI discomfort.

◆ Tell patients to maintain daily fluid intake sufficient to ensure a daily urinary output of at least 2 L; this may require an intake of 2500 ml per day (about 10 8-oz glasses of fluid).

Continued.

NURSING IMPLICATIONS SUMMARY—cont'd

◆ Warn patients to avoid driving or operating hazardous equipment and to notify the physician if dizziness occurs. Warn patients that flushing may occur after drug ingestion. Caution patients to avoid analgesics containing salicylates without the physician's approval.

◆ Remind patients to inform all health-care providers of all drugs they take. Probenecid may interfere with the desired effect of other prescribed drugs.

◆ Alkalinization of urine helps prevent crystallization of uric acid. Sodium bicarbonate, potassium citrate, or other alkalinizing agent may be prescribed concurrently.

◆ Review Dietary Consideration: Purine on p. 372.

◆ Patients should limit the intake of alcoholic beverages.

◆ Some products contain colchicine and probenecid. Review side effects of both drugs with patients.

Sulfinpyrazone
Drug administration

◆ Assess for development of tinnitus and changes in hearing or GI distress. Inspect for skin changes or rash.

Patient and family education

◆ Review anticipated benefits and possible side effects of drug therapy. Instruct patients to report bruising, bleeding, nosebleeds, blood in stool, fever, sore throat, malaise, or tinnitus. GI discomfort is common. Encourage patients to notify the physician of any GI discomfort. Administer oral doses with milk, meals, or snacks to reduce gastric irritation.

◆ Tell patients to maintain daily fluid intake sufficient to ensure daily urinary output of at least 2 L; this may require an intake of 2500 ml/day (about 10 8-oz glasses of fluid).

◆ Caution patients to avoid the use of analgesics containing salicylates without obtaining the physician's approval.

◆ Remind patients to inform all health-care providers of all drugs they take. Sulfinpyrazone may interfere with the desired effect of other drugs taken.

◆ Review Dietary Consideration: Purine on p. 372.

◆ Intake of alcoholic beverages should be limited.

CHAPTER REVIEW

◆ KEY TERMS

analgesic, p. 357
antipyretic, p. 358
gout, p. 370
Reye's syndrome, p. 360
rheumatoid arthritis, p. 368
salicylism, p. 360

◆ REVIEW QUESTIONS

1. List the three pharmacologic actions characteristic of aspirin.
2. How do the nonnarcotic analgesics produce analgesia?
3. What is the mechanism of antipyresis?
4. Why is acetaminophen considered safer than aspirin? Why should children not take aspirin?
5. What are the side effects of acetaminophen?
6. What is the mechanism of acetaminophen toxicity?
7. What is the dosage difference between aspirin taken for analgesia-antipyresis and for an antiinflammatory response?
8. How does aspirin affect the stomach? How does aspirin affect platelets? Describe nursing care considerations related to these effects.
9. What factors determine the metabolism and excretion of salicylate?
10. Describe salicylism. Describe aspirin toxicity.
11. What pharmacologic actions are characteristic of the NSAIDs?
12. Why is phenylbutazone used for 2 weeks or less?
13. What are the major side effects of indomethacin?
14. Describe the uses of NSAIDs.
15. Which four drugs are used to induce a remission in progressive rheumatoid arthritis?
16. Describe the role of colchicine in treating gout.

17. Describe the mechanisms of allopurinol, probenecid, and sulfinpyrazone for lowering the uric acid concentration of the body.

18. Develop a nursing care plan for a patient receiving one or more of the drugs in this chapter.

SUGGESTED READING

Abramson SB, Weissmann G: The mechanism of action of nonsteroidal antiinflammatory drugs, *Arthritis Rheum* 32(1):1, 1989.

Blake GJ: Methotrexate for rheumatoid arthritis, *Nurs 91* 21(2):26, 1991.

Brassell MP: Pharmacologic management of rheumatic disease, *Orthop Nurs* 7(2):43, 1988.

Brucker MC: Management of common minor discomforts in pregnancy: II. Managing minor pain in pregnancy, *J Nurse Midwife* 33(1):25, 1988.

Gever MP: Top 25 discharge drugs, *Nurs 91* 21(6):53, 1991.

Kremer JM: Severe rheumatoid arthritis: current options in drug therapy, *Geriatrics* 45(12):43, 1990.

Lynn MM, Holdcroft C: Preventing NSAID-induced ulcers: the use of misoprostol, *Nurse Pract* 15(10):38, 1990.

McGuire L: Administering analgesics: which drugs are right for your patient, *Nurs 90* 20(4):34, 1990.

CHAPTER 24

Antihistamines

LEARNING OBJECTIVES

After studying this chapter, you should be able to do the following:

- Describe localized and generalized allergic responses.
- Discuss the role of histamine in allergic responses.
- Describe the common side effects of antihistamines, including the anticholinergic effects.
- Develop a nursing care plan for a patient taking an antihistamine.

CHAPTER OVERVIEW

- **Histamine** is a naturally occurring amine that is formed from the amino acid histidine. Histamine is found in mast cells, which are numerous in the lung and skin, and basophils, the counterparts of mast cells in the blood. The histamine released from the mast cells causes many of the symptoms associated with allergic reactions. It is also found in the gastrointestinal (GI) tract, where histamine is a potent stimulant for the secretion of acid in the stomach. Histamine is also found in parts of the brain, where it is believed to be a neurotransmitter. At present, the role of histamine in the brain is speculative but may involve regulating the level of arousal. This chapter focuses on the role of histamine in allergic reactions and the drugs available to treat these reactions. The role of histamine in the stomach is discussed in Chapter 13.

Nursing Process Overview

ANTIHISTAMINES FOR ALLERGIC REACTIONS

Assessment

Assess vital signs, respiratory and cardiovascular status, relevant history of previous allergy, exposure to possible allergens, subjective symptoms, and objective data such as the extent and type of rash. Anaphylaxis is an emergency; the more delayed and chronic response may represent a source of annoyance to the patient but may never progress to an acute phase.

Nursing Diagnoses

High risk for injury secondary to drowsiness related to antihistamine therapy

Possible altered bowel elimination: constipation related to antihistamine use

Management

The acute allergic reaction anaphylaxis requires immediate diagnosis and treatment, usually with 1:1000 epinephrine injected subcutaneously or intramuscularly, followed by parenteral antihistamines. Supportive care is symptomatic and based on rapid assessment of the cardiovascular and respiratory response. Management of the less acute allergic response is not an emergency. Monitor the vital signs, respiratory status, cardiovascular status, platelet count, and white blood cell count. Observe for side effects of drug therapy, especially drowsiness; monitor fluid intake and output to check for urinary retention; and monitor the frequency of bowel movements to assess for constipation.

Evaluation

Before discharge, determine that patients can explain why and how to take the prescribed medication, what side effects may appear and which of these to report immediately, and what to do for specific side effects such as dry mouth, constipation, hypotension, and drowsiness. If specific allergens are identified, patients should be able to name them. Verify that patients understand the importance of wearing a medical identification tag or bracelet listing specific allergens.

HISTAMINE AND ANTIHISTAMINES
Allergic Responses and Histamine
Histamine release and metabolism

Histamine in mast cells and basophils is complexed with heparin and stored in granules. The typical allergic reaction such as hay fever or contact dermatitis involves the release of these granules in response to an antigen. Antibodies of the immunoglobulin E (IgE) class fix to the mast cells and basophils. When an antigen binds to the fixed IgE, the cells degranulate, releasing histamine, heparin, and other compounds, which alter capillary permeability and attract phagocytes to degrade the bound antigen. This process is illustrated in Figure 24-1.

In addition to antigen-induced degranulation, many drugs and venoms cause degranulation. These include drugs and dyes that carry a positive charge,

large molecules that occur in animal sera and dextran solutions, and venoms and enzymes that damage tissue.

Once histamine is released, it is metabolized to inactive compounds in 5 to 15 min. One of the degradative pathways is inhibited by aspirin so that histamine may persist. This is the mechanism for one type of aspirin sensitivity.

Allergic responses explained by the action of histamine

Local allergic responses involving histamine are as follows:

Angioedema: Swelling caused by plasma leakage and blood vessel dilation in the skin or mucous membranes ("giant hives")

Anaphylaxis: Systemic. Onset is usually indicated by a generalized itching and tingling sensation and a feeling of apprehension. Profound hypotension leading to shock may follow, and the bronchioles are constricted, causing a choking sensation

Asthma: Spasm of the bronchial smooth muscle

Eczema: Inflamed areas of skin

Purpura: Red spots on the skin caused by the leakage of blood from small vessels

Rhinitis: Inflammation of the nasal mucous mem-

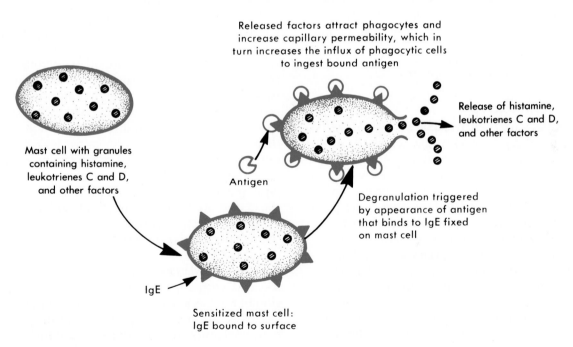

FIGURE 24-1
Immunologic mechanism underlying release of histamine from mast cells. Antibodies of IgE class are bound to surface of mast cells. Binding of antigen to IgE triggers degranulation of mast cell, releasing histamine and leukotrienes C and D. Histamine is responsible for many allergy and asthma symptoms.

branes that allows fluid to escape

Urticaria: Hives, which are large wheals caused by leakage of plasma and are accompanied by severe itching

Two actions of histamine are prominent in explaining allergic responses. Histamine is a potent dilator of arterioles and renders the capillaries more permeable so that fluid and protein are lost into the extravascular space. This explains the bump that appears after an insect sting. Initially, a red spot reflects the dilation of the small blood vessels, and as fluid leaks into the extravascular space, the bump, representing local edema, appears. Histamine also stimulates the contraction of smooth muscle, particularly the bronchial smooth muscle. When mast cells are degranulated in the lung, as in asthma, the airway is narrowed and patients have difficulty breathing.

Histamine released systemically causes anaphylaxis, characterized by a profound fall in blood pressure resulting from vasodilation and severe constriction of the bronchioles making breathing difficult. The loss of fluid from circulation resulting from the increased capillary permeability causes the shock that develops in an untreated anaphylactic response. Edema in the mucous tissue of the upper windpipe (laryngeal edema) can block the airway altogether. Epinephrine is the drug of choice for anaphylactic shock. Epinephrine constricts blood vessels to raise the blood pressure and relieve laryngeal edema and dilates the bronchioles, actions that reverse those of histamine (see Chapter 14).

Antihistamines as H-1 Receptor Antagonists

General pharmacology

Antihistamines have been available for over 50 years. Although these drugs block some actions of histamine, they do not block the histamine-mediated secretion of acid in the stomach. There are two types of histamine receptors, the H-1 receptors, acting principally on blood vessels and the bronchioles, and the H-2 receptors, acting mainly on the GI tract. The older antihistamines are specific antagonists for the H-1 receptors. Antagonists specific for the H-2 receptor are cimetidine (Tagamet), famotidine (Pepcid), nizatidine (Axid), and ranitidine (Zantac). These drugs, used primarily to decrease stomach acid, are discussed in Chapter 13. In this chapter, the term *antihistamine* refers to drugs that specifically block the H-1 receptors.

Absorption and fate. Antihistamines are given orally and are absorbed well. Their action is seen in 10 to 30 min and lasts for 4 to 6 hr. Timed-release forms are active for 8 to 12 hr. Antihistamines are metabolized to inactive compounds by the liver and kidneys.

Other pharmacologic actions. Although the antihistamines are so named because they specifically compete with histamine for the H-1 receptors, they have other pharmacologic properties. The main secondary action is an anticholinergic or atropinelike action. This is the origin of side effects such as inhibition of secretions, blurred vision, urinary retention, fast heart rate (tachycardia), and constipation. In the central nervous system (CNS) the anticholinergic effect can cause insomnia, tremors, nervousness, and irritability. These effects are particularly predominant in children. Sedation and drowsiness, the central antihistaminic effects, are more common in adults. The spectrum of antihistaminic and anticholinergic properties depends on the drug, the dose, and the individual.

Most antihistamines have a local anesthetic effect, which might relieve the itching of skin rashes. Antihistamines are rarely used for this purpose because they tend to be good antigens, thereby causing skin rashes themselves. Other clinically important pharmacologic actions are limited to a few antihistamines. Some antihistamines prevent nausea and vomiting, particularly from motion sickness. A few antihistamines prevent vertigo (the feeling of movement, particularly rotational movement, when there is none). Antihistamines that suppress the tremors of Parkinson's disease are discussed in Chapter 35.

Toxic effects. Antihistamine overdose can cause CNS depression or stimulation, the latter being more common in children. The atropinelike symptoms (i.e., a flushed skin and fixed, dilated pupils) are also prominent. Treatment maintains an airway and treats hypotension. In children a high temperature is common, which can be reversed with ice packs and sponge baths. If the antihistamine is not a phenothiazine, vomiting is induced, gastric lavage is carried out, and cathartics are used to empty the GI tract of remaining drug. Vomiting should not be induced with phenothiazines, since they can cause uncoordinated movements of the head and neck, which would cause aspiration of vomitus. Antihistamines that are phenothiazine derivatives are identified in the drug tables.

Drug interactions. The main drug interaction associated with antihistamines is the additive depression of the CNS when taken with alcohol, hypnotics, sedatives, antipsychotics, antianxiety drugs, or narcotic analgesics. Because of their atropinelike effects, antihistamines should be used with caution in patients with glaucoma, hyperthyroidism, cardiovascular disease, or hypertension.

Contraindications. Antihistamines are contraindicated for nursing mothers because the drugs are secreted in milk. Antihistamines taken by young children can cause paradoxic excitement, whereas elderly patients are sensitive to the sedative actions.

Antihistamines and allergic reactions

Antihistamines used to control allergic reactions are listed in Table 24-1. Antihistamines are primarily effective in decreasing the discomfort of acute allergic reactions that involve the upper respiratory system, such as hay fever, or the skin, such as hives. Hay fever is most successfully treated when the antihistamine therapy is begun while the pollen count is still low. Sneezing, runny nose, and swollen eyes are reduced in more than 70% of patients. Antihistamines reduce the swelling and itching (pruritus) of urticaria and related conditions.

Antihistamines do not prevent or treat colds effectively, although they are present in many over-the-counter (OTC) cold remedies. Because most antihistamines have anticholinergic actions, they can dry up a runny nose and relieve the symptoms of a cold. Antihistamines do not treat asthma, probably because substances other than histamine are responsible for the prolonged bronchiole constriction characteristic of asthma. Since the drugs have a drying effect because they inhibit bronchial secretions, they can aggravate asthma.

Antihistamines do not affect histamine receptors on their own. Because of this, some allergic responses are not effectively treated with antihistamines. Anaphylaxis represents a true emergency for which an

Table 24-1   Antihistamines for Allergies

Generic name	Trade name	Administration/dosage	Comments
Astemizole	Hismanal*	ORAL: *Adults*—10 mg once a day, taken on an empty stomach. *Children*—2 mg/10 kg body weight once a day, taken on an empty stomach.	Nonsedating antihistamine Does not cause sedation.
Azatadine maleate	Optimine*	ORAL: *Adults*—1 to 2 mg twice daily. *Children*—not established. FDA Pregnancy Category B.	Drowsiness is the most common side effect.
Brompheniramine maleate	Dimetane*‡ Various others	ORAL: *Adults*—4 to 8 mg 3 to 4 times daily or 8 to 12 mg of sustained-release form 2 to 3 times daily. *Children*—over 6 years, ½ adult dose; under 6 years, 0.5 mg/kg daily divided into 3 to 4 doses. FDA Pregnancy Category B.	Drowsiness is the most common side effect.
Carbinoxamine maleate	Clistin	ORAL: *Adults*—4 to 8 mg 3 to 4 times daily or 8 to 12 mg of sustained-release form 2 to 3 times daily. *Children*—over 6 years, 4 mg 3 to 4 times daily; 3 to 6 years, 2 to 4 mg 3 to 4 times daily; 1 to 3 years, 2 mg 3 to 4 times daily. FDA Pregnancy Category B.	Low incidence of drowsiness. Anticholinergic effect is weak.
Chlorpheniramine maleate	Aller-Chlor‡ Chlortab Chlor-Trimeton‡ Teldrin‡ Various others	ORAL: *Adults*—4 mg 3 to 4 times daily or 8 to 12 mg of sustained-release form 2 to 3 times daily. *Children*—6 to 12 years, 2 mg 3 to 4 times daily or 8 mg of sustained-release form once daily; 2 to 6 years, 1 mg 3 to 4 times daily.	Low incidence of drowsiness. A common ingredient in cold remedies.
Clemastine Sumarate	Tavist*	ORAL: *Adults*—2.68 mg 3 times daily. Not intended for children.	Low incidence of drowsiness. Very weak anticholinergic effects.

*Available in Canada and United States.
†Available in Canada only.
‡Available without a prescription.

Continued.

Table 24-1   Antihistamines for Allergies—cont'd

Generic name	Trade name	Administration/dosage	Comments
Cyproheptadine hydro-chloride	Periactin	ORAL: *Adults*—4 to 20 mg daily, not more than 0.5 mg/kg. Dose is started at 4 mg 3 times daily. *Children*—7 to 14 years, 4 mg 2 to 3 times daily to a maximum of 16 mg daily; 2 to 6 years, 2 mg 2 to 3 times daily to a maximum of 12 mg daily. FDA Pregnancy Category B.	Used to relieve itching. Drowsiness is the most common side effect.
Dexchlorpheniramine maleate	Polaramine*	ORAL: *Adults*—1 to 2 mg 3 or 4 times daily or 4 to 6 mg 2 times daily or 6 mg of timed-release form 3 times daily. *Children*—under 12 years, 0.15 mg/kg daily divided into 4 doses. FDA Pregnancy Category B.	Drowsiness is the most common side effect.
Diphenhydramine hydrochloride	Benadryl Hydrochloride‡ Various others	ORAL: *Adults*—25 to 50 mg 3 to 4 times daily. *Children*—over 20 lb, 2.5 to 25 mg 3 to 4 times daily; under 12 years, 5 mg/kg in 4 divided doses each day.	High incidence of drowsiness with little paradoxic stimulation in children. Also used to treat motion sickness and mild parkinsonism. Also used as an antitussive. May be used with epinephrine in treating an anaphylactic reaction.
Diphenylpyraline hydrochloride	Hispril	ORAL: *Adults*—2 mg every 4 hr or 5 mg of sustained-release form every 12 hr. *Children*—over 6 years, 2 mg every 6 hr or 5 mg of sustained-release form once daily; 2 to 6 years, 1 to 2 mg every 8 hr.	
Doxylamine succinate	Unisom	ORAL: *Adults*—12.5 to 25 mg every 4 to 6 hr. *Children*—6 to 12 years, 75 mg divided into 4 to 6 doses daily; under 6 years, 2 mg/kg body weight divided into 4 to 6 doses daily. Decapryn available without prescription.	High incidence of drowsiness. Often included in nonprescription sleep aids.
Loratadine	Claritin†	ORAL: *Adults*—10 mg once a day.	New drug for seasonal rhinitis.
Methdilazine hydro-chloride	Tacaryl	ORAL: *Adults*—8 mg 2 to 4 times daily. *Children*—over 3 years, 4 mg 2 to 4 times daily.	A phenothiazine derivative used primarily to relieve itching. Incidence of drowsiness is less than with other phenothiazines.
Phenindamine tartrate	Nolahist	ORAL: *Adults*—25 mg every 4 to 6 hr as needed. *Children* (6 to 12 years)—12.5 mg every 4 to 6 hr.	Used for seasonal rhinitis.

*Available in Canada and United States.
†Available in Canada only.
‡Available without a prescription.

Table 24-1   Antihistamines for Allergies—cont'd

Generic name	Trade name	Administration/dosage	Comments
Pyrilamine maleate	Nisaval	ORAL: *Adults*—25 to 50 mg 4 times daily. *Children*—6 to 12 years, ½ adult dose. Available without prescription.	Low incidence of drowsiness.
Terfenadine	Seldane*	ORAL: *Adults*—60 mg every 8 to 10 hr as needed. FDA Pregnancy Category C.	New nonsedating antihistamine.
Trimeprazine tartrate	Panectyl† Temaril	ORAL: *Adults*—2.5 mg 4 times daily or 5 mg of sustained-release form every 12 hr. *Children*—over 3 years, 2.5 mg at bedtime or up to 3 times daily (children over 6 years can take 5 mg of sustained-release form once a day); 6 months to 3 years, 1.25 mg at bedtime or up to 3 times daily.	A phenothiazine derivative. Drowsiness is the most common reaction. Used primarily to relieve the itching of neurodermatitis, contact dermatitis, and chickenpox.
Tripelennamine citrate or hydrochloride	PBZ-SR Pyribenzamine† Hydrochloride† Various others	ORAL: *Adults*—25 to 50 mg every 4 to 6 hr or 100 mg of sustained-release form every 12 hr. *Children*—over 5 years, 50 mg of sustained-release form every 12 hr; children and infants, 5 mg/kg daily divided into 4 to 6 doses.	Dizziness is a common side effect.
Triprolidine hydrochloride	Alleract† Actidil* Myidil	ORAL: *Adults*—2.5 mg 3 to 4 times daily. *Children*—over 6 years, ½ adult dose; under 6 years, 0.3 to 0.6 mg 3 to 4 times daily. FDA Pregnancy Category B.	Low incidence of side effects, with drowsiness being the most common.

*Available in Canada and United States.
†Available in Canada only.

antihistamine is inadequate because it neither acts fast enough nor reverses the histamine reactions. Epinephrine acts rapidly, and its pharmacologic actions reverse those of histamine.

Antihistamines as sedatives

Sedation is a common side effect of antihistamines, some of which are used principally for this purpose. Many OTC sleeping aids use an antihistamine as the active agent. The antihistamines approved as sleep-aid ingredients are pyrilamine, doxylamine succinate, and diphenhydramine. Hydroxyzine (Vistaril, Atarax) is an antihistamine often used as an antianxiety agent (see Chapter 27).

Antihistamines to control vomiting

Antihistamines used to control vomiting are listed in Table 13-3. Antihistamines prevent the nausea of motion sickness, but the drug must be taken before the motion starts. Cyclizine (Marzine), meclizine (Antivert, Bonine), and dimenhydrinate (Dramamine) are the antihistamines most effective in preventing motion sickness. Diphenhydramine (Benadryl) causes considerable sedation.

Nausea and vomiting caused by factors acting on the chemoreceptor trigger zone are best treated with the antipsychotic drugs, the phenothiazines. These drugs are chemically related to the antihistamines but also block the dopamine receptor in the chemoreceptor trigger zone.

Drug administration

- Monitor blood pressure, pulse, and intake and output. Auscultate breath sounds. Inspect for development of rash. Monitor complete blood count, white blood cell count and differential, and platelets count. Supervise ambulation, especially of elderly patients. Keep side rails up and a nightlight on. Monitor smoking. Assess for urinary retention (difficulty initiating voiding and feeling of incomplete bladder emptying). Palpate the bladder.

INTRAMUSCULAR ADMINISTRATION

- Use large muscle masses (see Chapter 6). Record and rotate injection sites. Aspirate before injecting medication to prevent accidental intravenous (IV) administration. Warn patients that IM injection of antihistamine may burn as the medication is injected.
- Read labels carefully. Some forms are for IM use only and should not be used for IV administration. Antihistamines may be prescribed with narcotic analgesics for pain relief. They may decrease nausea and may potentiate central nervous system (CNS) depression, but they do not enhance the analgesic effect of the narcotic. It may be necessary to lower the dose of one of the drugs because of the hypotension, sedation, and other side effects that may occur when both drugs are used.

INTRAVENOUS BROMPHENIRAMINE

- It may be given undiluted, but further dilution is preferred. Check with the pharmacist regarding compatibility with other drugs. Administer a single bolus injection over at least 1 min.

INTRAVENOUS CHLORPHENIRAMINE

- It may be given undiluted. Administer at a rate of 10 mg over 1 min or longer if possible.

INTRAVENOUS DIMENHYDRINATE

- Dilute 50 mg of drug in 10 ml of sodium chloride injection. Administer at 25 mg/min.

INTRAVENOUS DIPHENHYDRAMINE

- It may be given undiluted. Administer at 25 mg/min or longer if possible.

INTRAVENOUS PROMETHAZINE

- Dilute to at least 25 mg/ml, preferably to 2.5 to 5 mg/ml. Administer at 25 mg/min. Slightly yellow solutions may be safely used; discard highly discolored solutions.

Patient and family education

- Warn patients to avoid driving or operating hazardous equipment if drowsiness, blurred vision, or dizziness occurs. Notify physician if blurred vision develops.
- Review Patient Problems: Constipation on p. 182, Dry Mouth on p. 166, Orthostatic Hypotension on p. 234, and Photosensitivity on p. 629.
- Instruct patients to report fever, sore throat, rash, unexplained bleeding, or bruising, since these may be signs of rare but serious hematologic side effects. Instruct patients to take oral doses with meals or a light snack to decrease gastric irritation.
- Patients should swallow sustained-release forms whole, without crushing or chewing. Scored tablets may be broken before swallowing. Capsules may be opened and contents poured into soft food for ease in taking. Patients should chew gum forms for 15 min or longer (see manufacturer's literature). For motion sickness, doses should be taken 30 to 60 min before beginning travel.
- Patients traveling by car should face forward in the center of the front seat if possible.
- Patients should avoid the use of alcohol and other CNS depressants.
- Remind patients to keep all health-care providers informed of all medications being used, even OTC preparations. Regular use of antihistamines may mask side effects developing from other drugs in use, especially ototoxic effects.
- Teach patients to read labels of OTC preparations carefully. Patients using remedies for colds, hay fever, insomnia, and other problems may be taking unnecessary drugs or taking the same drug in two or more combination products. Consult the pharmacist for assistance.
- Remind patients that antihistamines may also cause allergies. Encourage patients to report any unexpected sign or symptom to the physician.
- Encourage patients with allergies to wear a medical identification tag or bracelet indicating the nature of the allergies. Pregnant women should not take any medication without the approval of the physician. Remind patient to keep these and all drugs out of the reach of children.
- A potentially fatal drug interaction exists between terfenadine and ketoconazole. Remind patients to inform all health-care providers of all medications being used.

CHAPTER REVIEW

◆ KEY TERMS

anaphylaxis, p. 381
angioedema, p. 381
antihistamine, p. 382
asthma, p. 381
eczema, p. 381
histamine, p. 380
purpura, p. 381
rhinitis, p. 381
urticaria, p. 381

◆ REVIEW QUESTIONS

1. Describe the origin, location, and role of histamine.
2. What factors mediate histamine release?
3. What are five pharmacologic actions of antihistamines?
4. What are the drug interactions and contraindications for the antihistamines?
5. Describe three clinical uses of the H-1 receptor antihistamines.
6. How does cimetidine differ from the H-1 receptor antihistamines?

SUGGESTED READING

Brucker MC: Management of common minor discomforts in pregnancy: I. Managing upper respiratory infections in pregnancy, *J Nurse Midwife* 32(6):349, 1987.

Dolan B: Rapid desensitization, *Am J Nurs* 82(10):1532, 1982.

Druce HM, Kaliner MA: Allergic rhinitis, *JAMA* 259(2):260, 1988.

Pepper GA: OTCs vs. Rx for allergic rhinitis, *Nurse Pract* 12(6):58, 1987.

CHAPTER 25

Bronchodilators and Other Drugs to Treat Asthma

LEARNING OBJECTIVES

After studying this chapter, you should be able to do the following:

- Discuss the role of the nonselective and selective beta-adrenergic bronchodilators, xanthines, cromolyn, ketotifen, glucocorticoids, and ipratropium in treating asthma.

- Describe the alpha, beta-1, beta-2 and central nervous system (CNS) effects of sympathomimetic bronchodilators.

- Discuss the role of alpha-1 proteinase inhibitor in the treatment of chronic obstructive pulmonary disease.

- Discuss the role of surfactant in infants with respiratory distress syndrome.

- Develop a nursing care plan for patients receiving one or more of the groups of drugs discussed in this chapter.

CHAPTER OVERVIEW

- Drugs that dilate the bronchioles (**bronchodilators**) and other drugs that are used to treat asthma are discussed in this chapter. Asthma affects about 10 million Americans. Treatment has focused on dilating the constricted bronchioles and relieving the wheezing, difficult breathing, and coughing that occur during an asthma attack. Theophylline or a beta-adrenergic bronchodilator have been used. Recently attention has focused on inflammation in asthma. Inhaled steroids or cromolyn sodium decrease inflammation. This chapter also introduces the new surfactant drugs used to prevent lung collapse in premature infants.

Nursing Process Overview
BRONCHODILATORS
Assessment

Perform a general assessment of the patient. The focus is often on the respiratory system. Check the vital signs, the amount and characteristics of secretions, and the level of fatigue; auscultate breathing sounds; determine arterial blood gas levels and vital capacity; assess subjective complaints and patient's ability to perform and tolerate activities of daily living; and obtain relevant history regarding issues such as smoking, exposure to irritants, infection, and stress.

Nursing Diagnoses

Anxiety related to difficult breathing, air hunger, tachycardia, and drug side effects.

Possible complication: hypertension secondary to bronchodilator use.

Management

Monitor vital signs; an acute care unit may be appropriate for the patient in acute respiratory distress. Monitor fluid intake and output, level of consciousness, blood gas levels, vital capacity, and treatment of any infectious process. Use an infusion control device for intravenous (IV) drugs. Monitor serum xanthine levels and blood glucose level in patients receiving xanthine therapy.

Evaluation

These drugs are successful if the patient's condition is subjectively and objectively improved. The vital capacity should increase, arterial blood gas levels should be closer to normal values, the respiratory rate should decrease, and the patient should appear to be in a less respiratory distress. Subjectively, the patient should report easier breathing, less shortness of breath, less fatigue, and better tolerance for activities of daily living. Before discharge, verify that the patient can explain which drugs are to be taken and how to take them correctly, what situations require notification of the physician because of exacerbation of the disease process or because of effects resulting from drug therapy, how to perform measures such as exercises for respiratory management, and how to use oxygen correctly. Determine that the patient can demonstrate correct use of any equipment such as intermittent positive-pressure breathing (IPPB) machines or drug administration devices such as inhalers or nebulizers. Finally, check that the patient can explain which respiratory irritants should be avoided.

ASTHMA

Asthma is a disease of reversible obstruction of the bronchioles. About 12 million Americans have asthma and about 5000 die of severe asthma attacks each year. An asthma attack involves not only constriction of the bronchioles but also edema of the bronchial mucosa and excess secretion of mucus, combining to restrict the caliber of the airway, as diagrammed in Figure 25-1. Asthma is classified as *extrinsic asthma* if an allergic response is the primary stimulus for bronchial constriction. When no such response can be identified, asthma is classified as *intrinsic asthma*.

Mechanisms in Extrinsic Asthma

Extrinsic asthma involves an immunologic mechanism. The mast cells play a major role in precipitating the attack. In the lung, mast cells are primarily located in the epithelial layer and exposed to the surface. Immunoglobulin E (IgE) antibodies bind to mast cells, and when an antigen appears it binds to the IgE. The formation of the antigen-antibody complex causes the mast cells to degranulate, releasing several substances, including histamine and leukotrienes C and D.

The leukotrienes are potent bronchoconstrictors, chemically related to the prostaglandins. Histamine, also a bronchoconstrictor, additionally induces vasodilation and increased capillary permeability, which results in the mucosal edema characteristic of asthma.

Adrenergic Mechanisms in Asthma

Recently much has been learned about the molecular pharmacology of the bronchial smooth muscle and the mast cell. This knowledge has led to an understanding of some of the mechanisms involved in reversible airway obstruction. As diagrammed in Figure 25-2, the beta-adrenergic system affects relaxation of

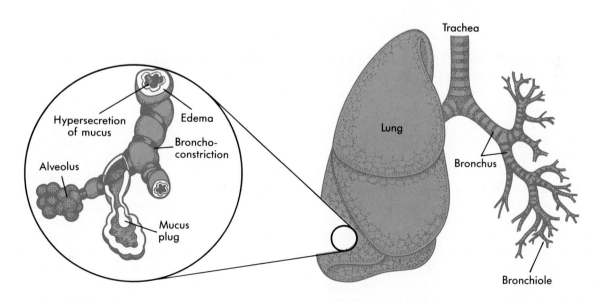

FIGURE 25-1

Factors restricting airway include hypersecretion of mucus, mucosal edema, and bronchoconstriction. Mucous plugs may form in alveoli.

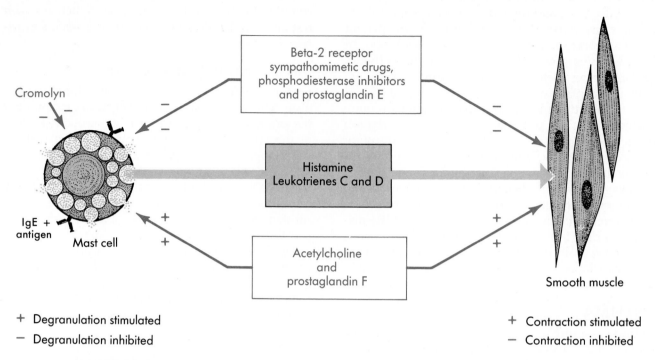

Cromolyn

Beta-2 receptor
sympathomimetic drugs,
phosphodiesterase inhibitors
and prostaglandin E

Histamine
Leukotrienes C and D

IgE +
antigen

Mast cell

Acetylcholine
and
prostaglandin F

Smooth muscle

+ Degranulation stimulated

− Degranulation inhibited

+ Contraction stimulated

− Contraction inhibited

FIGURE 25-2

Histamine and leukotrienes C and D released from mast cells stimulate smooth muscle contraction to produce bronchoconstriction. Mast cell degranulation and smooth muscle contraction are stimulated by acetylcholine and prostaglandin F. Smooth muscle relaxation and inhibition of mast cell degranulation are promoted by beta-2 receptor agonists, phosphodiesterase inhibitors, and prostaglandin E.

bronchial smooth muscle and inhibits degranulation of the mast cells. Activation of the beta-2 receptor stimulates an enzyme, adenylate cyclase, to synthesize more cyclic adenosine 3′,5′-monophosphate (cyclic AMP), which is a second messenger for the beta-2 receptor (see Chapter 10). Cyclic AMP activates intracellular pathways, resulting in relaxation of smooth muscle, inhibition of mast cell degranulation, and stimulation of the ciliary apparatus to remove secretions more effectively. Drugs that increase cyclic AMP are bronchodilators, inhibitors of mast cell degranulation, and promoters of secretion flow in the bronchioles. These drugs include beta-adrenergic agonists, which stimulate the beta-2 receptor, and phosphodiesterase inhibitors, which inhibit the breakdown of cyclic AMP. Xanthine compounds are used clinically as bronchodilators because they inhibit phosphodiesterase. Prostaglandins E_1 and E_2 also stimulate adenylate cyclase, but currently no drugs are available clinically that mimic these prostaglandins.

Cholinergic Mechanisms Controlling Bronchioles

There is little, if any, direct innervation of the bronchioles by the sympathetic nervous system. However, there is indirect involvement, since sympathetic nerve terminals in pulmonary blood vessels release norepinephrine, which can act on the beta-2 receptors in the bronchioles. Norepinephrine is not a potent stimulant of beta-2 receptors. The beta-2 receptors are activated by epinephrine released from the adrenal medulla in response to stress. Acetylcholine, the neurotransmitter of the parasympathetic nervous system, acts on muscarinic receptors to cause bronchoconstriction through the intracellular second messenger, cyclic 3′,5′-guanyl monophosphate (cyclic GMP). Mast cell degranulation is also promoted by agents that stimulate the formation of cyclic GMP. Intrinsic asthma is believed to arise from direct stimulation of the enzyme guanyl cyclase, which synthesizes cyclic GMP. Irritants such as noxious gases can stimulate guanyl cyclase. Asthmatic individuals respond to low doses of inhaled methacholine, a cholinomimetic drug, with bronchospasm, whereas high doses are needed to induce bronchospasm in nonasthmatic individuals. Intrinsic asthma may therefore primarily involve a parasympathetic response, mediated by cyclic GMP, to inhaled bronchial irritants. Blocking the muscarinic receptor with atropine or scopolamine causes bronchodilation, but muscarinic antagonists do not currently play a major role in asthma treatment.

Prostaglandin F_{2a} is another potent bronchoconstrictor that stimulates synthesis of cyclic GMP. The factors causing the release of prostaglandin F_{2a} are not well understood, and it is not clear whether prostaglandin F_{2a} affects asthma.

OTHER AIRFLOW OBSTRUCTION DISEASES

Obstruction of airflow is a component of many pulmonary diseases. Chronic obstructive pulmonary disease (COPD) describes conditions in which the common feature is limitation of airflow. In long-standing pulmonary disease, irreversible changes take place so that the elastic smooth muscle tissue is replaced with inelastic scar tissue. This can occur in the bronchioles in chronic bronchitis or in the alveoli in emphysema. These irreversible changes cannot be modified with drugs. However, since the early stages of chronic bronchitis and emphysema often involve reversible bronchospasm, bronchodilators can provide some relief. The atropinelike drug, ipratropium, is a bronchodilator that appears to treat chronic bronchitis.

DRUG THERAPY FOR ASTHMA

Drug therapy for asthma aims to prevent bronchospasm and to control the hyperactivity of the bronchioles. Mild asthma involves brief episodes of wheezing. These episodes are commonly managed with a beta-adrenergic inhalant bronchodilator for prompt relief. Cromolyn sodium is of value as a prophylactic treatment, since it prevents the mast cells from degranulating to start an asthma attack. Moderate asthma is characterized by wheezing and difficulty in breathing to a degree that interferes with daily activities. Theophylline, a long-acting oral bronchodilator, is widely used as daily therapy for moderate-to-severe asthma, with an inhalant beta-adrenergic bronchodilator for acute attacks. However, inhaled steroids are preferred by asthma specialists over theophylline as daily therapy for moderate-to-severe asthma to control the disease with fewer side effects.

Antihistamines are sometimes administered to prevent mild episodes. Because antihistamines have a drying effect that turns the excess mucus into hard plugs, they are contraindicated for patients with severe asthma.

BRONCHODILATORS
Beta-Adrenergic Agonists

Mechanism of action. The beta receptors of the bronchial smooth muscle are beta-2 receptors, whereas cardiac beta receptors are beta-1 receptors. The goal

Table 25-1 Bronchodilators' Specificity for Adrenergic Receptors*

Drug	Alpha effects	Beta-1 effects	Beta-2 effects
Albuterol	0	0	+
Bitolterol	0	0	+
Cyclopentamine	+	0	0
Ephedrine	+	+	+
Epinephrine	+	+	+
Ethylnorepinephrine	0	0	+
Fenoterol	0	0	+
Isoetherine	0	0	+
Isoproterenol	0	+	+
Metaproterenol	0	(±)	+
Phenylephrine	+	0	0
Pirbuterol	0	0	+
Procaterol	0	0	+
Terbutaline	0	0	+

ALPHA EFFECTS

Vasoconstriction
1. Systemic: increased blood pressure.
2. Inhaled: decreased bronchial congestion, increased duration of action for coadministered beta-2 drug.

BETA-1 EFFECTS
1. Stimulation of heart, increasing rate, force of contraction, and rate of repolarization. Overstimulation causes palpitations and arrhythmias.
2. Increased breakdown of fat (lipolysis).
3. Relaxation of gastrointestinal (GI) tract.

BETA-2 EFFECTS
1. Bronchiole dilation.
2. Stimulation of skeletal muscle to cause a tremulous or shaky feeling.
3. Vasodilation (mainly in blood vessels supplying muscle).
4. Breakdown of stored glucose (glycogenolysis).

CNS EFFECTS

Stimulation, causing nervousness, anxiety, insomnia, irritability, dizziness, and sweating.

*0, No stimulation; +, stimulation; ±, modest stimulation.

has been to develop drugs that stimulate only beta-2 receptors, since stimulation of the heart is not desirable and can limit the use of the drug. In theory, stimulation of alpha receptors causes vasoconstriction of the blood vessels around the bronchioles, limiting the edema, a desirable action. However, systemic constriction of alpha receptors can cause an undesirable increase in blood pressure. Alpha receptors may constrict bronchiolar smooth muscle, at least in disease states. Table 25-1 summarizes the alpha, beta-1, and beta-2 activities of the adrenergic drugs used as bronchodilators.

Administration and fate. Also important to the selection of a bronchodilator is the route of administration and the onset and duration of action. Table 25-2 summarizes these points. Inhalation is a partic-

ularly effective route of administration for the bronchodilators. Not only are epinephrine, isoproterenol, and isoetharine degraded if swallowed, but inhalation also places the drug near the site of action. When inhalation is the route, alpha-agonist activity reduces congestion and limits systemic absorption of the drug. Cyclopentamine or phenylephrine, which stimulate alpha but not beta receptors, are included in inhalation preparations of isoproterenol to relieve congestion and to slow systemic absorption, thereby limiting cardiac effects while increasing the duration of action of the beta agonist.

Many bronchodilators are administered by inhalation. This requires that the drug be in a solution contained in a nebulizer or pressurized cartridge (aerosol), which disperses the drug solution in tiny

Table 25-2   Bronchodilators: Onset and Duration of Action

Generic name	Trade name	Administration	Onset (min)	Duration (hr)
Albuterol	Proventil	Inhalation Oral	30	4 to 6
Bitolterol	Tornalate	Inhalation	3	5 to 8
Ephedrine	Ventolin	Oral	15	2 to 4
Epinephrine hydrochloride		Subcutaneous Inhalation	5 2	1 to 3 2 to 3
Epinephrine suspension	Sus-Phrine	Subcutaneous	15	Up to 8
Ethylnorepinephrine	Bronkephrine	Subcutaneous	10	1 to 2
Fenoterol	Berotec	Inhalation Oral	5 30 to 60	2 to 3 6 to 8
Isoetharine	Bronkometer Bronkosol Dilabron	Inhalation	2	1
Isoetharine and phenylephrine	Bronkosol-2	Inhalation	2	2
Isoproterenol	Isuprel Vapo-Iso	Inhalation	2	½ to 2
Isoproterenol and cyclopentamine	Aerolone Compound Aludrine	Inhalation	2	3½
Isoproterenol and phenylephrine	Nebu-Prel	Inhalation	2	3½
Metaproterenol	Alupent Metaprel	Inhalation Oral	2 15	2 to 4 3 to 4
Pirbuterol	Maxair	Inhalation	5	5
Procaterol	ProAir	Inhalation	5	6 to 8
Terbutaline	Bricanyl Brethine	Oral Subcutaneous	10 15	4 to 7 2 to 4

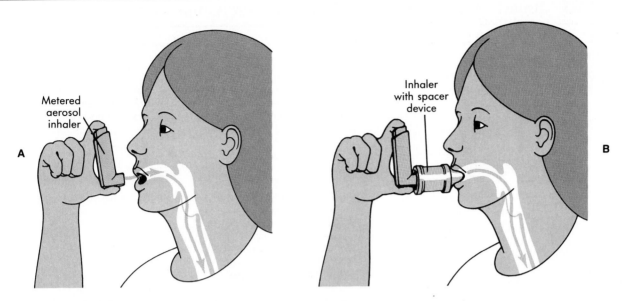

FIGURE 25-3

Inhaled drugs commonly used in asthma treatment include beta-adrenergic bronchodilators, cromolyn sodium, and aerosol glucocorticoids. Metered aerosol inhaler **A,** should not be put in mouth, but held about two finger widths (1½ inch) front of mouth. Alternatively, spacer device **B,** can be used. Patients should breathe deeply once before activating the inhaler, and then continue breathing in for about 5 sec. Patients should then hold the breath for 10 to 15 sec before breathing out slowly. If second dose is needed, patients should wait 1 to 2 min before taking another dose.

drops to be taken into the lungs by deep inhalation. Metered-dose aerosols are easy to use and deliver a measured dose with each push of the cartridge (Figure 25-3). The disadvantage is that the inert carrier substances may irritate the bronchioles and cause bronchospasm. Patients must also be instructed in inhalation therapy to ensure that the drug is inhaled and that there is no gagging and swallowing of the drug.

In a severe attack, patients may not be able to inhale the drug. Subcutaneous injection of epinephrine or terbutaline is then appropriate. An orally or subcutaneously administered bronchodilator is preferred if there is a great deal of mucosal edema and bronchoconstriction, which would limit the access of the inhaled drug.

Nonselective Beta-Adrenergic Bronchodilators

The older beta-adrenergic bronchodilators, ephedrine, epinephrine, and isoproterenol, are not selective for the beta-2 adrenergic receptor. They have a range of side effects resulting from their nonselective action. These drugs are listed in Table 25-3.

Epinephrine

Epinephrine (Asmolin, Medihaler-Epi, Adrenalin, and others) can be administered subcutaneously to relieve an acute asthmatic attack. The drug causes bronchodilation and vasoconstriction to relieve bronchial edema. Given subcutaneously, an aqueous suspension of epinephrine (Sus-Phrine) lasts 8 hr; the hydrochloride salt lasts only 3 hr. Epinephrine is also available in metered-dose inhalers as an aerosol or in solution for use in a nebulizer.

Common side effects of epinephrine are increased heart rate, muscle tremors, and stimulation of the CNS to produce anxiety, nervousness, or excitability. Large doses can produce an acute hypertensive episode and cardiac arrhythmias.

Ephedrine

Ephedrine (Ephed II) acts like epinephrine but is effective orally. Ephedrine is a weaker bronchodilator than epinephrine and is of no use for an acute asthma attack. It is used as a prophylactic for patients with mild-to-moderate asthma. Several formulations combine ephedrine with theophylline and a sedative in a single pill.

Text continued on p. 397.

Table 25-3   Bronchodilators and Other Drugs to Treat Asthma

Generic name	Trade name	Administration/dosage	Comments
BETA-RECEPTOR AGONISTS			
Albuterol (salbutamol) sulfate	Novosalmol† Proventil Ventolin*	INHALATION: *Adults and children over 12 years*—one or two inhalations every 4 to 6 hr. ORAL: *Adults and children over 12 years:* 2 to 4 mg three or four times daily. Federal Drug Administration FDA Pregnancy Category C.	Relatively selective for beta-2 (bronchial) receptors. May cause fine finger tremor. Injectable form available in Canada.
Bitolterol	Tornalate*	INHALATION: *Adults*—two inhalations every 8 hr for prophylaxis. To treat an attack, one inhalation followed by a second after 1 to 3 min; then two inhalations every 4 hr or three inhalations every 6 hr. FDA Pregnancy Category C.	A new beta-2 selective bronchodilator
Ephedrine sulfate	Ephed II*	ORAL: *Adults*—25 to 50 mg every 3 to 4 hr as needed. FDA Pregnancy Category C. *Children*—6 to 12 years, 6.25 to 12.5 mg every 4 to 6 hr; 2 to 6 years, 0.3 to 0.5 mg/kg every 4 to 6 hr.	Oral or parenteral administration only. CNS stimulation is a common side effect. Not selective for beta-2 receptors.
Epinephrine (base)	Sus-Phrine* (1:200)	INTRAMUSCULAR, SUBCUTANEOUS: *Adults*—For 1:200 solutions, 0.1 to 0.3 ml not more often than every 4 hr, maximum test dose, 0.1 ml. FDA Pregnancy Category C. *Children*—For 1:200 solutions, 0.005 ml/kg body weight not more than every 4 hr, maximum test dose, 0.15 ml.	Long-acting suspension. Effect may persist for 8 to 10 hr.
	Asmolin (1:400)	For 1:400 solutions, double above volumes.	
Epinephrine bitartrate	Asthma Haler Medihaler-Epi* Primatene Mist Various others	INHALATION: Aerosol nubulizers metered to deliver 0.2 mg epinephrine (0.1 mg for Medihaler-Epi) with each inhalation. Allow 1 to 2 min between inhalations.	Overuse can cause serious adverse effects, leading to death. Reduce dose if bronchial irritation or CNS stimulation arises. For symptomatic relief only.
Epinephrine (racemic)	Vaponefrin*	As for epinephrine bitartrate.	
Epinephrine hydrochloride	Adrenalin Chloride* (1:1000)	SUBCUTANEOUS: *Adults*—0.2 to 0.5 mg every 2 hr as needed for an acute asthma attack. *Children*—0.01 mg/kg body weight, maximum, 0.5 mg, every 4 hr as needed for an acute asthma attack. For severe acute attacks, may repeat initial dose every 20 min for three doses.	Short-acting injection. Do not expose drug to light. Do not use if brown or contains a precipitate. Reacts with many compounds.

*Available in Canada and United States.
†Available in Canada only.

Table 25-3   Bronchodilators and Other Drugs to Treat Asthma—cont'd

Generic name	Trade name	Administration/dosage	Comments
BETA-RECEPTOR AGONISTS—cont'd			
Epinephrine hydro-chloride—cont'd	Adrenalin Chloride (1:100)* Vaponephrin (2.25%)*	INHALATION: Solutions for nebuli-zation. Allow 1 to 2 min between inhalations.	Excessive use causes bronchial inflammation and stimulation of the heart and CNS.
Ethylnorepinephrine	Bronkephrine*	INTRAMUSCULAR, SUBCUTANEOUS: *Adults*—1 to 2 mg. FDA Pregnancy Category C. *Children*—0.2 to 1 mg.	A new beta-2 selective bronchodilator.
Fenoterol	Berotec†	INHALATION: *Adults*—one or two inhalations every 6 hr as needed.	A beta-2 selective bronchodilator. Not available in the United States.
Isoetharine hydro-chloride	Bronkosol* Various others	INHALATION: nebulized solution; three to seven inhalations. FDA Pregnancy Category C.	A beta-2 selective drug. Phenylephrine is included to relieve congestion and prolong the duration of action.
Isoetharine mesy-late	Bronkometer*	INHALATION: aerosol; one to four inhalations every 3 to 6 hr, maximum 12 inhalations daily.	
Isoproterenol hydrochloride	Isuprel Hydrochloride* Various others	SUBLINGUAL: *Adults*—10 mg initially. No more than 15 mg four times daily or 20 mg three times daily. FDA Pregnancy Category C. *Children*—5 to 10 mg, not exceeding 30 mg daily. INTRAVENOUS: *Children only*—initial infusion rate is 0.1 μg/kg/min. Increase by 0.1 μg/kg/min every 15 min until heart rate exceeds 180 bpm or clinical improvement is seen or infusion rate is 0.8 μg/kg/min.	Sublingual absorption is unreliable. Patients should not swallow saliva until tablet has completely disintegrated. This route of administration is used only in pediatric intensive care units for children in respiratory failure.
	Isuprel Mistometer* Norisodrine Aerotrol*	INHALATION: (solution for nebulization, 0.5% to 1%): *Adults*—one or two deep inhalations, repeated no more than every 4 hr.	Excessive use has caused refractory bronchial obstruction and tolerance to the drug. In some individuals inhalation precipitates a severe, prolonged asthma attack.
Isoproterenol sulfate	Medihaler-Iso*	INHALATION (aerosol metered dose): *Adults*—one or two deep inhalations repeated once or twice at 5- to 10-min intervals if necessary. Repeat after 4 hr. *Children*—five to 15 deep inhalations of 1:200 aerosol repeated in 10 to 30 min if necessary.	

*Available in Canada and United States.
†Available in Canada only.

Continued.

Table 25-3   Bronchodilators and Other Drugs to Treat Asthma—cont'd

Generic name	Trade name	Administration/dosage	Comments
BETA-RECEPTOR AGONISTS—cont'd			
Metaproterenol sulfate	Alupent* Metaprel	ORAL: *Adults*—10 mg 3 or 4 times daily initially, increased to 20 mg three or four times daily over 2 to 4 weeks. FDA Pregnancy Category C. *Children*—6 to 9 years, 10 mg three or four times daily; over 9 years or over 60 lb, 20 mg three or four times daily. INHALATION (metered aerosol): *Adults and children over 12 years only:* two to three inhalations every 3 to 4 hr not to exceed 12 inhalations daily.	Longer acting than isoproterenol. Patients are less likely to develop tolerance to metaproterenol than to isoproterenol.
Pirbuterol	Maxair	INHALATION: *Adults*—one or two inhalations every 6 hr as needed. FDA Pregnancy Category C.	Beta-2 selective bronchodilator.
Procaterol	ProAir†	INHALATION: *Adults*—2 inhalations 3 times/day.	Beta-2 selective bronchodilator. Available in Canada but not in the United States.
Terbutaline sulfate	Brethine Bricanyl*	SUBCUTANEOUS: *Adults*—0.25 mg repeated in 15 to 30 min if necessary, with no more than 0.5 mg administered in any 4-hr period. FDA Pregnancy Category B. *Children*—0.01 mg/kg body weight to a maximum of 0.25 mg. ORAL: *Adults*—initially 2.5 mg every 8 hr, increased to 5 mg every 8 hr three times daily over 2 to 4 weeks. Dose may be lowered to 2.5 mg if side effects are too disturbing. *Children 12 years and younger*—1.25 to 2.5 mg three times daily during waking hours.	Shakiness is the most frequent side effect.
	Brethaire	INHALATION (metered aerosol): *Adults and children over 12 years*—two inhalations 1 min apart, every 4 to 6 hr.	Side effects are mild. Headache, nausea, and GI upset are the most common.
XANTHINES			
Aminophylline (theophylline ethylenediamine)	Sold mainly under generic name	For acute asthma attack: INTRAVENOUS: Solutions should be diluted to 25 mg/ml and injected no more rapidly than 25 mg/min to avoid circulatory collapse. Loading dose, 5.6 mg/kg over 30 min. Maintenance dose, no more than 0.9 mg/kg/hr by continuous infusion. Dose is determined by age, cardiac and liver status, and smoking history.	85% theophylline, so 116 mg of aminophylline is equivalent to 100 mg theophylline. Watch for nausea, wakefulness, restlessness, and irritability as early symptoms of toxicity. Serious toxic effects of IV include delirium, convulsions, hyperthermia, and circulatory collapse.

*Available in Canada and United States.
†Available in Canada only.

Table 25-3   Bronchodilators and Other Drugs to Treat Asthma—cont'd

Generic name	Trade name	Administration/dosage	Comments
XANTHINES—cont'd			
Aminophylline—cont'd		RECTAL: *Adults*—250 to 500 mg one to three times daily. FDA Pregnancy Category C. *Children*—5 mg/kg not more often than every 6 hr. ORAL: *Adults*—500 mg for an acute attack. Maintenance dose, 200 to 250 mg every 6 to 8 hr. *Children*—7.5 mg/kg for an acute attack. Maintenance dose, 5 mg/kg every 6 hr.	
Dyphylline	Dilor* Dyflex* Lufyllin* Neothylline*	ORAL: *Adults*—200 to 800 mg every 6 hr. FDA Pregnancy Category C. *Children*—2 to 3 mg/lb/24 hr given in divided doses every 6 hr. Maximum dose, 15 mg/kg every 6 hr. INTRAMUSCULAR: *Adults*—250 to 500 mg.	Not a theophylline salt. Has a short half-life (2½ hr) and is not excreted in the urine without being metabolized.
Oxtriphylline (choline theophyllinate)	Protophylline† Choldeyl* Novotriphyl†	ORAL: *Adults*—200 mg every 6 hr. FDA Pregnancy Category C. *Children 2 to 12 years*—100 mg/60 lb every 6 hr.	64% theophylline, so 156 mg is equivalent to 100 mg theophylline.
Theophylline	Many names, elixirs, syrups, tablets, capsules, timed-release preparation, and suppositories	ORAL: *Adults*—Initial dose, 3 to 5 mg/kg every 6 hr. For maintenance: *Adults*—100 to 200 mg every 6 hr FDA Pregnancy Category C. *Children*—50 to 100 every 6 hr. RECTAL: *Adults*—250 to 500 mg every 8 to 12 hr. *Children*—10 to 12 mg/kg/24 hr. Administered no more frequently than every 6 hr.	Headache, dizziness, nervousness, nausea, vomiting, and epigastric pain are the most common side effects of oral administration. Therapeutic levels are 10 to 20 mg/ml serum.
Theophylline sodium glycinate	Synophylate*	ORAL: *Adults*—330 to 660 mg every 6 to 8 hr after meals. *Children*—over 12 years, 220 to 300 mg; 6 to 12 years, 165 to 220 mg; 3 to 6 years, 110 to 165 mg; 1 to 3 years, 55 to 110 mg every 6 to 8 hr after meals.	49% theophylline, so 198 mg is equivalent to 100 mg theophylline.

*Available in Canada and United States.
†Available in Canada only.

Ephedrine releases stored norepinephrine from sympathetic neurons, an indirect sympathomimetic effect that explains the weak bronchodilator action. The major metabolite is phenylpropanolamine, an active alpha-adrenergic drug frequently used as a decongestant.

The most common side effect of ephedrine is stimulation of the CNS manifested as nervousness, excitability and insomnia. The development of orally active, beta-2 selective bronchodilators is making ephedrine obsolete.

Ethylnorepinephrine

Ethylnorepinephrine (Bronkephrine) acts on beta-1 and beta-2 adrenergic receptors. It also exerts some vasoconstrictive activity that reduces bronchial congestion. Ethylnorepinephrine is available only for subcutaneous or intramuscular (IM) administration.

Isoproterenol

Isoproterenol (Isuprel Hydrochloride, Vapo-Iso, Medihaler-Iso, and Norisodrine Sulfate) was the first widely used adrenergic drug with selectivity for beta rather than alpha receptors. It is not selective for beta-2 receptors and therefore stimulates the heart. Isoproterenol is primarily given by inhalation and relieves bronchoconstriction for up to 2 hr. If swallowed, it is degraded in the gut wall. It is available as a sublingual tablet, but absorption is so erratic that this route is not often used.

Side effects are related to stimulation of the heart and include palpitation, tachycardia, and arrhythmias. Isoproterenol can also cause tremors, headache, nervousness, and hypotension. Excessive inhalation can cause bronchial constriction for which the drug no longer has a bronchodilator effect. Drug effectiveness returns when the drug is discontinued for a few days.

Selective Beta-Adrenergic Bronchodilators

The newer beta-adrenergic bronchodilators are relatively selective for the beta-2 receptor, the adrenergic receptor mediating bronchodilation. Because of this selective action, these drugs are less likely to cause unwanted cardiac effects or breakdown of liver glycogen to glucose. Patients with hypertension, cardiac disease, or diabetes can better tolerate the selective beta-adrenergic bronchodilators. Occasionally, nervousness or restlessness are side effects.

Many of the new bronchodilators are available in metered aerosol form so that one inhalation delivers a given amount of a drug. These include bitolterol, fenoterol, isoetharine, metaproterenol, pirbuterol, procaterol, and terbutaline (see Table 25-3). If more than one inhalation is administered, patients should wait a minute or so between inhalations. The metered-dose inhaler has emerged as the standard for aerosol therapy. The correct use of the inhaler is illustrated in Figure 25-3. Since only about 10% of the delivered drug is deposited in the lung, the likelihood of overdosing is small. However, recent studies indicate that overuse of inhalers (more than one incident per month) may be associated with an increased death rate.

Albuterol, fenoterol, metaproterenol, and terbutaline are available in oral forms. Although oral administration is convenient, especially for children, the patient is exposed to more side effects with oral administration than with aerosol administration.

Albuterol

Albuterol (Proventil and Ventolin) is available in forms for oral and inhalation administration for treatment of acute asthma or for prophylaxis in chronic asthma. The inhalation forms include a metered aerosol and a solution. The solution is administered by nebulizer or IPPB. The onset of action is 5 to 15 min, and the duration of action 3 to 6 hr. For oral administration, albuterol is available as a syrup, tablets, or extended-release tablets. The onset of action is 15 to 30 min, and the duration of action is 8 hr. In Canada an injectable form is also available with a duration of action of 12 hr. Albuterol is metabolized by the liver to an inactive form and excreted in the urine.

Bitolterol

Bitolterol (Tornalate) is available in metered aerosol form for treatment of acute asthma or for prophylaxis in chronic asthma. The onset of action is 3 to 4 min, and the duration of action is 5 to 8 hr. Bitolterol is conjugated and excreted in the urine.

Fenoterol

Fenoterol (Berotec) is available in metered aerosol form, solution, and as tablets for the treatment of acute asthma or for prophylaxis in chronic asthma. Although available in Canada, fenoterol is not available in the United States.

Isoetharine

Isoetharine (Bronkometer, Bronkosol, and others) is available in metered aerosol form and as a solution for the treatment of acute asthma or for prophylaxis in chronic asthma. The onset of action is 1 to 6 min, and the duration of action is 1 to 4 hr. Isoetharine is metabolized by the liver and excreted in the urine.

Metaproterenol

Metaproterenol (Alupent and Metaprel) is available as a metered aerosol and as a solution for inhalation administration and as a syrup and tablet for oral administration. Metaproterenol is used for treatment of acute asthma or for prophylaxis in chronic asthma. The aerosol form has an onset of action of 1 min and a duration of action of 1 to 5 hr. The solution, administered by hand-bulb nebulizer or IPPB, has a slower onset of action, 5 to 30 min, and a duration of action of 2 to 6 hr. Oral forms are effective in 15 to 30 min for up to 4 hr. Metaproterenol is metabolized by the liver and excreted in the urine.

Pirbuterol

Pirbuterol (Maxair) is available as a metered aerosol for the treatment of acute asthma or for prophylaxis in chronic asthma. The onset of action is 5 min, and the duration of action is 5 hr. Pirbuterol is conjugated and excreted in the urine.

Procaterol

Procaterol (ProAir) is available as a metered aerosol for asthma but is available only in Canada. The onset of action is 5 min, and the duration of action is 6 to 8 hr.

Terbutaline

Terbutaline (Bricanyl and Brethine) is available in metered aerosol, tablets, and as an injection for the treatment of acute asthma or for prophylaxis in chronic asthma. Inhaled terbutaline is effective in 5 to 30 min and has a duration of action of 3 to 6 hr. With oral administration, the onset of action is 1 to 2 hr and the duration of action 4 to 8 hr. When injected, onset of action is within 15 min and the duration of action ½ to 4 hr. Terbutaline is metabolized by the liver and excreted in the urine.

XANTHINES

Theophylline and related drugs are listed in Table 25-3.

Theophylline

Mechanisms of action. Theophylline is the prototype of the xanthines used to treat asthma. Like beta-adrenergic agonists, theophylline is thought to act by increasing cellular cyclic AMP concentrations, which relaxes bronchial smooth muscle and inhibits mast cell degranulation. Theophylline and the other xanthines accomplish this by inhibiting the degradation of cyclic AMP by the enzyme phosphodiesterase. This action complements that of the beta agonists, and the two kinds of agents may be included in therapy when the effect of either drug alone is insufficient to control bronchospasm. However, theophylline has side effects, and asthma specialists prefer inhaled steroids over theophylline as prophylaxis for moderate-to-severe asthma.

Administration and fate. Theophylline is an effective bronchodilator that can be given intravenously (as aminophylline) to control acute bronchospasm in status asthmaticus or orally to control the bronchospasm of mild, moderate, or severe asthma. Theophylline is not highly water soluble, and there are many formulations to improve the solubility. Studies have shown that theophylline tablets are well absorbed, with more than 96% of the drug appearing in the plasma within 2 hr. Aminophylline, the most common soluble form of theophylline, is the only form that can be administered intravenously.

Several soluble salts of theophylline are available, and dosage is determined by the theophylline conent. The drug is also available in slow- and fast-release preparations, alcoholic or aqueous solutions, and suppositories. Only the suppository is erratically absorbed and therefore unreliable. Rectal solutions are well absorbed. Theophylline is combined with ephedrine and a sedative in several combination products for treating asthma. Most clinicians prefer to individualize doses of each ingredient to minimize side effects while maximizing therapeutic effects and therefore do not favor combination drugs. Theophylline is not effective when administered by inhalation. IM injections of theophylline are not used because they are painful.

Variability of plasma levels. Theophylline is metabolized by the liver into inactive compounds excreted in the urine. There is a wide variability among individuals as to the plasma half-life of theophylline. In normal, nonsmoking adults the plasma half-life is about 6 hr but can vary from 3 to 12 hr. In smokers and children the plasma half-life is shorter, whereas in elderly patients, premature infants, and patients with liver disease or congestive heart failure with pulmonary edema, the plasma half-life is prolonged.

Side and toxic effects. The most common side effects of theophylline after oral administration are nausea and epigastric pain. Headache, dizziness, and nervousness are also common. The effectiveness of theophylline is determined by its plasma concentrations, and the therapeutic range is 10 to 20 µg/ml. Agitation, exaggerated reflexes, and mild muscle tremors (fasciculations) are often seen when plasma levels are 20 to 30 µg/ml. Seizures and cardiac arrhythmias may occur when plasma levels exceed 30 µg/ml but occasionally occur with plasma concentrations between 20 and 30 µg/ml.

Other actions of theophylline seen in the therapeutic dose range are dilation of blood vessels and mild diuresis resulting from the increased renal blood flow and glomerular filtration. Stomach acid secretion is increased, which may be a problem for a patient with an ulcer. Stimulation of the medullary centers of respiration may occur, which is beneficial if the asthmatic patient is hypoxic. Theophylline treats Cheyne-Stokes respiration, in which the medullary sensitivity to hypoxia is decreased. Theophylline stimulates respiration in newborns who do not breathe well.

Dyphylline

Dyphylline (Airet, Dilor, Lufyllin, and Neothylline) is related to theophylline but is less potent and shorter acting. Dyphylline has a half-life of 2½ hr and is eliminated largely unchanged in the urine.

OTHER DRUGS

Drugs in this section are listed in Table 25-4.

Cromolyn sodium

Cromolyn sodium (Intal and Fivent) is a prophylactic drug that acts by inhibiting mast cell degranulation

Table 25-4   Other Asthma Drugs

Generic name	Trade name	Administration/dosage	Comments
Beclomethasone dipropionate	Beclovent* Becotide† Vanceril*	INHALATION (metered dose inhaler): each dose is 50 μg. *Adults*—two inhalations 3 to 4 times daily. *Children 6 to 12 years*—one to two inhalations 3 to 4 times daily.	Inhaled glucocorticoid. Patients transferring from oral glucocorticoids to beclomethasone must be carefully monitored because adrenal function is impaired and may require months to begin functioning adequately.
Cromolyn sodium	Intal* Fivent†	INHALATIONS: *Adults and children over 5 years*—20 mg capsule inhaled 4 times daily. (Spinhaler); two inhalations four times daily (inhalation aerosol). FDA Pregnancy Category B.	Prophylactic drug used to inhibit mast cell degranulation. Cough or bronchospasm is occasionally experienced after inhaling the dry powder.
Dexamethasone sodium	Decadron Respihaler*	INHALATION (metered dose inhaler): each dose is 84 μg. *Adults*—three inhalations 3 or 4 times daily. *Children*—two inhalations three or four times daily.	Inhaled glucocorticoid. See warnings for beclomethasone.
Flunisolide	AeroBid*	INHALATION (metered dose inhaler): each dose is 250 μg. *Adults and children over 6 years*—two inhalations two times daily initially. Patients over 15 years may increase dose to four inhalations twice daily if necessary.	Inhaled glucocorticoid. See warnings for beclomethasone.
Ipratropium	Atrovent*	INHALATION (metered dose inhaler): each dose is 18 μg. *Adults*—one or two inhalations three or four times daily. FDA Pregnancy Category B.	New anticholinergic bronchodilator.
Ketotifen	Zaditen†	ORAL—*Children 3 years of age and older*—1 mg two times daily with morning and evening meals.	Prophylactic for asthma in children.
Triamcinolone	Azmacort*	INHALATION (metered dose inhaler): each dose is 100 μg. *Adults*—two sprays three or four times daily, up to 12 to 16 sprays daily. *Children 6 to 12 years*—one or two sprays three or four times daily, up to 12 sprays daily for severe cases.	Inhaled glucocorticoid. See warnings for beclomethasone.

*Available in Canada and United States.
†Available in Canada only.

and the release of bronchospastic agents caused by immunologic (antigen IgE) or nonimmunologic (exercise or hyperventilation) stimulation. Cromolyn does not treat an ongoing asthma attack or prevent asthma attacks brought on by vagal reflexes rather than by mast cell degranulation. By itself, cromolyn does not have bronchodilator or antiinflammatory activity.

Cromolyn can be administered by inhalation using a "spinhaler," a hand-held, hand-operated device that when activated punctures a capsule, releasing a dry powder. This powder is dispersed by the air current from a small rotor blade and enters the lungs during deep inhalation.

Cromolyn is also available as a metered inhalation aerosol, which will probably replace the spinhaler. In addition, cromolyn is formulated for nasal administration (Nasalcrom and Rynacrom), as prophylaxis for allergic rhinitis, and for ophthalmic administration (Opticrom and Vistacrom) for allergic conjunctivitis.

Given orally or parenterally, cromolyn is so rapidly excreted in the urine that effective drug levels cannot be maintained. Because of this rapid clearance, cromolyn is practically nontoxic. The major side effect that can limit use is bronchospasm caused by the dry powder in sensitive individuals. Some individuals become allergic to cromolyn.

Cromolyn is usually added to bronchodilator therapy to avoid the use of glucocorticoids, especially in children, or to allow the gradual reduction in dose of glucocorticoids. No tolerance develops to the drug. Cromolyn is more effective in treating children than adults for asthma.

Ketotifen

Ketotifen (Zaditen) is an antihistamine with cromolynlike activity. It can be taken orally and has a duration of action of 12 to 24 hr. This drug may cause prophylaxis of asthma and relief of the sneezing and eye irritation from allergies. Side effects include sedation, dizziness, nausea, headache, and dry mouth. Asthma and bronchospasm may be aggravated.

Glucocorticoids

Oral glucocorticoids (corticosteroids) treat asthmatic patients with severe symptoms that are not controlled by bronchodilator therapy. Initially, very high doses (up to 1 gm of methylprednisolone) of a glucocorticoid may be administered for as long as 5 days to bring a severe asthma attack under control when IV aminophylline and sympathomimetics have proved inadequate. As discussed in Chapter 51, high doses of glucocorticoids can be tolerated for short periods, but cause many severe side effects on a long-term basis. Few patients with asthma require glucocorticoids even after an acute attack. The mechanisms by which these drugs act to alleviate asthma are not known, but they do potentiate the action of the bronchodilators. To minimize the long-term toxic effects of glucocorticoids, they are administered in small doses (20 mg) every other day. This schedule minimizes suppression of adrenal function and also avoids excessive use, which could cause Cushing's syndrome (characteristic of excessive glucocorticoid administration; see Chapter 51).

Aerosol glucocorticoids. Aerosol glucocorticoids have been developed that can be inhaled daily without producing adrenal suppression or Cushing's syndrome. Asthma specialists now advocate the use of aerosol glucocorticoids over theophylline in the daily management of moderate-to-severe asthma. As with other aerosol medications, the patient must be carefully instructed in the administration of the aerosol glucocorticoids (see Figure 25-3). The aerosol cannot be used during an episode of acute bronchospasm because the powder causes further irritation and the bronchospasm prevents adequate inhalation. An oral glucocorticoid is indicated instead. Patients using these aerosols should gargle after use to prevent the drug trapped in the throat from being swallowed and absorbed systemically and to avoid a candidal infection (a fungal infection) in the mouth or throat. Glucocorticoids available as aerosols include beclomethasone, dexamethasone, flunisolide, and triamcinolone.

Ipratropium

Ipratropium bromide (Atrovent) is the first anticholinergic drug available to treat asthma and conditions such as chronic bronchitis and emphysema in which bronchoconstriction is present. It opens narrowed breathing passages by blocking vagal nerve impulses that tighten the muscles in the walls of the bronchial tubes. Mucus secretion is also reduced. Ipratropium is not appropriate for treating acute asthma. The onset of action is 5 to 15 min, and the duration of action is 3 to 6 hr. The drug is primarily excreted unchanged in the feces. It has negligible cardiovascular effects. Atropinelike side effects are rare with inhalation administration.

CHRONIC OBSTRUCTIVE PULMONARY DISEASE

Alpha-1 proteinase inhibitor in COPD

Chronic bronchitis and emphysema are referred to as *chronic obstructive pulmonary disease (COPD)*. Patients with COPD commonly have some degree of reversible airflow obstruction. As with asthma, bronchodilators and corticosteroids play a major role in supportive therapy.

Lung damage in COPD results from the destruction of elastin, a major structural protein of the lung. Elastin is destroyed when there is an imbalance between the lung proteinase, elastase, which breaks down elastin, and alpha-1-proteinase inhibitor (also called *alpha-1 antitrypsin*), a protein that inhibits elastase. Smoking depresses alpha-1-proteinase inhibitor, which can account for the high association between smoking and COPD. Some people have a genetic defect that results in low levels of alpha-1-proteinase inhibitor (Table 25-5). Alpha-1-proteinase inhibitor (Prolastin) is available for replacement therapy in patients with a congenital deficiency of alpha-1-proteinase inhibitor. This drug is currently purified from human plasma and administered intravenously. The recommended dosage is 60 mg/kg body weight administered once weekly.

Table 25-5   Miscellaneous Drugs for Pulmonary Conditions

Generic name	Trade name	Administration/dosage	Comments
Alpha$_1$ Proteinase Inhibitor, Human	Prolastin*	INTRAVENOUS: *Adults*—60 mg/kg body weight, administered at a rate of 0.08 m/kg of body weight per min, once a week.	For emphysema caused by a deficiency of alpha-$_1$-antitrypsin.
Beractant	Survanta	INTRATRACHEAL: *Neonates*—100 mg immediately after birth. Doses may be repeated every 6 hr, up to 4 doses.	Pulmonary surfactant for respiratory distress syndrome of neonates.
Colfosceril palmitate, Cetyl alcohol, and Tyloxapol	Exosurf	INTRATRACHEAL: *Neonates*—80 mg/kg just after birth and again at 12 and 24 hr for high-risk infants. For infants with respiratory distress syndrome, 2 doses of 80 mg/kg at 12 hr intervals.	Pulmonary surfactant for respiratory distress syndrome of neonates.

*Available in Canada and United States.

RESPIRATORY DISTRESS SYNDROME

Infants born after less than 37 weeks gestation are at risk for **respiratory distress syndrome,** also called *hyaline membrane disease.* This condition is a collapse of the tiny air sacs of the lung secondary to a deficiency of surfactant. Surfactant is a lipoprotein material coating the air sacs in mature lungs, lowering the surface tension and thereby allowing ready inflation of the lungs. About 60,000 to 70,000 American premature infants develop respiratory distress syndrome each year, with 6000 to 10,000 of those affected dying. In addition, about half of the 150,000 adult Americans who develop respiratory distress syndrome as a result of injuries or blood infections die.

Surfactant Preparations

Recently, surfactant preparations have become available that diminish the mortality from respiratory distress syndrome (see Table 25-5). It is not clear whether it is preferable to give surfactant for prophylaxis or as treatment only. Dosing schedules are still being refined.

Beractant or surfactant TA (Survanta) is derived from cow's lungs. For high-risk infants weighing 600 to 1250 gm, beractant is administered prophylactically in a single 100-mg dose immediately after birth. For infants with respiratory distress syndrome, 100-mg doses are given no more than every 6 hr, up to 4 doses. All doses are administered intratracheally.

Colfosceril palmitate, cetyl alcohol, and tyloxapol (Exosurf) is a synthetic mixture. The colfosceril palmitate is the lipid and active ingredient. Cetyl alcohol is a spreading agent, and tyloxapol is a nonionic detergent that serves as a dispersing agent. For high-risk infants weighing less than 1350 gm, 80 mg/kg is given shortly after birth and again at 12 and 24 hr. For infants with respiratory distress syndrome, two doses of 80 mg/kg are given at 12-hr intervals. All doses are administered intratracheally.

NURSING IMPLICATIONS SUMMARY

General Guidelines for Bronchodilator Therapy

Drug administration

◆ Review side effects discussed in the text and the information in Tables 25-1 to 25-3.

◆ Monitor pulse, blood pressure, and respiratory rate. Auscultate lung sounds. The frequency of monitoring varies with the drug, dose, route of administration, and patient condition. During IV administration, monitor vital signs every 5 to 15 min until stable. With subcutaneous and inhalation administration, monitor every 15 min.

◆ Monitor all patients requiring bronchodilators carefully but especially elderly patients and those with cardiovascular or hypertensive disease or diabetes mellitus.

◆ Monitor acutely ill patients in the intensive care setting. Monitor electrocardiogram (ECG).

◆ Anxiety, insomnia, fear, and other emotional responses may aggravate bronchospasm and air hunger. Maintain a calm but efficient attitude in caring for patients. Do not leave patients unattended for long periods. Keep the call bell within easy reach.

◆ With subcutaneous or IM injection, aspirate before administering dose to avoid inadvertent IV administration.

◆ For continuous IV infusion, use an infusion control device and usually microdrip tubing. Monitor intake and output and vital signs.

◆ Monitor blood glucose level of diabetic patients carefully, since these drugs may produce hyperglycemia.

Patient and family education

◆ Review the common side effects of the prescribed drugs. Wait until patients are out of acute respiratory distress.

◆ If tachycardia is a problem, suggest that patients limit caffeine intake.

◆ Tell patients with respiratory problems to stop smoking.

◆ Before discharge, check that patients can describe or demonstrate the correct way to take ordered medication including frequency, route of administration, and use of devices, and know under what circumstances to return to the physician or emergency room if the drugs are not effective. Caution patients to use these drugs only as prescribed and not to increase dose size or frequency unless directed

to do so by the physician. Patients who find relief with metered-dose inhalers may begin using them more often than prescribed. These drugs soon become ineffective, or patients suffer significant side effects.

◆ Warn diabetic patients to monitor blood glucose levels carefully, especially when changing doses of bronchodilator.

◆ Patients should let sublingual tablets dissolve under the tongue. Instruct patients not to swallow saliva until the tablet is completely dissolved.

◆ Instruct patients to take oral doses with meals or snacks to lessen gastric irritation.

◆ Make certain patients can use the metered-dose inhaler correctly when using it for the first time. Review manufacturer's instruction sheet with patients. Have patients assemble the inhaler and shake the canister. Patients should exhale deeply, then put the mouthpiece into the mouth with the opening directed to the back of the throat. Patients should grasp the mouthpiece with the teeth and lips. They should inhale deeply while depressing the aerosol container or activating the spray mechanism. Then they should hold the breath as long as possible before exhaling. Instruct patients to wait several minutes before taking a second dose (if prescribed). For children, it may be necessary to hold the nose shut. When finished, tell patients to wash and dry the mouthpiece (see Figure 25-3). For additional information about drugs via inhalation, see Chapter 6.

◆ Special devices can help children use inhalation medications if they are having difficulty using the metered-dose inhaler; examples include the InspirEase and Inhal-Aid devices. Consult the pharmacist.

◆ When two drugs are ordered via inhalation, patients should use the bronchodilator first, then take the second drug such as beclomethasone.

◆ Teach patients to check the supply of drug on hand to avoid running out at inopportune times. To check the amount in a canister, drop the canister into water (without mouthpiece). Full containers sink to the bottom, and half-full containers float with part of the container out of the water. The empty container floats on its side, half submerged (see p. 101). Consult the manufacturer's literature for additional information.

Continued.

♦ Remind patients to inform all health-care providers of all drugs being taken. Remind patients to avoid over-the-counter (OTC) drugs unless first approved by the physician. Many decongestants and cold remedies contain products that duplicate the effects of the bronchodilators, causing increased side effects.

♦ Instruct patients to keep these and all drugs out of the reach of children.

♦ No drugs should be used during pregnancy or lactation unless first approved by the physician.

Nonselective Beta-Adrenergic Bronchodilators

Drug administration

♦ Epinephrine hydrochloride (adrenalin chloride) is used via subcutaneous injection or IM injection to treat anaphylactic allergic reactions. The dose is 0.1 to 0.5 mg (0.1 to 0.5 ml) of 1:1000 injection.

♦ See general guidelines. Monitor the pulse and blood pressure carefully.

♦ Sus-Phrine is a suspension. Rotate the vial between the hands to mix the suspension before preparing the dose, and administer immediately so the drug does not settle out of suspension.

♦ See Chapter 14 for a discussion of use of these drugs in shock.

Patient and family education

♦ Review the general guidelines.

♦ Review Patient Problems: Dry Mouth on p. 166 and Orthostatic Hypotension on p. 234.

Selective Beta-Adrenergic Bronchodilators

Patient and family education

♦ Review the general guidelines.

♦ Review Patient Problems: Dry Mouth on p. 166 and Orthostatic Hypotension on p. 234.

♦ Sustained-release formulations should be swallowed whole, without chewing or crushing. If there is a question about a specific product, consult the pharmacist.

Xanthines

Drug administration

♦ Review the general guidelines for bronchodilator therapy.

♦ Monitor the vital signs and blood pressure, and auscultate lung sounds. Hypotension may be pronounced. Supervise ambulation. Keep side rails up. Monitor serum theophylline levels.

INTRAVENOUS AMINOPHYLLINE

♦ Only the concentration of 25 mg/ml may be given undiluted, by direct IV push, at a rate of 20 mg/min. Usually, aminophylline is diluted in at least 100 to 200 ml of 5% dextrose in water and given as an infusion, based on serum levels or patient's response. It is available prediluted. It is incompatible with many drugs, so you should not usually administer it "piggyback"; start and maintain a separate IV for replacement fluids and other drugs.

Patient and family education

♦ Review the general guidelines for bronchodilator therapy.

♦ Review Patient Problem: Orthostatic Hypotension on p. 234.

♦ Warn patients to avoid driving or operating hazardous equipment if dizziness, light-headedness, or vertigo develop; notify the physician.

♦ Teach patients to read drug prescriptions and labels carefully. Many of these drugs are available in regular and sustained-release formulations; they cannot be interchanged on the same dosing schedule. See Chapter 6 for a discussion of sustained-release products.

♦ Instruct patients to limit or avoid the use of coffee, tea, chocolate, and other methylxanthines, since they may affect xanthine metabolism.

♦ Tell patients to avoid smoking cigarettes or marijuana, which may alter serum levels.

INHALED GLUCOCORTICOIDS

Drug administration

♦ See Chapter 51 for a detailed discussion of glucocorticoid therapy. Systemic side effects with inhaled forms are uncommon but may occur. See the general guidelines for bronchodilator therapy for a discussion of the use of metered-dose inhalers. Teach patients to gargle and rinse the mouth after each use of the inhaler to help prevent fungal infections.

Cromolyn

Patient and family education

♦ See the general guidelines for bronchodilation therapy for a discussion of metered-dose inhalers. The spinhaler is packaged with detailed instructions, which should be reviewed with the patient.

♦ Teach patients the importance of taking this drug as ordered, on a regular basis. This drug is useful for prophylactic treatment of asthma but will not control an acute attack of asthma.

◆ See Patient Problem: Dry Mouth on p. 166.
◆ Side effects are rare, but encourage patients to report unexpected signs or symptoms.

Ketotifen
Patient and family education
◆ Teach patients the importance of taking this drug as ordered, on a regular basis. This drug is useful for prophylactic treatment of asthma.
◆ Instruct patients to avoid driving or operating hazardous equipment if sedation or dizziness occur, and to notify the physician.
◆ See Patient Problem: Dry Mouth on p. 166.

Ipratropium
Patient and family education
◆ See the general guidelines for a discussion of metered-dose inhalers.
◆ Review Patient Problems: Dry Mouth on p. 166 and Constipation on p. 182. See Chapter 13 for a detailed discussion of anticholinergics.

Alpha-1-Proteinase Inhibitor
Drug administration
◆ Consult the manufacturer's literature for current guidelines.
◆ Store the drug in the refrigerator before reconstitution and at room temperature after reconstitution, and administer within 3 hr.
◆ Patients may also be immunized against hepatitis B since the drug is prepared from pooled human plasma.

◆ Monitor vital signs. Administer IV at 0.08 ml/kg/min.

Surfactant Preparations
Drug administration
◆ Protocols for administration of these agents are being developed and refined. Check hospital protocol for guidelines.
◆ Rotate vial to suspend or resuspend drug in diluent.
◆ Dosage is based on weight. Inject drug intratracheally via endotracheal tube. The manufacturer of Exosurf provides an endotracheal tube adapter to permit injection.
◆ Suction the infant before administration of surfactant, but avoid suctioning, if possible, for at least 2 hr after administration of the drug and for as long as 6 hr, if tolerated by infants.
◆ To distribute the drug throughout the lungs, it may be necessary to gently rotate the infant from side to side or to ventilate the infant manually with a resuscitation bag after administration of the drug.
◆ Monitor clinical appearance, pulse oximetry, partial pressure of oxygen (PO_2), carbon dioxide partial pressure (PCO_2), arterial blood gases, lung sounds, and cardiac monitoring.
◆ Keep mother and family informed of the infant's condition.

CHAPTER REVIEW

◆ **KEY TERMS**

asthma, p. 389
bronchodilators, p. 388
chronic obstructive pulmonary disease (COPD), p. 401
extrinsic asthma, p. 389
intrinsic asthma, p. 389
respiratory distress syndrome, p. 402

◆ **REVIEW QUESTIONS**

1. What three components restrict the airway in extrinsic asthma?
2. Contrast the mechanisms responsible for extrinsic and intrinsic asthma.
3. What is the mechanism of action of the bronchodilators (beta-adrenergic receptor agonists and theophylline)? List three beneficial responses attributed to this mechanism.
4. Which beta-adrenergic agonists used as bronchodilators are relatively specific for the beta-2 receptor?
5. What side effects are associated with bronchodilators?
6. How does cromolyn treat extrinsic asthma? What is its mechanism of action?
7. How does beclomethasone treat extrinsic asthma? What is its mechanism of action?
8. How does alpha-1 proteinase inhibitor treat COPD? What are the nursing considerations in its administration?
9. For what are surfactant preparations used? How would you administer them?

SUGGESTED READING

Brim S: A quick guide for home use of inhalant medications, *Pediatr Nurs* 15(1):87, 1987.

Cutie AJ, Sciarra JJ: Therapeutic inhalation aerosols in the treatment of asthma, *J Pract Nurs* 40(4):41, 1990.

Dickerson M: Anaphylaxis and anaphylactic shock, *Crit Care Nurs Q* 11(1):68, 1988.

Ellis P: Asthma: meeting the demand for rapid relief. Drugs and inhalation devices, *Prof Nurs* 6(2):76, 1990.

Ellis P: A new direction for asthma relief? Alternatives to MDI inhalers, *Prof Nurs* 6(3):145, 1990.

Ioli JG, Richardson MJ: Giving surfactant to premature infants, *Am J Nurs* 90(3):59, 1990.

Janson-Bjerklie S: Status asthmaticus, *Am J Nurs* 90(9):52, 1990.

Lindell KO, Mazzocco MC: Breaking bronchospasm's grip with MDIs, *Am J Nurs* 90(3):34, 1990.

Nemec MA: Inhalation medications for chronic asthma, *J Pediatr Health Care* 1(4):223, 1987.

Paynton A: Synthetic surfactant, *Nurs 91* 21(3):64, 1991.

Renaud MT: On the horizon: surfactant replacement therapy, *AACN Clin Issues Crit Care Nurs* 1(2):422, 1990.

CHAPTER 26

Drugs to Control Bronchial Secretions

LEARNING OBJECTIVES

After studying this chapter, you should be able to do the following:

◆ Discuss the action of the alpha-adrenergic agonists, the imidazolines, and the antihistamines in relieving nasal congestion.

◆ Differentiate between expectorants, antitussives, and mucolytic agents in treating a cough.

◆ Develop a nursing care plan for a patient receiving a nasal decongestant or a drug to treat a cough.

CHAPTER OVERVIEW

◆ Many of the drugs covered in this chapter are available over-the-counter (OTC) for treatment of colds and coughs. Nasal decongestants are covered in the first section, and drugs to treat a cough are covered in the second section.

Nursing Process Overview

DRUGS MODIFYING RESPIRATORY SECRETIONS

Assessment

Perform a general assessment of the patient in addition to focusing on subjective complaints. An appropriate history asks about the onset of symptoms, possible irritants for symptoms, times of the day when symptoms are worse (e.g., a cough that is more troublesome at night), therapies used by the patient that have successfully relieved the symptoms, and the history of irritants or environmental conditions that may aggravate the symptoms. Objective data include the respiratory rate, vital signs, character and quantity of secretions, examination of the nose, throat, and ears, and assessment of the lungs.

Nursing Diagnoses

Ineffective airway clearance related to suppressed ability to cough

Potential altered health maintenance related to misuse or overuse of nasal decongestants

Management

Monitor symptoms, vital signs, and in some patients, fluid intake and output. Identify nonmedical solu-

tions for troublesome symptoms. For patients receiving mucolytic agents, have a suction machine at the bedside if there is doubt that the patient can adequately handle secretions.

Evaluation

These drugs are successful if symptoms are relieved. Before discharge, determine that patients can explain how to take the drugs correctly, what side effects might occur that would require notification of the physician, why the drugs should be discontinued after symptoms have improved, and what actions to take if the symptoms return or do not improve.

DRUGS TO TREAT NASAL CONGESTION

Alpha-Adrenergic Agonists

Mechanism of action

Nasal congestion results when the blood vessels in the nasal passage become dilated as a result of infection, inflammation, allergy, or emotional upset. Dilation increases capillary permeability and allows fluid to escape into the nasal passage. Drugs that stimulate alpha receptors cause blood vessels to constrict, thereby relieving the congestion. These drugs are termed *alpha-adrenergic agonists* because they mimic the action of the neurotransmitter norepinephrine (see Chapter 10).

Topical Nasal Decongestants

Several alpha-adrenergic agonists are applied topically as drops or sprays. Because these nasal decongestants have immediate and direct contact with the nasal mucosa, they act rapidly and provide temporary symptomatic relief by opening the nasal passages. However, when the effect of the drug wears off, the congestion reappears (**rebound congestion**). If nasal decongestants are used with increasing frequency, they have less and less effect. The drug ultimately irritates the nasal passages and causes the congestion to become worse rather than better. For this reason, decongestants are most effective when used only occasionally and for no longer than 3 to 5 days. Nasal decongestants are available without a prescription.

Administration of nose drops

When a nasal decongestant is applied as drops into the nostril, the patient should be lying on a bed with the head hanging over the edge and turned to one side. The drops are instilled into the upper nostril. After a few seconds the head is turned to allow administration to the other nostril. Use of this lateral, head-low position allows the drops to coat the nasal mucosa without being immediately swallowed. The drops may cause a stinging or burning sensation or induce sneezing.

With repeated use of a nasal decongestant, more of the drug is absorbed, and systemic effects become possible. The symptoms of an overdose are those expected from a sympathomimetic drug (See Chapter 10); including nervousness, dizziness, palpitation, and transient high blood pressure readings. Children are especially vulnerable to overdoses of nasal decongestants and may have reactions that include sweating, drowsiness, shock, or coma.

Orally Active Decongestants

Alpha-adrenergic agonists most commonly found in cold remedies include phenylpropanolamine, phenylephrine, and pseudoephedrine. Cold remedies are syrups, tablets, or capsules that may also include an antihistamine, an analgesic, or other miscellaneous ingredients. Cold remedies are discussed in Chapter 4.

Drug interactions

Patients with hyperthyroidism, diabetes mellitus, hypertension, or heart disease are vulnerable to the sympathomimetic side effects of nasal decongestants and should avoid these drugs. A hypertensive reaction to a nasal decongestant may occur in patients taking a monoamine-oxidase inhibitor. Patients receiving tricyclic antidepressants are vulnerable to the cardiac effects of sympathomimetic agents.

Specific Sympathomimetic Drugs

These drugs are listed in Table 26-1.

Phenylephrine

Phenylephrine (Coricidin, Neo-Synephrine, and others) is a potent alpha-adrenergic agonist that is administered orally or topically. It is available both alone and in many combination cold preparations.

Phenylpropanolamine

Phenylpropanolamine (Propadrine) is used mainly in oral combination cold remedies. It is an alpha-adrenergic agonist and acts indirectly, releasing norepinephrine from nerve terminals.

Pseudoephedrine

Pseudoephedrine (Novafed, Sudafed, and others) is included in many oral combination cold remedies. It is a beta and an alpha agonist.

Propylhexedrine

Propylhexedrine (Benzedrex) is a volatile drug that stimulates alpha receptors. It causes little stimulation of the central nervous system (CNS) and is therefore generally safer than some of the other nasal decongestants.

Imidazolines

The imidazolines include four chemically related nasal decongestants (See Table 26-1). These drugs stimulate the alpha-adrenergic receptors to produce vasoconstriction. They are potent, and only xylometazoline is considered safe for young children. All are used topically. Naphazoline and xylometazoline react with aluminum and should not be used in atomizers with aluminum parts.

Naphazoline

Naphazoline (Privine) is an effective nasal decongestant but can produce a severe rebound congestion resulting from irritation and swelling of the nasal mucosa. Overdosage of naphazoline has reportedly produced coma in children and systemic effects such as hypertension, sweating, cardiac arrhythmias, and drowsiness in adults.

Oxymetazoline

Oxymetazoline (Afrin) is a relatively long-lasting nasal decongestant that has not been implicated in as many severe systemic effects as naphazoline. However, rebound congestion occurs with repeated use.

Table 26-1 Nasal Decongestants

Generic name	Trade name	Administration/dosage	Comments
Epinephrine hydrochloride	Adrenalin Chloride*	TOPICAL: 0.1% aqueous solution as a spray or 1 to 2 drops every 4 to 6 hr. Not recommended for children under 6 years.	Short acting. Frequently causes rebound congestion. Can cause CNS stimulation, headaches, and palpitations.
Ephedrine sulfate	Ectasaale Epedsol	ORAL: *Adults*—25 to 50 mg every 3 to 4 hr. *Children*—3 mg/kg body weight daily in 4 to 6 divided doses. TOPICAL: *Adults and children*—3 to 4 drops of a 1% or 3% solution in each nostril every 3 to 4 hr, no more than 4 times daily. Also may apply as a pack or tampon.	Can cause CNS stimulation, transient hypertension, and palpitations, so contraindicated for patients with heart disease, diabetes, hypertension, and hyperthyroidism. Rebound congestion is common.
Naphazoline hydrochloride	Privine Hydrochloride*	TOPICAL: 0.05% and 0.1% solutions. Two drops in each nostril no more than every 3 hr or 2 sprays every 4 to 6 hr.	An imidazoline. Can cause rebound congestion. Systemic effects from overuse include arrhythmias, transient hypertension, slowing of the heart rate, and drowsiness. Do not use in an atomizer with aluminum parts.
Oxymetazoline hydrochloride	Afrin* Nafrine†	TOPICAL: *Adults*— 2 to 4 drops or 2 to 3 sprays of 0.05% solution in each nostril at morning and at bedtime. *Children*—over 6 years, as for adults; 2 to 5 years, 0.025% solution is used as above.	An imidazoline. Long acting. Side effects are mild and generally safe.
Phenylephrine hydrochloride	Coricidin Decongestant Nasal Mist Neo-Synephrine hydrochloride* Super Anahist nasal spray	TOPICAL: *Adults*—drops of 0.25% to 1% solution in each nostril (head in lateral, head-low position) every 3 to 4 hr. Nasal spray or jelly may be used. *Children over 6 years*—as for adults. *Infants and young children*—0.125% solution is used as above.	Less potent and longer action than epinephrine. No CNS stimulation, but can cause transient hypertension, headaches, and palpitations.
Phenylpropanolamine hydrochloride	Various combination drugs	ORAL: *Adults*—25 mg every 3 to 4 hr or 50 mg every 6 to 8 hr. *Children 8 to 12 years*—20 to 25 mg 3 times daily. Not recommended for children under 8 years.	Similar to ephedrine but with less CNS stimulation.
Propylhexidrine	Benzedrex	TOPICAL (inhalation): 2 inhalations in each nostril as needed.	A volatile drug safe for adult use; children should be supervised. Inhaler should be warmed by the hands if cold.
Pseudoephedrine hydrochloride	Novafed Sudafed* Robidrine†	ORAL: *Adults*—60 mg every 6 to 8 hr. *Children*—4 mg/kg body weight in 4 divided doses.	The stereoisomer of ephedrine with a lesser incidence of CNS stimulation and hypertension than ephedrine. Useful for relief of a runny nose or congestion leading to an earache.
Pseudoephedrine sulfate	Afrinol Repetabs	As for pseudoephedrine hydrochloride.	

*Available in Canada and United States.
†Available in Canada only.

Continued.

Table 26-1   Nasal Decongestants—cont'd

Generic name	Trade name	Administration/dosage	Comments
Tetrahydrozoline hydrochloride	Tyzine	TOPICAL: *Adults*—2 to 4 drops of a 0.1% solution in each nostril. Do not repeat more frequently than every 3 hr. *Children*—6 years and over, as for adults; 2 to 6 years, 2 to 3 drops of a 0.05% solution in each nostril every 4 to 6 hr.	An imidazoline. Adverse reactions can be severe and include hypertension, drowsiness, sweating, rebound hypotension, bradycardia, and cardiac arrhythmias. May cause high fever and coma in young children. Rebound congestion may persist a week after discontinuing.
Xylometazoline hydrochloride	Neo-Synephrine II, Long-acting Otrivin-Spray* Sinutab Long-Lasting Sinus Spray	TOPICAL: *Adults*—2 to 3 drops of 0.1% solution or 1 to 2 inhalations of 0.1% spray in each nostril every 8 to 10 hr. *Children*—6 months to 12 years, 2 to 3 drops of 0.05% solution in each nostril every 4 to 6 hr. *Infants*—1 drop of 0.05% solution in each nostril every 6 hr.	An imidazoline. A relatively safe, long-acting decongestant but should not be used excessively or for more than a few days. Do not use in atomizers with aluminum parts.

*Available in Canada and United States.
†Available in Canada only.

Tetrahydrozoline

Tetrahydrozoline (Tyzine) is an effective nasal decongestant similar to naphazoline in its adverse effects.

Xylometazoline

Xylometazoline (Neo-Synephrine II, Sinutab Long-Lasting Spray, and others) is similar to oxymetazoline in its effects.

Other Drugs to Relieve Nasal Congestion

Nasal congestion is common in allergies such as hay fever. As discussed in Chapter 24, antihistamines treat hay fever because they block the receptors for histamine on the blood vessels and thereby prevent the dilation that causes nasal congestion. Antihistamines are also frequently included in cold remedy preparations. The anticholinergic action characteristic of antihistamines aids in reversing the vasodilation of the nasal blood vessels.

EXPECTORANTS, ANTITUSSIVES, AND MUCOLYTIC DRUGS
Origin of Secretions

Respiratory secretions in the trachea, bronchi, and bronchioles originate from the goblet cells and bronchial glands (Figure 26-1). The goblet cells lie on the surface, making up part of the epithelial layer. The tracheal epithelium consists of about 20% goblet cells, and the bronchiolar epithelium consists of 2%

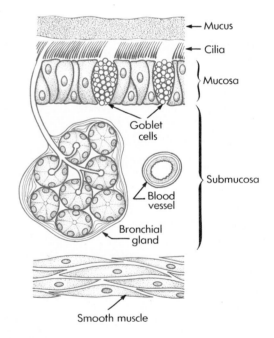

FIGURE 26-1
Mucous layer at top is lumen of airway. Relative position of goblet cells and bronchial glands, secretions of which make up the mucous, are shown. Mucous layer is normally swept up toward throat by cilia to cleanse airway.

goblet cells. These cells produce a gelatinous mucus that they periodically secrete. It is not known what factors normally control the goblet cells, but chronic exposure to irritants increases their size, number, and activity. An example is the phlegm coughed up by smokers. The bronchial glands lie several layers beneath the epithelium. The grapelike (acinar) cells are controlled by the cholinergic nervous system, and when stimulated these cells secrete a plentiful watery fluid into a duct that empties onto the surface.

The secretions of the goblet cells and bronchial glands combine to form a mucus called the *respiratory tract fluid.* Much of the water in the respiratory secretions evaporates to humidify the air taken into the lungs. If too much water is lost to humidification, the mucus forms thick plugs that cannot be readily eliminated. Normally, the respiratory tract fluid forms a lining that is swept upward by the action of the ciliary hairs into the throat (pharynx), where it is swallowed. This activity, the **mucociliary escalator,** provides a cleansing mechanism for the lungs, since any foreign particles or bacteria are trapped in this viscous layer and eliminated. If the ciliary hairs are paralyzed by tobacco smoke or alcohol, secretions cannot be cleared naturally and give rise to the "smoker's cough."

Cough

A **cough** is a protective reflex initiated by irritation in the airway. As long as material is being brought up by the cough, it is beneficial. Several situations cause an unproductive cough. The air of heated rooms can dry the airway enough to cause irritation. A sore throat can produce an unproductive cough and can be self-perpetuating when the cough further irritates the throat. A cough can result from irritants responsible for asthma or pulmonary edema, which also stimulate the cough receptors. Congestion of the nasal mucosa results in postnasal drip. which irritates the throat and produces the cough associated with a cold or the flu.

When a cough is not productive and disrupts sleep and rest, relief is sought. Therapy for a cough depends on the cause. If the air is dry, a vaporizer or steamer may sufficiently liquefy the secretions so that they do not become irritating. A dehydrated state limits respiratory secretions, so having the patient drink plenty of fluids prevents or overcomes the dehydration that accompanies common illnesses. Patients with sore throats can suck hard candies to increase saliva flow to coat the throat. If these simple measures do not eliminate the cough, expectorants may be used. An **expectorant** increases the output of respiratory tract fluid to coat the trachea and bronchi. In addition, a cough suppressant or **antitussive** drug may be taken.

Expectorants and antitussive drugs are widely available as OTC drugs.

Expectorants

Although many drugs are used as expectorants (Table 26-2), no expectorant has proved effective. Iodide, usually given as potassium iodide, is one widely used expectorant. After entering the bloodstream, potassium iodide is believed to stimulate the bronchial glands to secrete more fluid. Use of iodides is associated with a high incidence of adverse effects. Potential side effects include skin rash, hypothyroidism, and a mumpslike swelling of the parotid glands, presumably a result of stimulation of the glands. Iodides are seldom used today.

Another mechanism that stimulates the secretion of respiratory tract fluid is the reflex activity carried by the vagal nerve and characteristic of nausea. Some drugs used as expectorants are believed to initiate this reflex by irritating the stomach when swallowed. One such drug is guaifenesin (glycerol guaiacolate), a widely used expectorant for which there is some evidence of efficacy. Other drugs acting by this mechanism include syrup of ipecac and ammonium chloride. Potassium iodide is believed to act in part by this latter mechanism and by the secretory mechanism. Syrup of ipecac is more commonly used to induce vomiting (emesis) than as an expectorant. Other agents added as expectorants to cough suppressant mixtures include terpin hydrate, citric acid, sodium citrate, iodinated glycerol, and calcium iodide.

Antitussives

Tussis is the Latin word meaning cough, and cough suppressants are called antitussives. These drugs are listed in Table 26-3.

Codeine and hydrocodone

Codeine and hydrocodone are good antitussives, but they are opiates and therefore are capable of producing drug dependence. Hydrocodone has a greater potential for producing drug dependence than codeine. Most preparations containing codeine or hydrocodone are prescription drugs. Some preparations are available as Schedule V drugs and may be obtained by signing for them with a registered pharmacist. The opiates suppress a cough by directly inhibiting the medullary center for the cough reflex. The doses required to suppress a cough are less than those to produce analgesia or respiratory depression. Side effects at antitussive doses are uncommon but include nausea, dizziness, and constipation.

Nonopiate antitussives include dextromethorphan, diphenhydramine, and benzonatate.

Table 26-2 Expectorants§

Generic name	Trade name	Administration/dosage	Comments
Guaifenesin (glycerol guaiacolate)	Anti-tuss Glycotuss Nortussin Robitussin* Various others	ORAL: *Adults*—200 to 400 mg every 3 to 4 hr. *Children*—6 to 12 years, 100 mg every 3 to 4 hr; 2 to 6 years, 50 mg every 3 to 4 hr.	Use for symptomatic relief of a dry, unproductive cough. Occasionally causes nausea or drowsiness. Available without prescription.
Iodinated glycerol	Organidin*	ORAL: *Adults*—20 drops of solution (50 mg) or a 60 mg tablet or 5 ml elixir (60 mg) 4 times daily. *Children*—no more than ½ adult dose daily.	See potassium iodide.
Potassium iodide	Potassium Iodide SSKI Pima Iodo-Niacin	ORAL: *Adults*—300 mg every 4 to 6 hr. *Children*—60 to 500 mg daily, divided in 2 to 4 doses.	Contraindicated for patients with hyperkalemia, hyperthyroidism, or hypersensitivity to iodide. Symptoms of hypersensitivity include skin rash. Iodism (overdose of iodide) causes a metallic taste in the mouth, fever, skin eruptions, nausea, vomiting, mucous membrane ulcerations, and salivary gland swelling.

§Only those expectorants available alone are listed. Other drugs included in cough or cold mixtures as an expectorant include potassium guaiacolsulfonate, ammonium chloride, terpin hydrate, ipecac, calcium iodide, and citric acid.
*Available in Canada and United States.

Table 26-3 Antitussives

Generic name	Trade name	Administration/dosage	Comments
Chlophedianol	Ulo Ulonet	ORAL: *Adults*—25 mg 3 or 4 times daily. *Children 6 to 12 years*—12.5 to 25 mg 3 or 4 times daily. *2 to 6 years*—12.5 mg 3 or 4 times daily.	Prescription drug. Side effects include drowsiness and nausea.
Codeine, codeine phosphate, codeine sulfate		ORAL: *Adults*—10 to 20 mg every 4 to 6 hr, no more than 120 mg in 24 hr. *Children 6 to 12 years*—½ adult dose. *2 to 6 years*—¼ adult dose.	Schedule II drug. Codeine is included in some Schedule III and Schedule V combination formulations, usually including a decongestant, an antihistamine, and an expectorant. For adverse effects, see Chapter 31.
Dextromethorphan hydrobromide	Coughettes Sucrets cough control lozenge Romilar CF Various others	ORAL: *Adults*—10 to 20 mg every 4 hr or 30 mg every 6 to 8 hr. *Children 6 to 12 years*—½ adult dose; *2 to 6 years*—¼ adult dose.	Nonnarcotic, available without prescription. No tolerance develops. Has no analgesic or hypnotic effect and does not depress respiration. Does not cause constipation as readily as codeine.
Diphenhydramine hydrochloride	Benylin Cough Syrupt Benadryl*	ORAL: *Adults*—25 mg every 4 hr, no more than 100 mg in 24 hr. *Children 6 to 12 years*—½ adult dose. *2 to 5 years*—¼ adult dose.	An antihistamine. Side effects include drowsiness and a drying effect.
Hydrocodone bitartrate	Codone Dicodid Robidonet	ORAL: *Adults*—5 to 10 mg every 6 to 8 hr. *Children*—0.6 mg/kg body weight daily in divided doses.	Schedule II drug. Hydrocodone is included in some Schedule III and Schedule V combination formulations, usually including a decongestant, an antihistamine, and an expectorant. For adverse effects, see Chapter 31.

*Available in Canada and United States.
†Available in Canada only.

Dextromethorphan hydrobromide

Dextromethorphan hydrobromide is the most widely used antitussive in OTC cough mixtures. It is related to the opiates but has no analgesic effect and causes no drug dependence. Dextromethorphan is an effective cough suppressant that inhibits the medullary center for the cough reflex. It is well tolerated and only occasionally causes drowsiness or dizziness.

Chlophedianol

Chlophedianol (Ulone) is a centrally acting antitussive with some local anesthetic and anticholinergic action. Use of this drug may cause some patients to become excited and hyperirritable. Large doses cause sedation. Chlophedianol is available in Canada but not the United States.

Diphenhydramine

Diphenhydramine (Benylin) is an antihistamine with antitussive action. Adverse effects include drowsiness common to the antihistamines and the anticholinergic drying effect that hinders a productive cough.

Mucolytic Drug

Water, taken as liquid or inhaled as vapor, keeps the mucus from becoming too viscous. Expectorants stimulate the watery secretion of the bronchial glands. **Mucolytics** break up viscous mucus so that it can be coughed up or otherwise drained. Viscous mucus is most likely to occur in the patient with a pulmonary infection or with chronic obstructive lung disease in which the normal mechanisms for clearing the lungs are compromised. Table 26-4 lists dosages and administration of the mucolytic drug currently available.

Acetylcysteine

Acetylcysteine (Mucomyst) is a sulfhydryl compound that can break disulfide bonds. Viscous mucus has long molecules linked by disulfide bonds; when these disulfide bonds are broken, the molecules separate, reducing the viscosity.

Acetylcysteine is administered by nebulizer through a face mask, mouthpiece, or tracheostomy. Acetylcysteine has a rotten egg odor and may irritate the nasal passages.

Table 26-4 Mucolytic

Generic name	Trade name	Administration/dosage	Comments
Acetylcysteine	Mucomyst* Airbront	NEBULIZATION USING FACE MASK, MOUTHPIECE, OR TRACHEOSTOMY: 1 to 10 mg of a 20% solution or 2 to 20 ml of a 10% solution every 2 to 6 hr. DIRECT INSTILLATION: 1 to 2 ml of a 10% or 20% solution as often as every hour.	Has the odor of rotten eggs, which may cause gastrointestinal (GI) upset. Solutions can be diluted with sterile water for nebulization. Reacts with iron, copper, and rubber, so nebulization equipment should not contain these materials.

*Available in Canada and United States.
†Available in Canada only.

NURSING IMPLICATIONS SUMMARY

Nasal Decongestants

Drug administration

◆ Monitor blood pressure and pulse. Monitor blood glucose levels in diabetic patients.
◆ Assess for GI symptoms. Persistent or severe GI symptoms indicate a need to change drug or dose.

Patient and family education

◆ Review side effects with the patient. Teach patients to choose OTC remedies appropriate for their symptoms and to read product labels. Patients should use products only as directed. Consult the pharmacist in choosing an appropriate remedy for a specific problem.
◆ Remind patients to keep all health-care providers informed of all drugs being used, even OTC preparations. In particular, patients with thyroid disease, diabetes mellitus, hypertension, or heart disease should use nasal decongestants only with physician approval.

Continued.

NURSING IMPLICATIONS SUMMARY—cont'd

◆ Remind patients to keep all drugs out of the reach of children, even nasal sprays and drops. Only pediatric preparations and pediatric doses should be used for children.

◆ Review Chapter 6 for information about using nose drops and nose sprays correctly. To prevent contamination of equipment, family members should not share droppers or spray applicators. Rinse and dry applicators after each use.

◆ To prevent insomnia, instruct patients to take the last dose of the day around the time of the evening meal. If photophobia occurs, instruct patients to avoid brightly lit areas and to wear sunglasses.

◆ Instruct patients how to use nasal jelly (phenylephrine and others). First, blow the nose. Wash hands. Place a pea-sized amount of jelly in each nostril. Sniff well to move jelly back into nose. Wipe off the tip of the tube with a tissue and replace the cap.

Expectorants and Antitussives

Patient and family education

◆ Teach patients about the difference between an antitussive and an expectorant.

◆ Remind patients to read labels carefully on OTC preparations to avoid taking unnecessary medications. Consult the pharmacist for assistance as needed.

◆ Remind patients to keep these and all drugs out of the reach of children. Only products for pediatric use and in pediatric doses should be administered to children.

◆ Remind patients to avoid driving or operating hazardous equipment if drowsiness is a problem.

◆ Tell patients with a cough to stay well hydrated (daily fluid intake of at least 2500 ml for an adult), avoid smoking, and keep the room air moist by using a vaporizer or humidifier.

◆ For preparations containing iodide, question patients about history of allergy to iodine or shellfish before administering. Teach patients to swallow enteric-coated tablets whole, without chewing or crushing, and take them with a full glass of liquid. Liquid preparations should be diluted with water, milk, or juice. Teach patients to take doses with meals or a snack to reduce gastric irritation. Discuss signs of chronic iodine poisoning such as headache, swelling of eyelids, metallic taste in the mouth, nausea, vomiting, diarrhea, skin changes, and mouth ulcers. Remind patients to report any unexpected sign or symptom to the physician.

◆ Codeine and hydrocodone have the same potential for side effects as all narcotics; see Chapter 44.

Mucolytic Agents

Drug administration

◆ Supervise patients receiving acetylcysteine during and after treatment to see that the airway is still patent in the presence of increased pulmonary secretions. Have a suction machine at the bedside of patients who are elderly, immobilized, or intubated, or anyone who may not be able to handle secretions.

◆ Before using a mucolytic agent with a patient for the first time, review the purpose and desired effects of the drug. Tell patients to cough up and expectorate loosened secretions.

◆ Supervise patients with asthma who are receiving acetylcysteine, since it may cause bronchospasm. If bronchospasm develops, discontinue nebulization; if severe, notify the physician. Assess for other common side effects including stomatitis, rhinorrhea, and nausea.

◆ Acetylcysteine is administered orally to treat acetaminophen overdose. The dose is based on the time since acetaminophen ingestion and the serum level of acetaminophen. The regimen involves a loading dose, followed by 17 doses at 4-hr intervals. Dilute doses in juice or cola beverages before administering. If the patient vomits within 1 hr after receiving a dose, the dose should be repeated; consult the physician.

CHAPTER REVIEW

◆ KEY TERMS

antitussive, p. 411

cough, p. 411

expectorant, p. 411

mucociliary escalator, p. 411

mucolytics, p. 413

rebound congestion, p. 408

respiratory tract fluid, p. 411

◆ REVIEW QUESTIONS

1. Explain how alpha-adrenergic agonists relieve nasal congestion.
2. Describe the technique for administering topical nasal decongestants.
3. What are the side effects, drug interactions, and contraindications for nasal decongestants?
4. What is rebound congestion?
5. Categorize the drugs used as nasal decongestants as topical sympathomimetics, oral sympathomimetics, and imidazolines.
6. Describe the origin and function of mucus.
7. List expectorants and their mechanisms of action.
8. Describe the mucolytic drug and its mechanism of action.
9. List antitussives and their mechanisms of action.
10. What are the nonmedicinal approaches for treating a cough?

SUGGESTED READING

Brown LH: The effective cough, *Crit Care Nurse* 8(2):77, 1988.

Thurkauf GE: Acetaminophen overdose, *Crit Care Nurse* 7(1):20, 1987.

DRUGS AFFECTING THE IMMUNE SYSTEM

This section presents the pharmacology of the immune system. Chapter 27, Basic Function of the Immune System, relates the basic functions of the immune system so that the rationale for pharmacologic intervention can be understood. Chapter 28, Immunomodulators, discusses drugs intended to enhance or block immune responses. The situations in which these drugs are indicated are also discussed.

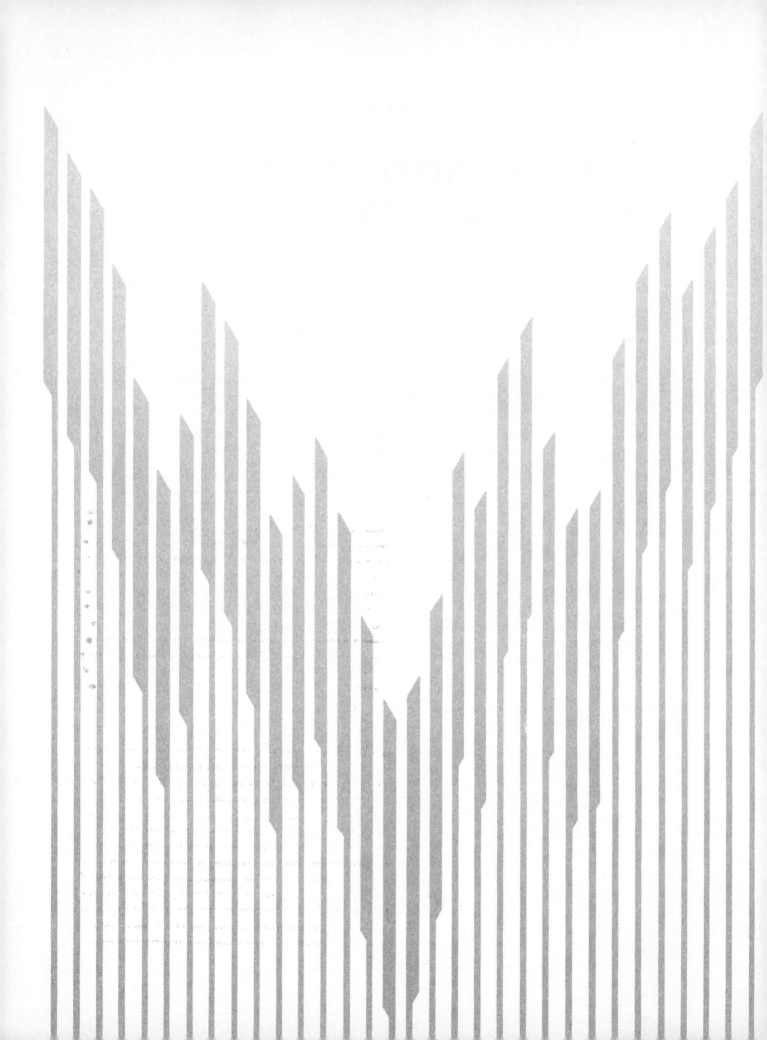

Basic Function of the Immune System

STEPHEN HATFIELD

LEARNING OBJECTIVES

After studying this chapter, you should be able to do the following:

- Discuss the organs and cells of the immune system.
- Discuss the general function of cytokines.
- Describe the classes of immunoglobulins.
- Describe the uses of colony stimulating factors.

CHAPTER OVERVIEW

- The immune system allows us to live safely in a world full of dangerous organisms that could invade the body and cause disease. This chapter describes the components of the immune system. Understanding the function and regulation of the various cells and organs in the immune system creates a foundation for understanding how medical manipulations can influence this vital body system.

IMMUNE SYSTEM

The immune system is a complex and diffuse system that is present throughout the body. It protects the body from damage caused by foreign environmental agents. Foreign agents include invading microorganisms such as bacteria, fungi, parasites, and viruses, as well as foreign tissue such as transplanted kidneys, hearts, and livers. Any foreign agent capable of inducing an immune response is termed an *antigen*. The immune system also protects the body, ridding it of malignant cells as they arise and preventing it from acting against its own tissues. Like all other body systems, the immune system can exhibit pathology and abnormal responses.

Innate and Acquired Immunity

Immunity is innate or acquired. **Innate immunity** is derived from all elements with which a person is born and that are always available on short notice to protect the body from challenges by foreign materials. Innate immunity is conferred by physical, cellular, and chemical barriers. Physical barriers include skin, mucous membranes, and the cough reflex. Phagocytic cells make up the cellular barrier. **Phagocytosis** is ingestion and destruction of foreign particles such as bacteria by individual cells of the immune system. Biologically active substances that include degradative enzymes, toxic free radicals, lipids, and low pH are chemical barriers to invasion by foreign agents.

Acquired immunity is not present at birth but develops as the individual grows and matures. Although a person has the capacity at birth for developing acquired immunity, it is not exhibited until the person has had two sequential exposures to the same foreign agent. Acquired immunity has two main arms, the humoral and the cellular immune response. Humoral immunity involves production of antibodies, which are soluble proteins present in normal serum. Cellular immunity consists of responses such as the delayed type of hypersensitivity, which are mediated by cells rather than by soluble substances. **Lymphocytes** are the main providers of acquired immunity.

Organs and Cells of the Immune System

The immune system is comprised of six white blood cell types: lymphocytes, monocytes and macrophages, polymorphonuclear leukocytes (PMNs), basophils, mast cells, and eosinophils. All of these, as well as red blood cells and platelets, are derived from a common precursor cell type found in the bone marrow. This precursor cell type is the stem cell.

Monocytes and macrophages represent different states of cell maturation. Monocytes circulate freely within the body; with differentiation, they become macrophages. Macrophages may be fixed within the tissues, where they may persist for years; some, however, recirculate through secondary lymphoid organs.

Fixed or recirculating macrophages can assist lymphocytes in generating immune responses and can phagocytize foreign particles. Macrophages can become activated to kill tumor cells.

Lymphocytes are subdivided into the thymus-derived or T cells and the bone-marrow–derived or B cells. The B lymphocytes produce antibodies. T lymphocytes are further subdivided into helper T cells and cytotoxic T cells. Helper T cells assist B cells in responding to an antigen and mediate the delayed type of hypersensitivity. Cytotoxic T cells reject grafts and destroy virus-infected cells. The ratio of helper cells to cytotoxic cells normally ranges from 1.2 : 1 to 2 : 1. In the acquired immunodeficiency syndrome (AIDS), this ratio is usually reversed and can be as low as 0.2 (1 : 5).

Polymorphonuclear leukocytes (PMNs) are the predominant phagocytes within the circulation. They are usually the first cells to arrive at the site of an infection. Besides phagocytosis, the PMN has two other means of killing foreign invaders. The oxidative burst of the PMNs leads to release of superoxide dismutase and hydrogen peroxide. Antimicrobial substances including lysozyme, lactoferrin, cathepsin G, and defensins, are contained within azurophil granules and are released on activiation of the PMNs.

Basophils participate in allergic and inflammatory responses. These cells contain densely staining granules in their cytoplasm. Within these granules are mediators of allergic and inflammatory responses such as histamine, complement components, and leukotrienes C and D. Degranulation occurs when antigen interacts with immunoglobulin E (IgE) molecules bound to the cell surface of the basophil.

Eosinophils participate in allergic reactions but also kill parasites. Contained within the cytoplasmic granules of the eosinophil are some of the same mediators found in basophil granules, such as leukotrienes C and D, and a number of proteins toxic to parasites. Eosinophils can also cause histamine to be released from mast cells and basophils. Eosinophils are also phagocytic, but their role as phagocytes is not as important as is that of the PMNs.

In addition to these circulating white blood cells, mast cells are also important in immunity and especially in certain pathologic disorders. Like basophils, mast cells can participate in allergic reactions and inflammation and are thought to affect asthma. Mast cell granules contain histamine and a number of protease enzymes. Like basophils, mast cells can also synthesize leukotrienes C and D, as well as prostaglandin D2. Also like basophils, mast cells degranulate when antigen interacts with IgE molecules bound to the cell surface. High numbers of mast cells can be found in the skin, lung, and intestinal mucosa. Subtypes of mast cells have been classified based on the types of proteases found within their granules. The tryptase-containing, or mucosal, mast cells are mainly located in mucosal areas as the name implies. Tryptase-chymase–containing, or connective tissue, mast cells are found in the skin. The connective tissue subtype contains more histamine than the mucosal variety. Depending on the microenvironment, mast cells can interconvert.

Organs of the immune system are classified as primary or secondary. The primary lymphoid organs are the thymus and the bone marrow. Maturation of lymphocytes occurs in these structures. The spleen, lymph nodes, and Peyer's patches are the secondary lymphoid organs. Peyer's patches are clusters of lymphocytes spread throughout the lining of the intestinal wall, tonsils, and appendix. Secondary lymphoid tissues trap and concentrate foreign substances and are the main sites of antibody production and generation of antigen-specific T lymphocytes.

IMMUNE RESPONSES

Generation of humoral or cellular immunity requires (1) activation, (2) proliferation, and (3) differentiation. Activation of T lymphocytes requires that antigen be processed and presented by specialized cells called *antigen-presenting cells*. The antigen-presenting cells also secrete soluble factors necessary for the proliferation of T cells. The major antigen-presenting cells are monocytes and macrophages. Other cells that can also present antigen include dermal Langerhans' cells, dendritic cells in various locations, and hepatic Kupffer cells. The antigen-presenting cells take up antigen, process it, and then express it on the cell surface with histocompatibility antigens. T lymphocytes are activated by interaction with this complex of processed and histocompatibility antigen on the surface of the antigen-presenting cells. B lymphocytes are activated by interacting directly with unprocessed antigen via antibody molecules on their surface.

Once activated, T and B lymphocytes express receptors for growth factors synthesized and released primarily by activated helper T cells. In response to these growth factors the T and B cells proliferate. Having undergone proliferation, B and T cells can then respond to other soluble mediators secreted by activated helper T cells and will differentiate into functional effector cells. B lymphocytes differentiate into antibody-secreting plasma cells. T lymphocytes differentiate into cells capable of mediating a delayed type of hypersensitivity or killing virus-infected cells. Generation of humoral and cellular immune responses is summarized in Figure 27-1.

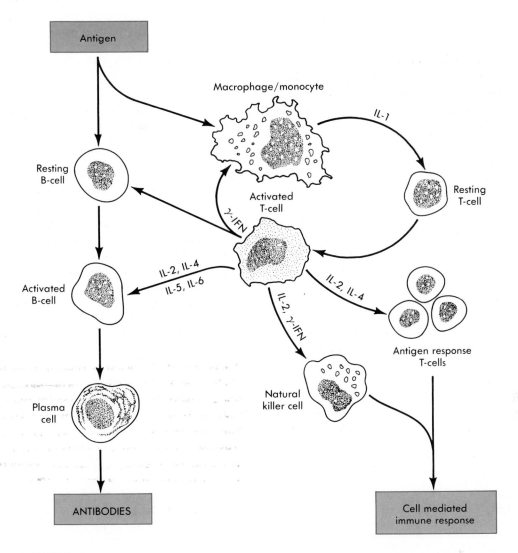

FIGURE 27-1

Generation of immune response. Key features of immune reaction include factors responsible for humoral immunity shown on left and factors responsible for delayed, cell-mediated immunity shown on right.

Soluble Mediators Involved in Immune Responses

Communication within the immune system occurs mainly through release of soluble factors by the cells that respond to the foreign agent. In addition, certain immune functions are also mediated by soluble factors. Most of these soluble factors are named *interleukins* because they allow one type of leukocyte to influence the function of other leukocytes. Some of these mediators can act on or be produced by cells outside of the immune system. The genes for most of these factors have been cloned so that they can be produced outside the body in large amounts. These recombinant DNA techniques have made using those factors in clinical trials in humans possible. The names and major actions of the soluble factors are summarized in Table 27-1. Overproduction of some of these agents can lead to pathologic states, as in the production of tumor necrosis factor in shock.

Immunoglobulins, the soluble mediators of humoral immunity, are divided into five classes: IgM, IgG, IgA, IgE, and IgD (Table 27-2). The immunoglobulin molecule is comprised of two light chains and two heavy chains. Figure 27-2 is a schematic diagram of an antibody molecule. The light chain is made up of a variable region (V) and a constant

Table 27-1   Properties of Human Cytokines

Cytokine	Biologic properties
Interleukin-1 (IL-1)	Activates resting T cells; is a cofactor for hemopoietic growth factors; stimulates synthesis of cytokines; increases natural killer cell activity; chemotaxin for neutrophils, lymphocytes, and macrophages.
Interleukin-2 (IL-2)	Growth factor for activated T cells; induces cytokine production by T cells; activates cytotoxic T cells; increases natural killer cell activity; induces lymphokine-activated killer cells.
Interleukin-3 (IL-3)	Supports the growth of pluripotent bone marrow stem cells; growth factor for mast cells.
Interleukin-4 (IL-4)	Growth factor for activated B cells; induces class II histocompatibility antigens on B cells; growth factor for T cells; growth factor for mast cells; induces IgE synthesis.
Interleukin-5 (IL-5)	Induces differentiation of eosinophils; increases IgM and IgG secretion by activated B cells.
Interleukin-6 (IL-6)	Induces differentiation of activated B cells into plasma cells; with IL-1 activates T cells.
Interleukin-7 (IL-7)	Induces proliferation of immature lymphoid cells; cofactor for T cell growth with IL-2; induces lymphokine-activated killer cells.
Interleukin-8 (IL-8)	Chemoattraction and activation of PMNs; weak chemoattraction and activation of basophils.
Interleukin-9 (IL-9)	Enhances the proliferation of IL-3 dependent mast cells; promotes survival of mast cells; growth factor for T cells.
Interleukin-10 (IL-10)	Inhibits production of gamma-interferon and other cytokines by T cells; inhibits production of cytokines by monocytes; cofactor for T cell growth; cofactor for mast cell growth.
Interferon-gamma (gamma-IFN)	Exerts antiviral activity; induces expression of class II histocompatibility antigens on macrophages; decreases IgE synthesis by B cells; increases natural killer cell activity.
Tumor Necrosis Factor (TNF)	Directly cytotoxic to some tumor cells; stimulates synthesis of cytokines; activates macrophages; mediates inflammation and septic shock.
Granulocyte-Macrophage Colony Stimulating Factor (GM-CSF)	Stimulates growth of trilineage bone marrow progenitors; inhibits migration of PMNs; induces TNF and IL-1 production by monocytes and macrophages; enhances PMNs, eosinophil, and monocyte and macrophage mediated antibody-dependent cellular cytotoxicity.

Table 27-2   Major Classes of Immunoglobulins

Class	Distribution	Biologic properties
IgG	Intravascular and extravascular	Majority of secondary response to most antigens; activation of complement, opsonin; sensitize target cells for destruction by killer cells; neutralization of toxins and viruses; can pass placenta; immobilization of bacteria.
IgM	Mostly intravascular	First class produced during primary immune response; activates complement well; efficient agglutinating antibodies; natural isohemagglutinins.
IgA	Intravascular and secretions	Most common antibody in secretions where it protects mucous membranes; bactericidal in presence of lysozyme; efficient antiviral antibody.
IgE	On basophils and mast cells; in saliva and nasal secretions	Mediates hypersensitivity and allergic reactions; protects against parasite infections.
IgD	On surface of B lymphocytes; trace in serum	Serves as antigen-specific receptor on B cells; may be involved in differentiation of B lymphocytes.

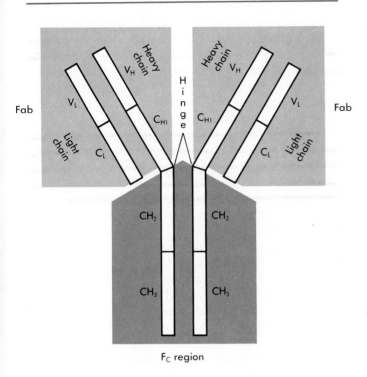

FIGURE 27-2

Schematic diagram of antibody molecule. Heavy and light chains composed of variable (V_H, V_L) regions and constant (C_H, C_L) regions. The Fab portions of molecule are responsible for antigen binding, and Fc portion mediates biologic activity.

region (C). Heavy chains contain three or four constant regions and the variable region. Each variable portion of the immunoglobulin molecule includes three hypervariable regions, which vary widely in amino-acid composition. The combination of these hypervariable regions makes up the antibody-combining site of the immunoglobulin molecule. This portion of the molecule binds the antigen against which the antibody was generated. Each antibody molecule has two combining sites. Five different constant regions define the major immunoglobulin classes. IgG is the major immunoglobulin in serum and has four subclasses. Two subclasses of IgA molecules exist. IgG, IgE, and IgD are monomeric, each composed of one antibody molecule. IgM is composed of five antibody molecules and IgA is composed of two. A protein, the J chain, joins the five basic molecules that make up the IgM molecule. Secretory component, synthesized by epithelial cells, connects the two IgA molecules that compose the dimer. Table 27-2 summarizes the immunoglobulin classes and their functions.

Growth and differentiation of stem cells into mature cells within the immune system is directed by several of the same soluble mediators generated during immune responses. This function of these proteins is called *colony stimulating activity*. Table 27-3 summarizes the major colony stimulating factors and the cells that develop from their action. The development of some immune cells can be directed by more than one of these factors.

Table 27-3   Colony-Stimulating Factors

Factor	Produced by	Colony-stimulating activity
Granulocyte-Macrophage Colony Stimulating Factor (GM-CSF)	T cells; macrophages; fibroblasts; endothelial cells; keratinocytes; thymic epithelium; mesothelium; and uroepithelium	Stimulates colonies of PMNs, monocyte/macrophages, and eosinophils from trilineage bone marrow progenitors.
Granulocyte Colony Stimulating Factor (G-CSF)	Monocytes; macrophages; fibroblasts; endothelial cells; keratinocytes; thymic epithelium; mesothelium; and uroepithelium	Stimulates colonies of PMNs from trilineage bone marrow progenitors; stimulates early pluripotent stem cells to accelerate entry into the cell cycle; synergizes with IL-3 to support proliferation of early pluripotent stem cells.
Macrophage Colony Stimulating Factor (M-CSF)	Monocytes; fibroblasts; and endothelial cells	Stimulates colonies of monocyte and macrophage precursors.
Interleukin-3 (IL-3)	T cells and mast cells	Stimulates colonies of pluripotent stem cells; promotes proliferation and maturation of committed granulocyte and macrophage, eosinophil, and basophil progenitors.
Interleukin-5 (IL-5)	T cells and mast cells	Promotes growth and differentiation of eosinophil progenitors.

COMPLEMENT SYSTEM

The complement system is a group of enzymes found in serum. Its major functions include mediating inflammatory responses and opsonization, or coating, of antigenic particles (including microorganisms), which causes damage to the membrane of pathogens and often results in lysis of the pathogen. Nineteen distinct proteins make up the complement system. Proteins of the complement system interact such that the products of one reaction form the enzyme needed for the next step in the enzyme cascade. A small stimulus can be amplified to activate large amounts of complement.

Complement can be activated by the classical and the alternate pathway. The pathways share many components but differ in the ways they become activated. The classical pathway is activated by antigen-antibody complexes. The alternate pathway is activated by suitable surfaces or molecules, including cell walls of some bacteria, cell walls of yeast, endotoxin derived from cell walls of gram-negative bacteria, and aggregated IgA. Several steps in the complement cascade result in the release of a fragment of some of the proteins of the complement system. These small molecules are very potent mediators of a number of reactions. C3a and C5a are chemotaxins and anaphylatoxins. Chemotaxins cause phagocytic cells to migrate from an area where there is less chemotaxin to an area of higher concentration. Anaphylatoxins cause mast cell degranulation, smooth muscle contraction, and increased capillary permeability. C3b opsonizes anything to which it binds. C3b and C5b activate the lytic pathway, leading to the formation of the membrane attack complex, a series of proteins with detergent properties that produce "holes" in the target cell membrane, resulting in lysis of the target cell.

IMMUNE SYSTEM DISORDERS AND PATHOLOGY

The immune system is tightly regulated to ensure optimal function. Disorders in the development of immune cells during the generation of immune responses or in the synthesis of the products of the immune system may cause immunologic disorders ranging in severity from mild to fatal. The disorders can be classified into deficiencies of immune cells or their soluble products and overproduction of immune cells or their products. Immune deficiencies are primary or secondary. **Primary immune deficiencies** are diseases in which the immune deficiency is the cause of the disease; they may be hereditary or acquired. Secondary immune deficiencies result from diseases. These patients invariably suffer from recurrent infections; this development often leads to the diagnosis of an immune deficiency.

Primary Immune Deficiencies

B cell deficiencies can result in the absence of one or all immunoglobulin classes. Persons with B cell deficiencies suffer mainly from recurrent bacterial infections. Although immunoglobulin-replacement therapy may maintain them for as long as 20 to 30 years, the prognosis is poor, and many succumb to chronic lung disease.

T cell deficiencies affect not only cell-mediated immune responses but also synthesis of antibody, since T cells are necessary for most antibody responses. Patients with T cell disorders are extremely susceptible to fungal, viral, and protozoal infections.

Severe combined immunodeficiencies result from defects in both T and B cells. These disorders are very serious. Untreated infants rarely survive beyond 1 year of age. These patients are susceptible to every type of infection. Treatment with drugs alone is ineffective. Infants can be cured by bone marrow transplantation, provided the transplantation is done before irreversible complications of the disease arise.

Phagocytic cell dysfunctions also cause severe disorders because these cells affect both innate and acquired immunity. Defects may result from deficiencies of antibody, lymphokines, or complement deficiencies, and can also result from cell defects.

Abnormalities in the complement system can lead to immunodeficiencies. Not only is the complement system important in fighting infections, but an intact complement system prevents diseases characterized by inappropriate response to the body cells and tissues. These diseases are termed *autoimmune diseases*. Genetic defects affecting nearly all of the individual components of the complement system have been documented.

Secondary Immune Deficiencies

Secondary immunodeficiencies occur as complications of other diseases. The most common cause of these disorders is the deliberate immune suppression associated with the use of chemotherapeutic agents in cancer treatment or the immunosuppressive drugs used to prevent rejection of transplanted organs. The best known secondary immune deficiency is the acquired immunodeficiency syndrome (AIDS). This disease is caused by infection with human lymphotropic virus III, now called *human immunodeficiency virus* (HIV). The immune deficiency associated with AIDS is largely due to the loss of helper T cells. These cells are not the only immune cells affected by the virus, since the profound immune suppression associated with AIDS cannot be explained only on the basis of loss of helper T cells. Patients with secondary immunodeficiencies suffer severe recurrent infections by opportunistic organisms normally not pathogenic.

Gammopathies

Several neoplastic diseases arise from abnormal proliferation of B cells and plasma cells. These diseases are termed *gammopathies*. The principal gammopathies are multiple myeloma, macroglobulinemia, and heavy chain disease.

Multiple myeloma is the most common of the gammopathies, resulting from the malignant proliferation of plasma cells. It is characterized by synthesis of large amounts of a given isotype of immunoglobulin and may be accompanied by the production of free light chains (called *Bence Jones proteins*). Multiple myeloma involves multiple organ systems resulting from infiltration of them by malignant plasma cells. Patients are susceptible to recurrent bacterial and viral infections due to suppression of the synthesis of normal antibodies.

Macroglobulinemia occurs because of synthesis of large amounts of IgM. The excess immunoglobulin leads to increased viscosity of serum, which leads to decreased blood flow, thrombosis, disorders of the central nervous system (CNS), and bleeding. Decreased synthesis of the other immunoglobulin classes is observed, leading ultimately to hypogammaglobulinemia.

Heavy chain disease is characterized by the appearance of large amounts of protein in the serum and urine resembling the Fc portion of the immunoglobulin molecule. This disorder is uncommon. Patients have recurrent bacterial infections, anemias, and enlarged lymphoid organs.

CHAPTER REVIEW

◆ KEY TERMS

acquired immunity, p. 419
antigen, p. 419
gammopathies, p. 425
immunoglobulins, p. 421
innate immunity, p. 419
lymphocytes, p. 419
phagocytosis, p. 419
primary immune deficiencies, p. 424
secondary immune deficiencies, p. 424

◆ REVIEW QUESTIONS

1. What is innate immunity?
2. Define acquired immunity.
3. What are the forms of acquired immunity?
4. What white blood cell types are responsible for phagocytosis?
5. What are T cells? Where are they formed?
6. What are B cells? Where are they formed?
7. What cell type forms antibodies?
8. What cell type produces the delayed type of hypersensitivity?
9. What are interleukins?
10. What are the five classes of antibodies?
11. What are the primary functions of each class of antibody?
12. What is the complement system?
13. What are the two major functions of the complement system?
14. Define primary and secondary immunodeficiency.
15. Define gammopathy.

SUGGESTED READING

Benjamini E, Leskowitz S: *Immunology: a short course*, New York, 1988, Alan R Liss.

Delafuente JC: *Immunodeficiency diseases*. In DiPiro JT and others, editors, *Pharmacotherapy: a pathophysiologic approach*, New York, 1989, Elsevier.

Dinarello CA, Mier JW: Current concepts: lymphokines, *N Engl J Med* 317(15):940, 1987.

Fonger PA and others: Nursing care of the child with severe combined immune deficiency (SCIDS), *J Pediatr Nurs* 2(6):373, 1987.

Male D: *Immunology: an illustrated outline*, London, 1986, Gower.

O'Garra A and others: B-cell factors are pleiotropic, *Immunol Today* 9(2):45, 1988.

O'Garra A: Peptide regulatory factors. I. Interleukins and the immune system, *Lancet* 1:943, 1989.

O'Garra A: Peptide regulatory factors. II. Interleukins and the immune system, *Lancet* 1:1003, 1989.

Pohl LR and others: The immunologic and metabolic basis of drug hypersensitivities, *Ann Rev Pharmacol* 28:367, 1988.

Reckling JB, Neuberger GB: Understanding immune system dysfunction, *Nurs 87* 17(9):34, 1987.

Tartaglione TA, Collier AC: *Principles and management of the acquired immunodeficiency syndrome*. In DiPiro JT and others, editors, *Pharmacotherapy: a pathophysiologic approach*, New York, 1989, Elsevier.

CHAPTER 28

Immunomodulators

STEPHEN HATFIELD

LEARNING OBJECTIVES

After studying this chapter, you should be able to do the following:

♦ Discuss the difference between passive and active immunity.

♦ Describe the clinical application of interleukins and interferons.

♦ Describe the clinical application of immunosuppressive agents.

♦ Develop a nursing care plan for the patient receiving an immunomodulator.

CHAPTER OVERVIEW

♦ Immunization, a way of modulating the action of the immune system to medical advantage, has been known for a long time. Other ways to alter function of the immune system have been more difficult to develop; only recently have new approaches become available. This chapter describes the classic immunostimulants used for immunization and also explains the use of interferons, interleukins, and colony-stimulating factors. Finally, this chapter covers immunosuppressants used primarily in conjunction with organ transplantation. Additional immunosuppressants are covered in Chapters 39 and 51.

Nursing Process Overview
IMMUNOMODULATORS
Assessment

Perform a baseline assessment based on the age of the patient, severity of presenting problems, acuity level, and planned drug intervention.

Nursing Diagnoses

Possible complication: immunosuppression and risk of infection
Possible complication: serum sickness

Management

Monitor vital signs, temperature, and appropriate lab work including the complete blood count, white blood cell differential, and platelet count. The frequency and extent of monitoring depends on how severely ill the patient is. Immunotherapy is changing rapidly, and new guidelines for many drugs may be available; consult manufacturer's literature for updated information.

Evaluation

Before discharge, teach patients about anticipated benefits and possible side effects of immunomodulators. Encourage patients to call if questions arise or new signs or symptoms develop.

IMMUNOSTIMULANTS

Immunostimulants enhance or stimulate the immune system.

Enhancement of the immune system can be accomplished by two methods linked to acquired immunity. Active acquired immunity involves administration of substances such as **vaccines** that stimulate the immune system to respond against a foreign material. Vaccines usually contain killed or attenuated bacteria or viruses, but protection can also be conferred with immunogenic proteins or toxoids from the pathogen in question (Tables 28-1 and 28-2). Once the immune response has occurred, specific cells in the immune system "remember" the response, and

Table 28-1   Vaccines to Prevent Bacterial and Rickettsial Diseases

Disease	Vaccine characteristics	Vaccine administration
Bubonic plague	Inactivated *Yersinia pestis* confers immunity.	Administered during outbreaks or to persons heavily exposed.
Cholera	Killed strains of *Vibrio cholerae* confer resistance.	Used in persons entering a country where cholera exists.
Diphtheria, tetanus, and pertussis (whooping cough)	This combination, known as *DTP*, contains absorbed toxoids and a vaccine to protect against all three diseases.	Given routinely to children between the ages of 2 months and 7 years. In event of injury, additional protection against tetanus may be needed.
Haemophilus influenzae type B	Based on polysaccharide from the organism.	Recommended for all children 2 years of age or older.
Meningitis	Meningococcal polysaccharide mixtures give protection against group A, group C, or both.	Used only in outbreaks or in exposed persons who also receive antibiotics to protect against infections by serogroup B.
Pneumococcal pneumonia	Mixed capsular material from cultured pneumococci confers resistance to lobar pneumonia and bacteremia caused by one of the strains used as a source of capsular material.	Given only to high-risk patients, weak convalescents, or patients over 50 years of age.
Tetanus and diphtheria	Mixed absorbed toxoids are used in patients over 6 years of age.	Used for routine prophylaxis in patients who have not received DTP.
Tetanus toxoid	Absorbed tetanus toxoid confers immunity.	May be used for routine immunization but DTP is preferred. Most commonly given after an injury that poses risk of tetanus infection.
Tuberculosis	Attenuated strain of *Mycobacterium bovis* confers variable temporary immunity.	Given to exposed but uninfected patients who cannot receive drug therapy.
Typhoid	Killed *Salmonella typhosa* gives prolonged protection.	Used in exposed persons or persons traveling where typhoid is endemic.
Typhus	Killed *Rickettsia prowazekii* confers resistance.	Given to persons traveling to areas where exposure to the louse-borne disease is likely.

a secondary immune response occurs rapidly on a subsequent encounter with the antigen. This principle is illustrated in Figure 28-1. Active immunity usually persists for years.

Passive acquired immunity involves administration of preformed substances such as immune serum or antibodies that can immediately combat the foreign agent to which they are directed. The passive immunity conferred by immune sera, antibodies, or globulins lasts only weeks.

Immunizations

The fetus is protected from bacterial and viral infections and from microbial toxins by maternal Immunoglobulin G (IgG) antibodies, which pass to the fetus through the placenta to confer passive immunity. IgG is the only antibody that can cross the placenta. Newborn infants do not have a fully functional immune system; human milk, however, contains factors that aid the newborn response against infectious agents. Some of these factors enhance the growth of beneficial intestinal flora, and others nonspecifically inhibit the growth of harmful microorganisms. The inhibitory factors include lysozyme, lactoferrin, interferon, and leukocytes. Antibodies are also found in breast milk and are especially abundant in colostrum (first milk). Immunizations can begin when the infant is 2 months of age and can mount an effective immune response on its own. Table 28-3 indicates the recommended schedule for active immunizations.

Table 28-2 Vaccines to Prevent Viral Diseases

Disease	Characteristics of vaccine
Poliomyelitis	Oral vaccine containing attenuated live poliovirus mimics natural form of the disease without risk of central nervous system (CNS) involvement.
Rubella (German measles)	Attenuated live rubella vaccine confers long-term resistance.
Measles (rubeola)	Attenuated live virus vaccine stimulates protective antibodies in 95% of children receiving vaccine.
Mumps	Attenuated live virus vaccine stimulates protective antibodies in 95% of those receiving vaccine.
Influenza	Inactivated viruses of types causing recent outbreaks are used. Vaccine differs yearly.
Smallpox	Success of vaccination is judged by response at vaccination site.
Yellow fever	Live attenuated virus confers resistance to most persons receiving vaccine.
Rabies	Killed, fixed virus confers resistance to most patients exposed to infection.
Hepatitis	It is developed from surface antigens from hepatitis B virus.

Table 28-3 Active Immunization Schedule

Age	Vaccine
2 months	Diphtheria, tetanus, and pertussis (DTP-1) and trivalent oral polio (TOP-1)
4 months	DTP-2 and TOP-2
6 months	DTP-3 and TOP-3
15 months	Measles, mumps, and rubella
18 months	DTP-4, TOP-4, and *Haemophilus influenzae* Type B
4 to 6 years	DTP-5 and TOP-5
14 to 16 years (and each 10 years thereafter)	Tetanus toxoid and reduced adult dose of diphtheria toxoid
18 to 24 years	Measles, mumps (especially for susceptible males), and rubella
25 to 64 years	Measles (for persons born after 1956), mumps (especially for susceptible males), and rubella (for females up to 45 years)
>65 years	Influenza and pneumococcus

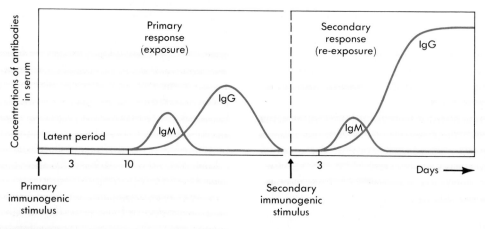

FIGURE 28-1

Time course of antibody release on first exposure versus subsequent exposure.

Absorption and fate of immunostimulants

Intramuscular (IM) injection is the usual route of administration of the immune serums and globulins (Table 28-4). Oral administration is not usually possible with these agents, since the degradative processes in the digestive tract would render them inactive before they could be absorbed. Distribution is fairly rapid after IM injection, but if very rapid therapy is required, these agents can be given intravenously, resulting in immediate distribution. The immunity provided by immune globulins and serums lasts from 1 to 6 weeks. Once injected, the antibodies interact with the entire organism against which they were generated, thus facilitating phagocytosis of the organism by monocytes or macrophages and polymorphonuclear leukocytes (PMNs). Antibodies made against toxins of pathogenic microorganisms form complexes with the toxin, and these immune complexes are also cleared by phagocytes. Immunity is lost when the injected antibodies are cleared from the system.

Vaccines are administered by either IM or subcutaneous injection (see Table 28-4). Exceptions to these routes are smallpox vaccine, which is given intradermally, and oral poliovaccine. Duration of protection is usually from 1 to 10 years. Since vaccines stimulate the immune system to respond actively rather than passively, protection persists after the injected agent has disappeared. The fate of vaccines is similar to that of immune globulins. Since vaccines are antigens and not antibodies, they are taken up and processed by antigen-presenting cells (see Chapter 27) for the generation of immune responses. Some of the injected agent will be metabolized in this manner. Once antibodies have been produced, any remaining injected material can be complexed with the antibodies and cleared by phagocytes.

Side effects and toxicity

Many side effects of immune serum or globulin injections are dose-related. Patients may have pain at the injection site, mild chest pain, and chills. Less common side effects include malaise, headache, nausea and vomiting, dyspnea, syncope, and back pain. Hepatitis B immune globulin can also cause urticaria and angioedema. Varicella zoster immune globulin injections can cause a mild rash, usually observed 10 to 14 days after immunization.

Immune sera, especially those using nonhuman proteins, can cause anaphylaxis in patients with a history of hypersensitivity reactions to immune globulin injections. This serum sickness results from an immune response directed against proteins in the injected serum. Massive immune complex formation occurs, followed by deposition of these complexes in the kidney and circulatory system, leading to nephritis and arteritis. The deposited immune complexes also initiate mediator release from platelets, basophils, and PMNs. This massive mediator release can be life-threatening. A local deposition of insoluble immune complexes at the site of injection produces the Arthus reaction, in which redness and edema occur near blood vessels. Use caution when repeating injections of foreign serum. Other signs of serum sickness include arthralgia, lymphadenopathy, and pruritus. In serious cases, abdominal pain, fever, headache, and malaise may occur. Use of immune sera may be contraindicated in patients with thrombocytopenia, since excessive bleeding may occur at the injection site. Live virus vaccines should not be used in patients receiving immunosuppressive therapy, since these vaccines can cause progressive disease in immunocompromised patients. Live virus vaccines are also contraindicated in pregnant women, because they can damage the fetus.

Drug interactions

There are no known drug interactions associated with the use of passive immunostimulants, immune serum, and globulins. All immunosuppressive agents can interfere with the generation of active immunity induced by vaccines and toxoids. Corticosteroids, azathioprine, cyclosporine, and some agents used in cancer chemotherapy fall in this category.

Interferons and Interleukins

The **interferons** and **interleukins**, especially interleukin-2 (IL-2), are new forms of therapy whose use is growing rapidly. Both interferons and interleukins are used to treat cancer; the interferons are also used to treat certain viral infections. The anticancer effects of interleukin-2 are indirect. Interleukin-2 stimulates a population of lymphocytes to become killer cells capable of destroying tumor cells. Leukocytes are removed from the patient by leukophoresis and cultured with IL-2 in the laboratory under sterile conditions. The leukocytes are grown until at least 1 billion cells are available. These cells are reinjected into the patient. IL-2 is then introduced into the patient to maintain these lymphokine-activitated killer cells in the body to allow them to kill cancer cells.

Interferon has been approved by the Food and Drug Administration (FDA) for use in five clinical situations with approval for a sixth use pending as of January 1992. Interferon does not exhibit direct antiviral action but acts indirectly within virus-susceptible cells to mediate its antiviral effects. Interferon binds to specific cell surface receptors, resulting in signal transduction through the membrane and ultimately protein synthesis. Over 24 proteins have

Table 28-4 Immunostimulants

Generic name	Route	Duration of effect	Contraindications
Antirabies serum	IM	3 weeks	Allergy to equine serum
Cholera vaccine	IM, SC	6 months	Previous allergic reaction to vaccine
Crotaline antivenin, polyvalent	IV	3 weeks	Allergy to equine serum
Digoxin immune Fab	IV; ID: for allergy testing	1 week	Allergy to sheep or serum products
Diphtheria antitoxin	IV, IM	3 weeks	Allergy to equine serum; pregnancy
Diphtheria toxoid, adsorbed	IM: *Children 6 weeks to 6 years;* second dose 6 to 8 weeks after first; third dose 1 year after second dose	10 years	CNS disease; not used in adults
Diphtheria and tetanus toxoids	IM: adults only	10 years; boosters required	History of neurologic reaction to diphtheria-tetanus toxoids
Diphtheria and tetanus toxoids and adsorbed pertussis vaccine	IM: *Children 6 weeks to 6 years*—4 doses at 2, 4, 6, and 18 months; booster at 4 to 6 years	10 years; boosters required for tetanus toxoid	Encephalopathy, seizures, or other signs of CNS damage; not used in adults
H. influenzae type B vaccine	SC: *Children 1½ to 4 years*	Not clearly known	Children younger than 1½ years or older than 5 years; not used in adults
Hepatitis B vaccine	IM, SC: 3 doses; second dose 1 month after first; third 6 months after first dose	At least 5 years	Severe cardiovascular disease with pulmonary dysfunction; pregnancy
Immune globulin	IV, IM	4 weeks; more often if needed	Selective IgA deficiency; thrombocytopenia; pregnancy
Influenza virus vaccine	IM: *Adults and children over 12 years*—single dose; *Children 3 to 12 years*—2 doses 4 or more weeks apart	1 year	Allergy to eggs or chicken; history of Guillain-Barré syndrome; pregnancy
Measles virus vaccine live	SC	8 years or longer	Immune deficiencies; febrile seizures or cerebral trauma; pregnancy; women should not become pregnant within 3 months after vaccination
Mumps virus vaccine live	SC	Permanent immunity (develops in only 75% to 90% of patients receiving vaccine)	Immune deficiencies; pregnancy; women should not become pregnant within 3 months after vaccination
Pertussis immune globulin	IM	3 weeks	Hypersensitivity to IgG; not used in adults
Pneumococcal vaccine polyvalent	IM, SC	Months to years, exact duration not known	Recent pneumococcal pneumonia; children under 2 years; pregnancy

ID, intradermal; IM, intramuscular; IV, intravenous; SG, subcutaneous

Table 28-4   Immunostimulants—cont'd

Generic name	Route	Duration of effect	Contraindications
Poliovirus vaccine inactivated	SC: 4 doses; *Adults*—first 2 doses at least 4 weeks apart; third and fourth doses a few months apart; children—first 3 doses at 4 to 8 week intervals; final dose 6 to 12 months after third dose	Years, exact duration not known	Acute febrile illness; pregnancy
Poliovirus vaccine live oral	ORAL: *Adults*—single dose, but adults should receive inactivated vaccine; *Children*—3 doses; two schedules—6 to 12 weeks, 8 weeks later, and 8 to 12 months after second dose or at 2, 4, 18 months	Years, exact duration not known	Elderly patients and pregnancy, except single doses may be given when rapid immunization is needed
Rabies immune globulin	IM	3 weeks	Thrombocytopenia
Rabies vaccine	IM	Years; boosters may be required	None
Rh$_o$ (D) immune globulin	IM	3 weeks; treatment required after each subsequent pregnancy	RH$_o$ (D) positive blood type and elderly patients
Rubella virus vaccine live	SC	Years; boosters not recommended although exact duration not known	Immune deficiencies; recent treatment with blood products or immune globulins; pregnancy; women should not become pregnant within 3 months after vaccination
Smallpox vaccine	ID	Complete protection for 1 to 3 years; significant protection for 20 years	Viral diseases other than smallpox; pregnancy
Tetanus antitoxin	IM, SC	3 weeks	Allergy to equine serum; pregnancy
Tetanus immune globulin	IM	32 days	Allergy to immune globulins; pregnancy
Tetanus toxoid	IM, SC: tetanus toxoid only if SC	10 years; boosters required	Prior reactions to tetanus toxoid preparations; children under 6 weeks of age; pregnancy
Typhoid vaccine	SC, ID: 2 doses 4 weeks apart	3 years; boosters can be given when needed	Severe febrile illness; pregnancy
Varicella-zoster immune globulin	IM	3 to 4 weeks	Allergy to immunoglobulin; pregnancy
Yellow fever vaccine	SC	10 years; boosters may be given when needed	Allergy to eggs or chicken; immune deficiencies; pregnancy

been found whose synthesis is induced by interferon. These proteins include a protein kinase that interferes with translation of viral proteins, a protein that enzymatically degrades viral RNA, and a protein that glycosylates viral proteins that affect virus packaging and release. Interferon has direct and indirect antitumor actions. The primary direct effect involves a cytostatic mechanism of slowing tumor cell growth by increasing the time it takes the tumor cell to go through the cell cycle. Inteferons also have a direct cytotoxic action on the tumor cell to enhance their lysis. Indirect antitumor actions of interferon are mediated by host cytotoxic cells and immune responses such as antibodies directed against the tumor cell.

The indications for which interferons have been approved include two viral infections, one inherited immune disease, and two forms of cancer (see Chapter 39). Alpha-interferon is very effective in treating hairy-cell leukemia. More than 90% of patients with this disorder treated with alpha-interferon experience remissions. Treatment involves subcutaneous injection of 2 million units/M^2 of body surface three times weekly. Although treatment is continued for several years, long-term remissions have occurred with as little as 1 year of therapy. Alpha-interferon is also used to treat epidemic Kaposi's sarcoma in AIDS patients. Effective treatment requires higher doses of alpha-interferon (18 to 36 million units/day) and therefore an increase in adverse reactions is seen. This is acceptable in these patients, since the morbidity and mortality associated with Kaposi's sarcoma in AIDS patients is quite high. Response rate is 25% to 45%. Treatment of basal cell carcinoma with alpha-interferon (1.5 million units injected intralesionally 3 times weekly for 3 weeks) awaits FDA approval.

Condyloma acuminatum (genital warts) and non-A, non-B hepatitis (hepatitis C) are viral infections for which use of alpha-interferon has been approved. Doses of 1 to 5 million units 3 times weekly for 3 to 8 weeks eliminates all visible lesions in 60% to 70% of patients treated. Non-A, non-B hepatitis previously had no effective treatment before approval of alpha-interferon for this use. Two million units 3 times weekly for 6 months results in the normalization of liver enzymes and improvements in liver histology in 48% of patients. However, relapse is frequent, and patients may require further treatment.

Chronic granulomatous disease is the final indication for which interferon is approved. Chronic granulomatous disease is an inherited immune disease in which patients have many severe, recurrent infections of skin, lymph nodes, liver, lungs, and bones caused by impairment of phagocytes. Gamma-interferon is the first agent other than antibiotics approved for treatment of chronic granulomatous disease. Pro-

Table 28-5   Toxic Effects of Interleukin-2 and Interferons

Immunomodulator	Common effects
Alpha-interferon	Neurotoxicity (fatigue and lethargy) Hematologic (leukopenia, neutropenia, and thrombocytopenia) Allergic (skin reaction, fever, and chills) Gastrointestinal (anorexia, diarrhea, and nausea) Other (tachycardia, headache, myalgia, and arthralgia)
Beta-interferon	As for alpha-interferon but fever, gastrointestinal side effects, and less thrombocytopenia
Gamma-interferon	Similar to beta-interferon
Interleukin-2	Cardiovascular and renal (fluid retention and elevated serum creatinine level) Neurotoxicity (fatigue and lethargy) Hematologic (anemia) Hepatic (hyperbilirubinemia) Pulmonary (interstitial edema and dyspnea)

phylactic treatment with gamma-interferon reduced the risk of serious infection in these patients by 70%, representing a significant breakthrough in the treatment of this disease.

Since therapy with these agents can be life-threatening, it warrants special consideration. These agents were not expected to have significant toxicity, since they are natural human substances; however, in early trials, four cancer patients treated with alpha-interferon died. This event led to a careful examination of how interferons and interleukins affect human subjects. Though these substances occur naturally in the body at very low concentrations, therapy usually involves administration of high doses, which leads to a wide range of adverse reactions. Their toxic effects are summarized in Table 28-5. These reactions refer to IV administration. No toxic effects have been reported after local injection into tissue. In the trials the major dose-limiting effect of the interferons was severe fatigue. Marked fluid retention caused by a generalized increase in vascular permeability is the most serious adverse reaction of IL-2 therapy.

Colony Stimulating Factors

Since **colony stimulating factors** induce the production of granulocytes in vivo, especially PMNs, they are good candidates as adjuncts to cancer chemotherapy and bone marrow transplantation. Colony stimulating factors in cancer chemotherapy are used to reduce toxicity and morbidity, as well as to allow the dose of chemotherapeutic agents to be increased.

Patients treated with subcutaneous injection of granulocyte-macrophage colony stimulating factor (GM-CSF) along with chemotherapy had significantly less severe neutropenia, or the duration of neutropenia was shortened considerably. Dose-escalation studies have also been performed with GM-CSF. Treatment with GM-CSF allows increased doses of chemotherapy to be used in patients refractory to the standard chemotherapy regimens with up to 40% of patients responding to the higher levels of chemotherapeutic agents. In some of these studies, morbidity was not reduced despite the decrease in neutropenia. In one study, two patients died from sepsis with GM-CSF treatment although none of the patients receiving chemotherapy alone died. Since GM-CSF can induce the production of TNF and IL-1, these cytokines may act synergistically with endogenous endotoxin to cause profound septic shock.

Granulocyte colony stimulating factor (G-GSF) has been used in similar studies. Patients treated with G-CSF showed significant rises in PMNs and a reduction in the period of absolute neutropenia. There was no change in the level to which the PMN count fell in some studies, but in others PMN counts were less depressed. Severe infections decreased as did the requirement for antibiotics. Dose-escalation studies with G-CSF showed a return of PMN levels to normal in 12 to 14 days compared with the 19 to 21 days in patients not receiving G-CSF.

Bone marrow transplantation has a significant mortality rate caused by the severe and prolonged pancytopenia and also requires long hospital stays. Colony stimulating factors have been used to reduce the length of pancytopenia. GM-CSF and G-CSF decreased the time to recovery of PMN counts. A decreased incidence of bacterial and fungal infections and a decrease in the febrile response to chemotherapy occured. Overall, earlier discharge from the hospital occured with patients receiving therapy with colony stimulating factors.

Pharmacokinetics of GM-CSF and G-CSF were different for the two cytokines. The elimination of GM-CSF is reportedly independent of dose. Elimination half-times for intravenous G-CSF depended on dose. A single bolus of 10 μg/kg administered subcutaneously yielded peak serum levels in 4 hr with levels remaining detectable for 9 hr or longer. Continuous subcutaneous infusion of 10 μg/kg/day for 5 days saw serum G-CSF levels fall drastically over the last 2 days instead of maintaining a plateau as expected, since the rate of infusion was constant. A new mechanism of clearance had apparently become activated. The dramatic increase in clearance was not observed if a high output of PMN was not achieved by the G-CSF treatment.

Colony stimulating factors have also been used in clinical trials for the treatment of myelodysplastic syndrome; leukemia and lymphoma; cyclic, congenital, and idiopathic neutropenia; aplastic anemia; and acquired immunodeficiency syndrome (AIDS).

Side effects of GM-CSF and G-CSF are much less severe than those with clinical use of the interleukins and interferons. There are currently no known dose limiting effects seen with the use of G-CSF. Dose limiting toxicities of GM-CSF are fluid retention, pericarditis, and pleural and peritoneal effusions (because of capillary leak syndrome). Bone pain, rash at the site of injection, and transient hypotension are seen with G-CSF and GM-CSF. Fever, chills, headache, nausea and vomiting, weakness, and fatigue are the most common complaints reported with GM-CSF.

IMMUNOSUPRESSANTS

Immunosuppressants lessen or prevent an immune response. Immunosuppressive drugs are used in organ transplantation and autoimmune diseases. Patients who have received kidney, heart, liver, bone marrow, or skin allografts require immunosuppressive agents to prevent rejection of the foreign graft by their immune system. Combinations of these agents are sometimes necessary during a rejection episode. Certain immunosuppressive drugs are used only immediately after transplantation. The major immunosuppressive drugs in clinical use are listed in Table 28-6.

Corticosteroids are used to treat autoimmune disorders such as rheumatoid arthritis. Prednisone was the drug of choice for maintenance immunosuppression in organ transplantation before the advent of cyclosporine. Methylprednisolone and azathioprine were routinely used during a rejection episode. Steroid immunosuppressive drugs are thought to bind to cytoplasmic receptors and to be carried into the cell's nucleus, where they alter cellular metabolism. These drugs markedly reduce certain populations of lymphocytes (see Chapter 51).

Certain anticancer agents are also used as immunosuppressants. Cyclophosphamide, methotrexate, and mercaptopurine are used to severely suppress immune function or to aid in complete destruction of the immune system before bone marrow transplantation. These drugs block proliferation of cells of the immune system. When used in this manner, they are usually combined with whole body irradiation or total lymphoid irradiation (see Chapter 39).

Antithymocyte globulin (ATG) or serum and antilymphocyte globulin (ALG) or serum are used in

Table 28-6 Major Immunosuppressants in Clinical Use

Generic name	Route	Half-life	Contraindications
Antithymocyte globulin	IV: daily for 14 days then alternate days for 14 days; ID: for allergy testing	6 days	Previous allergy to equine materials or serum products; pregnancy
Antihuman lymphocyte globulin	IM, IV: single dose with prednisone before transplantation, daily after transplantation for 4 weeks, alternate days for weeks 5 and 6, every third day until patient leaves hospital	6 days	Known allergy to equine materials or serum products; pregnancy
Azathioprine sodium	ORAL: daily for transplantation until patient leaves hospital; IV: until patient can tolerate oral dose	In plasma-1 hr	Renal impairment; pregnancy
Cyclosporine	ORAL: single daily dose, first dose preceding transplantation; IV: single dose by infusion until patient can tolerate oral dose	19 to 27 hr	Allergy; pregnancy
Muromonab-CD3	IV: daily by rapid injection for 10 to 14 days	Effect lasts for 1 week	Recent exposure to chickenpox or herpes zoster; fluid overload or pulmonary edema; fever above 37.8° C; pregnancy; dose in children not established

ID, intradermal; IM, intramuscular; IV, intravenous

organ transplantation, usually during the first 14 to 28 days after surgery or during an acute rejection episode. Antibodies in these preparations bind to lymphocytes, leading to their destruction or to inhibition of their actions. These agents are usually produced in horses, although goats and rabbits may be used if allergic reactions to the equine material occur.

Muromonab-CD3 is a monoclonal antibody directed against the CD-3 molecule present on the surface of all T lymphocytes. Monoclonal antibodies are much more specific than antibodies prepared against whole lymphocytes, since the antibody can bind only to cells that express the CD-3 molecule. Other cells of the immune system are thus spared the effects of the antibody preparation. Muromonab-CD3 prepares bone marrow before infusion, rids the marrow of immunocompetent cells, and increases the likelihood that only stem cells will be injected. This process aids in preventing graft-versus-host disease, a common and possible fatal outcome of bone marrow transplantation. Muromonab-CD3 is also used during graft rejection when other therapy has proved ineffective.

Azathioprine functions similarly to other antiproliferative drugs. Although this drug exerts effects in its native form, it can be converted in the body to mercaptopurine, which may account for its immunosuppressive action.

Cyclosporine is becoming the drug of choice for immunosuppression in organ transplantation. Originally isolated from fungi found in soil, it is currently being made synthetically. Cyclosporine, unlike most of the other immunosuppressive agents, is relatively selective for cells of the immune system, especially the helper subset of T lymphocytes. Myelosuppression, a common problem with many immunosuppressive drugs, is not seen with cyclosporine. Cyclosporine may prevent synthesis of IL-2 by activated helper T lymphocytes. It can maintain immunosuppression in kidney transplantation without the need for any other agents and is combined with low doses of corticosteroids in liver and heart transplantation.

Absorption and fate

Absorption and fate of the corticosteroids are discussed in detail in Chapter 51, and the anticancer agents are discussed in Chapter 39.

The usual route of administration of antilymphocyte globulin and antithymocyte globulin is by IV infusion. Distribution is therefore immediate. The half-life of equine IgG is 6 days. Small amounts of these preparations can be given intradermally to test for allergic responses. A wheal with localized erythema and edema observed within 60 min of injection indicates a positive test and may prohibit safe administration of the globulin.

Muromonab-CD3 is given by rapid IV injection. Immediately on administration, the antibody binds to CD-3 positive T lymphocytes. Its effects persist for about 1 week after therapy is discontinued.

Azathioprine is usually given orally but can be given by IV injection immediately after surgery until the patient is able to tolerate oral dosing. The drug is readily absorbed orally, is distributed rapidly throughout the tissues, and is metabolized extensively. Metabolites of azathiprone, including the antiproliferative compound mercaptopurine, are excreted by the kidney.

Cyclosporine is available as an oral and an IV solution. As with azathioprine, IV injections can be given until the patient can take oral doses. Bioavailability after oral doses of cyclosporine is variable. Maximum absorption is about 30%. Peak plasma levels are observed 3½ hr after an oral dose. Because of its relatively high lipid solubility, cyclosporine is distributed to most tissues and fluids including the fetus and breast milk. It is extensively metabolized by the liver, and a first-pass effect is observed after oral administration. The elimination half-time for cyclosporine is variable, ranging from 19 to 27 hr. Metabolized drug appears in the bile, but little is seen in urine.

Side effects and toxicity

Increased incidence of infections and of certain cancers, predominantly lymphomas, are complications shared by virtually all immunosuppressant drugs. The increased incidence of infection is especially noteworthy since many of these infections are unusual and difficult to treat. The risk of developing cancer is confirmed when patients are carefully monitored over months and years, and their incidence of cancer is compared with that of age-matched controls.

Antithymocyte globulin and antilymphocyte globulin share certain side effects. Lymphocytopenia is the desired action of these drugs, but a more general leukocytopenia may develop. Thrombocytopenia may also occur. The incidence of leukocytopenia and thrombocytopenia can be as high as 20%. Fever and malaise are common and should be expected during the early phases of therapy. Allergic reactions ranging from local skin reactions to serum sickness and anaphylaxis may be observed in 15% of patients. Gastrointestinal (GI) upset, marked by diarrhea, nausea, vomiting, and abdominal distention, can result from treatment with antithymocyte globulin. Cardiovascular problems, including hypotension, hypertension, tachycardia, generalized and pulmonary edema, and chest pain have occured with antithymocyte globulin therapy. Hypoglycemia is possible, and diabetic patients should be monitored closely. CNS involvement is less common but can include seizures.

Azathioprine therapy is limited by a number of side effects. Bone marrow suppression is the most common toxic effect that limits use of the drug. Indications of bone marrow suppression include leukocytopenia, macrocytic anemia, pancytopenia, and thrombocytopenia, which can lead to unexplained bleeding and bruising. Anorexia, nausea, vomiting, and diarrhea occur, especially with large doses. Toxic hepatitis with biliary stasis leading to jaundice may be observed in renal transplantation patients. Allergic reactions can accompany azathioprine therapy. Rashes, fever, and serum sickness may arise.

Complications associated with cyclosporine therapy involve nearly every physiologic system. Nephrotoxicity is the dose-limiting toxic effect of cyclosporine. This toxicity is dose related, with up to 38% of patients showing elevated BUN and serum creatinine levels. Tremor develops in up to 50% of treated patients. Less common are confusion, headaches, flushing, and seizures. Hypertension also occurs in up to 50% of patients and may require treatment with antihypertensives. Anemia, leukopenia, and thrombocytopenia are rare. GI symptoms include diarrhea, nausea, vomiting, and GI bleeding. Hirsutism develops in a quarter to nearly half of patients, and acne may also appear. Hepatotoxicity is seen in a small percentage of patients; it is usually reversed when doses are lowered. Cyclosporine may induce lymphomas, especially when given in conjunction with other immunosuppressive agents. Gingival hyperplasia develops in 30% of treated patients.

Muromonab-CD3 has several toxic effects associated with the first dose that seldom recur on subsequent doses. Trembling and shaking of hands, chest pain, diarrhea, nausea, and vomiting fall in this category. Allergic symptoms are also common after the first dose, but persistence of these symptoms should be investigated. Causes include infection, severe pulmonary edema, and fluid overload.

Drug interactions

Treatment with immunosuppressive drugs in general decreases effectiveness of any therapy that enhances immunity. Live vaccines are contraindicated with most immunosuppressants, since their use can lead to serious, even fatal, disease instead of immunity. Combination therapy with two or more immunosuppressive agents can profoundly impair normal host defense mechanisms, progressing to increased risk of infection or development of malignancies, especially lymphomas.

Antithymocyte globulin or antilymphocyte globulin administration can enhance other immunosuppressive agents given at the same time, which further impairs host defenses. This may be life-threatening or may lead to blood dyscrasias.

Allopurinol interferes with the metabolism of azathioprine, leading to accumulation of azathioprine and thus increasing the risk of bone marrow suppression.

Cyclosporine-induced nephrotoxicity precludes the use of aminoglycoside antibiotics. Amphotericin B should similarly be avoided. Administration of corticosteroids and ketoconazole may increase the serum level of cyclosporine by diminishing the normal hepatic metabolism of the latter.

Immunotoxins

With recombinant DNA technology a new class of agents has been developed that may allow for more selective therapy in organ transplantation, treatment of cancer, and treatment of AIDS. **Immunotoxins** contain a highly toxic agent coupled to a protein that selectively binds to the cells rejecting transplanted organs, cancer cells, or cells infected with the human immunodeficiency virus (HIV).

Early immunotoxins were monoclonal antibodies to tumor antigens, coupled chemically to ricin, an agent that inactivates ribosomes, thereby preventing protein synthesis and leading to cell death. One molecule of ricin was sufficient to kill a cell. Animal studies showed limited success with the immunotoxins. A critical problem with monoclonal antibodies directed against tumor antigens is that they frequently cross-react with normal tissue. New immunotoxins were developed to overcome this problem. Pseudomonas exotoxin is composed of domains for binding to the cell, for translocating into the cell, and for inactivating elongation factor 2 and preventing protein synthesis. By joining the DNA sequences for the translocation and toxic domains of the exotoxin with DNA sequences that code for proteins targeting the immunotoxin, agents have been produced that are highly and selectively toxic against human cells. Similarly, diphtheria toxin has been used in animal studies. This toxin cannot be administered in humans once they are immunized against diphtheria. In mice, toxin coupled to interleukin-2 (IL-2) prolongs survival of transplanted hearts. The cells that reject the graft express receptors for IL-2, which can bind the immunotoxin, can be killed by the toxin. In mice, this toxin has also prevented the delayed type of hypersensitivity. Coupling the toxin to transforming growth factor alpha generates a toxin capable of killing cells that express a high number of epidermal growth factor receptors, such as in certain types of cancer. Lastly, the exotoxin has been coupled to CD4, a cell surface molecule expressed on T cells, which is recognized by HIV. A cell infected with HIV expresses on its surface a protein that binds CD4. The CD4-exotoxin protein eliminates HIV-infected cells in vitro but does not kill noninfected cells. At this writing, clinical trials with this agent are under way.

NURSING IMPLICATIONS SUMMARY

Vaccines

- ◆ Any serum product containing proteins can cause acute allergic reactions and serum sickness. Review signs and symptoms of serum sickness with the patient, and instruct the patient to notify the physician if it develops. Note that serum sickness may not develop for up to 6 to 12 days after immunization.
- ◆ Have available epinephrine 1:1000 solution in settings where protein-containing products are administered. Have drugs, equipment, and personnel available to treat acute allergic reactions.
- ◆ Question women about the possibility of pregnancy before administering vaccines. Live virus vaccines are contraindicated in pregnant women.

- ◆ For IM administration, use anatomic landmarks in selecting injection sites. Use the deltoid muscle for administration of most vaccines and similar medications in older children and adults. Usually, avoid the injection sites in the gluteal area unless large-volume doses must be divided into two or more injections or the patient is receiving two or more drugs that cannot be administered in the same site. Use the vastus lateralis muscle in infants and small children. Aspirate before injecting drug to avoid inadvertent IV administration; if blood is aspirated, withdraw needle, discard syringe and needle, and prepare a fresh dose.
- ◆ Review manufacturer's instructions when preparing unfamiliar medications.

◆ Sensitivity tests may be ordered on patients before administering the full dose of antirabies serum, crotaline antivenin (snakebite antivenin), diphtheria antitoxin, and tetanus antitoxin. Consult the physician.

Patient and family education

◆ Review anticipated benefits and possible side effects of drug therapy with patients. With small children, if regular immunizations usually cause a fever, suggest that the mother use acetaminophen to treat this side effect. Consult the physician.
◆ Warn patients to avoid scratching injection sites. Brief application of an ice pack may lessen irritation.
◆ When appropriate, review with patients the schedule for additional doses of immunizations.
◆ Refer patients to the local health department if appropriate.
◆ Instruct patients who manifest an allergic response to wear a medication identification tag or bracelet listing the allergic response and to be cautious in taking vaccines or immunomodulators without consulting the physician.

Interferons

Drug administration

◆ Review the side effects listed in Table 28-5.
◆ Assess for development of side effects. Be alert to signs of depression including insomnia, weight loss, withdrawal, anorexia, and lack of interest in personal appearance.
◆ Monitor pulse and blood pressure. Auscultate lung and heart sounds. Monitor intake, output, and weight.
◆ Monitor hematocrit or hemoglobin level, platelet count, white blood cell differential, and liver function tests.
◆ Keep patients well hydrated to lessen symptoms from hypotension.

Patient and family education

◆ Review anticipated benefits and possible side effects of drug therapy.
◆ Review the dosing schedule, and discuss with patients what to do if a dose is missed, if they are self-administering these drugs. Make certain they can inject the dose correctly.
◆ Warn patients to avoid driving or operating hazardous equipment if fatigue or dizziness develops.
◆ These drugs often cause a flulike reaction, with fever, chills, and headache. Consult the physician about appropriate instructions for the patient related to notifying the physician and self-medicating with antipyretics.
◆ Do not change to other brands of interferon without consulting the physician.
◆ Avoid other drugs that may also cause drowsiness or fatigue, unless specifically approved by the physician; this includes alcohol.
◆ Review Patient Problems: Depressed White Blood Cell Count on p. 560 and Bleeding Tendencies on p. 570.
◆ Take doses at night to lessen daytime fatigue.

Interleukins

◆ Review the information given in Table 28-5 for interferons.
◆ Monitor weight, and assess for edema. Monitor blood pressure.
◆ Consult manufacturer's literature for current guidelines.

Colony Stimulating Factors

◆ Review side effects.
◆ Assess for fluid retention, and monitor weight.
◆ Auscultate lung sounds. Monitor blood pressure.
◆ Tell patients receiving GM-CSF that fever, chills, headache, nausea and vomiting, weakness, and fatigue may occur. If persistent or severe, notify the physician.
◆ Review insert supplied by manufacturer.

Glucocorticoids

◆ See Chapter 51.

Antilymphocyte Globulin

Drug administration

◆ Assess blood pressure, temperature, and pulse. Inspect for skin changes.
◆ Monitor complete blood count and differential.
◆ See manufacturer's literature for current guidelines.

Patient and family education

◆ Review anticipated benefits and possible side effects of drug therapy. Note that serum sickness may develop. Teach patients that serum sickness may not develop for up to 10 to 14 days after drug therapy.
◆ See Patient Problems: Depressed White Blood Cell Count on p. 560 and Bleeding Tendencies on p. 570.

Continued.

Antithymocyte Globulin

Drug administration

◆ Monitor blood pressure and pulse. Auscultate lung sounds. Assess for jugular venous distention. Monitor intake, output, and weight, and inspect for skin changes.

◆ Monitor complete blood count and differential, platelet count, blood glucose level, and serum electrolyte level.

◆ Thrombophlebitis is common. Assess the IV line for patency before administering. Instruct the patient to report pain or redness at the IV site.

◆ Fistulas or shunts may clot in some patients. Assess fistulas or shunts according to agency procedure (through palpation or auscultation) at least every 2 hr while the patient is receiving this drug. If the patient knows how to assess shunts or fistulas, engage the patient in monitoring also.

◆ Since this drug may cause allergic reaction, monitor patients closely, and have available drugs, equipment, and personnel to treat allergic reaction.

Patient and family education

◆ Review anticipated benefits and possible side effects of drug therapy. Note that serum sickness may develop. Teach patients that serum sickness may not develop for up to 10 to 14 days after drug therapy.

◆ Instruct diabetic patients to monitor blood glucose levels carefully, since antithymocyte globulin may cause changes in blood glucose levels.

◆ See Patient Problems: Decreased White Blood Cell Count on p. 560 and Bleeding Tendencies on p. 570.

Muromonab-CD3

◆ Monitor blood pressure and pulse. Remain with the patient for 15 to 30 min after the first dose. Chest pain may follow the first dose but is rare thereafter.

◆ Assess for side effects that commonly occur such as fever, chills, dyspnea, wheezing, nausea, vomiting, tremor, headache, and tachycardia.

◆ Forewarn the patients that trembling and shaking of the hands after the first dose is common.

◆ Monitor intake, output, and weight. Auscultate breath sounds.

◆ See manufacturer's literature for current guidelines.

Azathioprine

Drug administration

◆ Wear gloves, and prepare doses in laminar flow hoods to avoid inadvertent contamination with drug.

◆ Monitor intake, output, and weight. Assess for skin changes.

◆ Monitor complete blood count and differential, platelet count, and liver function tests.

◆ Assess for signs of hepatitis including right upper quadrant abdominal pain, jaundice, fever, malaise, nausea, vomiting, and anorexia. Tell patients to report these signs and symptoms if they develop.

INTRAVENOUS ADMINISTRATION

◆ Reconstitute as directed on the vial. Administer correctly diluted solution over 30 to 60 min.

Patient and family education

◆ Review the benefits and possible side effects of drug therapy.

◆ Tell patients that weeks to months of therapy with this drug may be necessary for full benefit.

◆ Warn patients that serum sickness may occur but may not develop for 10 to 14 days after taking a dose.

◆ See Patient Problems: Decreased White Blood Cell Count on p. 560, Bleeding Tendencies on p. 570, and Stomatitis on p. 561

◆ Take oral doses after meals to lessen gastric irritation.

◆ Avoid having immunizations while taking this drug, unless approved by the physician.

Cyclosporine

Drug administration

◆ See information on side effects.

◆ Monitor blood pressure and pulse. Monitor intake, output, and weight. Inspect teeth and gums regularly.

◆ Monitor complete blood count and differential, liver function tests, and BUN and serum creatinine levels.

NURSING IMPLICATIONS SUMMARY—cont'd

◆ Review manufacturer's instructions when preparing oral doses, since doses must be measured with a dropper, then diluted in a glass container.

INTRAVENOUS ADMINISTRATION

◆ Review manufacturer's instructions regarding preparation. Infuse properly diluted doses over 2 to 6 hr. Monitor vital signs.

Patient and family education

◆ Review the anticipated benefits and possible side effects of drug therapy.

◆ Warn patients that tremor may develop.
◆ Warn patients to avoid driving or operating hazardous equipment if confusion develops; notify the physician.
◆ Instruct patients not to stop therapy without consulting the physician.
◆ Reinforce the importance of regular dental hygiene including flossing, brushing, and visiting the dentist.
◆ Avoid immunizations while taking cyclosporine unless approved by the physician.

CHAPTER REVIEW

◆ **KEY TERMS**

colony stimulating factors, p. 432
immunostimulants, p. 426
immunosuppressants, p. 433
immunotoxins, p. 436
interferons, p. 429
interleukins, p. 429
vaccines, p. 426

◆ **REVIEW QUESTIONS**

1. Explain active acquired immunity and how it is achieved. How long does it last?
2. Explain passive acquired immunity and how it is achieved. How long does it last?
3. What immune protection does the fetus have?
4. What is a common side effect of immune serums? How should you assess this and teach patients about it?
5. Name a pharmacologic role for interferons and for interleukin-2?

6. What are the colony stimulating factors and in what major clinical areas are they used?
7. What are the clinical indications for immune suppressants?
8. How do corticosteroids cause immune suppression?
9. How do anticancer drugs such as cyclophosphamide or mercaptopurine produce immune suppression?
10. How do antithymocyte globulin and antilymphocyte globulin act?
11. What is the mechanism of action of muromonab-CD3?
12. What is the mechanism of action of azathioprine?
13. What is the mechanism of action of cyclosporine?
14. Name two important side effects of immunosuppressant drugs. How should you assess for these?
15. Why must live vaccines not be given to patients receiving immunosuppressant drugs?
16. What are immunotoxins? How do they act?

SUGGESTED READING

Baron S and others: The interferons: mechanisms of action and clinical applications, *JAMA,* 266(10):1375, 1991.

Benjamin, E and Leskowitz S: *Immunology: a short course*, New York, 1988, Alan R Liss.

Bertino JS and Chiarello LA: Vaccines, toxoids, and other immunobiologics, In DiPiro, JT. and others, editors, *Pharmacotherapy: a pathophysiologic approach*, New York, 1989, Elsevier.

Burlingame MB and Delafuente JC: Systemic lupus erythematosus, In DiPiro JT and others, editors, *Pharmacotherapy: a pathophysiologic approach*, New York, 1989, Elsevier.

Chaudhary VK and others: Selective killing of HIV-infected cells by recombinant human CD4-pseudomonas exotoxin hybrid protein, *Nature* 335(6188):369, 1988.

Cress NB, Owens BM, and Hill FH: ImuVert™ therapy in the treatment of recurrent malignant astrocytomas: nursing implications, *J Neurosci Nurs* 23(1):29, 1991.

Dault LA, Nagy C, and Collins JA: Reversing cardiac transplant rejection with orthoclone OKT3, *Am J Nurs* 89(7):953, 1989.

Fedric TN: Immunosuppressive therapy in renal transplantation, *Crit Care Nurse Clin North Am* 2(1):123, 1990.

Fent K and Zbinden G: Toxicity of interferon and interleukin, *Immunol Today* 8(3):100, 1987.

Jordan K: Interferon: clinical uses in nursing implications, *J Intravenous Nurs* 13(6):388, 1990.

Matas AJ and others: ALG treatment of steroid-resistant rejection in patients receiving cyclosporine, *Transplantation* 41(5):579, 1986.

Mitsuyasu RT: The enhanced potential use of recombinant alpha interferon in the treatment of AIDS-related Kaposi's sarcoma, *Oncol Nurs Forum* 16(6):5, 1989.

Moir EJ: Nursing care of patients receiving Orthocline OKT 3 ... Orthoclone OKT 3 (muromonab-CD3) is an antirejection drug, *AANA J,* 16(5):327, 1989.

Moore MAS: The clinical use of colony stimulating factors, *Annu Rev Immunol* 9:159, 1991.

Ortho Multicenter Transplant Study Group: A randomized clinical trial of OKT3 monoclonal antibody for acute rejection of cadaveric renal transplants, *N Engl J Med* 313(6):337, 1985.

Pastan I, Willingham MC, and FitzGerald DJP: Immunotoxins, *Cell* 47(5):641, 1986.

Ponticelli C and others: Clinical experience with Orthoclone OKT3 in renal transplantation, *Transplant Proc* 18(4):942, 1986.

Pezze JL and Whiteman K: FK 506: transplantation's newest weapon, *Am J Nurs* 91(10):40, 1991.

Ptachcinski RJ, Venkataramanan R and Burckart GJ: Drug therapy in transplantation, In DiPiro JT and others, editors, *Pharmacotherapy: a pathophysiologic approach*, New York, 1989, Elsevier.

ANTIINFECTIVE AND CHEMOTHERAPEUTIC AGENTS

This section discusses drugs that act as selective poisons against certain organisms or types of cells. Chapter 29, Introduction to Use of Antiinfective Agents, introduces the principle of selective toxicity that underlies all the information in the remaining chapters and focuses on the use of selective poisons to treat disease caused by bacteria or closely related microorganisms. Chapters 30 through 35 discuss specific antiinfective agents, grouping drugs into chapters on the basis of similar mechanisms of action (Chapters 30 to 32), similar toxic reactions and side effects (Chapter 33), and similar uses (Chapters 34 and 35).

Chapters 36 to 38 consider several types of drugs. Each chapter not only discusses specific drugs but also delineates the differences between therapy of diseases produced by viruses, fungi, or eucaryotic parasites from the therapy of bacterial disease.

Chapter 39, Drugs to Treat Neoplastic Diseases, presents individual antineoplastic agents and information on the nature of neoplastic disease to clarify the rationale behind the use of these agents. The mechanism of drug action is emphasized so that toxicity may be more readily understood. Understanding the mechanism of action allows the clinical properties of these drugs to be more easily appreciated and puts the nursing management into perspective.

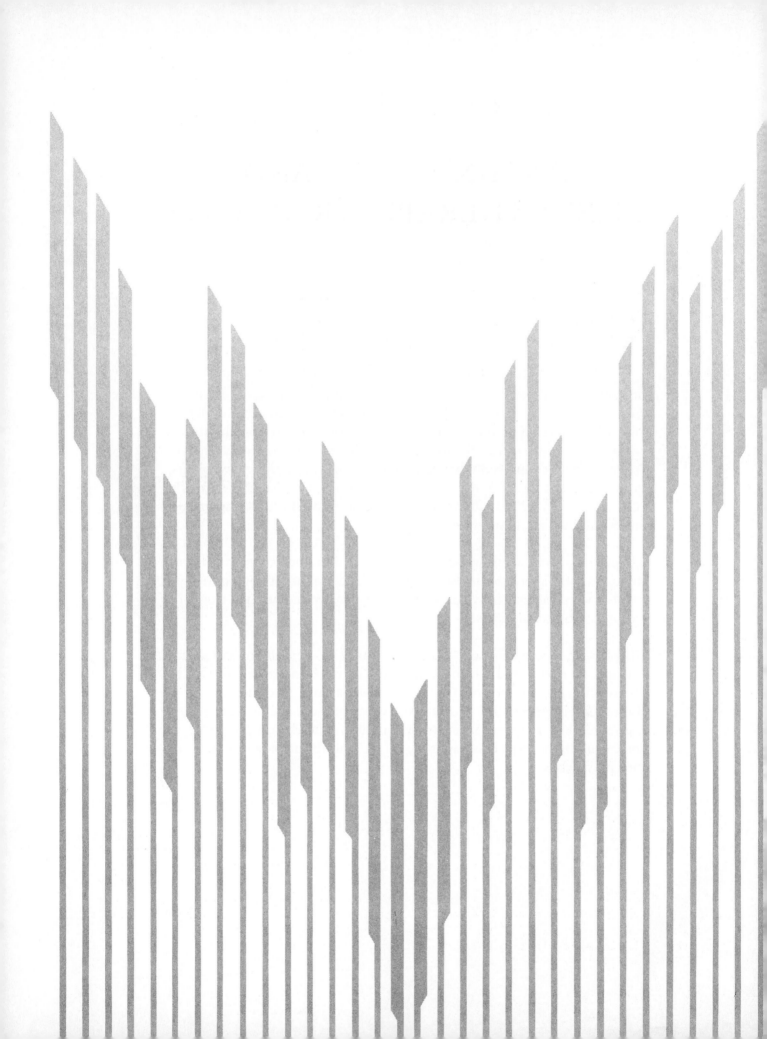

CHAPTER 29

Introduction to Use of Antiinfective Agents

LEARNING OBJECTIVES

After reading this chapter, you should be able to do the following:

- Discuss the principle of selective toxicity.
- Describe the difference between bactericidal and bacteriostatic agents.
- Discuss the influence of plasmids on antibiotic resistance.
- Describe factors that influence the outcome of antibiotic therapy.
- Explain why antibiotics should not be discontinued until the therapy prescribed is complete.
- Outline important patient teaching points relating to general use of antiinfective agents.

CHAPTER OVERVIEW

◆ Preceding chapters presented the use of drugs intended to alter processes occurring naturally in the body. For example, cardiotonic drugs alter existing patterns of ion flow in heart cells; the therapeutic goal of increasing contractility of the heart is achieved by this direct action of the drug. Similarly, a direct action on normal physiologic functions can be cited for each drug discussed previously. In contrast the drugs considered in this section ideally do not directly affect any physiologic process in the patient. The antiinfective agents may be considered selective poisons, since the goal of therapy with these drugs is to poison invading, pathogenic microorganisms without poisoning the patient.

◆ This introductory chapter presents concepts important in understanding antibiotic therapy. Microbiologic principles that make antibiotic therapy effective are reviewed, general mechanisms by which these drugs act are discussed, and major problems associated with antimicrobial therapy are presented.

Nursing Process Overview
ANTIINFECTIVE THERAPY
Assessment
Perform a complete physical assessment. Assess for fever, purulent drainage, elevation of the white blood cell count, and signs of inflammation such as redness, swelling, or tenderness. Check culture results. Monitor vital signs. Obtain history of any exposure to infecting organisms and preexisting medical conditions.

Nursing Diagnoses
Altered bowel elimination: diarrhea and cramping secondary to antiinfective use
High risk for vaginal superinfection with *Candida*

Management
Obtain additional data relevant to the antibiotic prescribed, such as renal function of liver function studies, and assessment of ototoxicity. Monitor vital signs, blood count, culture reports, and the patient's subjective and objective signs of infection. Maintain adequate nutritional and fluid intake, and use other appropriate therapies such as warm soaks, debridement of infected areas, and special wound-cleaning procedures. Use agents for patient comfort such as antipyretics for fever or bladder analgesics for bladder discomfort. Assess for side effects and for *Candida* overgrowth.

Evaluation

Before discharge, ascertain that patients can explain why and how to take the prescribed drug, why it is necessary to continue the course of therapy as prescribed, what side effects may occur and which ones warrant contacting the physician, and what symptoms indicate that the medication is not effective.

HISTORIC OVERVIEW

Although the microbial world was discovered by Anton Van Leeuwenhoek in 1676, the impact of these tiny organisms on human destiny was not appreciated until the last third of the nineteenth century. During this period, Louis Pasteur and Robert Koch, working in separate laboratories and on different microorganisms, showed that bacteria could cause human disease. After these discoveries, two subsequent developments became almost inevitable. Microbiologists and physicians began to classify human diseases in terms of the organism that produced the disease. By the early twentieth century, microorganisms that cause cholera, typhoid, bubonic plague, gonorrhea, leprosy, malaria, syphilis, and other diseases were isolated and identified.

This new knowledge put therapy of microbially induced diseases on a more rational basis. The first attempts at controlling diseases caused by microorganisms involved immunization. This approach allowed certain diseases to be prevented. However, immunization was not effective for all diseases nor effective once the disease was established. Thus chemists sought out agents that could eradicate invading pathogens in a living patient. A leader in this area was Paul Ehrlich, who in 1912 introduced salvarsan, a drug specific for syphilis. Salvarsan and a related drug, neosalvarsan, established the validity of the principle of selective toxicity. In 1935 a synthetic agent was discovered that could cure streptococcal infections, and in 1939 development was begun on an extract of culture fluid from the mold *Penicillium*. These discoveries marked the beginnings of the sulfonamides and penicillin. The search for more effective antimicrobial agents has not ceased. As subsequent chapters illustrate, that search has been extraordinarily fruitful.

MICROBIOLOGIC BASIS FOR ANTIINFECTIVE AGENTS

Many similarities exist in the chemical processes all life forms. Deoxyribonucleic and ribonucleic acids (DNA and RNA) carry the genetic information for all living things, and all use the same code to translate DNA and RNA into proteins. Proteins, or enzymes, carry out all the metabolic transformations required for life.

Some important differences in chemical or molecular organization exist among living things. Based on these differences, life forms are divided into two categories: procaryotes and eucaryotes. **Procaryotic cells** have genetic material that exists free within the cell protoplasm, whereas **eucaryotic cells** have membrane-bounded nuclei that contain the genetic material. Other distinguishing characteristics exist. For example, procaryotes possess cell walls composed in part of peptidoglycan, a complex molecule containing amino acids and sugars. Eucaryotic cells from multicelled organisms usually have no cell wall but only a cell membrane. Single-celled eucaryotic organisms such as algae and fungi may possess complex, rigid cell walls, but these walls do not contain peptidoglycan.

Procaryotes and eucaryotes also differ in certain internal functions. For example, ribosomes in eucaryotes are larger than those in procaryotes, and the two forms differ in their response to certain chemicals (see Chapters 31 to 33). Likewise, folic acid metabolism may differ. Many procaryotes cannot use folic acid from the environment but must synthesize the vitamin from simpler starting materials. In contrast, eucaryotes cannot synthesize folic acid but must absorb it from the diet.

The structural and metabolic differences in procaryotes and eucaryotes form the basis for selective toxicity. **Selective toxicity** is the selective poisoning of an invading, disease-causing organism by means of an agent that has no effect on the person in whom the disease exists.

An ideal antimicrobial agent would have no effect on the patient's tissue but would destroy the pathogens causing disease. However, no drug yet approaches that ideal, and every antiinfective agent causes some direct effect on the host. We must therefore consider some way to evaluate the degree of selective toxicity that may be achieved with a drug. One way to do this is by means of the therapeutic index (TI) (see Chapter 1). The **therapeutic index** is the ratio of the dose of a certain drug that kills 50% of the test animals to the dose of that drug that is effective in 50% of the animals (TI = LD50/ED50). A drug that is relatively nontoxic may be given in very large doses before it kills animals. If the drug is also potent, it may require small doses to achieve the desired clinical effect, which in this case is to cure the infection. Such a drug would have a large TI and would be considered to display good selective toxicity: it attacks the pathogen at doses well below those that are dangerous to the host. In contrast a drug with low TI would not have good selective toxicity. A drug with a TI of 1 would be equally toxic to the bacteria and to the patient.

The TI is derived from studies performed on laboratory animals. Since correlating animal studies with the clinical effectiveness of a drug is sometimes difficult, other indices of selective toxicity have been used to indicate clinical experience with a drug. For example, the safety margin of a drug is the percentage increase above the standard therapeutic dose that is required to produce serious toxic reactions in a certain percentage of patients. This evaluation is based entirely on clinical experience. A drug with a large TI and a wide safety margin may be given to patients in larger than normal doses without causing significant toxicity in most patients. To illustrate this principle, consider the antibiotics gentamicin and penicillin G. Gentamicin must be given in carefully controlled doses because it can damage the kidneys if the concentration in the bloodstream becomes too high. Gentamicin has a low TI and a narrow safety margin. Increasing the dose by 50% may cause significant toxicity (see Chapter 33). In contrast, penicillin G, which was the first clinically useful penicillin, has a very wide safety margin and a high TI. Direct toxicity with this drug is low, and doses 3 or 4 times the standard dose may be administered with little risk of toxic reactions in most patients (see Chapter 30).

HOW ANTIBIOTICS ACHIEVE SELECTIVE TOXICITY

Most antibiotics act on microorganisms in one of the following five ways: they inhibit cell wall formation, block protein synthesis, disrupt cell membranes, interfere with nucleic acid synthesis, or prevent synthesis of folic acid. Each mechanism of action exploits a biochemical difference between eucaryotic and procaryotic cells.

In addition to categorizing antibiotics by specific mechanisms, they may be broadly categorized as bacteriostatic or bactericidal drugs. **Bactericidal drugs** directly kill bacterial cells. For example, several antibiotics, by interfering with cell wall synthesis, may cause the bacterial cell to explode, since the osmotic forces generated within the cytoplasm can no longer be contained by the defective cell wall. Likewise, antibiotics that disrupt the bacterial cell membrane allow the cytoplasmic contents of the cell to leak out, and the cell dies.

Bacteriostatic drugs may not directly kill the bacterial cell but rather halt the cell's growth and reproduction. With bacteriostatic drugs, bacteria removed from exposure to the drug can resume growth. These drugs do not directly cause death of the bacteria. The host's immune system must attack, immobilize, and eliminate the pathogens for therapy with bacteriostatic drugs to achieve a long-term cure. In theory, cures can be effected with bactericidal drugs independent of the immune system. Such cures are not easily achieved; any cure of bacterial disease in normal persons depends strongly on immunologic factors. In immunosuppressed patients, cures of bacterial infections are much more difficult to achieve, even with appropriately prescribed bactericidal drugs.

To classify a drug as exclusively bactericidal or bacteriostatic is misleading. Many antibiotics are bacteriostatic or bactericidal depending on dose, site of infection, and the causative organism. For example, consider sulfonamides, which prevent folic-acid synthesis in sensitive bacteria. These drugs might be considered bacteriostatic for a systemic infection but, because of the high drug concentration in urine, may be bactericidal in urine. Other examples are cases in which two types of microorganisms differ greatly in sensitivity to a certain antibiotic. For the more sensitive organism, the serum and tissue levels achievable with normal dosage may be sufficient for bactericidal action, whereas the more resistant organism may sim-

Table 29-1 Microbial Pathogens of Humans

Organisms	Common diseases produced
VIRUSES	
Influenza	Flu and upper respiratory tract infection
Herpes simplex	Skin, eye, and brain infections
CHLAMYDIA	Psittacosis; eye and genital infections
RICKETTSIA	Typhus, Q fever, and Rocky Mountain spotted fever
SPIROCHETES	Syphilis and yaws
EUBACTERIA, GRAM NEGATIVE	
Haemophilus	Meningitis
Escherichia	Urinary tract infections
Proteus	Urinary tract infections
Klebsiella	Urinary tract infections and pneumonia
Pseudomonas	Urinary tract infections and meningitis
Neisseria	Meningitis and gonorrhea
Salmonella	Typhoid and gastroenteritis
Shigella	Dysentery
EUBACTERIA, GRAM POSITIVE	
Staphylococcus	Soft tissue infections
Streptococcus	Upper respiratory tract infections
MYCOBACTERIA	Tuberculosis and leprosy
ACTINOMYCETES	Organ lesions and abscesses
FUNGI	
Candida	Minor skin, mild respiratory, and severe systemic infections
Cryptococcus	
Histoplasma	
Blastomyces	

ply suffer growth inhibition, a bacteriostatic effect, at that same antibiotic concentration.

The **antimicrobial spectrum** of drugs is the range of microorganisms against which the drug is effective. Table 29-1 lists common pathogenic microorganisms according to criteria established by microbiologists. A drug effective against only a few of these organisms has a narrow spectrum, such as penicillin G, which is primarily effective against gram-positive bacteria. In contrast a drug that can be used against several groups of organisms has a broad spectrum, such as tetracycline, which is effective against gram-positive and gram-negative bacteria, as well as against *Rickettsia* and *Chlamydia*.

Minimum inhibitory concentration (MIC) and **minimum bactericidal concentration (MBC)** relate to the concept of the antimicrobial spectrum. For each antibiotic and microorganism, it is possible to determine in the laboratory the amount of that drug required to halt the growth of the organism and the amount required to kill the organism. The concentrations are the lowest ones at which growth inhibition or cell death can be observed. A consideration of these figures and determination of safe blood levels for an antibiotic help determine an effective therapeutic regimen. For example, a blood concentration above the MBC is desirable, but whether that concentration can be obtained depends on the pharmacologic properties governing drug absorption and elimination and the threshold for toxicity produced by the drug in the host.

MICROBIAL RESISTANCE TO ANTIBIOTICS

Not all microorganisms are sensitive to all antibiotics. Resistance to antibiotics may be inherent or acquired. **Inherent resistance** to an antibiotic is unrelated to prior exposure of the microbe to the drug. For example, the first time a culture of *Pseudomonas aeruginosa* was exposed to penicillin G, it was resistant; penicillin resistance was an inherent quality of the microorganism.

In contrast, **acquired resistance** depends on prior exposure of the microbe to the drug. For example, when penicillin G was first tested against *Staphylococcus aureus*, the organism was extremely sensitive. If the organism was exposed to sublethal doses of the drug for long periods, however, more and more penicillin-resistant microbes began to appear. The population of a strain of *S. aureus* can be converted from penicillin sensitivity to penicillin resistance by continuous low-level exposure to the drug, which allows genetic variants displaying penicillin resistance to proliferate. This phenomenon is called *acquired resistance*. Not only can acquired resistance be demon-

strated in the laboratory, but it also occurs clinically. *S. aureus* is again a good example, since strains isolated from clinical infections during the 1940s were almost always penicillin sensitive, whereas today clinically isolated *S. aureus* strains are mainly penicillin resistant.

Plasmids are small, circular pieces of DNA found separate from the chromosome in bacteria. Many genes for antibiotic resistance reside on plasmids. Since plasmids may be rapidly passed between bacterial cells, antibiotic resistance can spread rapidly through an entire bacterial population. This mechanism for acquired resistance usually results in serious therapeutic difficulty, since resistance to several antibiotics may occur simultaneously.

The precise mechanisms by which microorganisms achieve resistance to an antibiotic may be divided into three categories. Actual destruction of the antibiotic by the microorganism usually involves enzymes that chemically alter and thereby inactivate the antibiotic. Examples of this process include penicillinase, which destroys penicillin, and the acetylase, phosphorylase, and adenylating enzymes that inactivate the aminoglycoside antibiotics.

Bacteria may also achieve antibiotic resistance by reducing the uptake of the drug into the bacterial cell. Many antibiotics freely enter and in some cases are concentrated within bacterial cells. Resistance is achieved by blocking this uptake. An example of this type of resistance is tetracyclines, which can freely enter sensitive bacteria but not resistant strains.

The third mechanism for resistance involves a mutation or an alteration in the target of the antibiotic in the microorganism. For example, erythromycin inhibits protein synthesis by binding to certain sites on the bacterial ribosome. Certain resistant microorganisms form altered ribosomes that do not bind erythromycin and are therefore resistant to its inhibitory action. Some types of streptomycin resistance may occur through similar means. A clinically important example of this type of resistance is methicillin-resistant *S. aureus*.

FACTORS AFFECTING THE OUTCOME OF ANTIBIOTIC THERAPY

In antibiotic therapy the first step is proper identification of the microorganism causing the disease. In some infections the symptoms are sufficiently clear to allow accurate diagnosis with a physical examination only. In other cases, culturing must be done to identify the organism. In some institutions, nursing personnel are trained to take specimens for culture, whereas in others laboratory personnel or physicians perform this function.

The second step in treatment is the selection of the

proper antibiotic, a process that depends on knowledge of the pathogen involved. This decision may be based entirely on clinical experience or may be aided by antibiotic sensitivity testing carried out in the microbiology laboratory on the pathogen isolated from the patient.

Even when the proper drug has been selected, several factors influence the effectiveness of therapy. One is the site of infection. For example, meningitis is difficult to treat partly because many antibiotics do not penetrate the blood-brain barrier very well, making an effective drug concentration at the infection site difficult to obtain. Similarly, many abscesses or soft tissue infections are not easily treated, since the areas of infections are poorly perfused, and many drugs do not penetrate well into these areas. Healing is frequently hastened by surgical drainage.

Other drugs the patient is receiving may influence the outcome of antibiotic therapy. Immunosuppressant drugs, for example, limit antibiotic effectiveness by depressing immune mechanisms. Large doses of glucocorticoids cause significant immunosuppression. Other specific interactions may occur and are mentioned with individual drug classes in subsequent chapters.

Finally, the patient's clinical status can alter the outcome of antibiotic therapy. In particular, renal function is important, because many available antibiotics are excreted by the kidney. If renal function is impaired, drugs eliminated through the kidney may accumulate. Likewise, hepatic disease may cause accumulation of drugs that are eliminated primarily by liver mechanisms. Patients with insufficiencies in these organ systems must be watched closely for signs of drug toxicity, which may occur at lower doses than would be expected in normal persons.

PROBLEMS IN ANTIBIOTIC THERAPY

Side Effects of Antibiotics

Direct drug toxicity is observed with many classes of antibiotics. Each antibiotic should be considered for its potential toxicity to the patient when it is administered. These direct toxic effects are frequently highly characteristic. For example, any aminoglycoside antibiotic can cause kidney damage and loss of hearing or equilibrium. When these drugs are given, patients should be observed closely for these toxic signs. Even drugs with a high therapeutic index occasionally cause direct toxic reactions such as penicillin's effects on the central nervous system. Nursing personnel should be alert to these signs. Many direct toxic reactions to antibiotics are dose dependent and would be expected to be more frequent and serious when high doses of drugs are given or when drug accumulation occurs in patients with renal or hepatic impairment.

Allergies occur frequently with several antibiotics. The penicillins can produce allergic reactions ranging from simple rashes to anaphylactic shock. Allergies occur in patients who have previously been exposed to the antibiotic, in the medical setting or in the environment. Although in theory animals intended for immediate slaughter may not be treated with antibiotics also used in humans, meat occasionally has contained sufficient quantities of antibiotics to sensitize some people who consumed the meat.

Superinfections are infections that arise during antibiotic therapy. By definition, they involve microorganisms resistant to the antibiotic originally used; thus superinfections are often serious and difficult to treat. Such infections are more common with broad-spectrum than narrow-spectrum antibiotics. This observation is based on the fact that broad-spectrum antibiotics eliminate much more of the natural bacterial flora and upset the ecologic controls that normally keep the resistant pathogens in check. With tetracyclines, for example, yeasts such as *Candida* are often involved in superinfections.

Misuse of Antibiotics

Antibiotics are often misunderstood and misused. One common misconception is that antibiotics can cure any type of infectious disease, including those caused by viruses. No effective drugs exist to treat minor viral infections such as colds. As discussed in Chapter 37, few drugs are available for use in any viral infections, and certainly none of the commonly used antibiotics are effective in viral diseases.

Many infectious diseases resolve quickly once appropriate antibiotics are administered. Thus it is tempting for patients to discontinue medication much earlier than the physician planned, namely as soon as they feel better. This practice is dangerous for several reasons. Antibiotics with bacteriostatic action inhibit growth of bacteria, but cells remain viable, at least until the immune system can eliminate them. Therefore, if therapy is discontinued too early, these organisms may again proliferate and relapse may occur. Not only does this prolong recovery, but it may also make the disease more difficult to treat. If we consider that the organisms most resistant to the drugs being used are the ones that probably survive longest, we can appreciate that these resistant organisms may cause the relapse. Therapy may therefore be difficult, because some degree of drug resistance has occurred.

One excuse frequently given when patients discontinue antibiotic therapy early is that they wish to have the medication on hand in case they ever need it again. This practice is dangerous not only for the reasons just discussed but also because it assumes that patients can diagnose future illnesses accurately. Self-medication with old, unused antibiotic prescriptions may delay proper medical attention and prolong or worsen the patient's disease. Once medication has been started, culture results become relatively unreliable and proper diagnosis may be impossible. Thus patients should be discouraged from saving previously prescribed antibiotics to take them "just until I can get to the doctor."

Many drugs require special storage conditions and do not remain active for long when exposed to the warm, humid environment of most bathroom medicine cabinets. Drugs stored for weeks or months under such conditions may be inactive or may convert to forms that are more toxic. Penicillin in solution tends to form polymers that have been implicated in increased incidence of anaphylactic episodes. Tetracyclines tend to be light-sensitive and break down to toxic compounds.

Any drug that remains in the household may be a hazard to children. Proper use and disposal of drugs is important to protect children from accidental poisoning. In addition, young children may be much more sensitive to certain antibiotics than adults. Antibiotics should never be given to children without first consulting a physician.

NURSING IMPLICATIONS SUMMARY

Antiinfective Agents

Drug administration

◆ Assess for history of allergy to antibiotics or antiinfectives before administering dose. Phrase questions appropriately. For example, "Are there any medicines you should not take and why?" may elicit more information than "Are you allergic to any antibiotics?" Have patients describe previous problems. A gastric upset is probably a side effect; the development of hives is probably an allergic reaction. If there is a question whether the patient is allergic to a medication, consult the physician before administering the dose.

◆ Label the patient's health record, chart, medication kardex, and armband (per agency procedure) if the patient is allergic to any medications. In some hospitals, patients with allergies wear a second specially marked or colored identification bracelet indicating allergies.

◆ Observed all patients receiving antiinfective agents for possible allergic reactions. Monitor vital signs. Have available equipment and personnel to treat acute allergic reactions. Have drugs available to treat allergic reactions such as epinephrine, antihistamines, and steroids.

◆ Nurses who are allergic to any antiinfective agent should wear gloves when preparing or administering doses of that drug.

◆ Read orders and labels carefully. Within a class of antiinfectives, there may be several drugs with similar names.

◆ Reconstitute parenteral forms as directed by the label or in the manufacturer's literature. Date and initial the vial if some of the drug will be saved for later use. Do not use undated reconstituted medications. Observe expiration dates.

◆ For IM administration, use large muscle masses (see Chapter 6). Aspirate before administering to prevent inadvertent IV administration. Record and rotate injection sites. If the ordered dose is a large volume of medication, divide the dose and administer in two injections.

Patient and family education

◆ Review anticipated benefits and possible side effects of drug therapy with the patient. Instruct patients to report the development of any unexpected sign or symptom.

◆ Encourage patients with a known allergy to any drug to wear a medical identification tag or bracelet indicating allergies.

◆ Instruct patients to take antiinfective agents for as long as prescribed (usually 1 week to 10 days), even if they begin to feel better. Do not share drugs with other family members. Do not save remaining doses to treat later infections.

◆ Antiinfectives work best when taken at evenly spaced intervals throughout the day. Discuss with patients an appropriate dosing schedule based on the prescribed drug frequency.

◆ Tell pregnant or lactating women not to take any antiinfective agents without consulting the physician.

◆ Shake suspensions thoroughly before pouring dose. Use the same spoon or same size medicine cup to ensure the same dosage each time.

◆ Some oral liquids are dispensed in bottles with droppers, although the medicine is to be taken orally.

◆ Patients should chew and swallow chewable tablets for best effect.

NURSING IMPLICATIONS SUMMARY—cont'd

◆ Tell patients to swallow enteric-coated preparations whole, without crushing or chewing. Consult the pharmacist if in doubt.

◆ Review with patients any restrictions about taking the drug with meals, milk, or a snack and special storage considerations such as refrigeration. Pharmacists usually label drugs that must be refrigerated.

◆ If a dose is missed, tell patients to take it as soon as remembered, unless close to the next dose, in which case the forgotten dose should be omitted. Exact guidelines vary, depending on the frequency of doses. Do not double up for missed doses.

◆ Remind parents to keep drugs out of the reach of children. Pediatric dosage forms are often disguised in pleasant-tasting syrups and diluents, and children may want to take more than ordered doses. Tell parents to give children only drugs and doses prescribed for children.

◆ Instruct patients to keep all health-care providers informed of all drugs being taken. Review all drugs a patient is taking. If questions about drug incompatibilities arise, consult the physician or pharmacist.

CHAPTER REVIEW

◆ KEY TERMS

acquired resistance, p. 446

antimicrobial spectrum, p. 446

bactericidal drugs, p. 445

bacteriostatic drugs, p. 445

eucaryotic cells, p. 444

inherent resistance, p. 446

minimum bactericidal concentration (MBC), p. 446

minimum inhibitory concentration (MIC), p. 446

plasmids, p. 446

procaryotic cells, p. 444

selective toxicity, p. 444

superinfections, p. 447

therapeutic index (TI), p. 444

◆ REVIEW QUESTIONS

1. What is the principle of selective toxicity?
2. Why is selective toxicity possible to achieve?
3. How is selective toxicity achieved? How is it measured?
4. What is the difference between a bacteriostatic and a bactericidal drug?
5. What is the antimicrobial spectrum of a drug?
6. Define minimum inhibitory concentration (MIC) and minimum bactericidal concentration (MBC).
7. What is the difference between inherent and acquired resistance?

8. What are the three types of mechanisms by which microorganisms become resistant to antibiotics?
9. Name five factors that influence the outcome of antibiotic therapy.
10. What are three general types of problems that may arise during antibiotic therapy? How would you assess for superinfections?
11. What are some of the common misuses of antibiotics? What should you teach patients to help avoid these problems?
12. What are the dangers associated with premature cessation of antibiotic therapy? What would you teach patients about this problem?
13. What two dangers are associated with saving leftover antibiotics in the home?

SUGGESTED READING

Farrington E: Pediatric drug information . . . recommended concentration of antibiotics for intravenous administration, *Pediatr Nurs* 16(3):310, 1990.

Gleckman RA, Czachor JS: Reviewing the safe use of antibiotics in the elderly, *Geriatrics* 44(7):33, 1989.

Kirby DF: Antibiotic prophylaxis: the who, when, where, why and with what! *Gastroenterol Nurs* 13(1):9, 1990.

Ma M: Brush up on antibacterial agents, *Nurs 89* 19(1):76, 1989.

Rowland MA: When drug therapy causes diarrhea, *RN* 52(12):32, 1989.

Walters JE: How antibiotics work: nucleic acid synthesis, *Prof Nurs* 5(12):641, 1990.

Wilkowske CJ: General principles of antimicrobial therapy, *Mayo Clin Proc* 66(9):931, 1991.

CHAPTER 30

Penicillins, Cephalosporins, and Related Drugs

LEARNING OBJECTIVES

After studying this chapter, you should be able to do the following:

- Explain the specific antibacterial effect of penicillins and cephalosporins.
- Describe the classes of penicillins.
- Explain the mechanism of resistance bacteria develop to penicillins and cephalosporins.
- Describe the most common reaction to penicillins.
- Describe the most common reactions to cephalosporins, aztreonam, and imipenem.
- Develop a nursing care plan for a patient receiving one of the drugs discussed in this chapter.

CHAPTER OVERVIEW

◆ This chapter introduces the most widely used family of antibiotics in medical practice today, the **beta-lactam antibiotics**, of which penicillins and cephalosporins are the most important representatives. We first discuss the properties common to all members of this family of antibiotics and then consider the features of individual agents.

Nursing Process Overview
PENICILLINS, CEPHALOSPORINS, AND RELATED DRUGS

See Chapter 29 for general guidelines.

Assessment

Assess patients, and monitor for clinical signs of infection. Pay special attention to subjective data suggesting the patient has a history of allergy to penicillins or to related drugs. Monitor renal function.

Nursing Diagnoses

Possible complication: allergic reaction
Possible complication: gastrointestinal (GI) distress

Management

Observe patients closely for possible allergic response for 20 to 30 min after the first dose is administered. Have available drugs and equipment for resuscitation. In preparation for discharge, review with pa-

tients the need to take the prescribed drug for the full course of therapy and to try to space doses evenly throughout the 24-hr day.

Evaluation

These drugs seldom cause long-term side effects. Before discharge, ascertain that patients can judge improvement in the infection and describe possible side effects and situations that warrant consulting the physician.

PROPERTIES COMMON TO ALL PENICILLINS AND CEPHALOSPORINS
Mechanism of Action and Bacterial Resistance

Pencillins and cephalosporins are irreversible inhibitors of a bacterial enzyme called *transpeptidase*. This enzyme cross-links parallel strands of cell wall material called *peptidoglycan*. When cross-linking occurs, peptidoglycan becomes rigid and is an effective cell wall. When cross-linking is blocked by penicillin or cephalosporin, cell wall synthesis continues without cross-linking. Ultimately the unreinforced strands formed cannot resist the osmotic forces within the bacterial cell. The bacterium may explode. Since exposed bacteria may be directly killed, beta-lactam antibiotics are classified as *bactericidal drugs*. However, even at doses below those required to kill bacteria, penicillins and cephalosporins are effective in some circumstances. Minimum disruption of the bacterial cell wall by these drugs may make the bacterium more liable to elimination by the immune system of the host.

Penicillins and cephalosporins do not destroy existing bacterial cell wall; these drugs instead prevent formation of new, intact cell wall. Thus penicillins and cephalosporins are most effective against actively multiplying bacteria.

Resistance to penicillins and cephalosporins develops in microorganisms. The most common mechanism for resistance involves enzymes called *beta-lactamases*. These enzymes are usually referred to as *penicillinases* or *cephalosporinases*, depending on which type of drug the enzyme is most effective against. These enzymes destroy the penicillin or cephalosporin nucleus (Figure 30-1), rendering the drug inactive. Some organisms possess these enzymes as part of their normal metabolic makeup and therefore are intrinsically resistant to beta-lactam antibiotics. Other organisms may acquire the enzyme and thus be converted from antibiotic sensitivity to resistance. Clinically important examples of acquired penicillin resistance are *Staphylococcus aureus* and *Neisseria gonorrhoeae*. Although 25 years ago both organisms could routinely be considered sensitive to penicillin G, today significant resistance to penicillin G exists for both organisms. In some hospitals, more that 90% of *S. aureus* strains are resistant.

Though resistance to penicillins is most commonly acquired by developing beta-lactamase, other important forms of resistance are known. The most clinically relevant example may be methicillin-resistant *S. aureus* (MRSA). In this organism, resistance is conferred by altered penicillin targets.

Excretion

Penicillins, except nafcillin, and most cephalosporins are excreted by the kidney, primarily by active secretion. Exceptions are cefotaxime and ceftriaxone, which are metabolized by the liver, and cefoperazone, which is excreted in bile.

Toxicity of Penicillins and Cephalosporins

Allergies are the most common adverse reaction to the penicillins. Many patients experience skin rashes or urticaria, but anaphylaxis is a much more dangerous allergic response. Whereas allergic rashes and

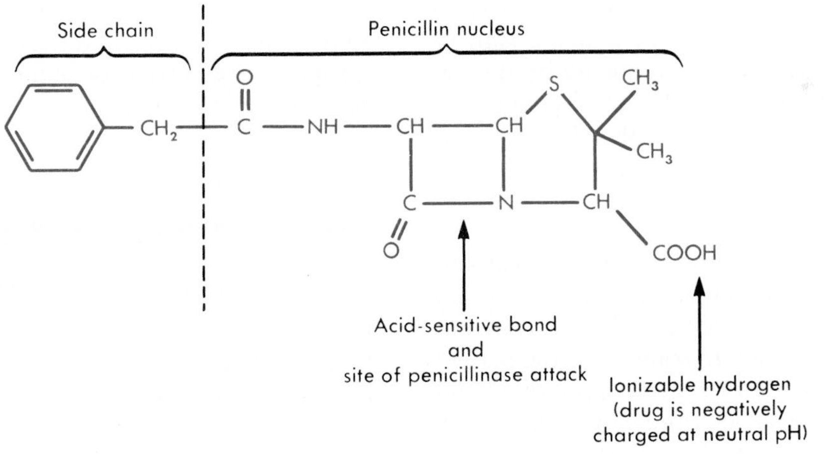

FIGURE 30-1

Structure of penicillin G. All penicillin antibiotics contain the penicillin nucleus shown. Chemical disruption of the nucleus, such as that produced by acid or penicillinase, results in loss of antibiotic activity. Ionizable hydrogen may be replaced with sodium or potassium ion without affecting drug activity. Alterations of side chain of penicillin affect acid stability, penicillinase resistance, and antimicrobial spectrum of drug. Penicillins used clinically differ in their side-chain structures. Cephalosporins contain a slightly different nucleus and side chains than penicillins.

drug fevers usually appear after several days of therapy, the onset of anaphylaxis is nearly always within 10 min. Injections of penicillin are responsible for most anaphylactic episodes, but any form of exposure to penicillin may produce anaphylaxis in sensitive individuals.

A patient beginning penicillin therapy should remain under medical supervision for 30 min after a penicillin injection so that if anaphylaxis develops, help is immediately available. If anaphylaxis occurs, medical personnel first should administer subcutaneous epinephrine. Anaphylaxis involves profound vasomotor collapse, and laryngeal edema may further complicate resuscitation efforts. Steroids may be required, as well as a tracheostomy and oxygen under positive pressure. All these emergency supplies should be on hand in any clinical setting where antibiotics are administered.

Some physicians perform a skin test before administering penicillins to try to identify allergic patients. An estimated 3% to 5% of the population is allergic to penicillin; about 10% of those who have previously received penicillin in a medical setting may be allergic. Patients about to receive penicillin must be asked if they have ever been given penicillin before and if they have ever had a rash or other allergic symptom during penicillin therapy. This information, although necessary, is somewhat unreliable, because many patients who report past allergy to penicillin do not experience allergic reactions when reexposed. This may be because the original reaction was not a true penicillin allergy. Ampicillin, for example, may cause a benign macular eruption rather than a urticarial reaction. This toxic rash is not a sign of allergy but may be reported as an allergy by the patient. Another explanation for apparent changes in sensitivity to penicillins is that some patients are allergic to contaminants present in early penicillin preparations but absent from the more purified modern preparations.

Some patients who report no previous allergies to penicillin and some who claim never to have received penicillin may still experience an allergic response when they receive the drug. In some cases the patient might be unaware of what drug was prescribed and thus may not be a reliable source. Although rare, some persons have become sensitized by being exposed to penicillin in the environment or in the food chain. For example, animals destined for human food use can be treated with penicillins by the feed lot owner, although sufficient time should be allowed before slaughter so that the drug can be removed from the animal's system.

Cephalosporins are good allergens much like penicillins, and many patients suffer allergic reactions to the drugs. Rashes are most common, but anaphylaxis is possible. Many patients who are allergic to penicillins are also allergic to cephalosporins and vice versa.

Direct drug toxicity with penicillin is low; massive doses have been given with no ill effects. The tissue most sensitive to direct effects is the central nervous system (CNS). Intrathecal injection (into the subarachnoid space or cerebrospinal fluid) may produce convulsions. Convulsions also occur occasionally in patients given high doses intramuscularly or intravenously, especially if some renal impairment occurs and the drug accumulates. A relatively high concentration in the cerebrospinal fluid must be achieved before convulsions occur. This complication could occur in an elderly patient being treated for a serious infection such as streptococcal endocarditis. This patient may receive 25 to 40 million units of penicillin daily to maintain continuous bactericidal drug concentrations. Whereas normal persons can readily eliminate these large amounts through their kidneys, elderly persons may have diminished renal function (see box). Therefore drug accumulation may occur, and penicillin may enter the CNS. The first sign may be loss of consciousness or myoclonic movements. Generalized seizures may follow.

Another group of patients with reduced ability to excrete penicillin are newborn infants. Because of this, neonates receive carefully adjusted penicillin doses based on their body weight and reduced clearance of penicillin.

Cephalosporins also are excreted primarily by the kidney and, as with the penicillins, may accumulate in patients with impaired renal function. Hence cephalosporin dosage may be reduced when renal function is lower than normal.

GERIATRIC CONSIDERATION: PENICILLINS AND CEPHALOSPORINS

THE PROBLEM

Most beta-lactam antibiotics are excreted primarily through the kidneys, with biliary excretion as an alternative route. If renal function is impaired, excretion may be slowed, and the drug can accumulate. Healthy geriatric patients may have significantly lower renal function than younger adults and may need to be considered as renally impaired.

SOLUTIONS

When administering these drugs to elderly patients, it is important to monitor renal function. Adjust doses for renal function as prescribed or as described in the package insert.

Oral penicillin preparations cause GI distress in some patients. Reactions include irritation and inflammation of the upper GI tract, nausea, vomiting, and diarrhea. Orally administered cephalosporins also cause gastric irritation, nausea, and vomiting.

Several penicillin and cephalosporin preparations contain sufficient sodium or potassium to alter electrolyte balance in some patients. For example, 1 million units of penicillin G and penicillin V may contain 1.5 mEq of potassium. Given in high enough doses for long enough periods, potassium intoxication and cardiac arrhythmias may occur. Carbenicillin and some preparations of penicillin G contain high concentrations of sodium, which may cause difficulties in patients with preexisting cardiac or renal dysfunction.

Penicillins and cephalosporins require care in handling and diluting for intramuscular (IM) or intravenous (IV) therapy. Many penicillins require properly buffered solutions for best stability, and thus not all are compatible with common IV fluids. Check the package insert or ask the pharmacist before adding penicillins or cephalosporins to any IV fluid.

Probenecid is sometimes used with penicillins to increase their effective duration of action by slowing excretion in the kidney. Probenecid may cause toxic reactions that are difficult to distinguish from a penicillin reaction. For example, probenecid may produce chills, fever, rash, GI irritation, and anemia. Probenecid also blocks renal excretion of some cephalosporins.

PENICILLINS
Penicillin G

Absorption

Penicillin G was the first penicillin adopted for widespread clinical use. This drug is one of several natural penicillins, formed spontaneously by the *Penicillium* mold and released into the culture fluid. Of these naturally occurring compounds, penicillin G has the most potent antibacterial action. The structure of penicillin G differs from the other penicillins only in the side chain (see Figure 30-1). The penicillin nucleus is found in all clinically useful penicillins.

The penicillin nucleus must remain intact to retain antibacterial activity. At least one bond in the nucleus is sensitive to acid, which explains the lability of penicillin G in the stomach (see Figure 30-1). Approximately 30% of an orally administered dose is absorbed, the rest being destroyed in the stomach or retained in the intestine and destroyed by bacteria in the large bowel. Because of the incomplete and somewhat variable absorption of penicillin G by this route, oral doses of penicillin G are not recommended.

Penicillin G is rapidly and completely absorbed after IM injection (Figure 30-2). Serum concentrations reach a peak 20 to 30 min after injection. This peak concentration persists for only a short time, primarily because the kidney so efficiently removes penicillin from the bloodstream. Within 2 to 3 hr after IM injection, about 60% of the penicillin dose appears in urine. The drug in urine is unchanged and still possesses antibacterial activity. Penicillin enters urine by active secretion in the renal tubule. This process involves a specific transport system for which several drugs may compete. Physicians may take advantage of this trait by using a drug such as probenecid to block penicillin excretion, thereby increasing peak penicillin concentration in the serum and increasing its effective duration.

Distribution

Penicillin G is generally well distributed throughout many body tissues, with high concentrations found in blood, liver, kidney, and bile. Virtually none is found in brain or cerebrospinal fluid in normal persons. If the meninges are inflamed, as in meningitis, penicillin can penetrate the CNS in significant amounts.

Uses

Penicillin G is a narrow-spectrum antibiotic; the organisms against which it is effective are summarized in Table 30-1. Most of the sensitive organisms are gram-positive bacteria. These bacteria are characterized by thick, peptidoglycan-rich cell walls, which react with the Gram's stain. Some of these gram-positive organisms such as *S. aureus*, *Streptococcus* species, and *Streptococcus pneumoniae* cause common infections of the upper respiratory tract and soft tissues, as well as more serious infections. Other rare gram-positive organisms, such as the ones that cause anthrax, gas gangrene, tetanus, and diphtheria, are also sensitive to penicillin.

Among gram-negative organisms, clinically significant sensitivity to penicillin G is seen only with *N. meningitidis* (meningococcus) and *N. gonorrhoeae* (gonococcus). Other common gram-negative organisms normally found in the bowel and those frequently responsible for urinary tract infections are clinically resistant to penicillin G. In the laboratory, some of these gram-negative bacteria can be affected by high doses of penicillin G, but these high drug levels cannot routinely be achieved in patients. Although penicillin G is not effective against common pathogens in routine urinary tract infections, it is effective against syphilis and gonorrhea. Syphilis, caused by a spirochete, and gonorrhea, caused by *N. gonorrhoeae*, are frequently treated effectively with single-dose penicillin therapy.

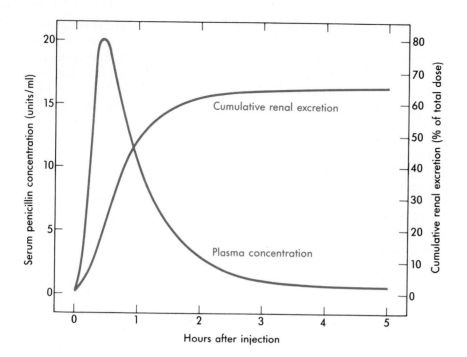

FIGURE 30-2
Serum concentration and urinary excretion of IM dose of penicillin G. Penicillin G is efficiently and rapidly absorbed after IM injections. Peak plasma concentrations of drug appear 20 to 30 min after injection. Penicillin G is actively secreted by renal tubules accounting for rapid elimination half-time of about 20 to 30 min. Most of drug dose ends up in urine as unaltered penicillin.

Table 30-1   Antimicrobial Spectrum of Penicillin G

Organism	Typical infections
GRAM-POSITIVE BACTERIA	
Streptococcus, selected strains	Upper respiratory infections, endocarditis, and bacteremia
Streptococcus pneumoniae	Abscesses, bronchitis, meningitis, pneumonia, and bacteremia
Staphylococcus aureus, nonpenicillinase	Skin and soft tissue infections, bronchitis, endocarditis, otitis, pneumonia, meningitis, and bacteremia
Bacillus anthracis	Anthrax
Corynebacterium diphtheriae	Diphtheria
Clostridium tetani	Tetanus
Clostridium perfringens	Gas gangrene
GRAM-NEGATIVE BACTERIA	
Neisseria gonorrhoeae	Gonorrhea
Neisseria meningitidis	Meningitis
SPIROCHETE	
Treponema pallidum	Syphilis

Repository Penicillins: Procaine Penicillin G and Benzathine Penicillin G

Absorption

One disadvantage of penicillin G is its short duration of action. Repository penicillins were designed to slow absorption from IM injection sites and thereby prolong the duration of action. Along with slower absorption comes a lower peak serum concentration (see Chapter 2). Once the drug is absorbed from the depot sites, it is hydrolyzed to release penicillin G, which is the active form of the drug.

The repository penicillins are procaine penicillin G and benzathine penicillin G. Procaine penicillin G reaches its peak serum concentration 3 to 4 hr after injection, and significant serum concentrations may persist for up to 48 hr. With a single dose of 300,000 units of aqueous penicillin G, peak serum levels for penicillin may reach 6 to 8 units/ml, whereas for procaine penicillin G at that same dose, the peak concentration will be only 1 to 2 units/ml. Benzathine penicillin G is absorbed even more slowly and reaches maximum concentration 8 hr after injection. This concentration decreases very slowly, and significant serum levels are observed for 2 weeks or longer. A common adult dose of 1.2 million units produces peak serum levels of only 0.1 to 0.3 units/ml (Table 30-2).

Table 30-2 Common Dosages of Representative Penicillins

Generic name	Trade name	Administration/dosage
BIOSYNTHESIZED PENICILLINS		
Penicillin G	Crystapen† Megacillin† Pentids Pfizerpen	ORAL: *Adults*—200,000 to 500,000 units every 6 to 8 hr administered ½ hr before or 2 hr after meals. *Children*—25,000 to 90,000 units/kg body weight daily in 3 to 6 doses. INTRAMUSCULAR: *Adults*—1 million to 5 million units daily in divided doses. *Children*—50,000 to 250,000 units/kg body weight daily divided among 6 doses. INTRAVENOUS: *Adults and children*—same as for IM. Higher doses have been used for severe infections.
Penicillin V	Pen-Vee-K V-Cillin K* Veetids	ORAL: *Adults*—125 to 500 mg every 4 to 6 hr. *Children*—25 to 50 mg/kg body weight daily in divided doses.
REPOSITORY PENICILLINS		
Benzathine penicillin G	Bicillin* Megacillin†	ORAL: *Adults*—400,000 to 600,000 units (base) every 4 to 6 hr. *Children*—25,000 to 90,000 units/kg daily, divided into 3, 4, or 6 doses. INTRAMUSCULAR: *Adults*—600,000 to 1.2 million units every 2 to 4 weeks. *Children*—50,000 units/kg body weight once.
Procaine penicillin G	Crysticillin Duracillin A.S. Wycillin*	INTRAMUSCULAR: *Adults and children*—600,000 to 1.2 million units every 12 to 24 hr. For uncomplicated gonorrhea, 4.8 million units in 1 dose divided between two sites. *Infants*—50,000 units/kg body weight once daily.
PENICILLINASE-RESISTANT PENICILLINS		
Cloxacillin	Orbenin† Tegopen	ORAL: *Adults*—0.25 to 1 gm every 4 to 6 hr. *Infants*—25 to 50 mg/kg body weight daily divided into 4 doses. Administer 1 hr before or 2 hr after meals.
Dicloxacillin	Dycill Dynapen* Pathocil*	ORAL: *Adults*—0.125 to 1 gm every 4 to 6 hr. *Children*—12.5 to 25 mg/kg body weight daily divided into 4 doses. Administer 1 hr before or 2 hr after meals.
Methicillin	Staphcillin	INTRAMUSCULAR: *Adults*—1 gm every 4 to 6 hr. *Children*—100 to 200 mg/kg body weight daily divided into 4 to 6 doses. INTRAVENOUS: *Adults*—1 to 2 gm diluted into 50 ml sodium chloride injection USP injected at a rate of 10 ml/min every 4 to 6 hr. *Children*—same as for IM.
Nafcillin	Nafcil Nallpen Unipen*	ORAL: *Adults*—0.25 to 1 gm every 4 to 6 hr. *Children*—50 to 100 mg/kg body weight daily divided into 4 doses. *Neonates*—30 to 40 mg/kg body weight daily divided into 3 or 4 doses. INTRAMUSCULAR: *Adults*—500 mg every 4 to 6 hr. *Children*—40 to 100 mg/kg body weight daily divided into 4 doses. INTRAVENOUS: *Adults*—0.5 to 1 gm every 4 hr. *Children*—150 mg/kg body weight daily divided into 4 doses.
Oxacillin	Bactocill Prostaphlin	ORAL: *Adults*—0.5 to 1 gm every 4 to 6 hr. *Children*—50 to 100 mg/kg body weight daily divided into 4 doses. Administer 1 hr before or 2 hr after meals. INTRAMUSCULAR: *Adults*—0.25 to 2 gm every 4 to 6 hr. *Children*—50 to 100 mg/kg body weight daily divided into 4 to 6 doses. INTRAVENOUS: *Adults*—same as for IM. The drug should be diluted to 20 mg/ml or less before injection.
EXTENDED SPECTRUM PENICILLINS		
Amoxicillin	Amoxil* Polymox	ORAL: *Adults*—250 to 500 mg every 8 hr. *Infants and children 8 to 20 kg*—20 to 40 mg/kg body weight daily divided into 3 doses.
Amoxicillin + K clavulanate	Augmentin Clavulin†	ORAL: *Adults*—250 or 500 mg amoxicillin + 125 mg K clavulanate every 8 hr. FDA Pregnancy Category B. *Infants*—amoxicillin 20 to 40 mg/kg body weight + 5 to 10 mg K clavulanate daily divided into 3 doses.

*Available in Canada and United States.
†Available in Canada only.

Continued.

Table 30-2   Common Dosages of Representative Penicillins—cont'd

Generic name	Trade name	Administration/dosage
EXTENDED SPECTRUM PENICILLINS—cont'd		
Ampicillin	Ampicin† Omnipen Penbritin† Polycillin Principen Totacillin	ORAL: *Adults*—250 to 500 mg every 6 hr. *Infants*—50 to 100 mg/kg body weight daily divided into 4 doses. INTRAMUSCULAR: *Adults*—same as for oral. *Infants*—100 to 200 mg/kg body weight daily divided into 4 doses. INTRAVENOUS: *Adults*—same as for oral. *Infants*—same as for IM. Higher doses have been administered for serious infections.
Ampicillin + sulbactam	Unasyn	INTRAMUSCULAR, INTRAVENOUS: *Adults*—1 to 2 gm ampicillin and 0.5 to 1 gm sulbactam every 6 hr. FDA Pregnancy Category B.
Bacampicillin	Penglobe† Spectrobid	ORAL: *Adults*—400 to 800 mg every 12 hr (400 mg bacampacillin = 280 mg ampicillin). FDA Pregnancy Category B. *Children*—25 mg/kg every 12 hr.
Cyclacillin	Cyclacillin	ORAL: *Adults*—250 to 500 mg every 6 hr. *Children*—125 to 250 mg every 8 hr.
ANTI-*PSEUDOMONAS* PENICILLINS		
Azlocillin	Azlin	INTRAVENOUS: *Adults*—3 gm every 4 hr or 4 gm every 6 hr by slow injection. Up to 24 gm may be given daily for life-threatening infections. FDA Pregnancy Category B.
Carbenicillin	Geocillin Geopen* Pyopen†	INTRAMUSCULAR: *Adults*—1 to 2 gm every 6 hr. Doses increased for life-threatening infections but should not exceed 40 gm daily. *Children*—50 to 200 mg/kg body weight daily divided into 4 to 6 doses. INTRAVENOUS: *Adults and children*—same as for IM.
Carbenicillin indanyl ester	Geocillin	ORAL: *Adults*—382 to 764 mg (1 or 2 tablets) every 6 hr.
Mezlocillin	Mezlin	INTRAMUSCULAR, INTRAVENOUS: *Adults*—3 to 4 gm every 4 to 6 hr. Severe infections may be treated with up to 24 gm daily in equally divided doses. FDA Pregnancy Category B. *Children*—50 mg/kg body weight every 4 hr.
Piperacillin	Pipracil*	INTRAMUSCULAR, INTRAVENOUS: *Adults*—3 to 4 gm every 4 to 6 hr. IV doses by slow injection. Up to 24 gm may be given daily for life-threatening infections. FDA Pregnancy Category B.
Ticarcillin	Ticar*	INTRAMUSCULAR: *Adults*—1 gm every 4 to 6 hr. *Children*—50 to 100 mg/kg body weight daily divided into 3 or 4 doses. INTRAVENOUS: *Adults and children*—200 to 300 mg/kg body weight daily in 4 to 6 doses. Drug should be infused over 10 to 20 min.
Ticarcillin + clavulanate	Timentin*	INTRAVENOUS: *Adults*—as for ticarcillin, based on ticarcillin content of preparation. FDA Pregnancy Category B.

*Available in Canada and United States.
†Available in Canada only.

Toxicity

Repository penicillins are intended for deep muscular injections. Both preparations are stabilized suspensions of relatively insoluble forms of penicillin and contain up to about 2% weight/volume of emulsifying agents in addition to buffers. Such preparations should never be given by IV routes. Care must be taken on IM injection to prevent the accidental entry of these preparations into blood vessels, since occlusion of blood vessels may result.

Uses

Repository penicillins are not appropriate for serious infections when high serum concentrations of drug are required. Rather, these drugs are appropriate to maintain modest serum levels for relatively long periods. These conditions occur when very sensitive organisms are involved in mild to moderately serious infections or when prophylaxis is required.

Procaine penicillin G is associated with CNS toxicity because of the procaine. After injection, procaine may be released in significant amounts into the bloodstream and may produce anxiety, lowered blood pressure, respiratory depression, and convulsions. These CNS reactions to procaine are usually transient, lasting less than 1 hr.

Phenoxy Penicillins: Penicillin V

Absorption

Attempts to improve the oral absorption of penicillin G led to the development of phenoxy derivatives of penicillin. The most useful member of this class is penicillin V. Penicillin V is more acid stable and thus more efficiently absorbed from the GI tract than penicillin G, but is less potent as an antibacterial agent.

Uses

The uses of penicillin V are restricted to those circumstances in which oral antibiotic therapy is appropriate. Mild to moderately serious infections caused by penicillin-sensitive organisms may be treated with penicillin V. Penicillin V also may be used in prophylaxis, especially in patients who have had rheumatic fever. In these patients, penicillin V prophylaxis may prevent recurrent streptococcal infections, which could lead to heart or kidney damage.

Besides being better absorbed orally, penicillin V resembles penicillin G. Penicillin V has the same antimicrobial spectrum, pattern of distribution and excretion, and toxicity as penicillin G. Penicillin V should be given 1 hr before or 2 hr after meals, because food can interfere with absorption.

Penicillinase-Resistant Penicillins: Methicillin

Absorption

Methicillin is not acid stable and therefore must be administered parenterally.

Toxicity

Methicillin can cause significant blood dyscrasias and interstitial nephritis. These reactions are uncommon with other penicillins. Methicillin is also unusual in that resistance to the drug involves cell tolerance rather than the penicillinase development. When methicillin resistance does occur, the organism also becomes resistant to penicillin G, cephalosporins, other penicillinase-resistant penicillins, and other antibiotics.

Uses

Methicillin was the first penicillin developed to be resistant to attack by penicillinase. This breakthrough in pharmaceutic development allowed penicillin therapy of penicillinase-producing staphylococcal infections. Methicillin is best used only to treat infections caused by this pathogenic organism; in all other penicillin-sensitive infections penicillin G is preferred, because it is more potent than methicillin.

Acid-Stable, Penicillinase-Resistant Penicillins: Nafcillin, Oxacillin, and Dicloxacillin

Absorption and excretion

This group combines two of the most useful features of penicillin derivatives: acid stability, which allows oral dosage; and resistance to staphylococcal penicillinase, which allows the drugs to be used against many penicillin G-resistant organisms. Nafcillin is unique among all the penicillins, since it is excreted primarily in the bile. All other penicillins are excreted primarily by the kidney. Although nafcillin is occasionally used orally, it is not as well absorbed as the other members of this class—oxacillin, cloxacillin, and dicloxacillin. With these latter drugs, oral absorption can be approximately doubled by fasting. These drugs are all more potent than methicillin but less potent than penicillin G.

Uses

This group of drugs is primarily used in initial therapy when a penicillinase-producing organism is suspected. If the infection is later demonstrated by culture results to be caused by a nonpenicillinase-producing organism, frequently patients may be switched to penicillin V or penicillin G. One of the dangers in too frequent use of these drugs is that the unusual drug-tolerance type of resistance may develop in more and more bacterial populations. As discussed for methicillin, this type of resistance then affects all beta-lactam antibiotics and makes the resistant organism quite dangerous and difficult to eradicate.

Extended Spectrum Penicillins: Ampicillin, Amoxicillin, Bacampacillin, and Cyclacillin

Absorption

Ampicillin may be administered orally, but only 35% to 50% of an oral dose is absorbed. Bacampacillin and cyclacillin are prodrug forms that were designed to be more rapidly and completely absorbed than ampicillin but also to release ampicillin on breakdown in the body. Amoxicillin is chemically related to ampicillin but is more acid stable and therefore better absorbed orally.

Uses

All the penicillins discussed previously have relatively narrow antimicrobial spectra, being primarily useful against gram-positive bacteria. The development of ampicillin and related drugs significantly broadened the penicillin spectrum to include several common gram-negative pathogens. These drugs penetrate gram-negative cell walls better and are therefore more effective against these organisms than penicillin G. The extended-spectrum penicillins are not resistant to penicillinase and so may not be effective against *S. aureus* strains resistant to penicillin G.

Ampicillin is available in a fixed combination with sulbactam, and amoxicillin is available in fixed combination with clavulanic acid. Sulbactam and clavulanic acid are inhibitors of penicillinases. Inclusion of these inhibitors in the fixed combinations protects the active drugs from destruction, allowing their use against some organisms that would otherwise be resistant.

Anti-*Pseudomonas* Penicillins: Azlocillin, Carbenicillin, Mezlocillin, Piperacillin, and Ticarcillin

Absorption

These drugs must be administered parenterally. For carbenicillin, an indanyl ester is available, which allows the drug to be used orally. However, indanyl carbenicillin does not produce high enough serum levels of carbenicillin to make the drug effective for most infections. Therefore it is reserved for use in urinary tract infections, because the drug does accumulate to high concentrations in urine after oral dosage.

Uses

One pathogenic organism that is not sensitive to ampicillin or amoxicillin is *Pseudomonas aeruginosa*. This gram-negative bacterium is responsible for certain urinary tract infections, bacteremias, and infections in burn patients and is unusually resistant to many antibiotics. Thus the anti-*Pseudomonas* drugs were developed specifically for use against this organism.

Anti-*Pseudomonas* penicillins may be used with gentamicin (see Chapter 33) to treat severe *Pseudomonas* infections. Gentamicin must never be directly mixed in the syringe or IV bottle with these agents, since these penicillins inactivate gentamicin.

CEPHALOSPORINS

The **cephalosporins** are divided into three subgroups, referred to as *generations*. Among the first-generation cephalosporins, cephalothin and cefazolin are the most widely used parenteral agents, and cephalexin is the most widely used oral agent, although other members of this class differ little from these three. Second-generation cephalosporins differ from the first-generation drugs by having slightly extended activity against gram-negative bacteria. For example, the second-generation drug cefamandole has better

activity than first-generation cephalosporins against *Enterobacter*. Other second-generation cephalosporins are especially active against *Haemophilus*. Third-generation cephalosporins generally have lower activity against gram-positive organisms than first-generation drugs, but third-generation cephalosporins have significant activity against the gram-negative pathogen *P. aeruginosa*. They are the only cephalosporins to possess such activity. In addition, several third-generation cephalosporins are distributed reliably into the CNS.

Absorption

Several cephalosporins are currently available for oral use (Table 30-3). These preparations are well absorbed and produce effective serum concentrations of antibiotic. Absorption of cephalosporins from the GI tract is slowed by food in the stomach, but about the same amount of drug is ultimately absorbed as in a fasting patient.

Most cephalosporins are given parenterally, because they are well absorbed from IM sites. The elimination half-times of all these drugs are about twice as long as that of penicillin G and are roughly equivalent to those of ampicillin or the penicillinase-resistant penicillins.

Distribution

Cephalosporins are distributed in the body in a manner similar to that of penicillins, except that first-generation and most second-generation cephalosporins do not penetrate the CNS well enough to be used in meningitis. Cephalosporins, with the exception of cefoperazone and ceftriaxone, are excreted primarily by the kidney and are highly concentrated in urine, making them useful in treating several common types of urinary tract infections.

Toxicity

Many cephalosporins cause pain at the injection site. When given intravenously, these drugs cause phlebitis or thrombophlebitis and pain along the affected vein. Orally administered cephalosporins may cause gastric irritation, nausea, and vomiting.

Interstitial nephritis occasionally has been observed with these drugs. There is danger of synergistic nephrotoxicity when any cephalosporin is given with other nephrotoxic agents such as the antibiotics gentamicin, kanamycin, and polymyxin or the diuretics furosemide and ethacrynic acid.

Uses

The primary usefulness of cephalosporins is based on the differences in the antimicrobial spectra of penicillins and cephalosporins. First-generation cephalosporins resemble ampicillin in their effectiveness

Table 30-3   Common Dosages of Representative Cephalosporins

Generic name	Trade name	Administration/dosage
FIRST GENERATION		
Cefadroxil	Duricef* Ultracef	ORAL: *Adults*—1 to 2 gm daily in divided doses. FDA Pregnancy Category B. *Children*—30 mg/kg body weight daily divided into 2 equal doses.
Cefazolin	Ancef* Kefzol*	INTRAMUSCULAR, INTRAVENOUS: *Adults*—250 mg every 8 hr, up to 1.5 gm every 6 hr. FDA Pregnancy Category B. *Children*—25 to 50 mg/kg body weight total daily dose in 3 or 4 divided doses.
Cephalexin	Ceporex† Keflex*	ORAL: *Adults*—1 to 4 gm daily. FDA Pregnancy Category B. *Children*—25 to 100 mg/kg body weight total daily dose divided into 4 doses.
Cephalothin	Ceporacin† Keflin*	INTRAMUSCULAR, INTRAVENOUS: *Adults*—1 to 2 gm every 4 to 6 hr. FDA Pregnancy Category B. *Children*—80 to 160 mg/kg body weight total daily dose.
Cephapirin	Cefadyl*	INTRAMUSCULAR, INTRAVENOUS: *Adults*—500 mg to 1 gm every 4 to 6 hr. FDA Pregnancy Category B. *Children*—40 to 80 mg/kg body weight total daily dose.
Cephradine	Anspor Velosef*	ORAL, INTRAMUSCULAR, INTRAVENOUS: *Adults*—1 to 6 gm total daily dose. FDA Pregnancy Category B. *Children*—25 to 100 mg/kg body weight divided into 4 daily doses.
SECOND GENERATION		
Cefaclor	Ceclor*	ORAL: *Adults*—1 to 4 gm daily. FDA Pregnancy Category B. *Children*—20 to 40 mg/kg body weight, not to exceed 1 gm daily.
Cefamandole	Mandol*	INTRAMUSCULAR, INTRAVENOUS: *Adults*—500 mg to 2 gm every 4 to 6 hr. FDA Pregnancy Category B. *Children*—50 to 100 mg/kg body weight daily divided into 3 to 6 doses.
Cefixime	Suprax*	ORAL: *Adults*—200 mg every 12 hr or 400 mg once daily. FDA Pregnancy Category B. *Children*—4 mg/kg body weight every 12 hr or 8 mg/kg body weight once daily.
Cefonicid	Monocid	INTRAMUSCULAR, INTRAVENOUS: *Adults*—1 to 2 gm once daily. No more than 1 gm should be given at a single IM site. FDA Pregnancy Category B. *Children*—safety and effectiveness have not been established.
Ceforanide	Precef	INTRAMUSCULAR, INTRAVENOUS: *Adults*—0.5 to 1 gm twice daily. FDA Pregnancy Category B. *Children*—20 to 40 mg/kg body weight daily in 2 equally divided doses.
Cefotetan	Cefotan*	INTRAMUSCULAR, INTRAVENOUS: *Adults*—1 to 2 gm every 12 hr. Do not exceed 6 gm daily. FDA Pregnancy Category B. *Children*—Safe dosage not established.
Cefoxitin	Mefoxin*	INTRAMUSCULAR, INTRAVENOUS: *Adults*—3 to 12 gm daily in 3 or 4 equal doses. FDA Pregnancy Category B. *Children*—50 to 150 mg/kg body weight daily divided into 4 to 6 doses.
Cefsulodin	Cefomonil†	INTRAVENOUS: *Adults*—2 to 12 gm total daily dose, divided into 4 equal doses.
Cefuroxime axetil	Ceftin	ORAL: *Adults*—250 to 500 mg every 12 hr. FDA Pregnancy Category B. *Children*—125 mg every 12 hr.
Cefuroxime	Kefurox Zinacef*	INTRAMUSCULAR, INTRAVENOUS: *Adults*—0.75 to 1.5 Gm every 6 to 8 hr. FDA Pregnancy Category B. *Infants to 3 months*—30 to 100 mg/kg divided into 2 or 3 daily doses. *Children over 3 months*—75 to 120 mg/kg body weight daily divided into 3 equal doses.
THIRD GENERATION		
Cefoperazone	Cefobid*	INTRAMUSCULAR, INTRAVENOUS: *Adults*—2 to 4 gm daily divided into 2 equal doses. More severe infections may require up to 12 gm daily divided into 2 to 4 doses. FDA Pregnancy Category B. *Children*—safe use has not been established.
Cefmetazole	Zefazone	INTRAVENOUS: *Adults*—2 gm (base) every 6 to 12 hr for 5 to 14 days.
Cefotaxime	Claforan*	INTRAMUSCULAR, INTRAVENOUS: *Adults*—3 to 4 gm daily divided into 3 or 4 equal doses. More severe infections may require up to 12 gm daily. FDA Pregnancy Category B. *Children*—50 to 180 mg/kg body weight doses have been used.

*Available in Canada and United States.
†Available in Canada only.

Continued.

Table 30-3   Common Dosages of Representative Cephalosporins—cont'd

Generic name	Trade name	Administration/dosage
THIRD GENERATION—cont'd		
Ceftazidime	Fortaz* Tazicef	INTRAMUSCULAR, INTRAVENOUS: *Adults*—0.5 to 2 gm every 8 to 12 hr. FDA Pregnancy Category B. *Children*—30 to 50 mg/kg body weight every 8 to 12 hr.
Ceftizoxime	Cefizox	INTRAMUSCULAR, INTRAVENOUS: *Adults*—3 gm daily divided into 2 equal doses. Severe infections may require up to 12 Gm daily, divided into 3 doses. FDA Pregnancy Category B. *Children*—safety and effectiveness have not been established.
Ceftriaxone	Rocephin	INTRAMUSCULAR, INTRAVENOUS: *Adult*—1 to 2 gm as a single dose or divided into 2 doses daily. FDA Pregnancy Category B. *Children*—50 to 75 mg/kg body weight daily, divided into 2 doses.
Moxalactam	Moxam*	INTRAMUSCULAR, INTRAVENOUS: *Adults*—2 to 4 gm daily divided into 3 equal doses. FDA Pregnancy Category C. *Children*—50 mg/kg body weight every 6 to 8 hr.

*Available in Canada and United States.

Table 30-4   Clinical Summary of Aztreonam and Imipenem

Generic name	Trade name	Administration/dosage
Aztreonam	Azactam	INTRAMUSCULAR, INTRAVENOUS: *Adults*—1 to 8 gm daily, divided into 2 to 4 equal doses. FDA Pregnancy Category B.
Imipenem-cilastatin	Primaxin*	INTRAVENOUS: *Adults*—1 to 4 gm daily, divided into 3 or 4 equal doses. FDA Pregnancy Category C.

*Available in Canada and United States.

against gram-negative bacteria. Unlike ampicillin, cephalosporins resist the action of staphylococcal penicillinase and can be used when the organism is resistant to penicillin G. Second- and third-generation cephalosporins are used for specific, serious infections cause by gram-negative bacteria.

RELATED BETA-LACTAM ANTIBIOTICS

Beta-lactam antibiotics related to penicillins and cephalosporins are available for clinical use. These include aztreonam (a monobactam) and imipenem (a carbapenem).

Aztreonam

Aztreonam (Table 30-4) has a mechanism of action similar to that of other beta-lactam antibiotics, interfering with bacterial cell wall synthesis. Unlike most penicillins and cephalosporins, aztreonam inhibits or destroys primarily gram-negative aerobic bacteria and has little effect on gram-positive or anaerobic bacteria. Aztreonam must be administered parenterally to obtain useful concentrations in plasma. The drug is distributed well to many body tissues and fluids, but is relatively low in cerebrospinal fluid. Excretion is primarily via the kidneys, and only minor amounts of drug are eliminated by hepatic mechanisms.

The principal adverse reactions to aztreonam include pain or phlebitis at the injection site in up to 2.4% of patients. GI symptoms including nausea, diarrhea, or vomiting occur in up to 1.3% of patients. Rash and other symptoms of allergic reactions can occur, as with all beta-lactam antibiotics.

Aztreonam is given to treat urinary tract infections, septicemia, infections of the lower respiratory tract, intraabdominal or gynecologic infections, and soft-tissue infections. These infections are typically caused by gram-negative bacteria, including *Pseudomonas*.

Imipenem

Imipenem (see Table 30-4) is an extremely potent inhibitor of bacterial cell wall synthesis. The mechanism of action resembles that of other beta-lactam antibiotics. Imipenem has a broad antimicrobial spectrum that includes gram-positive, gram-negative, and anaerobic bacteria. Imipenem is effective against penicillinase-producing *S. aureus*.

Imipenem is well distributed to many tissues but is low in cerebrospinal fluid. Excretion is through the kidney. When given alone, imipenem is hydrolyzed in the kidneys and excreted as inactive products. The clinical preparation includes cilastatin, an agent chemically related to imipenem but with no antibacterial activity. Cilastatin inhibits destruction of imipenem in the kidneys and allows active imipenem to accumulate in renal tissue and urine.

Imipenem can cause mild-to-serious allergic reactions, as can other beta-lactam antibiotics. Imipenem can also cause rare CNS reactions, which may include seizures. Pseudomembranous colitis can also occur.

Because imipenem has such a broad antimicrobial spectrum, it is used to treat a variety of infections at many sites. *P. aeruginosa* is usually sensitive, but resistant strains may occur.

Table 30-5   Direct Infusion Rate for Penicillins, Cephalosporins, and Related Drugs

Drug	Recommended dilution*	Rate of administration†
Ampicillin	500 mg/at least 5 ml diluent	1 dose/10 to 15 min
Ampicillin + sulbactam	1.5 gm/4 ml diluent	1 dose/15 to 30 min
Azlocillin	1 gm/10 ml diluent	3 to 5 min
Carbenicillin	Dilute as directed on vial, then further dilute each gram in at least 10 ml diluent	1 gm/5 min
Methicillin	500 mg reconstituted drug in at least 25 ml diluent	10 ml/min
Mezlocillin	1 gm in at least 10 ml diluent	1 dose/3 to 5 min
Nafcillin	Desired amount of drug in 15 to 30 ml diluent	500 mg/5 to 10 min
Oxacillin	1 gm/10 ml diluent	1 ml/min
Piperacillin	1 gm/5 ml diluent	1 dose/3 to 5 min
Ticarcillin	1 gm in at least 4 ml diluent, then further diluted to 1 gm/10 ml	1 gm/5 min
Ticarcillin + clavulanate	3.1 gm/13 ml diluent; further dilute in 50 to 100 ml of fluid	1 dose/30 min
Cefamandole	1 gm/10 ml diluent	1 gm/3 to 5 min
Cefazolin	1 gm/10 ml diluent	1 gm/5 min
Cefmetazole	Dilute as directed on vial	1 dose/3 to 5 min.
Cefonicid	0.5 gm/2 ml diluent	1 dose/3 to 5 min
Cefoperazone	1 gm/5 ml diluent	1 dose/3 to 5 min
Ceforanide	0.5 gm/5 ml diluent	1 dose/3 to 5 min
Cefotaxime	1 dose/10 ml diluent	1 dose/3 to 5 min
Cefotetan	1 gm/10 ml diluent	1 dose/3 to 5 min
Cefoxitin	1 gm/10 ml diluent	1 gm/3 to 5 min
Cefpiramide	1 gm/9.4 ml diluent; check drug insert	1 dose/3 to 5 min
Ceftazidime	0.5 gm/5 ml	1 dose/3 to 5 min
Ceftizoxime	1 gm/10 ml diluent	1 dose/3 to 5 min
Ceftriaxone	250 mg/2.4 ml; further dilute in 50 to 100 ml of fluid	1 dose/30 min
Cefuroxime	750 mg/9 ml diluent	1 dose/3 to 5 min

Continued.

Table 30-5   Direct Infusion Rate for Penicillins, Cephalosporins, and Related Drugs—cont'd

Drug	Recommended dilution*	Rate of administration†
Cephalothin	1 gm/10 ml diluent	1 gm/3 to 5 min
Cephapirin	1 gm/10 ml diluent	1 gm/5 min
Cephradine	500 mg/5 ml diluent	1 gm/3 to 5 min
Moxalactam	1 gm/10 ml diluent	1 dose/3 to 5 min
Aztreonam	1 dose/6 to 10 ml diluent	1 dose/3 to 5 min
Imipenem and cilastatin	1 dose/10 ml diluent; further dilute in 100 ml fluid	1 dose/20 to 30 min

*For information about appropriate diluents, preparations for constant infusion, compatibilities with infusion fluids, storage conditions, and other questions, consult the pharmacist and the manufacturer's information. Because the cephalosporins are so irritating to the vein, diluting these drugs more than is indicated in the table is preferable, when possible.
†These rates are for direct IV line unless otherwise noted. When diluted in 50 to 100 ml or more, the rate is determined in part by the total volume.

NURSING IMPLICATIONS SUMMARY

Penicillins, Cephalosporins, and Related Drugs

Drug administration

◆ Review the Nursing Implications Summary in Chapter 29.
◆ Assess for history of allergy before administering these drugs.
◆ Monitor vital signs and temperature. Inspect for rash.
◆ Monitor serum creatinine and blood urea nitrogen (BUN) levels, liver function tests, complete blood count (CBC), and differential count. Monitor serum electrolyte level of patients with hypertensive, renal, or cardiovascular disease and in patients receiving drugs high in potassium or sodium.
◆ For IV administration, consult the manufacturer's literature or Table 30-5 for the approximate rate of IV push administration. Too-rapid administration of penicillins has resulted in the occurrence of seizures. Too-rapid administration of the cephalosporins contributes to venous irritation and patient discomfort.
◆ Warn patients that IM injection may be painful. Use large muscle masses. Record and rotate injection sites. See Chapter 6 for a description of IM injection sites.

◆ Read labels and orders carefully. Products containing procaine, benzathine, or a combination of these are never given by IV routes. Occasional patients are sensitive to procaine; symptoms include anxiety, confusion, agitation, fear of impending doom, and convulsions.

Patient and family education

◆ Review the Nursing Implications Summary in Chapter 29.
◆ The following drugs should be taken on an empty stomach, 1 hr before or 2 hr after meals, with a full glass (8 oz) of water: ampicillin, liquid bacampicillin, carbenicillin, cloxacillin, dicloxacillin, methicillin, nafcillin, oxacillin, and penicillin G.
◆ The following drugs can be taken with food: amoxicillin, amoxicillin and clavulanate, the tablet form of bacampicillin, penicillin V, and oral cephalosporins.
◆ Cefuroxime axetil should be taken with food or snack and may be crushed and mixed with food to ease taking and to help disguise the taste.
◆ The penicillins, cephalosporins, and related drugs may cause false-positive reactions with copper sulfate urine-glucose tests. Check with the physician before changing insulin or diet. Instruct patients to monitor blood glucose levels.

NURSING IMPLICATIONS SUMMARY—cont'd

- ◆ Warn the patient that amoxicillin, amoxicillin and clavulanate, ampicillin, bacampicillin, penicillin G, and penicillin V may cause the tongue to discolor or darken during therapy, but this is not significant.
- ◆ If chewable tablets are prescribed, tell patients to chew or crush the tablets before swallowing them.
- ◆ These drugs may cause diarrhea. If severe or persistent, notify the physician. For mild diarrhea, only medicines containing kaolin or attapulgite should be used.

- ◆ Warn patients taking cefamandole, cefoperazone, cefotetan, or moxalactam to avoid the use of alcohol while taking these drugs and for several days after completing the course of therapy. Ingestion of alcohol may cause a disulfiram type of reaction (see Patient Problem: Disulfiram Reaction on p. 614).
- ◆ Warn females taking ampicillin, bacampicillin, or penicillin V that oral contraceptives containing estrogen may not work during the course of antiinfective drug therapy. Females should use an alternate or additional form of birth control while taking these antiinfectives; consult the physician or pharmacist.

CHAPTER REVIEW

◆ KEY TERMS

beta-lactam antibiotics, p. 450
beta-lactamases, p. 451
cephalosporins, p. 458
penicillin G, p. 453

◆ REVIEW QUESTIONS

1. What is the mechanism of action of penicillins and cephalosporins?
2. What is the effect of beta-lactam antibiotics on existing bacterial cell walls?
3. How do most bacteria gain resistance to beta-lactam antibiotics?
4. What is the mechanism of excretion for most penicillins and cephalosporins?
5. What is the most common toxic reaction to penicillins and cephalosporins? What should you watch for?
6. What is the purpose of skin tests for penicillin allergies?
7. What is the effect of penicillin on the CNS?
8. Name two groups of patients most at risk of accumulating penicillins given at normal doses.
9. What patient would be most at risk from the potassium and sodium contained in many penicillin and cephalosporin preparations? What tests should you monitor?
10. Why is probenecid sometimes administered with penicillin G?
11. What is the effect of destroying the penicillin nucleus?
12. Why is penicillin G absorbed erratically from the GI tract?
13. When does the peak concentration of penicillin G appear in the bloodstream after an IM dose of the drug?
14. What is the elimination half-time for penicillin G in normal patients?
15. How does the penetration of penicillin G into the cerebrospinal fluid differ in normal patients and in those with meningitis?
16. Why do procaine penicillin G and benzathine penicillin G have longer durations of action than penicillin G?
17. What is the danger to patients of accidentally administering the repository penicillins by IV routes?
18. Which would produce a higher serum concentration of antibiotic, 1 million units of penicillin G or 1 million units of procaine penicillin G?
19. What advantage does penicillin V have over penicillin G?
20. Why is methicillin useful in treating infections caused by penicillinase-producing *S. aureus*?
21. How do bacteria become resistant to methicillin?
22. What is the route of excretion of nafcillin?
23. What advantages do oxacillin, cloxacillin and dicloxacillin have over methicillin?
24. How does the antimicrobial spectrum of ampicillin and amoxicillin differ from that of penicillin G?
25. What advantage does amoxicillin possess over ampicillin?
26. Why is clavulanic acid or sulbactam included in fixed combination with ampicillin, amoxicillin, or ticarcillin?

27. Infections caused by what pathogen are appropriately treated with carbenicillin or ticarcillin?

28. How does indanyl carbenicillin differ from carbenicillin?

29. Why are first-generation cephalosporins not useful in treating meningitis?

30. What is the most common reaction expected from most cephalosporins when administered by IV routes?

31. How does the antimicrobial spectrum of the cephalosporins differ from that of penicillin G?

32. What is the antimicrobial spectrum of aztreonam?

33. What is the antimicrobial spectrum of imipenem?

34. Why is imipenem given with cilastatin?

35. What teaching points are important for patients receiving one of the antiinfectives in this chapter?

36. What are the main points of a nursing care plan for patients receiving drugs discussed in this chapter?

SUGGESTED READING

Childs SJ, Bodey GP: Aztreonam: a review of its pharmacologic, microbiologic, and clinical properties, *Pharmacotherapy* 6(4):138, 1986.

Gustaferro CA, Steckelberg, JM: Cephalosporin antimicrobial agents and related compounds, *Mayo Clin Proc* 66(10):1064, 1991.

Shovein J, Young MS: MRSA [Methicillin-resistant *Staphylococcus aureus*]: Pandora's box for hospitals, *Am J Nurs* 92(2):48, 1992.

Wright AJ, Wilkowske CJ: The penicillins, *Mayo Clin Proc* 66(10):1047, 1991.

CHAPTER 31

Erythromycin, Clindamycin, and Miscellaneous Penicillin Substitutes

LEARNING OBJECTIVES

After studying this chapter, you should be able to do the following:

- Explain the common indications for erythromycin, azithromycin, clindamycin, vancomycin, and spectinomycin.
- Explain why bacitracin is not given systemically.
- Describe common side effects of erythromycin, clindamycin, and vancomycin.
- Explain why erythromycin is not administered intramuscularly.
- Develop a nursing care plan for a patient receiving a drug discussed in this chapter.

CHAPTER OVERVIEW

◆ This chapter introduces several antibiotics with antimicrobial spectra similar to those of narrow-spectrum penicillins. Because of this property, these drugs are sometimes grouped together as **penicillin substitutes**. The mechanisms of action, modes of bacterial resistance, absorption properties, drug distribution and excretion, and the unique toxic reactions these drugs may induce are discussed.

Nursing Process Overview
PENICILLIN SUBSTITUTES

Refer to Chapter 29 for general guidelines for the nursing process with antibiotic therapy.

Assessment

Perform a thorough patient assessment, with emphasis on the sites of infection. Monitor other clinical signs of infection.

Nursing Diagnoses

Possible complication: pseudomembranous colitis
Possible complication: ototoxicity

Management

In addition to baseline data, check on organs known to be affected by the prescribed drug. Monitor liver function tests for patients taking erythromycin and renal function tests for patients receiving spectino-

mycin. Teach patients taking clindamycin to report diarrhea to the physician.

Evaluation

Before discharge, verify that the patient can explain what drug reactions might be expected and when to notify the physician.

ERYTHROMYCIN AND OTHER MACROLIDES
Mechanism of Action and Bacterial Resistance

Erythromycin and other **macrolides** bind to bacterial ribosomes and thus prevent bacterial protein synthesis. At low concentrations, this effect is bacteriostatic, but at high concentrations the drugs may be bactericidal.

Bacteria become resistant to erythromycin by one of two mechanisms. Gram-negative organisms seem to be relatively impermeable to erythromycin and are therefore intrinsically resistant. Cell wall–deficient forms of these bacteria (L-forms) are permeable to erythromycin and are highly sensitive to the drug. Gram-positive organisms acquire resistance by chemically altering their ribosomes so that the ribosomes no longer bind erythromycin; thus protein synthesis is not inhibited. This ribosomal alteration is catalyzed by an enzyme that is synthesized from genes carried on a bacterial plasmid. Plasmids are discrete circular molecules of deoxyribonucleic acid (DNA) that are separate from the bacterial chromosome (see Chapter 43). These plasmids can be transferred directly from one bacterial cell to another. Therefore resistance to erythromycin may spread rapidly throughout a bacterial population.

The mechanism of resistance to other macrolides such as azithromycin and clarithromycin is similar to that of erythromycin, but the spread of resistance has not yet been assessed for these newer drugs.

Absorption

Erythromycin is sensitive to acid and therefore may be extensively degraded in the stomach. Thus erythromycin base is formulated with acid-resistant coatings so that the drug will pass intact through the stomach and be dissolved and absorbed in the small intestine. This tactic is based on the knowledge that the pH of the duodenum is near neutrality (see Chapter 1).

Certain chemical forms of erythromycin are used clinically primarily because of their increased resistance to acid and their better oral absorption. These compounds are the stearate, ethylsuccinate, and estolate esters of erythromycin (Table 31-1). Erythromycin stearate and erythromycin ethylsuccinate are absorbed more rapidly and completely from the gastrointestinal (GI) tract than erythromycin base. Free erythromycin apparently is absorbed from the duodenum with these agents after hydrolysis of the esters. With erythromycin estolate, much better absorption of drug is achieved, and serum levels may be four times higher than with other forms of erythromycin. However, with erythromycin estolate, most of the drug in the serum is actually the ester, and controversy exists regarding whether this form of the drug has biologic activity. Many physicians prefer erythromycin estolate because of the high tissue and blood levels and note that many tissues and bacteria can hydrolyze the ester form of the drug to release free erythromycin at the infection site.

Food may interfere with the oral absorption of most erythromycin preparations. Erythromycin estolate and erythromycin ethylsuccinate are exceptions, being well absorbed even when food is present.

Erythromycin is available as the lactobionate or the gluceptate for intravenous (IV) injection (see Table 31-1). These water-soluble products may be diluted with sterile water for injection but should not be diluted in sterile water containing preservatives. Erythromycin lactobionate or erythromycin glucceptate may be rapidly inactivated if added to fluids below pH 5.5. This sensitivity to extremes of pH makes erythromycin incompatible in solution with a number of other drugs. Before adding erythromycin to any other drug solution, compatibility of the agents should be verified with the pharmacist. Erythromycin lactobionate and erythromycin glucceptate should be infused slowly into the vein to avoid pain.

Intramuscular (IM) administration of erythromycin is avoided because injections are extremely painful.

Azithromycin and clarithromycin are well absorbed orally. Azithromycin is much more resistant to stomach acidity than is erythromycin.

Distribution and Excretion

Erythromycin readily enters body tissues, and tissue concentrations of drug may persist well beyond when it can be detected in the serum. Erythromycin is especially concentrated in the liver and spleen. It enters fluids of the middle ear and pleural fluids but not cerebrospinal fluid, unless the meninges are inflamed. The drug does cross the placenta, but fetal blood levels are less than 20% of maternal blood levels. Erythromycin also enters breast milk, in which the concentrations may equal that of maternal serum.

Azithromycin and clarithromycin are more strongly concentrated in tissues than is erythromycin and therefore persist longer in the body. Azithromycin in particular concentrates in the lungs and other organs but like erythromcyin does not accumulate in normal brain tissue.

The liver is the major excretory organ for erythromycin and other macrolides. A large percentage of orally administered drug is concentrated in bile and excreted in feces. Some reabsorption from the intestine occurs in a process called *enterohepatic circulation* (see Chapter 1). Another significant proportion of erythromycin is apparently inactivated in the liver. Less than 10% of orally administered erythromycin appears as active drug in urine. With IV dosage, about 15% of the dose appears in urine. Because of the relative importance of the liver and the kidney in drug excretion, patients with mild renal insufficiency might be expected to receive normal doses of erythromcyin, whereas a patient with hepatic insufficiency might require reduced drug doses.

Table 31-1 Summary of Macrolides

Generic name	Trade name	Drug form	Administration/dosage
Azithromycin	Zithromax	Tablets	ORAL: *Adults and children over 16 years*—500 mg on the first day, then 250 mg once daily.
Clarithromycin	Biaxin	Tablets	ORAL: *Adults and children over 12 years*—250 mg every 12 hr. FDA Pregnancy Category C.
Erythromycin base	E-Mycin* Erythromid† Robimycin	Enteric or film-coated tablets	ORAL: *Adults*—250 mg 4 times/day (15 to 20 mg/kg body weight/day, not to exceed 4 g daily.) *Children*—30 to 100 mg/kg per day in 3 or 4 doses.
Erythromycin base	Staticin*	Gel, solution, or swabs	TOPICAL: *Adults and children*—Apply to skin twice daily.
Erythromycin base	Ilotycin*	Ophthalmic ointment	TOPICAL: *Adults and children*—Apply to conjunctiva once daily.
Erythromycin stearate	Erythrocin Stearate Wyamycin-S	Film-coated tablets and oral suspension	ORAL: *Adults and children*—same as for erythromycin base.
Erythromycin estolate	Ilosone* Novorythro†	Tablets, capsules, suspension, and chewable tablets	ORAL: *Adults and children*—same as for erythromycin base.
Erythromycin ethyl-succinate	E.E.S.*	Drops, suspension, chewable tablets, and film-coated tablets	ORAL: *Adults*—400 mg 4 times/day. *Children*—same as for erythromycin base.
Erythromycin ethyl-succinate + sulfisoxazole	Eryzole Pediazole*	Oral suspension	ORAL: *Children*—12.5 mg erythromycin/kg body weight every 6 hr.
Erythromycin lacto-bionate Erythromycin gluceptate	Erythrocin* Ilotycin*	Powder stabilized with benzyl alcohol; to be reconstituted with diluent suggested by manufacturer	INTRAVENOUS: *Adults and children*—15 to 20 mg/kg body weight/day not to exceed 4 gm daily, preferably by continuous infusion; intervals between doses for intermittent therapy should be 6 hr or less.

*Available in Canada and United States.
†Available in Canada only.

Toxicity

The most common patient complaint with oral erythromycin is some form of GI difficulty. Abdominal discomfort and cramping are dose-related reactions to these drugs. At normal doses, nausea, vomiting, and diarrhea are apparently less frequent than with oral penicillins or tetracyclines.

Allergic reactions to erythromycin have occurred, although these are rare. Reactions ranging from urticaria to anaphylaxis have been noted. Rarely, patients who receive more than 4 gm of erythromycin lactobionate/day experience hearing loss.

The most significant toxicity occurs with erythromycin estolate. This drug damages the liver by direct drug toxicity or by an immune reaction. This reaction, called *cholestatic hepatitis*, usually appears 10 to 12 days after therapy is begun but may appear earlier in patients previously exposed to the drug. These patients may experience severe abdominal pain, liver enlargement, fever, and jaundice. When the drug is discontinued, these symptoms rapidly disappear in most patients.

Drug Interactions

Erythromycin is metabolized in the liver and may therefore compete with other drugs for the limited metabolic capacity of the liver. For example, alfentanil, carbamazepine, warfarin, and theophylline must be eliminated by hepatic mechanisms. When erythromycin is given concurrently, the aforementioned drugs are eliminated more slowly, serum levels rise, and the drugs may accumulate. Because all of these drugs have dose-related toxicity, erythromycin not only increases serum levels but also increases the risk of serious toxicity.

Rarely, erythromycin may cause hepatotoxicity, especially when used at high doses or for long periods. The risk of liver damage is increased if erythromycin is given concurrently with other hepatoxic agents such as acetaminophen (high dose), anabolic steroids, androgens, estrogens, isoniazid, ketoconazole, phenothiazines, rifampin, azlocillin, mezlocillin, piperacillin, sulfonamides, or valproic acid.

Erythromycin and other macrolides can antagonize the antibacterial effects of lincomycin or clindamycin because they share the same target in bacteria and may displace each other from from the target. Erythromycin should not be used concurrently with clindamycin or lincomycin.

Uses

Erythromycin has a similar antimicrobial spectrum to penicillin G but is chemically unrelated to penicillins and is not cross-allergenic with them. Therefore it is a useful substitute in patients allergic to penicillins. In addition, since penicillins and erythromycin act by entirely different mechanisms, bacteria that become resistant to one of these drugs are still sensitive to the other. The newer macrolides have equal or improved activity over erythromycin toward gram-positive organisms.

Erythromycin is the drug of choice for some conditions, including atypical pneumonias such as those caused by *Mycoplasma pneumonia* and *Legionella pneumophila* (Legionnaires' disease). Azithromycin and clarithromycin have equal or better activity against these organisms and in addition display activity toward other serious pathogens such as *Borrelia burgdorferi* and *Campylobacter pylori*. Erythromycin may be preferred over penicillin G for diphtheria, since it eradicates the diphtheria carrier state. Erythromycin also may be useful in relapsing urinary tract infections; the relapse is frequently caused by L-forms of gram-negative organisms such as *Escherichia coli* and *Proteus mirabilis*. These L-forms lack cell walls and are therefore resistant to penicillins. The L-form bacteria remain latent during penicillin therapy, revert to normal, and again produce disease when penicillin therapy is stopped. Since erythromycin penetrates these L-forms and blocks protein synthesis, the infection may be eradicated.

Clinical studies suggest that pregnant women have variable absorption of oral erythromycin, and many do not achieve effective serum concentrations of the drug. Because of this lack of effect and because erythromycin can accumulate over long periods in fetal livers, it may not be recommended during pregnancy.

CLINDAMYCIN AND LINCOMYCIN
Mechanism of Action and Bacterial Resistance

Clindamycin and lincomycin inhibit the action of bacterial ribosomes in a manner analogous to that of erythromycin. These drugs halt bacterial protein synthesis and may be bacteriostatic or bactericidal, depending on drug concentrations. Bacterial resistance to lincomycin and clindamycin apparently develops in several ways. Some organisms may become impermeable to the drugs. Others alter the ribosome so that it does not bind lincomycin or clindamycin. With this latter mechanism, organisms may become resistant to lincomyin and erythromycin. In practice, most clinically observed resistance to clindamycin and lincomycin develops slowly and in a gradual, stepwise manner.

Absorption

Lincomycin may be administered by oral, IM, or IV routes (Table 31-2). When given orally, peak serum concentrations occur about 4 hr after the dose is administered. Food significantly hinders lincomycin absorption and results in serum levels much lower than those observed in the fasting state. Thus the drug should be administered between meals so that no food is eaten for 1 to 2 hr before and after the drug.

In contrast to lincomycin, clindamycin absorption is not significantly impaired by food. Clindamycin is more rapidly absorbed orally than is lincomyin and produces higher blood concentrations, at least during the first few hours of therapy. Clindamycin palmitate is also available as flavored granules to be used in suspension for oral administration. The palmitate is apparently rapidly removed to release active clindamycin.

Lincomycin or clindamycin-2-phosphate may be injected by IM routes. Clinical reports suggest that local pain after injection may occur with clindamycin-2-phosphate, but this has rarely been reported for lincomycin. Absorption of drug by this route is good, with serum peaks being achieved 30 to 60 min after injection. These drugs are also suitable for IV use. By this route, clindamycin-2-phosphate causes pain and phlebitis, whereas this reaction has not been observed with lincomycin. Clindamycin-2-phosphate is inactive as an antibiotic but is rapdily converted to clindamycin in the body.

Distribution and Excretion

Clindamycin and lincomycin are well distributed to most body tissues, with the exception of the central nervous system (CNS). Lincomycin does not appear in the cerebrospinal fluid of normal patients but may enter the CNS when the meninges are inflamed by infection. Clindamycin does not appear in the cerebrospinal fluid even when meningitis is present. Lincomycin and clindamycin appear in the milk of lactating females treated with these drugs.

Clindamycin and lincomycin are extensively bio-

Table 31-2   Summary of Lincomycin and Clindamycin

Generic name	Trade name	Drug form	Administration/dosage
Clindamycin	Cleocin HCl Dalacin C†	Capsules (hydrochloride hydrate)	ORAL: *Adults*—150 to 450 mg 4 times daily. *Children*—2 to 5 mg/kg body weight every 6 hr.
Clindamycin palmitate	Cleocin Pediatric Dalacin C†	Granules in suspension	ORAL: *Children*—8 to 25 mg/kg body weight/day in 3 or 4 doses for children over 10 kg. Smaller children should receive 37.5 mg 3 times daily.
Clindamycin phosphate	Cleocin Phosphate Dalacin C†	Solution with benzyl alcohol, disodium edetate, and hydrochloric acid or sodium hydroxide	INTRAMUSCULAR, INTRAVENOUS: *Adults*—300 to 600 mg every 6 to 8 hr to an upper limit of 2.4 gm/day (no more than 0.6 gm/injection site intramuscularly). *Children over 1 month*—15 to 40 mg/kg body weight daily in 3 or 4 doses.
Clindamycin phosphate	Cleocin T	1% topical gel or solution	TOPICAL: *Adults and children*—for acne vulgaris, apply thin film to affected area twice daily.
Lincomycin	Lincocin*	Capsules and syrup	ORAL: *Adults*—500 mg 3 or 4 times daily. *Children over 1 month*—30 to 60 mg/kg body weight/day in 3 or 4 divided doses.
		Solution with 0.9% benzyl alcohol	INTRAMUSCULAR: *Adults*—600 mg once or twice daily. *Children over 1 month*—10 mg/kg body weight once or twice daily. INTRAVENOUS: *Adults*—600 mg to 1 gm 2 or 3 times daily; to an upper limit of 8.4 gm/day. *Children over 1 month*—10 mg/kg body weight once or twice daily.

*Available in Canada and United States.
†Available in Canada only.

degraded in the body; the liver is the primary site of biotransformation. Since less than 20% of the total drug administered shows up as active antibiotic in urine or feces, these drugs are used at normal dosages in patients with renal insufficiency or failure. Neither lincomycin nor clindamycin is removed by hemodialysis.

Toxicity

The most serious reaction to lincomycin or clindamycin is colitis. Symptoms range from mild diarrhea to a severe, life-threatening condition called *pseudomembranous colitis*. Any increase in frequency of bowel movements or softness of the stools may be reason to discontinue the drug, especially in elderly patients. Significant diarrhea should prompt discontinuation of the drug and may be relieved by that measure alone. The appearance of blood or mucus in the stool may signal severe colitis.

Pseudomembranous colitis is caused by a toxin produced by *Clostridium difficile*. Overgrowth of this organism in the bowel can result from antibiotic disturbance of the bacterial flora in the bowel. This superinfection and its associated colitis may be treated with vancomycin. Fluid and electrolyte replacement and other supportive therapy also may be required. Agents that slow peristaltic action may worsen the condition or prolong it; thus opiates or diphenoxylate with atropine are not appropriate for use in these patients.

In addition to colitis, clindamycin and lincomycin may produce GI irritation ranging from nausea and vomiting to glossitis and stomatitis.

Allergies to clindamycin and lincomycin range from mild rashes to drug fever and anaphylactic shock. These reactions may occur in any patient but are more common in those with other allergies. The appearance of any allergic response is cause for discontinuing the drug.

Some reports suggest that blood dyscrasias and liver dysfunction occur during lincomycin or clindamycin therapy. A direct cause-and-effect relationship between the drugs and these reactions has not been demonstrated.

Lincomycin administered by IV routes has caused hypotension in a few patients. Cardiopulmonary arrest has occurred. These reactions are apparently related to a too-rapid IV injection. Lincomycin should be administered in an IV solution no more concentrated than 1 gm/100 ml at a rate no more rapid than 100 ml/hr. Clindamycin should be administered in an IV solution no more concentrated than 0.6 gm/100 ml at a rate no more rapid than 100 ml/20 min.

Drug Interactions

Lincomycin is incompatible in solution with the antibiotics novobiocin and kanamycin. Clindamycin is incompatible with aminophylline, ampicillin, barbiturates, calcium gluconate, magnesium sulfate, and phenytoin.

Since clindamycin and lincomycin have neuromuscular blocking properties, they may enhance the action of various neuromuscular blocking agents and inhalation anesthetics.

The absorption of oral doses of lincomycin may be decreased by food and other agents. The use of kaolin-pectin—antidiarrheal agents given at the time oral lincomycin is ingested markedly lowers the serum concentrations of lincomycin.

Uses

Clindamycin and lincomycin have antimicrobial spectra similar to those of penicillin G or erythromycin, being primarily effective against gram-positive organisms. Lincomycin and clindamycin are not as effective as penicillin against *Neisseria gonorrhoeae* or other gram-negative cocci. Clindamycin is effective against several anaerobic organisms, particularly *Bacteroides fragilis*. Infections caused by these organisms are a major indication for clindamycin.

The dangers of severe colitis have largely restricted the use of clindamycin and lincomycin to cases in which patients are allergic to safer drugs or the pathogenic organism is demonstrated by the microbiology laboratory to be sensitive to these agents. Clindamycin is more effective and less toxic than lincomycin and is much more commonly used.

VANCOMYCIN
Mechanism of Action and Bacterial Resistance

Vancomycin prevents synthesis of bacterial cell walls by blocking peptidoglycan strand formation. This site of action is different from the sites sensitive to penicillin and other antibiotics interfering with cell wall synthesis.

Resistance to vancomycin is relatively uncommon and tends to develop slowly. As the drug is used clinically, it is a rapidly bactericidal agent, which may partly explain the low incidence of bacterial resistance to vancomycin.

Absorption

Vancomycin is a complex glycopeptide that may be positively or negatively charged, depending on the pH. Therefore vancomycin does not easily cross biologic membranes and is not absorbed significantly after oral administration (Table 31-3). Vancomycin is most often administered IV by intermittent infusion; 500 mg may be dissolved in 10 ml of sterile

Table 31-3   Summary of Miscellaneous Penicillin Substitutes

Generic name	Trade name	Drug form	Administration/dosage
Vancomycin	Lyphocin Vancocin*	Powder to be reconstituted with sterile water	INTRAVENOUS: *Adults*—500 mg 4 times daily. *Children*—40 mg/kg body weight/day in divided doses.
Vancomycin	Vancocin*	Powder	ORAL: same as for IV. Note this route is for intestinal infections only.
Bacitracin	Altracin	Tablets	ORAL: *Adults*—50,000 IU (2 tablets) 4 times daily.
Bacitracin		Ointment for ophthalmic or skin application; also contains neomycin and polymyxin	TOPICAL: *Adults and children*—ointments contain 500 units of antibiotic/gm. Application may be every 3 hr or less frequently, depending on the infection.
Spectinomycin	Trobicin*	Powder to be reconstituted with diluent	INTRAMUSCULAR: *Adults*—2 to 4 gm in a single dose.

* Available in Canada and United States.
† Available in Canada only.

water and then added to 100 to 200 ml of 0.9% sodium chloride injection or 5% dextrose in water for infusion over 20 to 30 min. This regimen may be repeated every 6 hr.

Vancomycin may rarely be given by mouth for intestinal infections. Bactericidal concentrations of the drug are not obtained in the systemic circulation under this circumstance.

Distribution and Excretion

Vancomycin is well distributed throughout the body and reaches clinically effective concentrations in various body fluid compartments such as pericardial, synovial, and pleural fluids. It does not penetrate normal cerebrospinal fluid but does enter the CNS when the meninges are inflamed.

The kidney is the major excretory organ for vancomyin. The drug appears in very high concentrations in urine and is in the active form when excreted.

Vancomycin elimination by nonrenal routes is limited. In patients with renal insufficiency, vancomycin may accumulate unless drug doses are reduced to compensate for loss of excretory efficiency. In patients who lack kidney function, vancomycin is usually administered only once between dialyses. Less-frequent intervals may be required for individual anephric patients. Vancomycin is not cleared from the body by hemodialysis.

Toxicity

Vancomycin causes deafness in some patients, especially when serum concentrations exceed 80 μg/ml serum. Since patients with impaired renal function and elderly patients are more likely than normal persons to show drug accumulation (see box), these patients should be closely watched for ringing in the ears (tinnitus) or hearing loss. Some patients have regained some hearing acuity when vancomycin was discontinued. For others, hearing loss may continue even after the drug is stopped.

Nephrotoxicity may occur. Blood and protein in urine occasionally have been noted. Allergies manifested by urticarial rashes may also occur.

IV infusion of vancomycin has produced nausea, flushing, and itching. These reactions are more likely when undiluted vancomycin is dripped directly into a running IV line rather than being properly diluted beforehand. If vancomycin inadvertently enters muscle or skin around the IV site, local tissue necrosis may develop.

Drug Interactions

Vancomycin is compatible with many common IV fluids. The major consideration in combining vancomycin use with another drug should be to avoid administering another ototoxic drug such as an aminoglycoside antibiotic, bumetanide, ethacrynic acid, or furosemide. Combined use of ototoxic drugs may result in additive toxic effects and may severely impair hearing.

Uses

Vancomycin is primarily effective against gram-positive organisms and most often is used in staphylococcal or streptococcal infections. Since the drug is chemically unrelated to penicillins and has a different mechanism of action, it acts against organisms that resist penicillins, including methicillin-resistant staphylococci. Since vancomycin and penicillin are not cross-allergenic, vancomycin is useful in patients allergic to penicillins. Vancomycin also has special utility in treating antibiotic-induced colitis, which arises from a superinfection with *C. difficile* in the bowel.

BACITRACIN

Mechanism of Action and Bacterial Resistance

Bacitracin blocks the regeneration of a lipid carrier that transports cell wall material through the bacterial cell membrane. This site of action is different from that of penicillins or other antibiotics that inhibit cell wall formation. In addition to this action, the drug interferes with bacterial cell-membrane function.

Inherent resistance to bacitracin exists in gram-negative organisms, but acquired resistance among the gram-positive organisms in uncommon. Organisms resistant to bacitracin are not necessarily resistant to other antibiotics.

GERIATRIC CONSIDERATION: VANCOMYCIN

THE PROBLEM

Patients over 60 years of age have reduced renal function and therefore excrete vancomycin more slowly than do younger adults. The drug may accumulate because alternative paths of elimination are limited. Older adults also have some hearing loss because of their age.

SOLUTIONS

◆ Lower doses to avoid accumulation
◆ Monitor serum vancomycin concentrations
◆ Monitor renal function tests
◆ Perform baseline auditory function tests; repeat during therapy

Absorption, Distribution, and Excretion

Bacitracin is well absorbed from IM injection sites and penetrates all body organs. The kidney eliminates the drug, primarily by glomerular filtration.

The most common route of administration is topical, on the skin or in the eye (see Table 31-3). When applied to the body surface or when used to lavage the peritoneal cavity, the drug is not absorbed to any significant degree.

Toxicity

Bacitracin is extremely nephrotoxic. Glomerular and tubular necrosis have occurred. Protein may appear in urine, and azotemia (excess urea and other nitrogen-containing compounds in the blood) may develop. Because of the great risk of permanent kidney damage, bacitracin is not used systemically. Other less toxic drugs can usually be substituted. When used topically, the drug is practically nontoxic.

Uses

Bacitracin is effective against gram-positive bacteria, especially staphylococci. The most common use of bacitracin is as a topical ointment for superficial skin infections. The drug may be obtained alone or in combination with various other antibiotics in several nonprescription preparations. Special formulations of bacitracin exist for use in the eye.

SPECTINOMYCIN

Mechanism of Action, Bacterial Resistance, and Clinical Use

Spectinomycin inhibits bacterial protein synthesis. Both gram-positive and gram-negative bacteria may be affected, but the ability of spectinomycin to inhibit *N. gonorrhoeae* is the basis for its clinical usefulness. On this basis, it is classified as a penicillin substitute. Resistance to spectinomycin may occur.

Absorption, Distribution, and Excretion

Spectinomycin is administered by IM injection to treat gonorrhea (see Table 31-3). Absorption produces high serum concentrations of drug and maintains those concentrations long enough after a single injection to eradicate *N. gonorrhoeae* from the infection site. Within 2 days, nearly all of the injected drug appears in active form in urine.

Toxicity

Single doses of spectinomycin have caused nausea, chills, and dizziness. Patients may report pain at the injection site, urticaria, or fever. Urine output may be diminished, but renal damage has not been verified.

NURSING IMPLICATIONS SUMMARY

Erythromycin and Other Macrolides

Drug administration

◆ See Nursing Implications Summary in Chapter 29.
◆ Assess for history of allergy before administering drug.
◆ Assess baseline hearing acuity. Assess for GI symptoms and signs of liver dysfunction. Monitor intake and output and weight.
◆ Monitor liver function tests.

INTRAVENOUS ERYTHROMYCIN LACTOBIONATE OR GLUCEPTATE

◆ Dilute each 500 mg with 10 ml of sterile water for injection, and further dilute as instructed in drug insert. Administer at a rate of 1 gm diluted in 100 ml over 20 to 60 min. Monitor vital signs.

Patient and family education

◆ See Nursing Implications Summary in Chapter 29.

◆ Instruct patients to report tinnitus or hearing loss, malaise, fever, jaundice, right upper quadrant abdominal pain, and change in the color or consistency of stools.
◆ Patients should take oral doses with meals or a snack to reduce gastric irritation.

Clindamycin and Lincomycin

Drug administration

◆ See Nursing Implications Summary in Chapter 29.
◆ Assess for history of allergy before administering drug.
◆ Assess for diarrhea or GI distress. Monitor intake and output and weight.
◆ Monitor complete blood count (CBC) and differential, platelet count, liver function tests, and serum electrolyte level.

INTRAVENOUS CLINDAMYCIN

◆ Dilute each 300 mg with at least 50 ml suitable diluent; see drug insert. Administer at a

NURSING IMPLICATIONS SUMMARY—cont'd

rate of 300 mg or less over at least 10 min. Do not administer too rapidly. Monitor vital signs. Supervise ambulation.

INTRAVENOUS LINCOMYCIN

◆ Dilute 1 gm with at least 100 ml of suitable diluent; see drug insert. Administer at a rate of 1 gm or less/hr. Monitor vital signs. Do not administer too rapidly. Supervise ambulation.

Patient and family education

◆ Instruct patients to report diarrhea and not to self-medicate to treat diarrhea without first checking with the physician.
◆ Teach patients to take oral doses of clindamycin with a full glass (8 oz) of fluid, with or without meals.
◆ Patients should take oral lincomycin with a full glass (8 oz) of fluid on an empty stomach, 1 hr before or 2 hr after meals or a snack.
◆ For topical administration, apply carefully, avoiding the eyes, nose, mouth, or mucous membranes.

Vancomycin

Drug administration

◆ See Nursing Implications Summary in Chapter 29.
◆ Assess for history of allergy before administering drug.
◆ Assess baseline hearing acuity.
◆ Monitor serum creatinine level, blood urea nitrogen (BUN) level, CBC, and differential count. Monitor urinalysis.

INTRAVENOUS VANCOMYCIN

◆ Dilute each 500 mg with 10 ml of sterile water for injection. Further dilute with compatible fluid; see drug insert. Administer each diluted dose over 60 min. Monitor vital signs. Too-rapid IV administration may be associated with hypotension, cardiac arrest, or "red man's syndrome" or "red-neck syndrome":

maculopapular or erythematous rash of the face, head, chest, and arms; and fever, chills, fainting, nausea, vomiting, tachycardia, or itching.

Patient and family education

◆ See Nursing Implications Summary in Chapter 29.
◆ Instruct patients to report tinnitus or hearing loss.
◆ Patients should not take oral doses within 4 hr of cholestyramine or colestipol.
◆ If vancomycin is prescribed to treat diarrhea caused by other antibiotics, avoid antidiarrheal medicine unless first approved by the physician.

Bacitracin

Drug administration and patient and family education

◆ See Nursing Implications Summary in Chapter 29.
◆ Topical use of this drug is rarely associated with side effects.

Spectinomycin

Drug administration and patient and family education

◆ See Nursing Implications Summary in Chapter 29.
◆ Caution patients to avoid driving or operating hazardous equipment if dizziness develops; notify the physician.
◆ Warn patients that IM injections may cause burning at the injection site. Use diluent supplied by the manufacturer. Dilute as directed on the vial label.
◆ If given to treat gonorrhea, warn patient that the sexual partner may also need treatment to avoid passing the organism back and forth. Also, teach patients about sexually transmitted diseases as appropriate. Caution patients that the male sexual partner should wear a condom to prevent transmission of infection.

CHAPTER REVIEW

◆ **KEY TERMS**

macrolides, p. 465
penicillin substitutes, p. 465

◆ **REVIEW QUESTIONS**

1. Why are erythromycin, clindamycin, vancomycin, bacitracin, and spectinomycin called penicillin substitutes?

2. What advantages do the esters of erythromycin have over erythromycin base?

3. Which of the erythromycin esters is best absorbed orally and may be taken with meals?

4. Which forms of erythromycin can be used parenterally?

5. What property limits parenteral use of erythromycin?

6. What is the major route of excretion of macrolides?

7. What is the most common adverse reaction to macrolides?

8. What toxic reaction is unique to erythromycin estolate?

9. How does azithromycin differ from erythromycin in distribution in the body and in antibacterial spectrum?

10. Bacterial resistance to clindamycin is associated with resistance to which other antibiotic?

11. How do clindamycin and lincomycin differ in oral absorption?

12. What form of clindamycin is appropriate for parenteral use?

13. How is clindamycin eliminated from the body?

14. What is the limiting toxicity to clindamycin? What implications does this have for nursing care?

15. How is clindamycin-induced colitis best treated?

16. Why is bacterial resistance to vancomycin relatively rare?

17. By what route is vancomycin usually administered?

18. What is the major route of excretion of vancomycin?

19. What toxic reactions are most common with vancomycin?

20. Name three clinical uses for vancomycin.

21. By what route is bacitracin usually administered?

22. What is the primary clinical indication for spectinomycin?

23. What pharmacologic property of spectinomycin makes it a useful replacement of penicillin in treating gonorrhea?

24. Develop a nursing care plan for a patient receiving a drug discussed in this chapter.

SUGGESTED READING

Foxworth J: Toxicities of antimicrobial agents used in the intensive care arena, *Crit Care Nurs Q* 11(4):1, 1989.

Smilack JD, Wilson WR, Cockerill FR III: Tetracyclines, chloramphenicol, erythromycin, clindamycin, and metronidazole, *Mayo Clin Proc* 66(12):1270, 1991.

Washington JA II, Wilson WR: Erythromycin: I. Microbial and clinical perspective after 30 years of clinical use, *Mayo Clin Proc* 60(3):189, 1985.

Washington JA II, Wilson WR: Erythromycin: II. Microbial and clinical perspective after 30 years of clinical use, *Mayo Clin Proc* 60(4):271, 1985.

Wilhelm, MP: Vancomycin, *Mayo Clin Proc* 66(11):1165, 1991.

CHAPTER 32

Tetracyclines and Chloramphenicol

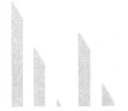

LEARNING OBJECTIVES

After studying this chapter, you should be able to do the following:

◆ Describe how the antimicrobial spectra of tetracyclines and chloramphenicol differ from those of erythromycin (see Chapter 31) and penicillin G (see Chapter 30).

◆ Name the most common route of administration for tetracyclines and chloramphenicol.

◆ Explain how doxycycline and minocycline differ from other tetracyclines.

◆ Describe common side effects of tetracyclines.

◆ Describe the serious side effects of chloramphenicol.

◆ Develop a nursing care plan for a patient receiving a tetracycline or chloramphenicol.

CHAPTER OVERVIEW

◆ This chapter introduces antibiotics with very broad antimicrobial spectra: tetracyclines and chloramphenicol. The **tetracyclines** are a large family of chemically related compounds, many of which are clinically useful. Chloramphenicol is the only member of its chemical class approved for use in the United States.

Nursing Process Overview

TETRACYCLINES AND CHLORAMPHENICOL

Refer to the Nursing Implications Summary in Chapter 29 for general guidelines.

Assessment

Carry out a thorough patient assessment. Monitor liver and kidney function. Monitor signs of clinical infection.

Nursing Diagnoses

Possible complication: gastrointestinal (GI) distress
Possible complication: bone marrow depression

Management

Monitor renal and liver function. Assess for GI distress. Adjust timing of ordered doses to allow for interactions with food or other drugs (especially with tetracycline).

Evaluation

Before discharge, ascertain that patients can take drugs as ordered and can explain signs and symptoms warranting consultation with the physician.

TETRACYCLINES

Mechanism of Action and Bacterial Resistance

The tetracyclines block bacterial growth by preventing ribosomes from binding messenger RNA, thereby preventing the initiation of protein synthesis. Members of this drug family are therefore bacteriostatic rather than bactericidal.

For tetracyclines to be effective, they must first be

transported into the bacterial cell. Antibiotic uptake is accomplished by an energy-dependent–transport system. Resistant bacteria lose the ability to transport tetracyclines into the bacterial cell, and the antibiotic does not come in contact with its intracellular target. Much observed tetracycline resistance involves a plasmid (see Chapter 29) that is transmitted from bacterium to bacterium and may therefore spread rapidly throughout bacterial populations. For example, families of patients treated on a long-term basis with low doses of tetracyclines may show a conversion of the normal tetracycline-sensitive bacterial flora to tetracycline-resistant forms. Cross-resistance between the older tetracyclines is complete. The newer tetracyclines minocycline and doxycyline are more lipid soluble than the other drugs and are transported into the bacterial cell by different mechanisms than the older drugs. These drugs may therefore penetrate bacterial cells that do not concentrate the older tetracyclines. For example, strains of *Staphylococcus aureus* resistant to tetracycline do not accumulate tetracycline but may accumulate minocycline and may be sensitive to it.

Absorption

Tetracyclines are administered primarily by the oral route (Table 32-1). They are frequently administered as a hydrochloride or as a phosphate salt to increase solubility and thereby increase absorption.

Tetracyclines are variably absorbed from the GI tract. Absorption is influenced by acid lability, water solubility, and lipid solubility. All the tetracyclines, with the exception of doxycycline and minocycline, are acid labile and are partly destroyed by stomach acid. Tetracyclines are not highly water soluble, and this solubility may be further reduced by complex formation with metal ions or with solid material in the intestine. In these insoluble forms, drugs are not absorbed but remain in the intestine and are excreted in the feces. Doxycycline and minocycline are the exceptions, being highly lipid soluble; both drugs pass freely through GI membranes and are much more completely and rapidly absorbed than most of the other tetracyclines.

Absorption of tetracyclines from intramuscular (IM) sites is generally poor and frequently causes local tissue irritation and pain at the injection site. IM use of tetracyclines is therefore limited.

Tetracyclines may be used intravenously in serious infections. Tetracycline, oxytetracycline, doxycycline, and minocycline can be obtained in a form suitable for intravenous (IV) use. These drugs have relatively low water solubility and must be diluted extensively before use by this route. When used intravenously, tetracyclines may cause thrombophlebitis. Improper dilution of the drug or repeated infusion into the same vein increases the likelihood of thrombophlebitis.

Table 32-1   Clinical Summary of Tetracyclines

Generic name	Trade name	Administration/dosage
Tetracycline HCl	Achromycin* Tetracyn* Achromycin IM Tetracyn IM Achromycin IV Tetracyn IV	ORAL: *Adults*—1 to 2 gm/day in 2 to 4 doses. *Children over 8 years*—25 to 50 mg/kg/day in 2 to 4 doses. INTRAMUSCULAR: *Adults*—300 to 800 mg/day in divided doses. *Children over 8 years*—15 to 25 mg/kg not to exceed 250 mg/dose. INTRAVENOUS: *Adults*—250 to 500 mg every 12 hr. *Children over 8 years*—15 to 25 mg/kg/day in 2 doses.
Oxytetracycline HCl	Terramycin*	ORAL, INTRAMUSCULAR, INTRAVENOUS: As for tetracycline.
Methacycline HCl	Rondomycin	ORAL: *Adults*—600 mg/day in 2 or 4 doses. *Children over 8 years*—10 mg/kg/day in 4 doses.
Demeclocycline HCl	Declomycin*	ORAL: *Adults*—600 mg to 1 gm/day in 4 doses. *Children over 8 years*—6 to 12 mg/kg/day in 2 to 4 doses.
Doxycycline	Vibramycin*	ORAL: *Adults*—100 to 200 mg/day in 2 doses. *Children over 8 years*—2 to 4 mg/kg/day in 2 doses. INTRAVENOUS: As for oral route.
Minocycline HCl	Minocin* Minocin IV	ORAL: 200 mg initially, then 100 mg every 12 hr. INTRAVENOUS: As for oral route.

*Available in Canada and United States.

Distribution and Excretion

Tetracyclines are well distributed in most body tissues and fluids, appearing in liver, spleen, bone marrow, bile, and cerebrospinal fluid even in the absence of inflammation. The drugs pass the placental barrier and enter fetal circulation in appreciable amounts. Tetracyclines also appear in the milk of nursing mothers.

Differences in lipid solubility among the tetracyclines affect their elimination. The more polar or water-soluble drugs are eliminated through the kidney in greater amounts than are the lipid-soluble tetracyclines. All tetracyclines enter urine by passive glomerular filtration. However, lipid-soluble drugs are more completely reabsorbed from the kidney tubule than drugs that are charged at the acid pH of the tubular fluid. This high degree of reabsorption is reflected in the longer elimination half-life for doxycycline and minocycline (12 to 15 hr) than those of less lipid-soluble tetracyclines such as oxytetracycline, tetracycline, or chlortetracycline (6 to 9 hr).

The second major route of elimination is by biliary excretion. Tetracyclines are concentrated in the liver and bile and carried into the intestine, where they may be reabsorbed by enterohepatic circulation. The liver is also the site for biotransformation of several tetracyclines. In general the more lipid-soluble drugs penetrate the liver cells and are more extensively biotransformed. In particular, minocycline is extensively biotransformed. The high lipid solubility of doxycycline and its tendency to form insoluble complexes with intestinal solids account for an unusual mode of elimination for this drug. It seems to diffuse directly into the intestine, where the drug is sequestered by complex formation with fecal material. Because of this unusual mechanism for excretion, doxycycline does not accumulate in renal failure.

Toxicity

Tetracyclines cause a wide variety of adverse reactions. The most common complaint is GI irritation. Many patients suffer nausea, vomiting, or pain with oral tetracyclines. Diarrhea may occur as a result of irritation by unabsorbed tetracycline remaining in the bowel. Diarrhea may also result from changes in the intestinal flora. Occasionally the effects of these broad-spectrum drugs on intestinal flora are so extensive that overgrowth of drug-resistant bacteria occurs. Staphylococcal enterocolitis may result and may be life-threatening, producing bloody diarrhea and extensive damage to the intestinal epithelium. *Candida* superinfections of the throat, vagina, and bowel also occur occasionally.

Allergies to tetracyclines are uncommon. Urticaria, morbilliform rashes, and dermatitis occur, as do more serious reactions such as asthma, angioedema, and anaphylaxis.

Tetracyclines are not entirely specific for bacterial ribosomes and may inhibit mammalian protein synthesis to a small degree. This may explain their toxic effect on various tissues. For example, kidney function may be impaired by tetracyclines, and the effects may be worse in a kidney already damaged by disease or by trauma. Renal function should therefore be carefully watched in patients receiving these drugs. Likewise the liver is sensitive to tetracyclines. Hepatotoxicity may progress to jaundice, fatty liver, and death unless the drug is discontinued at the first sign of difficulty. Pregnant women are most sensitive to this complication and should rarely, if ever, be given tetracyclines. Elderly patients who are extremely debilitated or patients recovering from extensive surgery or traumatic injuries may suffer metabolic derangement when given tetracyclines. These patients commonly show negative nitrogen balance. This reaction is thought to result from tetracycline inhibition of mammalian protein synthesis.

Tetracyclines also delay blood coagulation. The exact mechanism for this reaction is not known, but it may involve binding the calcium that is required in coagulation.

The ability of tetracyclines to bind calcium also leads to their deposition in bones and teeth. In adults, this binding produces little visible effect, but in children under 8 years of age the newly formed permanent teeth may be stained by the drug. This staining is irreversible. Binding of tetracyclines to bones may slow bone growth visibly in fetuses or young children. Infants may also display increased intracranial pressure with bulging fontanelles when given tetracyclines.

Specific tetracyclines may cause unique adverse reactions. Minocycline can damage vestibular function, thereby impairing balance. No other tetracyclines produce this effect, although other antibiotics do. Another specific reaction to a single tetracycline is the phototoxic effect of demeclocycline. All tetracyclines can be degraded to toxic products by exposure to light, but demeclocycline is most effective in producing these reactions. The drug is broken down by the action of ultraviolet light on the skin, and the toxic products released cause an intense sunburn reaction. Since tetracyclines other than demeclocycline can cause this reaction, it is prudent to suggest that patients receiving these drugs limit their exposure to direct sunlight, especially in subtropical or tropical climates.

Outdated tetracycline preparations have been implicated in occasional severe adverse reactions, apparently caused by toxic breakdown products of the drugs. A reaction called the *Fanconi syndrome* has been observed, in which the patient loses amino acids, proteins, and sugar in urine and suffers polyuria and polydipsia, acidosis, nausea, and vomiting. These reactions slowly disappear after the drug is discontinued. In other cases, patients show symptoms reminiscent of systemic lupus erythematosus.

Drug Interactions

Several tetracycline interactions with other drugs result from the ability of tetracyclines to form insoluble complexes with metal ions. For example, oral tetracyclines frequently cause gastric irritation, and for this reason, patients may wish to take antacids along with the antibiotic. This practice should be discouraged, since common antacids include magnesium and aluminum salts, which complex with tetracyclines and prevent their absorption from the GI tract. Therefore the antacids reduce the antibacterial effect of the antibiotic. Likewise, iron-containing preparations such as vitamin or mineral supplements may prevent tetracycline absorption. Milk and other dairy products are high in calcium and also impair absorption. Sodium bicarbonate taken with a tetracycline tablet may impede tablet dissolution in the stomach and thereby reduce absorption of the drug.

Food in the stomach impairs absorption of oral tetracyclines, with the exception of doxycycline and minocycline. These lipid-soluble tetracyclines are absorbed well even in the presence of food or milk products in the stomach.

Several tetracyclines, especially doxycycline and minocycline, are metabolized to some degree by the liver. Drugs such as barbiturates, which increase hepatic drug-metabolizing enzymes, shorten the duration of action of doxycycline and minocycline. This action may decrease the antibacterial effectiveness of these agents.

The bacteriostatic mechanism of action of tetracyclines leads to interactions with immunosuppressants and penicillins. Immunosuppressant drugs such as glucocorticoids depress the host defense mechanisms against bacterial infections. Since tetracyclines are bacteriostatic, they depend on the patient's immune system to eliminate the pathogen. If this elimination cannot occur, bacteria may overcome the inhibitory effects of the tetracycline, causing the effect of the drug to be lost. Penicillins given with tetracyclines may be less effective than penicillin given alone. Penicillins are bactericidal and act against actively multiplying bacteria. Tetracyclines inhibit bacterial growth, thereby making them resistant to the action of penicillins.

Tetracycline nephrotoxicity may become significant and dangerous when these antibiotics are given with other nephrotoxic agents. One example involves the anesthetic methoxyflurance (Penthrane). This anesthetic gas is nephrotoxic; when given to patients receiving tetracyclines, it may exacerbate kidney damage.

Uses

Tetracyclines are clinically important because of their wide antibacterial spectrum. Most gram-positive organisms are sensitive to tetracyclines; however, most infections caused by these organisms are best treated by other agents because penicillins, cephalosporins, erythromycin, and clindamycin are equally or more effective against these organisms and are less toxic. Nevertheless, when laboratory results confirm the organism to be sensitive to tetracyclines, these drugs can be used in some gram-positive infections.

Gram-negative bacteria found in the bowel are usually sensitive to tetracyclines, but resistance does develop. *Serratia, Proteus,* and *Pseudomonas* strains are usually resistant.

Neisseria gonorrhoeae is sensitive to tetracyclines. Clinically, tetracyclines are used to treat gonorrhea only when penicillin is contraindicated. Tetracyclines are clinically effective for a number of bacterial infections that are relatively rare in the United States including chancroid (*Haemophilus ducreyi*), rabbit fever or tularemia (*Francisella tularensis*), black plague (*Yersinia pestis*), brucellosis (*Brucella* species), and cholera (*Vibrio cholerae*).

Tetracyclines are highly effective for diseases caused by rickettsiae (tick fever, Rocky Mountain spotted fever, typhus, and Q fever), chlamydia (parrot fever or psittacosis, trachoma, lymphogranuloma venereum), and *Mycoplasma pneumoniae* (atypical or "walking" pneumonia).

Tetracyclines are useful in treating Lyme disease (*Borrelia burgdorferi*), relapsing fever (*Borrelia recurrentis*), syphilis (*Treponema pallidum*), and yaws (*Treponema pertenue*), which are all caused by spirochetes. Tetracyclines may have a useful role in treating amebic dysentery. Minocycline in particular may be useful in nocardial infections.

Tetracyclines are widely used to treat acne. Relatively low doses may be prescribed over long periods of time. Although this treatment is effective for many patients, questions arise as to long-term adverse effects of the drugs and to the contribution this practice makes to the development of tetracycline-resistant bacterial populations.

Pharmaceutic formulations of tetracyclines are quite varied. These antibiotics are available in 100- to 500-mg tablets or capsules, syrups for pediatric use, ophthalmic ointments or drops, and various forms for topical use.

CHLORAMPHENICOL
Mechanism of Action and Bacterial Resistance

Chloramphenicol inhibits bacterial protein synthesis. The mechanism of action is different from that of tetracyclines in that chloramphenicol inhibits late rather than early steps in ribosomal function. Like tetracyclines, chloramphenicol is bacteriostatic rather than bactericidal.

Bacterial resistance to chloramphenicol nearly always involves destruction of the antibiotic by bacterial enzymes. These enzymes are not always present but may be induced by exposure of potentially resistant bacteria to sublethal doses of chloramphenicol. The genes required for synthesizing this enzyme are usually carried on small DNA molecules called *plasmids,* which may exist separately from the bulk of genetic material in the cell. Plasmids may be transmitted from bacterium to bacterium, and resistance to chloramphenicol may thereby be transmitted widely throughout bacterial populations.

Absorption, Distribution, and Excretion

Chloramphenicol is nearly completely absorbed from the GI tract after oral administration. The peak serum concentration achieved by an oral dose is about the same as that produced by an equivalent dose given by IV, although attainment of peak serum concentration is somewhat delayed with oral administration (Table 32-2). IM injection produces lower blood levels than oral administration and for this reason is not recommended. Seriously ill patients should receive chloramphenicol intravenously, since oral absorption may be impaired in these patients. The succinate form of chloramphenicol is used for IV administration only, whereas the parent drug, chloramphenicol, is used orally.

Chloramphenicol is well distributed throughout body tissues and fluids. Significant and effective concentrations of the drug enter the eye, joint (synovial), and pleural fluids. Unlike many other antibiotics, chloramphenicol enters cerebrospinal fluid relatively easily, even when the meninges are not inflamed. Chloramphenicol also easily crosses the placenta and appears in human milk.

Most of a dose of chloramphenicol is inactivated in the liver. The drug is conjugated with glucuronic acid to form chloramphenicol glucuronide. This inactive drug form may be excreted in the kidney by tubular secretion, whereas unaltered chloramphenicol is excreted solely by glomerular filtration. The actual concentration of active chloramphenicol in urine is high enough to be antibacterial, but active chloramphenicol in urine is only a small fraction of the total drug excreted via this route.

Toxicity

Chloramphenicol is an effective antibiotic, but its clinical use is limited by its potential for bone marrow toxicity. A reversible form of bone marrow depression causes a reduction of reticulocytes and leukopenia. These symptoms usually resolve quickly when chloramphenicol is discontinued. Patients receiving chloramphenicol should have routine blood tests performed during therapy to detect early signs of this toxic reaction.

Chloramphenicol may also induce an irreversible bone marrow depression, which leads to aplastic anemia, a condition with high mortality. This condition is usually characterized by pancytopenia (loss of all

Table 32-2   Clinical Summary of Chloramphenicol

Generic name	Trade name	Administration/dosage	Comments
Chloramphenicol	Chloromycetin Novochlorocap†	ORAL: *Adults*—50 to 100 mg/kg/day in 4 doses. *Children*—25 to 50 mg/kg/day or less, depending on liver function.	Blood levels should ordinarily not exceed 20 μg/ml.
Chloramphenicol	Chloroptic*	OPHTHALMIC: *Adults and children*—Apply to conjunctiva every 3 hr or more frequently.	Solution or ointment may be used.
Chloramphenicol	Chloromycetin* Pentamycetin*	OTIC: *Adults and children*—Apply 2 or 3 drops to ear canal every 6 to 8 hr.	For external infections.
Chloramphenicol palmitate	Chloromycetin	ORAL: *Children*—as for other oral forms.	This tasteless suspension is intended for pediatric use.
Chloramphenicol succinate	Chloromycetin*	INTRAVENOUS: As for oral.	Should be administered as a 10% solution and injected slowly into the vein.

*Available in Canada and United States.
†Available in Canada only.

forms of blood cells), but in some cases, one or more of the major blood cells continues to be formed. Aplastic anemia, although rare, may appear weeks or months after chloramphenicol therapy. This time lag between drug administration and appearance of aplastic anemia complicates the accurate calculation of drug-associated risk, especially considering that most patients have received more than one other drug during the interim between chloramphenicol therapy and development of aplastic anemia. Best estimates of the actual incidence suggest that roughly one in 30,000 chloramphenicol-treated patients will develop aplastic anemia. Although this incidence is low, the frequently fatal outcome is sufficient cause to restrict the use of chloramphenicol to the treatment of very serious infections.

Less severe problems also occur with chloramphenicol therapy. Allergies of various types and GI irritation may occur. Long-term therapy has been associated with neuritis, which may involve the optic nerve. Blindness has occurred in a few patients. Central nervous system (CNS) symptoms are also seen in some patients including headache, mental confusion, depression, or delirium.

Patients with reduced liver function are at risk of severe toxic reactions because of drug accumulation. The liver normally converts over 90% of administered chloramphenicol, which is toxic, to the glucuronide, which is nontoxic. Therefore any reduction in the liver's ability to detoxify the drug may result in accumulation of the toxic drug in the body, unless dosages are appropriately reduced. Newborn infants are especially at risk for this complication. Neonates have an immature liver that lacks the enzyme to form the glucuronide. When these infants are given a weight-adjusted dosage based on adult doses, many develop a condition termed the *gray syndrome*. Drug accumulation proceeds without symptoms for 3 to 4 days, after which time the infant may develop abdominal distention, emesis, progressive pallid cyanosis, and irregular respiration. In a high percentage of cases, vasomotor collapse and death result. Infants receiving

smaller doses are less likely to develop these symptoms. If early signs of the condition are noted by alert health-care personnel and the drug is discontinued, most infants recover.

Chloramphenicol crosses the placenta and may concentrate in the fetal liver. For this reason the drug is not given to pregnant women near term.

Drug Interactions

Chloramphenicol can inhibit drug-metabolizing enzymes of the liver. This property may lead to dangerous interactions with drugs that have a relatively low therapeutic index and a major route of elimination by microsomal enzymes of the liver. The three drugs that fall into this category are phenytoin, tolbutamide, and coumarin anticoagulants. When a patient receiving one of these drugs on a long-term basis is given chloramphenicol, these liver-metabolized drugs tend to accumulate. As a result, well-controlled diabetic patients may become hypoglycemic, successfully anticoagulated patients may develop spontaneous bleeding, and controlled epileptic patients may develop phenytoin toxicity.

Since chloramphenicol is rarely used, these interactions are rare. In the unusual case in which these drugs must be combined the early signs of drug interactions should be anticipated.

Uses

Because of dangerous toxic reactions, chloramphenicol is used only in serious infections. Chloramphenicol is the drug of choice for typhoid fever. In addition, life-threatening infections such as bacteremias or meningitis may be treated with chloramphenicol when the pathogen has been tested and has proved sensitive to the drug. The antibacterial spectrum of chloramphenicol is similar to that of tetracyclines and is especially effective against gram-negative bacteria (except *Pseudomonas aeruginosa*), rickettsiae, and chlamydia. Chloramphenicol is especially effective against the important anaerobic pathogen *Bacteroides fragilis*.

NURSING IMPLICATIONS SUMMARY

Tetracyclines

Drug administration

◆ See Nursing Implications Summary in Chapter 29.
◆ Assess for allergy before administering drug.

◆ Assess for dizziness and vertigo in patients receiving minocycline. Inspect for bruising, bleeding, and blood in stool.
◆ Monitor blood urea nitrogen (BUN) level, serum creatinine level, liver function tests, complete blood count (CBC) and differential, and platelet count.

NURSING IMPLICATIONS SUMMARY—cont'd

◆ Palpate the fontanelles of infants every 4 hr; report bulging to the physician.

◆ Do not administer drug to children under 8 years of age unless absolutely necessary.

◆ Warn patients that IM injections are painful.

◆ Administer IV doses slowly, and well diluted, to lessen the chance of venous irritation and phlebitis. Make certain IV is patent before administering drug to avoid extravasation.

INTRAVENOUS OXYTETRACYCLINE AND TETRACYCLINE

◆ Dilute as directed in drug insert. Administer at a rate of 100 mg or less over at least 5 min.

INTRAVENOUS DOXYCYCLINE

◆ Dilute each 100 mg with 10 ml sterile water for injection or normal saline. Further dilute as directed in drug insert with 100 to 1000 ml of compatible fluid. Administer at a rate of 100 mg over 1 to 4 hr.

INTRAVENOUS MINOCYCLINE

◆ Dilute as directed in drug insert. Final dilution is in a volume of 500 to 1000 ml. Administer at an appropriate rate for the volume.

Patient and family education

◆ See Nursing Implications Summary in Chapter 29.

◆ Tell patients to take oral doses with a full glass (8 oz) of water.

◆ Usually, patients should take oral tetracyclines on an empty stomach, 1 hr before or 2 hr after meals. However, if the drug causes stomach upset, the physician may permit it to be taken with meals or a snack. Doxycycline and minocycline may be taken on a full or an empty stomach.

◆ Tell patients not to take tetracyclines within 1 to 2 hr of having milk, milk products, formula, or any of the following medications: antacids, calcium supplements, choline and magnesium salicylate combinations, magnesium salicylate, magnesium-containing laxatives, or sodium bicarbonate. Review other prescribed medications with patients to clarify these instructions.

◆ Instruct patients not to take iron or vitamin preparations containing iron within 2 to 3 hr of taking a tetracycline.

◆ Warn patients that tetracyclines may cause the tongue to become darkened or discolored. This effect is not significant and clears when the drug is stopped.

◆ Contraceptive pills containing estrogen may not be effective while patients are taking tetracyclines; other forms of birth control should be used. Discuss this effect with the physician or pharmacist.

◆ This drug may cause patients to develop photosensitivity (see Patient Problem: Photosensitivity on p. 629).

◆ Demeclocycline may be used to treat the syndrome of inappropriate antidiuretic hormone (SIADH) and, when used for this, functions as a diuretic. This diuretic action is effective in patients with SIADH but is not satisfactory in other patients who may require diuresis.

◆ When tetracyclines are used in children under 8 years of age, discoloration of the teeth may occur. Notify the physician if this happens.

◆ Teach patients to observe expiration dates on all medications but especially tetracyclines. Use of outdated preparations or those that have deteriorated or changed color may cause severe adverse reactions.

◆ Warn patients taking minocycline to avoid driving or operating hazardous equipment if vertigo or dizziness occurs; notify the physician.

◆ Tell diabetic patients that tetracyclines may contribute to false results in urine glucose tests. Consult physician before changing diet or insulin. Monitor blood glucose level.

◆ Teach patients to take the capsule form of doxycycline whole, without crushing or breaking.

Chloramphenicol
Drug administration

◆ See Nursing Implications Summary in Chapter 29.

◆ Assess for history of allergy before administering drug.

◆ Assess visual acuity before beginning therapy and at regular intervals. Assess for GI side effects, skin changes, and signs of hematologic side effects.

◆ Monitor infants for appearance of the gray syndrome. Assess for failure to feed, abdominal distention, progressive pallid cyanosis, and irregular respiration. Note that the gray syndrome can develop in infants of women who received chloramphenicol during labor or the last few days of pregnancy.

◆ Monitor serum drug levels, CBC and differential, platelet count, BUN level, serum creatinine level, and liver function tests.

Continued.

NURSING IMPLICATIONS SUMMARY—cont'd

INTRAVENOUS CHLORAMPHENICOL

◆ Dilute 1 gm with 10 ml of sterile water of 5% dextrose in water. It may be further diluted with 50 to 100 ml of compatible solution; see drug insert. Administer IV push at a rate of 1 g over at least 1 min. For infusion, administer volume of 50 to 100 ml over 30 to 60 min. Warn patients that they may experience a bitter taste in the mouth after IV administration that should resolve after a few minutes.

Patient and family education

◆ See Nursing Implications Summary in Chapter 29.
◆ Instruct patients to report unexplained bruis-

ing or bleeding, nosebleed, bleeding from gums, or blood in stools and fever, sore throat, malaise, fatigue, or symptoms of infection. Tell the patient to report these symptoms even if they develop after the drug has been stopped.
◆ Instruct patients to take oral doses with a full glass (8 oz) of water on an empty stomach, 1 hr before or 2 hr after meals for best effect.
◆ Caution patients to avoid driving or operating hazardous equipment if confusion or visual changes occur.
◆ Warn diabetic patients that chloramphenicol may cause false results with urine glucose tests. Consult the physician before changing diet or diabetes medications. Monitor blood glucose levels.

CHAPTER REVIEW

◆ **KEY TERMS**

chloramphenicol, p. 479
tetracyclines, p. 475

◆ **REVIEW QUESTIONS**

1. What is the mechanism of action of tetracycline antibiotics?
2. What is the mechanism by which bacteria become resistant to tetracyclines?
3. What factors influence the oral absorption of tetracycline antibiotics? What are some teaching implications?
4. How does the absorption of minocycline and doxycycline differ from that of other tetracyclines?
5. What factors limit the IM use of tetracyclines?
6. What precautions are necessary for using tetracyclines by IV routes?
7. What are the three main routes of excretion for the tetracyclines?
8. Are minocycline and doxycycline eliminated in the same way as other tetracyclines?
9. What are the main toxic reactions common to all tetracycline antibiotics?
10. What toxic reaction is especially associated with demeclocycline?
11. What toxic reaction is especially associated with minocycline?

12. What toxicity is associated with outdated tetracycline preparations?
13. What is the effect of administering tetracyclines with antacids? What is the teaching implication?
14. Why do immunosuppressant drugs interfere with the clinical effect of tetracyclines?
15. Why do tetracyclines interfere with the antimicrobial action of penicillins?
16. Name three groups of organisms against which the tetracyclines are effective.
17. What is the mechanism of action of chloramphenicol?
18. What is the mechanism by which bacteria become resistant to chloramphenicol?
19. Which routes of administration give the most rapid and complete absorption of chloramphenicol?
20. Does chloramphenicol efficiently enter the cerebrospinal fluid?
21. What is the primary route of elimination of chloramphenicol?
22. What is the most dangerous toxic reaction associated with chloramphenicol?
23. What is the gray syndrome?
24. Name a clinical indication for chloramphenicol.
25. Develop a nursing care plan for a patient receiving one of the drugs discussed in this chapter.

SUGGESTED READING

Smilack JD, Wilson WR, Cockerill FR III: Tetracyclines, chloramphenicol, erythromycin, clindamycin, and metronidazole, *Mayo Clin Proc* 66(12):1270, 1991.

CHAPTER 33

Aminoglycosides and Polymyxins

LEARNING OBJECTIVES

After studying this chapter, you should be able to do the following:

♦ Explain why aminoglycosides are administered only by parenteral routes.

♦ Describe the toxicity associated with aminoglycoside use.

♦ Explain why aminoglycosides are sometimes used along with penicillins for serious infections.

♦ Explain why polymyxins have limited clinical uses.

♦ Develop a nursing plan for a patient receiving an aminoglycoside or a polymyxin.

CHAPTER OVERVIEW

♦ In this chapter, two groups of antibiotics with primary usefulness against gram-negative bacteria are introduced. The aminoglycosides are antibiotics composed of three or four amino sugars held together in glycosidic linkage. Great variability in structure is possible in these component sugars, and as a result, several antibiotics of this type exist. Polymyxins are peptide antibiotics created by a spore-forming bacillus found in the soil. These groups of drugs are considered together, since they have similar antimicrobial spectra and share certain toxic properties.

Nursing Process Overview
AMINOGLYCOSIDES AND POLYMYXINS

Refer to Chapter 29 for general guidelines on the nursing process with antibiotic therapy. The additional material in this chapter relates specifically to the aminoglycosides and polymyxins.

Assessment

Perform a full assessment with a focus on the signs and symptoms of infection. Assess renal function, hearing acuity, and vestibular function. Note other medications the patient is receiving.

Nursing Diagnoses

Possible complication: ototoxicity secondary to aminoglycoside therapy

Possible complication: renal damage or failure secondary to aminoglycoside therapy

Management

Once the decision is made to administer aminoglycosides or polymyxins, gather the proper supplies for proper administration by the parenteral route chosen. Note whether the patient has received any other neuromuscular blocking agents or whether the patient has any other condition such as myasthenia gravis that would predispose the patient to respiratory paralysis. Have available equipment to deal with respiratory paralysis if it occurs. Ensure that the medications are administered at the times prescribed. If samples are being taken for the measurement of blood levels of these drugs, obtain samples as ordered, since the timing is critical for proper interpretation of the information.

Evaluation

Monitor vital signs closely, and assess objective and subjective signs and symptoms. Hearing loss caused by aminoglycosides and polymyxins may progress during and after therapy. Continue to evaluate the patient for this symptom and for any loss of control of equilibrium as evidenced by difficulty in walking, staggering, or dizziness.

AMINOGLYCOSIDES
Mechanism of Action and Bacterial Resistance
The **aminoglycosides** inhibit early steps in bacterial protein synthesis by binding to bacterial ribosomes. Under certain conditions, bacterial protein synthesis may continue in the presence of aminoglycosides but with a greatly increased error rate. Defective proteins formed may damage the bacterial cell. Aminoglycosides also have a somewhat delayed effect on the bacterial cell membrane. Aminoglycosides are more bactericidal than many other antibiotics that inhibit bacterial protein synthesis.

Resistance to aminoglycosides occurs as a result of decreased antibiotic uptake, changes in antibiotic binding to the ribosome, or enzymatic destruction of the aminoglycosides. By far the most common mechanism for resistance involves antibiotic destruction. Many sites for enzymatic attack exist on the amino sugar components of aminoglycosides. Several different enzymes exist that modify the aminoglycosides by different mechanisms. The primary sites of attack are amino and hydroxyl groups on the sugars. Amino groups may be acetylated, and hydroxyl groups may have a phosphate or an adenylate group added. Any of these substitutions may render the aminoglycoside inactive. At least 13 separate enzymes catalyzing these reactions have been identified. Aminoglycosides differ in susceptibility to degradation, ranging from kanamycin, which is destroyed by at least six different enzymes, to amikacin, which is sensitive to only two enzymes.

Rarely, bacterial resistance may result from reduced drug uptake. This mechanism has been observed especially with amikacin. An equally rare mechanism of resistance involves lowering drug binding to the ribosome. Occasional streptomycin-resistant strains arise by this mechanism.

Absorption
Aminoglycosides are polycationic molecules at physiologic pH. As a result of being charged, these drugs do not penetrate mammalian membranes readily and are not absorbed orally. Therapy with aminoglycosides is therefore by intramuscular (IM) or intravenous (IV) routes and usually involves hospitalized patients suffering from moderate-to-severe infections. Absorption of aminoglycosides from IM injections sites is rapid, and peak serum concentrations occur between 1 and 1½ hr after injection.

GERIATRIC CONSIDERATION: AMINOGLYCOSIDES

THE PROBLEM
Patients over 60 years of age have reduced renal function and therefore may excrete aminoglycosides more slowly than younger adults. In the elderly, aminoglycosides may accumulate because alternative paths of elimination are limited. Older adults also have some hearing loss because of their age and may therefore be more susceptible to drug-induced hearing loss.

SOLUTIONS
◆ Lower doses to avoid accumulation
◆ Monitor serum aminoglycoside concentrations
◆ Monitor renal function tests
◆ Perform baseline auditory function tests; repeat during therapy

---

Distribution and Excretion
Aminoglycosides do not enter the central nervous system (CNS) to any significant extent in normal persons. Some drug does appear in cerebrospinal fluid when meningitis is present. Aminoglycosides enter most other body fluids and tissues with the exception of bile. These drugs cross the placenta and achieve significant concentrations in the fetus.

Aminoglycosides are excreted by glomerular filtration in the kidney. Active drug is concentrated in the urine. Since the kidney is the primary site for elimination of these drugs, any reduction in renal function may lower the excretion sufficiently to cause aminoglycoside accumulation. The approximate half-time for elimination of these drugs is 2 to 4 hr but in renal failure may be greatly prolonged. Excretion is also lower in neonates, who have immature kidneys, and in elderly patients, whose renal function is diminished simply as a function of age (see box).

Toxicity
The aminoglycosides exert significant toxicity of three major types: ototoxicity, renal toxicity, and neuromuscular blockade (Table 33-1). Ototoxicity may cause hearing loss, loss of equilibrium control, or both. Hearing loss in some patients continues even after the drug is discontinued. Loss of equilibrium may be less obvious than hearing loss but can usually be revealed by appropriate tests. Nausea or dizziness may signal disturbance of equilibrium. Ototoxicity is usually more severe when serum concentrations of aminoglycosides exceed 8 to 10 μg/ml. Total dose administered may also be a factor, since some patients treated over long periods may display these symptoms in spite of never having excessively high serum levels of the drug. Amino-

Table 33-1   Aminoglycoside Toxicity

Drug	Ototoxicity Vestibular	Ototoxicity Hearing	Renal toxicity	Neuromuscular blockade
Amikacin	Lower incidence than hearing impairment.	From 3% to 11% of treated patients may show measurable hearing impairment.	More patients show rise in serum creatinine level than with gentamicin. Up to 20% of patients may be affected.	Expected from animal studies.
Gentamicin	About 2% of treated patients suffer permanent mild to severe vestibular damage.	Less frequent than vestibular damage, and usually involves high-tone hearing loss.	Acute renal failure has occurred. Blood urea and creatinine levels may rise; proteinuria may occur. Damage is usually but not always reversible.	May occur, but is less common than with kanamycin, neomycin, and streptomycin.
Kanamycin	Vertigo or other symptoms of vestibular damage affect about 7% of patients receiving high doses.	Up to 30% of patients receiving high doses suffer detectable hearing loss; fewer patients develop complete deafness.	Blood urea and creatinine levels may rise; hematuria and other signs of renal irritation may occur. Most signs of damage disappear when drug is discontinued.	Occurs after peritoneal lavage; usually not reversed by neostigmine, and occasionally not reversed by calcium.
Neomycin	Not common.	Irreversible hearing loss progressing to complete deafness is common.	Reversible, progressive kidney toxicity causes an increase in blood urea.	Occurs after peritoneal lavage; usually reversed by neostigmine.
Netilmicin	Possible but less likely than hearing loss.	About 1% to 2% of treated patients show hearing impairment.	From 3% to 8% of treated patients show some sign of changes in renal function.	May be twice as potent as gentamicin in producing blockade.
Streptomycin	May affect 75% of patients receiving 2 gm daily for 2 to 4 months and 25% of patients receiving 1 gm daily.	Loss usually partial but may be complete; affects 4% to 15% of patients receiving drug longer than 1 week.	Not common unless high drug doses are used and the urine is acidic.	May occur after peritoneal lavage; reversed by neostigmine or calcium.
Tobramycin	From 1% to 11% of treated patients show measurable impairment.	Incidence is the same as for vestibular damage.	Serum creatinine level may be elevated, but the incidence may be less than with gentamicin or amikacin.	Expected from animal studies.

glycosides may damage both tubules and glomeruli in the kidney, especially when high doses are given. This toxic potential can cause a rapid clinical deterioration, since renal damage can cause drug accumulation, which in turn causes further damage to the kidney. This cycle of accumulation and increasing renal damage can destroy kidney function. Patients who accumulate the drug because of renal dysfunction are also more prone to ototoxicity.

The third characteristic toxic reaction to aminoglycosides is neuromuscular blockade. This reaction is usually observed in surgical patients when an aminoglycoside is used in peritoneal lavage. Neuromuscular blockade usually is manifested by respiratory paralysis, since the muscles of the chest involved in breathing are prevented from functioning. Some of the aminoglycosides produce a competitive neuromuscular blockade, which may be reversed by neostigmine. Others such as kanamycin produce an irreversible blockade, which neostigmine does not affect, although calcium may relieve the blockade in some cases. Patients who have recently received muscle relaxants are more prone to suffer neuromuscular blockade with aminoglycosides. Patients with myasthenia gravis are also more sensitive to this effect.

Less common adverse reactions include effects on a variety of organ systems. Blood dyscrasias, while rare, may occur with any aminoglycoside. Likewise, rare neurotoxicity may be manifested by headaches, paresthesias, tremor, confusion, and disorientation. The aminoglycosides are also somewhat irritating and may cause pain at the injection site.

Drug Interactions

The ototoxicity and nephrotoxicity of aminoglycoside antibiotics may be enhanced by a variety of agents. For example, if a patient who is receiving an aminoglycoside is also given a nephrotoxic drug such as a cephalosporin or methoxyflurane (Penthrane), the risk of kidney damage is increased. Likewise, ototoxic drugs such as ethacrynic acid may enhance ototoxicity in a patient receiving an aminoglycoside antibiotic. All aminoglycosides possess neuromuscular blocking activity. This action has led to enhancement of agents used for neuromuscular blocking action during surgery.

Gentamicin is frequently combined with an anti-*Pseudomonas* penicillin to treat *Pseudomonas aeruginosa* infections. Although these drugs may be used in the same patient, they should never be physically mixed, since penicillins chemically inactivate gentamicin in solution.

Aminoglycosides are many times more effective at the slightly alkaline pH of normal serum (pH 7.4) than at the acidic pH of normal urine (pH 5). Therefore, in the treatment of urinary tract infections with these drugs, a therapeutic advantage may be gained by alkalinizing urine.

Oral neomycin causes mucosal alterations in the bowel, which may in extreme cases lead to malabsorption syndrome. Oral neomycin may also impair absorption of orally administered drugs. This potential interaction has been documented with penicillin V, digoxin, and vitamin B_{12}. If these drugs must be given to a patient receiving oral neomycin, extra care should be taken to ensure that adequate amounts of the other orally administered medications are being absorbed.

Uses

The clinical use of these drugs is limited by their toxic potential. As a general rule the aminoglycosides are reserved for serious infections caused by aerobic gram-negative bacteria or by mycobacteria (see Chapter 35). Individual drugs in this family differ in specific uses as a result of differences in relative toxicity and antibacterial activity. Table 33-2 lists the most important clinical uses of individual aminoglycosides. Streptomycin is most useful today in combination with other agents to treat infections in which strict bactericidal action is required for most effective therapy. Examples of these infections are bacterial endocarditis and tuberculosis (see Chapter 35). Neomycin is too toxic for parenteral use but may be administered orally with the intent that the drug will remain in the bowel and lower the bacterial population. This effect may be useful before bowel surgery or in hepatic coma. Certain specific infections of the

Table 33-2   Aminoglycoside Antibiotics Use

Drug	Indications
Amikacin	Serious infections resulting from aerobic gram-negative bacteria including *Pseudomonas aeruginosa*
Gentamicin	Serious infections resulting from aerobic gram-negative bacteria including *P. aeruginosa*.
Kanamycin	Serious infections resulting from aerobic gram-negative bacteria other than *Pseudomonas*.
Neomycin	Oral use for reducing bacterial population of the bowel.
Netilmicin	Serious infections resulting from aerobic gram-negative bacteria including *P. aeruginosa*.
Streptomycin	Used alone to treat tularemia (rabbit fever) and bubonic or black plague. Used in combination with other antibiotics to treat bacterial endocarditis (with penicillin G), tuberculosis (with isoniazid or other antituberculosis agents), brucellosis (with tetracyclines), and *Listeria* infections (with ampicillin or penicillin G).
Tobramycin	Primarily for *P. aeruginosa* infections; may also substitute for gentamicin in other infections.

bowel may also respond to this therapy. Kanamycin may occasionally be used orally in a manner similar to neomycin; however, it is most useful for serious systemic infections.

One difference among aminoglycosides is their different degree of activity against *P. aeruginosa*. Amikacin, gentamicin, and tobramycin are most effective against this pathogen. Kanamycin usually is not effective. Amikacin differs from other aminoglycosides in being less sensitive to common aminoglycoside-degrading enzymes. Amikacin is therefore active against some bacterial strains that are resistant to other aminoglycosides.

Table 33-3 lists common dosages for aminoglycosides used in patients with normal renal function. When renal function is significantly impaired or is in question, it is necessary to monitor serum levels of these drugs to prevent intoxication.

POLYMYXINS

Mechanism of Action and Bacterial Resistance

Polymyxins alter the permeability of bacterial cell membranes, causing the loss of required small molecules and ions from the cell. This action is made possible by the combination of highly ionic groups

Table 33-3 Aminoglycoside Antibiotics

Generic name	Trade name	Administration/dosage
Amikacin	Amikin*	INTRAMUSCULAR, INTRAVENOUS: *Adults, children, and infants*—15 mg/kg body weight daily in 2 or 3 doses. Do not exceed 1.5 gm daily. IV doses are given by slow infusion. FDA Pregnancy Category D.
Gentamicin	Cidomycin† Garamycin*	INTRAMUSCULAR, INTRAVENOUS: *Adults*—3 to 5 mg/kg daily in 3 doses. FDA Pregnancy Category C. *Children*—6 to 7.5 mg/kg daily in 3 doses. *Neonates*—5 mg/kg daily in 2 or 3 doses.
Kanamycin	Kantrex	INTRAMUSCULAR, INTRAVENOUS, INTRAPERITONEAL: *Adults and children*—not to exceed 15 mg/kg daily, divided into 2 or 3 doses. FDA Pregnancy Category D.
Neomycin	Mycifradin*	ORAL: *Adults*—4 to 8.4 gm daily in up to 6 doses. *Children*—Up to 4.8 gm/M² daily divided into 4 doses. Not used for systemic infections. TOPICAL: *Adults and children*—commonly used as 0.35% creams and ointments. Also used in numerous combinations with other antibiotics.
Netilmicin	Netromycin*	INTRAMUSCULAR, INTRAVENOUS: *Adults*—4 to 6.5 mg/kg daily divided into 3 equal doses. FDA Pregnancy Category D. *Children*—5.5 to 8 mg/kg daily divided into 2 or 3 doses. *Neonates to 6 weeks*—adult dose.
Streptomycin	Streptomycin	INTRAMUSCULAR, INTRAVENOUS: *Adults*—1 to 4 gm daily in 2 or 3 doses (15 to 25 mg/kg daily). Elderly patients may require less drug. Lower doses are used for long-term treatment of mild tuberculosis. IV route rarely used. FDA Pregnancy Category D. *Children*—20 to 40 mg/kg daily in 2 doses.
Tobramycin	Nebcin*	INTRAMUSCULAR, INTRAVENOUS: *Adults, infants*—3 to 5 mg/kg daily divided into 3 doses. FDA Pregnancy Category D. *Children*—6 to 7.5 mg/kg daily divided into 2 or 3 doses.

*Available in Canada and United States.
†Available in Canada only.

along with lipid-soluble hydrocarbon chains all within the same molecule. The positively charged portion of the polymyxin molecule is attracted to the negatively charged surface of the bacterial membrane. Membrane disruption occurs when the hydrocarbon chain portion of the polymyxin is inserted into the lipid-rich bacterial membrane. Bacterial cell death results from the loss of cell nutrients and cofactors required for energy production. Polymyxins affect actively growing or static bacterial cells.

Polymyxins are of clinical interest because of their bactericidal action on gram-negative bacteria. With the exception of *Proteus, Neisseria,* and *Bacteroides,* most gram-negative organisms including *P. aeruginosa* are sensitive to the polymyxins. Gram-positive organisms are usually considered resistant to the polymyxins.

Clinical resistance to polymyxins has not increased since the drugs were introduced into clinical practice in 1947. Organisms that are naturally resistant to these drugs apparently possess barriers that prevent polymyxin from contacting the cell membrane.

Absorption, Distribution, and Excretion

Polymyxins are not absorbed from the gastrointestinal (GI) tract, but effective systemic concentrations of the drugs can be achieved by parenteral administration (see Table 33-3). Peak blood levels are ordinarily reached about 2 hr after IM injection, but severe pain may result with this route of administration.

IV administration of the polymyxins is by relatively slow infusion. These drugs should never be given rapidly by IV, since the resulting high blood levels can produce respiratory paralysis in some patients.

Polymyxins are bound to various tissues and persist at those sites for up to 3 days after therapy is stopped. Significant concentrations of polymyxins appear in fetuses when these drugs are administered to the mother.

Excretion of polymyxins is primarily by the kidney. The serum half-life for polymyxins in the body is 2 to 3 hr in a patient with normal renal function.

Toxicity

Since the detergent-like action of polymyxins on cell membranes is nonspecific, this family of drugs has a low therapeutic index. Significant neurotoxicity, nephrotoxicity, and neuromuscular blockade can be produced.

Neuromuscular blockade is caused by a curarelike action of polymyxin at the neuromuscular junction. This effect is most often observed clinically as respiratory paralysis. Calcium chloride may relieve the blockade in some patients but neostigmine does not.

Nephrotoxicity, manifested by decreased glomerular filtration rates and increased serum creatinine and BUN levels, occurs when polymyxin concentrations in the blood exceed recommended levels. Nephrotoxicity is usually reversible. However, patients in whom renal toxicity is not recognized may suffer a rapid deterioration in clinical status because of the cycle of drug accumulation, increasing renal deterioration, further drug accumulation, and additional drug toxicity.

Neurotoxicity of polymyxins is manifested by symptoms of numbness, tingling of the extremities, generalized pruritus, and dizziness. Paresthesias are observed fairly commonly. At higher doses or in patients suffering drug accumulation, more severe symptoms may be observed. These symptoms include giddiness or mental confusion, slurring of speech, ataxia, convulsions, or coma. The signs of neurotoxicity usually disappear when polymyxins are discontinued.

Drug Interactions

The most important clinical interaction of polymyxins occurs with muscle-relaxing agents. In some patients, unexpected neuromuscular blockade and respiratory paralysis have occurred when the patient received both polymyxin and another antibiotic with curarelike action. Potential for this interaction exists with kanamycin, streptomycin, neomycin, and probably other aminoglycoside antibiotics.

The muscle-relaxing agents used in conjunction with surgery are the drugs most commonly involved in drug interactions with polymyxins. These curariform muscle relaxants include ether, tubocurarine, succinylcholine, gallamine, and decamethonium. Patients who are receiving or have recently received these drugs should be most carefully observed for development of respiratory paralysis if polymyxins must be administered.

Uses

Because of their relatively narrow antimicrobial spectrum and relatively high toxicity, the uses for these drugs are limited. Specific indications for the individual members of this drug class are listed in Table 33-4.

Polymyxins are also used in various ointments and creams intended for topical application. For this purpose, they are frequently combined with neomycin and bacitracin.

Table 33-4   Polymyxins

Generic name	Trade name	Administration/dosage	Clinical use
Colistimethate sodium (colistin methane sulfonate)	Coly-Mycin M	INTRAMUSCULAR, INTRAVENOUS: *Adults and children*—2.5 to 5 mg/kg body weight daily in 2 to 4 doses up to 300 mg daily. Dosage must be reduced if renal impairment exists.	Reserve drug for treatment of *Pseudomonas aeruginosa*.
Polymyxin B sulfate	Aerosporin	INTRAVENOUS: *Adults and children*—15,000 to 25,000 units/kg daily by infusion in 300 to 500 ml 5% dextrose. INTRATHECAL: *Adults*—50,000 units in single daily dose. *Children under 2 years*—20,000 units in single daily dose.	Reserve drug for treatment of *P. aeruginosa*. Reserve drug for treatment of *P. aeruginosa* meningitis.

NURSING IMPLICATIONS SUMMARY

Aminoglycosides

Drug administration

◆ See Nursing Implications Summary in Chapter 29.
◆ Assess for history of allergy before administering drug.

◆ Review Table 33-1 for a summary of toxicity observed with these drugs. Assess for changes in hearing and balance and for development of tinnitus and buzzing.
◆ Monitor intake and output and weight. Assess for increased thirst, nausea, vomiting, loss of appetite, and increase or decrease in frequency of urination.

NURSING IMPLICATIONS SUMMARY—cont'd

◆ Monitor vital signs, and auscultate lung sounds.

◆ Monitor serum creatinine level, BUN level, urinalysis, liver function tests, serum electrolyte level, complete blood count and differential, and platelet count.

◆ Monitor serum drug levels. Peak and trough levels may be available. Peak levels indicate serum levels after a dose is given and reflect the highest serum level for that patient at that dose. Trough levels are drawn shortly before a dose is given and reflect the lowest serum level for that patient at that dose. If peak and trough levels are ordered, notify the laboratory of the time a dose will be given, so blood specimens can be obtained at the necessary times for drug level calculations.

◆ Have available neostigmine and calcium chloride in settings where aminoglycosides are used with high-risk patients such as in the operating room, recovery room, and intensive care units. Monitor respiratory status. Have available a suction machine at the bedside.

◆ A separate form of gentamicin without preservatives is available for intrathecal administration.

◆ Do not mix aminoglycosides in a syringe with other medications.

◆ For pediatric doses and dilutions, consult the manufacturer's literature.

◆ Because of the possibility of hypotension or vertigo, keep side rails up. Supervise ambulation.

◆ Neomycin may be ordered orally or via enema to inhibit ammonia-forming bacteria in the GI tract of patients with hepatic encephalopathy.

◆ Streptomycin may cause peripheral neuritis. Assess for burning of face, numbness, and tingling.

INTRAMUSCULAR STREPTOMYCIN

◆ Dilute as directed on the label of the vial. Use a large muscle mass. This drug is not administered by IV.

INTRAVENOUS AMIKACIN

◆ Dilute 500 mg in 100 to 200 ml of normal saline or 5% dextrose in water, and administer over 30 to 60 min.

INTRAVENOUS GENTAMICIN

◆ Dilute a single dose in 50 to 200 ml of normal saline or 5% dextrose in water. The concen-

tration should not exceed 0.1% (1 mg/ml). Administer each dose over 30 to 60 min. Prepared dilutions are available.

INTRAVENOUS KANAMYCIN

◆ Dilute the prescribed dose in normal saline, 5% dextrose in normal saline, or 5% dextrose in water to a concentration of 500 mg in 100 to 200 ml. Administer over 30 to 60 min.

INTRAVENOUS NETILMICIN

◆ Dilute a single dose in 50 to 200 ml of diluent; see drug insert. Administer over 30 min to 2 hr.

INTRAVENOUS TOBRAMYCIN

◆ Dilute dose in 50 to 100 ml of 5% dextrose in water or normal saline, and administer over 20 to 60 min.

Patient and family education

◆ See Nursing Implication Summary in Chapter 29.

◆ Instruct the patient to report hearing loss, nausea, dizziness or vertigo, decreased urinary output, nausea, vomiting, loss of appetite, and increased thirst.

◆ Streptomycin is often given in combination with other drugs in long-term therapy for tuberculosis. Streptomycin may cause false results in urine glucose tests. Warn diabetic patients about this. Monitor blood glucose level if possible.

◆ Streptomycin may cause peripheral neuritis. Caution patients to report changes in vision, burning, numbness, or tingling.

◆ With topical preparations, systemic side effects are rare but can occur. Factors that influence the likelihood of toxicity include the frequency of application, the size of the area to which the preparation is being applied, whether the skin surface was intact, and the amount and kind of other ototoxic or nephrotoxic drugs the patient might be receiving concomitantly.

◆ Photosensitivity has been reported with topical preparations (see Patient Problem: Photosensitivity on p. 629).

Polymyxins

Drug administration

◆ See Nursing Implications Summary in Chapter 29.

◆ Assess for history of allergy before administering drug.

Continued.

NURSING IMPLICATIONS SUMMARY—cont'd

◆ Review toxicity observed with use of these drugs. Assess for confusion, slurred speech, and ataxia. Monitor intake and output and weight. Monitor vital signs, and auscultate lung sounds.

◆ Monitor serum creatinine level, BUN level, urinalysis, liver function tests, serum electrolyte level, complete blood count and differential, and platelet count.

◆ Have available calcium chloride in settings where polymyxins are used with high-risk patients such as in the operating room, recovery room, and intensive care units. Monitor respiratory status. Have available a suction machine at the bedside.

◆ Warn patients that IM injections may cause pain at the injection site.

INTRAVENOUS COLISTIMETHATE

◆ Dilute the 150 mg vial with 2 ml sterile water for injection. Further dilute each dose with 20 ml sterile water for injection. Administer at a rate of 75 mg or less over 5 min. May also be further diluted and administered as an infusion; see drug insert.

INTRAVENOUS POLYMYXIN B

◆ Dilute 500,000 units of powder with 5 ml sterile water or normal saline for injection. Further dilute dose in 300 to 500 ml compatible fluid. Administer diluted dose over 60 to 90 min. For intrathecal use, dilution is different; consult literature. Monitor vital signs, especially respirations.

Patient and family education

◆ See Nursing Implications Summary in Chapter 29.

◆ Caution patients to avoid driving or operating hazardous equipment if dizziness, vertigo, confusion, ataxia, or blurred vision develop; notify the physician.

CHAPTER REVIEW

◆ **KEY TERMS**

aminoglycosides, p. 484
polymyxins, p. 486

◆ **REVIEW QUESTIONS**

1. What is the mechanism of action of aminoglycoside antibiotics?
2. What is the most common mechanism for bacterial resistance to aminoglycosides?
3. Which routes of administration are appropriate for aminoglycosides?
4. What is the primary route of excretion of aminoglycosides?
5. What effect may aminoglycoside antibiotics have on the ear?
6. How do aminoglycoside antibiotics affect the kidneys? How should you assess for these effects?
7. What groups of patients might be more prone to aminoglycoside ototoxicity and nephrotoxicity?
8. How do aminoglycosides affect the neuromuscular junction?
9. What groups of patients are most likely to develop respiratory paralysis after therapeutic use of aminoglycoside antibiotics? How should you monitor these patients?
10. What special precautions must be taken when gentamicin and carbenicillin are used together?
11. What drugs may be poorly absorbed when neomycin is used orally?
12. Name three clinical uses of streptomycin.
13. Name one clinical indication for neomycin.
14. How does the clinical indication for the use of kanamycin differ from the indications for gentamicin, tobramycin, netilmicin, and amikacin?
15. What is the mechanism of action of polymyxins?
16. By what routes are polymyxins best administered?
17. How is polymyxin eliminated?
18. What are the three most common toxic reactions to polymyxins?
19. What patients are most at risk of neuromuscular blockade with polymyxins?
20. Given a patient receiving one or more drugs listed in this chapter, develop a nursing care plan.

SUGGESTED READING

Edson RS, Terrell CL: The aminoglycosides, *Mayo Clin Proc* 66(11):1158, 1991.
Foxworth J: Toxicities of antimicrobial agents used in the intensive care arena, *Crit Care Nurs Q* 11(4):1, 1989.
Matthews A and others: Clinical pharmacokinetics, toxicity and cost effectiveness analysis of aminoglycosides and aminoglycoside dosing services, *J Clin Pharm Ther* 12:(5):273, 1987.
Roach AC: Antibiotics therapy in septic shock, *Crit Care Nurs Clin North Am* 2(2):179, 1990.

CHAPTER 34

Sulfonamides, Trimethoprim, Quinolones, and Nitrofurantoins

LEARNING OBJECTIVES

After studying this chapter, you should be able to do the following:

- Explain why trimethoprim is given in fixed combination with a sulfonamide.
- Explain the unique mechanism of action of quinolone antibiotics.
- Discuss the limited indications for nitrofurantoins.
- Develop a nursing care plan for patients receiving drugs discussed in this chapter.

CHAPTER OVERVIEW

- This chapter focuses on drugs used mainly to treat urinary tract infections (see box on p. 492). Four separate chemical families are represented: (1) sulfonamides, (2) trimethoprim, (3) quinolones, and (4) nitrofurantoins. The antimicrobial mechanisms and pharmacokinetic properties that make these drugs useful in a variety of other infections are also considered.

Nursing Process Overview

SULFONAMIDES, QUINOLONES, AND NITROFURANTOINS

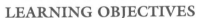

Refer to Chapter 29 for general guidelines on the nursing process with antibiotic therapy. The additional material relates specifically to the sulfonamides, quinolones, and other drugs discussed in this chapter.

Assessment

The drugs described in this chapter are used mainly to treat urinary tract infections (UTIs). Focus assessment on renal function. Monitor other clinical signs of infection. Include objective data such as blood tests, history of allergies, and mental function.

Nursing Diagnoses

Possible altered home maintenance management related to the need to increase fluid intake to 1500 ml or more/day
Possible complication: blood dyscrasias

Management

Monitor progress of treatment for UTIs by assessing clinical signs such as relief of pain and itching and by culturing urine. Ascertain that urine samples are appropriately collected to prevent trivial contamination, which renders the culture results meaningless. Blood tests may be required for patients receiving sulfonamides. Encourage adequate fluid intake to maintain good urine flow. Teach patients about the signs of blood dyscrasias for those receiving sulfonamides, signs of pulmonary distress and peripheral neuropathy for those receiving nitrofurantoins, and signs of central nervous system (CNS) distress for those receiving nalidixic acid or cinoxacin. These side effects are usually sufficient cause for the physician to discontinue medication.

Evaluation

Ascertain that patients can explain how to take the prescribed medication and can point out which side effects are sufficient reason to call the physician.

PATIENT PROBLEM: URINARY TRACT INFECTIONS

THE PROBLEM

Urinary tract infections (UTIs) are more common in females than in males, since the urethra is shorter in females. They are also more common in patients wearing urinary retention catheters (Foley catheters) and in patients requiring intermittent catheterization or urinary tract manipulation. Drugs may be prescribed when an infection develops, prophylactically when genitourinary examination or manipulation is planned, or when a history of chronic UTI exists.

SIGNS AND SYMPTOMS

Burning on urination, frequent urination, irritation, itching in the area of the urinary meatus, fever, and malaise.

PATIENT AND FAMILY EDUCATION

◆ Instruct patients to drink sufficient fluids to ensure a daily urine output of 1500 to 2000 ml. Usually, this means drinking at least 6 to 8 full glasses (8 oz) of fluid for adults.

◆ Instruct females to always wipe from front to back after voiding or defecating to avoid accidental contamination of the urinary meatus with bacteria from the anal region.

◆ Instruct patients to avoid bubble baths. Some patients, especially females, may have to eliminate all baths and shower only.

◆ Wash soap off the perineal region completely to avoid irritation from the soap. Some patients may have to wash with water only.

◆ Instruct patients to void immediately after sexual intercourse.

◆ Some drugs for UTIs are most effective if urinary pH is changed. This is difficult to do through diet alone, so other drugs may be prescribed by the physician. If sodium bicarbonate or other drugs are prescribed, instruct patients to take as ordered for best treatment of the UTI.

◆ Patients should take drugs for the full prescribed dose (often 7 to 10 days); they should not stop when symptoms begin to subside.

FOR PATIENTS WITH URINARY CATHETERS

◆ Secure catheter well, so there is minimal pulling on the meatal area.

◆ Wash the catheter insertion area with soap and water, but avoid rough scrubbing. Rinse well.

◆ Avoid opening the drainage system unless necessary.

◆ Clean the tubing and bag as directed (unless replacing them with a new device), usually with a dilute bleach solution or as instructed by the discharge nurse.

◆ In the hospital, use sterile technique to insert catheters. In the home, use clean technique as instructed.

◆ Maintain a good fluid intake.

SULFONAMIDES AND TRIMETHOPRIM
Mechanism of Action and Bacterial Resistance

Sulfonamides are metabolic inhibitors that block bacterial synthesis of folic acid, a vitamin required for the synthesis of amino acids and nucleic acids (Figure 34-1). The metabolically active form of folic acid, tetrahydrofolic acid (THFA), is synthesized in bacteria from simple precursor molecules. Two of the enzymes involved in these conversions have been exploited as targets of antibacterial drugs. Dihydropteroate synthetase, which converts para-aminobenzoic acid (PABA) and other small molecules to dihydropteroate, is the target for sulfonamides. The sulfonamides competitively inhibit this enzyme. The second target in this pathway is dihydrofolic acid reductase, the enzyme that forms THFA.

Sulfonamides are selectively toxic to organisms that must form folic acid from PABA and the other precursors. Fortunately, humans are not sensitive to this action, because we cannot synthesize folic acid but must absorb it preformed in our diet. Sulfonamides are primarily bacteriostatic against those organisms they affect.

Trimethoprim inhibits dihydrofolic acid reductase and thereby also prevents THFA formation in bacteria. Dihydrofolic acid reductase functions in humans and in bacteria, since much of the vitamin in the mammalian diet is converted to dihydrofolic acid. Therefore trimethoprim might be expected to be toxic to humans and to bacteria. This is not the case, however, because dihydrofolic acid reductase in humans is relatively resistant to the action of trimethoprim, and the drug may be given at doses that inhibit this enzyme in bacteria but not in humans.

Sulfonamides are potentially active against a wide range of gram-positive and gram-negative organisms, as well as *Nocardia, Chlamydia,* and *Actinomyces.* Bacterial resistance to sulfonamides has become widespread and has reduced the clinical usefulness of these drugs. Some bacteria such as pneumococci acquire an altered dihydrofolic acid synthetase, which is less sensitive to sulfonamides. Overproduction of PABA is a common mechanism of resistance for several pathogens, including staphylococci, pneumococci, and gonococci. Since sulfonamides are only competitive inhibitors of PABA incorporation into folic acid, excess PABA overcomes the sulfonamide inhibition.

Trimethoprim has a spectrum of antimicrobial ac-

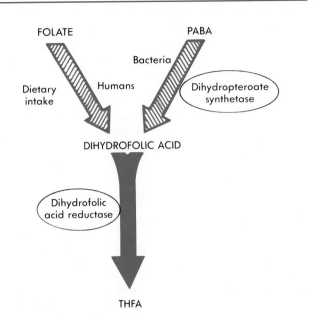

FIGURE 34-1

Synthesis of tetrahydrofolic acid (THFA) in bacteria and humans. THFA is vitamin required for nucleic acid and amino acid synthesis. Many bacteria form this vitamin from paraaminobenzoic acid (PABA) and other small molecules. Two enzymes involved in this synthesis have proved useful in chemotherapy, dihydropteroate synthetase and dihydrofolic acid reductase. Sulfonamides inhibit dihydropteroate synthetase, thereby blocking THFA synthesis in bacteria. Humans are immune from this action, since preformed folate and dihydrofolic acid are supplied in diet. Dihydrofolic acid reductase in bacteria is inhibited by trimethoprim.

tivity similar to that of the sulfonamides with some exceptions. Trimethoprim is more active against the gram-negative bacteria *Proteus, Klebsiella,* and *Serratia.* It is not useful alone against *Chlamydia* or *Nocardia.* Trimethoprim resistance has not yet become widespread. Trimethoprim is used in the United States most commonly in combination with a sulfonamide. A preparation of trimethoprim alone is available for use in UTIs.

Absorption, Distribution, and Excretion

Sulfonamide antibacterial agents with a wide variety of pharmacokinetic properties are available (Tables 34-1 to 34-3). Some of these drugs are not absorbed from the GI tract and are intended to remain within the bowel and to reduce the bacterial population there. Some systemic absorption of these agents can occur through ulcerated regions of the bowel. Systemic absorption can likewise occur when sulfonamides are used on extensive areas of burned skin.

The sulfonamides used to treat systemic infections are well absorbed from the GI tract. Distribution of these drugs to body tissues including brain is good. Concentrations of sulfonamides in cerebrospinal and other body fluids may approach those of serum. Sulfonamides also pass the placental barrier and enter the fetus.

Elimination of sulfonamides from the body involves the liver and the kidneys. The liver converts a portion of the sulfonamide in the bloodstream to an acetylated derivative, which is usually bacteriologically inactive. Acetylated and free drug are eliminated by the kidney, primarily by glomerular filtration. Tubular reabsorption is significant for some sulfonamides. Since absorbed sulfonamides are excreted by the kidney in part in the free, unacetylated form, antibacterial activity occurs in urine. Excretion of the sulfonamides is favored by alkalinizing urine. This procedure increases the solubility of these drugs in urine and also converts the drugs to a charged form that does not undergo renal tubular reabsorption.

The use of trimethoprim in fixed combination with sulfamethoxazole (see Table 34-2) represents an exploitation of drug properties for therapeutic effect. These drugs are administered in tablets with a 1:5 trimethoprim/sulfamethoxazole ratio. Both drugs are well absorbed from the GI tract. Serum concentrations of the free drug not bound to serum proteins are usually in a 1:20 trimethoprim/sulfamethoxazole ratio. At this concentration ratio, the drugs have maximum antibacterial activity. The combination is synergistic, that is, more effective in combination than would be expected from the action of either drug alone. Synergy may result because both drugs ultimately starve sensitive bacteria for THFA, but the drugs work on two different enzymes in the sequence of reactions leading to THFA. The sequential blockade of this metabolic pathway is much more effective than blockade of a single step by one drug at high concentrations.

Trimethoprim has synergistic effects with any systemically effective sulfonamides. Sulfamethoxazole was chosen for use in the fixed combination with trimethoprim because the kinetics of elimination of the two drugs are similar. Therefore use of this fixed combination does not lead to accumulation of either of the drugs.

Trimethoprim penetrates body tissues better than sulfamethoxazole. Trimethoprim concentrations in breast milk, bile, prostatic fluid, vaginal fluids, liver, spleen, skin, and kidneys may exceed plasma concentrations of the drug. Penetration into other tissues is adequate, including the CNS.

Trimethoprim appears in urine at a concentration approximately 100 times the plasma concentration, with most of the drug in the active form. Sulfa-

Table 34-1   Summary of Sulfonamides: Single Component Formulations

Generic name	Trade name	Administration/dosage	Clinical use
Sulfacytine	Renoquid	ORAL: *Adults*—500 mg loading dose, then 250 mg 4 times daily. Not for children under 14 years.	UTIs.
Sulfadiazine	Microsulfon	ORAL: *Adults*—single loading dose of 2 to 4 gm, then 2 to 4 gm daily in 3 to 6 doses. *Children over 2 months*—75 mg/kg body weight to load, then 150 mg/kg daily in 4 to 6 doses.	Nocardiosis and rheumatic fever prophylaxis.
Sulfamethoxazole	Gantanol*	ORAL: *Adults*—single 2 gm loading dose, then 1 gm 2 or 3 times daily. *Children over 2 months*—50 to 60 mg/kg loading dose, then 25 to 30 mg/kg twice daily, not to exceed 75 mg/kg daily.	Conjunctivitis, nocardiosis, otitis media, trachoma, and UTIs.
Sulfapyridine	Dagenan† Sulfapyridine*	ORAL: *Adults*—500 mg 4 times daily. Reduce by 500 mg increments as improvement allows.	Dermatitis herpetiformis.
Sulfasalazine	Azulfidine Salazopyrin*	ORAL: *Adults*—3 to 4 gm daily in divided doses. *Children over 2 years*—40 to 60 mg/kg daily in 3 to 6 doses.	Two thirds of oral dose remains in bowel for treatment of ulcerative colitis.
Sulfisoxazole	Gantrisin Novosoxazole†	ORAL: *Adults*—2 to 4 gm loading dose, then 4 to 8 gm daily in 3 to 6 doses. *Children over 2 months*—75 mg/kg loading dose, then 150 mg/kg daily in 4 to 6 doses.	UTIs and systemic infections caused by sensitive organisms and nocardiosis.

*Available in Canada and United States.
†Available in Canada only.

Table 34-2   Summary of Sulfonamides: Fixed Combinations for Oral Use

Components of combination	Drug form	Trade name	Dosage	Clinical use
Sulfamethoxazole—400 mg Trimethoprim—80 mg	Tablet	Bactrim* Cotrim Roubac† Septra*	*Adults*—2 tablets every 12 hr. For pneumocystis pneumonia, 25 mg/kg sulfamethoxazole and 5 mg/kg trimethoprim every 6 hr. *Children over 2 months*—4 to 6 mg/kg trimethoprim and 20 to 30 mg/kg sulfamethoxazole daily in 2 doses.	UTIs, otitis media, enteritis caused by sensitive *Shigella*, pneumocystis pneumonia.
Sulfadiazine—410 mg Trimethoprim—90 mg	Tablet	Coptin†	*Adults*—1 tablet every 12 hr. *Children 3 months to 5 years*—¼ to ½ tablet every 12 hr. *Children 5 to 12 years*—½ to 1 tablet every 12 hr.	UTIs.
Sulfadoxine—500 mg Pyrimethamine—25 mg	Tablet	Fansidar*	*Adults*—for treatment, 2 to 3 tablets as single dose; or 1 tablet for chemoprophylaxis. *Children 2 months to 4 years*—¼ tablet once every 7 days for chemoprophylaxis. *Children 5 to 8 years*—½ tablet once every 7 days for chemoprophylaxis. *Children 9 to 14 years*—¾ tablet once every 7 days for chemoprophylaxis.	Malaria.
Sulfamethoxazole—500 mg Phenazopyridine—100 mg	Tablet	Azo-Gantanol UroGantanol†	*Adults*—4 tablets to load, then 2 tablets every 12 hr for 2 days.	UTIs only.
Sulfisoxazole—500 mg Phenazopyridine—50 mg	Tablet	Azo-Gantrisin*	*Adults*—4 to 6 tablets to load, then 2 tablets every 6 hr for 2 days.	UTIs only.

*Available in Canada and United States.
†Available in Canada only.

Table 34-3   Summary of Sulfonamides: Topical Agents

Generic name	Trade name	Application form	Clinical use	Comments
Mafenide acetate	Sulfamylon*	Cream: 85 mg mafenide acetate/gm.	Treatment of second- and third-degree burns.	Drug is effective against a broad spectrum of pathogens, including *Pseudomonas aeruginosa*. Drug may be absorbed through burned tissues.
Silver sulfadiazine	Silvadene Flamazine† Thermazene	Cream: 10 mg/gm	Treatment of second- and third-degree burns.	Drug is effective against a broad spectrum of pathogens, including *P. aeruginosa* and certain yeasts. Drug may be absorbed through burned tissues.
Sulfacetamide	Bleph Liquifilm* Cetamid* Sulamyd*	Solution: 10%, 15%, or 30% Ointment: 10%	Ophthalmic only. For conjunctivitis, corneal ulcer, and trachoma.	Drug allergy may develop in sensitive patients.
Sulfisoxazole diolamine	Gantrisin Ophthalmic	Solution: 4% Ointment: 4%	Ophthalmic only. For conjunctivitis, corneal ulcer, and trachoma.	Drug allergy may develop in sensitive patients.

*Available in Canada and United States.
†Available in Canada only.

methoxazole in urine is mostly in the acetylated form, and the urinary concentration is about five times the plasma concentration.

Sulfonamides may be combined with phenazopyridine to treat UTIs (see Table 34-2). The sulfonamide component supplies antibacterial activity and the phenazopyridine, which is excreted in urine, exerts an analgesic effect on the mucosa of the urinary tract. The added phenazopyridine therefore relieves the pain, burning, and itching associated with the UTI.

Sulfonamide preparations are available for vaginal application, but no evidence of effectiveness exists. Moreover, sensitization may be produced.

Toxicity

Sulfonamides induce allergic reactions in a significant proportion of patients receiving the drugs. The most common reactions are skin rashes and pruritus, but drug fever and other more serious reactions may occur. Anaphylaxis has been reported. Since sulfonamides are chemically related to the thiazide diuretics, acetazolamide, and oral hypoglycemic agents, a patient who becomes allergic to a sulfonamide may also become allergic to one or more of these agents (see boxes).

GI disturbances also occur with the sulfonamides. In addition to nausea, vomiting, and diarrhea, pancreatitis, hepatitis, and stomatitis may occur. CNS alterations have also been observed, including headache, ataxia, hallucinations, and convulsions.

Deaths from aplastic anemia and other blood dyscrasias, although rare, have been connected with sul-

---

GERIATRIC CONSIDERATION: SULFONAMIDES

THE PROBLEM

Elderly patients are more likely to suffer severe blood and skin reactions to sulfonamides than younger adults. Diuretics, commonly taken by elderly patients for high blood pressure, compound the risk.

SOLUTIONS

◆ Monitor blood tests for signs of bone marrow depression
◆ Watch for bleeding or reduced platelet counts
◆ Inspect carefully for rash or purpura
◆ Ascertain if the patient is taking thiazide diuretic, either alone or as a component of other preparations

---

PEDIATRIC CONSIDERATION: SULFONAMIDES

THE PROBLEM

Sulfonamides displace bilirubin from serum proteins. In neonates, who typically have elevated bilirubin, this displacement may be sufficient to produce kernicterus.

SOLUTIONS

◆ Avoid sulfonamides in pregnancy near term
◆ Avoid sulfonamides in infants younger than 1 month of age

fonamide therapy. Sore throat, fever, or pallor may signal a serious blood dyscrasia.

Renal toxicity was of great concern with sulfonamides in use before 1960. Most of the renal damage associated with these older agents was produced by drug precipitation or crystallization in urine. These drugs precipitated because of their low solubility in normal acidic urine. Newer sulfonamides are much more soluble under these conditions, and drug precipitation is seldom a problem. However, patients should receive sufficient fluids to produce at least 1 L of urine daily while receiving sulfonamides. Solubility of the sulfonamides in urine may be increased by alkalinizing urine. Sulfamethizole and sulfasalazine produce a yellow-orange coloration in alkaline urine. This coloration, also observable in skin, is not harmful.

Patients with preexisting renal or hepatic disease may be more prone to develop toxic reactions, since these organs are the primary means of removal of sulfonamides from the body. Patients with a known genetic deficiency of glucose 6-phosphate dehydrogenase (G6PD) are also at greater risk of hemolytic anemia induced by sulfonamides. The highest frequency of G6PD deficiency is observed among blacks and Mediterranean populations; patients from these groups should be watched carefully for signs of anemia.

Trimethoprim appears to be less toxic than the sulfonamides, although it may affect the bone marrow. When trimethoprim is used in combination with sulfamethoxazole, patients should be observed for all signs of sulfonamide toxicity.

Drug Interactions

Certain sulfonamides are highly bound to serum proteins and may therefore displace other drugs from protein binding sites. This displacement can occur with oral anticoagulants, sulfonylureas (oral hypoglycemic agents), and the antineoplastic agent methotrexate.

PABA may interfere with the action of sulfonamides. Procaine, a local anesthetic that is derived from PABA, may also block the action of sulfonamides in dihydrofolic acid synthetase (see Figure 34-1).

QUINOLONES
Mechanism of Action and Bacterial Resistance

Quinolones interfere with DNA replication in bacteria by inhibiting the proper functioning of DNA gyrase. DNA gyrase is the enzyme that allows bacterial DNA to unwind (relax) so that replication may proceed. The quinolones block this action and lead to breaks in the double-stranded DNA. At achievable clinical concentrations, these agents are bactericidal. Ciprofloxacin, norfloxacin, and ofloxacin have broad antibacterial spectra, with activity toward aerobic gram-positive and gram-negative bacteria, including *Pseudomonas aeruginosa*. Cinoxacin and nalidixic acid have more restricted spectra, covering many common gram-negative pathogens but not *P. aeruginosa*. Enoxacin also has restricted activity against *P. aeruginosa* and is not as effective as other quinolones against gram-positive bacteria but is active against pathogens causing common UTIs and gonorrhea.

Resistance to these drugs can occur, but plasmid-mediated resistance is not yet significant. One mechanism of resistance may involve blockage of antibiotic transport into the bacterial cell.

Absorption, Distribution, and Excretion

Quinolone and related antibiotics (Table 34-4) are generally well absorbed when given orally. Portal circulation carries absorbed drug directly to the liver, where metabolism occurs. Nalidixic acid is the most extensively metabolized drug of this group, with glucuronide and hydroxylated derivatives being formed. The hydroxylated form of nalidixic acid is biologically active and comprises a significant proportion of the active drug in the bloodstream and in urine. Over 90% of nalidixic acid in the bloodstream is bound to serum proteins. Little enters most body tissues. The only organ in which drug concentration exceeds the plasma concentration is the kidney. Nalidixic acid has the lowest plasma concentration of any drug in this group.

Ciprofloxacin, norfloxacin, enoxacin, and cinoxacin are less extensively metabolized than nalidixic acid. From 30% to 60% of an oral dose of these drugs appears unchanged in urine. Tissue penetration and persistance in plasma is greater with ciprofloxacin, enoxacin, ofloxacin, and norfloxacin than with cinoxacin or nalidixic acid.

Doses of quinolones may need to be adjusted in patients with renal impairment because the kidneys are the primary organ of excretion of active drug or metabolites. Ciprofloxacin is also eliminated by trans-intestinal transport, with about 15% of each dose appearing in feces.

Toxicity

Quinolones have two major side effects. The first involves the CNS. Symptoms range from headache, dizziness, tinnitus, insomnia, shakiness, and changes in vision to seizures. These drugs should not be given to patients with preexisting CNS disease because they

Table 34-4   Quinolone and Related Antibiotics

Generic name	Trade name	Administration/dosage	Comments
Cinoxacin	Cinobac	ORAL: *Adults*—250 mg every 6 hr or 500 mg every 12 hr. FDA Pregnancy Category C.	For UTIs
Ciprofloxacin	Cipro	ORAL: *Adults*—500 to 750 mg every 12 hr. FDA Pregnancy Category C. INTRAVENOUS: *Adults*—400 mg every 12 hr for 7 to 14 days.	Bone and soft tissue infections, pneumonia, and bacterial diarrhea may respond
Enoxacin	Penetrex	ORAL: *Adults*—200 to 400 mg every 12 hr.	UTIs and gonorrhea
Nalidixic acid	NegGram*	ORAL: *Adults*—1 gm 4 times daily for 1 to 2 weeks	UTIs only; emergence of resistant bacterial strains commonly causes treatment failure
Norfloxacin	Noroxin*	ORAL: *Adults*—400 mg every 12 hr for 3 to 21 days. FDA Pregnancy Category C.	Currently indicated primarily for UTIs
Ofloxacin	Floxin	ORAL, INTRAVENOUS: *Adults*—200 to 400 mg every 12 hr. FDA Pregnancy Category C.	UTIs, gonorrhea, pneumonia, and soft tissue infections.

*Available in United States and Canada.
†Available in Canada only.

PEDIATRIC CONSIDERATION: QUINOLONES

THE PROBLEM

Quinolones, including nalidixic acid and cinoxacin, have damaged cartilage in tests in young animals, leading to permanent joint impairment.

SOLUTIONS

◆ Avoid quinolone use in children
◆ Remind adults not to share drugs with children, even if symptoms appear to be the same; some drugs should not be used in children.

---

can exacerbate the problem. The second side effect shared by the quinolones is a tendency to damage cartilage, especially in the young (see box). This reaction has been observed in the young of several animal species and has led to permanent damage and lameness. For this reason, quinolones are not given to children.

Drug Interactions

Antacids containing aluminum or magnesium compounds can block absorption of ciprofloxacin and norfloxacin. Lower plasma and urinary concentrations of antibiotic and loss of antibacterial effectiveness result.

Sodium bicarbonate, citrates, carbonic anhydrase inhibitors, and antacids containing calcium may alkalinize urine, which renders ciprofloxacin less soluble. The drug may crystallize in the urinary tract, causing pain and obstruction. Avoiding these agents and maintaining an adequate fluid intake lessen the risk of crystalluria developing.

Ciprofloxacin use lowers hepatic clearance of theophylline, which can cause theophylline to accumulate. As serum theophylline levels increase, so does the risk of CNS toxicity; nausea, vomiting, tremors, restlessness, agitation, and palpitations may occur.

NITROFURANTOIN
Mechanism of Action and Bacterial Resistance

Nitrofurantoin apparently inhibits certain bacterial enzymes required for metabolism of sugar and perhaps other compounds. It is effective against some gram-positive and gram-negative organisms, including most common pathogens of the urinary tract. *Pseudomonas* and *Proteus* species are, however, usually intrinsically resistant. Development of resistance to nitrofurantoin therapy is not a significant problem.

Absorption, Distribution, and Excretion

Many compounds that are effective antibacterial agents in the laboratory are ineffective when used to

Table 34-5   Nitrofurantoin and Trimethoprim

Generic name	Trade name	Administration/dosage	Comments
Nitrofurantoin	Furadantin Furalan	ORAL: *Adults*—50 to 100 mg 4 times daily. *Children*—5 to 7 mg/kg daily in 4 divided doses. The drug should not be given to children under 3 months of age.	Gastric irritation may be minimized by administering the drug with food or milk.
Nitrofurantoin macrocrystals	Macrodantin*	As for nitrofurantoin.	Large crystal size minimizes gastric irritation.
Trimethoprim	Proloprim* Trimpex	ORAL: *Adults*—100 mg every 12 hr. FDA Pregnancy Category C. *Children*—3 mg/kg body weight twice daily has been used.	Blood changes can occur with this drug.

*Available in Canada and United States.

treat systemic infections because of the unfavorable pharmacokinetics of the drugs. One example of such a compound is nitrofurantoin (Table 34-5). This drug, in spite of being well absorbed from the small intestine, never achieves satisfactory blood levels. Low blood levels result from a rapid excretion of the drug in the kidney. Removal of the drug from the system occurs so quickly that it fails to accumulate in the bloodstream. Therefore despite its broad antibacterial spectrum, it is ineffective against systemic infections. However, nitrofurantoin is concentrated in the kidney and achieves antibacterial concentrations in urine. In the renal tubule, it diffuses into kidney tissues so that the final concentration in the kidney is much greater than would be expected from the very low blood concentrations of the drug. These properties make the drug effective against UTIs.

Toxicity

One of the more common reactions to nitrofurantoin is gastric irritation, with anorexia, nausea, and emesis. This reaction apparently lessens if the drug is administered as large crystals (e.g., Macrodantin, see Table 34-5) rather than in the original microcrystalline form. The large crystals are more slowly absorbed, but this does not interfere with clinical effectiveness.

Rashes, allergies, and reversible blood dyscrasias have been observed with nitrofurantoin. Hemolytic anemia similar to that seen with sulfonamides may also be seen. Infants under 3 months of age have undeveloped enzyme systems that make them especially susceptible to hemolytic anemia induced by nitrofurantoin. It should be used with care in pregnant patients.

Oral suspensions may stain the teeth. Nitrofurantoin also causes urine to turn brown, but this is harmless. Occasionally, patients may suffer hair loss while receiving the drug.

Peripheral neuropathy is one of the most serious toxic effects of nitrofurantoin. If detected early, the condition disappears after discontinuation of the drug. Damage may be permanent if the drug is continued after signs of peripheral neuropathy have developed. As with any drug that is excreted primarily by the kidney, nitrofurantoin may accumulate in patients with renal failure. These patients are more likely to suffer from significant side effects of nitrofurantoin therapy. Vitamin B deficiency, common in alcoholics, may also predispose a patient to peripheral neuropathy. Diabetes mellitus, a disease that may cause peripheral neuropathy, may produce added risk of neural complications.

Patients receiving nitrofurantoin for long periods should be observed for pneumonitis or pulmonary fibrosis, which may develop gradually or may appear as an acute illness.

Nitrofurantoin is used clinically to treat certain types of UTIs, especially when the causative organism is a sensitive strain of *Escherichia coli*.

NURSING IMPLICATIONS SUMMARY

Sulfonamides and Trimethoprim

Drug administration

◆ Review Nursing Implications Summary in Chapter 29.

◆ Question patients about history of allergy to other sulfonamides, thiazide diuretics, acetazolamide, or oral hypoglycemic agents before administering sulfonamides.

◆ Inspect for rashes or skin changes and GI distress. Monitor temperature.

◆ Monitor complete blood count (CBC) and differential, platelet count, blood urea nitrogen (BUN) level, serum creatinine level, liver function tests, and urinalysis.

◆ Topical sulfonamide preparations are used to treat burns (see Table 34-3). Wear sterile gloves when applying medication. The drugs are most effective when the area is cleaned of debris and pus. Dressings are not necessary but may be used. Medicate for pain before redressing wounds. Monitor serum drug and serum electrolyte levels, in addition to blood work noted previously.

INTRAVENOUS TRIMETHOPRIM AND SULFAMETHOXAZOLE

◆ Dilute each 5-ml ampule in 125 ml 5% dextrose in water. Administer diluted dose over 60 to 90 min. Flush tubing well after administration. For patients on fluid restriction, see package insert.

Patient and family education

◆ Review Nursing Implications Summary in Chapter 29.

◆ Review the benefits and possible side effects of drug therapy. Instruct patients to report fever, sore throat, unexplained bleeding or bruising, malaise, jaundice, rashes, and skin changes.

◆ Review Patient Problem: Urinary Tract Infections on p. 492.

◆ Tell patients receiving sulfasalazine that this drug may turn urine or skin a yellow-orange color.

◆ Tell patients taking combination products that contain phenazopyridine that this compound turns urine reddish orange in color. In addition, this dye may produce false results with urine glucose tests. Tell diabetic patients about this effect. Instruct such patients not to change insulin dose or diet without discussing this with the physician. Monitor blood glucose level.

◆ Patients should take doses with a full glass (8 oz) of water or other liquid.

◆ Do not give sulfonamide drugs to children under 12 years of age unless specifically prescribed by a physician.

◆ Review Patient Problem: Photosensitivity on p. 629 with patients.

◆ Caution patients to avoid driving or operating hazardous equipment until the effects of this medication are known. Report dizziness to the physician.

◆ Sulfonamides are available for ophthalmic use. See Chapter 6 for a discussion of application of drops and ointment.

◆ Sulfonamides are available for intravaginal use. Make certain the patient can apply the ordered dose correctly (see Patient Problem: Treatment of Vaginal Infections on p. 518).

◆ Remind patients to inform all health-care providers of all drugs being used.

Quinolones

Drug administration

◆ See Nursing Implications Summary in Chapter 29.

◆ Assess for history of allergy before administering drug.

◆ Assess for CNS side effects such as headache, dizziness, tinnitus, insomnia, shakiness, and changes in vision.

◆ Monitor CBC and differential, platelet count, BUN level, serum creatinine level, and liver function tests.

Patient and family education

◆ See Nursing Implications Summary in Chapter 29.

◆ Review anticipated benefits and possible side effects of drug therapy. Instruct patients to report any new sign or symptom.

◆ Reinforce the importance of not giving quinolones to children.

◆ Take oral doses with a full glass (8 oz) of water or fluid.

◆ See Patient Problems: Urinary Tract Infections on p. 492, Photosensitivity on p. 629, and Dry Mouth on p. 166.

◆ Note the drug interactions. Take ciprofloxacin or norfloxacin 1 hour before or 2 hours after antacids containing aluminum or magnesium. Review the patient's other medications, and counsel as necessary. Remind patients to inform all health-care providers of all drugs being used.

Continued.

NURSING IMPLICATIONS SUMMARY—cont'd

◆ Caution patients to avoid driving or operating hazardous equipment if CNS symptoms develop. Report dizziness, tinnitus, and visual changes to the physician.

◆ If photophobia develops (eyes have increased sensitivity to light), instruct patients to wear sunglasses and to avoid bright lights or sunlight.

◆ Tell diabetic patients taking nalidixic acid that the drug may interfere with urine glucose results. Do not change diet or insulin dose without consulting the physician. Monitor blood glucose level.

Nitrofurantoin

Drug administration

◆ See Nursing Implications Summary in Chapter 29.

◆ Assess for GI disturbance, skin changes, and peripheral neuropathy. Assess lung sounds and respiratory rate. Monitor weight.

◆ Monitor CBC and differential and liver function tests.

Patient and family education

◆ See Nursing Implications Summary in Chapter 29.

◆ Review anticipated benefits and possible side effects of drug therapy. Instruct patients to report any new sign or symptom.

◆ Review Patient Problem: Urinary Tract Infections on p. 492.

◆ Take oral doses with meals or a snack to reduce gastric irritation. Warn patients that oral suspensions may stain teeth. Dilute doses of suspension with milk or juice before taking.

CHAPTER REVIEW

◆ **KEY TERMS**

nitrofurantoin, p. 497
quinolones, p. 496
sulfonamides, p. 492
urinary tract infections (UTIs), p. 492

◆ **REVIEW QUESTIONS**

1. What is the mechanism for the antibacterial effect of sulfonamides?

2. Why are sulfonamides not equally toxic to humans and bacteria?

3. By what routes may sulfonamides be administered?

4. Do sulfonamides enter the cerebrospinal fluid from the bloodstream?

5. What is the route of elimination of sulfonamides?

6. What is the purpose of combining sulfonamides with phenazopyridine to treat UTIs? What should you teach patients about this?

7. What are the major toxic reactions to sulfonamides?

8. How has the renal toxicity of the sulfonamide preparations used clinically changed since the early 1940s?

9. What is the mechanism for the antibacterial effect of trimethoprim?

10. Why is trimethoprim not equally toxic to humans and bacteria?

11. Why are trimethoprim and sulfamethoxazole combined to treat UTIs and infections at other sites?

12. What is the mechanism of the antibacterial effect of quinolones?

13. By what route are quinolones given?

14. What is the major clinical use of nalidixic acid, cinoxacin, enoxacin, and norfloxacin?

15. What is the major route of excretion of the quinolones?

16. What type of toxicity is associated with quinolones?

17. Why are quinolones not used in children?

18. Why is nitrofurantoin not effective for systemic infections?

19. By what route is nitrofurantoin administered?

20. What reactions to nitrofurantoin are commonly encountered with short-term therapy?

21. What reactions to nitrofurantoin are associated with long-term therapy?

22. Develop a nursing plan for a patient receiving one of the drugs discussed in this chapter.

SUGGESTED READING

Cockerill FR III, Edson RS: Trimethoprim-sulfamethoxazole, *Mayo Clin Proc* 66(12):1260, 1991.

Fiorelli RL: Recurrent urinary tract infections in women: pathogenesis and treatment, *J Urol Nurs* 7(4):510, 1988.

Glatt AE: Treating *P. carinii* pneumonia in patients with AIDS, *Drug Therapy* 19(4):69, 1989.

Karb VB: Two new fluoroquinolones: ciprofloxacin and norfloxacin, *J Neurosci Nurs* 20(5):327, 1988.

Manzo M: Ciprofloxacin and norfloxacin—potent oral antiinfectives, *Nurs 89* 19(2):30, 1989.

Millette-Petit JM: Urinary tract infections in older adults, *Nurse Pract* 13(12):21, 1988.

Osborne S: Ciprofloxacin—a new fluoroquinolone antimicrobial agent, *J Urol Nurs* 7(4):505, 1988.

Todd B: Treating UTIs, *Geriatr Nurs* 11(2):95, 1990.

Walker RC, Wright AJ: The fluoroquinolones, *Mayo Clin Proc* 66(12):1249, 1991.

Wilhelm MP, Edson RS: Antimicrobial agents in urinary tract infections, *Mayo Clin Proc* 62(11):1025, 1987.

CHAPTER 35

Drugs to Treat Tuberculosis and Leprosy

LEARNING OBJECTIVES

After studying this chapter, you should be able to do the following:

◆ Explain why therapy of tuberculosis and leprosy must continue for years.

◆ Describe the use of isoniazid, and identify types of patients most at risk of severe reactions to the drug.

◆ Describe the use of dapsone.

◆ Discuss why drug combinations are commonly used for tuberculosis and leprosy.

◆ Develop a nursing care plan for a patient receiving drug therapy for tuberculosis or leprosy.

CHAPTER OVERVIEW

◆ Tuberculosis and leprosy are diseases produced by *Mycobacterium* infections. Both diseases have been known since ancient times and are among the earliest examples of diseases that were recognized as infectious. Tuberculosis, or the white plague, was a major cause of death in Europe and the Orient throughout the Middle Ages and until recent times. Leprosy, although less common, was greatly feared because of the disfigurement it caused. This grim picture changed in the early 1940s when the first effective antituberculosis agent, streptomycin, was discovered. Around the same time a sulfone was discovered to be effective in controlling leprosy. With these and other more recently discovered agents, both diseases may now be treated effectively in most patients. Patients with acquired immunodeficiency syndrome (AIDS) who also have *Mycobacterium avium* complex face a poor prognosis. In this chapter the clinical features of *Mycobacterium* infections, which make treatment more difficult than that of most other bacterial diseases, are considered. Second, the properties of the drugs used to treat these diseases and the ways they are used are covered.

Nursing Process Overview

TREATMENT OF TUBERCULOSIS

Assessment

Antituberculosis therapy is used in patients diagnosed with active tuberculosis, those whose tuberculosis skin tests convert from negative to positive, or in some instances those receiving high doses of adrenocortical steroids. In the latter group of patients the concern is that high doses of steroids will alter the patient's ability to resist infection from tuberculosis or will cause reactivation of earlier tubercular infections. Perform a thorough total assessment, emphasizing subjective complaints, possible history of tuberculosis in the patient and family, and recent activities such as travel or moving that might have influenced exposure to the disease. Tuberculosis can appear in other organs besides the lungs (e.g., tuberculosis meningitis). The focus of the assessment would be different if the patient had a nontraditional form of tuberculosis.

Nursing Diagnoses

Anxiety related to the diagnosis and long-term drug therapy

Possible altered home maintenance management related to lack of knowledge about how to incorporate drug therapy into daily activities

Management

As soon as diagnosis is made, begin patient education. If unsure of the local standards regarding care of tuberculosis patients, contact the local health department or hospital-infection control department. Place hospitalized patients in isolation until no longer infectious. Remember that many tuberculosis patients are diagnosed and treated entirely on an outpatient basis.

Evaluation

Noncompliance is a major cause of treatment failure. Before they begin self-management, ascertain that patients can explain why and how to take the drugs ordered, possible side effects, ways to treat minor side effects such as nausea associated with taking medication, and side effects that require notification of the physician. Verify that patients can explain when and why to return for evaluation of laboratory work and other patient data. Also check that patients can demonstrate measures to take to decrease the possibility of spreading the disease to others.

Because exposure to tuberculosis may occur any time the nurse provides care for a patient, nurses should have regular tuberculosis skin tests.

TUBERCULOSIS

Clinical Features

Tuberculosis is produced by *Mycobacterium tuberculosis* or less commonly by other mycobacteria harbored by cattle or birds. Three features of *M. tuberculosis* are especially important to recall in considering how disease is produced in humans by these organisms. First, mycobacteria are strict aerobic organisms, which means that they must live in an oxygen-rich environment and may explain why the first site of infection in humans is usually along the alveoli of the lung. Second, mycobacteria induce activity of macrophages, causing these cellular immunity factors to phagocytize *M. tuberculosis*. Rather than helping prevent infection, this action actually may enhance survival and spread of the disease-causing organisms because *M. tuberculosis* resists the acids and enzymes that usually destroy bacteria within macrophages. *M. tuberculosis* reproduces within macrophages at a near-normal rate and may be carried by them throughout the body. Third, mycobacteria are slow-growing organisms relative to other bacteria. The time required for tubercle bacilli to reproduce is 10 to 12 hr compared with 20 to 30 min for other bacteria such as *Escherichia coli* or *Pseudomonas aeruginosa*. This slow growth contributes to the difficulty encountered in treating the disease because it is during active growth that the organism is most susceptible to metabolic interference.

The disease may pass through several phases. The initial or primary infection usually occurs in the lung as a result of inhaling droplets containing live *M. tuberculosis*. These infective aerosols are generated when a patient with an established active case of tuberculosis coughs or sneezes. Once in the alveoli, *M. tuberculosis* is phagocytized and begins to multiply. Infected macrophages may remain in the lung, but a significant number enter the lymphatic system, and a few enter the bloodstream and are carried throughout the body. In response to the increasing number of tubercle bacilli in the lung a pneumonialike condition may develop within a few weeks. This inflammatory response to the infection may continue for a few weeks, but in most people, this process is ultimately halted by the delayed immune reaction provoked by the infection. This acquired cellular immunity results in increased effectiveness of macrophages in destroying *M. tuberculosis*. Lesions within the lungs resolve when infective loci become calcified. Living tubercle bacilli no longer appear in sputum at this stage, and the disease is said to be inactive. Living *M. tuberculosis* remains within the body, however, and relapses may occur months or years after the initial infection. When relapse occurs, localized areas again become sites of active multiplication of tubercle bacilli. Local necrosis develops while the cellular immunity factors attempt to isolate the infection. Necrosis may spread as a result of this inflammatory response and may cause large cavities within the lungs or other tissues.

M. tuberculosis, like most other bacteria, can acquire resistance to drugs. Development of resistance is common when patients are treated with a single drug. To minimize this therapeutic complication, multiple drug therapy is used. The rationale for this therapy is that since mutations are required for the development of resistance to a drug, if two drugs that have different mechanisms of action are administered concurrently, the organism must acquire two independent mutations to become resistant to both drugs. Since mutations are rare, the likelihood of simultaneously acquiring two specific mutations is small. The probability of developing resistance is further reduced by using three drugs with independent mechanisms of action.

The traditional method of chemotherapy for established tuberculosis has been to administer a combination of drugs for 2 years or longer. Treated patients rapidly cease to be infectious, but chemotherapy must be continued for long periods to eliminate most of the dormant tubercle bacilli. Frequency of relapse seems inversely proportional to the duration of therapy. Recent clinical studies in Great Britain and the United States have suggested that shorter treatment periods may be used if three drugs are used continuously for the first 2 months of therapy followed by an additional 6 to 9 months with two of the drugs. Clinical trials are also being conducted with intermittent therapy in which drugs are administered twice weekly. Intermittent therapy seems best suited to patients who do not reliably take their medication without direct medical supervision. For these patients the drugs may be administered by a visiting nurse.

Many drugs are now available for tuberculosis. These agents differ in potency, spectrum of activity, and toxicity. The most commonly used drugs are isoniazid, rifampin, streptomycin, and ethambutol. The remaining drugs are used in combinations or as reserve drugs. The properties and uses of antituberculosis agents are considered in the following sections.

Properties of Individual Agents

Isoniazid

Clinical use. Isoniazid is considered to be the best antituberculosis drug available. It is the only antituberculosis agent used alone routinely for prophylaxis. The drug is available as a single agent formulation (Table 35-1) and in combination with other antituberculosis agents (Table 35-2).

Table 35-1 Antituberculosis Drugs

Generic name	Trade name	Administration/dosage	Clinical use	Patient populations with increased risk of toxicity
Amikacin	Amikin*	INTRAMUSCULAR, INTRAVENOUS: *Adults*—15 mg/kg daily, not to exceed 1.5 gm daily for 10 days.	Atypical mycobacterial infections.	Elderly or renally-impaired patients have increased risk. See Chapter 33.
Aminosalicylate sodium	Nemasol† Tubasal	ORAL: *Adults*—10 to 12 gm daily in 3 or 4 doses. *Children*—200 to 300 mg/kg daily in 3 or 4 doses.	Combination therapy of pulmonary or extrapulmonary tuberculosis.	Patients with active hypertension or other diseases in which sodium overload is undesirable may be unable to tolerate the sodium load with this drug.
Capreomycin	Capastat*	INTRAMUSCULAR: *Adults*—1 gm daily in single dose. FDA Pregnancy Category C. Not recommended for children.	Retreatment of tuberculosis.	Patients with hearing impairment, renal function impairment, or muscle weakness may suffer exacerbations of their condition.
Cycloserine	Seromycin	ORAL: *Adults*—15 mg/kg daily in 2 doses up to maximum daily dose of 1 gm. FDA Pregnancy Category C. *Children*—5 to 20 mg/kg in divided doses.	Retreatment of tuberculosis; urinary tract tuberculosis.	Central nervous system toxicity, including seizures, is more likely in alcoholics or patients with prior seizure disorders.
Ethambutol	Etibi† Myambutol*	ORAL: *Adults*—initially 15 mg/kg in a single daily dose or 25 mg/kg in a single daily dose for 2 months, after which dose may be reduced to 15 mg/kg daily. *Children under 13 years*—should not receive drug. ORAL: *Adults*—45 to 50 mg/kg twice weekly with isoniazid.	In multidrug initial therapy of tuberculosis. In multidrug intermittent therapy of tuberculosis.	Patients with reduced renal function require reduced drug doses. Patients with preexisting visual defects may be difficult to evaluate for drug-induced visual changes.

*Available in Canada and United States.
†Available in Canada only.

Table 35-1 Antituberculosis Drugs—cont'd

Generic name	Trade name	Administration/dosage	Clinical use	Patient populations with increased risk of toxicity
Ethionamide	Trecator SC	ORAL: *Adults*—0.5 to 1 gm daily in 1 to 3 doses. *Children*—4 to 5 mg/kg every 8 hr.	Any form of tuberculosis when primary drugs are inappropriate; retreatment.	Patients also receiving cycloserine are at greater risk for seizures.
Isoniazid (INH)	Isotamine† Laniazid	ORAL: *Adults*—300 mg daily maximum. FDA Pregnancy Category C. *Children*—10 to 20 mg/kg daily.	In multidrug therapy for active tuberculosis. Alone for prophylaxis.	Older patients or patients also receiving rifampin have an increased risk of drug-induced hepatitis.
	Nydrazid	INTRAMUSCULAR: As for oral.	As for oral form.	Malnourished patients, alcoholics, and diabetics may suffer vitamin B_6 depletion and are therefore more at risk of peripheral neuropathies. Alcoholics and patients with impaired liver function have greater risk of hepatotoxicity. Fetuses and neonates are at risk during therapy of mother.
Pyrazinamide	Pyrazinamide* Tebrazid†	ORAL: *Adults*—20 to 35 mg/kg daily up to 3 gm. *Children*—15 to 30 mg/kg of body weight daily.	Combined with other drugs for treatment of tuberculosis.	Hepatotoxicity; increased blood concentrations of uric acid (hyperuricemia).
Rifampin	Rifadin* Rimactane* Rofact†	ORAL: *Adults*—600 mg daily in 1 dose. FDA Pregnancy Category C. *Children*—10 to 20 mg/kg up to 600 mg daily.	In multidrug initial therapy or retreatment for pulmonary tuberculosis.	Patients with prior liver disease and alcoholics are more likely to suffer drug-induced hepatotoxicity. Pregnant women or nursing mothers should be observed to see if rifampin is harming the fetus or the nursing infant.
	Rifadin IV	INTRAVENOUS: *Adults*—As for oral.	As for oral.	Patients also receiving isoniazid have an increased risk of drug-induced hepatitis.
Streptomycin	Streptomycin	INTRAMUSCULAR: *Adults*—1 gm daily for 2 to 4 months or longer. Dosage may then be reduced to 1 gm 2 or 3 times weekly. *Children and elderly patients*—may require smaller doses.	In multidrug therapy for all forms of tuberculosis.	Patients with renal insufficiency are more prone to accumulate streptomycin and to develop ototoxicity. Elderly patients are more sensitive to ototoxic effects of streptomycin.

*Available in Canada and United States.
†Available in Canada only.

Table 35-2 Fixed Combinations Used in Treating Tuberculosis

Generic name	Trade name	Administration/dosage	Clinical use
Rifampin and isoniazid	Rifamate	ORAL: *Adults*—600 mg of rifampin and 300 mg of isoniazid (2 tablets) once daily.	Treatment of pulmonary tuberculosis after dose of separate drugs has been established.
Rifampin, isoniazid, and pyrazinamide	Rifater	ORAL: *Adults*—As for individual components.	Short-course treatment of tuberculosis. This preparation is an orphan drug product.

Mechanism of action. Although isoniazid alters several metabolic processes in mycobacteria, it is not yet known which of these actions are critical for destruction of the microorganism in vivo. Isoniazid is a potent inhibitor of an enzyme involved in cell wall synthesis and also blocks pyridoxine (vitamin B_6) utilization in a number of intracellular enzymes. Isoniazid is bactericidal and affects both intracellular (within macrophages) and extracellular mycobacteria.

Whatever the precise mechanism of action of isoniazid, mycobacteria can rapidly acquire resistance to it. In early trials, when isoniazid was used alone to treat active pulmonary tuberculosis, 11% of the patients carried isoniazid-resistant strains at the end of 1 month of therapy. At the end of 3 months, 71% of these patients harbored resistant *Mycobacterium*. Observations such as these have led to the clinical practice of combining isoniazid therapy with one or two other drugs. Combined drug therapy successfully suppresses the appearance of resistant organisms in most patients.

Isoniazid is used alone for prophylaxis. The drug is prescribed for persons exposed to tuberculosis or patients who have recently converted from negative to positive reactions in the skin test for tuberculosis. The latter patients usually have smaller numbers of *Mycobacterium* than would be found in an active, symptomatic case of tuberculosis, and for them the use of isoniazid alone is usually successful.

Isoniazid is most effective against *M. tuberculosis,* inhibiting the growth of over 90% of tested strains at a concentration of 0.2 mg/ml. Evidence suggests that resistant strains of *M. tuberculosis* are less pathogenic than sensitive strains. For this reason, isoniazid therapy may be continued even after isoniazid-resistant strains are cultured. *Mycobacterium kansasii,* which rarely causes disease in humans, is less sensitive to isoniazid than is *M. tuberculosis.* Other mycobacteria are resistant to the drug.

Absorption, distribution, and excretion. Isoniazid is well absorbed after oral administration, achieving peak serum levels in 1 to 2 hr. The drug enters body tissues relatively efficiently, and bactericidal concentrations are found in most tissues, including pleural fluids and caseous exudates surrounding active loci of tuberculosis infections in the lung.

Isoniazid undergoes a number of metabolic conversions in the liver, most resulting in inactive drug, which is excreted primarily in the kidney. The major metabolite is an acetylated form of isoniazid. The rate of drug acetylation differs markedly among populations, and two genetically determined types may be distinguished. Rapid acetylators inactivate isoniazid two to three times as rapidly as slow acetylators. As would be expected, rapid acetylators have lower blood concentrations of active drug than slow acetylators. Nevertheless, both types of patients respond well to standard therapeutic doses administered once daily. Increasing the drug dose or the frequency of administration in slow acetylators is not wise, since these patients tend to accumulate the acetylated metabolite, which is hepatotoxic.

Slow acetylators include 45% to 65% of Northern European and American white or black populations. Oriental and Eskimo populations contain predominantly rapid acetylators.

Toxicity and drug interactions. Isoniazid is a relatively nontoxic drug. Nevertheless, as with any drug, untoward reactions can occur in a small percentage of treated patients. The most commonly encountered toxic reaction is peripheral neuropathy. Diabetic patients, alcoholics, and malnourished persons are more prone to this complication than the general population. At least some of these reactions are related to low vitamin B_6 levels and may be prevented by administration of 5 mg of the vitamin daily. Peripheral neuropathies are more likely to occur in slow acetylators.

Hepatotoxicity is the most serious side effect associated with isoniazid. Fatalities resulting from liver failure have been noted, even among persons receiving the drug prophylactically. Hepatitis caused by isoniazid is rare among patients under 20 years of age and occurs in patients 20 to 34 years of age at a rate of approximately 3 cases/1000 patients. After age 50, the incidence increases to 23 cases/1000 patients. Patients also have an increased risk of hepatitis if they are rapid acetylators of isoniazid, if they ingest ethanol daily, or if they also receive the drug rifampin. Liver function should be monitored in all patients receiving isoniazid and most carefully watched in those patients at high risk. Various other reactions have occasionally been reported with isoniazid, including allergies, blood dyscrasias, gastric distress, and metabolic acidosis.

Patients receiving phenytoin for convulsive disorders may require dosage adjustment because isoniazid decreases the metabolism of phenytoin. Isoniazid may also enhance metabolism of the antifungal drug ketoconazole and may reduce effectiveness of the agent. In contrast, carbamazepine metabolism is inhibited by isoniazid, and serum concentrations of this drug may increase when isoniazid is given.

Ethambutol

Clinical use. Ethambutol is an effective antituberculosis drug that is chemically unrelated to other antituberculosis drugs or antibiotics. It is apparently effective only against mycobacteria and no other bacteria, viruses, or fungi tested. Ethambutol, a first-line drug in conventional antituberculosis therapy, is frequently used as one of the drugs in intermittent therapeutic programs.

Mechanism of action. The precise antibacterial action of ethambutol is unknown. The drug interferes with the formation of several cellular metabolites and cell walls of *Mycobacterium;* bacterial death follows in about 24 hr. Nearly all strains of *M. tuberculosis* are sensitive to the drug. Nearly all strains of *M. avium* are resistant. Other mycobacteria have intermediate sensitivity to ethambutol.

Resistance to ethambutol develops in vivo if the drug is used alone in therapy. Since ethambutol is chemically unrelated to other antituberculosis drugs and presumably has a different mechanism of action, it does not induce cross-resistance to other antituberculosis agents.

Absorption, distribution, and excretion. Ethambutol is administered orally and is well absorbed from the gastrointestinal (GI) tract in either the presence or the absence of food. Peak serum concentrations are observed 2 to 4 hr after an oral dose. Ethambutol is less extensively metabolized than isoniazid, and up to 50% of the drug excreted in urine is in the unaltered active form. Up to 15% of the drug in urine is in the form of a metabolite. Fecal concentrations of the drug represent unabsorbed material.

Ethambutol has been detected in cerebrospinal fluid after oral therapy, although the levels are below those found in plasma. The drug is also known to concentrate in erythrocytes.

Toxicity. Ethambutol has become a first-line antituberculosis drug because of its relatively wide spectrum of activity against *Mycobacterium* species and its relatively low toxicity. These advantages have outweighed the disadvantage that it is somewhat less potent than several other antituberculosis agents.

The most commonly reported toxic reaction to normal therapeutic doses of ethambutol is visual disturbance. Some patients report changes in color vision, whereas others suffer a more prominent loss of visual acuity. These signs are cause to terminate ethambutol use. If the drug is discontinued when these visual signs appear, the changes are reversible, although full recovery may take months.

Other reactions to ethambutol appear rarely. Allergic reactions have occasionally been reported. Peripheral neuritis can occur with higher doses. Some reactions attributed to ethambutol may actually have been caused by other drugs administered concomitantly. Elevated uric acid levels have been reported in patients receiving ethambutol, although evidence linking this action directly to ethambutol is scanty.

Rifampin

Clinical use. Rifampin, originally developed as an antibacterial drug, was observed to be effective against *Chlamydia,* some viruses, and mycobacteria. Rifampin is as potent as isoniazid against mycobacteria and has the broadest spectrum of activity of any antituberculosis agent against species of mycobacteria. These advantages have placed rifampin in the group of first-line–antituberculosis agents. The disadvantages of the drug include its expense and its tendency to cause increased toxicity when administered intermittently.

Rifampin is available as a single-ingredient formulation (see Table 35-1) and in fixed combination with other antituberculosis drugs (see Table 35-2).

Mechanism of action. Rifampin inhibits DNA-dependent–RNA polymerase in sensitive organisms. As a result, gene transcription halts, and protein synthesis is prevented. Metabolic activity in the *Mycobacterium* stops, and the cell ultimately dies or is eliminated by host defenses.

Resistance to rifampin can occur when the drug is used alone against *Mycobacterium.* Resistant strains have an altered DNA-dependent RNA polymerase that is no longer inhibited by the drug. Cross-resistance to other antituberculosis drugs does not occur.

Absorption, distribution, and excretion. Rifampin is absorbed orally in adequate amounts in the presence or absence of food. The slightly slower absorption observed in the presence of food is apparently not clinically important.

Rifampin is a relatively lipid-soluble agent. This property explains why it is found in higher concentrations in body tissues than in serum. Its lipid solubility also explains its ability to penetrate white blood cells and to attack *Mycobacterium* living there.

Roughly 40% of a dose of rifampin is excreted in the bile and a little less in urine. The drug is also deacetylated by the liver, and the deacetylated metabolite is excreted via the bile into feces.

Toxicity and drug interactions. Rifampin can cause a variety of mild reactions such as GI upset and central nervous system (CNS) disturbances. The drug also turns body fluids such as tears, sweat, saliva, and urine an orange-red color, which might be mistaken for blood. This coloration is harmless.

Liver abnormalities seem to be the most common reaction observed with rifampin. Mild abnormalities in liver function may return to normal without discontinuing the drug, but increases in alkaline phosphatase or the appearance of jaundice signals that the drug should be discontinued.

High doses given intermittently may cause an immune reaction that is associated with a variety of symptoms. This flulike syndrome may progress from chills, fever, vomiting, diarrhea, and myalgia to acute renal failure. Deaths have occurred. Since these symptoms occur when therapy is resumed, patients should be advised not to miss doses of rifampin, especially if they are receiving relatively high doses. Some treatment centers have significantly lowered rifampin dosage for intermittent therapeutic programs and have reduced these immune reactions (see Table 35-1 and Appendix A).

Rifampin also seems to be an immunosuppressant in humans, producing delayed effects on the immune system. The implication of this action on the clinical effectiveness of rifampin is unknown.

Rifampin induces liver enzymes involved in drug and hormone metabolism in humans. This action leads to several drug interactions. Patients receiving coumarin anticoagulants, oral hypoglycemic agents, methadone, or digitalis may require adjustment of the dosage of these agents because rifampin induces the liver microsomal enzymes that degrade these drugs. Patients receiving oral contraceptives or replacement doses of cortisol may lose the effectiveness of these agents because rifampin accelerates breakdown of the steroids. Patients receiving isoniazid along with rifampin have an increased risk of drug-induced hepatitis.

Streptomycin

Clinical use. The first of the antituberculosis drugs to be discovered, streptomycin is still a reliable agent. Streptomycin is frequently used as part of a three-drug regimen for initial therapy (see Table 35-1). It is usually discontinued after the number of infective organisms has been greatly reduced, usually after 2 to 4 months. The patient may continue to receive the remaining two drugs throughout the treatment period. Streptomycin has also been used as part of intermittent treatment programs in which the drug is given two or three times a week for the first 2 months of therapy.

Mechanism of action. Streptomycin inhibits protein synthesis in sensitive bacteria (see Chapter 33) and in mycobacteria. The drug is highly effective against most types of pathogenic mycobacteria with the exception of *M. avium.*

Resistance to streptomycin may develop when the drug is used alone. When streptomycin is used in combination with isoniazid or another first-line agent, development of resistance is minimized.

Absorption, distribution, and excretion. Streptomycin is not absorbed orally and must be administered by IM injection for routine clinical use (see Chapter 33). This property restricts its use to the hospital setting or to a well-supervised outpatient program. Because of the difficulties of daily injections, patients are frequently taken off streptomycin after 2 to 4 months of therapy, if bacteriologic improvement is obvious. Therapy is continued in these cases with other antituberculosis drugs.

Streptomycin is well distributed in the body and may be used to treat tuberculosis meningitis and other forms of nonpulmonary tuberculosis. The excretion of streptomycin is discussed in Chapter 33.

Toxicity and drug interactions. Streptomycin can produce any toxic reaction seen with other aminoglycoside antibiotics (see Chapter 33), but ototoxicity is the most commonly encountered reaction in tuberculosis patients. Careful attention to maintaining dosage within safe limits (see Table 35-1) prevents the reaction in most patients. Patients with renal insufficiency, elderly patients, and patients receiving long-term streptomycin therapy are more prone to develop toxic reactions.

Because streptomycin causes ototoxicity, it should not be combined with other ototoxic drugs such as the diuretic ethacrynic acid. Patients receiving muscle relaxants along with streptomycin may suffer excessive muscle relaxation because streptomycin is a weak neuromuscular blocking agent.

Alternate Drugs Used in Tuberculosis Therapy

Aminosalicylate

Clinical use. Aminosalicylate (PAS) in the past was included in the standard three-drug regimen for tuberculosis in which streptomycin, isoniazid, and PAS were administered for 3 to 4 months. After active mycobacteria had disappeared from sputum and other fluids, PAS and isoniazid were continued for another 2 years. Currently, treatment protocols are more likely to include ethambutol or rifampin than PAS. PAS is not effective in short-course regimens and is considered an alternate drug.

Mechanism of action. PAS inhibits mycobacterial growth by interfering with folic acid metabolism. The mechanism is probably similar to sulfonamide inhibition of bacterial growth. Mycobacteria can develop resistance to PAS, and the drug is never used alone in therapy. *M. tuberculosis* is usually sensitive to PAS, but other types of mycobacteria are generally resistant.

Absorption, distribution, and excretion. PAS is efficiently absorbed by the oral route and is well distributed to most body tissues. It does not enter the cerebrospinal fluid in the absence of inflamed meninges. Excretion is primarily via the kidney, but PAS is also acetylated in the liver and inactivated.

Toxicity. PAS is not well tolerated by most patients. Nearly all patients receiving the drug report GI irritation. Taking the drug with food or antacids prevents some of the irritation produced by the large amount of drug contained in a normal dose (see Table 35-1). Allergic symptoms have also been reported with PAS, including exfoliative dermatitis and severe organ damage. Low patient acceptance of PAS and availability of better tolerated and more effective agents have combined to restrict the use of PAS.

Amikacin, capreomycin, cycloserine, ethionamide, and pyrazinamide

The major properties of other alternate drugs used to treat tuberculosis are summarized in Table 35-1. The wide use of these drugs is limited by various factors. As a group, the reserve drugs are more toxic than the first-line drugs. Moreover, many of the reserve drugs are not as potent as the more commonly used drugs. Nevertheless, these reserve agents are useful when strains of mycobacteria resistant to first-line drugs appear or when a patient develops intolerable toxic reactions to these drugs.

Nursing Process Overview
TREATMENT OF LEPROSY
Assessment

In the United States the diagnosis of leprosy is unusual. Perform a thorough total assessment, with special emphasis on subjective and objective deviations from normal.

Nursing Diagnoses

Anxiety related to diagnosis and long-term drug therapy

Possible complication: depression related to change in skin color secondary to drug side effect

Management

The diagnosis of leprosy causes a great deal of fear and anxiety in patients. Refer to appropriate agencies for education and support, and begin patient and family education. Appropriate agencies include the health department and the Centers for Disease Control in Atlanta. Continue regular total patient assessment, with a focus on identifying possible toxic and side effects of the drugs prescribed.

Evaluation

Therapy for leprosy is often continued for 4 years or longer. Before discharging the patient, ascertain that the patient can explain why and how to take the drugs prescribed, and possible side effects, side effects that require notification of the physician, and possible ways to treat more commonly seen side effects. Any additional measures that may be prescribed related to the stage of the disease as it was diagnosed should be discussed. Report the diagnosis of leprosy to the local health department for family follow-up.

LEPROSY

Leprosy, like tuberculosis, is currently found primarily in developing countries and is rarely encountered in the United States or Canada. Also like tuberculosis, leprosy is curable with appropriate drug therapy. Patients are usually treated for at least 4 years, and some must be treated for life. Long-term treatment is required because *Mycobacterium leprae,* the causative agent of leprosy, is a slow-growing organism and may remain dormant for long periods in humans.

The primary drug used to treat leprosy is the sulfone dapsone, but alternatives are now available. Clofazimine seems as effective as dapsone. Moreover, strains of *M. leprae* that acquire resistance to dapsone remain sensitive to clofazimine. The antituberculosis drugs rifampin and more rarely ethionamide have also been used to treat leprosy.

Resistance to dapsone is appearing more frequently today than in previous years. Therefore combination therapy has become the accepted policy in the United States because combining of drugs lessens the likelihood that resistance will occur and increases the likelihood that all mycobacteria will be eradicated, and a permanent cure will be achieved. Rifampin is combined with dapsone or clofazimine for the first 6 months to 3 years, after which dapsone or clofazimine alone may be continued for as long as is necessary. Patients with dermatitis herpetiformis may be placed on a gluten-free diet (see box). The properties of drugs used to treat leprosy are summarized in Table 35-3.

DIETARY CONSIDERATION: GLUTEN-FREE DIET

Gluten, which is found in many grains, is restricted in the management of several health problems, including celiac disease (nontropical sprue) and dermatitis herpetiformis. Food items to avoid on a gluten-free diet include cereal grains such as wheat, barley, oats, rye, bran, graham, millet, wheat germ, bulgur, and malt and products containing these grains. Products made with gluten-containing grains include prepared meats, thickened stew, breaded vegetables, root beer, pasta, macaroni products, gluten stabilizer, brewer's yeast, flour (when the source is not indicated), and pizza.

The following foods are permitted: rice, corn, flours made from soybeans, buckwheat, lima beans, gluten-free wheat starch, cornmeal, and hominy.

Encourage patients to read labels carefully.

Refer patients as needed to the dietitian.

Table 35-3 Drugs to Treat Leprosy

Generic name	Trade name	Administration/dosage	Toxicity	Comments
Dapsone	Avlosulfon† Dapsone*	ORAL: Adults—100 mg daily for 4 years to life, with rifampin for first 6 to 36 months. FDA Pregnancy Category C. Children—1.4 mg/kg daily.	Serum sickness reactions are possible	Patients with G6PD deficiency are more prone to hemolytic reactions and must receive reduced doses
Ethionamide	Trecator-SC	ORAL: Adults—250 mg every 8 to 12 hr.	Hepatitis, peripheral neuritis, CNS effects	Not approved for this use in the United States
Clofazimine	Lamprene	ORAL: Adults—50 to 100 mg daily for 4 years to life, with rifampin for first 6 to 36 months. FDA Pregnancy Category C.	GI distress; discoloration of the skin is an expected, reversible side effect	Primary use is for dapsone-resistant leprosy
Rifampin	Rifadin* Rimactane* Rofact†	ORAL, INTRAVENOUS: Adults—600 mg once a month for 24 months, with dapsone or clofazimine.	Liver toxicity; abdominal distress	Not approved for this use in the United States

*Available in Canada and United States.
†Available in Canada only.

NURSING IMPLICATIONS SUMMARY

General Guidelines for Patients with Tuberculosis or Leprosy

◆ Provide emotional support for patients and their families when a diagnosis of tuberculosis or leprosy is made. Both diseases may be associated with patient fears and misunderstandings. Teach patients and families about the diseases, their spread, and control and about drug therapy.

◆ Review anticipated benefits and possible side effects associated with drug therapy.

◆ Emphasize the importance of long-term therapy for best effect.

◆ Encourage patients to return as scheduled for follow-up appointments. Blood work must be monitored to rule out side effects.

◆ Refer patients to the local health department for teaching and for follow-up.

◆ Emphasize the importance of taking drugs on a regular basis. Review guidelines for missed doses, which are to be taken as soon as remembered, unless shortly before the next dose. Do not double up for missed doses.

◆ Health-care personnel should obtain a routine tuberculosis screening test annually.

◆ Inform all health-care providers of all drugs being taken.

◆ Some of these drugs are contraindicated during pregnancy or breast feeding. Tell female patients to consult with their physicians before getting pregnant, if possible.

Drug administration and patient and family education

◆ See general guidelines for patients with TB.

◆ Take oral doses with meals or a snack to lessen gastric irritation. Provide positive reinforcement. This drug is difficult to take. A 10 gm/day dose requires 20 500-mg tablets, divided into three or four doses.

◆ Discard discolored tablets, and obtain a fresh supply.

◆ To prevent crystalluria, maintain a fluid intake of 2000 to 2500 ml/day.

◆ For the powder form of the drug, dissolve contents of the package in a glass of water and stir well. Drink all of the fluid to obtain the full dose.

◆ Do not take aminosalicylates within 6 hr of doses of rifampin.

◆ Do not take aminosalicylate calcium within 1 to 3 hr of when tetracycline doses are taken.

◆ If photophobia develops, wear sunglasses, and avoid areas of bright lights or sunlight.

NURSING IMPLICATIONS SUMMARY—cont'd

◆ Warn diabetic patients that aminosalicylates may cause false urine glucose results. Do not change diet or insulin dose without consulting the physician. Monitor blood glucose level if possible.

Capreomycin

Drug administration and patient and family education

◆ Review the general guidelines.
◆ This drug is only available for IM administration. Reconstitute as directed on label. If for home management, instruct patients in proper administration technique.
◆ Give cautiously with other drugs known to cause renal impairment or ototoxicity. Examples include aminoglycosides, furosemide, and cisplatin.
◆ Monitor renal function including blood urea nitrogen (BUN) level and serum creatinine level.
◆ Assess for ototoxicity including hearing acuity and balance.
◆ Avoid driving or operating hazardous equipment if drowsiness or dizziness occurs; notify the physician.

Cycloserine

Drug administration and patient and family education

◆ Review general guidelines.
◆ Assess for signs of depression including malaise, lack of interest in personal appearance, insomnia, withdrawal, and weight gain or loss.
◆ Avoid driving or operating hazardous equipment if drowsiness or dizziness occurs; notify the physician.
◆ Avoid alcoholic beverages while taking this drug.

Ethambutol

Drug administration

◆ See general guidelines for patients with tuberculosis and the Nursing Implications Summary in Chapter 29.
◆ Assess for visual changes and peripheral neuropathy.
◆ Monitor complete blood count (CBC) and differential and uric acid levels.

Patient and family education

◆ Review general guidelines.

◆ Take oral doses with meals or a snack to lessen gastric irritation.
◆ Report changes in vision to the physician.
◆ Avoid driving or operating hazardous equipment until the effects of this medication are known; it may cause drowsiness or dizziness.

Ethionamide

Drug administration and patient and family education

◆ See general guidelines for patients with tuberculosis and the Nursing Implications Summary in Chapter 29.
◆ Assess for peripheral neuropathy including numbness, tingling, paresthesia, and feelings of heaviness of the fingers, arms, and legs.
◆ Pyridoxine may also be prescribed with this drug. Emphasize the importance of taking both drugs. See Dietary Consideration: Vitamins on p. 275.
◆ Report changes in vision to the physician.
◆ Avoid driving or operating hazardous equipment until the effects of this medication are known; it may cause drowsiness or dizziness.
◆ Assess for depression including malaise, lack of interest in personal appearance, insomnia, withdrawal, and weight gain or loss.

Isoniazid

Drug administration

◆ Review Nursing Implications Summary in Chapter 29.
◆ Assess for peripheral neuropathy including numbness, tingling, paresthesia, and feelings of heaviness of the fingers, arms, and legs.
◆ Monitor CBC and differential, platelet count, liver function tests, and blood glucose level.
◆ IM injection may produce pain at the injection site; warn patients about this.

Patient and family education

◆ Review general guidelines.
◆ Instruct patients to report any new sign or symptom.
◆ Emphasize to patients the importance of taking pyridoxine if prescribed. Review Dietary Consideration: Vitamins on p. 275 for information about dietary sources of pyridoxine.
◆ Avoid the use of alcohol while taking isoniazid.
◆ Take oral doses with meals to avoid gastric irritation.
◆ See Patient Problem: Dry Mouth on p. 166.

Continued.

- Caution patients to avoid driving or operating hazardous equipment if dizziness, ataxia, tinnitus, or vision changes occur; notify the physician.
- Ingestion of fish or cheese by patients taking isoniazid may cause a reaction. Symptoms include headache, flushing, nausea, vomiting, tachycardia, itching skin, and light-headedness. Tell patients to limit or avoid cheese or fish. Notify the physician if these symptoms develop.
- Tell diabetic patients that isoniazid may cause false results in urine glucose tests. Do not change diet or insulin dose without contacting the physician. Monitor blood glucose level if possible.
- Do not take aluminum-containing antacids within 1 hr of taking isoniazid.

Pyrazinamide

Drug administration and patient and family education

- Review Nursing Implications Summary in Chapter 29 and general guidelines.
- Monitor liver function tests and serum uric acid level.
- Warn diabetic patients that this drug may alter results of urine ketone tests; monitor blood sugar level.

Rifampin

Drug administration

- See general guidelines for patients with TB and the Nursing Implications Summary in Chapter 29.
- Assess CBC and differential, platelet count, and liver function tests.

Patient and family education

- Review general guidelines.
- If tolerated, take rifampin on an empty stomach, 1 hr before or 2 hr after meals. Take with meals if gastric irritation is severe when taken on an empty stomach.
- Warn patients that body fluids (tears, sweat, feces, and urine) may turn orange-red while on rifampin therapy. Soft contact lenses may be permanently stained.
- It is especially important not to miss rifampin doses. Take regularly, as prescribed, for best results.
- Do not take doses of rifampin within 6 hr of doses of PAS.
- Avoid driving or operating hazardous equipment if drowsiness, dizziness, or visual changes occur; notify the physician.
- Avoid alcoholic beverages while taking rifampin.

- Contraceptive pills may not be effective in patients who are also taking rifampin. Instruct patients to use another means of birth control while taking rifampin; consult the physician.
- Capsules may be opened, and the contents may be mixed with applesauce or jelly for ease in taking.
- A suspension can also be made; consult the pharmacist.

Streptomycin

- Streptomycin is discussed in Chapter 33.

Dapsone

Drug administration and patient and family education

- See general guidelines for patients with TB and leprosy.
- Assess for skin changes and peripheral neuropathy.
- Monitor CBC and differential, platelet count, BUN level, and serum creatinine level. Monitor urinalysis.
- Take ordered doses with meals or a snack to lessen gastric irritation.
- If insomnia occurs, take once-daily doses in the morning.
- Avoid driving or operating hazardous equipment if dizziness or light-headedness occurs; notify the physician.
- Patients with dermatitis herpetiformis may be placed on a gluten-free diet (see Dietary Consideration: Gluten-free Diet on p. 509).

Clofazimine

Drug administration and patient and family education

- Take oral doses with meals or a snack to lessen gastric irritation.
- Warn patients that this drug may cause red-to-brown pigmentation of the skin and eyes. Assess for discoloration. If skin changes produce depression or extreme sadness, notify the physician.
- See Patient Problem: Photosensitivity on p. 629.
- Clofazimine may discolor feces, sputum, sweat, tears, and urine. It may also produce black, tarry, or bloody stools; notify the physician.
- Use lotion or skin cream to treat dry, scaly skin.
- Avoid driving or operating hazardous equipment if drowsiness or dizziness occurs; notify the physician.

CHAPTER REVIEW

◆ KEY TERMS

leprosy, p. 509
tuberculosis, p. 503

◆ REVIEW QUESTIONS

1. What properties of mycobacteria make controlling tuberculosis more difficult than many other bacterial diseases?
2. During what phase of tuberculosis is the disease contagious?
3. Why is tuberculosis usually treated by multiple drug therapy? What implications are there for patient assessment and teaching?
4. What is the duration of therapy for tuberculosis?
5. What is the mechanism of action of isoniazid?
6. What is the outcome of using isoniazid alone to treat active tuberculosis?
7. When is isoniazid used alone in tuberculosis therapy?
8. How is isoniazid administered in tuberculosis therapy?
9. What is the fate of isoniazid in the body?
10. What toxicity is associated with isoniazid?
11. What is the mechanism of action of ethambutol?
12. How is ethambutol administered in tuberculosis therapy?
13. What toxicity is associated with ethambutol?
14. What is the mechanism of action of rifampin?
15. How is rifampin administered in tuberculosis therapy?
16. How may the timing of rifampin therapy influence the toxicity it produces?
17. What is the mechanism of action of streptomycin?
18. How is streptomycin administered?
19. What toxicity is associated with streptomycin?
20. What is the mechanism of action of PAS?
21. How is PAS administered in tuberculosis therapy?
22. What toxicity is associated with PAS?
23. Why are certain drugs classified as alternate drugs in tuberculosis therapy?
24. What drugs are most useful in treating leprosy?
25. How long must therapy continue for control of leprosy?
26. Given one or more drugs discussed in this chapter, develop a nursing care plan for your patient.

SUGGESTED READING

Cohn JP: Leprosy: out of the dark ages, *FDA Consum* 23(7):24, 1989.

Cornell C: tuberculosis in hospital employees, *Am J Nurs* 88(4):484, 1988.

Gangadharam PRJ: Antimycobacterial drugs, *Antimicrobial Agents Annual* 3:15, 1989.

Hastings RC, Franzblau SG: Chemotherapy of leprosy, *Ann Rev Pharm Tox* 28:231, 1988.

Jacobson RR: Antibiotic therapy for leprosy, *Antimicrobial Agents Annual* 3:41, 1989.

Lancaster E: tuberculosis on the rise, *Am J Nurs* 88(4):484, 1988.

Mathewson HS: Treatment of pulmonary mycobacterial infections, *Respir Care* 35(5):427, 1990.

Todd B: Treating tuberculosis, *Geriatr Nurs* 9(4):250, 1988.

Van Scoy RE, Wilkowske CJ: Antituberculous agents, *Mayo Clin Proc* 67(2):179, 1992.

CHAPTER 36

Antifungal Agents

LEARNING OBJECTIVES

After studying this chapter, you should be able to do the following:

- Explain the mechanism of action of amphotericin B and imidazole antifungal drugs.
- Discuss the dose-limiting toxicity of amphotericin B.
- Explain why drugs too toxic for systemic use may be used for local fungal infections.
- Develop a nursing care plan for the patient receiving one of the parenteral, oral, or topical antifungal agents discussed in this chapter.

CHAPTER OVERVIEW

- Fungal diseases range from mild infections in localized areas of the skin to grave systemic infections. Diseases of various types may be produced by a wide range of fungi, and to a great extent the seriousness of the infection is determined by the nature of the infective organism and the immune status of the host. In this chapter, some of the more common and the more serious fungal diseases are examined, and the drugs that are used to control these specific infections are considered.

Nursing Process Overview
FUNGAL INFECTIONS
Assessment

Fungal infections are relatively common and can occur in patients of any age. Perform a thorough total assessment, with a focus on the specific subjective complaints or objective signs that indicate possible fungal infection. Include as part of the history recent use of drugs that may alter the patient's immune response and measures the patient has tried for eradication of the problem. Patients most likely to have fungal infections include those receiving cancer chemotherapy, immunotherapy, antibiotic therapy, or drugs that alter the normal pH of areas such as the vagina; those receiving nutritional support via peripheral or central venous catheters; and those taking high doses of adrenocortical steroids.

Nursing Diagnoses

Possible altered comfort: nausea and vomiting as a side effect of drug therapy
Possible complication: renal damage and failure

Management

Teach the patient about the drugs prescribed, the infection, and possible ways to limit the spread of the infection and to prevent its recurrence. Treatment of systemic fungal infections is more serious. Monitor the vital signs and appropriate laboratory work to evaluate possible side effects.

Evaluation

Before discharge, ascertain that the patient can explain why the drug is being used, how it should be used and under what circumstances, what to do if side effects should occur, and which side effects require notification of the physician.

SELECTIVE TOXICITY IN THE TREATMENT OF FUNGAL DISEASES

Although the **fungi** that cause disease in humans are single-celled organisms, they are eucaryotes (see Chapter 29) and therefore resemble human cells more than bacteria in their biochemical properties. These biochemical similarities to human cells present therapeutic problems. For instance, none of the antibiotics that inhibit bacterial protein synthesis affect that process in fungi because fungal ribosomes resemble those in humans and are sensitive to the same drugs. Therefore selective toxicity cannot be achieved by this mechanism. Moreover, fungal cells do not contain a peptidoglycan cell wall, which renders them resistant to all antibiotics that block peptidoglycan synthesis (e.,g., penicillins). For these reasons the antimicrobial agents discussed in previous chapters cannot be used to treat fungal diseases.

Design of new antifungal agents is limited by the number of known biochemical differences between fungal and mammalian cells. The only systematically exploited difference lies in the outer membranes of the cells. Human cells contain cholesterol in their membranes, whereas those of fungi contain **ergosterol.**

This feature of membrane structure is the basis of action of the polyene antifungal drugs. Polyene antifungal agents have a greater affinity for ergosterol than for cholesterol and therefore somewhat selectively react with ergosterol from fungal cell membranes. This action destroys the integrity of the cell membrane and causes cytoplasmic components to be lost and the cell to die. However, the selectivity of these drugs is not so great as that of most drugs used for treating bacterial infections. Imidazole antifungal agents inhibit the synthesis of ergosterol. This action also impairs the function of the fungal cell membrane.

Fungal cells possess many cell surface antigens, which ultimately provoke host immune responses. Most fungal infections resolve in this way, many times without the host ever being aware of an active disease. This pattern is especially common with the fungal diseases spread by breathing in spores from contaminated soil. Examples of diseases of this type are histoplasmosis, blastomycosis, coccidioidomycosis, cryptococcosis, and aspergillosis. Several of these diseases are concentrated in specific geographic areas. For example, coccidioidomycosis is most common, or endemic, in the southernmost portions of California, Nevada, Utah, Arizona, New Mexico, and Texas, whereas histoplasmosis is endemic in the states bordering the Mississippi and Ohio rivers. Blastomycosis is endemic in isolated areas along the Mississippi and Ohio Rivers, around the Great Lakes, along the St. Lawrence River, and in the Carolinas.

Some fungal diseases are spread by contact with soil contaminated with bird droppings. Birds are not necessarily affected by these diseases, but they do frequently carry the organisms. Cryptococcosis frequently follows exposure to high concentrations of pigeon droppings. Histoplasmosis is associated with avian excreta such as chicken or starling droppings or bat guano.

Although pulmonary forms of these diseases are usually mild and limited by effective development of immunity in the victim, in rare cases the fungus may become disseminated and invade other body tissues. A notorious example is the yeast *Cryptococcus neoformans,* which can cause meningitis, pulmonary disease, and infections at many other sites. The disseminated, or systemic, fungal diseases are most likely to develop in patients whose immune system is depressed by disease or drug therapy, especially with glucocorticoids or immunosuppressant antineoplastic agents.

The yeast *Candida* may cause a range of infections from serious systemic disease to annoying mucous membrane infections. Since *Candida* is normally found on the skin and mucous membranes of healthy persons, the growth of *Candida* to cause disease usually represents an opportunistic infection. *Candida* infections are therefore most common in persons receiving broad-spectrum antibacterial drugs such as tetracyclines (see Chapter 29) or in persons with suppressed immune systems. *Candida* infections are very common in patients with acquired immunodeficiency syndrome (AIDS).

Dermatophytes are fungi whose growth is almost always restricted to the skin of humans. These fungi cause the annoying infections commonly known as *ringworm* and *athlete's foot,* as well as several others. This group of infections is frequently referred to as *tinea.* Drugs used for these superficial infections are not the same as those used for systemic fungal infections. Many of the drugs used topically are not absorbed extensively through the skin. Therefore more toxic agents may be used, and selective toxicity is achieved against many dermatophytes.

DRUGS TO TREAT SYSTEMIC FUNGAL INFECTIONS

Systemic fungal infections pertain to the whole body. Table 36-1 summarizes drugs used to treat systemic fungal infections.

Amphotericin B

Mechanism of action

Amphotericin B is a polyene antifungal drug whose action depends on selectively damaging membranes containing ergosterol, that is, fungal membranes. This membrane-disruptive effect is not entirely selective, and some of the cholesterol-containing membranes of mammalian cells are also damaged. Nevertheless, amphotericin B can be used to treat a broad spectrum of fungal diseases, including those caused by *Histoplasma, Blastomyces, Cryptococcus,* and *Aspergillus.* Amphotericin B may also treat systemic *Candida* and *Coccidioides* infections. Although a topical preparation of amphotericin B exists, it is not rec-

Table 36-1   Drugs to Treat Systemic Fungal Infections

Generic name	Trade name	Administration/dosage	Clinical use	Principal toxic reactions
Amphotericin B	Fungizone*	INTRAVENOUS: *Adults and children*—0.25 to 1 mg/kg/day infused at 0.1 mg/ml in 5% dextrose over 6 hr. Total drug course usually less than 4 gm. FDA Pregnancy Category B.	Disseminated, symptomatic fungal disease caused by *Histoplasma, Blastomyces, Coccidioides, Cryptococcus, Aspergillus, Candida,* and others.	Initial headache, nausea, vomiting, and fever. Progressive nephrotoxicity, anemia, and renal electrolyte imbalance.
Fluconazole	Diflucan*	ORAL, INTRAVENOUS: *Adults*—200 to 400 mg once daily. FDA Pregnancy Category C.	Meningitis caused by *C. neoformans;* and systemic, esophageal, or oropharyngeal candidiasis.	Gastrointestinal (GI) disturbances. Exfoliate skin disorders, hepatotoxicity, or thrombocytopenia are rare serious reactions.
Flucytosine	Ancobon Ancotil†	ORAL: *Adults and children*—50 to 150 mg/kg daily in 4 doses. Lower drug doses are required when renal function is impaired. FDA Pregnancy Category C.	Disseminated fungal infections caused by sensitive *Candida* strains, cryptococcal meningitis, and other infectitons; usually combined with amphotericin B.	Nausea and diarrhea are relatively common. Blood dyscrasias are also possible.
Itraconazole	—	ORAL: *Adult*—200 mg daily. Investigational agent.	Dermatophytoses, vaginal candida, histoplasmosis, coccidioidomycosis, and cryptococcosis.	GI disturbances. Sexual impotence has been reported.
Ketoconazole	Nizoral*	ORAL: *Adults*—200 to 400 mg once daily. FDA Pregnancy Category C. *Children over 2 years*—3.3 to 10 mg/kg once daily.	Disseminated infections caused by *Histoplasma, Paracoccidioides,* and *Candida.* Also used topically (see Table 36-2).	Nausea, pruritus, headache, and GI disturbances. Gynecomastia occurs in about 10% of treated males. Rare fatal hepatic necrosis.
Miconazole nitrate	Monistat-IV	INTRAVENOUS: *Adults*—200 mg to 3.6 gm, divided into 3 equal doses, may be indicated, depending on the causative organism. *Children*—total daily dose 20 to 40 mg/kg with no single infusion exceeding 15 mg/kg.	Systemic infections caused by *Candida, Cryptococcus,* and *Aspergillus.* Also used topically (see Table 36-2).	Thrombophlebitis, GI distress, blood dyscrasias, and allergic reactions have been reported.

*Available in Canada and United States.
†Available in Canada only.

ommended for this application because other topical agents such as ciclopirox, clotrimazole, econazole and miconazole are more effective.

Absorption, distribution, and excretion
Amphotericin B is not absorbed orally and must be administered intravenously, although the drug irritates vascular tissue and frequently causes phlebitis. The drug, which is lipid soluble, is administered as a colloidal suspension stabilized with small amounts of the detergent desoxycholate. Amphotericin B must be infused at a concentration of less than 0.1 mg/ml in a 5% dextrose solution. Higher drug concentrations cause precipitation of the drug in the intravenous (IV) solution and endanger the patient.

Amphotericin B has a high affinity for lipids and therefore tends to bind to tissues rather than remain in the bloodstream. The elimination half-life of the drug is about 12 hr after a single IV dose. During long-term therapy, only a fraction of the daily dose can be recovered in urine or feces. The unrecovered drug is apparently held in tissues, since amphotericin B continues to appear in urine for long periods after therapy is halted. The tissue-binding properties and the relative water insolubility of amphotericin B prevent the drug from entering body fluids efficiently. For this reason, concentrations of the drug in the cerebrospinal fluid or in ocular fluid may not be high enough to effectively eliminate infections at those sites. To overcome this problem, amphotericin B may be injected intrathecally (into the cerebrospinal fluid) in meningitis.

Toxicity

Most patients are begun on low doses of amphotericin B, and the dosage is increased as tolerance to the ensuing toxic reactions develops. Headache, fever, nausea, and vomiting may occur after the first few injections, but these side effects usually subside as therapy continues. Renal damage progresses with length of therapy and may become irreversible when total doses of amphotericin B approach 4 gm. Anemia also develops with time, as do a number of electrolyte disturbances including acidosis and hypokalemia (low blood potassium).

Amphotericin B therapy must be continued for long periods to attempt to cure disseminated fungal disease. No firm guidelines for therapy exist, although physicians try to limit the total drug dose to under 4 gm. Even with doses approaching this limit, cures are not always obtained. For many patients, therapy must be discontinued early because of toxic effects of the drug.

Amphotericin B has been experimentally administered encapsulated in liposomes (lipid vesicles). Patients whose therapy was ineffective with the standard preparation responded to the liposomal form of the drug. This experimental method of administration may also reduce the drug's toxicity. Development of this technique continues.

Flucytosine

Mechanism of action

Flucytosine is a pyrimidine analogue that is apparently converted to the cytotoxic agent 5-fluorouracil in sensitive fungi. Because this metabolite is not freely formed in humans, a degree of selective toxicity is achieved. A relatively narrow range of fungi are sensitive to the drug, including *Cryptococcus*, *Candida*, and a few other rarely encountered pathogenic fungi. Intrinsic resistance to flucytosine may exist in a significant number of clinically encountered *Candida* strains, and resistance to the drug may be acquired

by *Cryptococcus* during therapy. This pattern of resistance has limited the drug's usefulness.

Absorption, distribution, and excretion

Flucytosine is a water-soluble drug that is well absorbed from the GI tract and well distributed into body fluids. Drug concentration in cerebrospinal fluid may be 50% to 70% of serum levels, in contrast to amphotericin B, for which cerebrospinal fluid levels are less than 5% of serum levels. The primary organ of excretion for flucytosine is the kidney. More than 90% of an oral dose can be recovered intact in urine, in which concentrations of the drug are high. The elimination half-life is about 6 hr.

Toxicity

Flucytosine therapy is usually continued for several weeks to months. Unlike the situation with amphotericin B, few patients are forced to discontinue medication because of toxic reactions. Nausea and diarrhea appear in roughly a fourth of patients. Blood dyscrasias and transient liver abnormalities have been reported. Because it is frequently administered with amphotericin B, it may be difficult to distinguish which toxic reactions are caused by flucytosine.

The rationale for combining flucytosine and amphotericin B therapy for serious infections caused by fungi is twofold. The combination allows the dose of amphotericin B to be lowered somewhat, thereby reducing toxicity. The resistance to flucytosine is minimized by combination chemotherapy.

Imidazole Antifungals

Mechanism of action

Imidazole antifungals inhibit synthesis of ergosterol. As a result, the function of the fungal cell membrane is impaired. Development of invasive hyphae by fungal cells may be retarded, enhancing the ability of the host immune system to eliminate the fungi.

Imidazole antifungal agents are used to treat a variety of fungal infections. Fluconazole is indicated for cryptococcal meningitis and for systemic, esophageal, or oropharyngeal candidiasis. Ketoconazole is used against *Histoplasma* and *Paracoccidioides*. It may also be effective in certain patients with disseminated candidiasis, blastomycosis, coccidioidomycosis, and cryptococcosis. Itraconazole has been tested against many of these infections and others. Miconazole may be used against systemic coccidioidomycosis, cryptococcosis, and candidiasis but is primarily used as a topical agent. Clotimazole has been used topically, vaginally, and as a troche to be dissolved in the mouth to treat oral candidiasis. Econazole is used topically for tinea and vaginally for *Candida*. Terconazole is used only for vaginal infections caused by *Candida* (see box).

PATIENT PROBLEM: VAGINAL INFECTIONS

THE PROBLEM

The dark, moist environment of the vagina is prone to infection by a variety of organisms. Some chronic health problems such as diabetes mellitus increase susceptibility to vaginal infection. Treatment with some groups of drugs such as antibiotics may increase susceptibility to fungal superinfection. Finally, some invading organisms are passed as venereal diseases. Treatment of vaginal infection may be messy and difficult. It is difficult to reach all mucosal surfaces, and, since the woman is upright during most of the day, medications drain out because of gravity.

SOLUTIONS

◆ Use prescribed agents for the full course of therapy; do not stop when symptoms disappear.

◆ Do not wear tampons during therapy. Wear sanitary napkins to prevent staining of clothing.

◆ Continue therapy through the menstrual period.

◆ Wash hands carefully before and after using prescribed medications.

◆ Use once-daily doses of vaginal medication in the evening, before retiring. Insert vaginal suppository, ointment, or cream just before going to bed to allow the medication to remain in the vaginal area as long as possible.

◆ If douching is prescribed, wash douche equipment carefully after each use and dry it.

◆ Depending on the infecting agent, it may be necessary to treat the sexual partner also; consult the physician.

◆ Usually, avoid sexual intercourse during the course of therapy. If not possible, the sexual partner should wear a condom.

TO HELP PREVENT VAGINAL INFECTION

◆ Wear clean underwear daily, preferably of cotton material. Synthetic fabrics do not allow air to circulate as well and thus keep the vaginal area more moist than normal. Avoid pantyhose for the same reason.

◆ Wipe from front to back after voiding or defecating.

◆ Do not douche unless prescribed by the physician. Do not douche between doses of vaginal medications.

◆ Avoid bubble baths and soaps that may irritate vaginal mucosa. Wash the vaginal area gently, and rinse soap off well. Some women may need to wash with water only, if soap is irritating to the vaginal area.

◆ Use water-soluble lubricants, if needed, in the vagina. Do not use oil-based products such as petroleum jelly.

Absorption, distribution, and excretion

Ketoconazole is adequately absorbed orally, but bioavailability depends on sufficient stomach acidity. Ketoconazole is best absorbed on an empty stomach and should not be administered within 2 hr of administration of antacids or H-2-histamine receptor blocking drugs such as cimetidine. Ketoconazole is not well distributed to all tissues and is especially low in cerebrospinal fluid. Elimination is primarily by the liver, which forms inactive metabolites and excretes the drug into bile.

Fluconazole is well absorbed orally, with a bioavailability of about 90%; absorption does not depend on stomach acidity as much as with ketoconazole. Fluconazole is well distributed to most body tissues, including the cerebrospinal fluid. Little hepatic metabolism of fluconazole occurs, and most of the drug is excreted unchanged in urine. The half-life of the drug in patients with normal renal function is 30 hr.

Itraconazole is relatively lipid soluble and is absorbed after oral administration, but miconazole must be administered intravenously in systemic infections. Miconazole metabolites are formed in the liver and excreted in urine.

Toxicity

Ketoconazole is relatively nontoxic for many patients. Nausea and pruritus occur in less than 5% of treated patients. Dizziness, nervousness, and headache have been reported less frequently. Ketoconazole may inhibit testosterone and cortisol synthesis. Gynecomastia (excessive development of mammary glands) has been noted in about 10% of males receiving ketoconazole. Liver changes have also been noted, which in rare cases progresses to hepatitis or fatal hepatic necrosis.

Fluconazole may cause side effects in up to 13% of treated patients. GI disturbances such as nausea or diarrhea and headaches are the most common complaints. Thrombocytopenia, which produces unusual bleeding or bruising, and hepatotoxicity are more serious rare effects. Rarely, patients may develop dangerous allergic reactions such as Stevens-Johnson syndrome or exfoliative skin disorders.

Miconazole may produce rashes, itching, redness at the injection site, or phlebitis. Reversible platelet dysfunction, thrombocytopenia, and anemia may also occur with systemic administration.

Itraconazole appears to cause less hepatic toxicity than does ketoconazole and alters platelet function less than miconazole. Further clinical experience is required to fully assess the side effects.

DRUGS TO TREAT LOCALIZED OR TOPICAL FUNGAL INFECTIONS

In this section, drugs that are used to treat **localized fungal infections,** or those restricted to skin, mucous membranes, or GI tract, are considered. The properties of specific drugs are listed in Table 36-2. Most of these agents are used strictly locally, being applied at the site of infection. For example, tolnaftate is used to treat simple cases of tinea, but the effectiveness is limited by the accessibility of locally applied drug to

Table 36-2 Drugs to Treat Topical Fungal Infections

Generic name	Trade name	Administration/dosage	Clinical use	Cautions
Benzoic and salicylic acids	Whitfield's ointment	TOPICAL: *Adults and children*—6% benzoic and 3% salicylic acids, or double strength, applied 2 or 3 times daily.	OTC—Ringworm.	Keratolytic ointment may cause local tissue irritation.
Butoconazole	Femstat	INTRAVAGINAL: *Adults*—2% cream applied once daily for 3 days. FDA Pregnancy Category C.	Rx—Vaginal infections caused by *Candida*.	Vaginal burning is possible; has been used by pregnant women.
Calcium undecylenate	Caldesene Cruex	TOPICAL: *Adults and children*—10% powder applied as needed.	OTC—Tinea cruris (jock itch); also used for diaper rash or other skin irritations of groin area.	Powder should not be inhaled or allowed to contact eyes or mucous membranes. Diabetics and others with impaired circulation should use only with physician's advice.
Carbolfuchsin (Castellani paint)	Castel Plus	TOPICAL: *Adults and children*—Solution swabbed over affected area 1 to 3 times daily.	Rx—Athlete's foot and ringworm.	Contact sensitivity may cause reactions; poisonous if ingested.
Ciclopirox olamine	Loprox*	TOPICAL: *Adults*—1% cream applied twice daily. FDA Pregnancy Category B.	Rx—Tinea infections including tinea versicolor and cutaneous candidiasis.	May cause redness, itching, and stinging of skin. Avoid eyes.
Clioquinol (iodochlorhydroxyquin)	Torofor Vioform*	TOPICAL: *Adults and children*—3% cream, ointment, or powder applied 2 or 3 times daily.	Rx—Localized dermatophytoses.	Irritation of skin usually mild, but avoid eyes. Can cause a false-positive result in the ferric chloride test for phenylketonuria (PKU) and can alter iodine content of blood.
Clotrimazole	Canesten† Lotrimin Mycelex	TOPICAL: *Adults and children*—1% cream, lotion, or solution applied twice daily. FDA Pregnancy Category B.	Rx—Tinea and cutaneous *Candida*.	Skin irritation, pruritus, and urticaria may occur; avoid eyes.
	Canesten† Gyne-Lotrimin Myclo†	INTRAVAGINAL: *Adults*—tablets or creams containing 100 mg inserted once daily. FDA Pregnancy Category B.	Rx—Vulvovaginal candidiasis.	
	Mycelox	ORAL: *Adults and children over 4 years*—10 mg lozenge dissolved in mouth 5 times daily. FDA Pregnancy Category C.	Rx—Candidiasis, oropharyngeal.	
Econazole	Ecostatin† Spectazole	TOPICAL: *Adults and children*—1% cream applied to skin 1 or 2 times daily. FDA Pregnancy Category C.	Rx—*Candida*, mucocutaneous; tinea.	May cause skin irritation; avoid eyes.

OTC, over the counter; Rx, prescription.
*Available in Canada and United States.
†Available in Canada only.

Continued.

Table 36-2 Drugs to Treat Topical Fungal Infections—cont'd

Generic name	Trade name	Administration/dosage	Clinical use	Cautions
Econazole—cont'd	Ecostatin†	VAGINAL: *Adults*—single 150 mg suppository inserted once daily for 3 days.	Rx—*Candida* vulvovaginal.	Vaginal irritation may occur.
Gentian violet	Genapax	INTRAVAGINAL: *Adults*—One tampon (Genapax) inserted once or twice daily for 12 days. FDA Pregnancy Category C.	Rx—*Candida* infections of vagina.	Irritation of vagina can be damaging. This dye stains skin and clothing.
Griseofulvin	Fulvicin* Grifulvin Grisactin Gris-PEG	ORAL: *Adults*—500 mg microcrystalline form in single or divided dose. Avoid during pregnancy. *Children*—5 to 10 mg/kg daily.	Rx—Tinea infections with exception of tinea versicolor. Not for *Candida*.	Headache occurs early in treatment. GI disturbances, neuritis, allergies, and hepatotoxicity may occur. Warfarin anticoagulant activity blocked. Barbiturates decrease griseofulvin activity.
Haloprogin	Halotex	TOPICAL: *Adults and children*—1% cream or solution applied twice daily. FDA Pregnancy Category B.	Rx—Tinea and other superficial fungal infections.	Local tissue irritation may occur; avoid eyes.
Ketoconazole	Nizoral	TOPICAL: *Adults and children*—2% cream applied once daily. FDA Pregnancy Category C.	Rx—Tinea and cutaneous *Candida*.	Irritation is rare; avoid eyes.
Miconazole nitrate	Micatin Monistat-Derm Monistat*	TOPICAL: *Adults and children*—2% cream, lotion, or aerosol applied twice daily. INTRAVAGINAL: *Adults*—2% cream, tampon, or suppositories applied once daily.	Rx—Dermatophytoses or *Candida* infections.	Local tissue irritation may occur; avoid eyes.
Naftifine	Naftin	TOPICAL: *Adults and children*—1% cream, applied to skin twice daily. FDA Pregnancy Category B.	Rx—Tinea.	Local irritation may occur. Avoid contact with mucous membranes.
Natamycin	Natacyn	OPHTHALMIC: *Adults and children*—5% ophthalmic suspension, 1 drop every 2 to 6 hours.	Rx—Fungal blepharitis, conjunctivitis, or keratitis.	Eye irritation may occur with this chemical relative of amphotericin.
Nystatin	Mycostatin* Nadostine† Nilstat* Nystex	ORAL: *Adults and children*—0.5 to 1 million units 3 times daily. *Infants*—0.1 to 0.2 million units 4 times daily.	Rx—oropharyngeal *Candida* infections.	Nausea, vomiting, or diarrhea may occur. Drug is not absorbed from intestinal tract.

*Available in Canada and United States.
†Available in Canada only.

Table 36-2   Drugs to Treat Topical Fungal Infections—cont'd

Generic name	Trade name	Administration/dosage	Clinical use	Cautions
Nystatin—cont'd		TOPICAL: *Adults and children*—ointments, creams, and lotions (0.1 million units/g) applied twice daily.	Rx—*Candida* infections of skin.	Irritation of skin may occur.
		INTRAVAGINAL: *Adults*—tablets, 0.1 to 0.2 million units daily.	Rx—*Candida* infections of vagina.	Irritation is rare. Relief of symptoms is rapid, but dosage should be continued for 2 weeks or longer if necessary.
Sodium thiosulfate	—	TOPICAL: *Adults and children*—25% lotion or solution applied twice daily for weeks.	OTC—Tinea versicolor.	Irritation is possible; avoid eyes.
Terconazole	Terazol	VAGINAL: *Adults*—5 gm 0.4% cream or 80 mg suppository applied once daily. FDA Pregnancy Category C.	Rx—*Candida* vulvovaginal.	Vaginal burning may occur.
Tolnaftate	Aftate Tinactin*	TOPICAL: *Adults and children*—1% cream, gel, solution, powder, or aerosol applied twice daily.	OTC—Tinea infections only; not effective against *Candida*.	Rarely causes irritation or sensitization. Avoid eyes; 2 to 3 weeks of therapy is usually sufficient.
Undecylenic acid	Desenex Ting Undecylenic compound Unde-Jen	TOPICAL: *Adults and children*—ointment (5%, with 20% zinc undecylenate), powder (2%, with 20% zinc undecylenate), 10% solution, or 2% soap applied twice daily.	OTC—Athlete's foot and ringworm in areas other than around nails or hairy areas.	Avoid eyes and mucous membranes. Diabetics and others with impaired circulation should use only with physician's advice.

*Available in Canada and United States.
†Available in Canada only.

the infective fungi. For this reason, tinea infections around nails and heavily keratinized skin are hard to eradicate.

Griseofulvin is effective against several types of dermatophytic infections. It is administered orally rather than topically. For this reason, griseofulvin is especially useful for treating fungal infections of the scalp. The usefulness of this drug as an oral agent depends on its ability to localize in the skin after oral absorption. Those skin cells containing high concentrations of griseofulvin are resistant to infection by dermatophytes. Ultimately, all infected cells will be lost through the natural sloughing off of skin cells, and the disease will be cured. This process takes a considerable period of time and, accordingly, griseofulvin therapy may need to be continued for several weeks or months, depending on the site and the severity of the infection.

Nystatin is sometimes administered orally to treat intestinal fungal infections. This treatment may be considered topical, since nystatin is not absorbed orally and is retained in the intestinal tract. Nystatin is also used to treat vaginal infections such as those caused by *Candida*. This treatment is also local, since the drug is administered intravaginally and is not significantly absorbed from that site. Nystatin is too toxic to be used for systemic infections.

Numerous over-the-counter preparations are available for treating fungal infections of the skin. Some of these preparations contain useful antifungal agents, whereas others are practically useless. The most effective preparations appear in Table 36-2.

Antifungal agents are also available in combination with various antibacterial drugs. The rationale for these combinations is that many infections diagnosed as fungal are mixed bacterial and fungal infections. Full resolution of symptoms may therefore require treatment with an antibacterial and an antifungal agent. However, this therapy is best accomplished by using two separate preparations so that the most effective drugs for the specific infection may be chosen. Moreover, dosage adjustment is easier with separate preparations.

NURSING IMPLICATIONS SUMMARY

Amphotericin B

Drug administration

◆ Side effects with topical preparations are uncommon. The cream form may stain skin. Fabric discoloration from lotion or cream can be removed with soap and water. Discoloration from ointment can be removed with cleaning fluid. The remaining comments about amphotericin B focus primarily on parenteral administration.

◆ Assess for side effects such as nausea, vomiting, chills, phlebitis, headache, anemia, and electrolyte imbalances.

◆ Monitor temperature, vital signs, intake and output, and weight.

◆ Monitor complete blood count (CBC) and differential, platelet count, and serum creatinine, BUN, and serum electrolyte levels.

◆ Use an infusion monitoring device to assist in regulating the rate. Too-rapid infusion may be associated with cardiac toxicity.

◆ To prevent side effects, corticosteroids may be administered before or during therapy or may be added to the infusion.

◆ Monitor blood glucose levels.

◆ Antiemetics may be given 30 min before starting the infusion to help prevent nausea and vomiting.

◆ Acetaminophen may be administered before or during infusion to treat fever or headache. Codeine or other analgesics may also be used to treat headache.

◆ Other drugs may be administered to prevent or treat side effects. Heparin may be added to infusions to help prevent thrombophlebitis; IV meperidine may be used to treat rigors (shaking chill); and diphenhydramine may be administered to prevent chills.

◆ There is disagreement about the need to cover the tubing and fluid reservoir containing amphotericin B. Follow agency custom; most agencies still cover the bag with a plastic or paper bag.

◆ Keep side rails up and call bell within easy reach. Do not leave patient unattended for long periods.

◆ Use of IV filters is controversial. If an IV filter is used, it must be at least 1.0 micron in diameter.

◆ Prepare IV doses as directed in the package insert. Dissolve doses in sterile water with no bacteriostatic agent. Further dilute to desired volume in 5% dextrose in water; no other diluent may be used. Do not administer other IV medications via the amphotericin B line without flushing well before and after the dose with 5% dextrose in water. If other IV medications are to be administered during amphotericin B infusion, start and maintain a separate IV access line.

◆ The diluted drug is a suspension. Gently agitate the bag or bottle regularly during the infusion to promote uniform dilution.

Patient and family education

◆ See package insert for instructions for preparing intrathecal doses.

◆ Review anticipated benefits and possible side effects of drug therapy. Patients may need not only teaching, but also continued emotional support, since IV therapy is continued for weeks to months. Some patients are suitable candidates for home therapy. Assess the patient, and consult the physician.

◆ Instruct the patient to report any new sign or symptom.

◆ Refer home therapy patients to a community-based nursing care agency.

◆ Monitor serum electrolyte level and hematocrit and hemoglobin counts.

◆ Provide instruction on dietary sources of sodium, potassium, and iron as indicated.

◆ Warn patients to avoid driving or operating hazardous equipment if visual changes occur; notify the physician.

◆ Remind patients to inform all health-care providers of all drugs being used.

Flucytosine

Drug administration

◆ Inspect patient for bruising, bleeding, or other signs and symptoms of blood dyscrasias. Assess for GI side effects. Monitor weight.

◆ Monitor BUN and serum creatinine levels, CBC and differential, platelet count, and liver function tests.

◆ Check stools for blood and guaiac regularly.

Patient and family education

◆ Review anticipated benefits and possible side effects of drug therapy. Tell the patient to report any new sign or symptom.

◆ Provide emotional support as needed; weeks to months of therapy may be needed for adequate treatment.

NURSING IMPLICATIONS SUMMARY—cont'd

◆ Instruct patients to take oral doses with meals or a snack to lessen gastric irritation. Take doses over 15 min to lessen gastric irritation.

◆ Warn patients to avoid driving or operating hazardous equipment if vertigo or sleepiness occurs; notify the physician.

Ketoconazole

Drug administration

◆ Monitor for side effects such as central nervous system (CNS) effects and GI distress.

◆ Monitor liver function tests.

◆ A potentially fatal drug interaction between ketoconazole and terfenadine has been reported. Inform all health care providers of all drugs being used.

Patient and family education

◆ Review anticipated benefits and possible side effects of drug therapy. Tell patients to report any new sign or symptom.

◆ Warn patients to avoid driving or operating hazardous equipment if dizziness or lethargy develops; notify the physician.

◆ Do not take H-2 receptor blocking drugs (e.g., cimetidine and ranitidine) or antacids within 2 hr of ketoconazole doses.

◆ Avoid alcoholic beverages while taking ketoconazole.

◆ If photophobia develops (sensitivity of the eyes to light), wear sunglasses, and avoid bright lights and sunlight.

◆ Absorption of this drug requires an acid pH in the stomach. For patients with achlorhydria, dissolve each 200 mg of ketoconazole in 4 ml of 0.2 N HCl solution. Administer the solution through a straw to avoid contact with the teeth. Follow the dose with a full glass of water. Consult the pharmacist and physician as needed.

Fluconazole

Drug administration

◆ Monitor BUN level, serum creatinine level, and liver function tests.

◆ Monitor for side effects including exfoliative skin disorders, hepatotoxicity, thrombocytopenia, GI distress, and headache.

Patient and family education

◆ Review anticipated benefits and possible side effects of drug therapy. Tell patients to report any new sign or symptom.

◆ Review Patient Problem: Bleeding Tendencies on p. 570.

Miconazole

Drug administration

◆ Perform neurologic assessment regularly. Monitor vital signs and weight. Inspect injection site for phlebitis and pruritus.

◆ Monitor CBC and serum electrolyte level.

INTRAVENOUS MICONAZOLE

◆ Dilute dose in 200 ml of normal saline or 5% dextrose in water. Administer dose over 30 to 60 min. Monitor vital signs with IV doses, and do not administer too rapidly.

Patient and family education

◆ Review anticipated benefits and possible side effects of drug therapy. Instruct patients to report any new sign or symptom. Provide emotional support as needed, since therapy may be needed for weeks to months.

Itraconazole

Drug administration and patient and family education

◆ Consult drug insert for current information.

◆ Monitor liver function tests.

◆ Instruct the patient to report any new sign or symptom.

Topical Antifungal Agents

Patient and family education

◆ For best effect, these agents must be used regularly, as prescribed.

◆ With ointments and creams, apply dose as directed, and gently rub into the area. Do not cover with a dressing unless instructed to do so.

◆ With aerosol powders or solutions, shake well before using. Hold spray opening 6 to 10 inches away from area to be treated, and spray well. Do not inhale powder or solution, and avoid the eyes.

◆ With powder forms, sprinkle liberally on the affected area such as the toes and feet.

◆ When treating toes and feet, make certain drug reaches area between toes and on bottom of feet. Sprinkle or spray onto socks or in shoes, if directed to do so.

◆ See Patient Problem: Vaginal Infections on p. 518.

◆ Remind women that no medications, even topical ones, should be used during pregnancy or lactation without prior consultation with the physician.

Continued.

NURSING IMPLICATIONS SUMMARY—cont'd

Griseofulvin

Drug administration and patient and family education

◆ Assess for side effects.
◆ Monitor CBC and differential, liver function tests, serum creatinine level, and urinalysis.
◆ Take oral doses with meals or a snack to lessen gastric irritation.
◆ Review Patient Problem: Photosensitivity on p. 629.
◆ Avoid drinking alcoholic beverages while taking griseofulvin.
◆ Warn patients to avoid driving or operating hazardous equipment if dizziness or sleepiness occurs; notify the physician.
◆ Oral contraceptives may be ineffective if taken concurrently with griseofulvin. Other forms of birth control should be used. Consult the physician.

Nystatin

Drug administration and patient and family education

◆ Side effects are uncommon. Tell patients to report any new sign or symptom.
◆ With nystatin suspension, the drug may be dispensed with a dropper; use this to measure the dose. Place half the dose in one side of the mouth, and the other half in the other side. Hold, swish, and gargle for as long as possible before swallowing.
◆ With nystatin powder, add dose (about 1/8 tsp) to 4 to 5 oz of water, and stir well. Take a mouthful of the suspension, hold, swish, and gargle for as long as possible before swallowing. Repeat with another mouthful until the entire dose has been taken.
◆ With lozenge form, allow the lozenge to dissolve slowly in the mouth, which may take 15 to 30 min. Swallow the saliva as needed. Do not chew or break the lozenge. Do not let children under 5 years have lozenges, since they may choke on them.

CHAPTER REVIEW

◆ KEY TERMS

dermatophytes, p. 515
ergosterol, p. 515
fungi, p. 514
localized fungal infections, p. 518
systemic fungal infections, p. 515

◆ REVIEW QUESTIONS

1. Why are fungi resistant to drugs such as penicillins and tetracyclines?

2. What animal species commonly spreads fungal diseases to humans?

3. What types of infections are commonly caused by *Candida*? What are signs and symptoms of these infections?

4. What are dermatophytes?

5. What is the mechanism of action for the polyene antifungal agent amphotericin B?

6. By what route is amphotericin B administered? What are nursing care activities associated with the administration of amphotericin B?

7. What types of fungal infections are properly treated with amphotericin B?

8. How does the lipid solubility of amphotericin B influence its tissue distribution?

9. What are the characteristic toxic reactions associated with systemic use of amphotericin B?

10. What is the mechanism of action of flucytosine?

11. May flucytosine be used as an oral agent?

12. What is the main route of excretion of flucytosine?

13. What toxic reactions occur with the use of flucytosine?

14. Why are flucytosine and amphotericin B sometimes combined for antifungal therapy?

15. What is the mechanism of action of fluconazole, ketoconazole, and related drugs?

16. By what route are fluconazole and ketoconazole administered?

17. What type of fungal infections respond to fluconazole?
18. What side effects may occur with fluconazole and ketoconazole? How should you assess for these?
19. What is the mechanism of action of griseofulvin?
20. How is griseofulvin administered?
21. Is therapy with griseofulvin long or short term?

SUGGESTED READING

Amantea MA, Drutz DJ, Rosenthal JR: Antifungals: a primary care primer, *Patient Care* 24(18):58, 1990.

Bailey EM, Krakovsky DJ, Rybak MJ: The triazole antifungal agents: a review of itraconazole and fluconazole, *Pharmacotherapy* 10(2):146, 1990.

Lynn MM, Holdcroft C: Treatment for fungal skin infections: an update, *Nurse Pract* 14(8):64, 1989.

Mathewson HS: Systemic antifungal agents, *Respir Care* 35(10):987, 1990.

Terrell CL, Hughes CE: Antifungal agents used for deep-seated mycotic infections, *Mayo Clin Proc* 67(1):69, 1992.

Wack EE, Galgiani JN: The azoles: miconazole, ketoconazole, itraconazole, *Antimicrobial Agents Annual* 3:251, 1989.

CHAPTER 37

Treatment of Viral Diseases

LEARNING OBJECTIVES

After studying this chapter, you should be able to do the following:

♦ Explain why acyclovir is selectively active against virus-infected cells.

♦ Discuss the basis of anti-HIV activity of zidovudine and didanosine.

♦ Develop a nursing care plan for a patient receiving an antiviral agent.

♦ What points should the nurse teach the patient about topical treatment of genital herpes?

CHAPTER OVERVIEW

♦ Viral diseases are among the most common infections in humans, but the prevention and treatment of these diseases has lagged far behind the ability to control bacterial infections. This chapter discusses the properties of viral diseases that make them difficult to prevent or treat and the mechanisms of action of antiviral drugs that have been developed.

Nursing Process Overview
ANTIVIRAL AGENTS

Assessment

Use of antiviral agents is limited to patients in whom supportive therapy has not been helpful or who have viruses known to be particularly virulent or frequently fatal. Perform a thorough total assessment. Emphasize the subjective and objective complaints related to the virus. Assess laboratory work, cultures, and other studies that would help monitor the progress of the disease.

Nursing Diagnoses

Possible complication: blood dyscrasias secondary to drug therapy

Possible complication: injury related to ataxia as a drug side effect

Management

Monitor appropriate laboratory work, vital signs, and other objective data that help chart the progress of the disease. Monitor for side effects known to occur with the drug used. If the patient will receive antiviral drug therapy after discharge, instruct the patient and family about possible side effects. If the virus is known to be virulent, isolate the patient during the hospitalization phase. For information about specific viruses, consult the infection control department, the local health department, or the Centers for Disease Control in Atlanta. Many serious viral illnesses should be reported to the local health department, since this information is used for epidemiologic charting of viral spread; examples include polio and rabies. Finally, immunize family members and health-care team members if appropriate.

Evaluation

Before discharge, ensure that patients can explain how to take the drug correctly, can identify side effects that may occur, and can describe situations that require consultation with the physician.

NATURE OF VIRAL DISEASE

Viruses cause a wide variety of clinical disease, including some conditions that have only recently been recognized as viral in origin. Viral diseases may be acute, chronic, or slow. Acute illnesses include the common cold, influenza, and various other respiratory tract infections. These illnesses frequently resolve quickly and leave no latent infections or sequelae. Chronic infections are those in which the disease runs a protracted course with long periods of remission interspersed with reappearance of the disease. An example is herpes infection of the conjunctiva, skin, or genitalia in which active disease alternates with latent periods during which the virus remains dormant in nervous tissue. Slow virus infections progress over a number of months or years, causing cumulative damage to body tissues and ending in death of the host. Diseases that involve infection with slow-acting viruses include multiple sclerosis amyotrophic lateral sclerosis, Alzheimer-Pick disease, and various other degenerative diseases of the central nervous system (CNS). Infection with the retrovirus **human immunodeficiency virus (HIV)** is followed by a symptom-free period that may last several years. During this latent period, the viral DNA exists within the host cell genome, in a form called the *provirus*. As the disease enters the active phase, virus particles are produced from the previously infected cells. The progressive destruction of immune function caused by HIV ultimately produces **acquired immune deficiency syndrome (AIDS).**

Viruses may attack specific cell types within the host. For example, several viruses affect only the tissues of the respiratory tract. For these diseases, symptoms develop as the infection spreads from the original site to immediately adjacent cells. The severity of symptoms depends in part on how many host cells are affected. The rabies virus specifically attacks nervous tissue, traveling along nerves and eventually invading the brain, causing the characteristic symptoms of rabies. HIV has an affinity for T-lymphocytes, attacking those cells specifically because the virus attaches to the characteristic cell surface receptor CD4. This infection has such devastating effects because the cells attacked by HIV are critical for immune function.

Some viruses have the potential for more generalized invasion of tissues throughout the body by a mechanism called *viremic spread*. Viremic spread is detailed in Table 37-1. Clinical symptoms do not appear in most diseases spread in this manner until very late in the disease, when the secondary viremia occurs. At this stage, most viral infections are self-limiting and resolve even without medical attention. However, certain viruses can attack the brain after the secondary viremia. An example is the poliovirus, which causes relatively mild disease during the respiratory phase and secondary viremic stage but becomes life-threatening when it invades the CNS. Even with polioviruses, invasion of the CNS is rare, and most infections end with the secondary viremia.

With infections caused by bacteria, symptoms oc-

Table 37-1   Viremic Spread in Mammalian Body

Site	Symptoms
PRIMARY SITE OF INFECTION	
For example, lung in pox, measles, and mumps; and GI tract in polio	First wave of replication produces no symptoms.
BLOODSTREAM	
Viruses free or bound to blood cells	Primary viremia produces no symptoms.
SECONDARY SITES OF INFECTION	
For example, liver, spleen, bone marrow, or lymphoid tissue	Second wave of replication may produce mild symptoms for some viral diseases.
BLOODSTREAM	
Viruses free or bound to blood cells	Secondary viremia may produce fever, rashes, and other symptoms whose severity depends on the number of viruses released.
CENTRAL NERVOUS SYSTEM	Although rarely involved, infections at this site are serious.

cur during the period of most active bacterial reproduction; therefore therapy can begin relatively early in the disease and may include bactericidal agents. With viral diseases, this is not the case. Symptoms occur after most of the virus particles have reproduced, and therapy would be instituted late in the disease. Unfortunately, the antiviral drugs currently available inhibit reproduction but do not kill viruses. For these reasons, therapy with antiviral drugs is generally expected to limit further progression of the disease but not to eradicate latent viruses or proviruses.

VACCINES TO PREVENT VIRAL DISEASES

The external surface of viruses contains antigenic substances that promote antibody production. These humoral factors limit the spread of many types of viral disease and allow the body to eliminate the virus. Infected cells are also changed sufficiently in many viral diseases so that these cells are also eliminated.

Many viral diseases are best controlled by inducing antibodies in healthy individuals before exposure to the viral disease. This prophylaxis is successful for many diseases (see Table 28-2).

Vaccines cannot be produced efficiently for all viral diseases, however. One example is rhinoviruses, which cause respiratory disease. Among these viruses, there are approximately 100 strains, which each induce a specific antibody in humans; however, no antibody attacks more than one of the serotypes. Therefore successful immunization would require an antibody to be developed against each of the 100 pathogenic strains. Such a program is not feasible.

Influenza viruses illustrate another difficulty in immunizing against viral diseases. With influenza the antigenic properties shift every few years so that those persons who were immunized naturally or artificially against the prevalent strain of the virus are unprotected when the new viral type arises. Therefore influenza immunizations are effective only for a specific viral strain and should not be expected to carry over when new strains appear. Rapid antigenic shift is also a characteristic of HIV.

The most successful immunization programs are for those viral diseases in which few pathogenic strains exist and with which antigenic properties do not change. The vaccine for poliovirus fits these criteria. The oral vaccine is directed against the three major viral strains; these strains have not shifted in antigenic properties.

In addition to the traditional immune responses to viral infection, the body has another mechanism by which it limits the spread of viral diseases. This mechanism is the production of glycoproteins called *interferons* (see Chapter 27). Interferons, released from virus-infected cells, alter the metabolism of uninfected cells to prevent the virus from attacking these new cells. This mechanism prevents the spread of the viral disease to new cells and allows the immune system to eliminate the viruses and infected cells.

Interferons are **host specific** and not virus specific. This property means that interferons induce resistance to several types of viruses at once. Host specificity of interferons determines that only human interferon prevents viral disease in humans. In the past, this host specificity limited development of interferons for clinical use because no ready source of the material was available. Today, human proteins of many kinds are made by recombinant DNA technology, which allows human interferons to be produced in large quantities by recombinant organisms.

The protection offered by interferons may be transient. Long-term protection does not develop as with antibody production. To overcome this problem, inducers of interferons have been tested. Although compounds have been developed that successfully induce interferons, the protection produced is again transient. Moreover, cells exposed to the inducers become refractory to further induction for a period of time, making it impossible to continuously maintain high interferon levels.

Interferons are not used as routine antiviral agents but have a few specific indications (see Chapter 28).

They are also used as anticancer agents because they limit cell proliferation (see Chapter 39).

SELECTIVE TOXICITY IN THE TREATMENT OF VIRAL DISEASES

Because viral reproduction is carried out mostly by host cell enzymes and ribosomes, targets for selective toxicity are difficult to identify. Virus reproduction can be divided into four steps (Table 37-2). Study of the details of these processes has revealed more potential for selective toxicity than was originally thought. It is now known that a few viral enzymes help form viral nucleic acid. Viral enzymes or processes that occur only in virus-infected cells are likely points for attack with selectively toxic agents. Many agents have been tested as antiviral drugs, but only a few meet the test of effective action against virus-infected cells with low toxicity to uninfected host cells.

Development of anti-HIV drugs is proceeding rapidly. A variety of approaches are being explored, including blocking specific absorption of the virus to its target cells, inhibiting virus-specific proteases re-

Table 37-2   Sequence of Events in Virus Reproduction in Mammalian Cells

Step in reproduction	Biochemical events	Drugs that block process
1. Adsorption	Initial ionic, dissociable association becomes irreversible adsorption of virus to cell surface.	No clinically useful drugs block this process
2. Penetration and uncoating	Virus particles enter the cell and the outer coats dissolve, releasing the viral genetic material (DNA or RNA).	Amantadine
3. Replication and transcription	All viruses synthesize new messenger RNA and, using host ribosomes, synthesize viral proteins.	Acyclovir Didanosine Ganciclovir Foscarnet Idoxuridine (IUdR) Trifluridine Vidarabine (ara-A) Zidovudine
4. Assembly and release	Viral nucleic acids and proteins are assembled to form mature viruses, which are then released by budding off from infected cell or by lysis of infected cell.	No clinically useful drugs block this process

quired for maturation of the virus, and developing other inhibitors of reverse transcriptase similar to zidovudine and didanosine. Agents that can improve immune function in AIDS patients are also being tested. Imuthiol (sodium diethyldithiocarbamate), isoprinosine (inosine pranobex), and ampligen (Poly I: Poly C12U) influence the immune system and may have direct inhibitory effects on the virus.

The status of these investigational agents changes very quickly. Current information can be obtained by consultation with the AIDS section at the National Institutes of Health or by consulting current publications devoted to AIDS research. Drugs approved as of March, 1992, are included in the next section.

SPECIFIC ANTIVIRAL DRUGS

Table 37-3 summarizes specific antiviral drugs.

Acyclovir

Mechanism of action

Acyclovir is one of the most highly selective of the antiviral agents in use in the United States. The drug is activated by viral thymidine kinase, an enzyme found only in virus-infected cells. The activated form of the drug preferentially and irreversibly inhibits the viral DNA polymerase present in infected cells, effectively halting virus production. Much higher concentrations of acyclovir are required to halt normal human cell metabolism. Therefore effective doses for antiviral activity are relatively nontoxic to normal host cells.

Acyclovir is used to treat initial lesions or recurrences of genital herpes, mucocutaneous herpes simplex infections in immunocompromised patients, herpes simplex encephalitis, and herpes zoster infections.

Absorption, distribution, and excretion

Acyclovir is used intravenously to treat mucocutaneous herpes simplex in immunocompromised patients and to treat severe genital herpes or herpes simplex encephalitis. Oral administration of acyclovir leads to incomplete absorption, but this route is effective when used for mild-to-moderate genital herpes. Once absorbed, acyclovir is widely distributed to tissues. The topical ointment may be useful in mild herpes infections, but parenteral routes are more effective and usually preferred.

Excretion is by renal mechanisms. Little metabolism of acyclovir occurs in the liver. The drug is eliminated with a half-life of about 2½ hr in patients with normal renal function.

Side effects

Acyclovir is relatively nontoxic for most patients. Nephrotoxicity, including crystallization of drug in the renal tubule, can be minimized by giving the drug as a slow infusion rather than as a rapid bolus. Increasing water intake also helps. Phlebitis at the injection site may also occur with acyclovir administered intravenously.

Rarely, patients receiving parenteral acyclovir may suffer coma, confusion, seizures, or tremors. Light-headedness is common. Oral administration can cause GI disturbances.

Amantadine

Mechanism of action

Amantadine appears to block uncoating of influenza type A viruses (see Table 37-2). This drug has a narrow antiviral spectrum, being effective only against influenza type A. Amantadine is most effective at preventing the disease. There is limited clinical evidence that if the drug is administered by a nebulizer so that it is breathed into the lungs, it may help reduce the severity of the symptoms and the duration of influenza type A infections. At present, the drug is limited to prophylaxis in elderly patients or others in whom influenza is likely to lead to life-threatening complications.

Absorption, distribution, and excretion

Amantadine is well absorbed orally and distributes well to tissues. The concentrations in lung tissue may exceed serum concentrations. The concentrations of amantadine that reaches the epithelial surfaces of lung tissues is the determining factor in protecting against influenza A infections. Nearly all elimination of the drug is by renal mechanisms. The half-life for elimination is about 15 hr in patients with normal renal function, 24 to 29 hr in the elderly, and 7 to 10 days in renally impaired patients.

Toxicity

Toxicity with amantadine prophylaxis for viral diseases is ordinarily low, unless kidney failure is present, and the drug accumulates in the bloodstream. Amantadine can cause amphetamine-like stimulation of the CNS, lethargy, ataxia, slurred speech, and other symptoms. Because of these CNS effects, the drug should be used cautiously, if at all, in elderly patients with cerebral arteriosclerosis or in patients with a history of epilepsy (see box).

Amantadine has been used to treat Parkinson's disease (see Chapter 48). Since doses used for this purpose are about twice those for influenza prophylaxis, toxic reactions are more common.

Rimantadine, a chemical relative of amantadine, may be more concentrated in the lung than amantadine. Rimantadine may also have less CNS toxicity. This new drug has been extensively used in Russia and is under investigation in the United States.

Table 37-3   Drugs to Treat Viral Diseases

Generic name	Trade name	Administration/dosage	Clinical use	Principal toxic reactions
Acyclovir	Zovirax*	ORAL: *Adults*—200 mg 5 times daily. FDA Pregnancy Category C. INTRAVENOUS: *Adults*—5 mg/kg infused at a constant rate over 1 hr, repeated every 8 hr. *Children under 12 years*—250 mg/M^2 infused at a constant rate over 1 hr, repeated every 8 hr. TOPICAL: 5% ointment applied directly to initial lesions of genital herpes.	Mucosal and cutaneous herpes simplex infections in immunocompromised patients; severe initial episodes of genital herpes; and herpes zoster infections.	Renal toxicity; phlebitis; GI distress; and light-headedness.
Amantadine	Symadine Symmetrel*	ORAL: *Adults*—100 mg twice daily. *Geriatrics*—100 mg once daily. FDA Pregnancy Category C. *Children*—4.4 to 8.8 mg/kg, up to 150 mg daily.	Prophylaxis of influenza type A infections in high-risk patients.	CNS stimulation, ataxia, slurred speech, lethargy, loss of appetite, and nausea.
Didanosine	Videx	ORAL: *Adults*—200 mg tablet twice daily, body weight 50 to 74 kg; 125 mg twice daily, body weight 35 to 49 kg. *Children over 6 months*—200 mg/M^2 daily.	Treatment of patients with advanced HIV infection or those intolerant or unresponsive to zidovudine.	Acute pancreatitis and peripheral neuropathy.
Foscarnet	Foscavir	INTRAVENOUS: *Adults*—60 mg/kg 3 times daily for induction; 90 to 120 mg/kg daily for maintenance therapy.	Treatment of CMV retinitis in patients with AIDS.	Renal toxicity and electrolyte disturbances.
Gangciclovir	Cytovene*	INTRAVENOUS: *Adults*—5 mg/kg infused over at least 1 hr, every 12 hr for 14 to 21 days.	Treatment of CMV retinitis in immunosuppressed patients, including AIDS patients.	Granulocytopenia, thrombocytopenia, anemia, and phlebitis.
Idoxuridine	Herplex* Stoxil*	OPHTHALMIC: *Adults and children*—0.1% solution, 0.5% ointment used 5 times daily.	Topical use in the eye for herpes keratitis.	Local irritation and pitting defects in the cornea. Systemic toxicity is possible but rare by this route.
Ribavirin	Virazid Virazole*	INHALATION: *Children*—20 mg/ml in a Viratek small particle aerosol generator model SPAG-2 12 to 18 hr/day. FDA Pregnancy Category X.	Severe pneumonia caused by respiratory syncytial virus (RSV).	Few side effects when used by aerosol.
Trifluridine	Viroptic*	OPHTHALMIC: *Adults and children*—1% solution applied up to 9 times daily.	Topical use in the eye for herpes keratitis.	Local irritation.
Vidarabine	Vira-A*	OPHTHALMIC: *Adults and children*—3% ointment used 5 times daily. FDA Pregnancy Category C.	Topical use in the eye for herpes keratitis.	Local irritation, superficial punctate keratitis, and allergy.
Zidovudine	Retrovir*	ORAL: *Adults*—100 mg every 4 hr around the clock. FDA Pregnancy Category C.	HIV infection (AIDS and ARC).	Bone marrow depression may cause fever, chills, bleeding, tiredness, or weakness.

CMV, cytomegalovirus
*Available in Canada and United States.

Didanosine

Mechanism of action

Didanosine is a purine analogue that is activated by phosphorylation within cells and in this active form blocks synthesis of HIV DNA by inhibiting the virus-specific enzyme called *reverse transcriptase*. This mechanism of action is similar to that of the first drug approved for HIV infections, zidovudine.

Didanosine is currently indicated for the treatment of adults or children over 6 months of age who have advanced HIV disease and who are intolerant to zidovudine or have failed therapy with zidovudine.

Absorption, distribution, and excretion

Didanosine has a poor bioavailability in most patients because it is destroyed by stomach acid. Antacids or H-2 histamine receptor blockers may improve absorption by lowering acidity and preserving integrity of the drug. The average plasma half-life of didanosine is between ½ and 1⅓ hr, but the half-life within cells is longer than 12 hr. Therefore the drug is given every 12 hr. Excretion yields about 20% of a dose present in urine as active drug.

Toxicity

Peripheral neuropathy may occur in many patients receiving didanosine. Signs include tingling or aching in the legs or feet. Reflexes may also be diminished. Acute pancreatitis has also been noted. The risk for this latter reaction is increased in patients who also have received ganciclovir for cytomegalovirus (CMV) infections or rifampin and ethambutol for mycobacterial infections.

Foscarnet

Mechanism of action

Foscarnet inhibits viral DNA polymerases and reverse transcriptases. Because foscarnet is a chemical relative of inorganic phosphate, it does not require activation within cells. The drug has shown activity against HIV, herpesviruses, and hepatitis B but is presently indicated only for control of CMV retinitis in HIV-infected patients.

Absorption, distribution, and excretion

Foscarnet is poorly absorbed orally and must be given by IV injection or infusion. The drug distributes to tissues, including brain tissues, although levels are variable. As an analogue of inorganic phosphate, foscarnet seems to be incorporated into bone. Most of the remainder of the drug is excreted unchanged in urine.

Toxicity

Renal toxicity is the major concern with foscarnet. Signs of serious renal toxicity may occur in up to 25% of patients receiving the drug. Some protection may be afforded by assuring adequate hydration before administering foscarnet. Other neprotoxic drugs should be avoided during theapy with foscarnet.

Other side effects of foscarnet use include changes in calcium and phosphate concentrations in blood, nausea, seizures, and anemia.

Ganciclovir

Mechanism of action

Ganciclovir acts similarly to acyclovir, both drugs being readily activated within virus-infected cells to a form that inhibits virus reproduction. Unlike acyclovir, ganciclovir is also activated to a limited degree by normal cells.

Ganciclovir is indicated only for treatment of CMV retinitis in immunocompromised patients.

Absorption, distribution, and excretion

Ganciclovir is poorly absorbed orally, with a bioavailability of less than 5%. Administration is therefore by IV infusion. The drug distributes widely into tissues, including the eye. Ganciclovir is not biotransformed and is excreted unchanged in urine.

Toxicity

Ganciclovir causes granulocytopenia, marked by sore throat and fever, in about 40% of patients receiving the drug. Ganciclovir also causes thrombocytopenia, marked by bruising and unusual bleeding, in 20% of patients. These reactions are usually reversible. Anemia, allergies, and signs of CNS toxicity have also been reported less frequently.

Idoxuridine

Idoxuridine, also referred to as *5-iodo-2'-deoxyuridine* (IUdR) is an analogue of the thymidine normally found in DNA. Idoxuridine is incorporated into DNA in place of thymidine, thereby preventing normal DNA replication and halting virus formation.

Unfortunately, idoxuridine does not have a good therapeutic index and harms rapidly growing normal host and virus-infected cells. For this reason, its use is restricted to topical treatment of herpes simplex infections of the cornea, conjunctiva, and eyelids. These infections tend to recur, and idoxuridine does not prevent reappearance of the infection or scarring and resultant loss of sight in serious cases.

When used topically in the eye, little idoxuridine enters the systemic circulation. The drug can produce local reactions in the eye, the most serious being corneal defects. It may also interfere with corneal epithelial regeneration and healing. Idoxuridine is potentially mutagenic and carcinogenic.

Ribavirin

Ribavirin is a synthetic purine nucleoside that interferes with multiple steps leading to synthesis of viral nucleic acids. Because ribavirin blocks phosphorylation of nucleosides, it interferes with activation of zidovudine and therefore should not be given to patients receiving zidovudine. In the United States, ribavirin is indicated only for therapy of severe respiratory syncytial virus (RSV) in children, but in other parts of the world the drug has been used to treat various vial-induced hemorrhagic fevers.

Ribavirin is administered as an aerosol to treat respiratory viruses. In this way, drug levels in the lung are maximized, but systemic absorption is low, which minimizes side effects. Skin rashes can occur. Healthcare workers exposed during administration of the drug can suffer headaches and irritation of the eyes.

Trifluridine

Trifluridine, like idoxuridine, is activated by viral and host cell thymidine kinase to a form of drug that inhibits DNA polymerase. Trifluridine is not selective in its action, but it inhibits DNA polymerase in normal and virus-infected cells. Therefore trifluridine is not tolerated systemically.

Trifluridine is effective for topical therapy of herpes infections of the eye. This agent may be less damaging to the cornea than idoxuridine or vidarabine; nevertheless, burning of the conjunctiva and cornea can occur when the drug is placed in the eye. Swelling of the eyelids (palpebral edema) has also been noted.

Like idoxuridine and vidarabine, trifluridine is potentially mutagenic and carcinogenic. It is not clear how important this potential may be when these agents are used topically, since these drugs are not well absorbed from the eye into systemic circulation.

Vidarabine

Vidarabine inhibits viral DNA synthesis in a variety of DNA viruses. Vidarabine is activated by host cell enzymes to ara-ATP, a potent and selective inhibitor of viral DNA polymerase. Clinically important selectivity of action is achieved against herpes virus-infected cells.

Vidarabine is used topically in eye infections caused by herpes in much the same way as idoxuridine and trifluridine. Vidarabine is teratogenic and potentially carcinogenic. Ophthalmic use is not usually associated with serious side effects, but local irritation and sensitivity of the eyes to light may occur.

Zidovudine

Mechanism of action

Zidovudine is used in AIDS and in **AIDS-related complex (ARC)**, conditions caused by infection with HIV. HIV is a retrovirus that has had several names, including LAV (lymphadenopathy-associated virus) and HTLV-III (human T-cell lymphotropic virus type III). **Retroviruses** use RNA as their genetic material and must therefore convert RNA into DNA within the host cell for viral replication to take place. This unusual reaction, which does not normally occur in the host cell, is catalyzed by the enzyme, reverse transcriptase. Zidovudine inhibits reverse transcriptase. In addition, some of the drug may be incorporated into viral DNA, in which it causes premature chain termination. Both actions block viral replication. Zidovudine does not cure AIDS or ARC, but, by slowing replication of HIV, it may delay damage to the immune system and lower the incidence of opportunistic infections in these patients.

Absorption, distribution, and excretion

Absorption of zidovudine from the GI tract is rapid and nearly complete, but the drug is quickly metabolized to an inactive glucuronide on first pass through the liver. These factors give zidovudine a half-life of only 1 hr. For this reason, it is taken every 4 hr around the clock to maintain virustatic concentrations.

To be effective, zidovudine must be administered continuously throughout life. The short half-life and toxicity of the drug make this ideal difficult to achieve.

Toxicity

Nearly all patients suffer toxicity from zidovudine. The most common reactions are granulocytopenia and anemia. Routine blood monitoring is extremely important. Withdrawal from zidovudine may be necessary to allow recovery from drug-induced blood dyscrasias. Neurotoxicity has also been reported but may be difficult to distinguish from the neural effects of HIV infection.

Drug interactions may occur with zidovudine and other drugs often used in immunosuppressed patients. Ganciclovir and zidovudine combine to produce severe hematologic toxicity. Ribavirin interferes with the activation of zidovudine within the virus-infected cell and thereby blocks the anti-HIV effect of zidovudine.

NURSING IMPLICATIONS SUMMARY

Acyclovir

Drug administration

- Assess for GI symptoms and CNS side effects. Inspect for skin rashes.
- Monitor intake and output and weight.
- Monitor complete blood count (CBC) and differential and platelet count.

INTRAVENOUS ADMINISTRATION

- Dilute as directed in the drug insert. Administer dose over 1 hr. Use an infusion control device or microdrip tubing to help regulate infusion rate. Inspect IV site frequently, and question patient regarding symptoms of phlebitis or irritation. Because excretion is via kidneys, and drug half-life is about 2½ hr, patients should be well hydrated during IV infusion to prevent precipitation of the drug in the renal tubules.

Patient and family education

- Review anticipated benefits and possible side effects of drug therapy.
- Warn patients to avoid driving or operating hazardous equipment if dizziness, fatigue, or vertigo develop; notify the physician.
- Teach patients taking oral or IV doses to increase fluid intake to 2500 to 3000 ml/day.
- For topical application, use a glove or finger cot to apply ointment to avoid contamination of the finger. Avoid contact with the eyes. Use the drug on a regular basis, as prescribed, for best effect. Consult the physician if there is no improvement within a week.
- Teach the patient with genital herpes how to lessen the chance of spreading the virus by avoiding sexual activity when open lesions or scabs are present. Male partners should wear condoms. Acyclovir will not prevent the spread of herpes.
- Keep areas of infection clean and dry. Wear loose-fitting garments. Do not use other creams or ointments on viral lesions unless prescribed by the physician.
- Encourage women with genital herpes to have regular Pap smears to check for cervical cancer.
- Oral doses may be taken with meals.

Amantadine

- See Nursing Implications Summary in Chapter 48.

Rimantidine

See drug package insert for current information.

Didanosine

Drug administration and patient and family education

- Check drug insert for current information.
- Administer with antacids or within 1 hr of administration of H-2 histamine receptor blockers, if ordered.
- Assess for peripheral neuropathy including numbness or tingling of fingers and extremities. Assess deep tendon reflexes.
- Assess for pancreatitis including epigastric or left upper quadrant abdominal pain, nausea, vomiting, and fever. Monitor white blood cell count, amylase level, serum glucose level, and blood urea nitrogen (BUN) level.

Foscarnet

Drug administration and patient and family education

- Check drug insert for current information.
- Assure adequate hydration before administering drug to lessen the chance of renal toxicity.
- Monitor intake and output, weight, and BUN level.
- Monitor serum electrolyte level and CBC.
- Assess for nausea.

Ganciclovir

Drug administration

- See drug insert for preparation guidelines.
- Administer each dose over 1 hr as an infusion. Use microdrip tubing and an infusion monitoring device.
- Monitor CBC and platelet count, liver function tests, and BUN level.
- Monitor intake and output.

Patient and family education

- See Patient Problem: Bleeding Tendencies on p. 570.
- Instruct patients to use measures for contraception during treatment and for at least 90 days after treatment.
- Encourage patient to have an ophthalmic examination at the start of therapy and to report any changes in vision.

Idoxuridine

Drug administration and patient and family education

- See the general guidelines for use of eye medications in Chapter 12.

Continued.

◆ Warn the patient that photophobia may develop, which would cause the patient to find bright lights uncomfortable to the eyes. Instruct the patient to avoid bright light and to wear sunglasses.

◆ Teach the patient correct technique for administering eye medications (see Chapter 6).

◆ Warn the patient that blurred vision may occur for the first few minutes after drug administration.

◆ Consult the physician if itching, severe redness, clouding of vision, or photophobia develops.

Ribavirin

Drug administration and patient and family education

◆ Review anticipated benefits and possible side effects of drug therapy with the patient and family. Encourage the patient or family to report new signs or symptoms.

◆ Auscultate lung sounds and assess respiratory status. Monitor temperature and vital signs.

◆ Check drug package insert for current information. Do not administer simultaneously with other aerosolized medications. Use only the aerosol generator specified by the manufacturer.

◆ Health-care workers should avoid contact with the drug if possible, since it may cause eye irritation or headaches.

Trifluridine

Drug administration and patient and family education

◆ See the general guidelines for use of eye medications in Chapter 12.

◆ Teach the patient correct technique for administering eye medications (see Chapter 6).

◆ Remind the patient to continue the medicine for the full course of therapy but not to use the drug longer or more often than ordered.

Vidarabine

Drug administration

◆ Assess for CNS and GI side effects.

◆ Monitor intake and output and weight.

◆ Monitor CBC and differential and platelet count.

INTRAVENOUS ADMINISTRATION

Review drug package insert for dilution guidelines. Administer diluted dose over 12 to 24 hr, at a constant rate. Use an infusion monitoring device or microdrip tubing to ensure correct rate. Use an in-line filter of 0.45 micron. Inspect infusion site, and assess patient for signs of phlebitis.

Patient and family education

◆ Review anticipated benefits and possible side effects of drug therapy with patients and family. Encourage the patient to report new signs or symptoms.

◆ Make certain the patient can apply eyedrops correctly if that route is ordered. See Chapter 6 for a discussion of administration of eyedrops.

◆ Warn the patient that photophobia may develop, which would cause the patient to find bright lights uncomfortable to the eyes. Instruct the patient to avoid bright light and to wear sunglasses.

◆ Warn the patient that blurred vision may occur for the first few minutes after administration of ophthalmic ointment.

◆ Consult the physician if itching, severe redness, clouding of vision, or photophobia develops.

Zidovudine

Drug administration

◆ Assess for headaches, anxiety, and confusion. Inspect for rashes. Monitor temperature and pulse.

◆ Monitor CBC and differential and platelet count.

Patient and family education

◆ Review anticipated benefits and possible side effects of drug therapy with the patient and family. Encourage the patient to report new signs or symptoms.

◆ See Patient Problem: Bleeding Tendencies on p. 570.

◆ Review drug package insert for current information.

CHAPTER REVIEW

◆ KEY TERMS

acquired immune deficiency syndrome (AIDS), p. 527
AIDS-related complex (ARC), p. 532
host specific, p. 528
human immunodeficiency virus (HIV), p. 527
retroviruses, p. 532
viruses, p. 526

◆ REVIEW QUESTIONS

1. Are antiviral drugs virucidal or virustatic?
2. Why does HIV specifically attack T-lymphocytes?
3. Why is immunization not possible against all viral diseases?
4. What are interferons?
5. What properties of interferons make them less than ideal as antiviral agents?
6. What is the mechanism of action of acyclovir?
7. How is acyclovir used to treat viral diseases?
8. What side effects are associated with acyclovir? How should you assess for these?
9. What is the mechanism of action of amantadine?
10. How is amantadine used to treat viral diseases?
11. How are ganciclovir and foscarnet used as antivirals?
12. How are idoxuridine, trifluridine, and vidarabine used as antivirals?
13. What side effects are associated with idoxuridine, trifluridine, and vidarabine? How should you assess for these?
14. What is the mechanism of action of ribavirin?
15. How is ribavirin used to treat viral disease?
16. What is the mechanism of action of zidovudine?
17. How is zidovudine used to treat viral disease?
18. What side effects are associated with zidovudine? How should you assess for these?
19. Why is zidovudine given every 4 hr around the clock?
20. How does didanosine differ from zidovudine?

SUGGESTED READING

Armstrong-Esther C, Hewitt WE: AIDS: the knowledge and attitudes of nurses, *Can Nurse* 85(6):29, 1989.

Beaufoy A, Goldstone I, Riddell R: AIDS: what nurses need to know, *Can Nurse* 84(7):16, 1988.

Cohn JA: Virology, immunology, and natural history of HIV infection, *J Nurse Midwife* 34(5):242, 1989.

Davis K: Genital herpes: an overview, *JOGNN* 19(5):401, 1990.

de Roin S, Winters S: Amantadine hydrochloride: current and new uses, *J Neurosci Nurs* 22(5):322, 1990.

Flaherty E: Amantadine attack on influenza A, *Geriatr Nurs* 11(5):253, 1990.

Keating MR: Antiviral agents, *Mayo Clin Proc* 67(2):160, 1992.

Matthews SJ, Cersosimo RJ, Spivack ML: Zidovudine and other reverse transcriptase inhibitors in the management of human immunodeficiency virus-related disease, *Pharmacotherapy* 11(6):419, 1991.

Nettina SM: When patients with genital herpes turn to you for answers, *Nurs 89* 19(8):61, 1989.

Postic B: Antiviral therapy: reviewing the use of amantadine, acyclovir, ganciclovir, and zidovudine, *Consultant* 30(6):43, 1990.

CHAPTER 38

Drugs to Treat Protozoal and Helminthic Infestations

LEARNING OBJECTIVES

After studying this chapter, you should be able to do the following:

- Discuss how the site of infestation may affect the success of drug therapy.
- Describe the type of patients in whom specific protozoal or helminthic diseases might be more likely.
- Explain hygienic measures that should accompany drug therapy in controlling pinworm infestations.
- Develop a nursing care plan for the patient receiving one of the drugs in this chapter.

CHAPTER OVERVIEW

- On a worldwide scale, chronic diseases caused by protozoal (single-cell organism) or helminthic (worm) infestations are the most common afflictions of humanity. Although these diseases flourish primarily in tropical regions, several are encountered in North America. In this chapter the discussion centers on the treatment of diseases that occur in the continental United States and Canada.

- Parasitic diseases are caused by higher organisms against which selective toxicity is sometimes difficult to achieve. The selection of an effective drug involves matching the tissue distribution of the drug with the sites of infestation of the parasite and choosing an agent that possesses intrinsic activity against the parasite. The first sections of this chapter relate individual drugs to specific diseases and explain the rationale for their use. The last section covers the pharmacologic properties of the drugs.

Nursing Process Overview

PROTOZOAL OR HELMINTHIC THERAPY

Assessment

Perform a baseline assessment of the patient. Include in the patient history questions related to travel within and outside the United States or Canada; recent exposure to new food or water supplies; possible exposure through family members or school or business contacts who have had a similar illness recently; and any previous history of infection with protozoal or helminthic agents. Once drug therapy is ordered, monitor appropriate laboratory work related to potential drug side effects.

Nursing Diagnosis

Possible altered home maintenance management related to drug treatment regimen

Management

Monitor the overall patient condition, with close attention to subjective and objective data related to the infection. It may be appropriate to monitor close family members for the appearance of the infection. Refer patients to the local health department for follow-up and for epidemiologic tracking of health problems.

Evaluation

Many of these drugs do not cause side effects when used for a single infestation and for a short period of time. Before discharge, ascertain that the patient can explain why and how to take the drug, what side effects may occur, what side effects require consultation with the physician, what symptoms indicate unsuccessful treatment or reinfestation, and what other measures to use to assist in eliminating the protozoa or helminth causing the problem.

TREATMENT OF DISEASES CAUSED BY PROTOZOANS

Amebic Disease

Amebic disease is caused by a microscopic, single-celled parasitic organism. *Entamoeba histolytica* is a frequent pathogen of humans, commonly passed from host to host by oral ingestion of fecally contaminated food or water. The organism is ingested as the cyst form. Cysts have thick walls and resist desiccation and the action of stomach acids. Once in the intestine, the nonmotile cysts change to a motile, sexually active form called a *trophozoite*. Trophozoites produce the active disease as they reproduce and invade various tissues. Homosexual males have a high incidence of infection with *Entamoeba*.

Amebic disease may be restricted to the intestinal lumen. However, trophozoites invade the intestinal lining in the course of the disease and may penetrate the intestinal wall and create abscesses in other tissues and organs. The liver and lung are most commonly affected in this way.

The choice of drug for treating amebic disease depends on the stage of the disease. For the acute colitis that occurs while the disease is limited to the intestinal tract, several drugs are available (Table 38-1). Antibiotics such as tetracycline may be used as adjuncts to therapy. For more extensive intestinal disease or for abscesses in other organs, metronidazole is the safest and most effective agent. Metronidazole therapy is usually followed by iodoquinol or diloxanide, drugs that more effectively destroy free amebae within the intestinal lumen. Alternative therapy is dehydroemetine followed by iodoquinol alone or iodoquinol and chloroquine.

Cryptosporidiosis

Cryptosporidia are small protozoans that can cause diarrhea in several species of animals and in humans. The most common form in human hosts is *Cryptosporidium parvum*. The organism infects the microvillus of host intestinal cells. This disease is passed from host to host by ingestion of thick-walled cysts, but within a single host, thin-walled cysts can release sporozoites, which are invasive forms that invade surrounding host cells. This recycling autoinfection is especially likely in severely immunocompromised patients. Many patients with acquired immunodeficiency syndrome (AIDS) suffer chronic, debilitating diarrhea in the late stages of their disease, and for many of these patients, *C. parvum* infection is a contributing factor to the diarrhea.

Cryptosporidium may be passed from human to human and has spread as a waterborne infection when sewage containing the highly resistant thick-walled cysts contaminates water supplies. Animals including calves, puppies, kittens, and rodents also harbor *Cryp-*

Table 38-1 Drugs to Treat Amebic Infestations

Disease form	Drug used	Administration/dosage
Asymptomatic	Iodoquinol	ORAL: *Adults*—650 mg 3 times daily for 3 weeks. *Children*—30 to 40 mg/kg divided in 3 doses daily for 3 weeks. Maximum daily dose 2 gm.
	Diloxanide furoate	ORAL: *Adults*—500 mg 3 times daily for 10 days. *Children over 2 years*—20 mg/kg daily in 3 divided doses for 10 days.
Intestinal symptoms only	Metronidazole	ORAL: *Adults*—750 mg 3 times daily for 10 days. *Children*—35 to 50 mg/kg divided into 3 doses daily for 10 days.
	+ iodoquinol	As above.
	Metronidazole	As above.
	+ Tetracycline	ORAL: *Adults*—250 to 500 mg every 6 hr. *Children*—6.25 to 12.5 mg/kg every 6 hr.
	Dehydroemetine	INTRAMUSCULAR (deep), SUBCUTANEOUS: *Adults*—1 mg/kg up to 60 mg daily in a single dose for 5 days.
	+ iodoquinol	As above.
Abscesses in liver or other organs	Metronidazole	As above.
	+ iodoquinol	As above.
	Dehydroemetine	As above.
	+ iodoquinol	As above.
	+ chloroquine phosphate	ORAL: *Adults*—250 mg 4 times daily for 2 days, then 250 mg twice daily for 2 or 3 weeks. *Children*—10 mg/kg up to 500 mg daily for 3 weeks.

Table 38-2   Drugs to Treat Selected Protozoal Infestations

Disease	Drug	Administration/dosage
Cryptosporidiosis	Spiramycin	ORAL: *Adults*—1 gm 3 times daily for 3 to 4 weeks. *Children*—50 to 100 mg/kg daily divided into 2 or 3 doses.
Giardiasis	Quinacrine	ORAL: *Adults*—100 mg 3 times daily for 5 to 7 days. *Children*—6 mg/kg daily in 3 divided doses for 5 days. Daily dose should not exceed 300 mg in children.
	Metronidazole	ORAL: *Adults*—250 to 500 mg 3 times daily for 5 to 7 days.
	Furazolidone	ORAL: *Adults*—100 mg 4 times daily for 5 to 7 days.
Pneumocystosis	Trimethoprim with sulfamethoxazole	ORAL, INTRAVENOUS: *Adults and children*—20 mg/kg trimethoprim and 100 mg/kg sulfamethoxazole daily divided into 4 doses.
	Pentamidine isethionate	INTRAVENOUS, INTRAMUSCULAR: *Adults and children*—4 mg/kg daily as a single dose for 12 to 14 days or longer. AEROSOL: *Adults*—approved for prophylaxis.
Toxoplasmosis	Pyrimethamine	ORAL: *Adults*—50 to 200 mg daily for 1 or 2 days, then 25 mg daily for up to 5 weeks. *Children*—1 mg/kg daily in 2 doses for 2 to 4 days. Continue 0.5 mg/kg for 30 days.
	+ sulfadiazine	ORAL: *Adults*—75 mg/kg up to 4 gm for 1 or 2 weeks, then 100 mg/kg daily divided into 2 or 3 doses. *Children*—150 mg/kg total divided into 4 to 6 daily doses after an initial dose equivalent to half the daily total.
Trichomoniasis	Povidone-iodine	VAGINAL: *Adults*—10% gel applied nightly; 10% douche applied every morning. Therapy continues for 2 weeks or longer.
	Metronidazole	ORAL: *Adults*—250 mg 3 times daily for 7 to 10 days.

tosporidium and may pass the organism to human handlers.

No effective therapy for *C. parvum* infections exists, although spiramycin has been somewhat helpful for some patients (see Table 38-2). Patients with intact immune systems generally recover well with only supportive therapy to maintain fluid and electrolyte balance. New drugs will be required to aid severely immunosuppressed patients.

Giardiasis

Giardiasis is an intestinal infection caused by the protozoan *Giardia lamblia*. This disease, which is passed between human hosts by ingestion of fecally contaminated food, may be asymptomatic in many patients. For others, it may be much more severe, producing diarrhea, gastrointestinal (GI) distress, and malabsorption.

Quinacrine is the most commonly recommended drug for giardiasis in adults (see Table 38-2). Children should receive metronidazole. Many adults now also receive metronidazole. Furazolidone is a secondary agent for giardiasis.

Malaria

Malaria is a serious infectious illness caused when an infected mosquito injects a species of *Plasmodium* into the bloodstream of a person. Four species of *Plas-*

modium produce human disease: *P. falciparum, P. vivax, P. ovale,* and *P. malariae.*

Plasmodia have complex life cycles. The form that enters the human bloodstream (sporozoites) travels immediately to the liver and may persist in the organ for prolonged periods. Clinical malaria is produced when merozoites, the plasmodial form produced in liver cells, are released into the bloodstream. The merozoites attack red blood cells and ultimately cause them to rupture, thus producing the fever, chills, and sweating characteristic of the disease. A few gametocytes are also formed, which means that the patient at this stage of the disease can transmit the parasites to mosquitoes and thence to other human hosts. Only gametocytes cause a mosquito to become infectious and capable of transmitting the disease.

Therapy for malaria depends on the stage of the disease and which plasmodial species is involved. *P. falciparum* and *P. malariae* do not seem to produce persistent tissue forms of the parasite. Therefore therapy that destroys blood forms of the protozoan will be curative. With *P. vivax* and *P. ovale*, therapy must include a drug that destroys the persistent tissue forms of *Plasmodium*. A drug such as chloroquine is quite effective against blood forms (Table 38-3). Using chloroquine phosphate plus primaquine phosphate allows radical cure of *P. vivax* and *P. ovale* malaria.

Table 38-3   Drugs to Treat Malaria

Disease form	Drug used	Administration/dosage
Blood forms causing clinical symptoms	Chloroquine phosphate	ORAL: *Adults*—600 mg initially; 300 mg at 6, 24, and 48 hr. *Children*—10 mg/kg initially; 5 mg/kg at 6, 24, and 48 hr.
	Chloroquine hydrochloride	INTRAMUSCULAR, INTRAVENOUS: *Adults*—3 mg/kg every 6 hr (maximum 800 mg/24 hr). *Children*—3.5 mg/kg repeated in 6 hr. Not for IV use in children under 7 years.
	Hydroxychloroquine sulfate	ORAL: *Adults*—620 mg initially (four 200 mg tablets of the sulfate equals 620 mg base); 310 mg at 6, 24, and 48 hr. *Children*—10 mg/kg initially; 5 mg/kg at 6, 24, and 48 hr.
	Quinine sulfate	ORAL: *Adults*—650 mg 3 times daily for 3 days. *Children*—25 mg/kg per day in 3 doses for 3 days.
Persistent tissue forms of *Plasmodia* (*P. ovale* and *P. vivax*) or gametocytes	Primaquine phosphate	ORAL: *Adults*—15 mg for 14 days after therapy with one of the drugs listed above. *Children*—0.39 mg/kg for 14 days after therapy with one of the drugs listed above.
Chloroquine-resistant *P. falciparum*	Quinine sulfate + pyrimethamine and sulfadoxine	As above. ORAL: *Adults and children over 4 years*—tablets contain 25 mg pyrimethamine and 500 mg sulfadoxine. One to 3 tablets as a single dose may be followed with quinine or primaquine.
	Mefloquine hydrochloride	ORAL: *Adults and children*—15 mg base per kg body weight, as a single dose.

Chloroquine has been a mainstay in treating malaria for a number of years. Unfortunately, chloroquine-resistant malaria has developed in several regions of the world. This disease is treated with the combination of quinine or mefloquine, and pyrimethamine and sulfadoxine. Pyrimethamine and sulfadoxine are synergistic in activity and are given together for maximum benefit.

Several of the drugs used to treat malaria may also be used for prophylaxis. Chloroquine, hydroxychloroquine, mefloquine, and pyrimethamine and sulfadoxine are given in once-weekly doses. Clindamycin, dapsone, doxycycline, and tetracycline have been included in treatment or prophylaxis regimens in other countries but are not officially recognized for this use in the United States.

Pneumocystosis

Pneumocystis carinii has been recognized as an opportunistic pathogen for several decades, but little is known about the life cycle of this organism. Long considered to be a protozoan, it has recently been recognized as more related to fungi, but the clinically effective drugs are antiprotozoal agents. *P. carinii* seldom causes disease in healthy humans, but it can produce severe pulmonary disease in patients receiving immunosuppressive drugs or suffering from AIDS. Young, malnourished children are also susceptible. As many as half of the patients who acquire this disease may die unless treated. Patients receiving immunosuppressive cancer chemotherapy or those receiving immunosuppressive drugs to prevent rejection of a transplanted organ usually respond well to the fixed combination of sulfamethoxazole and trimethoprim (see Chapter 34). Many of these patients may receive sulfamethoxazole and trimethoprim to prevent development of *P. carinii* pneumonia.

Sulfamethoxazole and trimethoprim may also be given to treat *P. carinii* pneumonia in AIDS patients, but these patients suffer an unusually high incidence of serious reactions to these drugs. Pentamidine isethionate is also effective against *P. carinii* pneumonia but can often cause serious toxicity. Experimental regimens in *P. carinii* pneumonia in AIDS patients include BW566C80, clindamycin with primaquine, dapsone with trimethoprim, and trimetrexate or piritrexim with leucovorin. Intermittent administration of aerosolized pentamidine is a popular method of prophylaxis. Because this area of medicine is changing so rapidly, nursing personnel should consult a current publication from the Centers for Disease Control or another official source for current information.

Toxoplasmosis

In the United States, toxoplasmosis is primarily acquired from ingestion of the oocyte of *Toxoplasma gondii*. The most common source of infection is cat feces. In adult humans the disease is usually mild and transitory, with symptoms resembling those of mild mononucleosis. Occasionally, the disease may involve the eyes or nervous system in adults.

One dangerous form of toxoplasmosis is congenital, resulting from infection in a pregnant woman. Congenital toxoplasmosis is usually fatal, causing severe damage to the eyes, brain, and other organs of the fetus. Because of the dangers this disease poses to fetuses, many obstetricians suggest that pregnant women not handle used cat litter and avoid close contact with cats.

Pyrimethamine and sulfadoxine or sulfadiazine are used in combination to treat this disease (see Table 38-2).

Toxoplasmosis is a common cause of death in AIDS patients, with encephalitis causing death. Aggressive therapy with pyrimethamine and sulfonamides is usually attempted, but for patients who cannot tolerate sulfonamides, other drugs such as clindamycin may be combined with pyrimethamine.

Trichomoniasis

Vaginal infections caused by *Trichomonas vaginalis* occur commonly. The disease is marked by watery discharge from the vagina and signs of tissue irritation. Trichomonas may be unnoticed in the urinary tract and in the rectum, but these sites can serve as sources of infection.

Vaginal **trichomoniasis** may be treated with local agents applied as gels or douches (see Table 38-2). Complete cure of the sites outside the vagina and of infections in the male urinary tract may require a systemic agent. Metronidazole is the drug of choice.

TREATMENT OF DISEASES CAUSED BY HELMINTHS

Helminths include flukes, tapeworms, and roundworms that can cause disease. Table 38-4 summarizes antihelminthic agents.

Ascariasis

Ascariasis, also called *roundworm infestation,* is produced by ingesting the eggs of *Ascaris lumbricoides.* This common disease is spread by fecally contaminated food and water. Larvae and adult worms migrate through the lungs, liver, gallbladder, and other organs and may cause severe damage. Ascaris infestations may be treated effectively with several agents, including mebendazole, pyrantel pamoate, and piperazine (see Table 38-4).

Enterobiasis

Enterobiasis is pinworm infestation. Pinworms are freely passed between individuals living in close prox-

imity. Constant reinfection occurs, since the eggs of these parasites are passed in great numbers and adhere to clothing, towels, and hands. The disease is usually mild and may be asymptomatic. However, patients may suffer pruritus ani and pruritus vulvae or more serious symptoms.

Since pinworms tend to stay within the intestinal tract, treatment of the disease is relatively simple. Mebendazole, pyrantel pamoate, and pyrvinium pamoate are all nearly 100% effective after a single dose. Piperazine is also effective, but therapy continues over a period of several days (see Table 38-4).

Whipworm Infestation

Whipworm infestation is usually asymptomatic, although large numbers of worms in small children may produce diarrhea, anemia, and cachexia. Whipworm infestations are easily and effectively treated with mebendazole (see Table 38-4).

Threadworm Infestation

Threadworm infestation, also called *strongyloidiasis,* is more serious than many infestations because the worms may reproduce in the human body. Larvae migrate from the wall of the intestine into systemic circulation and thence return to the intestine to mature and further increase the numbers of worms in the host. Malabsorption syndrome, diarrhea, and duodenal irritation may occur.

Most drugs used against worm infestations are ineffective against threadworms, since they live within the intestinal tissue. Thiabendazole is well distributed to the tissues where this parasite lives and eliminates the infestation. Ivermectin, a drug developed to treat river blindness and filariasis in tropical regions, is also useful against threadworms (see Table 38-4).

Hookworm Infestation

Hookworm infestation, called *necatoriasis,* occurs in the southern United States. Although two species of hookworms are known, most infestations encountered in the United States are caused by *Necator.* Therefore most patients may be treated with mebendazole or pyrantel pamoate. Another type of hookworm from dogs and cats produces a cutaneous lesion called *creeping eruption,* or *cutaneous larva migrans.* Thiabendazole, either topically or orally, may kill the parasites and limit the allergic responses, which cause itching, burning, and skin damage (see Table 38-4).

Trichinosis

Trichinosis, also known as *pork roundworm infestation,* is much less common today than it once was. Ingested cysts from raw or improperly cooked meat develop into adult worms in the human intestine. Larvae are

Table 38-4 Drugs to Treat Infestations by Helminths

Disease form	Drug used	Administration/dosage
Roundworms (ascariasis)	Pyrantel pamoate	ORAL: *Adults and children*—single dose of 11 mg/kg up to 1 gm.
	Mebendazole	ORAL: *Adults and children*—100 mg twice daily for 3 days.
	Piperazine	ORAL: *Adults*—2 gm 3 times in 12 hr. Repeat in 2 weeks. *Children*—75 mg/kg up to 3.5 gm once or twice in 12 hr; repeat in 2 weeks.
Pinworms (enterobiasis)	Mebendazole	ORAL: *Adults and children*—100 mg single dose.
	Pyrantel pamoate	ORAL: *Adults and children*—single dose of 11 mg/kg up to 1 gm.
	Pyrvinium pamoate	ORAL: *Adults and children*—single dose of 5 mg/kg.
	Piperazine	ORAL: *Adults and children*—65 mg/kg up to 2.5 gm once daily for 1 week.
Whipworms (trichuriasis)	Mebendazole	ORAL: *Adults and children*—100 mg daily for 3 days.
Threadworms (strongyloidiasis)	Thiabendazole	ORAL: *Adults and children*—25 mg/kg up to 3 gm twice daily for 1 or 2 days.
	Ivermectin	ORAL: *Adults*—up to 200 mg/kg body weight, as a single dose.
Hookworms (necatoriasis)	Mebendazole	ORAL: *Adults and children*—100 mg twice daily for 3 days.
	Pyrantel pamoate	ORAL: *Adults and children*—11 mg/kg up to 1 gm as a single dose for 3 days.
Cutaneous larva migrans	Thiabendazole	ORAL: *Adults and children over 13.6 kg*—25 mg/kg twice daily for 2 to 5 days plus topical application of suspension (500 mg/5 ml) 4 times daily for 5 days.
Pork roundworms (trichinosis)	Thiabendazole	ORAL: *Adults and children*—25 mg/kg up to 3 gm twice daily for 2 to 7 days.
Tapeworms (cestodiasis)	Niclosamide	ORAL: *Adults*—2 gm as a single dose. *Children weighing more than 34 kg*—1.5 gm as a single dose. *Children 11 to 34 kg*—1 gm as a single dose. For all patients, tablets should be thoroughly chewed and taken on an empty stomach. For treatment of dwarf tapeworm infestations, doses must be continued for 5 days and repeated 1 to 2 weeks after initial therapy.
	Praziquantel	ORAL: *Adults and children over 4 years*—10 to 25 mg/kg as a single dose.

released into the circulation and enter muscle to form cysts. Patients suffer GI upset, fever, muscle aches, and eosinophilia (accumulation of certain white cells in the blood).

Trichinosis cannot yet be effectively treated. Most patients receive therapy designed to minimize symptoms rather than produce a cure, since most patients survive the disease and carry the quiescent worms encysted in skeletal muscle for the rest of their lives. Thiabendazole and mebendazole have been used in selected cases to try to prevent the migration of the worms to the muscles (see Table 38-4).

Tapeworm Infestation

Tapeworms, or **cestodes,** of several types can infest humans. Beef, pork, fish, and dwarf tapeworms are all sensitive to niclosamide. Praziquantel, a drug used primarily in the tropics for schistosomiasis, may also be effective against tapeworms (see Table 38-4). All detected infestations are treated, even though they are mostly asymptomatic. Pork tapeworm infestations may become serious if reflux of eggs from the intestine allows them to reach the stomach and hatch into larvae that invade tissues.

PHARMACOLOGIC PROPERTIES OF SPECIFIC DRUGS

Chloroquine and Hydroxychloroquine

Mechanism of action

Chloroquine and hydroxychloroquine are members of a drug family called *4-aminoquinolines*. This family of drugs has been the mainstay of antimalarial therapy worldwide since the late 1940s. All effective members of this family can bind tightly to DNA in its double-stranded form, thereby altering the physical properties of DNA. These drugs may also inhibit metabolic processes in *Plasmodium.*

Absorption, distribution, and excretion

Chloroquine phosphate and hydroxychloroquine sulfate are satisfactorily absorbed from the GI tract. Chloroquine hydrochloride is available for intramuscular (IM) injection when oral dosage is impossible.

Drugs of the 4-aminoquinoline family are strongly concentrated in the liver, spleen, kidneys, and lungs. More important to the therapeutic usefulness, the drugs are also concentrated in red blood cells. Infected red blood cells may concentrate the drug up to 1000-fold over the drug concentration in plasma.

The 4-aminoquinolines may be metabolized in the liver by microsomal enzymes; some of the metabolites retain antiplasmodial activity. These drugs and metabolites are removed from the body by the kidneys. Renal excretion is enhanced by acidifying urine, which converts the drug to a charged form that is not reabsorbed.

Toxicity

Chloroquine and hydroxychloroquine are relatively safe drugs if care is taken to avoid overdose, prolonged use, or use in sensitive patients. Patients with glucose 6-phosphate dehydrogenase deficiency are more likely than normal patients to suffer hemolysis when treated with these drugs. Children are also more sensitive to these agents than are adults (see box). Patients with liver disease or retinal damage are also more at risk of severe toxic reactions.

At the doses commonly used in therapy, drugs of this family can produce nausea and other GI symptoms (Table 38-5). These symptoms may be minimized by administering the drug with meals.

Visual changes may be observed with 4-aminoquinolines. Blurred vision may signal reversible impairment of accommodation, but retinal or corneal changes are not reversible. Patients reporting misty vision, patchy vision, or foggy patches in the visual field may be developing serious eye damage. These complaints tend to arise in patients receiving the drugs for long periods.

Headache, dizziness, psychosis, and convulsions may be observed in patients treated with these drugs. In some patients, changes in heart function may be reported. Skin and blood changes may also occur.

The toxic reactions to 4-aminoquinolines are greatly increased when the drugs are used for prolonged periods such as with long-term malaria prophylaxis. When used in routine short-term treatment regimens for malaria (see Table 38-3), the drugs are better tolerated.

Dehydroemetine

Mechanism of action

Dehydroemetine is related to emetine, an alkaloid obtained from ipecac, which was used as an emetic. Dehydroemetine is similar to emetine but is thought to be less cardiotoxic. Dehydroemetine may block protein synthesis in eukaryotes. Therefore mammalian cells and the ameba may be sensitive.

Absorption, distribution, and excretion

Although dehydroemetine may be absorbed orally, the emetic and irritative properties of this drug cause it to be poorly tolerated by that route. Dehydroemetine is given by IM or subcutaneous injection. Intravenous (IV) injection is to be scrupulously avoided to prevent excessive toxicity to the heart. The drug may accumulate in various organs, including the liver, and may be slowly released.

Toxicity

Dehydroemetine is thought to be less cardiotoxic than emetine, but symptoms such as tachycardia (fast heart rate) and ECG changes signal that the drug should be discontinued to prevent further cardiac difficulty. Because of this potential for cardiac toxicity, every patient receiving dehydroemetine should be carefully monitored. Dehydroemetine may produce GI irritation, even when administered parenterally. Muscle weakness and skin lesions may also occur.

Diloxanide Furoate

Mechanism of action

Diloxanide eliminates *E. histolytica* from the intestine of persons mildly infected and who are passing cysts in their stools (see Table 38-1). The drug has little effect against acute colitis produced by this parasite and no effect on tissue abscesses. The mechanism of the ameba-destroying action of diloxanide is not known.

PEDIATRIC CONSIDERATIONS: CHLOROQUINE AND HYDROXYCHLOROQUINE

THE PROBLEM

Infants and children are more sensitive to 4-aminoquinolines than are adults. Children have died after swallowing as little as 750 mg of chloroquine. Severe reactions and sudden death have been reported with parenteral use.

SOLUTIONS

◆ Use minimal effective doses in children
◆ Do not give these drugs long-term to children
◆ Carefully observe children receiving these drugs
◆ Keep drugs out of easy reach of children
◆ Use childproof caps on medication containers
◆ Never refer to medication as candy

Table 38-5   Common Reactions to Antiparasitic Drugs

Generic name	Trade name	Toxicity	References for uses and dosages
Chloroquine	Aralen*	GI distress is most common. Vision changes, central nervous system irritability, and hemolysis can occur.	Malaria: treatment of clinical attacks or prophylaxis (see Table 38-3).
Dehydroemetine**		GI irritation and cardiac toxicity are common.	Amebiasis: severe colitis with or without tissue abscesses (see Table 38-1).
Diloxanide furoate**	Furamide	Flatulence is common. Other GI symptoms are rare.	Amebiasis: eliminates cysts; eradicates carrier state (see Table 38-1).
Hydroxychloroquine	Plaquenil sulfate*	As for chloroquine.	Malaria: treatment of clinical attacks or prophylaxis (see Table 38-3).
Iodoquinol (Diiodohydroxyquin)	Diodoquin† Diquinol Yodoxin*	GI upset and skin eruptions are most common. Blood levels of iodine may rise; optic neuritis may occur rarely.	Amebiasis: intestinal forms of disease (see Table 38-1).
Ivermectin**	Mectizan	Dizziness, fever, headache, and joint and muscle pain may occur.	Threadworms (see Table 38-4).
Mebendazole	Vermox*	Abdominal discomfort may occur. Mebendazole is teratogenic in rats. FDA Pregnancy Category C.	Roundworms, pinworms, whipworms, and hookworms (see Table 38-4).
Mefloquine	Lariam	Vomiting and other GI symptoms may occur. Central nervous system toxicity and visual disturbances have occurred.	Malaria: chloroquine-resistant (see Table 38-3).
Metronidazole	Flagyl* Protostat Trikacide†	GI distress, central nervous system effects, and pelvic discomfort may occur. FDA Pregnancy Category B.	Amebiasis: intestinal or tissue abscesses (see Table 38-1). Trichomoniasis and giardiasis (see Table 38-2).
Niclosamide	Niclocide	Mild GI upset on day of therapy. FDA Pregnancy Category B.	Tapeworms (see Table 38-4).
Pentamidine	Pentacarinat† Pentam	Hypoglycemia and hypotension may occur quickly. Blood dyscrasias, hyperglycemia, and diabetes mellitus are later reactions.	Pneumocystis pneumonia (see Table 38-2).
Piperazine	Entacyl†	GI upset may occur. Skin rashes and transient neurologic signs may be seen.	Roundworms and pinworms (see Table 38-4).
Povidone-iodine	Betadine*	Tissue irritation may occur with topically applied drug.	Trichomoniasis (see Table 38-2).
Praziquantel	Biltricide	GI distress, dizziness, or drowsiness may occur. FDA Pregnancy Category B.	Alternative drug for tapeworms (see Table 38-4) but a primary drug for schistosomiasis (snail fever).
Primaquine		GI distress can occur. Hemolysis may occur, especially when G-6-PD deficiency exists. Avoid during pregnancy.	Malaria: persistent tissue forms (see Table 38-2); pneumocystis pneumonia (see Table 38-2).
Pyrantel pamoate	Antiminth Combantrin†	Mild GI upset and transient changes in liver function occur. Headaches and dizziness are more rare.	Roundworms, pinworms, and hookworms (see Table 38-4).

*Available in Canada and United States.
†Available in Canada only.
**Available in United States through the CDC, Atlanta.

Continued.

Table 38-5   Common Reactions to Antiparasitic Drugs—cont'd

Generic name	Trade name	Toxicity	References for uses and dosages
Pyrimethamine	Daraprim*	Nausea, vomiting, and blood dyscrasias occur, especially with higher doses.	Malaria: with quinine and sulfadoxine (see Table 38-3). Toxoplasmosis: with sulfadiazine (see Table 38-2).
Pyrvinium pamoate	Vanquin†	Bright red drug stains teeth and intestinal contents.	Pinworms (see Table 38-4).
Quinacrine	Atabrine*	GI distress, dizziness, or headache may occur. Yellow discoloration of skin is harmless. Overdose may cause seizures and cardiovascular collapse.	Giardiasis (see Table 38-2).
Quinine	Quinamm Quiphile	Cinchonism is a dose-related sign of toxicity.	Malaria: with pyrimethamine and sulfadoxine (see Table 38-3).
Spiramycin	Rovamycine	Nausea, vomiting, diarrhea, and indigestion are common. FDA Pregnancy Category B.	Cryptosporidiosis (see Table 38-2).
Sulfadiazine	Microsulfon	GI, allergic, and blood reactions are possible (see Chapter 34).	Malaria: with pyrimethamine and quinine (see Table 38-3). Toxoplasmosis: with pyrimethamine (see Table 38-2).
Sulfadoxine and pyrimethamine	Fansidar*	Blood dyscrasias and allergic reactions as expected for sulfonamides (see Chapter 34) or for pyrimethamine may occur.	Malaria: prophylaxis or treatment of acute attack (see Table 38-3).
Sulfamethoxazole and trimethoprim	Bactrim* Septra*	Folic acid deficiency or sulfonamide toxicity may occur (see Chapter 34).	Pneumocystosis (see Table 38-2).
Tetracycline		GI distress is common (see Chapter 32).	Amebiasis: with iodoquinol for intestinal forms (see Table 38-1).
Thiabendazole	Mintezol	GI upset is common. Central nervous system effects and reduced liver function may be observed. FDA Pregnancy Category C.	Threadworms, hookworms, cutaneous larva migrans, and trichinosis (see Table 38-4).

*Available in Canada and United States.
†Available in Canada only.

Absorption, distribution, and excretion

Diloxanide is administered orally and is well absorbed by that route. Nevertheless, diloxanide is useful alone only for intestinal amebiasis. Excretion is primarily by the kidney.

Toxicity

Diloxanide is relatively safe, producing few systemic side effects. Flatulence (intestinal gas) is the most frequently reported side effect. Other GI disturbances such as nausea, diarrhea, and esophagitis may rarely be encountered.

Furazolidone

Mechanism of action

Furazolidone is a nitrofuran similar in action to the nitrofurans used to treat urinary tract infections (see Chapter 34). Furazolidone is an effective antimicro-

bial agent against many enteric microorganisms, including *G. lamblia* (see Table 38-2).

Absorption, distribution, and excretion

Furazolidone is administered orally to treat infections of the bowel. Like other nitrofurans, it does not achieve high serum concentrations.

Furazolidone is metabolized by the liver. One of the breakdown products is a potent inhibitor of monoamine oxidase (MAO). The inhibition of this enzyme lowers the ability of the body to eliminate catecholamines; therefore hypertension may result. In addition, this action makes drugs such as sympathomimetics (e.g., ephedrine, and phenylephrine in nasal decongestants), MAO inhibitors (e.g., pargyline), or foods rich in tyramine (e.g., cheese, beer, and wine) unsafe for patients receiving furazolidone.

Toxicity

Furazolidone may produce hemolytic reactions, especially in patients who have G-6-PD deficiency. Allergies and GI symptoms may also occur. Patients receiving furazolidone who also drink alcohol may exhibit a disulfiram-like reaction with flushing, difficulty in breathing, and a feeling of constriction in the chest (see Chapter 40).

Iodoquinol

Mechanism of action

Iodoquinol is an effective amebicidal agent (see Table 38-1) whose action is thought to relate to the iodine content of the drug.

Absorption, distribution, and excretion

Iodoquinol administered orally is not significantly absorbed from the intestine. Iodine is increased in the bloodstream, which suggests that some drug is absorbed or that the iodine is absorbed after breakdown of the drug in the gut.

Toxicity

Iodoquinol is relatively nontoxic. Skin eruptions may occur. Nausea and other GI symptoms have been reported. Iodoquinol can affect the thyroid gland and increae blood iodine levels. Prolonged high doses of iodoquinol may occasionally produce optic neuritis or atrophy and other signs of neuropathy.

Ivermectin

Mechanism of action

Ivermectin seems to act as an agonist at gamma-aminobutyric acid (GABA) receptors, which interferes with function of the nervous system in threadworms and other parasites. The paralyzed worms may die.

Absorption, distribution, and excretion

Ivermectin is given as a single oral dose that is effective for up to a year. The drug concentrates in the liver and fat tissue in the body. Excretion is primarily in feces, with little drug being found in urine.

Toxicity

Ivermectin may cause dizziness, fever, headache, arthralgia, myalgia, and swollen lymph nodes. Postural hypotension is rare.

Mebendazole

Mechanism of action

Mebendazole is an effective broad-spectrum antihelminthic agent (see Table 38-4). Mebendazole blocks glucose uptake in sensitive helminths. Since these organisms require externally supplied glucose to maintain energy levels, blockade of glucose absorption destroys the worms.

Absorption, distribution, and excretion

Mebendazole is used orally for its action against intestinal helminths. Very little of the drug is absorbed into systemic circulation. The small amount of drug that enters the bloodstream is metabolized by the liver and excreted by the kidneys.

Toxicity

Mebendazole produces few toxic reactions. A few reports of abdominal discomfort and diarrhea exist, but these symptoms may result from large masses of worms being expelled. Mebendazole is teratogenic in rats but has not produced birth defects in dogs, sheep, or horses. It is difficult to predict the effects in humans. Therefore physicians may limit the use of mebendazole, especially during pregnancy.

Mefloquine

Mechanism of action

Mefloquine is chemically related to quinine and, like quinine, acts only against the blood-borne forms of *Plasmodium* (see Table 38-3). The exact way in which the drug interferes with the parasite is unknown.

Absorption, distribution, and excretion

Oral absorption of mefloquine is usually in excess of 85%. The drug distributes well to many tissues, including cerebrospinal fluid and brain. Mefloquine is concentrated in red blood cells, which may contribute to the effect against the organisms harbored there.

Mefloquine is metabolized to a variable degree by the liver. Elimination is a slow process, with drug remaining in the body for 2 weeks to 1 month. This long elimination half-life allows the drug to be given as a single dose to treat malaria.

Toxicity

Mefloquine may cause GI distress, including vomiting. At higher doses, it may also cause central nervous system (CNS) effects such as dizziness, headache, anxiety, confusion, or seizures. Visual disturbances have also been noted. Slowing of the heart rate (bradycardia) is a rare side effect.

Metronidazole

Mechanism of action

Metronidazole attacks amebas at intestinal and other tissue sites (see Table 38-1). It has also been used to treat trichomoniasis (see Table 38-2). Metronidazole is most effective against anaerobes, being reduced in those organisms to a form that directly damages DNA.

Absorption, distribution, and excretion

Metronidazole is well absorbed after oral administration. The drug is metabolized by various pathways. Both metabolites and the unchanged drug appear in urine. Some patients observe a reddish brown discoloration of urine while receiving metronidazole. This discoloration is caused by a colored metabolite of metronidazole. Patients should be reassured that the discoloration is harmless.

Toxicity

Metronidazole can produce various GI symptoms. Some patients experience a sharp, metallic taste, as well as nausea, diarrhea, vomiting, epigastric pain, and abdominal cramping. Although annoying, these symptoms rarely necessitate stopping the medication.

Metronidazole can rarely cause changes in CNS function. Dizziness, ataxia (incoordination affecting walking), numbness, and paresthesias may occur. These symptoms may signal that metronidazole should be withdrawn. Metronidazole may also produce discomfort in the pelvic organs. Patients describe a sense of pressure in that region. Dysuria, cystitis, and dryness of the vagina may be experienced.

Metronidazole causes an alarming reaction when ethyl alcohol is ingested. Patients experience intense flushing, nausea, headaches, and abdominal cramps. This reaction is similar to that experienced by patients taking both disulfiram and ethyl alcohol (see Chapter 40). Metronidazole may potentiate the action of warfarin. Patients receiving both drugs should be carefully observed for signs of bleeding.

Because of its action on DNA, metronidazole may be mutagenic or carcinogenic in some experimental animals. This potential problem precludes the routine use of the drug in pregnant women.

Niclosamide

Mechanism of action

Niclosamide is effective against tapeworms. These segmented flatworms are killed by a single dose of niclosamide, which blocks their respiration and glucose uptake. The dead worm segments are frequently digested by proteolytic agents in the gut. For this reason, a cathartic may be given 1 or 2 hr after the drug has been administered to allow the dead-but-still-intact worm parts to be identified in the feces. This purge is a therapeutic necessity when the tapeworm infestation is caused by the pork tapeworm. With this organism, digestion of the dead worm segments releases living eggs, which can develop in humans and cause more serious, invasive disease. The purge removes the worm segments before they rupture and prevents this complication.

Absorption, distribution, and excretion

Niclosamide is not absorbed from the bowel and exerts all of its actions within the lumen of the bowel.

Toxicity

Niclosamide is almost without toxicity. Systemic toxicity is not a problem, since the drug is not absorbed. Some patients have mild GI symptoms on the day of therapy.

Pentamidine

Mechanism of action

The action of pentamidine against *P. carinii* (see Table 38-2) is not completely understood but involves an interference with DNA function.

Absorption, distribution, and excretion

Pentamidine is poorly absorbed orally and causes local tissue damage when given intramuscularly. For these reasons, the most common route of administration is IV. For prophylaxis of *P. carinii* pneumonia, pentamidine may be aerosolized. When properly administered by this route, the drug is carried into the lung in tiny droplets of a size carefully controlled to allow deposition into the alveoli, where *P. carinii* lodges. Therefore high concentrations are achieved at the site of infection, but because systemic absorption from the lung is very low, whole body toxicity is minimized.

Pentamidine is concentrated in renal tissue and is excreted primarily in urine. Little metabolism occurs. Complete elimination from the body is slow, with drug appearing in urine as long as 8 weeks after therapy stops.

Toxicity

Patients receiving pentamidine parenterally may suffer acute hypotension. Cardiac arrhythmias have also occurred and have caused deaths. Hypoglycemia may be severe. Long-term effects of pentamidine may include hyperglycemia or diabetes mellitus. Nephrotoxicity and blood dyscrasias can also develop. The incidence of side effects can vary, depending on the patient being treated. In general, AIDS patients suffer more of the major and minor reactions to pentamidine than do other patients.

Piperazine

Mechanism of action

Piperazine is effective against ascaris and pinworm infestations (see Table 38-4). The drug apparently blocks the action of acetylcholine on the muscles of these parasites. As a result, the worms are paralyzed and are eliminated from the bowel by normal peristaltic flow. The eliminated worms are alive.

Absorption, distribution, and excretion

Piperazine is well absorbed after oral administration. A portion of the drug is metabolized to various inactive products. The kidney is the primary route for excretion. Patients with impaired renal or hepatic function may be more sensitive to piperazine than other patients.

Toxicity

Piperazine produces few toxic effects at the doses routinely used to treat helminthic infestations. GI upset and occasional skin rashes have occurred. Transient neurologic signs ranging from headache and dizziness to ataxia, paresthesias, or convulsions have been seen, but these more severe reactions are more common with overdoses. The more severe reactions also occur in patients with renal dysfunction, who tend to accumulate the drug.

Povidone-Iodine

Mechanism of action

Povidone-iodine is a general antiseptic agent whose antiseptic effect is produced by the release of free iodine. The agent is widely used as a skin antiseptic in preparation for various medical procedures. In addition, povidone-iodine may be used topically to treat infections caused by *T. vaginalis* (see Table 38-2).

Absorption, distribution, and excretion

Povidone-iodine is used topically in the vagina. Absorption is usually minimal, but some patients display a rise in iodine levels in the blood.

Toxicity

Povidone-iodine may irritate tissues in some patients. Iodine toxicity is usually not a problem unless the patient is highly sensitive or is treated for extended periods.

Praziquantel

Mechanism of action

Praziquantel interferes with the function of suckers on cestodes and flukes, thereby causing these parasites to dislodge from tissue sites in the host. The drug may also interfere with muscle function in the parasites and can cause local destruction of the integument of these organisms.

Absorption, distribution, and excretion

Praziquantel is well absorbed after oral administration but undergoes extensive first-pass metabolism in the liver (see Chapter 1). The metabolites that are formed are excreted by the kidneys.

Toxicity

Praziquantel frequently causes mild and transient effects on the nervous system. Common signs are headache, dizziness, and malaise. Most patients also report GI distress.

Primaquine

Mechanism of action

Primaquine is an 8-aminoquinoline. The mechanism of action may be different from the related 4-aminoquinolines, but the exact mechanism by which primaquine kills certain forms of plasmodia is unknown (see Table 38-3).

Absorption, distribution, and excretion

Primaquine is well absorbed after oral doses. Drug concentrations in the plasma peak within 6 hr of the dose, but the drug is extensively metabolized and rapidly cleared from the bloodsteam.

Toxicity

Primaquine given at normal therapeutic doses produces little toxicity. Abdominal cramps and epigastric distress can occur, but these symptoms can usually be relieved by taking the drug with meals.

Primaquine may damage red blood cells. The drug blocks the production of an intracellular reducing agent, NADPH. In normal cells, this deficit is made up by glucose metabolism, and the cell continues to function normally. However, patients with reduced levels of glucose-6-phosphate dehydrogenase (G-6-PD) cannot use glucose rapdily enough to make up the deficit. The red blood cells in these patients accumulate oxidized products such as methemoglobin, which is not an efficient oxygen carrier. Cyanosis may result. Ultimately, these red blood cells may rupture. Hemolysis can be severe and signals that drug dosage should be reduced or that treatment should be terminated. One sign of hemolysis that may be seen easily is darkening of urine.

Primaquine toxicity is more severe in patients lacking G-6-PD. The lack of G-6-PD is genetically determined and exists in high proportions of certain populations such as Sardinians, Sephardic Jews, Greeks, and Iranians. Blacks are less prone to this deficiency than these groups but have a higher incidence than the white population of the United States. Patients discovered to have these increased sensitivities to primaquine may be given lower doses of the drug.

Pyrantel Pamoate

Mechanism of action

Pyrantel is a depolarizing neuromuscular blocking agent, similar in action to succinylcholine and decamethonium. Pyrantel causes spastic paralysis and gradual contraction of the muscle in worms (see Table 38-4). The parasites are then eliminated from the body by normal peristalsis. Pyrantel is effective, when given in short courses, against a variety of worms. Purges are not necessary adjuncts to therapy with this drug. Piperazine may antagonize the action of pyrantel.

Absorption, distribution, and excretion

Pyrantel is not absorbed from the GI tract to any great extent. What little drug is absorbed is excreted by the kidneys. Pyrantel produces its desired effects entirely within the lumen of the bowel.

Toxicity

Since pyrantel is not well absorbed after oral dosage, few systemic effects occur. Headache, muscle twitching, and dizziness may result from CNS effects of this drug. More commonly the drug causes mild GI upset and transient changes in liver function tests.

Pyrimethamine

Mechanism of action

Pyrimethamine inhibits the enzyme dihydrofolate reductase in plasmodia. Pyrimethamine therefore blocks the formation of tetrahydrofolic acid (THFA), a cofactor required for several metabolic transformations. The blocked enzyme normally converts dihydrofolic acid (DHA) to THFA. The formation of DHA may be blocked by sulfonamides (see Chapter 34). Combining pyrimethamine and a sulfonamide is an example of synergistic effects produced by drugs blocking sequential steps in a metabolic pathway. Another example is trimethoprim and sulfamethoxazole (see Chapter 34).

Absorption, distribution, and excretion

Pyrimethamine is well absorbed after oral administration. The drug is metabolized and appears in urine as metabolities. Pyrimethamine appears in the milk of nursing mothers.

Toxicity

Pyrimethamine, as it is normally used in treating chloroquine-resistant malaria, produces few side effects. In higher doses such as those used to treat toxoplasmosis the drug may impair host folic acid metabolism, leading to megaloblastic anemia and various other blood dyscrasias. Treatment with leucovorin (a folinic acid supplement) may be required. Large doses may also produce nausea and vomiting, which may be controlled partly by administering the drug with meals.

Pyrvinium Pamoate

Mechanism of action

Pyrvinium pamoate inhibits energy metabolism in facultative anaerobic organisms such as the intestinal parasitic worms. The drug is most effective against pinworm infestations (see Table 38-4), killing all the parasites in a large percentage of cases after a single dose.

Absorption, distribution, and excretion

Pyrvinium pamoate is not absorbed from the GI tract and is excreted in feces. Since the drug is a cyanine dye, it colors feces bright red.

Toxicity

Pyrvinium pamoate produces no dangerous toxicity. Older patients or patients receiving the drug in large doses or in suspension form may suffer intestinal distress, including emesis. Pyrvinium pamoate has a bright red color that can stain teeth and clothing. Patients should be cautioned not to chew the tablets. If emesis occurs, the vomitus may be red and capable of staining materials. The red color is not dangerous but makes therapy less tolerable.

Quinacrine

Mechanism of action

Quinacrine was first developed and used as an antimalarial agent but is now primarily used for giardiasis (see Table 38-2).

Absorption, distribution, and excretion

Quinacrine is well absorbed from the GI tract. However, when given orally, the drug induces vomiting in many patients because it is very bitter tasting. Quinacrine is well distributed throughout the body and seems to bind strongly to tissues. Patients may notice a yellow discoloration of the skin. The reaction is not a sign of jaundice but simply illustrates the distribution of this yellow-colored drug to the skin.

Toxicity

Quinacrine causes few serious side effects when used for short-term treatment courses. Dizziness and toxic psychosis are occasionally noted. Psoriasis may be exacerbated. Aplastic anemia has rarely been observed. The most common reactions to quinacrine are nausea and vomiting. Quinacrine crosses the placenta and should not be used in pregnant patients.

Quinine

Mechanism of action

Quinine is a plant alkaloid with many actions on various tissues. The exact mechanism of the antimalarial action of quinine is unknown. Although quinine is the oldest antimalarial agent known and was once the mainstay of therapy, today its use is restricted to treating chloroquine-resistant *P. falciparum* (see Table 38-3). Quinine should be combined with pyrimethamine and sulfadoxine for most effective action.

Absorption, distribution, and excretion

Quinine is rapidly absorbed after oral dosage. The drug is generally well distributed throughout the body, although it does not enter the cerebrospinal fluid to a significant degree. Quinine is extensively metabolized and excreted in urine. Excretion is enhanced in acidic urine.

Toxicity

Quinine can produce cinchonism (quinine comes from cinchona bark). Symptoms include ringing in the ears (tinnitus), altered hearing acuity, headache, blurred vision, and diarrhea. At the doses used today, these symptoms are usually mild. If the dosage is increased or if the patient is hypersensitive, severe cinchonism can arise. Various blood dyscrasias may occur as well.

Quinine is irritating and causes severe pain on subcutaneous or IM injections, which limits the use of these routes. Given intravenously, the drug can cause hypotension and circulatory failure.

Spiramycin

Mechanism of action

Spiramycin is a macrolide antibiotic related to erythromycin (see Chapter 31) and most likely affects bacterial ribosomes in the same way as erythromycin. The mechanism of action on *C. parvum* is unknown.

Absorption, distribution, and excretion

Oral absorption of spiramycin is variable but is less than 50% in most patients. The drug is distributed to many tissues but does not enter the cerebrospinal fluid to any significant degree. Spiramycin is concentrated in bile and excreted almost exclusively by that route. Very little drug appears in urine.

Toxicity

Nausea, vomiting, diarrhea, and indigestion are common side effects. Fatigue and altered sensation have also been reported.

Sulfadiazine

Sulfadiazine is a sulfonamide used in combination with pyrimethamine to treat toxoplasmosis. The fixed combination of pyrimethamine and sulfadoxine (Fansidar) (see Table 38-3) may be substituted. For a full description of the properties of sulfadiazine, see Chapter 34.

Sulfadoxine

Sulfadoxine is a sulfonamide frequently used in combination with pyrimethamine to treat chloroquine-resistant *P. falciparum* malaria (see Table 38-3). For a full description of the properties of sulfadoxine, see the previous discussion of pyrimethamine in this chapter and Chapter 34.

Sulfamethoxazole and Trimethoprim

Sulfamethoxazole and trimethoprim are used in combination to treat pneumocystosis (see Table 38-2). For a full description of these drugs, see Chapter 34.

Tetracycline

Tetracycline is a broad-spectrum antibacterial agent also used to treat amebic infestations (see Table 38-1). For a full description of this agent, see Chapter 32.

Thiabendazole

Mechanism of action

Thiabendazole is an extremely potent and specific anthelminthic agent (see Table 38-4). Its exact mechanism of action is unknown, but it is believed to attack a metabolic process essential in helminths but not found in humans.

Absorption, distribution, and excretion

Thiabendazole is well absorbed after oral administration, and peak blood levels may be expected within 1 hr of ingestion. Most of the drug is eliminated by hydroxylation in conjugation, these metabolites being the predominant forms of the drug excreted in urine. Very little unchanged drug appears in feces.

Toxicity

Thiabendazole can cause a wide variety of transient, dose-related toxic reactions. The most common reactions are anorexia, nausea, vomiting, and dizziness. A few patients experience more severe GI symptoms or CNS effects such as drowsiness, headache, or giddiness. Rarely, patients suffer tinnitus, abnormal sensations in the eyes, numbness, or metabolic derangements. Although these symptoms may incapacitate a patient, it is rare for the effect to persist beyond 48 hr, and most side effects subside much sooner.

Thiabendazole alters liver function in some patients. Therefore patients with preexisting liver disease should be more carefully observed for progressive liver damage.

Patients frequently report a strong, unpleasant urine odor after thiabendazole therapy. The odor is reminiscent of that produced when asparagus is ingested. Patients may be reassured that this odor is harmless and is caused by a metabolite of thiabendazole.

NURSING IMPLICATIONS SUMMARY

Drugs to Treat Protozoal and Helminthic Infestations

Patient and family education

◆ Review the information given in Table 38-5 about frequently encountered toxicities. Encourage patients to report any unexpected sign or symptom.

◆ Remind patients to keep these and all medications out of the reach of children. Many of the medications are available in pleasant-tasting syrups or chewable tablets, which may tempt young children.

◆ Many of the problems discussed in this chapter require treatment of an entire family. Doses of medication for children may be quite different than adult doses. Emphasize the importance of taking doses as prescribed.

◆ Remind patients to keep all health-care providers informed of all drugs being used or that have been used in the preceding 6 months.

◆ Most of these drugs are not recommended for use during pregnancy unless absolutely necessary and should not be used during lactation. Question female patients about possible pregnancy before administering drug.

◆ Reinforce to patients the need to continue the course of medication for as long as prescribed and to avoid discontinuing medications without notifying the physician.

◆ Remind patients to use medications only as directed. Many of these drugs are dispensed with patient information leaflets; review these with patients before discharge.

◆ Review with patients and families appropriate ways to treat or prevent the problem. Review as appropriate activities such as hand washing, sanitation, and cleaning infected bedding or clothing. Be nonjudgmental and supportive. Obtain information about diseases caused by protozoa and helminths from the local health department or the Centers for Disease Control in Atlanta. Refer patients as appropriate to the local health department for follow-up.

◆ Suggest to patients considering international travel that they may wish to contact the Centers for Disease Control about health hazards in countries they will be visiting.

◆ For patients taking antimalarial drugs for prophylaxis, make certain they understand the dosing schedule. Some drugs may be prescribed to be taken once a week.

Individual Drugs

Any drug not listed below is discussed fully in the text or is similar to others in its class.

4-Aminoquinolones (chloroquine and hydroxychloroquine)

Drug administration

◆ Assess patients for visual changes; signs of depression such as withdrawal, lack of interest in personal appearance, insomnia or anorexia; and hearing acuity.

◆ Monitor blood pressure and ECG (when patients are on long-term therapy), complete blood count (CBC) and differential, platelet count, serum creatinine level, and BUN level.

Patient and family education

◆ Review common side effects. Instruct patients to report signs of blood dyscrasia including pallor, malaise, sore throat, fever, and unexplained bleeding or bruising.

◆ Since many CNS side effects have been reported, including personality changes, teach family members to report any persistent personality changes, apathy, agitation, or irritation.

◆ Caution patients to avoid driving or operating hazardous equipment if visual changes occur; notify the physician. Encourage patients on long-term therapy to have periodic ophthalmic examinations.

◆ If hearing loss develops, notify the physician.

◆ Take doses with milk, meals or a snack to lessen gastric irritation. Report persistent or severe gastric irritation to the physician.

Dehydroemetine

Drug administration

◆ Review text for a discussion of side effects. Assess mental status and neurologic status; observe for signs of depression such as withdrawal, change in affect, lack of interest in personal appearance, and insomnia; and assess for skin changes and rashes. Monitor blood pressure and pulse. Monitor continuous ECG if possible, or at least serial ECG tracings. Monitor intake and output and weight.

◆ Monitor serum electrolyte, BUN, and serum creatinine levels and liver function tests.

Patient and family education

◆ Review with patients the anticipated benefits and possible side effects of drug therapy.

NURSING IMPLICATIONS SUMMARY—cont'd

◆ Consult with the physician, then review with the patient any limitations of activity.

Diloxanide

Patient and family education

◆ Instruct patients to report new signs and symptoms.
◆ If double vision or blurred vision develop, caution patients to avoid driving or operating hazardous equipment; notify the physician.
◆ If nausea and vomiting are severe or persistent, notify the physician.

Furazolidone

Drug administration and patient and family education

◆ Assess for nausea and vomiting. If persistent or severe, notify the physician.
◆ Review information on nitrofurans in Chapter 34.
◆ Review Patient Problem: Disulfiram-like Reactions on p. 614. Instruct patients to avoid alcohol while taking this drug and for 4 days after finishing therapy.
◆ Review Dietary Consideration: Tyramine on p. 642.
◆ Instruct diabetic patients to monitor blood glucose levels carefully; this drug may cause hypoglycemia.
◆ Tell patients that urine may be dark yellow or brown while taking this drug.
◆ Doses may be taken with food.

Iodoquinol

Drug administration

◆ Assess and monitor neurologic function. Assess for visual changes. Inspect for skin changes, rashes, and skin discoloration.
◆ Monitor intake and output and weight.

Patient and family education

◆ Review anticipated benefits and possible side effects of drug therapy.
◆ Tablets may be crushed and mixed with applesauce or chocolate syrup. Review with patients how to crush tablets, if necessary.
◆ Teach patients to take doses after meals.
◆ Because iodoquinol can interfere with thyroid function tests, remind patients to keep all health-care providers informed for at least 6 months after therapy with iodoquinol is completed that this drug has been taken.
◆ Caution patients to avoid driving or operating hazardous equipment if visual changes occur; notify the physician.

Ivermectin

Patient and family education

◆ Caution patients to avoid driving or operating hazardous equipment if visual changes occur; notify the physician.
◆ Review Patient Problem: Orthostatic Hypotension on p. 234.
◆ Instruct patients to notify the physician if any unexpected signs or symptoms develop.

Mebendazole

Patient and family education

◆ Tell patients to report any unexpected signs or symptoms.
◆ Warn patients to avoid driving or operating hazardous equipment if visual changes occur; notify the physician.
◆ Notify the physician if severe or persistent GI symptoms occur.
◆ Tablets may be chewed, swallowed whole, or crushed and mixed with food. Take doses with meals.

Mefloquine

Patient and family education

◆ Caution patients to avoid driving or operating hazardous equipment if visual changes, vertigo, or light-headedness occur; notify the physician.
◆ Take doses of mefloquine at least 12 hr after the last dose of quinidine or quinine, if both drugs are prescribed.

Metronidazole

Drug administration

◆ Assess for signs of depression such as withdrawal, change in affect, insomnia, anorexia, and lack of interest in personal appearance; assess and monitor neurologic status.

INTRAVENOUS METRONIDAZOLE

◆ Review manufacturer's instructions about reconstitution of IV doses. Do not use syringes with aluminum needles or hubs. Administer prepared dose over at least 1 hr; dose may also be given as a continuous infusion.
◆ Instruct the patient to report redness or pain in the extremity.
◆ Superinfection can occur. Assess for *Candida* overgrowth in mouth or vagina; assess for diarrhea.

Continued.

NURSING IMPLICATIONS SUMMARY—cont'd

Patient and family education

- Review anticipated benefits and possible side effects of drug therapy.
- Avoid drinking alcohol while taking metronidazole. See Patient Problem: Disulfiramlike Reactions on p. 614.
- See Patient Problems: Vaginal Infections on p. 518 and Dry Mouth on p. 166.
- For vaginal dryness, suggest that women use a commercially available lubricant designed for vaginal mucosa.
- Warn patients to avoid driving or operating hazardous equipment if visual changes or dizziness occur; notify the physician.
- Warn patients that urine may temporarily turn reddish brown because of the drug.
- Tactfully assess changes in libido. Provide emotional support as appropriate. Remind patients not to discontinue drug therapy without notifying the physician.

Niclosamide

Patient and family education

- Warn patients to avoid driving or operating hazardous equipment if visual changes occur; notify the physician.
- Instruct the patient to report any unexpected finding.
- Tell the patient to take doses after a light meal to avoid gastric upset.
- Instruct the patient to chew tablets well before swallowing. For small children, crush tablet and mix with water to form a paste.

Pentamidine

Drug administration

- With aerosolized doses, toxicity is less common. Monitor pulse, blood pressure, and respiratory rate. Auscultate lung sounds.
- With systemic administration, assess for signs of hypoglycemia such as pallor, perspiration, tachycardia, palpitations, nervousness, irritability, weakness, trembling, hunger, headache, blurred vision, cycloplegia, incoherent speech, emotional changes, and fatigue. Monitor blood glucose levels.
- Assess for skin changes.
- Monitor intake and output and weight.
- Monitor serum creatinine and BUN levels, CBC and differential, and serum electrolyte level.
- Warn patients that IM injections may cause a burning sensation and tenderness at the injection site. Use meticulous technique to avoid abscess formation.

PARENTERAL ADMINISTRATION

- Review manufacturer's insert for current guidelines. Keep patient supine. Monitor blood pressure before administering and at 5 to 15 min intervals. Monitor ECG if patient condition warrants it. Administer IV doses over 60 min. Monitor IV administration sites, and instruct patients to report pain or irritation.
- Have drugs, equipment, and personnel available to treat acute allergic reactions in the setting where pentamidine is administered.

Patient and family education

- Instruct patients to report any unexpected side effects.
- Review Patient Problems: Bleeding Tendencies on p. 570 and Depressed White Blood Cell Production on p. 560.

Piperazine

Drug administration and patient and family education

- Instruct patients to report any unexpected signs or symptoms.
- Notify physician if GI symptoms are severe or persistent.
- Take doses after meals or a snack to lessen gastric irritation.

Povidone-Iodine

Drug administration and patient and family education

- Assess for history of iodine allergy before administering drug.
- Ascertain that the patient knows how to administer a vaginal douche before discharging to home. Consult fundamentals of nursing tests. See Patient Problem: Vaginal Infections on p. 518.
- Povidone-iodine preparations will not stain the skin and should not stain clothing or bed linens. Patients may wish to wear a sanitary napkin, however, to keep the medication off linens or clothing. Instruct patients to change pad as needed or at least a couple of times daily.

Praziquantel

Patient and family education

- Warn patients to avoid driving or operating hazardous equipment if visual changes occur; notify the physician.

NURSING IMPLICATIONS SUMMARY—cont'd

◆ Tell patients not to chew tablets but to swallow them whole. Suggest that patients take doses during meals to avoid a bitter taste in the mouth.

◆ Instruct patients to notify the physician if unexpected signs or symptoms develop.

Primaquine

Drug administration and patient and family education

◆ Monitor CBC and differential and platelet count.

◆ Warn patients to avoid driving or operating hazardous equipment if visual changes occur; notify the physician.

◆ Instruct patients to take doses with meals or antacids to reduce gastric distress. Patients should notify the physician if gastric distress is severe or persistent.

◆ Tell the patient to report any new side effect.

Pyrantel Pamoate

Patient and family education

◆ Tell patients to notify the physician if new side effects develop.

◆ Instruct patients to take doses on a full or empty stomach, with or without beverages.

Pyrimethamine

Drug administration

◆ Assess and monitor neurologic status; assess for skin changes.

◆ Monitor CBC and differential and platelet count.

Patient and family education

◆ Remind patients to report any new side effects to the physician.

◆ Warn patients to avoid driving or operating hazardous equipment if excessive fatigue develops; notify the physician.

◆ See Patient Problem: Photosensitivity on p. 629.

◆ Instruct patients to take oral doses with meals, if desired. Tablets may be crushed to make a suspension; consult the pharmacist. If GI symptoms are severe or persistent, notify the physician.

◆ Leucovorin is discussed in Chapter 22.

Pyrvinium

Patient and family education

◆ Warn patients about the red discoloration of feces and vomitus.

◆ Warn patients not to chew the tablets but to swallow them whole.

◆ See Patient Problem: Photosensitivity on p. 629.

◆ Warn patients not to drive or operate hazardous equipment if dizziness develops; notify the physician.

◆ Instruct patients that all household members may have to be treated, and a second course of treatment may be needed to completely eradicate pinworm infection.

Quinacrine

Drug administration

◆ Assess and monitor mental status; assess for skin and vision changes.

◆ Monitor weight in patients on long-term therapy.

◆ Monitor CBC and differential, platelet count, and liver function tests.

Patient and family education

◆ Remind patients to report any new side effects.

◆ Warn patients to avoid driving or operating hazardous equipment if dizziness or confusion develops; notify the physician.

◆ Notify physician if GI symptoms are severe or persistent.

◆ Encourage patients to have regular ophthalmic examinations if recommended by the physician.

◆ Warn patients that this drug may cause a yellowish discoloration of the eyes, skin, or urine. This is harmless and will clear when the course of drug therapy is over. Review the drug package insert for information about treating tapeworms.

◆ Instruct patients to take doses after meals with a full glass (8 oz) of water, juice, or tea. Tablets may be crushed and mixed with jam, honey, chocolate syrup, or other sweet foods to mask the bitter taste. Mix with only a small amount, and take all of the dose as ordered.

Continued.

NURSING IMPLICATIONS SUMMARY—cont'd

Quinine

Drug administration

◆ Assess and monitor neurologic status; assess for cinchonism. Be alert to symptoms of hypoglycemia such as pallor, perspiration, tachycardia, palpitations, nervousness, emotional changes, weakness, trembling, hunger, headache, blurred vision, and incoherent speech. Monitor blood glucose levels.

◆ Monitor CBC and differential, platelet count, prothrombin time, partial thromboplastin time, and liver function tests.

INTRAVENOUS ADMINISTRATION
(QUINIDINE GLUCONATE)

◆ Dilute as directed. Administer a loading dose over 1 to 2 hr, while monitoring for hypotension and widening of the QRS interval. A constant infusion of a lower dose is administered after the loading dose. Keep the patient supine until blood pressure is stable. Keep side rails up. Monitor ECG.

Patient and family education

◆ Instruct patients to report any new side effects.

◆ Warn patients to avoid driving or operating hazardous equipment if visual changes occur; notify the physician.

◆ Take doses with meals or a snack to reduce gastric irritation. Warn diabetic patients to monitor blood glucose levels carefully.

Spiramycin

Drug administration and patient and family education

◆ Assess for side effects noted in the text.

◆ Review information about erythromycin in Chapter 31.

◆ Monitor liver function tests. Assess the following areas for hepatotoxicity: right upper quadrant abdominal pain, jaundice, nausea, vomiting, malaise, and fever.

◆ Take oral doses 2 hr before or 3 hr after meals.

Thiabendazole

Drug administration

◆ Monitor pulse and blood pressure.

◆ Monitor CBC and differential, serum creatinine and BUN levels, liver function tests, and blood glucose levels.

Patient and family education

◆ Instruct patients to report any new side effects.

◆ Warn diabetic patients to monitor blood glucose levels carefully.

◆ Warn patients to avoid driving or operating hazardous equipment if dizziness or visual changes occur; notify the physician.

◆ Take doses after meals or a snack to lessen gastric irritation.

◆ Tell patients that this drug may cause urine to have a temporary, harmless odor for up to 24 hr.

◆ For topical preparations, instruct patients to apply the medicine directly to the infected area and in a large circle around the area, up to 2 to 3 inches in each direction.

CHAPTER REVIEW

◆ KEY TERMS

amebic disease, p. 537
cestodes, p. 541
enterobiasis, p. 540
giardiasis, p. 538
helminths, p. 540
malaria, p. 538
trichomoniasis, p. 540

◆ REVIEW QUESTIONS

1. What are the main sites of amebic infection?
2. What are the two sites where plasmodia exist in the human body?
3. Where do trichomonas infections occur?
4. What type of disease is produced by *Giardia lamblia*? What patients are most at risk from toxoplasmosis?
5. What patient is most likely to contract pneumocystosis?
6. Why is threadworm infestation more serious than pinworm or whipworm infestation?
7. What is the fate of the pork roundworm in the human body?
8. What two forms of hookworm infestation occur?
9. How does the tissue distribution of the 4-aminoquinolones increase the usefulness of the drugs in treating malaria?
10. What toxicity is associated with the 4-aminoquinolones? How should you assess for these?
11. What is the major use of diloxanide?
12. What is the major use of dehydroemetine?
13. What toxicity is associated with dehydroemetine? How should you assess for this toxicity?
14. What is the mechanism of action of mebendazole?
15. How does the tissue distribution of mebendazole affect its use?
16. How does the tissue distribution of mefloquine affect its use?
17. What parasitic diseases are treated with metronidazole?
18. Why should patients receiving metronidazole avoid ethyl alcohol?
19. What is the mechanism of action of niclosamide?
20. What is the tissue distribution of orally administered niclosamide?
21. What two routes are used for pentamidine administration? Why?
22. What is the mechanism of action of praziquantel?
23. What toxicity is associated with primaquine?
24. What is the mechanism of action of pyrantel pamoate?
25. Is pyrantel pamoate absorbed from the intestinal tract?
26. What is the mechanism of action of pyrimethamine?
27. What toxicity is associated with pyrimethamine? How should you assess for it?
28. What is the mechanism of action of pyrvinium pamoate?
29. What harmless side effect of pyrivinium pamoate may be most distressing to patients?
30. What is the mechanism of action of quinacrine?
31. What reaction is common with oral administration of quinacrine?
32. What is cinchonism? How should you assess for this?
33. What transient effects follow thiabendazole administration?

SUGGESTED READING

Beck JW, Davies JE: *Medical parasitology,* ed 3, St Louis, 1981, Mosby–Year Book.

Drugs for parasitic infections, *Med Lett Drugs Ther* 34(865):March 6, 1992.

Mandell WF and others: Parasitic infections: therapeutic considerations, *Med Clin N Amer* 72(3):669, 1988.

Sheahan SL, Seabolt JP: Management of common parasitic infections encountered in primary care, *Nurse Pract* 12(8):19, 1987.

CHAPTER 39

Drugs to Treat Neoplastic Diseases

LEARNING OBJECTIVES

After studying this chapter, you should be able to do the following:

- Discuss why most anticancer drugs are toxic toward rapidly growing tissues, both normal and cancerous.

- Discuss the side effects common to most anticancer drugs.

- Discuss the risks anticancer drugs may pose to health-care personnel and how the risks can be minimized.

- Discuss the reasons for precautions to protect patients receiving anticancer drugs from exposure to infectious agents.

- Develop nursing care interventions for the patient with depressed white blood cell production, bleeding tendencies, or stomatitis.

- Develop a nursing care plan for the patient receiving one or more of the drugs discussed in this chapter.

CHAPTER OVERVIEW

◆ Neoplastic disease occurs when normal cells become transformed by chemicals, viruses, or unknown agents and thereby become resistant to normal regulation of cell division and other cellular processes. To understand cancer treatment, it is necessary to understand cell proliferation in normal and cancerous tissues. Therefore in this chapter the cell cycle and the principle of selective toxicity as applied to neoplastic disease, specific agents used in cancer therapy, and the rationale behind successful therapeutic regimens are discussed.

Nursing Process Overview
ANTINEOPLASTIC CHEMOTHERAPY
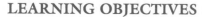
Assessment

Patients requiring chemotherapy may be of any age. Perform a thorough total assessment. Include as areas of focus probable drugs that will be used and their known side effects. Obtain a detailed history, especially if the patient has previously received chemotherapy. Previous response to chemotherapy will be a guide to anticipating response to a repeated dose of chemotherapeutic drugs. Assess laboratory work, including the hematocrit, hemoglobin, and blood count; liver function and renal function studies; and bone, liver, and other scans.

Nursing Diagnoses

Altered comfort: nausea and vomiting as drug side effect

Self-concept disturbance related to alopecia as a side effect of drug therapy

Fatigue

Management

Continue to monitor vital signs, body weight, and progress of anticipated side effects. When a side effect occurs with regularity, begin preventive or prophylactic measures as soon as possible. Monitor fluid intake and output. Monitor appropriate laboratory work, and institute nursing interventions based on that information. If medications are being adminis-

556

tered via constant infusion, use an infusion control device. Ensure that intravenous (IV) infusion lines are patent, and avoid extravasation. Investigate thoroughly any new signs or symptoms.

Evaluation

There are a few drugs that are used by the patient in the home for cancer treatment. For many patients, cancer chemotherapy is administered in the hospital or in the physician's office, since many of these drugs must be administered by IV. Before discharge, ascertain that the patient can explain how to take medications correctly, side effects that may occur, how to treat side effects, side effects that require notification of the physician, and any measures to be used to prevent complications caused by side effects. Because the nadir or most profound bone marrow suppression often occurs days to weeks after the drug is administered, the patient should know when to anticipate the side effects and what actions to take to deal with them. Teach all patients which situations require immediate notification of the physician.

THE CELL CYCLE

The cell cycle is the programmed sequence of events that occur during cell division. The cycle is divided into several segments according to the processes that occur during that phase. The first event in the cycle is a rapid increase in RNA synthesis compared to the low level of RNA formation in nonproliferating cells. RNA is formed from the sugar ribose, the purine bases adenine and guanine, and the pyrimidine bases uracil and cytosine. This phase during which RNA synthesis begins is called G_1 (Figure 39-1).

The next phase in the cell cycle is the S phase, during which DNA synthesis occurs. DNA is the nucleic acid that forms the chromosomes and contains the genetic information for the cell. DNA is formed from the same components as RNA, except that thymine is substituted for uracil, and deoxyribose is substituted for ribose.

When DNA synthesis is complete, the cell contains twice the amount of DNA found in a nondividing cell. At this point, RNA and protein synthesis increase, and the cell enters the G_2 phase. At the end of this phase the cell contains enough material to form two complete cells, and mitosis begins.

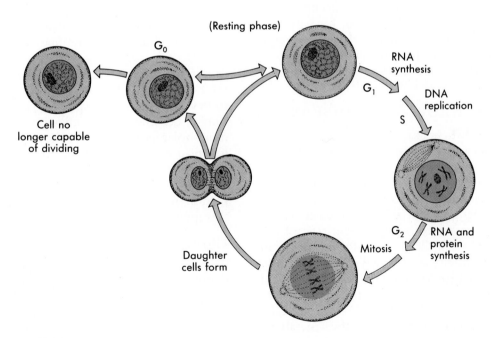

FIGURE 39-1

Proliferative cycle of mammalian cells. In actively dividing cells, metabolic processes required for cell division take place at different times during cycle. DNA synthesis precedes messenger RNA and protein synthesis; these processes must be complete before mitosis, or cell division, can occur. Because of metabolic differences, cells at different phases of cycle have different sensitivities to many drugs used to control cancer.

In **mitosis** the DNA condenses to form chromosomes. As mitosis begins the cell has two copies of each chromosome. To separate these pairs so that one copy of each chromosome goes into each daughter cell, the cell forms microtubules, which are organized into the mitotic spindle. Without the mitotic spindle to pull the chromosomes into opposite ends of the cell, reproduction would halt. Once the chromosomes have been successfully segregated into two complete sets, division is completed by closing the cell membrane to divide the mother cell into two daughter cells.

After cell division a cell may immediately reenter the reproductive cycle or may become temporarily nonreproductive. In this nonreproductive phase, called G_0, the cell does not carry out a large amount of nucleic acid or protein synthesis, although normal metabolic processes continue. A cell in the G_0 phase may become altered so that it is no longer capable of dividing, or it may, after a variable time, return to the proliferation cycle and enter phase G_1 (see Figure 39-1).

Most normal tissues have very few cells actively reproducing at any one time. Most of the cells are either temporarily or permanently incapable of division, but there are exceptions to this rule. For example, bone marrow is the site for formation of blood cells and as a result is constantly undergoing cell division. Lymphoid tissue is the site for formation of lymphocytes and monocytes and therefore has a high rate of cell division. The intestinal lining, testes, ovaries, and endometrium are all additional sites of rapid cell division.

NATURE OF NEOPLASTIC DISEASE
Origin of Cancer

Carcinogenesis is the process by which a normal cell is transformed into a cancerous cell. Agents called *carcinogens* may cause this transformation, but other factors are also involved. **Oncogenes** are altered regulatory genes that are associated with cancer. When these genes are expressed, normal regulation of cell growth is lost. As a result, the transformed cells can proliferate indefinitely, as opposed to most normal cells that do not proliferate or do so for a limited time. The altered metabolism of cancer cells reflects this commitment to proliferation. DNA and RNA synthesis is increased, along with other metabolic processes necessary for growth and cell division.

Spread of Cancer

Cancer cells lose the normal property called *contact inhibition.* Contact inhibition prevents normal cells from dividing once they have begun to be crowded together, but cancer cells continue to divide even when the pressure of the surrounding cell mass is considerable. Uncontrolled proliferation and loss of contact inhibition explain in part how a cancer develops in the human body. In certain tissues, as the cancer cell begins to proliferate in an uncontrolled manner, the cells form a solid mass and crowd surrounding normal tissue as the mass, or tumor, grows. In other tissues such as bone marrow, growth of the neoplastic cells is more diffuse, but ultimately normal tissue is overwhelmed and crowded out by the cancerous tissues.

Cancer cells can metastasize. In this process, cancer cells separate from the original mass and move directly or are carried by blood or lymph to distant sites. There the cells lodge in healthy tissue and begin to divide, thus producing a **metastasis** (secondary tumor). Tumors have been produced in experimental animals with single cancer cells. This property of cancer cells explains why cure of malignancies may require destruction of every cancer cell in the body.

Host Responses

In theory, one cancer cell left living after therapy is sufficient to cause recurrence of cancer in humans. This situation is quite different from that which occurs in antibacterial chemotherapy. With bacterial infections, therapy can be successful if the bacteria are stopped from growing long enough for the immune system to attack and eliminate the invaders. With neoplastic disease the immune system seems much less effective. One reason for this difference is that cancer cells are not easily recognized as foreign by the host immune system. Another factor that seems to lower the immune response to cancer is that as the tumors become massive, they produce a specific immune tolerance. Whatever the cause, chemotherapy for most cancers must proceed with little assistance from the host mechanism that so powerfully assists antibacterial agents. This factor helps explain why therapy for neoplastic diseases is less effective than therapy for bacterial infections.

Chemotherapy

Another difficulty in treating neoplastic diseases is that cancer cells offer fewer targets for selective toxicity than do bacterial cells. This similarity in structure and metabolic processes reminds us that cancer cells are derived from host cells. Some differences between normal and cancerous cells can be identified, but the differences are mostly quantitative rather than qualitative. Specific targets for selective toxicity are discussed with individual drug mechanisms.

Because cancer arises initially as a single transformed cell, diagnosis cannot be expected until much later in the course of the disease. A single cell after

10 cycles of cell division could be expected to produce at most 1024 cells, a mass far too small to be noticed. By the time the tumor weighs about 1 gm, it will have gone through about 30 division cycles. A 1 gm tumor is roughly 1 cm³ in volume or approximately the size of a small grape. In many locations within the body, a tumor this size may easily escape detection, yet in just 10 more cell divisions this tumor could exceed a mass of 1 kg (2.2 lb).

Most tumors do not grow nearly as rapidly as the theoretical example just cited, in which it was assumed that every cell formed immediately reentered the reproductive cycle. Certain cancers are rather slow growing and are described as having a low growth fraction. This description means that most of the tumor cells are temporarily or permanently incapable of division. Other tumors have a very fast growth rate with a high growth fraction.

Diseases Called Cancer

The public tends to think of cancer as a single disease, but it is a large family of related diseases. Cancers may be categorized according to the tissue of origin (Table 39-1). Within these large categories, many subdivisions are possible. For example, leukemias can arise from any of the various cells within the bone marrow. Therefore myelogenous leukemias (arising from myeloid tissue in the marrow), lymphocytic leukemias (arising from cells forming lymphocytes), and other forms of the disease exist.

Some tumors give rise to characteristic disease patterns. For example, Burkitt's lymphoma, Wilms' tumor, Hodgkin's disease, and choriocarcinoma all tend to strike a certain age and sex of patient (Table 39-2).

Table 39-1   Tissue of Origin for Types of Cancer

Cancer	Tissue of origin
Carcinoma	Epithelial cells (e.g., skin and mucous membranes of lung and gastrointestinal tract)
Leukemia	Blood-forming organ (e.g., bone marrow or lymphoid tissue)
Lymphoma	Lymphoid tissue
Melanoma	Pigmented skin cells
Myeloma	Bone marrow
Sarcoma	Connective tissue (e.g., bone, cartilage, and others)

Table 39-2   Selected Neoplastic Diseases

Disease	Characteristics
Burkitt's lymphoma	Rapidly growing tumor of lymphoid tissue; highly responsive to chemotherapy.
Choriocarcinoma (gestational trophoblastic tumors)	Rapidly growing tumor of embryonic cells; seeded in mother during abortion, childbirth, or after hydatidiform mole; highly responsive to chemotherapy.
Ewing's sarcoma	Rapidly growing tumor most frequently found in children; responsive to combination of surgery, radiation, and chemotherapy in early stages.
Hodgkin's disease	Tumor of the lymph nodes, spleen, and other lymphoid tissue; highly responsive to chemotherapy.
Kaposi's sarcoma	Highly malignant, metastasizing tumor usually noted on the skin of the extremities. A characteristic of AIDS patients, the tumor is also seen in older non-AIDS males.
Lymphocytic leukemia	Cancer of lymphoid tissue causing leukocytes in blood to be lymphocytes or lymphoblasts; response to therapy is best in acute form of the disease.
Myelogenous leukemia	Cancer of myeloid tissue leading to excess granular polymorphonuclear leukocytes in blood; response to therapy not as good as in lymphocytic leukemia.
Wilms' tumor	Rapidly growing tumor of children; highly responsive to combination of surgery, radiation, and chemotherapy.

SPECIFIC ANTINEOPLASTIC DRUGS
Agents that Directly Attack DNA

The genetic information necessary for cell reproduction resides in DNA. Although normal nucleated cells contain all the genetic information required to form new cells, this information is seldom expressed because normal cells in most tissues rarely divide. For this reason, damage to the DNA of many normal cells is undetectable because it is revealed only when the cell attempts to divide. This rationale explains the use of a large group of anticancer drugs called *alkylating agents*. These drugs form highly reactive compounds in the body that react with many chemicals including nucleic acids. The damage these chemicals do to DNA frequently makes the cell incapable of replication.

Alkylating agents may attack DNA in its double-stranded form, attaching various compounds to one strand or the other. Other agents may form cross-links, or chemical bonds, between the strands. Because the strands must unwind and separate during replication, cross-linking effectively blocks replication.

The specificity of agents that destroy nucleic acid is not great. All cells will suffer attack by these chemicals, although the action is lethal primarily when cells attempt division. Therefore normal tissues with high growth fractions will be expected to be most sensitive. Clinical symptoms to be expected include bone marrow suppression that produces **leukopenia** (low white cell counts) (see box), thrombocytopenia (low platelet counts) (see box), or other blood dyscrasias; mucocutaneous reactions including stomatitis (see box) or other signs; and gastrointestinal (GI) toxicity, including acute or delayed nausea and vomiting.

The alkylating agents chemically alter DNA and are mutagenic. Many of these drugs also have immunosuppressive activity. For these reasons, this class of agents can induce cancers of various types, which may show up years after exposure to the drug. Not every patient will develop a second cancer as a result of chemotherapy, but for patients exposed to alkylating agents, the risk is increased many times over

the normal low-incidence rate. The clinical properties of antineoplastic drugs that directly attack DNA are summarized in Table 39-3. Often-used drugs of this class are described more fully in the next sections.

Bleomycin

Mechanism of action. Bleomycin is a mixture of glycopeptides derived from cultures of *Streptomyces*. The drug is therefore an antibiotic (a compound produced by one life form with growth-inhibitory properties toward other life forms). Bleomycin produces breaks in DNA strands. The drug may also inhibit enzymes that normally repair damaged DNA. Bleomycin apparently attacks cells at several stages of the cell cycle. Bleomycin has been used against squamous cell carcinomas, testicular carcinomas, and lymphomas.

Absorption, distribution, and excretion. Bleomycin must be administered parenterally. Most tissues of the body rapidly inactivate bleomycin. Skin and lungs are exceptions, and the drug tends to concentrate at those sites and produce toxic reactions. Tumors tend not to inactivate bleomycin, so the drug is also concentrated there.

PATIENT PROBLEM: LEUKOPENIA

THE PROBLEM

Some drugs suppress the bone marrow, resulting in decreased production of white blood cells. With some drugs, this is a common side effect and is anticipated, as with many cancer chemotherapy drugs. With other drugs, this side effect is unexpected and occurs only occasionally. Several medical terms describe this effect including: agranulocytosis or granulocytopenia (severe reduction in granulocytes—basophils, eosinophils, and neutrophils) or neutropenia (reduction in neutrophils). The danger to the patient is the increased susceptibility to infection that results from a decreased supply of granulocytes.

SIGNS AND SYMPTOMS

Fever, sore throat, rash, malaise, chills, urinary frequency, dysuria, and altered level of consciousness. If the situation is untreated or unrecognized, the patient may develop a serious bacterial infection requiring IV drug therapy and hospitalization. The first line of treatment is to discontinue the drug causing the problem.

NURSING CARE

◆ Wash hands meticulously before caring for patients with suppressed white blood cell counts.
◆ Avoid putting patients with granulocytopenia into multibed rooms where other patients have infections. If possible, admit the patient to a private room.
◆ Use protective isolation only if necessary, since it isolates the patient from family and friends. Rather, screen visitors,

and do not permit visits from individuals with obvious colds, bronchitis, chicken pox, herpes simplex or herpes zoster, childhood infectious diseases, or any other infections.
◆ Avoid the use of rectal thermometers.
◆ Carefully assess patients who are also receiving steroids, since steroids may mask the symptoms of infection.
◆ Monitor the complete blood count (CBC), white blood cell differential, and hematocrit, hemoglobin, and platelet counts.

PATIENT AND FAMILY EDUCATION

◆ Notify the physician if symptoms develop.
◆ Monitor and record the temperature (if the patient is able).
◆ If a period of bone marrow suppression is anticipated with each course or dose of drug, find out when the nadir of bone marrow suppression will occur. The nadir is the period of greatest bone marrow suppression, or the period of lowest white blood count.
◆ If a period of suppressed white blood cell production is anticipated, as with cancer chemotherapy drugs, avoid contact with persons suffering from colds or infections during periods of greatest susceptibility.
◆ Wash hands carefully after using the bathroom and after contact with other persons. Ask family members and friends to wash hands carefully before contact with the patient.
◆ Do not bring cut flowers or fresh fruits and vegetables to the patient unless the latter are washed carefully.

PATIENT PROBLEM: STOMATITIS

THE PROBLEM

Mucosal cells lining the GI tract are sensitive to some drugs, especially many of the cytotoxic drugs used in cancer chemotherapy and gold preparations used in rheumatoid arthritis. As the mucosal cells are destroyed, there may be pain and inflammation along the entire GI tract, which is called **stomatitis.**

SIGNS AND SYMPTOMS

Inflamed oral mucous membranes, oral ulcers, areas of irritation in the mouth, pain on chewing and swallowing, anal discomfort, and pain on defecation.

PATIENT AND FAMILY EDUCATION

◆ If possible, have teeth professionally cleaned and dental caries repaired before starting drug therapy.
◆ If chewing and swallowing are painful, switch to a liquid diet, including milk shakes and ice cream. If discomfort is severe, try to maintain an intake of clear fluids of at least 2000 ml (approximately eight 8 oz glasses) per day to prevent dehydration.
◆ Try chilling food before eating it.
◆ If toothbrushing is irritating, try using swabs to clean your mouth. Avoid flossing when stomatitis is severe. Use water-spraying oral care devices on low setting only. Rinse your mouth after each meal with a mild solution of baking soda and water; baking soda, salt, and water; or hydrogen peroxide and water.
◆ Try painting your mouth with substrate of milk of magnesia up to four times per day. Allow the milk of magnesia to settle to the bottom of the bottle. Pour off the liquid portion at the top of the bottle, and paint the mouth with the white, pasty portion remaining.

◆ If a special mouthwash has been prescribed, use it as ordered. Many mouthwashes are effective only when used regularly, throughout the day. Over-the-counter (OTC) mouthwashes may be irritating because they contain alcohol; avoid them unless your doctor has prescribed them.
◆ Avoid spicy foods and foods with hard crusts or edges.
◆ Try keeping a humidifier running to keep the room air moist.
◆ Wear dentures or bridgework only while eating, and remove them at other times to decrease irritation.
◆ Keep the lips moist with lip balm or moisturizer.
◆ For anal irritation, avoid suppositories, enemas, and rectal thermometers. Try sitting in a tub of warm water several times daily. After bowel movements, clean the anal area completely; some patients find a baby wipe to be cooling for this purpose.
◆ If vaginal irritation is a problem, keep the vaginal area clean and dry, wipe from front to back, avoid soaps in the vaginal area, and pat dry. Avoid douching or using tampons. Notify the physician if vaginal discharge develops or change in the color, consistency, odor, or amount occurs. To decrease irritation during intercourse, use a commercially available, water-soluble lubricant; avoid hand lotion or petroleum jelly.

ADDITIONAL NURSING CARE MEASURES

◆ Assess the mouth of patients at high risk for stomatitis at least once each shift. In addition, inspect for oral fungal infections (thrush).
◆ Monitor intake and output.

Table 39-3 Anticancer Drugs That Directly Attack DNA

Generic name	Trade name	Administration/dosage‡	Comments
Altretamine	Hexalen	ORAL: *Adults*—260 mg/M² for 14 to 21 days/month.	Altretamine is used for ovarian carcinomas.
Bleomycin	Blenoxane*	INTRAMUSCULAR, INTRAVENOUS, SUBCUTANEOUS: *Adults and children*—0.25 to 0.50 units/ kg weekly or twice weekly initially; decreasing to 1 unit daily or 5 units weekly for maintenance.	Bleomycin is palliative therapy for lymphomas, squamous cell carcinomas, and testicular and ovarian carcinomas. Pulmonary toxicity, which may be fatal, occurs especially when the total dose exceeds 400 units.
Busulfan	Myleran*	ORAL: *Adults and children*—60 to 120 μg/ kg daily or 1.8 to 4.6 mg/M² body surface area daily. FDA Pregnancy Category D.	Busulfan may prolong survival in chronic myelocytic leukemia. Toxicity is mainly seen in bone marrow.
Carboplatin	Paraplatin*	INTRAVENOUS: *Adults*—infusion, 360 mg/M² once every 4 weeks. FDA Pregnancy Category D.	Carboplatin is palliative therapy in recurrent ovarian carcinoma. Carboplatin is similar to cisplatin but causes less renal toxicity.

*Available in Canada and United States.
†Available in Canada only.
‡The doses listed are representative. Very different doses and schedules may be indicated in specific diseases or protocols.

Continued.

Table 39-3 Anticancer Drugs That Directly Attack DNA—cont'd

Generic name	Trade name	Administration/dosage‡	Comments
Carmustine	BiCNU*	INTRAVENOUS: *Adults*—200 mg/M² as a single dose. Dose may be repeated no more frequently than every 6 weeks. FDA Pregnancy Category D.	Carmustine is palliative therapy for tumors of the central nervous system, myelomas, and lymphomas. Bone marrow suppression is delayed and may be severe.
Chlorambucil	Leukeran*	ORAL: *Adults and children*—0.1 to 0.2 mg/kg daily to treat, with smaller doses for maintenance. FDA Pregnancy Category C.	Chlorambucil is effective in treating lymphocytic leukemias and lymphomas. Bone marrow suppression is the most commonly encountered side effect.
Cisplatin	Abiplatin† Platinol* Platinol-AQ*	INTRAVENOUS: *Adults*—100 mg/M² once every 4 weeks, after heavy hydration to protect the kidneys. Doses are reduced when used in combinations.	Cisplatin is used to treat testicular cancer and carcinomas in many tissues. Renal damage may be severe. Nausea and vomiting, ototoxicity, neurotoxicity, and bone marrow suppression may occur.
Cyclophosphamide	Cytoxan* Neosar Procytox†	ORAL: *Adults and children*—1 to 5 mg/kg daily for maintenance. INTRAVENOUS: *Adults and children*—40 to 50 mg/kg total dose over 2 to 5 days for induction of remission; 3 to 5 mg/kg twice weekly for maintenance. FDA Pregnancy Category D.	Cyclophosphamide is effective in treating lymphomas, leukemias, myelomas, and certain solid tumors. Hemorrhagic cystitis, bladder fibrosis leukopenia, or cardiotoxicity may occur.
Dacarbazine	DTIC† DTIC-Dome	INTRAVENOUS: *Adults*—2 to 4.5 mg/kg for 10 days every month or 150 to 250 mg/M² for 5 days every month. FDA Pregnancy Category C.	Dacarbazine is used to treat malignant melanoma and lymphomas. Bone marrow suppression is maximal 16 to 20 days after therapy; painful tissue damage results if drug leaks from IV line into surrounding tissue.
Lomustine	CeeNU*	ORAL: *Adults*—130 mg/M² as a single dose. Repeated no more often than every 6 weeks.	Lomustine is similar in use and properties to carmustine.
Mechlorethamine or nitrogen mustard	Mustargen*	INTRAVENOUS: *Adults*—0.4 mg/kg total dose in 1 or several doses. Doses range from 6 to 10 mg/M², depending on the disease. INTRACAVITARY: *Adults*—0.2 to 0.4 mg/kg.	Mechlorethamine is used to treat Hodgkin's disease and other lymphomas; it may be palliative for some solid tumors and their pleural effusions. Bone marrow suppression begins soon after therapy; nadir is at 1 to 3 weeks.
Melphalan	Alkeran*	ORAL: *Adults*—0.15 mg/kg daily for 2 to 3 weeks or 0.25 mg/kg daily for 4 days. After recovery of the bone marrow for 1 month, 2 to 4 mg may be taken daily.	Melphalan is used to treat multiple myeloma and ovarian carcinomas. Bone marrow suppression is an expected, dose-related reaction.
Mitomycin	Mutamycin*	INTRAVENOUS: *Adults*—20 mg/M² as a single dose. Should be repeated no more frequently than every 6 to 8 weeks.	Mitomycin is used to treat GI tumors. Bone marrow suppression is gradual and progressive. Renal toxicity may occur.
Mitoxantrone	Novantrone	INTRAVENOUS: *Adults*—12 mg/M² daily for 2 or 3 days for consolidation or induction, with other drugs. FDA Pregnancy Category D.	Mitoxantrone is used in acute nonlymphocytic leukemia. Mitoxantrone causes severe myelosuppression and a high risk of infections.
Thiotepa (Triethyl-enethiophosphoramide)	Thiotepa*	INTRAVENOUS: *Adults*—0.3 to 0.8 mg/kg every 1 to 4 weeks. TOPICAL: *Adults*—30 to 60 mg in solution (sterile water) for application at tumor site	Thiotepa is palliative therapy for carcinomas and lymphomas. Bone marrow toxicity is dose related, appearing days or weeks after dose.

*Available in Canada and United States.
‡The doses listed are representative. Very different doses and schedules may be indicated in specific diseases or protocols.

Toxicity. Bleomycin often produces skin and mucous membrane changes, fever, chills, anorexia, and vomiting. Pulmonary reactions occur in 10% to 40% of treated patients, and 1% may die. Lung toxicity begins as pneumonitis and progresses to pulmonary fibrosis. Anaphylaxis may also occur. Bleomycin usually does not suppress the bone marrow.

Busulfan

Mechanism of action. Busulfan is an alkylsulfonate capable of cross-linking DNA and reacting with other substances. For reasons that are unclear, busulfan possesses a degree of selectivity that is unique among this class of drugs. Busulfan is a myelosuppressant at doses that do not significantly lower the levels of other blood cells, although platelets may be reduced. Because of this selectivity, busulfan is used in chronic myelocytic leukemia. The drug is not curative but prolongs life and improves its quality.

Absorption, distribution, and excretion. Busulfan is well absorbed orally and is used by this route in chronic intermittent therapy. The drug is highly reactive in blood and tissues and is rapidly broken down in the body to a variety of products that are excreted by the kidneys and other routes.

Toxicity. Busulfan may cause leukopenia, beginning usually 10 days after therapy. Hemorrhage may result if the drug is not discontinued. With long-term therapy, many body systems may show signs of toxicity. Busulfan may destroy large numbers of granulocytes during therapy. These dying cells release chemicals that may be converted to uric acid, excessively elevating blood levels of uric acid. To avoid the toxicity produced by uric acid, allopurinol may be given during busulfan therapy.

Carmustine and lomustine

Mechanism of action. Carmustine (BCNU) is a rapidly acting alkylating agent affecting numerous enzymes and nucleic acids. The drug can cross-link strands of DNA. Lomustine (CCNU) is chemically related to carmustine and similarly alkylates DNA and has widespread metabolic effects. One advantage carmustine and lomustine have over many other alkylating agents is that they penetrate the blood-brain barrier very well. They are therefore useful in controlling symptoms produced by tumors of the central nervous system (CNS), lymphomas, and multiple myeloma.

Absorption, distribution, and excretion. Carmustine is given by IV infusion. The drug is rapidly degraded so that only metabolites are detectable in blood or in tissues a few minutes after the dose is administered. Metabolites are excreted by the kidney for several days after therapy. These metabolites of carmustine may be the active form of the drug. Lo-

mustine is used orally, being well absorbed by that route. Once absorbed, it is metabolized and excreted similarly to carmustine.

Toxicity. Carmustine and lomustine cause a greatly delayed bone marrow suppression. After a single dose of drug, bone marrow function may fall for an extended period, reaching its lowest point 4 to 6 weeks after therapy. For this reason, doses must be given no more frequently than every 6 weeks or at more widely spaced intervals if the bone marrow does not promptly recover.

Pulmonary fibrosis may be an insidious side effect with these drugs. Cough or shortness of breath should be investigated quickly for cause. Nausea and vomiting are dose-related toxic reactions to carmustine and lomustine. Carmustine is highly irritating and may cause hyperpigmentation if it touches the skin. Pain during infusion of the drug is common. Patient discomfort can be reduced by slowing the rate of infusion of the drug and by properly diluting it before use.

Carmustine is a relatively unstable compound that decomposes in solution. The drug in the dry form in the unopened vial may also decompose at temperatures above 80° F (or 27° C). Only clear, colorless solutions freshly prepared (or stored for short periods in the cold) should be used. Lomustine capsules are relatively stable when stored at room temperature in sealed containers.

Chlorambucil

Mechanism of action. Chlorambucil is chemically related to mechlorethamine and is cytotoxic by the same mechanism. Chlorambucil is distinguished by being the slowest acting and the least toxic of the nitrogen mustard alkylating agents.

In addition to its cell cycle nonspecific cytotoxicity, chlorambucil displays a somewhat selective lympholytic action. The latter property makes chlorambucil an effective drug in treating chronic lymphocytic leukemia, Hodgkin's disease, and non-Hodgkin's lymphomas.

Absorption, distribution, and excretion. Chlorambucil is administered orally. Large doses (20 mg or more) may produce nausea and vomiting, but more common doses are well tolerated and reliably absorbed. The drug is commonly given 2 hr after the evening meal or in the morning at least 1 hr before breakfast. The drug is metabolized by the liver.

Toxicity. Chlorambucil commonly produces bone marrow suppression, although at normal doses the effects are usually mild and reversible. Chlorambucil can produce CNS stimulation, GI irritation, pulmonary fibrosis, liver toxicity, and skin reactions at high doses, but these responses are not commonly seen with normal clinical doses.

Uric acid in the blood can reach dangerous levels after chlorambucil treatment. Patients should be observed for this reaction and treated appropriately to avoid severe renal damage.

Chlorambucil is often very well tolerated when used at low doses for maintenance therapy.

Cisplatin and carboplatin

Mechanism of action. Cisplatin (CPDD) and carboplatin are platinum-containing complexes that act like alkylating agents. These drugs cross-link DNA and are not specific for cell cycle.

Cisplatin was first used to treat metastatic testicular tumors but is now also used in other genital and urinary tract tumors. Carboplatin is currently indicated only for palliative therapy in recurrent ovarian carcinoma. These drugs are investigational in other tumors.

Absorption, distribution, and excretion. Cisplatin and carboplatin must be administered intravenously. The effects of single doses last for weeks.

Toxicity. Cisplatin is a relatively toxic drug that almost always causes severe nausea and vomiting. The drug is also toxic to the renal tubule and may cause serious damage with high doses or too-frequent administration. Cisplatin causes hearing loss in the upper frequency ranges and ringing in the ears (tinnitus). Ototoxicity tends to progress with repeated doses. Myelosuppression manifested by lowered leukocyte and platelet counts persists for 3 weeks or longer after a single injection of cisplatin. Carboplatin causes dose-dependent bone marrow suppression, with leukopenia, neutropenia, thrombocytopenia, and anemia. Transfusion may be necessary.

Carboplatin causes less renal toxicity than does cisplatin and is less likely to cause severe nausea and vomiting, although most patients experience some degree of nausea with or without vomiting. Peripheral neuropathies may occur and may be irreversible with either drug. Loss of taste has also been reported. Anaphylactoid reactions may occur when cisplatin or carboplatin are given to patients who have previously received these platinum-containing agents.

Cyclophosphamide

Mechanism of action. Cyclophosphamide is a non-cytotoxic form of nitrogen mustard that must be activated by liver microsomal enzymes. Several metabolites of cyclophosphamide are formed in the liver, and at least one of these metabolites is a potent alkylating agent with activity similar to that of nitrogen mustard. Because the drug as administered is not active, it does not possess the strong vesicant activity (direct blistering and damage of tissues) seen with other nitrogen mustards. Cyclophosphamide is es-pecially effective against lymphoid or myeloid tissue proliferation. The drug is therefore useful to treat lymphomas, myeloma, and leukemias.

Absorption, distribution, and excretion. Cyclophosphamide may be used either orally or parenterally, which is a distinct advantage over most alkylating agents. Absorption by the oral route is good, with the absorbed drug passing through portal circulation directly to the liver where the drug is activated.

The metabolites of cyclophosphamide are excreted primarily in urine. The plasma half-life of the drug and metabolites is 4 to 6 hr. The metabolites are well distributed throughout the body and may enter the brain.

Toxicity. Cyclophosphamide produces all the expected side effects of nonspecific alkylating agents. Bone marrow suppression occurs and is frequently used to guide the physician in adjusting doses. In most patients the bone marrow begins to recover 7 to 10 days after the drug is discontinued.

GI toxicity with cyclophosphamide is common, usually consisting of nausea and vomiting although more severe reactions can occur. Hair loss or **alopecia** occurs with cyclophosphamide therapy much more commonly than with other drugs of this class. Most patients report regrowth of hair after therapy.

Immunosuppression is an expected side effect. The drug has been used directly for its immunosuppressive activity in rheumatoid arthritis and other nonneoplastic conditions.

Cyclophosphamide suppresses gonadal tissue, and the effects may be irreversible. Complete suppression of the menstrual cycles and of sperm formation have been reported.

Cyclophosphamide and its metabolites are excreted predominantly through the kidneys. The accumulation of these cytotoxic compounds in the bladder can produce hemorrhagic cystitis. Patients should receive ample fluids while this drug is being used and should be encouraged to void frequently to reduce damage to the bladder. Bladder fibrosis and carcinoma have increased in incidence in patients receiving long-term therapy with cyclophosphamide.

Several other drugs affect the metabolism and distribution of cyclophosphamide in the body. Allopurinol prolongs the plasma half-life of cyclophosphamide. Barbiturates induce the microsomal enzymes that activate cyclophosphamide, whereas corticosteroids and sex steroids may inhibit the enzymes and thereby lower the rate of formation of active metabolites of cyclophosphamide.

Dacarbazine

Mechanism of action. Dacarbazine apparently acts as an alkylating agent after being activated in the liver.

The drug may have other actions as well, but it clearly is cell cycle nonspecific. Dacarbazine is used to treat malignant melanoma and Hodgkin's disease.

Absorption, distribution, and excretion. Dacarbazine must be administered intravenously. The plasma half-life is about 30 min, and the drug appears to be concentrated in the liver. Dacarbazine is secreted by the renal tubule, with about half the drug dose excreted by this route. The remaining drug appears in the blood as a metabolite.

Toxicity. Dacarbazine causes delayed bone marrow toxicity (16 to 20 days after therapy). Many patients also report nausea and vomiting within a few hours after therapy. Tolerance to this symptom develops. Dacarbazine can cause severe pain and tissue damage if allowed to escape from the vein into surrounding tissues.

Mechlorethamine

Mechanism of action. Mechlorethamine (nitrogen mustard) is a potent alkylating agent that may attack DNA at one site or may cause cross-linking. Mechlorethamine is especially useful in lymphomas but may also be effective for lymphocytic or myelocytic leukemias, bronchogenic carcinoma, and malignant effusions.

Absorption, distribution, and excretion. Mechlorethamine is so highly unstable that it must be administered intravenously immediately after the solution is prepared. The drug is so highly reactive that it is destroyed within minutes of its injection into the bloodstream. No active drug appears in urine or is excreted by any other route.

Toxicity. Mechlorethamine is an extremely toxic agent with a very narrow margin of safety. Significant toxicity is to be expected in every treated patient.

Bone marrow suppression usually may be noted within a day of therapy and will progress to a nadir within 1 to 3 weeks. The platelet count may decrease sufficiently to cause bleeding gums and small subcutaneous hemorrhages. Recovery from the varied symptoms of bone marrow suppression may take several weeks.

Nausea and vomiting are acute toxic reactions commonly encountered with mechlorethamine and are thought to be triggered by a CNS mechanism. A short-acting barbiturate and an antiemetic may be required to control this reaction.

Germinal tissue may be severely damaged by mechlorethamine. Males may suffer complete arrest of spermatogenesis. Females may suffer menstrual irregularities. Fetuses of treated mothers are damaged by mechlorethamine.

Mechlorethamine may induce various malignancies. The drug is also an immunosuppressant and predisposes the patient to infections.

Mechlorethamine is a potent vesicant. Patients and medical personnel must be rigorously protected from improper contact with the drug. Because of its instability the drug must be dissolved immediately before use. The nurse or physician should wear surgical gloves for protection while the solution is being prepared and administered. Using a 10-ml sterile syringe, 10 ml of sterile water or saline should be injected into the vial. The vial should be shaken with the needle still in place and the appropriate amount of drug removed. This amount of the drug solution should be injected directly into a freely flowing IV line. This procedure avoids the danger of extravasation (leakage into tissues around the vein), which produces extreme pain and tissue destruction.

Melphalan

Mechanism of action. Melphalan (PAM, L-PAM, and phenylalanine mustard) is a derivative of nitrogen mustard that works very similarly to nitrogen mustard. Melphalan is therefore not specific for the cell cycle phase. Some difference in mechanism must exist between melphalan and cyclophosphamide, another alkylating agent, because cross-resistance between these drugs does not seem to occur. Melphalan is used for carcinomas of the reproductive tract and for multiple myeloma.

Absorption, distribution, and excretion. Melphalan is adequately absorbed orally in most patients. The drug persists in the blood longer than most alkylating agents, being detectable for up to 6 hr after a single dose.

Toxicity. Melphalan produces bone marrow suppression. Dosages are usually adjusted to produce mild leukopenia but no further damage. High doses can produce severe bone marrow depression, bleeding, and nausea and vomiting.

Mitomycin

Mechanism of action. Mitomycin is an antibiotic derived from cultures of *Streptomyces*. The drug is activated by enzymes in the body, so it becomes capable of alkylating DNA. Like other alkylating agents, mitomycin is nonspecific for cell cycle. Mitomycin seems most effective against tumors of the stomach, intestine, rectum, and pancreas, although it has been occasionally used against other tumors.

Absorption, distribution, and excretion. Mitomycin must be given intravenously because it is not absorbed orally and is highly irritating to skin and muscle. The drug apparently does not distribute to the brain.

Toxicity. Mitomycin produces severe and progressive myelosuppression. Leukopenia and thrombocytopenia occur within 3 to 8 weeks and may persist for up to 10 weeks or longer after therapy. Mitomycin should not be readministered until platelet and white cell counts show the bone marrow has recovered. Mitomycin also frequently causes nausea and vomiting, skin rashes, and alopecia. A few patients may also suffer renal failure with hemolysis, liver toxicity, and lung damage. Mitomycin also causes local necrosis if allowed to escape into cutaneous tissues during IV injection.

Mitoxantrone

Mechanism of action. Mitoxantrone reacts with DNA by an unknown mechanism. The drug is not specific for a particular phase of the cell cycle. Mitoxantrone is used in acute nonlymphocytic leukemia.

Absorption, distribution, and excretion. Mitoxantrone is available for IV use only. The drug is metabolized in the liver and excreted to some degree in bile. The small amount of drug or its metabolic products in urine add a blue-green color to urine for 24 hr after each dose.

Toxicity. Mitoxantrone is an extremely potent myelosuppressant, which limits its clinical utility. Up to two thirds of treated patients experience some signs of infection. Most patients also suffer GI irritation or distress. Approximately one third of patients experience cough or dyspnea. Cardiovascular toxicity is a risk, especially as the total dose exceeds 140 to 160 mg/kg.

Triethylenethiophosphoramide

Mechanism of action. Triethylenethiophosphoramide (Thiotepa) is the most widely used member of a class of compounds called *ethylenimines*. The drug is a nonspecific alkylating agent.

Thiotepa is not curative but may alleviate the symptoms of carcinomas, lymphomas, or malignant effusions. Because it is so nonselective, attempts are often made to apply the drug directly to the tumor when possible. For example, bladder carcinoma may be treated by instilling the drug directly into the bladder. This therapy allows high doses to be achieved at the tumor site, with lower doses escaping into systemic circulation. Because toxicity is dose related, such a treatment regimen minimizes systemic toxicity.

Absorption, distribution, and excretion. Thiotepa is administered only by parenteral injection or by topical application. The drug is relatively nonirritating and can be administered rapidly through IV lines. Impaired renal function may lower tolerance to thiotepa.

Toxicity. Thiotepa is primarily toxic to bone marrow. Because the drug produces its effects slowly, care must be taken not to excessively damage the bone marrow by too high a dose in the early stages of therapy. White blood cell counts may be used as an index of toxicity. The drug may also produce nausea and anorexia.

Agents that Block DNA Synthesis (S-phase Inhibitors)

The uncontrolled proliferation of cancerous cells is frequently expressed as rapid cell division or as a high growth fraction. This property distinguishes cancers from most normal tissues, in which a very low growth fraction is the rule. Because only cells in the S phase of the cell cycle synthesize DNA, they are most sensitive to agents that block DNA synthesis.

Drugs may block DNA synthesis in several ways. Some of the drugs in this section are specific enzyme inhibitors and prevent the action of an enzyme that is required for DNA synthesis. Other drugs that are chemically very similar to the natural purines and pyrimidines used to form DNA may be incorporated into DNA but make the DNA unstable and nonfunctional.

A cell that is not forming DNA will not be damaged by a drug that inhibits DNA synthesis. For this reason, nonproliferating cells or cells in resting phase are relatively insensitive to these drugs. These drugs are called *cycle-specific* or *phase-specific agents* because they affect primarily cells in S phase.

This property of phase specificity explains why these drugs must be given on a repeating schedule. In a single treatment, only the growing fraction of cells in the tumor will be affected. A recovery period with no drug given allows normal tissues with high growth fractions such as bone marrow to return to normal function. During this recovery period, many cells in the cancerous tissue will move from G_0 phase into the reproductive cycle. Other cells that were not in S phase during treatment continue to proliferate, and the tumor continues to grow. Repeated widely spaced doses of the drug give the maximum opportunity for the drug to catch the dividing cells in S phase when they will be sensitive.

Because the specificity of these drugs is toward any active DNA synthesis, many normal cells will be sensitive. At highest risk of toxicity are tissues with a high growth fraction. Bone marrow depression and suppression of lymphocyte formation are characteristic side effects of these drugs. Lowered lymphocyte formation reduces the ability of the patient to fight infection (immunosuppression), which may reduce the patient's chance for survival. GI mucosa also has a high growth fraction and is a target of serious toxic reactions to the drugs of this family.

The clinical properties of cycle-specific anticancer drugs are summarized in Table 39-4. Commonly used

Table 39-4   Anticancer Drugs That Block DNA Synthesis

Generic name	Trade name	Administration/dosage‡	Comments
Cytarabine, or Ara-C	Cytosar*	INTRAVENOUS BOLUS, INFUSION: *Adults and children*—100 mg/M² daily for 5 to 10 days. SUBCUTANEOUS: *Adults and children*—1 mg/kg once or twice per week. FDA Pregnancy Category D.	Cytarabine is used to induce and maintain remission in leukemia patients. Bone marrow suppression limits the use of this drug.
Floxuridine	FUDR	INTRAARTERIAL: *Adults*—0.1 to 0.3 mg/kg over 24 hr.	Floxuridine is palliative for solid tumors not treatable by other means. Toxicity as for fluorouracil.
Fludarabine	Fludara	INTRAVENOUS: *Adults*—25 mg/M² daily for 5 days; repeat monthly.	Fludarabine is used for chronic lymphocytic leukemia.
Fluorouracil, or 5-FU	Adrucil* Efudex* Fluoroplex	INTRAVENOUS: *Adults*—12 mg/kg for 4 days as initial therapy. Less frequent dosing is used for maintenance therapy. FDA Pregnancy Category D. TOPICAL: *Adults*—used as 1%, 2%, or 5% solution or cream.	Fluorouracil is palliative for solid tumors incurable by surgery or other means. GI and hematologic toxicity limit the use of this drug. Topical fluorouracil is used to treat multiple actinic (solar) keratoses. Local reactions include pain and dermatitis.
Hydroxyurea	Hydrea*	ORAL: *Adults*—doses range from 20 to 30 mg/kg daily up to 80 mg/kg every 3 days.	Hydroxyurea is used to treat melanoma, myelocytic leukemia, and carcinomas. Bone marrow suppression occurs.
Mercaptopurine	Puri-nethol*	ORAL: *Adults and children over 5 years*—2.5 mg/kg/day initially. May continue for weeks if toxicity does not supervene. FDA Pregnancy Category D.	Mercaptopurine produces remissions in leukemias. Delayed hematologic toxicity limits use of this drug; immunosuppression occurs.
Methotrexate*	Folex Mexate	ORAL: *Adults and children*—2.5 to 30 mg, dose and interval depending on disease. INTRAMUSCULAR: *Adults and children*—15 to 30 mg daily. INTRAVENOUS: *Adults*—0.4 to 2 mg/kg. INTRATHECAL: *Adults and children*—0.2 to 0.5 mg/kg up to 15 mg total. FDA Pregnancy Category X.	Methotrexate can cure choriocarcinoma; maintains remissions in lymphocytic leukemia; is palliative for lymphomas and carcinomas. GI toxicity frequently limits the use of this drug; bone marrow depression is also common, increasing susceptibility to infections.
Procarbazine hydrochloride	Matulane Natulan†	ORAL: *Adults*—2 to 4 mg/kg daily for 1 week; then 4 to 6 mg/kg daily until bone marrow toxicity occurs. On recovery of marrow, doses are 50 to 100 mg daily. *Children*—50 to 100 mg daily.	Procarbazine is palliative for Hodgkin's disease, lymphomas, and brain tumors. Bone marrow depression is used to guide dosage adjustments.
Thioguanine	Lanvis† Thioguanine	ORAL: *Adults*—2 mg/kg daily initially. May continue for weeks if toxicity does not supervene.	Thioguanine is used for myelocytic leukemia. Delayed hematologic toxicity occurs.

*Available in Canada and United States.
†Available in Canada only.
‡The doses listed are representative. Very different doses and schedules may be indicated in specific diseases or protocols.

drugs of this class are fully described in the following sections.

Cytarabine

Mechanism of action. Cytarabine is a chemical analogue of cytidine, a normal component of DNA. Cytarabine resembles cytidine well enough to interfere with the function of the enzyme DNA polymerase, which inserts cytidine into DNA but which cannot insert cytarabine. Therefore cytarabine slows or stops DNA synthesis. Although cytarabine has been tested in other tumors, it is used almost exclusively in leukemias. A related drug, fludarabine, is used in chronic lymphocytic leukemia (see Table 39-4).

Absorption, distribution, and excretion. Cytarabine must be injected, either subcutaneously, intrathecally, or intravenously. Subcutaneous injections are used only to maintain remissions and are given once or twice a week.

IV cytarabine may be given as a rapid bolus or as a slow continuous infusion. When it is given rapidly, higher doses may be tolerated, although nausea and vomiting are usually triggered. Infusion of the daily dose of the drug can take place over a 1-hr period or longer.

Cytarabine is rapidly inactivated by enzymes that deaminate the molecule. Blood and liver enzymes apparently contribute to this process.

Cytarabine does not easily pass into the cerebrospinal fluid. If it is administered intrathecally, it may persist in cerebrospinal fluid for several hours because that fluid has little of the deaminating enzyme that inactivates cytarabine.

Toxicity. Cytarabine is a potent bone marrow suppressant, acting on that tissue by the same mechanism effective in cancer cells. Most treatment programs call for increasing the dose of cytarabine until toxicity to the bone marrow becomes intolerable. Bone marrow depression is most profound 1 to 3 weeks after the drug is stopped. Recovery of marrow function takes at least 1 month for most patients and longer for those receiving the drug for extended periods. Cytarabine also causes significant GI toxicity in many patients. Some may suffer perforation or necrosis of the bowel. CNS toxicity is reported in up to 10% of treated patients.

Fluorouracil and floxuridine

Mechanism of action. Fluorouracil and floxuridine are synthetic pyrimidine bases that may be converted in the body to an active agent (floxuridine monophosphate). This active form of fluorouracil resembles the pyrimidine that is directly incorporated into RNA or that is converted to the pyrimidine thymi-

dylate. Thymidylate is used exclusively for DNA synthesis. Fluorouracil and floxuridine disrupt these pathways in at least two ways. First, the activated drug may enter RNA, creating a defective form of that nucleic acid that does not allow normal protein synthesis. Second, thymidylate synthase, the enzyme required to form thymidylate for DNA synthesis, is inhibited. With thymidylate synthase blocked, DNA synthesis halts. Therefore functionally both fluorouracil and floxuridine are S-phase inhibitors. Fluorouracil and floxuridine are used exclusively in solid tumors, and both must be considered palliative rather than curative.

Absorption, distribution, and excretion. Fluorouracil absorption by the oral route is erratic, and the drug is commonly given intravenously. For most patients, best results seem to be produced by giving loading doses intravenously for 4 consecutive days and then tapering to weekly maintenance doses.

Fluorouracil is extensively metabolized by the liver and other tissues. Less than 15% of the drug dose appears as active drug in the urine. Fluorouracil is cleared from the blood within 3 hr of an IV injection, but the effects persist longer.

The route of administration of floxuridine determines its metabolic fate and its effectiveness. If floxuridine is given intravenously by rapid injection, it is broken down to fluorouracil and thence to the normal breakdown products of fluorouracil. When floxuridine is given slowly by intraarterial infusion, metabolism to fluorouracil is minimized, and most of the drug is converted to floxuridine monophosphate. The intraarterial route requires a lower dose yet is more effective than IV administration.

Toxicity. Fluorouracil and floxuridine are highly toxic to the GI tract. Inflammation of the membranes of the mouth and pharynx may be an early sign of such toxicity. Nausea, vomiting, and diarrhea almost always occur, and if the drug is not discontinued, duodenal ulcers may occur and the bowel may perforate. Patients with preexisting poor nutritional status are at much greater risk with these drugs and are usually not considered candidates for therapy.

Blood dyscrasias also occur with fluorouracil and floxuridine and may cause termination of therapy. Leukopenia continues for 1 or 2 weeks after therapy is terminated. Various skin reactions and alopecia also occur but are not serious enough to cause the drug to be discontinued.

Hydroxyurea

Mechanism of action. Hydroxyurea inhibits the enzyme that converts ribonucleotide precursors of RNA to deoxyribonucleotides, which form DNA. Hydroxyurea inhibition of the enzyme blocks DNA synthesis. Hydroxyurea is specific for the S phase of the cell cycle. Hydroxyurea has been used to treat melanoma, myelocytic leukemias, and carcinoma of the ovary and has been combined with radiation therapy to treat head and neck carcinomas.

Absorption, distribution, and excretion. Hydroxyurea is well absorbed when given orally. The drug is excreted by the kidneys. Therefore patients with impaired renal function may be more sensitive to the drug than normal patients.

Toxicity. Hydroxyurea produces bone marrow suppression as the most common side effect. This reaction is reversible. GI disturbances, renal impairment, and skin reactions are reported less frequently.

Mercaptopurine and thioguanine

Mechanism of action. Mercaptopurine (6-Mercaptopurine and 6-MP) resembles adenine and guanine and blocks several points in the synthesis of these nucleic acid precursors. Thioguanine (TG and 6-TG) blocks two reactions, which are also sensitive to mercaptopurine. As a result of the blockade of purine synthesis, DNA synthesis is blocked by either drug. Therefore both mercaptopurine and thioguanine are S-phase specific inhibitors. Mercaptopurine is used for acute leukemias.

Absorption, distribution, and excretion. Mercaptopurine is adequately absorbed from the GI tract after oral dosage. The drug has a half-life of about 90 min in blood. Part of the dose is excreted by the kidney, but significant metabolic degradation also occurs. Mercaptopurine produces remissions in leukemias, being most effective in acute lymphoblastic leukemias of childhood. The properties of thioguanine are similar to those of mercaptopurine.

Toxicity. Bone marrow suppression may occur with mercaptopurine or thioguanine. Anemia may contribute to weakness and to fatigue.

Mercaptopurine is an immunosuppressant. This action of the drug may reduce host immune defenses and contribute to increased risk of infection in treated patients.

Mercaptopurine toxicity may be greatly increased by concomitant treatment with allopurinol. Allopurinol blocks uric acid synthesis and is frequently used to prevent toxic accumulation of that substance after extensive tumor cell destruction by chemotherapy. However, allopurinol also inhibits the metabolism of mercaptopurine. Therefore when the drugs are combined, more mercaptopurine persists in the bloodstream and in tissues for longer periods, and greater toxicity results. Thioguanine metabolism is not significantly affected by allopurinol.

Methotrexate

Mechanism of action. Methotrexate is commonly described as a folic acid antagonist because it prevents the regeneration of the metabolically active form of folic acid, tetrahydrofolate (THF). Without THF, cells cannot carry out carbon-transfer reactions, and normal metabolism is blocked at several points. One of these blockades prevents the formation of thymidylic acid, and another arrests adenine and guanine nucleotide synthesis in an early state. Without these precursors, DNA synthesis halts. Methotrexate is therefore specific for the S phase of the cell cycle.

Methotrexate is particularly effective in treating choriocarcinoma, an invasive tumor arising from disseminated fetal cells in new mothers. The drug is also used against a variety of other solid tumors. The most common current use is in maintaining remissions in various leukemias, especially acute lymphoblastic leukemia of childhood.

Absorption, distribution, and excretion. Methotrexate may be administered by oral, IM, IV, intra-arterial, or intrathecal routes. For many patients, the oral route is satisfactory because effective serum concentrations are reached within 1 hr. Parenteral administration results in a slightly faster absorption rate. The intrathecal route is required to treat leukemias that have penetrated the CNS. Methotrexate does not pass from the blood into cerebropsinal fluid in useful amounts.

Methotrexate is well distributed throughout the body and may accumulate to a degree in some tissues. Liver cells seem especially able to bind the drug for long periods. It also persists in the kidneys. These tissue sites of drug accumulation normally account for a small fraction of the total dose of methotrexate. Most of the drug is excreted directly in urine. The body apparently degrades methotrexate little, if at all, and the excreted drug is unchanged.

Toxicity. Methotrexate produces the classic signs of toxicity for drugs of this class. The rapidly dividing tissues of the GI mucosal lining are severely damaged. Stomatitis and diarrhea are common signs of toxicity that call for discontinuation of the drug. If therapy continues after these symptoms arise, severe GI damage, including perforation, can result.

Bone marrow function is also compromised with methotrexate. The result, as with other drugs of this class, is leukopenia. Other blood changes may occur and may ultimately produce uncontrolled bleeding (see box). Methotrexate is an immunosuppressant and may damage the body's ability to fight infection.

The effectiveness and toxicity of methotrexate may be affected by a variety of other drugs. Salicylates (e.g., aspirin), sulfonamides, phenytoin, tetracycline, and chloramphenicol all tend to increase methotrex-

---

PATIENT PROBLEM: BLEEDING TENDENCIES

May be caused by anticoagulant therapy or low platelet count (thrombocytopenia)

THE PROBLEM
The platelet level is low, so the patient bleeds easily, or the patient is receiving anticoagulant therapy to thin the blood.

SIGNS AND SYMPTOMS
Bruising; petechiae (minute, pinhead size hemorrhagic spots on the skin; seen only with reduced platelets); bleeding such as bleeding gums or nose bleeds (epistaxis); change in the color of urine which might indicate bleeding in the kidney; anal bleeding; and bleeding in stools.

PATIENT AND FAMILY EDUCATION
◆ Notify the physician if unexplained or excessive bleeding or bruising develops.
◆ Avoid using a razor with a blade; use an electric razor.
◆ If gums are bleeding, stop flossing teeth until gums no longer bleed. Use a soft-bristle toothbrush. If brushing causes bleeding, stop brushing and use a water-spraying oral-care device if available.
◆ Permit only experienced professionals to draw blood from your veins.
◆ Do not go barefoot, since foot injuries may be associated with excessive bruising or bleeding.
◆ Do not permit intramuscular (IM) injections if you are receiving anticoagulants or know your platelet count is below 60,000.
◆ Avoid getting constipated; drink plenty of fluids, stay active within the guidelines, drink fruit juices, and eat fruit and fiber. Do not use enemas unless told to do so by the physician.
◆ If you develop a headache or stiff neck, notify the physician.

◆ Wear a medical identification tag or bracelet identifying the medications you are receiving or that you have a low platelet count.
◆ Avoid using aspirin and OTC medications unless approved by the physician.

SPECIFICALLY FOR PATIENTS WITH LOW PLATELET COUNTS
◆ Keep track of platelet counts by maintaining close contact with the physician. When the platelet count is below 10,000 to 15,000, stop flossing teeth and use water-spraying oral care devices on low only. When the platelet count drops to 5000 to 10,000, stop brushing teeth, and clean the mouth with a swab or 4 × 4 gauze pad using a mild mouthwash or saline solution. Avoid mouthwashes containing alcohol or lemon-glycerin swabs.
◆ Consider limiting activities. The following is one regimen prepared by the American Cancer Society:
For platelet counts of 100,000 to 250,000, avoid contact sports; tennis, jogging, and basketball are permitted.
For platelet counts of 50,000 to 100,000, continue with moderate activity including walking, swimming, and usual activities of daily living.
For platelet counts below 50,000, only mild activities are permitted such as walking, light housework, or yardwork.

ADDITIONAL GUIDELINES FOR THE NURSE
◆ Check stools for occult blood, and monitor urinalysis.
◆ Inspect venipuncture sites for hematoma; apply pressure for at least 10 min after venipuncture to limit hematoma formation at venipuncture sites.
◆ Handle patients gently. Avoid restraints; if used, pad and inspect under restraints every 2 hr. Keep side rails padded.

---

ate toxicity by displacing methotrexate from plasma proteins. The increase in free plasma methotrexate frequently produces toxicity. Probenecid and other drugs excreted by renal tubular secretion may block the excretion of methotrexate and thereby increase toxicity of the drug.

Methotrexate produces its cytotoxic effects by blocking the regeneration of THF. It is therefore possible to prevent the action of the drug by supplying the body with THF. This use has been exploited for treating methotrexate overdose. Tumors such as osteosarcoma are now treated with massive doses of methotrexate. Under ordinary circumstances, these doses would destroy the bone marrow and would be lethal. However, if the patient receives IV leucovorin (citrovorum factor), an agent containing THF, and other forms of folic acid, the bone marrow can be protected. This type of therapy is called *citrovorum,* or *leucovorin, rescue.*

Procarbazine hydrochloride
Mechanism of action. Procarbazine has multiple effects on cellular enzyme systems and nucleic acids. It apparently oxidizes nucleic acids. In addition, nucleic acid synthesis is inhibited. Procarbazine is especially useful in Hodgkin's disease.

Absorption, distribution, and excretion. Procarbazine is well absorbed after oral administration. The drug rapidly equilibrates between plasma and cerebrospinal fluid, so it is potentially useful in brain tumors. Procarbazine is converted to an active metabolite by the liver and is excreted primarily by the kidneys.

Toxicity. Procarbazine frequently produces bone marrow depression and immune suppression. CNS stimulation or anemia may also occur.

Procarbazine inhibits monoamine oxidase. Patients should therefore not receive both procarbazine and drugs that elevate biogenic amine levels (e.g., sympathomimetics, tricyclic antidepressants, phenothiazines, and tyramine-containing food). Ethyl alcohol can produce a disulfiram-like reaction.

Agents that Block RNA or Protein Synthesis

The rapid proliferation of cancer cells can be inhibited by agents that block RNA formation or interfere with the use of RNA as a template for protein synthesis. These agents are not highly specific for cancer cells but rather interfere with RNA and protein synthesis in any rapidly dividing tissue. The exception to this rule is asparaginase, a drug with some selectivity for cancer cells. The clinical properties of these drugs are summarized in Table 39-5.

Asparaginase

Mechanism of action. Asparaginase is an enzyme that converts the amino acid asparagine to aspartic acid. The therapeutic effect of this agent arises because many types of cancer cells cannot form asparagine. The enzyme destroys circulating asparagine,

Table 39-5 Anticancer Drugs That Block RNA and Protein Synthesis

Generic name	Trade name	Administration/dosage‡	Comments
Asparaginase	Elspar Kidrolase†	INTRAMUSCULAR: *Children*—6000 i.u. (international units)/M² with other drugs. INTRAVENOUS: *Adults and children*—200 i.u./kg daily for 28 days. FDA Pregnancy Category C.	Asparaginase induces remissions in acute lymphocytic leukemia in children. Allergy to asparaginase occurs frequently and may include anaphylaxis.
Dactinomycin	Cosmegen*	INTRAVENOUS: *Adults*—0.5 mg/M² once weekly for 3 weeks. FDA Pregnancy Category C. *Children*—0.015 mg/kg or 0.45 mg/M² for 5 days.	Dactinomycin is used to treat choriocarcinoma, Wilms' tumor, sarcomas, and carcinomas. Bone marrow depression, GI irritation, and skin reactions are common.
Daunorubicin	Cerubidine*	INTRAVENOUS: *Adult*—45 mg/M² daily for 3 days. May be repeated every 3 to 6 weeks, but lifetime dose should not exceed 550 mg/M². FDA Pregnancy Category D. *Children*—25 mg/M² once weekly, with vincristine and prednisone.	Daunorubicin is used primarily for leukemias and neuroblastoma. Toxicity is as for doxorubicin.
Doxorubicin	Adriamycin*	INTRAVENOUS: *Adults*—60 to 75 mg/M² as a single injection repeated no more often than every 3 weeks. *Children*—30 mg/M² daily for 3 days; repeat every 4 weeks.	Doxorubicin is effective against leukemias, lymphomas, sarcomas, and carcinomas. Bone marrow depression and GI irritation are common. Heart toxicity occurs especially when total doses approach 500 mg/M².
Epirubicin	Pharmorubicin†	INTRAVENOUS: *Adults*—75 to 90 mg/M²; repeat every 3 weeks.	Epirubicin is used for carcinomas of the breast.
Idarubicin	Idamycin	INTRAVENOUS: *Adults*—12 mg/M² daily for 3 days. FDA Pregnancy Category D.	Idarubicin is used for acute myelocytic leukemia. Severe leukopenia and thrombocytopenia occur in all patients.
Plicamycin	Mithracin	INTRAVENOUS: *Adults*—0.025 to 0.050 mg/kg every other day for 8 doses. FDA Pregnancy Category X.	Plicamycin is used to treat embryonal cell carcinoma and metastatic bone tumors associated with hypercalcemia. Plicamycin produces GI, skin, liver, and kidney toxicity. Severe bleeding episodes may occur.

*Available in Canada and United States.
†Available in Canada only.
‡The doses listed are representative. Very different doses and schedules may be indicated in specific diseases or protocols.

starving the cancer cells for asparagine. Normal cells are spared because they can form asparagine internally.

To be most effective, asparagine starvation should occur in the G_1 phase of the cell cycle. If asparagine levels are kept low during that period, the asparagine-dependent cancer cell will be unable to carry out protein synthesis and, ultimately, RNA and DNA synthesis will cease. If asparagine starvation occurs later in the cell cycle after many critical proteins and nucleic acids have been formed, the cell may not die. Asparaginase is most effective in acute lymphocytic leukemia.

Absorption, distribution, and excretion. Asparaginase is a protein and must therefore be administered by parenteral routes. The drug persists in blood for extended periods and is slowly eliminated. It does not enter cerebrospinal fluid in useful amounts and is not excreted in urine.

Toxicity. Asparaginase produces a wide range of toxic reactions. Because the drug is a protein, it is an effective antigen and may provoke severe allergic reactions. Renal and hepatic function may be impaired, and some patients suffer bleeding episodes, since the drug suppresses various clotting factors. Hyperglycemia has also been observed. Many patients show signs of CNS toxicity, including depression, lowered consciousness, and coma. Asparaginase toxicity is increased by vincristine or prednisone. Nevertheless, these drugs are cautiously used together in certain combination treatment regimens.

Dactinomycin

Mechanism of action. Dactinomycin (actinomyin D) is an antibiotic derived from *Streptomyces*. The drug binds strongly to double-stranded DNA and prevents the DNA from serving as a template for RNA synthesis. The cell, unable to form messenger RNA, is thus unable to synthesize proteins and to complete cell division.

Dactinomycin produces remission of choriocarcinoma, Wilms' tumor, and specific carcinomas and sarcomas.

Absorption, distribution, and excretion. Dactinomycin is not well absorbed from the GI tract. The drug is also extremely corrosive to soft tissues and must therefore be given only by the IV route. Dactinomycin is rapidly cleared from blood, entering the liver and other tissues. The drug does not cross the blood-brain barrier in effective amounts. Excretion of dactinomycin is mainly into bile, with smaller amounts of unchanged drug also appearing in urine.

Toxicity. Dactinomycin is very toxic and must be administered with great care. The highly corrosive nature of the compound makes it imperative that IV

injection be given properly, with no leakage of drug into tissues surrounding the vein. Such extravasation can cause extensive tissue damage.

Dactinomycin causes significant hematologic changes, which may include aplastic anemia. These blood changes are most pronounced several days after therapy.

GI toxicity is severe with dactinomycin. Patients may experience extreme nausea and vomiting within hours of drug administration. Phenothiazine antiemetics may be required to control vomiting. Dactinomycin also irritates the lining of the entire GI tract. Patients commonly report lip inflammation (cheilitis), difficulty in swallowing (dysphagia), mouth sores (ulcerative stomatitis), inflammation of the pharynx (pharyngitis), abdominal pain, and anal inflammation (proctitis).

Dactinomycin also severely damages hair follicles, causing alopecia. The drug may cause reddening of the skin (erythema) and signs of inflammation, especially in an area also receiving irradiation.

Doxorubicin and daunorubicin

Mechanisms of action. Doxorubicin and daunorubicin are antibiotics derived from cultures of *Streptomyces*. These drugs bind strongly to double-stranded DNA and thus stop the formation of RNA. Cells are most markedly affected by these drugs during S and G_2 phases of the cell cycle.

Doxorubicin has a wide range of antitumor activity, including leukemias, lymphomas, sarcomas, genitourinary carcinomas, squamous cell carcinomas of the head and neck, and lung cancer. Daunorubicin has been used primarily in leukemias and neuroblastoma. Idarubicin, which has very similar properties to doxorubicin and daunorubicin, is used primarily for acute myelocytic leukemia. A related compound, epirubicin (Pharmorubicin), has been used in Canada for carcinoma of the breast.

Absorption, distribution, and excretion. These drugs are not well absorbed orally, are highly irritating to skin and soft tissues, and must therefore be given intravenously. The drug enters any tissues and organs, but it is the liver that metabolizes it rapidly and extensively. Active and inactive metabolites are formed. Most drug elimination occurs through the liver. These drugs do not readily enter the CNS.

Toxicity. Doxorubicin causes delayed leukopenia and other blood changes. Damage to bone marrow limits the amount of drug that may be used and the frequency of administration. Ordinarily, 21 days will be required for the bone marrow to recover. Toxicity to the heart also limits the total amount of drug that can be administered. Total doses of more than 550 mg/M^2 may produce irreversible toxicity to the heart, including ECG changes and congestive heart failure. Preexisting heart disease, prior irradiation to the region of the heart, or prior use of the cardiotoxic drugs cyclophosphamide, mitomycin, or dactinomycin may greatly increase the likelihood for heart damage with doxorubicin.

Because doxorubicin is metabolized and eliminated by the liver, patients with impaired liver function may suffer drug accumulation and increased toxicity unless doses are appropriately reduced. Some metabolites of doxorubicin and daunorubicin appear in urine of all treated patients and produce a harmless, red coloration of urine. Doxorubicin can cause severe tissue necrosis if allowed to escape from the vein during drug administration. Damage to veins may occur if the same vein is used repeatedly. Alopecia and GI irritation commonly occur with doxorubicin. Daunorubicin and idarubicin cause side effects similar to those of doxorubicin.

Plicamycin

Mechanism of action. Plicamycin is an antibiotic derived from *Streptomyces*. The drug binds DNA, thereby preventing RNA synthesis. Plicamycin also blocks parathyroid hormone activity on osteoclasts, thereby lowering the release of calcium into the bloodstream. This ability to lower blood calcium levels may be useful in patients suffering hypercalcemia as a result of metastatic cancer of the bone. Plicamycin also treats embryonal cell carcinoma of the testes.

Absorption, distribution, and excretion. Plicamycin must be given intravenously, since oral absorption is poor. It damages skin and muscle tissues.

Toxicity. Plicamycin is a very toxic drug whose use must be limited to specific neoplasms in which the beneficial results of therapy are known to outweigh the risks. Plicamycin produces anorexia, nausea, vomiting, skin changes, liver damage, kidney damage, and lowered blood concentrations of calcium, potassium, and phosphorus.

Plicamycin also produces an unusual syndrome involving episodes of bleeding from various sites. Nosebleed (epistaxis) frequently signals the onset of this syndrome. The condition may stabilize after a few episodes or may progress to extensive hemorrhage, usually within the GI tract, and death.

Agents that Arrest Mitosis

To segregate chromosomes, a dividing cell must form a mitotic spindle composed of microtubules. Microtubules normally function as part of the cytoplasmic transport systems in cells and are required for certain types of cell movement. The major component of microtubules is the protein tubulin.

The structure of microtubules can be disrupted by certain substances that bind to tubulin and cause it to be released from the microtubule. Breakdown of microtubular structure may not be lethal to a cell, unless it is in the process of forming the mitotic spindle. Cells exposed at this stage of division are arrested at that point, and reproduction cannot proceed. Ultimately, these cells die. Substances that act in this way are frequently referred to as *mitotic poisons*. The clinical properties of mitotic poisons and related compunds used to treat cancer are summarized in Table 39-6.

Vincristine

Mechanism of action. Vincristine (VCR) crystallizes microtubular and spindle proteins, halting cell division in the midst of mitosis. Vincristine, which is a complex alkaloid obtained from the periwinkle plant, is especially effective against lymphomas and lymphoblastic leukemias but is also used to treat various carcinomas and sarcomas. A related drug, vindesine (Eldisine), has been used in Canada against acute lymphocytic leukemia.

Absorption, distribution, and excretion. Vincristine must be administered intravenously. The drug does not cross the blood-brain barrier well enough to combat CNS spread of leukemia but is well distributed to other tissues. Vincristine is rapidly cleared from blood and is concentrated in the liver. This drug is excreted primarily by bile, with less than 5% of the drug appearing in urine. Biliary obstruction or liver impairment can dangerously impede elimination of vincristine.

Toxicity. Vincristine doses are usually limited by the peripheral neuropathy it produces. Many symptoms of nerve dysfunction may be observed, but loss of the Achilles tendon reflex is viewed as the first sign of neuropathy.

Vincristine is extremely irritating if it is allowed to escape from the vein into surrounding tissues during administration. Severe pain is produced, and necrosis may develop in the exposed tissue.

Vincristine produces alopecia in approximately 20% of treated patients. Many patients complain of constipation and abdominal pain, but these symptoms can usually be relieved with enemas and laxatives. Vincristine does not produce significant bone marrow depression.

Vinblastine

Mechanism of action. Vinblastine (VLB), like the related vinca alkaloid vincristine, is a cell cycle specific inhibitor of cells in mitosis. It causes breakdown of microtubules and prevents formation of the mitotic spindle. Vinblastine treats lymphomas and certain carcinomas.

Table 39-6 Anticancer Drugs That Block Mitosis

Generic name	Trade name	Administration/dosage‡	Comments
Etoposide VP-16	VePesid*	ORAL: *Adults*—100 mg/M² daily for 5 days. Repeat every 3 to 4 weeks. INTRAVENOUS: *Adults*—50 to 100 mg/M² daily for 3 to 5 days. Repeat at 3 to 4 weeks. FDA Pregnancy Category D.	Etoposide is used for refractory testicular tumors and small-cell lung carcinoma. Bone marrow suppression is the primary toxic reaction.
Teniposide	Vumon†	INTRAVENOUS: *Adults*—up to 180 mg/M², various schedules.	Tenoposide is used in lymphomas, acute lymphocytic leukemia, and neuroblastoma.
Vinblastine (VLB)	Velban Velbe† Velsar	INTRAVENOUS: *Adults*—doses must start at 0.1 mg/kg weekly and increase gradually. Range is usually 0.15 to 0.2 mg/kg weekly.	Vinblastine is palliative for lymphomas, carcinomas, and sarcomas. Dosage is limited by bone marrow suppression.
Vincristine (VCR)	Oncovin* Vincasar Vincrex	INTRAVENOUS: *Adults*—up to 1.4 mg/M² as a single dose. *Children*—up to 2 mg/M² as a single dose. FDA Pregnancy Category D.	Vincristine is used in acute leukemia, lymphomas, sarcomas, and Wilms' tumor. Peripheral neuropathy is common and limits the drug dose.
Vindesine sulfate	Eldisine†	INTRAVENOUS: *Adults*—3 mg/M² every 7 to 10 days, for 8 doses.	Vindesine is indicated for acute lymphocytic leukemia.

*Available in Canada and United States.
†Available in Canada only.
‡The doses listed are representative. Very different doses and schedules may be indicated in specific diseases or protocols.

Absorption, distribution, and excretion. Vinblastine must be administered intravenously. Like vincristine, vinblastine does not freely enter the CNS, is rapidly cleared from the blood, and is primarily excreted in bile.

Toxicity. Vinblastine produces neurologic toxicity similar to that produced by vincristine. Mental depression and headache may accompany the signs of peripheral neuritis or other peripheral neurologic disorders.

Vinblastine produces significant bone marrow suppression, primarily leukopenia. Leukopenia normally progresses to a low point 4 to 10 days after the dosage, but recovery usually occurs within 7 to 14 days. Nausea and vomiting are frequent, but this reaction can often be controlled with antiemetic agents. Stomatitis, diarrhea, or constipation can also occur.

Vinblastine can cause phlebitis and cellulitis if it is allowed to leak into the tissues during IV administration. Alopecia is common but often reverses even while the drug therapy is continued.

Etoposide

Mechanism of action. Etoposide (VP-16) is a podophyllotoxin derivative. Podophyllotoxins are microtubule or spindle poisons that are naturally found in the American mandrake, or mayapple plant. The semisynthetic derivative etoposide prevents the entry of cells into mitosis, rather than arresting cells in metaphase. The exact mechanism of action is unknown.

Etoposide is indicated for refractory testicular tumors. It also treats small-cell lung carcinoma. A chemical relative of etoposide, teniposide (VM-26), is sold in Canada under the trade name Vumon and is used for lymphomas, leukemias, and neuroblastoma.

Absorption, distribution, and excretion. Although about 50% of a dose may be absorbed orally, etoposide is administered primarily intravenously. The drug is highly protein bound and is slowly eliminated by the kidney, mostly as unchanged drug. Etoposide is lipid soluble but is poorly distributed to the CNS.

Toxicity. Etoposide produces bone marrow suppression, anorexia, nausea, vomiting, and alopecia.

Tissue-Specific Agents

Most of the anticancer drugs discussed to this point are not tissue specific in their cytotoxic action. For example, although chlorambucil is clinically useful because it attacks lymphoid tissue, it also attacks other tissues, especially at higher doses.

A few drugs are effective anticancer agents because they interact with specific receptors on or in certain cells. Most of these drugs are derivatives of hormones and interact with those cells bearing specific receptors for the hormone. For example, glucocorticoids suppress lymphoid tissue because of the specific receptors in that tissue for glucocorticoids.

The sex steroids (androgens, estrogens, and progestins) are also used in cancer chemotherapy. These steroid hormones enter sensitive cells and, complexed with specific receptor proteins, are transported to the cell nucleus. Within the nucleus, they alter RNA and protein synthesis, thereby changing the function of the cell. The use of these agents in cancer chemotherapy depends on a knowledge of the hormone dependence of certain tissues. For example, the prostate gland depends on androgens; without these hormones, the gland shrinks and loses function. Estrogens, hormones that produce feminization, antagonize the action of androgens on the prostate. Carcinoma of the prostate gland seems to retain a degree of this hormonal control, and tumor regression can frequently be produced by suppressing androgens and supplying excess estrogens.

Similar results can be achieved in many breast carcinomas in females by treating them with estrogens, antiestrogens, or androgens. To a certain extent, hormonal therapy of tumors of the reproductive tissues is empiric. The rationale behind all forms of this therapy is that (1) reproductive tissues proliferate in response to the proper balance of male and female hormones and (2) tumors of reproductive tissues tend to retain some dependence on hormones. Tumors in postmenopausal women respond to hormone therapy better than do those in premenopausal women. The clinical properties of these tissue-specific anticancer drugs are summarized in Table 39-7.

Androgens
Mechanism of action. Androgens interact with certain reproductive tissues, altering RNA and protein synthesis. This action is independent of the cell cycle. For estrogen-dependent tissues, androgens frequently interfere with estrogen function. Androgens can therefore cause involution of these tissues. This action forms the basis for the use of androgen to control some forms of breast cancer in postmenopausal women. Results of this form of therapy usually do not become evident until after 8 weeks of treatment or longer.

Absorption, distribution, and excretion. Androgens are in general not well absorbed orally, although a few synthetic androgens are exceptions (see Table 39-7). When given by injection, these oil-soluble substances are slowly absorbed from IM sites. Androgens are metabolized by the liver. Patients with impaired renal function may have difficulty eliminating the amounts of androgen used therapeutically and may suffer excessive toxicity.

Toxicity. Androgens produce varying degrees of virilization, which in females is observed as an unwanted side effect. Increased libido, edema, hypercalcemia, nausea, and pain on injection occur occasionally with one or more of the androgens used in cancer chemotherapy. Testolactone is used almost exclusively in cancer chemotherapy. Other androgens, used primarily in replacement therapy, may occasionally be used to treat specific cancers. These drugs include fluoxymesterone, methyltestosterone, testosterone enanthate, and testosterone propionate (see Chapter 54).

Antiandrogens
Mechanism of action. Flutamide blocks uptake of androgens into cells or the binding of androgens in cell nuclei.

Leuprolide, buserelin, and goserelin are synthetic analogues of luteinizing hormone-releasing factor (LHRH) that on continuous administration suppress secretion of gonadotropin-releasing hormone. The result is lower synthesis and release of testosterone. These three agents are able to produce the same low levels of male sex steroids produced by surgical castration.

Flutamide and one of the LHRH analogues are used in combination for metastatic carcinoma of the prostate, a tumor that often depends on androgens for its growth.

Absorption, distribution, and excretion. Leuprolide, buserelin, and goserelin are peptides and therefore cannot withstand the acidic environment of the stomach. These drugs are absorbed from subcutaneous sites. Flutamide is absorbed orally but undergoes extensive metabolism in the liver.

Toxicity. When given together, flutamide and an LHRH analogue reduce testosterone levels to those expected in castrated males. Many of the side effects are the result of low testosterone levels. Hot flashes are very common. About one third of patients report reduced libido or impotence. Gynecomastia occurs in about 9% of patients. Nausea and vomiting may also occur. Diarrhea is considered to be more related to flutamide than to leuprolide.

Estrogens
Mechanism of action. Estrogens can interact with certain reproductive tissues, altering RNA and protein synthesis. This action is independent of the cell cycle. For androgen-dependent tissues, estrogens frequently interfere with androgen function. Estrogens

Table 39-7   Drugs Used to Control Cancer of Specific Tissues

Generic name	Trade name	Administration/dosage	Comments
ANDROGENS			
Testolactone	Teslac	ORAL: *Adults*—250 mg 4 times daily for 12 weeks. FDA Pregnancy Category C.	Testolactone palliates symptoms of carcinomas of the breast in postmenopausal women. Hypercalcemia may occur.
ANTIANDROGENS			
Buserelin	Suprefact†	SUBCUTANEOUS: *Adults*—0.5 mg 3 times daily for 7 days, then 0.2 mg daily to maintain.	Buserelin is a synthetic analogue of LHRH (see Chapter 50) that suppresses FSH and LH, thereby ultimately lowering testosterone levels to those seen in castrated males.
Flutamide	Euflex*	ORAL: *Adults*—250 mg every 8 hr. FDA Pregnancy Category D.	Flutamide blocks the action of androgens on target cells. Flutamide is used with leuprolide for prostatic carcinoma.
Goserelin	Zoladex*	SUBCUTANEOUS IMPLANT: *Adults*—3.6 mg base every 28 days.	Goserelin has an action similar to that of buserelin.
Leuprolide	Lupron*	SUBCUTANEOUS: *Adults*—1 mg daily.	Leuprolide suppresses secretion of androgens. Leuprolide is used with flutamide for prostatic carcinoma.
ESTROGENS			
Chlorotrianisene	TACE	ORAL: *Adults*—12 to 25 mg daily.	Chlorotrianisene is a long-acting estrogen.
Diethylstilbestrol diphosphate	Stilphostrol Honvol†	INTRAVENOUS: *Adults*—500 mg in 250 ml of saline or 5% dextrose initially, then 1 gm/250 ml diluent for 5 days. Maintain with 250 to 500 mg once or twice weekly. ORAL: *Adults*—50 to 200 mg 3 times daily.	Diethylstilbestrol is palliative for carcinoma. Increased risk of thromboembolitic disease occurs with estrogen therapy; edema, hypercalcemia, mood changes, breast tenderness, and abdominal cramps may also occur.
Estramustine phosphate sodium	Emcyt*	ORAL: 14 mg/kg body weight daily in 3 or 4 doses.	Estramustine side effects include estrogen-like and nitrogen mustard-like adverse reactions.
ANTIESTROGENS			
Tamoxifen	Nolvadex* Tamofen†	ORAL: *Adults*—10 or 20 mg twice daily. FDA Pregnancy Category D.	Tamoxifen is palliative for advanced carcinoma of the breast. Hot flashes, nausea, and vomiting occur in many patients; vaginal discharge and menstrual disturbances may also occur.
PROGESTINS			
Medroxyprogesterone acetate	Depo-Provera*	INTRAMUSCULAR: *Adults*—400 to 1000 mg in weekly injections.	Medroxyprogesterone is palliative for advanced endometrial or renal carcinomas. Menstrual irregularities and thrombolytic disease may occur.
Megestrol acetate	Megace*	ORAL: *Adults*—40 to 320 mg daily in divided doses for at least 2 months for endometrial carcinoma; 160 mg daily, divided into 4 doses, for breast cancer.	Megestrol is palliative for advanced carcinoma of the breast. Thromboembolytic disease and breast cancer may be increased.

*Available in Canada and United States.
†Available in Canada only.

Table 39-7   Drugs Used to Control Cancer of Specific Tissues—cont'd

Generic name	Trade name	Administration/dosage	Comments
GLUCOCORTICOIDS			
Prednisone	Deltasone* Meticorten	ORAL: *Adults and children*—10 to 100 mg daily.	Prednisone is used to treat lympho-blastic leukemias and lymphomas. Long-term use may cause Cushing's syndrome.
ADRENAL ANTAGONIST			
Mitotane	Lysodren*	ORAL: *Adults*—6 to 15 mg/kg initially, daily in 3 or 4 doses. Daily dose may be increased gradually to 2 to 16 gm. FDA Pregnancy Category C.	Mitotane is used to control adrenal cortical carcinoma. Adrenocortical insufficiency occurs in most patients.
Trilostane	Modrastane	ORAL: *Adults*—initially 30 mg 4 times daily, increased slowly to 90 mg 4 times daily. FDA Pregnancy Category X.	Trilostane suppresses steroid production from adrenals and tumors.
BETA-CELL ANTAGONIST			
Streptozocin	Zanosar*	INTRAVENOUS: *Adults*—1 to 1.5 gm/M^2 weekly or 500 mg/M^2 daily for 5 days at 6-week intervals. FDA Pregnancy Category C.	Streptozocin is selectively taken up by pancreatic beta cells and is used for pancreatic tumors. Renal toxicity limits its use.
INTERFERONS			
Interferon alpha-2a, recombinant	Roferon-A	INTRAMUSCULAR or SUBCUTANEOUS: *Adults*—up to 36 million units daily at intervals. FDA Pregnancy Category C.	Drug is used for hairy cell leukemia, Kaposi's sarcoma, and other tumors.
Interferon alpha-2b, recombinant	Intron A	INTRAMUSCULAR or SUBCUTANEOUS: *Adults*—up to 30 million units/M^2 3 times weekly. FDA Pregnancy Category C.	Drug is used for hairy cell leukemia, genital warts, Kaposi's sarcoma, and other tumors.
Interferon alfa-n1 (LNS)	Wellferon†	INTRAMUSCULAR OR SUBCUTANEOUS: *Adults*—up to 3 million units/M^2 at intervals.	Drug is used for hairy cell leukemia, genital warts, carcinomas, leukemias, melanoma, and lymphomas.
Interferon alfa-n3	Alferon N	SUBCUTANEOUS: *Adults*—250,000 units intralesionally twice weekly for warts; antineoplastic doses not established. FDA Pregnancy Category C.	Drug is used for hairy cell leukemia, genital warts, and other tumors.

*Available in Canada and United States.
†Available in Canada only.

can therefore cause involution of these tissues. This action forms the basis for the use of estrogens to control prostatic carcinoma. Some carcinomas of the breast also respond to exogenous estrogen therapy, especially in postmenopausal women.

Absorption, distribution, and excretion. Natural steroid estrogens are not absorbed orally, but several of the synthetic, nonsteroidal estrogens may be given successfully by this route. Estrogens are also available for IM or IV injection. Estrogens are metabolized by the liver. Patients with marked liver impairment may accumulate these compounds.

Toxicity. Estrogens increase the risks of thromboembolytic disease. Estrogens also increase salt and water retention, alter mood in some patients, decrease glucose tolerance, elevate calcium levels, produce nausea and vomiting, and cause breast tenderness and abdominal cramps. Of these reactions, thromboembolytic disease, hypercalcemia, and edema are the most threatening for cancer patients.

Of the many estrogen preparations available, three are recommended primarily for use in prostatic carcinoma (see Table 39-7). Many of the estrogens discussed in Chapter 40 may also be used in palliative therapy for prostatic carcinoma or carcinoma of the female breast.

Estramustine phosphate sodium combines estradiol with a nitrogen mustard. The rationale for the combination is that the drug will be most concentrated in estrogen-sensitive tissues, including tumors. In those tissues the anticancer effects of the estradiol and the nitrogen mustard may be focused. The toxicity of the drug is largely caused by the estrogen component because release of the active nitrogen mustard into blood is low.

Tamoxifen

Mechanism of action. Tamoxifen is an antiestrogenic substance that blocks estrogen binding at receptor sites in cells. This action prevents estrogens from supporting the growth of estrogen-dependent cells. Tamoxifen is therefore most useful in palliating symptoms of breast carcinoma in which estrogen dependence of the tumor has been established. Tamoxifen acts throughout the cell cycle.

Absorption, distribution, and excretion. Tamoxifen is administered orally. The drug is extensively metabolized. Tamoxifen and its metabolites enter the bloodstream slowly, with peak blood concentrations occurring 4 to 7 hr after an oral dose. However, the drug persists in the bloodstream for days as a result of its entry into enterohepatic circulation. Most of the drug is slowly eliminated from the body in the feces. The kidney contributes little to the excretion of this drug.

Toxicity. Tamoxifen may produce cancer and birth defects in animals. It is not known whether tamoxifen produces these effects in humans. The drug seems less toxic than the estrogens and androgens used in anticancer therapy. It may occasionally alter platelet or white cell counts, but the changes observed are mild and usually innocuous. The most frequent reactions are nausea, vomiting, and hot flashes. Fewer patients report vaginal bleeding or discharge or menstrual irregularities. These reactions do not usually require discontinuance of the drug.

Patients who are started on tamoxifen therapy sometimes report an increase in pain at the tumor site and within metastases in bone. Tumor metastases within soft tissue may temporarily increase in size, and the surrounding tissue may become inflamed. This reaction, sometimes referred to as *disease flare,* may occur even when therapy is effective.

Progestins

Mechanism of action. Progestins normally establish secretory function in the estrogen-primed endometrium. The use of progestins as antineoplastic agents has been limited primarily to palliative therapy in endometrial carcinoma.

Absorption, distribution, and excretion. Progestins are available in various forms suitable for oral or IM administration. The drugs are metabolized primarily in the liver; derivatives of progestins appear in urine.

Toxicity. Progestins usually produce few toxic reactions. Patients should be observed for signs of thromboembolytic disease or sudden changes in vision. Fluid retention and disruption of normal menstrual cycles may also occur. Progestins that are injected may cause pain and tissue changes at the injection site.

Glucocorticoids: prednisone

Mechanism of action. Glucocorticoids are steroid hormones that regulate RNA and protein synthesis in various cells. This action is independent of cell cycle. Prednisone is the glucocorticoid most commonly used as an anticancer agent, although several of these agents are used for symptomatic relief. Prednisone is an effective anticancer agent because it attacks lymphoid tissue, causing regression of that tissue. Prednisone is therefore effective against lymphoid tumors and lymphoblastic leukemias, especially in children.

Absorption, distribution, and excretion. Prednisone is effectively absorbed orally and is metabolized to the active form of the drug, prednisolone. Liver disease may impair this process and thus interfere with the effectiveness of prednisone.

Toxicity. Prednisone may produce all the well-known signs of glucocorticoid excess, if given long enough at high doses. These symptoms are outlined in Table 39-7 and also in Chapter 53.

Mitotane

Mechanism of action. Mitotane is a derivative of the insecticide DDT. Toxicity studies with DDT insecticides showed specific effects on the adrenal cortex. Mitotane causes specific atrophy of the zona fasciculata and reticularis, the two inner layers of the adrenal cortex where the glucocorticoid cortisol is formed. Mitotane is not cell cycle specific and is not a general cytotoxic agent. Because of its unusual tissue selectivity, the drug is used to treat adrenal cortical carcinoma.

Absorption, distribution, and excretion. Mitotane is satisfactorily absorbed when given orally. The drug is metabolized by the liver before excretion. If liver function is impaired, the drug may accumulate, and toxic reactions may increase.

Toxicity. Mitotane causes anorexia, nausea, and vomiting in nearly every treated patient. Nearly half of those treated experience lethargy or dizziness. Dermatitis occurs in 20% of patients. Less frequent but serious reactions include abnormalities of the eye, changes in blood pressure, and hemorrhagic cystitis.

Trilostane

Mechanism of action. Trilostane is a competitive inhibitor of enzymes involved in steroid synthesis. In the adrenal gland, it blocks cortisol synthesis in the zona fasciculata, aldosterone synthesis in the zona glomerulosa, and androstenedione synthesis in the zona reticularis (see Chapter 51). The primary use of trilostane is in Cushing's syndrome, but the drug can also be used in various carcinomas, including breast carcinoma.

Absorption, distribution, and excretion. Trilostane is absorbed after oral administration and is biotransformed by the liver.

Toxicity. Trilostane produces signs of adrenocortical insufficiency, which may include darkening of the skin, fatigue, loss of appetite, and vomiting. These symptoms require medical attention. Diarrhea and stomach pains are also relatively frequent but are usually not severe.

Streptozocin

Mechanism of action. Streptozocin is a specific toxin for the beta (β) cells of the pancreatic islets. Other cells in islets are relatively insensitive to the drug. For this reason the drug is primarily used to treat insulin-secreting islet cell tumors of the pancreas. Other uses for streptozocin are being explored.

Absorption, distribution, and excretion. Streptozocin is relatively unstable and must be administered intravenously.

Toxicity. Streptozocin can destroy β cells. Therefore insulin production may cease. The drug is also toxic to the kidneys. Streptozocin does not ordinarily affect blood-forming cells, so blood dyscrasias are rarely encountered.

Interferons

Mechanism of action. Natural interferons are produced mainly by leukocytes and serve as part of the body's defense against viruses by blocking virus proliferation in infected cells. Interferons modulate the function of macrophages and lymphocytes and have a general antiproliferative activity. The recombinant interferons share these properties.

The interferons identified as recombinant are produced by genetic engineering, which uses microorganisms to produce human proteins. The nonrecombinant interferons are produced from cultures of human cells after stimulating interferon production with *Sendai* virus.

The anticancer activity of the interferons is not completely understood. The recombinant interferons, interferon alpha-2a and interferon alpha-2b, are administered in hairy cell leukemia, genital warts, and Kaposi's sarcoma in AIDS patients. In addition, these drugs are being investigated for their activity in various lymphomas, leukemias, and solid tumors. Interferons alfa n-1 and n-3 in general have the same uses, but not all interferons have been approved for all indications listed.

Absorption, distribution, and excretion. As proteins, these interferons cannot be administered orally. Absorption is adequate from IM or subcutaneous sites, producing peak serum concentration in 4 to 7 hr. These proteins are completely metabolized in the kidney and other tissues.

Toxicity. A flulike syndrome develops in most patients but resolves within 2 to 4 weeks, even when the drug is continued. Arrhythmias have been observed. Signs of neurotoxicity may involve the CNS (depression, nervousness, and insomnia) or the periphery (numbness or tingling in extremities). Loss of appetite builds during treatment with alpha-interferons and may persist for some time after therapy ends.

COMBINATION CHEMOTHERAPY

Few of the anticancer drugs discussed in this chapter are used alone. Experience has demonstrated that combinations of these drugs are much more effective than single agents. Several reasons for this increased success exist. First, combinations of drugs acting by different mechanisms are less likely to cause drug resistance. Like microbial cells, cancer cells can adapt and become drug resistant. This process occurs easily if only a single drug is used. If several are used, the cancer cell has greater difficulty in developing simultaneous resistance.

Second, drug combinations allow the physician to select agents that produce different patterns of toxicity and thereby reduce the damage directed at any one organ system. Most of the drugs discussed produce bone marrow suppression. Combining these suppressive drugs with drugs such as bleomycin, vincristine, or prednisone, which do not damage the bone marrow, allows more anticancer effect to be achieved with no added damage to the bone marrow.

Third, combining anticancer agents that act at different stages of the cell cycle allows for more tumor cells to be killed than would occur with the use of only one drug. For example, a drug like procarbazine is specific for the S phase of the cell cycle. Therefore tumor cells that pass into that phase while exposed to procarbazine die, but cells in resting phase survive. If an alkylating agent is added to the treatment regimen, we can expect a percentage of the cells that survive procarbazine treatment to be killed by the second drug. Adding a third drug with yet a different mechanism of action such as vincristine further reduces the number of surviving cancer cells.

Finally, if it is possible to add a tissue-specific drug to the regimen, even more anticancer effect may be

Table 39-8 Combination Chemotherapeutic Regimens

Regimen	Drugs included	Disease
ABVD	Doxorubicin (Adriamycin) Bleomycin (Blenoxane) Vinblastine (Velban) Dacarbazine (DTIC-Dome)	Hodgkin's disease
CHOP	Cyclophosphamide (Cytoxan) Doxorubicin (Adriamycin) Vincristine (Oncovin) Prednisone	Non-Hodgkin's lymphomas
CMF	Cyclophosphamide (Cytoxan) Methotrexate Fluorouracil	Breast carcinoma
CVP	Cyclophosphamide (Cytoxan) Vincristine (Oncovin) Prednisone	Non-Hodgkin's lymphomas
MOPP	Mechlorethamine (Mustargen) Vincristine (Oncovin) Procarbazine hydrochloride (Matulane) Prednisone	Hodgkin's disease
POMP	Prednisone Vincristine (Oncovin) Methotrexate Mercaptopurine (Purinethol)	Acute lymphocytic leukemia

gained. An established and effective treatment regimen such as has just been described exists for Hodgkin's disease. The regimen includes the alkylating agent mechlorethamine (Mustargen), the mitotic poison vincristine (Oncovin), the DNA synthesis inhibitor procarbazine (Matulane), and the lympholytic agent prednisone. This particular regimen is abbreviated MOPP. Many other established combination therapies exist for various types of cancer (Table 39-8).

Drugs Used in Supportive Therapy of Cancer Patients

Cancer patients require many drugs during the course of their disease. The drugs previously discussed attack the cancer directly. In addition to these agents, cancer patients frequently require other drugs to relieve symptoms of the disease or to ameliorate the side effects of the highly toxic antineoplastic drugs. A brief summary of drugs used in supportive care of cancer patients follows.

Allopurinol

Allopurinol may be included in treatment programs when large tumor masses are quickly destroyed by chemotherapy, releasing many breakdown products, including uric acid. Uric acid can severely damage kidney cells if it is allowed to increase unchecked. Allopurinol inhibits the formation of uric acid and therefore can prevent this complication. Allopurinol is also used to treat gout.

Analgesics

The pain associated with advanced cancer can be severe. Therefore hospitals and hospices specializing in care for the dying cancer patient have a policy of liberal use of narcotic analgesics. Frequent administration and high doses may be required to control pain. Addiction in this patient population is not a problem; therefore fear of addiction should not prevent adequate pain control in the terminal stages of the disease.

Antiemetics

Many of the drugs used to attack cancer cells also attack the GI mucosa. Nausea and vomiting are therefore very commonly encountered as side effects of cancer chemotherapy. With some of the anticancer drugs, vomiting is so severe that it must be treated to prevent electrolyte imbalance. In other cases, it is transient and less severe. Nevertheless, control of nausea and vomiting can greatly improve the patient's sense of well-being and aid in maintaining good nutritional status.

A variety of antiemetic agents are available (see Chapter 13). The severe nausea and vomiting encountered in cancer patients receiving cytotoxic drugs frequently requires the strong antiemetic action of phenothiazines. Patients may also be sedated to control nausea.

Control of hypercalcemia

Hypercalcemia can be a dangerous side effect of cancer chemotherapy, especially when tumor metastases exist in bone. Several agents are available to protect patients from this complication. Etidronate, pamidronate, and gallium nitrate block overproduction of calcium. Plicamycin helps with this symptom and in addition has anticancer activity, as described previously.

Isotopes

The use of radioactive isotopes is generally considered palliative therapy for cancer. These agents have their effect by virtue of the ionizing radiation they release. Sodium phosphate P^{32} (^{32}P) enters forming DNA, so it tends to be concentrated where that process is highest. Clinically, the use of this drug is to attempt to control proliferation of blood cells in polycythemia vera or in myelocytic leukemia. Gold Au 198 (^{198}Au) is used to control ascites. Ascites occurs when tumor cells are widely disseminated in the abdominal cavity, and large amounts of fluid accumulate. This condition differs from edema because ascitic fluid is free within the abdominal cavity and is not trapped in tissues. Pleural effusions may also be relieved by radioactive gold. The use of ^{131}I, a radioactive isotope of iodine, to destroy overactive thyroid tissue is discussed in Chapter 52.

NURSING IMPLICATIONS SUMMARY

General Guidelines for Patients Receiving Cancer Chemotherapy

Drug administration

◆ See Patient Problems: Stomatitis on p. 561, Bleeding Tendencies on p. 570, Constipation on p. 182, and Decreased White Blood Cell count on p. 560.
◆ Many patients receiving cancer chemotherapy develop anemia, which may be due in part to anorexia, poor nutrition, and bone marrow depression. The anemia may be caused by the drugs or by the cancer.

Nursing measures to decrease anemia

◆ Assess for malaise, fatigability, and pale skin color. Monitor hematocrit and hemoglobin counts, and check stools for occult blood.
◆ Obtain a dietary history. Teach about diet and counsel as appropriate. Iron-rich foods may be unappealing if anorexia or nausea is present; see Dietary Consideration: Iron on p. 347.
◆ Encourage frequent, small feedings. See interventions under anorexia.
◆ Suggest patients eat their largest meal in the morning, before increasing fatigue makes them too tired to eat late in the day.
◆ Encourage the use of iron preparations, if prescribed, although they may have limited value until chemotherapy is completed. Fluoxymesterone (Halotestin), an androgen, or other drugs, may also be prescribed to reverse anemia.

Nursing measures to decrease anorexia

◆ Anorexia may arise from drug therapy or may be caused by the underlying disease.
◆ Assess dietary intake; monitor weight.
◆ Avoid foods having a strong odor. Cool or cold foods may be more appealing than hot foods. Red meat may be less appealing than fish or chicken.
◆ Encourage small, frequent feedings. Instruct caregivers to fix small portions in an attractive manner.
◆ If the patient craves a specific food item, it is usually permissible for the patient to have it; the alternative may be a completely skipped meal.

◆ If food preparation is tiring to the patient, suggest that the patient prepare and freeze small portions of food on days he or she feels better so that when he or she is not feeling well, it is necessary only to thaw and eat the food. Encourage interested friends and family members to prepare individual servings for the patient also. Encourage snacking and nibbling during the day. Encourage the patient to keep available in the refrigerator high-protein beverages or snacks that may be appealing such as milk shakes, eggnogs, frozen yogurt, and ice cream. Obtain recipes for high-protein snacks from dietitians, the American Cancer Society, or the oncologist's office. Some patients may wish to purchase commercially prepared high-protein supplements that can be consumed as a drink or frozen and eaten as ice cream.
◆ Although a microwave oven is not a necessity, the patient may find it helpful to have one to quickly heat food. Explore this possibility with the patient and family and community resources.
◆ Some patients may find that a small glass of sherry or wine before dinner will stimulate their appetite. Consult the psysician and the patient.

Nursing measures to decrease diarrhea

◆ Certain drugs used for cancer chemotherapy cause diarrhea. This symptom may appear within 24 to 48 hr of receiving the drug or may be delayed for 5 to 10 days.
◆ Instruct patients to switch to a clear-liquid diet or a low-residue diet high in protein and calories. Patients should try to maintain a fluid intake of at least 2000 to 2500 ml per day. Caution patients to avoid foods known to be irritating to the GI tract such as fruit, fruit juices, spicy foods, raw vegetables, corn, and coffee.
◆ Review possible clear-liquid food the patient may like such as broth, gelatin, tea, popsicles, soft drinks, and water. The patient may be able to tolerate chicken noodle soup. Although electrolyte-containing drinks such as Gatorade are not required, they may provide a pleasant-tasting alternative less irritating than fruit juice.

Continued.

NURSING IMPLICATIONS SUMMARY—cont'd

◆ Instruct the patient to notify the physician if diarrhea is severe or persists longer than 2 to 4 days.

◆ Teach the patient that diarrhea can lead to electrolyte imbalance. When possible, monitor serum electrolyte level. In severe cases the patient may need to be admitted to the hospital for IV replacement of fluids and electrolytes.

◆ Instruct the patient not to use enemas, rectal suppositories, and rectal thermometers.

◆ If anal irritation occurs, suggest that the patient shower or sit in a warm tub of water several times per day. Wash the anal area with mild soap and water, and pat the area dry gently after each loose bowel movement. Some patients may find it easier or more comfortable to wash the area with prepackaged towelettes such as those used to clean infants during diaper changes or with preparations such as Tucks.

Nursing measures to decrease nausea and vomiting

◆ Nausea and vomiting may occur within hours of receiving a dose of chemotherapy or may be delayed for 5 to 10 days.

◆ Monitor response to chemotherapy. Record on the care plan actions that seem to contribute to or lessen the incidence of nausea and vomiting.

◆ Administer antiemetics, sedatives, and other drugs as ordered to decrease nausea. They are usually more effective if administered ahead of chemotherapy or at least before severe nausea and vomiting occur, rather than afterward.

◆ Consider the following interventions: Reschedule chemotherapy time in relation to meal times, either closer to or further from usual mealtimes. Limit oral intake to clear liquids on the day of or the evening before chemotherapy. Keep the environment odor free; do not wear perfume. Have the patient avoid spicy, fatty, or greasy foods the day of or before chemotherapy.

◆ Instruct the patient and family in relaxation techniques, hypnotism, guided imagery, or distraction techniques if they are interested.

◆ Instruct the patient to report severe or persistent vomiting occurring at home to the physician, since dehydration and electrolyte imbalance may develop.

Nursing measures to decrease alopecia

◆ Alopecia (hair loss) occurs when sensitive cells in the hair follicle are damaged by chemotherapy or radiation.

◆ Before starting chemotherapy, inform patients about the possibility of alopecia. Some patients may wish to invest in a wig resembling their own hair color and style before hair loss begins. In some communities the American Cancer Society has a "wig bank" from which cancer patients can borrow wigs during periods of alopecia. Explore this possibility. In addition, some insurance companies may reimburse patients for the cost of wigs.

◆ Point out that alopecia may involve eyebrows, eyelashes, nasal hair, and pubic hair, although hair loss may be patchy rather than total in these areas.

◆ Some drugs typically cause complete baldness, including cyclophosphamide, daunorubicin, doxorubicin, vinblastine, and vincristine. Some drugs cause a moderate degree of alopecia, including busulfan, etoposide, floxuridine, methotrexate, and mitomycin. Finally, some drugs cause only mild alopecia or sporadic thinning of hair. These drugs include bleomycin, carmustine, fluorouracil, hydroxyurea, and melphalan.

◆ Reassure patients that in most cases hair will grow back after the course of chemotherapy is finished. Some patients will begin to have hair growth before the course of chemotherapy is completed; this is variable from person to person. Usually, new hair is the same color and texture as the hair that was lost, but occasionally it is different.

◆ During alopecia, instruct the patient to wash hair infrequently, every 2 to 4 days. Use a mild shampoo but not necessarily "baby shampoo," which may be a little harsh. The patient's barber or hairdresser may be able to recommend a specific product. Use a cream rinse or conditioner. If the scalp is dry, apply a thin layer of baby oil, mineral oil, or A and D ointment. Brush and comb hair gently. Do not use dyes, tints, rinses, or any unnecessary chemicals on remaining hair.

◆ Suggest that patients use satin pillow covers.

◆ Avoid direct exposure to the sun either by wearing a hat or by using a maxiumu-protection sunscreen when out of doors (SPF 15 or greater). During cold weather, wear a hat when out of doors.

NURSING IMPLICATIONS SUMMARY—cont'd

◆ When appropriate, use a head tourniquet or ice cap to reduce alopecia. These are used only with IV drugs. The tourniquet limits IV spread of the chemotherapy drug to the vessels of the scalp that supply blood to the hair. The ice cap produces vasoconstriction of the blood vessels of the scalp. The ice cap is applied 15 to 30 min before the infusion, whereas the tourniquet can be applied just before the infusion. Both are left on for 15 to 45 min after the infusion. These devices should be avoided in patients with leukemia or lymphoma or any cancer that may migrate to or be found in the scalp; check with the physician when in doubt. Inform patients that some loss will probably occur, even with the use of the ice cap or tourniquet.

Nursing measures to decrease extravasation

◆ Many cytotoxic agents are highly irritating to normal tissues. When these drugs are administered intravenously, great care must be taken to prevent them from escaping into tissues surrounding the injection site. Pain, tissue damage, and necrosis can result.

◆ Assess for signs of extravasation when administering IV chemotherapy such as redness or swelling at the insertion site, decreased infusion rate, inability to obtain return of blood, pain, or resistance during injection of medication.

◆ Try to avoid extravasation of any IV drugs, but especially alert when the following drugs are administered because of tissue necrosis and sloughing that may occur: dactinomycin, mitomycin, carmustine, cisplatin, dacarbazine, daunorubicin, plicamycin, streptozocin, mitoxantrone, vincristine, and vinblastine.

◆ In the ideal situation, perform a fresh venipuncture for administering chemotherapy. Otherwise, ascertain that the infusion line to be used is patent beforehand.

◆ Use a forearm infusion site rather than the dorsum of the hand for infusion of drugs that may cause necrosis and sloughing if extravasation occurs. Extravasation in the forearm may be less severe than in the dorsum of the hand, where muscles and tendons that control hand movement and function may be affected. Remain with the patient during the infusion.

◆ If extravasation occurs, discontinue the infusion, but leave the needle or catheter in place. Attempt to aspirate any drug that can be retrieved. Follow agency procedures for managing the situation. A typical procedure would be to administer a corticosteroid subcutaneously in the area of extravasation or via the infusion catheter that is still in place, cover the area with a topical steroid, then cover with an occlusive dressing. Finally, apply ice compresses for 15 min four times a day, and keep the extremity elevated for 48 hr. Notify the physician. Use a fresh venipuncture site for infusion of any remaining chemotherapy drug.

◆ Medical orders for treatment of extravasation should be written before infusion is begun. These orders should be readily available to all persons who administer chemotherapy. Keep drugs ordered for treatment of extravasation readily available.

Safe handling of chemotherapeutic drugs

◆ Avoid direct contact with chemotherapeutic agents, since you may be exposed to drug toxicity through repeated skin or aerosolization contact.

◆ Prepare IV medications using a laminar airflow hood. Wash hands before and after handling chemotherapy drugs.

◆ Wear disposable gloves and long-sleeved gown during drug preparation. Wear gloves during drug administration.

◆ Use correct technique to avoid skin contact with prepared dosages. Use Luer-Lok fittings whenever possible to avoid inadvertent separation of syringe and needle. Establish and follow procedures for disposal of drug containers, contaminated gloves, syringes, and IV tubing.

◆ After drawing up dosages into the syringe, discard the needle, and attach a new sterile needle to avoid skin contact with any traces of medication that might be on the outside of the first needle.

◆ Check ordered doses carefully. Several drugs have similar names.

◆ Consult the manufacturer's literature for information about dilution and rate of administration.

◆ These drugs are highly toxic. Many agencies limit the number of persons who can administer these drugs to a few nurses who have had experience and additional training in their use.

Continued.

NURSING IMPLICATIONS SUMMARY—cont'd

◆ Allergic reactions have been reported with many of these drugs. Question patients about drug allergy before administering the drug. Have drugs, equipment, and personnel available to treat an acute allergic reaction in the setting where these drugs are administered. Assess patients frequently during IV administration. Do not leave patients unattended for prolonged periods during treatment.

◆ Monitor laboratory work on an ongoing basis including complete blood count (CBC) and differential, platelet count, blood urea nitrogen (BUN) and serum creatinine serum uric acid level, and liver function tests.

◆ These drugs are contraindicated during pregnancy. Counsel about contraceptive measures as appropriate. Menstrual irregularities are common in women receiving chemotherapy. Instruct women to keep a record of menstrual periods and to consult a physician immediately if pregnancy is suspected.

◆ Chemotherapy may cause diminished production or viability of sperm. Male patients may wish to arrange for deposit of sperm in a sperm bank before beginning chemotherapy.

Nursing measures to reduce uric acid levels

◆ Elevation of uric acid levels often accompanies administration of chemotherapy to patients with leukemia or some lymphomas. This is caused by the release of large quantities of breakdown products in these rapidly dividing forms of cancer. For this reason, chemotherapy orders may routinely be accompanied by orders for allopurinol. Monitor the uric acid levels. Keep the patient well hydrated (see Chapter 23).

Patient and family education

◆ Review with patients and families the anticipated benefits and possible side effects of drug therapy. Provide support to these patients who may be facing a difficult diagnosis and anticipating serious drug side effects.

◆ Encourage the patient to notify the physician if any new side effects develop.

◆ Encourage patients to return for follow-up visits as directed. Point out to patients that many side effects may not become evident for 2 to 3 weeks after the final dose of therapy.

◆ Remind patients to inform all health-care providers of all medications being taken. This is especially important because bone marrow suppression, stomatitis, and other side effects may not appear until after the drug has been administered.

◆ Remind patients not to use over-the-counter (OTC) preparations without first consulting the physician. Emphasize the importance of keeping these and all drugs out of the reach of children.

◆ Warn patients not to receive immunizations while taking cytotoxic drugs unless first approved by the physician. Before starting chemotherapy, some physicians recommend that patients receive flu shots or update immunizations; consult the physician.

◆ Inform patients that ridges in the fingernails may appear during chemotherapy; these reflect the effect of the drugs on the dividing cells of the nails.

◆ For information about the drugs, drug protocols, protocols to treat extravasation, oral gargles, mouthwashes, dietary supplements, snack recipes, patient teaching aids, and other information for patients, families, and healthcare providers, contact the chemotherapy department of local medical centers; the American Cancer Society; the Office of Cancer Communications at the National Cancer Institute, Bethesda, MD 20892, Telephone 1-800-4-CANCER [Spanish speaking staff members are also available]; the Department of Health and Human Services; or local oncologists' offices. Refer patients as appropriate to the local visiting nurse agencies or hospice.

◆ Unless additional teaching points are listed, points on patient and family education about the drugs discussed in this chapter are the same.

Bleomycin

Drug administration

◆ See Patient Problems: Bleeding Tendencies on p. 570 and Decreased White Blood Cell Count on p. 560.

◆ See general guidelines for information about nausea and vomiting, alopecia, and stomatitis.

◆ Assess for dyspnea and cough, and auscultate lung sounds. Tell patients to report shortness of breath or difficulty breathing.

◆ Encourage patients to stop smoking.

◆ Assess for skin changes; monitor blood pressure and pulse.

NURSING IMPLICATIONS SUMMARY—cont'd

◆ Monitor CBC and differential, platelet count, and urinalysis.

Busulfan

Drug administration

◆ See the general guidelines for information about thrombocytopenia, depressed white blood cell count, anemia, elevated uric acid levels, and alopecia.

◆ Auscultate lung sounds, and assess for dyspnea and cough. Monitor weight and blood pressure. Assess for skin changes.

◆ Monitor CBC and differential, platelet count, and liver function tests.

Carmustine (BCNU) and Lomustine (CCNU)

Drug administration

◆ See the general guidelines for information about depressed white blood cell count, thrombocytopenia, anemia, nausea, and vomiting.

◆ Assess for dyspnea and cough; auscultate lung sounds. Monitor weight. Inspect for skin changes and edema.

◆ Monitor CBC and differential, platelet count, liver function tests, BUN level, and serum creatinine level.

◆ Wear gloves when preparing or administering these drugs; hyperpigmentation may occur if the drug touches the skin.

Chlorambucil

Drug administration

◆ See the general guidelines for information about nausea and vomiting, depressed white blood cell count, thrombocytopenia, and high uric acid levels.

◆ Auscultate lung sounds, and assess for dyspnea and cough. Inspect for skin changes and rash.

◆ Monitor uric acid levels, liver function tests, CBC and differential, and platelet count.

Cisplatin and Carboplatin

Drug administration

◆ See the general guidelines for information about depressed white blood cell count, thrombocytopenia, anemia, and nausea and vomiting.

◆ Assess hearing acuity, and assess for tinnitus. Refer appropriate patients for audiograms; consult the physician.

◆ Assess for metallic taste in the mouth. Since this may affect nutritional intake, monitor weight.

◆ Monitor blood pressure and pulse; auscultate lung sounds.

◆ Monitor CBC and differential, platelet count, liver function tests, BUN and serum creatinine levels, serum electrolyte level, and uric acid levels.

◆ To limit the severe nausea and vomiting that frequently accompany cisplatin administration, the regimen may include administration of metoclopramide, antiemetics, sedative, steroids, and other drugs. In addition, to limit renal toxicity, the drug is often infused with large fluid volumes, such as 250 ml/hr for 4 hr. Monitor intake and output hourly for the first 6 to 8 hr, then every 12 to 24 hr.

Cyclophosphamide

Drug administration

◆ See the general guidelines for information about depressed white blood cell count, thrombocytopenia, anemia, nausea and vomiting, diarrhea, oral ulcers, high uric acid levels, and alopecia.

◆ Auscultate lung sounds; assess for cough and dyspnea. Assess pulse and blood pressure. Monitor weight.

◆ Monitor CBC and differential, platelet count, liver function tests, serum electrolyte levels, uric acid levels, and urinalysis.

Patient and family education

◆ See the general guidelines.

◆ Teach the patient to force fluids, up to eight 8-oz glasses of water daily and to notify the physician if there is blood in urine.

◆ Warn patients that temporary changes in skin pigmentation and nails may occur.

◆ Warn patients to avoid driving or operating hazardous equipment if blurred vision, confusion, or lethargy occurs; notify the physician.

Dacarbazine

Drug administration

◆ See the general guidelines for information about depressed white blood cell count, thrombocytopenia, anemia, nausea and vomiting, and extravasation.

◆ Assess for skin changes.

◆ Monitor the CBC and differential, platelet count, liver function tests, and BUN level.

Continued.

NURSING IMPLICATIONS SUMMARY—cont'd

◆ Monitor the infusion carefully to avoid extravasation.

Patient and family education

◆ See the general guidelines.
◆ See Patient Problem: Photosensitivity on p. 629.
◆ Warn patients to avoid driving or operating hazardous equipment if blurred vision, confusion, or lethargy occurs; notify the physician.

Mechlorethamine

Drug administration

◆ See the general guidelines for information about anemia, depressed white blood cell count, thrombocytopenia, nausea and vomiting, elevated uric acid level, amenorrhea, and azoospermia. Alopecia is a rare side effect.
◆ The nadir of bone marrow suppression occurs within 1 to 3 weeks.
◆ Assess and monitor neurologic function.
◆ With IV administration, if extravasation occurs, discontinue the infusion, and aspirate any remaining drug. Promptly infiltrate the area with sterile isotonic sodium thiosulfate injection, then apply cold compresses for 6 to 12 hr.
◆ If the drug comes in contact with the skin, wash immediately with copious amounts of water for 15 min, then rinse with a 2% sodium thiosulfate solution. If the drug comes in contact with the eye, irrigate immediately with 0.9% sodium chloride or balanced salt ophthalmic solution, then promptly consult an ophthalmologist.
◆ Wear protective gloves while applying topical application. Assess for rashes. Shower or wash the area before applying the solution or ointment. Make certain the skin surfaces are dry. Apply to the prescribed areas, but apply lightly to the axillary, perineal, inguinal and inframammary areas to avoid irritation. Do not shower again until before the next dose. Topical preparations may cause the skin to darken, but this should disappear when the drug is stopped.
◆ Prepare drug just before administration.

Patient and family education

◆ See the general guidelines. Warn patients to avoid driving or operating hazardous equipment if drowsiness, vertigo, weakness, or other neurologic symptoms develop; consult the physician.

Melphalan

Drug administration

◆ See the general guidelines for information about depressed white blood cell count, thrombocytopenia, nausea and vomiting, diarrhea, and stomatitis; alopecia is uncommon.
◆ Monitor pulmonary function; auscultate lung sounds. Assess for dyspnea and cough.
◆ Inspect for skin changes.
◆ Monitor CBC and differential and platelet count.

Mitomycin

Drug administration

◆ See the general guidelines for information about depressed white blood cell count, thrombocytopenia, anemia, anorexia, nausea and vomiting, and alopecia.
◆ Auscultate lung sounds, and assess for dyspnea and cough. Monitor intake and output and weight.
◆ Monitor CBC and differential, platelet count, serum creatinine level, and BUN level.

Mitoxantrone

Drug administration

◆ See the general guidelines for information about depressed white blood cell count, thrombocytopenia, nausea and vomiting, diarrhea, stomatitis, and alopecia.
◆ Monitor intake and output and weight. Auscultate lung sounds. Inspect for edema. Monitor vital signs.
◆ Monitor the CBC and differential, platelet count, and liver function tests.
◆ Tell patients that urine may be bluish green for a day or two after therapy.

Thiotepa

Drug administration

◆ See the general guidelines for information about depressed white blood cell count, thrombocytopenia, anemia, nausea and vomiting, and stomatitis.
◆ Assess for skin changes. Assess for urinary tract problems such as urgency, frequency, and change in urine color.
◆ Monitor CBC and differential, platelet count, and urinalysis.

NURSING IMPLICATIONS SUMMARY—cont'd

Cytarabine

Drug administration

◆ See the general guidelines for information about depressed white blood cell count, thrombocytopenia, anemia, anorexia, nausea and vomiting, diarrhea, elevated uric acid levels, and alopecia.

◆ Auscultate lung sounds, and assess for dyspnea and cough. Monitor pulse and blood pressure. Assess for skin changes, and inspect for edema.

◆ Assess for changes in vision, and instruct patients to report changes in vision.

◆ Intrathecal administration may be associated with CNS side effects. Use brands and diluents that do not contain benzyl alcohol as a preservative for intrathecal administration. Keep side rails up. Anticipate CNS effects.

◆ Monitor CBC and differential, platelet count, liver function tests, serum electrolyte level, serum creatinine level, BUN level, and serum uric acid level.

Fluorouracil and Floxuridine

Drug administration

◆ See the general guidelines for information about depressed white blood cell count, thrombocytopenia, anemia, nausea and vomiting, diarrhea, and stomatitis.

◆ Assess for ataxia, and assess mental status. Inspect for skin changes. See Patient Problem: Photosensitivity on p. 629.

◆ Monitor CBC and differential and platelet count.

Hydroxyurea

Drug administration

◆ See the general guidelines for information about depressed white blood cell count, thrombocytopenia, anorexia, diarrhea, stomatitis, nausea and vomiting, elevated uric acid levels, and alopecia.

◆ Assess neurologic and mental status. Monitor weight, and inspect for skin changes and edema.

◆ Monitor CBC and differential, platelet count, serum creatinine, BUN, and uric acid levels, and liver function tests.

Mercaptopurine and Thioguanine

Drug administration

◆ See the general guidelines for information about depressed white blood cell count, thrombocytopenia, anemia, anorexia, diar-

rhea, nausea and vomiting, stomatitis, and elevated uric acid levels.

◆ Assess for skin changes.

◆ Monitor CBC and differential, platelet count, serum uric acid, serum creatinine, and BUN levels, urinalysis, and liver function tests.

Methotrexate

Drug administration

◆ See the general guidelines for information about depressed white blood cell count, thrombocytopenia, anemia, nausea and vomiting, stomatitis, diarrhea, alopecia, and elevated uric acid levels.

◆ Monitor weight; inspect for skin changes and edema.

◆ Intrathecal administration is associated with CNS changes. Monitor mental status. Keep side rails up; supervise ambulation.

◆ Monitor CBC and differential, platelet count, urinalysis, liver function tests, and serum uric acid, serum creatinine, BUN, and blood glucose levels.

◆ See leucovorin rescue discussed also in Chapter 22.

Patient and family education

◆ See the general guidelines.

◆ Warn patients to avoid driving or operating hazardous equipment if blurred vision, drowsiness, dizziness, or ataxia develops; notify the physician.

◆ Review Patient Problem: Photosensitivity on p. 629.

◆ Instruct diabetic patients to monitor blood glucose levels, since methotrexate may cause an increase requiring a change in diet or insulin dose.

Procarbazine

Drug administration

◆ See the general guidelines for information about depressed white blood cell count, thrombocytopenia, anemia, nausea and vomiting, anorexia, diarrhea, and alopecia.

◆ Assess mental status, and monitor neurologic status. Anticipate CNS side effects. Keep side rails up, supervise ambulation, and keep a night light on.

◆ Monitor pulse and blood pressure. See Patient Problem: Orthostatic Hypotension on p. 234.

◆ Auscultate lung sounds. Assess for cough and dyspnea. Inspect for skin changes.

◆ Monitor CBC and differential, platelet count, blood glucose level, and urinalysis.

Continued.

NURSING IMPLICATIONS SUMMARY—cont'd

Patient and family education

- See the general guidelines.
- Warn patients to avoid the use of alcohol; see Patient Problem: Disulfiram-Like Reactions on p. 614.
- Warn patients to avoid foods containing tyramine (see Dietary Consideration: Tyramine on p. 642).
- Warn patients to limit intake of caffeine-containing foods such as chocolate, coffee, tea, or cola drinks.
- Tell diabetic patients to monitor blood glucose levels carefully; an adjustment in diet or insulin dose may be necessary.
- Warn patients to avoid driving or operating hazardous equipment if disorientation, dizziness, or unsteadiness develops; notify the physician.

Asparaginase

Drug administration

- See the general guidelines for information about depressed white blood cell count, bleeding tendencies, anorexia, and nausea and vomiting.
- Assess neurologic and mental status. Monitor blood pressure and pulse. Monitor weight. Assess for skin changes and edema. Check stools for guaiac or occult blood.
- Monitor CBC and differential, prothrombin time, partial prothrombin times, liver function tests, and serum creatinine, BUN, blood glucose, and serum amylase levels.

Dactinomycin

Drug administration

- See the general guidelines for information about depressed white blood cell count, thrombocytopenia, anemia, nausea and vomiting, stomatitis, diarrhea, alopecia, and extravasation.
- Monitor weight, blood pressure, pulse, and intake and output. Assess for edema. Auscultate lung sounds. Inspect for skin changes.
- Monitor CBC and differential and platelet count.

Doxorubicin and Daunorubicin

Drug administration

- See the general guidelines for information about depressed white blood cell count, thrombocytopenia, anemia, elevated uric acid levels, alopecia, nausea and vomiting, stomatitis, diarrhea, and extravasation.

- Monitor pulse and blood pressure. Assess for signs of congestive heart failure such as weight gain, edema of dependent areas, dyspnea, and jugular venous distention. Auscultate lung sounds, and monitor respiratory rate. Monitor serial ECGs.
- Monitor CBC and differential, platelet count, and serum uric acid level.
- Inform patients that urine may be reddish in color for 1 to 2 days after each dose.

Plicamycin

Drug administration

- See the general guidelines for information about depressed white blood cell count, thrombocytopenia, anorexia, diarrhea, nausea and vomiting, stomatitis, and extravasation.
- Monitor mental status. Warn patients to avoid driving or operating hazardous equipment if drowsiness, dizziness, fatigue or lethargy develops; notify the physician.
- Monitor CBC and differential, platelet count, serum creatinine, BUN, and serum electrolyte levels, and urinalysis.
- Assess for hypercalcemia and hypocalcemia. See Table 17-1 for a description of common electrolyte abnormalities.
- Warn patients that plicamycin may cause intense facial flushing.

Vincristine

Drug administration

- See the general guidelines for information about anemia, extravasation, diarrhea, nausea and vomiting, stomatitis, alopecia, and elevated serum uric acid level.
- Assess neurologic and mental status. Assess for peripheral neuropathy including depressed deep tendon reflexes, changes in gait, tingling of extremities (paresthesias), and other changes in the neurologic assessment.
- Monitor intake and output, blood pressure, pulse, and respiratory rate. Auscultate lung and bowel sounds. Monitor reflexes and gait.
- Monitor CBC and serum electrolyte and uric acid levels.

Vinblastine

Drug administration

- See the general guidelines for information about depressed white blood cell count, thrombocytopenia, anemia, nausea and vomiting, anorexia, diarrhea, stomatitis, alopecia, and extravasation.

NURSING IMPLICATIONS SUMMARY—cont'd

◆ Assess neurologic and mental status. Warn patients to avoid driving or operating hazardous equipment if dizziness or numbness develops; notify the physician.
◆ Assess for peripheral neuropathy including tingling or numbness of extremities. Assess for skin changes. See Patient Problem: Photosensitivity on p. 629.
◆ Monitor CBC and differential and platelet count.

Etoposide

Drug administration

◆ See the general guidelines for information about depressed white blood cell count, thrombocytopenia, anemia, anorexia, nausea and vomiting, and alopecia.
◆ Monitor pulse, blood pressure, and weight. Auscultate lung sounds; assess for dyspnea. Monitor ECGs at regular intervals. See Patient Problem: Orthostatic Hypotension on p. 234. Assess for skin changes.
◆ Monitor CBC and differential and platelet count.

Androgens and Estrogens

◆ Estrogens are discussed in Chapter 53; androgens are discussed in Chapter 54.

Flutamide and an LHRH Analogue

Drug administration

◆ See general guidelines for information about anorexia, nausea and vomiting, and diarrhea.
◆ Consult manufacturer's literature for current information.
◆ Assess for tingling of face, fingers, and toes.
◆ Monitor pulse, blood pressure, and weight. Inspect for edema. Monitor intake and output.
◆ Auscultate lung sounds.
◆ Allergic reactions have been reported. Have patients remain in the health-care setting for at least 15 min after doses. Have drugs, equipment, and personnel available to treat an acute allergic reaction.
◆ Monitor hematocrit and hemoglobin counts and serum creatinine and BUN levels.

Patient and family education

◆ Review anticipated benefits and possible side effects of drug therapy.

◆ Assess tactfully for impotence and decreased libido, since patients may not wish to discuss them. Provide emotional support as appropriate. Remind patients not to discontinue medications without consulting the physician. Reinforce to patients the importance of taking medications as prescribed for best effect.
◆ Warn patients that hot flashes may occur as a side effect; provide support as possible.
◆ Teach patients the appropriate technique for injecting subcutaneous medications at home.
◆ Buserelin is also available as a nasal spray; review patient instruction sheet provided.
◆ Warn patients to avoid driving or operating hazardous equipment if dizziness, blurred vision, lethargy, or memory disorders occurs; notify the physician.
◆ Warn patients to notify the physician if severe or persistent bone pain develops.
◆ Review the general guidelines.

Tamoxifen

Drug administration

◆ See the general guidelines for information about depressed white blood cell count, thrombocytopenia, nausea and vomiting, and anorexia.
◆ Assess for depression including withdrawal, change in affect, lack of interest in personal appearance, insomnia, and anorexia.
◆ Assess mental status and neurologic function.
◆ Assess for hypercalcemia; see Table 17-1 for a description of common electrolyte abnormalities.
◆ Monitor weight; assess for edema. Assess visual acuity.

Patient and family education

◆ Review anticipated benefits and possible side effects of drug therapy.
◆ Warn patients to avoid driving or operating hazardous equipment if confusion, dizziness, lassitude, or light-headedness develops; notify the physician.
◆ Teach patients to increase fluid intake to 2500 to 3000 ml/day to foster calcium excretion and to help prevent constipation.
◆ Warn patients that hot flases are common; provide support as appropriate.
◆ Tell patients to notify the physician if bone pain is severe or persistent.

Continued.

Glucocorticoids and Progestins

Glucocorticoids are discussed in Chapter 51. Progestins are discussed in Chapter 53.

Mitotane

Drug administration

◆ See the general guidelines for information about depressed white blood cell count, thombocytopenia, anemia, anorexia, diarrhea, nausea and vomiting, and alopecia.

◆ Assess for depression including anorexia, insomnia, lack of interest in personal appearance, and withdrawal.

◆ Monitor blood pressure and pulse. Assess for gynecomastia in males. Inspect for skin changes.

◆ Monitor the CBC and differential, platelet count, urinalysis, and serum cholesterol level.

Patient and family education

◆ Review anticipated benefits and possible side effects of drug therapy.

◆ Warn patients to avoid driving or operating hazardous equipment if confusion, somnolence, dizziness, fatigue, or other CNS side effects develop; notify the physician.

◆ Instruct patients to wear a medical identification tag or bracelet listing their medications. In the event of trauma or other injury, it is necessary to administer glucocorticoids.

◆ Instruct patients to contact the physician if they become sick, develop an infection, or are injured, since glucocorticoids may be necessary.

Trilostane

Drug administration

◆ See the general guidelines for information about nausea and vomiting and diarrhea.

◆ Assess for electrolyte abnormalities, including hypercalcemia and hyperkalemia. See Table 17-1 for a description of common electrolyte abnormalities.

◆ Assess for signs of possible adrenocortical insufficiency such as darkening of the skin, fatigue, loss of appetite, vomiting, and hypotension. Monitor serum cortisol level. Monitor blood pressure.

◆ Inspect for skin changes.

◆ Monitor serum cortisol level, serum electrolyte level, and liver function tests.

Patient and family education

◆ Review anticipated benefits and possible side effects of drug therapy.

◆ Instruct patients taking trilostane to wear a medical identification tag or bracelet listing their medications. In the event of trauma or other injury, it would be necessary to administer glucocorticoids.

◆ Instruct patients to contact the physician if they become sick, develop an infection, or are injured, since glucocorticoids may be necessary.

◆ See the general guidelines.

Streptozocin

Drug administration

◆ See the general guidelines for information about depressed white blood cell count, thrombocytopenia, anemia, extravasation, and nausea and vomiting.

◆ Assess mental status. Watch for depression including withdrawal, anorexia, insomnia, change in affect, and lack of interest in personal appearance.

◆ Monitor intake and output and weight.

◆ Monitor CBC, differential, platelet count, serum creatinine level, BUN level, serum electrolyte level, liver function tests, and blood glucose level.

Patient and family education

◆ Review anticipated benefits and possible side effects of drug therapy.

◆ Encourage patients to increase fluid intake to 2500 ml per day.

◆ Tell diabetic patients that streptozocin may alter glucose levels. Monitor blood glucose, and adjust diet or insulin as necessary.

◆ See the general guidelines.

Other Drugs

◆ Antiemetics are discussed in Chapter 13.

◆ Allopurinol is discussed in Chapter 23.

◆ Analgesics are discussed in Chapters 23 and 44.

◆ Interferons are discussed in Chapter 28.

CHAPTER REVIEW

◆ KEY TERMS

alkylating agents, p. 559
alopecia, p. 564
carcinogenesis, p. 558
contact inhibition, p. 558
leukopenia, p. 560
metastasis, p. 558
mitosis, p. 558
oncogenes, p. 558
stomatitis, p. 561

◆ REVIEW QUESTIONS

1. What are the phases of the cell cycle, and what events take place during each phase?
2. What is carcinogenesis?
3. What properties of cancer cells allow them to spread through the body?
4. How does the growth fraction of most normal tissues differ from that of most tumors?
5. On what property of cancer cells does most cancer chemotherapy depend?
6. What is the mechanism of action of alkylating agents used as anticancer medications?
7. What normal cells are especially vulnerable to attack by alkylating agents? How should you assess for these effects?
8. What type of toxicity is most common with the use of alkylating agents?
9. Which of the alkylating agents is not a strong vesicant as administered because it must be activated by liver microsomal enzymes?
10. Which drugs that directly damage the structure of DNA do not produce bone marrow suppression?
11. What is the mechanism of action of anticancer agents that block purine and pyrimidine formation or utilization?
12. Why are inhibitors of purine and pyrimidine formation or utilization considered phase-specific agents?
13. What type of toxicity is most common with drugs that inhibit DNA synthesis? How should you assess for these effects?
14. Which anticancer drug inhibits DNA synthesis by preventing regeneration of tetrahydrofolate (THF)?
15. What is the basis of the anticancer effect of drugs that block RNA or protein synthesis?
16. What toxicity is most common with anticancer drugs that inhibit RNA or protein synthesis? How should you assess for these effects?
17. What properties of asparaginase make it unique among anticancer drugs?
18. Which anticancer drugs that inhibit RNA formation have special toxicity toward the heart?
19. What is the basis of the anticancer effects of drugs that disrupt microtubule formation?
20. What toxicity is characteristic of mitotic poisons? How should you assess for these effects?
21. Which of the mitotic poisons is not associated with bone marrow suppression?
22. What is the basis for the anticancer effects of hormones such as androgens, antiandrogens, estrogens, progestins, and glucocorticoids?
23. What is the mechanism of action of tamoxifen?
24. Mitotane is effective against what specific type of cancer?
25. What is the rationale behind combination chemotherapy in the treatment of cancer?
26. Why is allopurinol frequently used in cancer treatment programs?
27. What principle governs the use of analgesics in treating cancer patients?
28. Why are antiemetics frequently used as adjuncts to cancer chemotherapy?
29. Why are drugs to lower blood calcium levels often required in cancer patients?

SUGGESTED READING

Birdsall C, Naliboff AR: How do you manage chemotherapy extravasation? *Am J Nurs* 88(2):228, 1988.

Brown-Daniels CJ, Blasdell A: Early stage breast cancer: adjuvant drug therapy, *Am J Nurs* 90(11):32, 1990.

Camp-Sorrell D: Controlling adverse effects of chemotherapy, *Nurs 91* 21(4):34, 1991.

Cawley MM: Recent advances in chemotherapy: administration and nursing implications, *Nurs Clin North Am* 25(2):377, 1990.

Doane LS, Fisher LM, McDonald TW: How to give peritoneal chemotherapy, *Am J Nurs* 90(4):58, 1990.

Fifield MY: Relieving constipation and pain in the terminally ill, *Am J Nurs* 91(7):18, 1991.

Fuller AK: Platelet transfusion therapy for thrombocytopenia, *Semin Oncol Nurs* 6(2):123, 1990.

Haynes AL: Clinical uses of interferons, interleukins, tumor necrosis factor, monoclonal antibodies, and growth factors in patients with cancer, *J Pediatr Oncol Nurs* 7(2):54, 1990.

Hockenberry-Eaton M, Benner A: Patterns of nausea and vomiting in children: nursing assessment and intervention, *Oncol Nurs Forum* 17(4):575, 1990.

Hogan CM: Advances in the management of nausea and vomiting, *Nurs Clin North Am* 25(2):475, 1990.

Lord J, Coleman EA: Chemotherapy for glioblastoma multiforme, *J Neurosci Nurs* 23(1):69, 1991.

Malloy J: Administering intraperitoneal chemotherapy: a new approach, *Nurs 91* 21(1):58, 1991.

Moshang T Jr, Lee MM: Late effects: disorders of growth and sexual maturation associated with the treatment of childhood cancer, *J Assoc Pediatr Oncol Nurses* 5(4):20, 1988.

Petros WP, Evans WE: Pharmacokinetics and pharmacodynamics of anticancer agents: contributions to the therapy of childhood cancer, *Pharmacotherapy* 10(5):313, 1990.

Phister JE, Jue SG, Cusack BJ: Problems in the use of anticancer drugs in the elderly, *Drugs* 37(4):551, 1989.

Schlesselman SM: Helping your patient cope with alopecia, *Nurs 88* 18(12):43, 1988.

DRUGS TO TREAT MENTAL AND EMOTIONAL DISORDERS

This section presents drugs that affect behavior. Chapter 40 includes drugs used to treat insomnia and anxiety. Although barbiturates are declining in use in favor of benzodiazepines, barbiturates remain an important example of how chemical structure determines drug disposition and tolerance. Benzodiazepines are discussed with respect to their favorable therapeutic index and low abuse potential. Other sedative-hypnotic, antianxiety drugs are not presented in detail. A major emphasis is the dependency potential of the drugs and their cross-tolerance. Alcohol is presented in detail because of these factors. The importance of alcohol as a source of drug interactions and abuse is noted.

Chapter 41 presents antipsychotic drugs, with emphasis on the antagonism of the central neurotransmitters dopamine, norepinephrine, and acetylcholine in explaining the various effects of these drugs. Chapter 42 presents the major classes of antidepressant drugs; the tricyclic antidepressants, the monoamine-oxidase inhibitors, and lithium. The role of these drugs in improving the neurotransmitter functions of norepinephrine and serotonin in the central nervous system (CNS) is emphasized. Chapter 43 concentrates on the therapeutic roles of CNS stimulants in treating narcolepsy, hyperactivity, and obesity and in improving deficient respiratory drive. The abuse of amphetamine, cocaine, and caffeine is also presented.

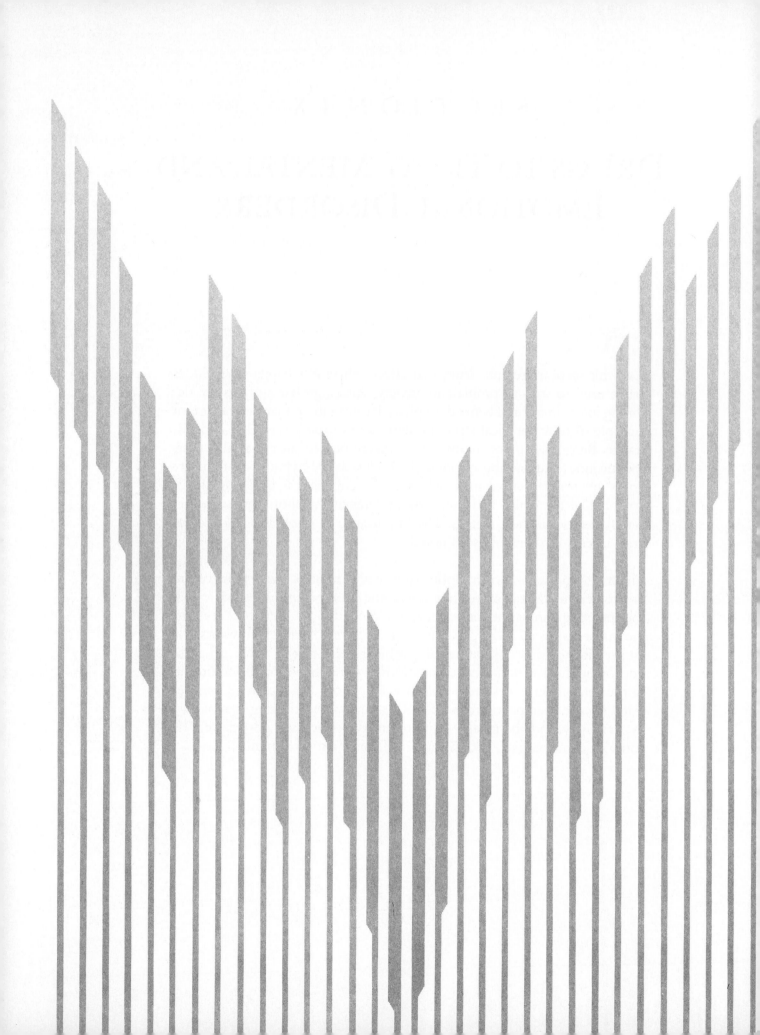

CHAPTER 40

Sedative-Hypnotic Agents, Antianxiety Agents, and Alcohol

LEARNING OBJECTIVES

After studying this chapter, you should be able to do the following:

◆ Discuss CNS depression, drug dependence and CNS depression, and the stages of sleep.

◆ Differentiate among sedatives, hypnotics, and antianxiety agents.

◆ Develop a nursing care plan for patients receiving benzodiazepines, barbiturates, or miscellaneous hypnotics or antianxiety agents.

◆ Describe the effects of alcohol ingestion on the body.

◆ Develop a teaching plan for the patient receiving disulfiram or a drug that may produce a disulfiram-like reaction when alcohol is ingested.

CHAPTER OVERVIEW

◆ Sedative-hypnotic drugs and antianxiety drugs are considered together because they are not different so much in their clinical action as in their historic origin. The term *sedative-hypnotic* is reserved for older drug classes, primarily barbiturates. Barbiturates are a class of chemically related drugs developed in the early 1900s, effective as sedatives and as hypnotics. A small dose to calm an anxious patient is called a **sedative**. A larger dose sufficient to induce sleep is a **hypnotic**.

◆ After the 1950s, drugs were developed specifically as hypnotics. Other drugs were developed as sedatives to treat anxiety. The benzodiazepines are the drug class most used today to treat anxiety. These drugs are referred to as *antianxiety drugs*. The older term was *minor tranquilizer*.

◆ An additional drug appropriate to this chapter is alcohol because it has the pharmacologic actions characteristic of a sedative-hypnotic or an antianxiety drug. The social use of alcohol is mainly as a self-prescribed antianxiety agent. Furthermore, drug abuse and dependence are discussed in this chapter. Alcohol, when recognized as a drug, is viewed as a major source of drug abuse and dependence.

Nursing Process Overview
SEDATIVE-HYPNOTIC AND ANTIANXIETY DRUGS

Assessment

Perform a systematic assessment, with attention to vital signs, level of consciousness, and emotional affect. Investigate fully any subjective complaints and other health problems.

Nursing Diagnoses

Possible complication: drug dependence or addiction
High risk for depressed level of consciousness

Management

The common denominator of the drugs discussed in this chapter is that they produce CNS depression. Assess level of consciousness, affect, vital signs, and blood pressure. Work with the patient to identify

595

nonmedicinal treatments that may help. For example, patients being treated with sedative-hypnotics to produce sleep may be aided by bedtime remedies such as warm milk, relaxing in a warm bath, or reading briefly. Monitor the ability of hospitalized patients to ambulate safely, and keep side rails up at night. If these drugs are being used by intravenous (IV) routes, have appropriate equipment for resuscitation and a suction machine available.

Evaluation

The success of these drugs depends on the original purpose for which they were being used. Before discharge, verify that patients can explain how to take the prescribed medication correctly, what symptoms may indicate too high a dose of medication, what to do if the medication is no longer effective, and when to return to the physician for follow-up. Determine that patients can list other drugs to avoid such as alcohol or other antianxiety drugs. Use judgement in indicating to patients that continued prolonged use of these drugs or use in increasing amounts can lead to drug dependence or addiction.

CENTRAL NERVOUS SYSTEM DEPRESSANTS
Behavioral Changes
Reticular activating system

The effects of a single dose of a sedative-hypnotic drug, an antianxiety drug, or alcohol are very similar. All these drugs act pharmacologically as general depressants of the CNS, since they depress the reticular activating system of the brain stem. The **reticular activating system** refers to neural pathways in which incoming signals from the senses (sight, sound, smell, touch, taste, and balance) and viscera are collected, processed, and passed on to the higher brain centers (Figure 40-1). Higher brain centers also have neural pathways to the reticular activating system to modulate activity. This system determines the level of awareness of the environment and therefore governs reactions to it.

Stages of depression

Depression of the reticular activating system by a general CNS depressant accounts for the behavioral changes seen in a person who has taken one of these drugs. The degree of depression depends on the amount of drug taken. At a low dose, sedation is produced, characterized by decreased physical and mental responses to stimuli. With an increased dose, disinhibition is the next level of depression reached. Disinhibition falsely appears as a stimulated state of

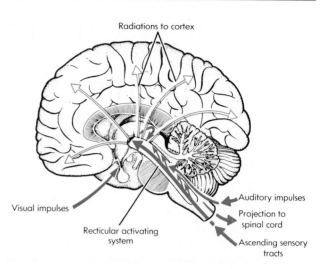

FIGURE 40-1

Awareness is a function of reticular activating system. Diagram illustrates reticular activating system as integration network. General CNS depressants act on reticular activating system, although mechanisms are not understood.

awareness. This is because neurons inhibiting arousal become depressed. The result of disinhibition may be euphoria, excitement, drunkenness, loss of self-control, and impaired judgment. Relief of anxiety produced by a general CNS depressant results from sedation or disinhibition. Loss of motor coordination (ataxia) and involuntary eye movements (nystagmus) are frequently seen at this level of depression and are clues when drug use is suspected. Pain can intensify disinhibition and can result in paradoxical excitement in postoperative patients who are given a sedative-hypnotic or an antianxiety drug. Increasing the drug dose further produces sleep (hypnosis). Anesthesia, the loss of feeling or sensation, is achieved at high doses of a general CNS-depressant drug.

The effect of a single dose of a sedative-hypnotic drug, an antianxiety drug, or alcohol therefore depends on the dose taken. In practice, not much distinction can be made in the sedative vs. hypnotic dose for drugs used primarily as hypnotics. Similarly, drugs most popular as sedative or antianxiety drugs are those that produce minimal sleepiness at an effective dose.

Drug Dependence
Origin

Continued administration of a general-CNS depressant drug can cause drug dependence. Drug dependence means that the body has adjusted to the continual CNS depression so that it now requires the presence of the drug to function. If administration is discontinued abruptly, the body experiences withdrawal symptoms. The symptoms of withdrawal from a general CNS depressant drug reflect CNS hyperactivity. Mild withdrawal symptoms include agitation, tremulousness, and insomnia, whereas the major withdrawal symptom is convulsions, a life-threatening emergency. The symptoms disappear when the drug is retaken.

Doses that produce dependence

It is not possible to state simply what dose produces drug dependence because great variation exists among individuals. In broad terms, general CNS-depressant drugs can produce drug dependence when taken at twice their prescribed doses for 2 to 8 weeks. The dependence potential varies among the drug classes somewhat, as is discussed more fully for each class. A thought-provoking observation is that each new sedative-hypnotic and antianxiety drug has been introduced with the conviction that it was not addicting, but no general CNS-depressant drug has turned out to be nonaddictive. The benzodiazepines, a class of drugs accounting for at least 15% of all prescriptions written in the United States, have only recently been widely recognized as capable of producing drug dependence. Now major questions are being raised about drug dependence with benzodiazepines.

Development of drug abuse

The time required for drug dependence to develop depends on the drug dose. Chronic use of low doses does not necessarily lead to drug dependence. Many people take low doses of barbiturates to control epilepsy and do not experience withdrawal symptoms if their medication is changed. Moderate alcohol consumption, even on a daily basis, does not necessarily lead to alcohol dependence. However, tolerance does develop to the sedative and euphoric effects of general CNS depressants. People abuse a drug when their reaction to this tolerance is to increase the amount of drug taken. As the drug dose increases, a point is reached at which failure to take the drug produces withdrawal symptoms. At this point, drug use may be continued as much to avoid withdrawal symptoms as to produce drug effects. This stage is referred to as *drug dependency* or *drug addiction.* The individual's life may become centered around the drug, and personal, family, and social interactions become less important.

Drug addiction cannot be explained merely by drug tolerance and physical dependence. In general, physical dependence can be overcome by decreasing the drug intake by 10% of the inital dose daily for 10 days. This gradual reduction prevents withdrawal symptoms from becoming severe. However, many patients revert to drug abuse after they have been withdrawn from drug dependence. Drug addiction therefore involves social and psychologic factors that underlie drug abuse.

Cross-tolerance

Tolerance to any sedative-hypnotic drug, antianxiety drug, or alcohol results in tolerance to any other of these general CNS depressants. This property is called *cross-tolerance* and is a major factor in drug abuse. The most common pattern of drug abuse is alcohol in combination with one or more sedative-hypnotic or antianxiety drugs. This combination works in an addictive fashion. One way an individual can avoid taking more of the same drug to overcome tolerance is by adding a second drug, usually alcohol. This can be lethal. Although someone drinking enough to die from alcohol alone is relatively uncommon, this becomes possible when another drug such as a sedative-hypnotic or an antianxiety drug is added. Moreover, because of cross-tolerance, a dose that would not lead to drug dependence by itself contributes to drug dependence when added to a second depressant.

MECHANISMS OF GENERAL CNS DEPRESSANTS FOR INSOMNIA AND ANXIETY

Sleep and Hypnotic Drugs

Stages of sleep

What determines sleep is not well understood. Current sleep research makes use of the brain-wave patterns and eye movements recorded during sleep, as shown in Figure 40-2. Four stages of sleep are defined by brain-wave patterns. Stage 1 represents the lightest level of sleep, accompanied by muscle relaxation and slowing of the heart rate (bradycardia). Stage 4 represents the deepest level of sleep, accompanied by marked muscle relaxation and bradycardia. During most of the sleep cycle the eye movements are not noticed under closed eyelids. However, during about 20% of the average adult sleep time the eyeballs move rapidly back and forth under the closed eyelids. This is called **REM sleep** (*r*apid *e*ye *m*ovement) and is superimposed on stage 1 or stage 2 sleep. The body is physiologically active during REM sleep so that the heart rate is increased, breathing is irregular, stomach acid is secreted, and the clitoris or penis becomes erect. Muscles lose their tone during REM sleep, however, so that only the mind and autonomic nervous system are active during this stage. Since dreaming occurs exclusively during REM sleep, this time is also called *dreaming sleep*. Many authorities believe that during REM sleep is when we integrate emotionally meaningful experiences.

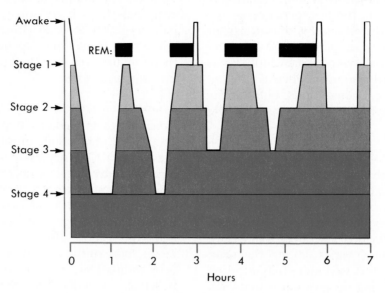

FIGURE 40-2

Normal sleep pattern. Sleep is cyclical. Deep sleep is more frequent during early than later cycles. Dreaming occurs during REM sleep and is associated with stage 1 and stage 2 sleep. Pattern shown is characteristic for adults. Children and elderly persons often awaken more frequently. Most hypnotics depress REM sleep.

Sleep cycles

As indicated in Figure 40-2, an individual normally cycles from stage 1 through stage 4 back to stage 1 about every 90 min. Deep sleep (stages 3 and 4) occupies more of the early sleep cycles, whereas dreaming occupies more of the late sleep cycles. Children spend more total time in deep sleep than adults, whereas the elderly may spend little time in deep sleep. With increasing age, it becomes more common to awaken at the end of a sleep cycle, particularly the early morning cycles.

Insomnia

Insomnia, inability to sleep, is the most common sleep complaint and can be characterized as either difficulty in getting to sleep or in waking up and being unable to get back to sleep. Insomnia is not a disease but a symptom of physical or mental distress. Several conditions in which insomnia is prominent are listed in Table 40-1.

Action of hypnotic drugs

Hypnotic drugs are taken to fall asleep faster or to sleep longer. Studies in sleep laboratories show that most hypnotic drugs suppress REM sleep. When the drug is discontinued, even after a single dose, there is a rebound in REM sleep with vivid dreams and increased awakening. Furthermore, after 3 weeks of

Table 40-1 Conditions Characterized by Insomnia

Condition	Characteristic type of insomnia
Depression	Early morning insomnia is common.
Chronic alcoholism	REM sleep and deep sleep are reduced.
Hyperthyroidism	Deep sleep is reduced.
Heart failure	Insomnia is an early complaint.
Pregnancy	Insomnia is common during the last trimester.
Renal insufficiency	
Many neurologic disorders	

continuous therapy, most hypnotic drugs are no longer effective in decreasing the time needed to fall asleep or the duration of sleep. Nevertheless, if the patient now discontinues the drug, worse insomnia and associated anxiety will be experienced because of the REM rebound. This reaction may lead the un-instructed patient to continue the drug, perhaps at an increased dose, to regain the hypnotic effect. This is the beginning of drug abuse with hypnotic drugs. Since hypnotic drugs can make insomnia worse rather than better, the cause of insomnia rather than the insomnia should be discovered and treated. Alcohol and antianxiety drugs can interfere with sleep patterns in a similar fashion if taken in large enough doses.

Anxiety and Drug Therapy

Anxiety means different things to different people. Many symptoms are associated with anxiety. These are listed in Table 40-2. An anxious individual will have some, but not all, of these physical symptoms. **Anxiety** may be generalized, in which the individual is unaware of a specific cause of anxiety and may even deny anxiety, or it may be anticipatory, in which the individual is well aware of its origin.

Specific types of anxiety states have also been identified. Phobic disorders are characterized by irrational fear of objects, activities, or situations and by the compelling desire to avoid them. Obsessive-compulsive disorder is characterized by persistent obsessive ideas, thoughts, or images or by compulsive behavior. Posttraumatic stress disorder follows a unique and psychologically traumatic experience.

Action of antianxiety drugs

The pharmacologic action of sedatives or antianxiety agents may be to decrease the general level of arousal by inhibiting the reticular activating system of the brain stem. This is not a cure for anxiety, although response is blunted. Rather, authorities agree that drug therapy for anxiety should be limited to a few weeks, and psychotherapy or behavior-modification

Table 40-2 Symptoms of Anxiety

Appearance	Complaints
Excessively alert	Cardiorespiratory: heart palpitations, fast heart rate, and breathlessness
Easily startled	
Constantly in motion or inhibited in motion	Gastrointestinal: abdominal cramps, nausea, vomiting, and diarrhea
Excessive and disjointed speech	
Eyes constantly scanning "Fussy" dress	Musculoskeletal: tension headaches, chest pain or tightness, and backache
Tremors, restlessness	General: fatigue, weakness, and insomnia
Dilated pupils	

therapy deals directly with the origin of the patient's anxiety. In part, this recommendation is based on tolerance to these drugs developing after a few weeks so that effective therapy requires larger doses, the first step in drug abuse. Patients taking sedative or antianxiety drugs should be told that drug therapy offers only limited relief.

Information about the regulation of anxiety is becoming more sophisticated. Current research suggests that reduction of anxiety can be achieved without sedation. In addition to the reticular activating system, two other integrating systems control anxiety, the limbic system and the hypothalamus. Although the reticular activating system allows information to enter the brain, the limbic system adds emotion and mediates a sequence of outgoing messages. The hypothalamus integrates the neuroendocrine response to stress, controlling the output of several hormones (see Chapter 36). The goal of current drug research is to identify drugs that affect anxiety without producing sedation. These drugs may act selectively in the limbic system.

Drugs Prescribed for Insomnia and Anxiety

Drugs prescribed for insomnia and anxiety are presented in three sections. The first section discusses benzodiazepines, the most popular drug class today for treating insomnia and anxiety. The second section presents barbiturates, an older class of drugs used as CNS depressants, from sedation to anesthesia. The third section discusses miscellaneous drugs occasionally prescribed for insomnia or anxiety.

BENZODIAZEPINES

Benzodiazepines were introduced clinically in the 1960s as antianxiety drugs. By the early 1970s, diazepam (Valium) was the most widely prescribed drug in the United States. The popularity of the benzodiazepines is due in part to their high therapeutic index. Overdoses of 1000 times the therapeutic dose have been reported not to result in death. At therapeutic doses, side effects beyond drowsiness and ataxia are uncommon. No drug interactions are prominent beyond the addictive effect with other CNS depressant drugs.

Mechanism of Action

Specific receptors for the benzodiazepines have been identified in the cerebral cortex and limbic system. Since the limbic system is a major integrating system governing emotional behavior associated with self-preservation, the presence of receptors for benzodiazepines in this system may account for their antianxiety action. Benzodiazepines increase the action of the inhibitory neurotransmitter, gamma-aminobutyric acid (GABA). Benzodiazepines and barbiturates help GABA open a chloride channel in the postsynaptic membrane of many neurons, which reduces the neuron's excitability.

Benzodiazepines have anxiety reducing (anxiolytic), sedative-hypnotic, muscle relaxing, and anticonvulsant actions. All benzodiazepines are schedule IV drugs. Estazolam (ProSom), flurazepam (Dalmane), lorazepam (Ativan), quazepam (Doral), temazepam (Resotril), and triazolam (Halcion) are effective as hypnotics. Clonazepam (Clonopin), clorazepate (Tranxene), and diazepam (Valium) have uses as anticonvulsants. Diazepam (Valium) is prescribed as a muscle relaxant. Alprazolam (Xanax), chlordiazepoxide (Librium), clorazepate (Tranxene), diazepam (Valium), halazepam (Paxipam), lorazepam (Ativan), oxazepam (Serax), and prazepam (Centrax) are widely used as antianxiety drugs.

Absorption and Distribution

The benzodiazepines are readily absorbed after oral administration. Only lorazepam is rapidly and completely absorbed after intramuscular (IM) injection. Chlordiazepoxide and diazepam may be administered by IV or IM routes, but chlordiazepoxide is not reliably absorbed after IM administration. Benzodiazepines are highly lipid soluble and therefore are widely distributed in body tissues. They are also highly bound to plasma protein, usually greater than 80%. No drug interactions have been described for protein binding, but it is reduced in patients with cirrhosis and renal insufficiency and in newborns. These patients often have impaired metabolism of benzodiazepines as well, making a reduction in dosage important.

Metabolism

The benzodiazepines are metabolized by the liver. Several benzodiazepines have active metabolites. N-desmethylated metabolites are active and have a longer duration of action than the parent compound. Lorazepam, oxazepam, temazepam, and triazolam do not have active metabolites to prolong their duration of action. These drugs are preferred for elderly patients and for patients with liver disease. Alprazolam is metabolized to weakly active compounds that are eliminated rapidly. The anticonvulsant clonazepam has only weakly active metabolites.

Side Effects

Side effects common with benzodiazepines include daytime sedation, ataxia, dizziness, and headaches. Tolerance commonly develops quickly to these side effects. The elderly are more likely to experience these side effects to a disabling degree. Moreover, they do not readily metabolize benzodiazepines, so the drug persists two to three times longer. For these reasons the drug dose is reduced for elderly patients and for patients who have impaired liver function. However, elderly patients are at risk for falling and injuring themselves while taking these drugs for sleep or anxiety. Less common side effects of benzodiazepines include blurred or double vision, hypotension, tremor, amnesia, slurred speech, urinary incontinence, and constipation.

Acute Toxicity

An acute overdose of benzodiazepines alone is seldom fatal. Patients frequently regain consciousness and normal vital signs with a large concentration of drug still in their bodies. Recently a benzodiazepine antagonist, flumazenil (Mazicon) has been released for clinical use. Flumazenil reverses symptoms of benzodiazepine overdose.

Abuse Potential and Withdrawal

Benzodiazepines are schedule IV drugs, since their abuse potential is considered low. Daily use of 30 mg of diazepam in the absence of alcohol or other depressant drugs for 3 months seldom produces dependence. Although tolerance to sedation and ataxia develops rapidly, tolerance to the antianxiety effect develops slowly. If dependence develops, the appearance of withdrawal symptoms after discontinuance will take several days for those benzodiazepines with active metabolites. An acute phase of chronic withdrawal symptoms, consisting of depression, insomnia, nightmares, agitation, and psychologic distress, can persist for 6 weeks. Withdrawal begins during the first week after discontinuance of the drug, with symptoms of agitation, nausea and vomiting, nervousness, sweating, and muscular cramps. Seizures are seldom seen unless high doses have been abused, but if seizures do occur, it is at the end of the first week.

Drug Interactions and Contraindications

Like the barbiturates, the sedative effect of the benzodiazepines is increased by other drug classes including alcohol and other general CNS depressants, tricyclic antidepressants, opiate analgesics, antipsychotics, and antihistamines. Unlike barbiturates, benzodiazepines have only slight effects on the liver microsomal enzymes. Patients over 50 years of age with a history of psychosis are the most likely to develop paradoxical excitement or aggression. Benzodiazepines may worsen glaucoma. Benzodiazepines are contraindicated for women in labor and for nursing mothers because of adverse depression of the infant. An increased incidence of cleft lip has been reported among infants whose mothers took diazepam (Valium) during early pregnancy. In general, benzodiazepines are associated with an increased incidence of congenital abnormalities in children whose mothers used the drugs during pregnancy.

Specific Benzodiazepines

These drugs are listed in Table 40-3.

Alprazolam

Alprazolam (Xanax) is indicated for the short-term relief of anxiety and may be effective in relieving anxiety associated with depression. Another use is to treat panic disorders. Alprazolam has a potential dependence liability with patients unable to give up use of the drug. Rebound panic, seizures, and delirium have been reported when the drug is rapidly discontinued.

Alprazolam is rapidly absorbed and is effective for about 12 hr. Although the drug is eliminated somewhat more slowly in the elderly than in young adults, the metabolites are only weakly active. Steady-state plasma levels are reached in 2 to 5 days with regular administration.

Bromazepam

Bromazepam (Lectopam) is prescribed as an antianxiety agent. It is available in Canada but not in the United States. Bromazepam has a short-to-intermediate half-life and does not tend to accumulate with multiple doses. The dose for elderly patients should be half the usual adult dose.

Chlordiazepoxide

Chlordiazepoxide (Librium) is prescribed as an antianxiety drug, as a preanesthetic medication for sedation, and to treat symptoms of alcohol withdrawal. Chlordiazepoxide is absorbed better orally than intramuscularly; care must be used with IV injections. Chlordiazepoxide is metabolized by the liver to an active metabolite to give a persistent effect.

Clonazepam

Clonazepam (Clonopin) is mainly used as an anticonvulsant (see Chapter 47). It also treats panic attacks.

Clorazepate

Clorazepate (Traxene) is prescribed for anxiety, panic attacks, the symptomatic relief of acute alcohol withdrawal, and as adjunctive therapy in the management of partial seizures.

Clorazepate is not absorbed orally until converted by stomach acid to an active metabolite. Any condition or medication such as antacids or cimetidine that reduce stomach acidity markedly interferes with clorazepate absorption. The metabolite persists in the body.

Diazepam

Diazepam (Valium) has many clinical uses in addition to treating anxiety and panic attacks. It relieves muscle spasticity in patients with cerebral palsy or other conditions and stops continued convulsions (status epilepticus). Diazepam is also used in the hospital as a preanesthetic medication for sedation. Alcohol withdrawal symptoms may be treated with diazepam.

Diazepam is well absorbed orally and is effective within 1 hr. Absorption from IM injection is erratic, and pain occurs at the injection site, so this route is seldom used. IV injection must be given slowly and carefully into a large vein to minimize irritation and swelling at the injection site, with possible phlebitis or thrombosis.

Estazolam

Estazolam (ProSom) is a new benzodiazepine prescribed for insomnia. It has a fast onset of action and is effective for 6 to 8 hr.

Flurazepam

Flurazepam (Dalmane) is prescribed as a hypnotic only. It suppresses stage 4 sleep but does not markedly depress REM sleep. Flurazepam is effective for more than 2 weeks. Also, it does not produce rebound insomnia when it is discontinued, probably because of the long half-life of its active metabolites. The persistence of active metabolites accounts for decreased mental alertness during the day, particularly after repeated use of flurazepam by elderly patients and by patients with decreased liver function.

Halazepam

Halazepam (Paxipam), an antianxiety drug, is well absorbed orally and is metabolized to an active metabolite with a long half-life. Cumulation of the drug and its metabolite occurs with repeated doses, particularly in the elderly or in patients with impaired liver function.

Ketazolam

Ketazolam (Loftran) is an antianxiety agent. It is available in Canada but not in the United States. Ketazolam has a long half-life and accumulates with multiple dosing.

Table 40-3 Sedative-Hypnotic and Antianxiety Drugs: Benzodiazepines

Generic name	Trade name	Administration/dosage	Comments
Alprazolam	Xanax*	ORAL: *Adults*—0.25 to 0.5 mg 3 times daily. Maximum daily dose: 4 mg. FDA Pregnancy Category D. *Elderly*—0.25 mg 2 or 3 times daily.	Used to treat anxiety. Metabolites are only weakly active. Schedule IV substance.
Bromazepam	Lectopam†	ORAL: *Adults*—6 to 30 mg daily in divided doses.	Used to treat anxiety.
Chlordiazepoxide	Libritabs Librium* Medilium† Novopoxide† Various others	ORAL: *Adults*—for anxiety, 15 to 100 mg divided in 3 to 4 doses or in 1 dose at bedtime. *Elderly*—5 mg 2 to 4 times daily. *Children*—0.5 mg/kg body weight daily in 3 to 4 doses. May be given intramuscularly. INTRAVENOUS: *Adults*—for alcohol withdrawal, 50 to 100 mg slowly over at least 1 min, then 25 to 50 mg every 6 to 8 hr, with the total dose not more than 300 mg.	Used to treat anxiety and alcohol withdrawal. Half-life is 24 to 48 hr. Metabolites are active. The hydrochloride salt is used for injection. Schedule IV substance.
Clonazepam	Klonopin Rivotril†	ORAL: *Adults*—Initially, 0.5 mg 3 times daily. Increase in increments of 0.5 mg to 1 mg every 3 days if necessary.	Primarily used as an anticonvulsant. Use to treat panic disorders is under investigation. Schedule IV substance.
Clorazepate	Tranxene* Novoclopate†	ORAL: *Adults*—13 to 60 mg divided into 2 to 4 doses or at bedtime. *Elderly*—6.5 to 15 mg daily.	Used to treat anxiety. Half-life is 30 to 200 hr. Metabolites are active. Schedule IV substance.
Diazepam	Valium* E-Pam† Various others	ORAL: *Adults*—4 to 40 mg divided into 2 to 4 doses or a single dose of 2.5 to 10 mg at bedtime. *Elderly*—2 to 2.5 mg once to twice daily. *Children*—0.12 to 0.8 mg/kg daily in 3 to 4 doses. INTRAVENOUS: administer no more than 5 mg/min. For severe anxiety, severe muscle spasm, status epilepticus, or recurrent seizures: *Adults*—5 to 10 mg initially, repeated in 3 to 4 hr if needed. *Children*—0.04 to 0.2 mg/kg initially, repeat in 3 to 4 hr if necessary. For basal sedation for cardioversion or endoscopic procedures: *Adults*—10 to 20 mg as required. For acute alcohol withdrawal symptoms: *Adults*—5 to 20 mg, then 5 to 10 mg in 3 to 4 hr if necessary.	Used to treat anxiety, severe muscle spasm, status epilepticus, and acute alcohol withdrawal symptoms and to provide sedation. Half-life is 48 to 200 hr. Metabolites are active. Schedule IV substance.
Estazolam	ProSom	ORAL: *Adults*—1 mg at bedtime; some patients may require 2 mg. Small or debilitated patients, 0.5 mg.	Used to treat insomnia. New drug.
Flurazepam	Dalmane* Durapam Somnol† Various others	ORAL: *Adults*—as hypnotic, 15 to 30 mg at bedtime. *Elderly*—15 mg. Onset: 20 to 45 min. Duration: 7 to 8 hr.	Used as a hypnotic only. Active metabolite is formed with half-life of 47 to 100 hr, so repeated use leads to cumulation of this metabolite, which may impair daytime activity. Schedule IV substance.
Halazepam	Paxipam	ORAL: *Adults*—20 to 40 mg 3 or 4 times daily. FDA Pregnancy Category D. *Elderly*—reduce dose to 20 mg 1 or 2 times daily.	Used to treat anxiety. Active metabolite with long half-life. Schedule IV substance.

*Available in Canada and United States.
†Available in Canada only.

Table 40-3 Sedative-Hypnotic and Antianxiety Drugs: Benzodiazepines—cont'd

Generic name	Trade name	Administration/dosage	Comments
Ketazolam	Loftran†	ORAL: *Adults*—15 mg to 1 to 2 times daily.	Used to treat anxiety.
Lorazepam	Alzapam Ativan* Nu-Loraz† Various others	ORAL: *Adults*—for anxiety, 1 to 2 mg 2 to 3 times daily, may increase dose to 10 mg maximum daily; as hypnotic, 2 to 4 mg at bedtime. FDA Pregnancy Category D. *Elderly*—½ adult dose.	Used to treat anxiety and insomnia. Repeated use for insomnia can cause rebound insomnia. Half-life is 15 hr, so little cumulation occurs. Metabolites are inactive. Schedule IV substance.
Nitrazepam	Mogadon†	ORAL: *Adults*—5 to 10 mg at bedtime. *Children* (anticonvulsant)—0.3 mg to 1 mg/kg body weight in 3 divided doses. May increase gradually if needed and tolerated.	Used as a sedative in adults and as an anticonvulsant in children.
Oxazepam	Serax* Ox-Pam† Zapex†	ORAL: *Adults*—for anxiety, 30 to 120 mg daily in 3 to 4 doses. *Elderly*—30 mg in 3 divided doses, increased if necessary to 45 to 60 mg.	Used to treat anxiety. Half-life is 3 to 21 hr, so little cumulation occurs. Metabolites are inactive. Schedule IV substance.
Prazepam	Centrax	ORAL: *Adults*—20 mg in a single dose, increased to 40 to 60 mg daily in divided doses or once at bedtime. *Elderly*—10 to 15 mg.	Used to treat anxiety. Half-life is 30 to 200 hr. Metabolites are active. Schedule IV substance.
Quazepam	Doral	ORAL: *Adults*—Initially, 15 mg. Reduce to 7.5 mg as needed.	Used to treat insomnia. Metabolites have a long half life. Schedule IV substance.
Temazepam	Razepam Restoril* Temaz	ORAL: *Adults*—30 mg at bedtime. FDA Pregnancy Category X. *Elderly*—reduce dose to 15 mg.	Used as a hypnotic only. Slowly absorbed. Metabolites are not active. Schedule IV substance.
Triazolam	Halcion* Novotriolam† Apo-Triazo†	ORAL: *Adults*—0.25 to 0.5 mg at bedtime. FDA Pregnancy Category X. *Elderly*—reduce dose to 0.25 mg.	Used as a hypnotic. May also be used as an antianxiety drug and an anticonvulsant. Metabolites are not active. Schedule IV substance.
Flumazenil	Mazicon	Reversal of conscious sedation or in general anesthesia: INTRAVENOUS: *Adults*—0.2 mg administered over 15 sec initially. Wait 45 sec for response. Further doses of 0.2 mg may be repeated at 60 sec intervals if needed, to a cumulative dose of 1 mg per treatment. Treatment may be repeated at 20 min intervals, with no more than 3 mg given in 1 hr. Management of suspected benzodiazepine overdose: INTRAVENOUS: *Adults*—0.2 mg is administered over 30 sec initially. If the desired level of consciousness is not seen after waiting 30 sec, a further dose of 0.3 mg is administered over another 30 sec. Further doses of 0.5 mg may be administered over 30 sec at 1 min intervals up to a cumulative dose of 3 mg. In the event of resedation, treatment may be repeated at 20 min intervals, with no more than 1 mg administered at one time and not more than 3 mg given in 1 hr.	New benzodiazepine atagonist for the reversal of benzodizaepine-induced sedation.

*Available in Canada and United States.
†Available in Canada only.

Lorazepam

Lorazepam (Ativan) is effective as a hypnotic and an antianxiety drug. It is well absorbed orally and intramuscularly. Parenteral lorazepam is sometimes given as a preanesthetic medication in adults. Lorazepam produces sedation, relieves anxiety, and decreases ability to recall events that day. The drug does not have active metabolites and therefore has a relatively short duration of action, about 15 hr.

Midazolam

Midazolam (Versed) is used as an IV anesthetic and is discussed in Chapter 45.

Nitrazepam

Nitrazepam (Mogadon) is a hypnotic. It is available in Canada but not in the United States. Nitrazepam has a short-to-intermediate half-life and has minimal accumulation with multiple dosing.

Oxazepam

Oxazepam (Serax) is effective as an antianxiety drug, especially in anxiety associated with depression, tension, agitation, and irritability in older patients. Oxazepam also reduces the anxiety associated with alcohol withdrawal.

Absorption is slow. The metabolites are not active; thus drug effects are not likely to be cumulative and do not persist for more than 24 hr.

Prazepam

Prazepam (Centrax), an antianxiety drug, is slowly absorbed orally. The metabolites are active; thus cumulative effects are seen with repeated administration.

Quazepam

Quazepam (Doral) is a new benzodiazepine used to treat insomnia. Its characteristics are much like flurazepam.

Temazepam

Temazepam (Restoril) is a hypnotic. Temazepam is slowly absorbed, and onset of sleep is not improved. The number of awakenings is decreased, however, and overall duration and quality of sleep improve. As with flurazepam, stage 4 sleep is suppressed but REM sleep is not. Unlike flurazepam, temazepam does not have active metabolites, and cumulation is not generally a problem.

Triazolam

Triazolam (Halcion) is a hypnotic, an antianxiety agent, and an anticonvulsant. It may have muscle-relaxant effects as well. Triazolam is rapidly absorbed.

Its metabolites are not active and are rapidly eliminated. Triazolam and alprazolam are closely related chemically.

The safety of triazolam has been questioned. However, the FDA determined that the incidence of severe side effects is not greater for triazolam than for flurazepam and temazepam, two other popular hypnotics, when compared at equivalent doses. Side effects include anxiety, restlessness, amnesia, aggression, and paranoia.

BENZODIAZEPINE ANTAGONIST

Flumazenil

Flumazenil (Mazicon) is the first benzodiazepine antagoist to be released for clinical use (see Table 40-3). Flumazenil binds to the benzodiazepine receptor competitively and thereby inhibits the action of benzodiazepines.

Two major clinical uses are anticipated for flumazenil. First, flumazenil is a diagnostic tool to confirm or exclude benzodiazepine intoxication. Flumazenil, administered intravenously, will reverse benzodiazepine intoxication in 5 min. Once benzodiazepine intoxication is confirmed, flumazenil can be given repeatedly to reverse the depression of the respiratory drive caused by benzodiazepine intoxication so that the need for endotracheal intubation and artificial ventilation is avoided or decreased. Second, flumazenil is used to reverse the sedative effects of benzodiazepines given during surgical procedures to induce conscious sedation or general anesthesia. Flumazenil is also beng tested as an agent to induce remission of functional CNS impairment, especially that of hepatic encephalopathy.

Flumazenil is generally well tolerated. Surgical patients are more likely to experience nausea and vomiting. Patients being treated for an overdose of benzodiazepines may experience agitation, restlessness, discomfort, and anxiety.

BARBITURATES

More than 50 derivatives of barbituric acid have been marketed for clinical use since the beginning of this century, and nine are still widely used. The **barbiturates** are classified according to their duration of action and have been traditionally divided into four classes: ultrashort-acting, short-acting, intermediate-acting, and long-acting. Although traditional, this classification was derived from animal data and is somewhat arbitrary in the clinical setting, where the variables of dose and patient expectations can modify the degree and duration of effectiveness. In particular the contrast between short-acting and intermediate-acting sedative-hypnotics is not as striking in clinical practice as in drug tables.

Onset and Duration of Action

The ultrashort-acting barbiturates are administered intravenously, but other barbiturates are usually given orally and are well absorbed. Differences in onset and duration of action among barbiturates depend on their lipid solubility and protein binding. These properties are determined by the chemical structure. The ultrashort-acting barbiturates are lipid soluble, and on IV administration the concentration reaching the brain, which has a high blood flow, is large because the barbiturates readily cross the blood-brain barrier and depress the reticular activating system. Their action is quickly terminated, however, because they are redistributed into organs with a lesser blood flow, so the concentration reaching the brain quickly drops. Ultrashort-acting barbiturates may persist in body fat because of their high lipid solubility and in muscle, reflecting their high degree of protein binding.

Metabolism

Barbiturates are released slowly from muscle and fat into the blood for eventual metabolism by the liver and excretion by the kidney. The persistence of low concentrations of barbiturates in the body is believed to account for the "hangovers" after the therapeutic effect has worn off. Short- and intermediate-acting barbiturates are redistributed less rapidly into body fat and muscle, thus acting longer. The long-acting barbiturate phenobarbital binds even less to protein and is much less lipid-soluble than the ultrashort-acting barbiturates. Although ultrashort-, short-, and intermediate-acting barbiturates must be metabolized by the liver to water-soluble metabolites for excretion by the kidney, 30% to 50% of a dose of phenobarbital is excreted unchanged in urine.

Side Effects and Toxicity

Mild withdrawal symptoms

As discussed for hypnotics in general, barbiturates are not effective as hypnotics after 2 weeks of use. Also, even a single dose suppresses REM sleep and leads to rebound REM when the barbiturate is discontinued. Mild withdrawal symptoms from short-term use of barbiturates include nightmares, daytime agitation, and a "shaky" feeling.

An acute overdose of barbiturates causes depression of the medullary centers controlling respiration and the cardiovascular system. The symptoms are a fast heart rate (tachycardia) and a fall in blood pressure (hypotension) that leads to shock. Reflexes disappear, and respiration is markedly depressed. The patient becomes comatose, and death may result from respiratory and cardiovascular collapse. No specific antagonist exists for barbiturates; thus treatment of barbiturate poisoning supports respiration and maintains blood oxygen levels.

Tolerance and Dependence

Metabolic tolerance

Administration of barbiturates for a few days activates the liver to synthesize more of the drug-metabolizing enzymes. This activation is called *enzyme induction*. Since these enzymes are located in the microsomal fraction of broken cell preparations, these drug-metabolizing enzymes usually are referred to as the *liver microsomal enzyme system*. After induction of the microsomal enzymes, the barbiturates are more rapidly metabolized, decreasing average blood levels after a given dose. This is a classic example of *metabolic tolerance*. Since many other drugs are also metabolized by the same microsomal enzymes, barbiturates can induce tolerance of other drugs. Examples are the coumarins (anticoagulants) and the anticonvulsant phenytoin (Dilantin).

Pharmacodynamic tolerance

In addition to drug-induced tolerance, pharmacodynamic tolerance also develops with repeated administration of the barbiturates. This is the tolerance described previously for all general CNS depressants, in which the nervous system adapts to the presence of the depressant. However, the medullary centers controlling respiration and the cardiovascular system do not adapt to general CNS depressants, since they are not affected at the usual doses taken. The lethal dose for barbiturates therefore does not increase with drug dependence; this accounts for the accidental death of individuals dependent on high doses of barbiturates, since these doses can be lethal. The lethal dose for barbiturates in nontolerant individuals is about 15 times the hypnotic dose.

Abuse

Barbiturates are a class of widely abused drugs (see box). As with other abused classes of drugs, individual drugs with the most rapid onset are the most abused. This is because the euphoric feeling or "rush" depends on a rapid rate of altering perception. Among the barbiturates, secobarbital, pentobarbital, and amobarbital are schedule II drugs (drugs having a high potential for abuse). Butabarbital is a schedule III drug (lesser abuse potential), whereas phenobarbital and mephobarbital are schedule IV (low abuse potential) drugs (see Chapter 2). With the schedule II barbiturates, a daily consumption of 400 mg leads to severe drug dependence in about 6 weeks. With larger doses, the time decreases.

Severe withdrawal symptoms begin within 24 hr after the drug is discontinued in an individual with

---

---

severe drug dependence. Grand mal convulsions and delirium are common symptoms; elevated temperature, coma, and death are less common. Because of the danger associated with barbiturate withdrawal, gradual withdrawal is used to detoxify a dependent person. Withdrawal is achieved by reducing the dose of the barbiturate to zero over 10 to 20 days. Sometimes the long-acting barbiturate phenobarbital is substituted for a short-acting barbiturate for once-a-day administration. Phenobarbital (30 mg) is substituted for 100 mg of secobarbital, pentobarbital, or amobarbital.

Drug Interactions

The depressant effect of barbiturates is not only additive with the other general CNS depressants but is also potentiated by antipsychotics and narcotic analgesics. These interactions are important to remember for the patient scheduled to undergo surgery. If secobarbital or pentobarbital is prescribed as the night-before sleeping pill, it should be given at least 8 hr before any of the major tranquilizers, narcotic analgesics, or general anesthetics are administered to avoid undue depression of the medullary control of respiration and the cardiovascular system.

Specific Barbiturates

These drugs are listed in Table 40-4.

Thiamylal, thiopental, and methohexital

Thiamylal (Surital), thiopental (Pentothal), and methohexital (Brevital) are ultrashort-acting barbiturates administered intravenously for the induction or maintenance of anesthesia. These barbiturates are discussed with the general anesthetics in Chapter 45.

Amobarbital, aprobarbital, pentobarbital, secobarbital, and talbutal

Amobarbital (Amytal), aprobarbital (Alurate), pentobarbital (Nembutal), secobarbital (Seconal), and talbutal (Lotusate) are used most frequently as hypnotic drugs. The combination of secobarbital and amobarbital is sold under the name Tuinal as a hypnotic. Although these barbiturates are effective hypnotics for a few days, they lose their effectiveness by the second week of use. Since barbiturates depress REM sleep, REM rebound occurs when they are discontinued. This REM rebound can lead to insomnia. Also, drug dependence can develop with the usual hypnotic doses within 2 months, although this does not lead to severe withdrawal symptoms unless the dose has been raised above 400 mg daily.

Butabarbital

Butabarbital (Butisol) is an intermediate-acting barbiturate prescribed for daytime sedation and less commonly for inducing sleep at night. It frequently is combined in sedative doses with other drugs used to treat conditions with psychogenic overtones such as allergies, ulcers, and inflammatory bowel disease.

Phenobarbital

Phenobarbital (Luminal) is the longest acting and most widely used of the barbiturates. Phenobarbital and mephobarbital (Mebaral) control some kinds of epilepsy (see Chapter 47). Phenobarbital is infrequently abused because it is slower in onset of action, and it does not give a rush. Peak blood levels occur 6 to 18 hr after an oral dose, and the half-life is 3 to 4 days. Phenobarbital is the barbiturate that most readily induces the liver microsomal enzyme system, thereby enhancing its own metabolism and those of many other drugs. Phenobarbital treatment enhances the degradation of bilirubin and is used in infants and children to lower elevated plasma bilirubin levels.

Phenobarbital may be substituted for other barbiturates or nonbenzodiazepine hypnotics when decreasing drug levels for withdrawal. Its longer action allows once-a-day therapy.

OTHER HYPNOTIC AND ANTIANXIETY DRUGS
General Comparisons with Barbiturates

The miscellaneous hypnotic and antianxiety drugs listed in Table 40-5 are more similar to the barbiturates than the benzodiazepines in that they are generally shorter acting, which makes them more readily

Table 40-4 Sedative-Hypnotic and Antianxiety Drugs: Barbiturates

Generic name	Trade name	Administration/dosage	Comments
Amobarbital‡	Amytal*	ORAL: *Adults*—as sedative, 50 to 300 mg daily in divided doses; as hypnotic, 65 to 200 mg at bedtime. *Children*—as sedative, 6 mg/kg body weight in 3 divided doses. INTRAMUSCULAR, INTRAVENOUS: *Adults*—65 to 200 mg as hypnotic dose; 30 to 50 mg as sedative dose. *Children*—2 to 3 mg/kg body weight as hypnotic dose; 3 to 5 mg/kg body weight as sedative dose. FDA Pregnancy Category D.	An intermediate-acting barbiturate that acts similarly to a short-acting barbiturate in humans. Used for daytime sedation, preanesthetic sedation, and hypnosis. Precautions are same as for secobarbital. Schedule II substance.
Aprobarbital	Alurate	ORAL: *Adults*—40 to 160 mg at bedtime. FDA Pregnancy Category D.	An intermediate-acting barbiturate. Used as a hypnotic. Reduce doses for elderly patients. Schedule III substance. Not available in Canada.
Butabarbital	Butalan Butisol Sodium* Sarisol	ORAL: *Adults*—as sedative, 50 to 120 mg/day in 3 or 4 divided doses; as hypnotic, 50 to 100 mg at bedtime. FDA Pregnancy Category D. *Children*—as sedative, 6 mg/kg in 3 divided doses daily.	An intermediate-acting barbiturate used for sedation or for insomnia when the need is to prolong sleep rather than to induce sleep. Schedule III substance.
Pentobarbital‡	Nembutal* Novopento-barb†	ORAL: *Adults*—as sedative, 30 mg 3 or 4 times daily or 100 mg in timed-release form in the morning; as hypnotic, 100 mg at bedtime. FDA Pregnancy Category D. *Children*—as sedative, 6 mg/kg in 3 divided doses daily. RECTAL: *Adults*—120 to 200 mg as required for sedation or hypnosis. *Children*—as sedative, 30 to 120 mg/day. INTRAMUSCULAR: *Adults*—as hypnotic, 150 to 200 mg. INTRAVENOUS: *Adults*—as hypnotic, 100 mg. After 1 min, can administer small increments, but no more than 500 mg total. *Children*—as hypnotic, 50 mg initially.	A short-acting barbiturate used principally for insomnia and preanesthetic sedation and occasionally for daytime sedation. Precautions are same as for secobarbital. Schedule II substance.
Phenobarbital‡	Luminal* Solfoton	ORAL: *Adults*—as sedative, 30 to 120 mg daily in 2 or 3 divided doses; as hypnotic, 100 to 320 mg at bedtime. FDA Pregnancy Category D. *Children*—as sedative, 6 mg/kg daily in 4 divided doses. INTRAMUSCULAR, INTRAVENOUS: *Adults*—as sedative, 30 to 120 mg; as hypnotic, 100 to 320 mg, with no more than 100 mg (2 ml of 5% solution)/min intravenously. Full effect lasts 15 min. RECTAL: *Children*—as sedative, 6 mg/kg divided in 3 doses.	A long-acting barbiturate used principally as a sedative. (For use as an anticonvulsant, see Chapter 34.) Not readily addictive. Schedule IV substance.

*Available in Canada and United States.
†Available in Canada only.
‡Also available as the sodium salt. Only the sodium salt is suitable for administration as a solution by the rectal, intramuscular, or intravenous route.

Continued.

Table 40-4   Sedative-Hypnotic and Antianxiety Drugs: Barbiturates—cont'd

Generic name	Trade name	Administration/dosage	Comments
Secobarbital	Seconal* Novosecobarb†	ORAL: *Adults*—as sedative, 30 to 50 mg; as hypnotic, 100 to 200 mg at bedtime; for preoperative sedation, 200 to 300 mg 1 to 2 hr before surgery. FDA Pregnancy Category D. *Children*—as sedative, 6 mg/kg in 3 divided doses; for preoperative sedation, 50 to 100 mg. RECTAL: *Adults*—120 to 200 mg as required for sedation or hypnosis. *Children*—15 to 120 mg. INTRAMUSCULAR: *Adults*—as hypnotic, 100 to 200 mg. *Children*—as hypnotic, 3 to 5 mg/kg, up to 100 mg. INTRAVENOUS: *Adults*—as hypnotic, 50 to 250 mg, inject only 50 mg in 15 sec.	A short-acting barbiturate used principally for insomnia and as preanesthetic sedative. Not indicated for repeated use because tolerance develops, rebound insomnia becomes marked, and the addiction potential is high. Schedule II substance.
Talbutal	Lotusate	ORAL: *Adults*—120 mg at bedtime. FDA Pregnancy Category D.	A short-acting barbiturate. Used as a hypnotic. Reduce doses for elderly patients. Schedule III substance. Not available in Canada.

*Available in Canada and United States.
†Available in Canada only.

abused. Discontinuance produces withdrawal symptoms resembling those described for the barbiturates. The degree of dependence is sometimes determined by giving 200 mg of pentobarbital every 2 hr until signs of intoxication appear. The patient is then detoxified with divided doses (4 to 6/day) of pentobarbital, and the total daily dose is decreased by 100 mg/day. This approach is possible because pentobarbital is cross-tolerant with these other drugs. Alternatively, the abused drug is decreased daily over a 10- to 20-day period, or phenobarbital is administered in decreasing daily doses.

In addition to these drugs, several antihistamines have a pronounced sedative effect, for which they are sometimes used (see Chapter 24).

Specific Drugs

Buspirone

Buspirone (BuSpar) is a newer antianxiety drug that is not a benzodiazepine. It does not cause the CNS depression characteristic of barbiturates and benzodiazepines. A lag time of 1 to 2 weeks is usual before a decrease in anxiety is noted. Little sedation or mental impairment is noted. However, at higher doses patients may experience sedation or a bad mood. Side effects are uncommon but include headaches, dizziness, nervousness, and light-headedness. Buspirone reportedly has little abuse potential. It is metabolized and excreted in urine.

Chloral hydrate

Chloral hydrate (Noctec) is the oldest of the currently used hypnotic drugs, introduced in the nineteenth century. Although it is not effective for more than 2 weeks, it does not suppress REM sleep and therefore does not cause REM rebound. Chloral hydrate and its active metabolite, trichlorethanol, have a half-life of only 8 hr, so no persistent effect occurs as does with flurazepam.

Chloral hydrate has an unpleasant taste and odor, which can be masked by taking the drug in capsules, as a chilled elixir or syrup, or as a suppository. The drug produces fewer side effects, particularly paradoxical excitement, among children or the elderly than other hypnotics, but it causes gastric irritation in some patients and displaces the coumarin anticoagulants from plasma protein. Drug dependence is produced by long-term use; an acute overdose can result in coma, with the patient having pinpoint pupils. In folklore, chloral hydrate added to an alcoholic beverage produces a "knockout" drink, the Mickey Finn, resulting from the additive effect of the two general CNS depressants.

Ethchlorvynol

Ethchlorvynol (Placidyl) was introduced in the 1950s as a hypnotic. The most frequent patient complaint is an aftertaste. Occasionally patients show exaggerated depression, with deep sleep and muscular weak-

Table 40-5   Miscellaneous Sedative-Hypnotic and Antianxiety Drugs

Generic name	Trade name	Administration/dosage	Comments
Buspirone	BuSpar	ORAL: *Adults*—initially, 5 mg 3 times daily. May increase by 5 mg daily every 2 to 3 days until desired response is obtained. Maximum daily dose: 60 mg. FDA Pregnancy Category B.	New antianxiety drug that causes less sedation. Does not react with alcohol or antidepressants.
Chloral hydrate	Noctec* Novochlor-hydrate†	ORAL, RECTAL: *Adults*—as sedative, 250 mg 3 times daily after meals; as hypnotic, 500 mg to 1 gm 15 to 30 min before bedtime. FDA Pregnancy Category C. *Children*—as sedative, 25 mg/kg body weight in 3 to 4 doses daily; as hypnotic, 50 mg/kg as a bedtime dose, not to exceed 500 mg.	A generally safe hypnotic. The unpleasant taste and odor can be masked by chilling the drug or using the capsule form. Schedule IV substance.
Ethchlorvynol	Placidyl*	ORAL: *Adults only*—as hypnotic, 500 mg to 1 gm at bedtime. FDA Pregnancy Category C.	Physical and psychologic dependence may occur. Schedule IV substance.
Ethinamate	Valmid	ORAL: *Adults only*—as hypnotic, 500 mg to 1 gm at bedtime. FDA Pregnancy Category C.	Physical and psychologic dependence may occur. Schedule IV substance.
Hydroxyzine hydrochloride, Hydroxyzine pamoate	Atarax* Vistaril Various others	ORAL: *Adults*—for anxiety, 75 to 400 mg daily in 4 divided doses. For allergic skin reactions: ORAL: *Adults*—25 mg 3 or 4 times daily. *Children under 6 years*—50 mg daily in 3 or 4 divided doses. *Adults*—for anxiety, 50 to 100 mg every 4 to 6 hr.	An antihistamine that has antiemetic and antianxiety properties. Used in treating allergic skin rashes and motion sickness and as a preanesthetic medication. Usual doses of barbiturates or narcotics must be cut by 50% if given concurrently.
Meprobamate	Equanil* Meprospan* Miltown* Various others	ORAL: *Adults*—for anxiety, 1.2 to 1.6 gm daily in 3 or 4 divided doses. *Children over 6 years*—for anxiety, 25 mg/kg daily in 2 or 3 divided doses.	Physical and psychologic dependence may occur. Schedule IV substance.
Methyprylon	Noludar	ORAL: *Adults*—as hypnotic, 200 to 400 mg at bedtime. FDA Pregnancy Category B.	Physical and psychologic dependence may occur. Schedule III substance.

*Available in Canada and United States.
†Available in Canada only.

ness. Some individuals have an idiosyncratic response of CNS stimulation that may be mild or hysteric. Ethchlorvynol is a schedule IV drug with a duration of action similar to that of the short-acting barbiturates.

Ethinamate

Ethinamate (Valmid) was introduced in the 1950s as a hypnotic. It has a shorter duration of action than the short-acting barbiturates and is a schedule IV drug.

Hydroxyzine

Hydroxyzine (Atarax and Vistaril), an antihistamine with sedative properties, is used as an antianxiety agent when it is desirable to have the antiemetic and antihistaminic properties for motion sickness or allergic skin reactions. Hydroxyzine is also used as a preanesthetic medication.

Meprobamate

Meprobamate (Equanil and Miltown) was introduced in the 1950s as the first widely prescribed antianxiety drug. Although physical dependence readily develops with abuse, meprobamate is a schedule IV drug. Withdrawal symptoms range from insomnia and anxiety to hallucinations and grand mal seizures. Meprobamate is sometimes used as a centrally acting skeletal muscle relaxant, although its effectiveness in this role is questionable.

Methyprylon

Methyprylon (Nolvdar) was introduced as a hypnotic in the 1950s. It is a schedule II drug used similarly to the short-acting barbiturates.

ALCOHOL

Alcohol is a widely used and abused drug. In this section the important actions of alcohol and its in-

teractions with other drugs are reviewed.

As a general CNS depressant, alcohol causes all the behavioral changes described in the overview: sedation, disinhibition, sleep, and anesthesia. As summarized in Table 40-6, the amount of alcohol in the blood, which can be predicted from the amount consumed, produces characteristic behavioral effects. Alcohol also enhances the sedative-hypnotic effects of other drug classes, including all the general CNS depressants discussed in this chapter and other drug classes with sedative side effects including the antihistamines, the phenothiazines, the narcotic analgesics, the tricyclic antidepressants, and the monoamine-oxidase inhibitors. This enhancement of CNS depression means that irreversible coma or death can occur when alcohol is taken concurrently with other

Table 40-6   Alcohol Intake and Its Behavioral Effects

Alcohol content (oz)	Beverage intake in 1 hr*	Blood alcohol level (mg/dl) in a 150-lb man	Behavioral effects
½	1 oz 100-proof spirits 1 glass wine 1 can beer	0.025	No noticeable effect
1	2 oz 100-proof spirits 2 glasses wine 2 cans beer	0.050	Lower alertness, impaired judgment, good feeling, and less inhibition
2	4 oz 100-proof spirits 4 glasses wine 4 cans beer	0.100	Slow reaction time, impaired motor function, and less cautious; should not drive; may activate vomiting reflex
3	6 oz 100-proof spirits 6 glasses wine 6 cans beer	0.150	Large increase in reaction times
4	8 oz 100-proof spirits 8 glasses wine 8 cans beer	0.200	Marked depression of sensory and motor abilities
5	10 oz 100-proof spirits 10 glasses wine 10 cans beer	0.250	Severe depression of sensory and motor abilities
6	12 oz 100-proof spirits 12 glasses wine 12 cans beer	0.300	Stuporous and unconscious of surroundings
7	14 oz 100-proof spirits 14 glasses wine 14 cans beer	0.350	Unconscious
8	16 oz 100-proof spirits 16 glasses wine 16 cans beer	0.400	Lethal dose in 50% of the population
12	24 oz 100-proof spirits 24 glasses wine 24 cans beer	0.600	Lethal dose in 95% of the population

*Since only ¼ to ⅓ oz of alcohol is metabolized each hour, alcohol rapidly accumulates.

drugs, a fact not widely enough appreciated in our society.

Alcohol as vasodilator. Acute ingestion of alcohol has effects in addition to those attributed to its general CNS depression. Rising levels of alcohol may activate the vomiting center. Alcohol acts centrally to produce vasodilation and a feeling of warmth. This vasodilation can produce a marked hypotensive response in persons taking guanethidine or nitroglycerin.

Factors affecting absorption. Alcohol is absorbed more readily from the small intestine than from the stomach. Absorption of alcohol therefore is decreased by food, which dilutes the alcohol and keeps it in the stomach longer. Alcohol in concentrations of 10% or less will stimulate gastric secretions, thereby aiding digestion, but larger concentrations inhibit gastric secretions and damage the cells lining the stomach. This irritation may make some people nauseated the day after heavy drinking and accounts for the inflammation of the stomach (gastritis) and ulcers frequently seen in alcoholics. Aspirin is another drug that readily damages the stomach lining. The combination of aspirin and alcohol can produce bleeding in the stomach.

Metabolism. More than 90% of ingested alcohol is oxidized by the liver, with the remainder being excreted in the breath and urine. The oxidation of alcohol to carbon dioxide and water means that alcohol is a source of calories. Alcoholics may get most of their calories from alcohol but may be malnourished because alcoholic beverages lack vitamins, minerals, and protein.

Two enzyme systems in the liver transform alcohol. The major enzyme for alcohol metabolism is alcohol dehydrogenase, which is also the enzyme that limits the rate of alcohol metabolism. In the average adult, the liver alcohol dehydrogenase can metabolize only about 10 ml of alcohol in 1 hr. This means that no matter how much someone has drunk, only 10 ml of alcohol can be metabolized in 1 hr, and alcohol readily accumulates in the body when this amount is exceeded. Neither coffee, fresh air, nor exercise will speed up alcohol metabolism to help someone "sober up".

The product of alcohol metabolism by alcohol dehydrogenase is acetaldehyde, a highly toxic compound. Ordinarily, acetaldehyde does not accumulate because it is metabolized further by aldehyde dehydrogenase. Disulfiram (Antabuse) and other drugs can inhibit this enzyme so that acetaldehyde accumulates and produces unpleasant symptoms, which include headache, nausea, and vomiting.

The liver microsomal enzyme system described for the barbiturates also can degrade alcohol but ordinarily with a very limited capacity. As with phenobarbital, alcohol can induce this enzyme system so that the liver can metabolize not only more alcohol but more of other drugs as well, and this is one source of drug interactions. Alcoholics are able to metabolize twice as much alcohol as those who do not drink chronically.

An elevated value of serum gamma glutamyl transpeptidase (GGTP) in the absence of other elevated enzymes is a good predictor of chronic alcohol or drug consumption. This enzyme is induced in the liver by alcohol and drugs and secreted into the circulation. An elevated GGTP is often the first biochemical sign of alcoholism and may occur before overt clinical signs and symptoms develop.

Drug interactions. Alcohol is a major source of drug interactions because it is so widely consumed. Alcohol particularly influences other CNS depressants, drug metabolism, gastric mucosal integrity, blood glucose levels, and vasodilation. These drug interactions are listed in Table 40-7. The importance of alcohol as a source of drug interactions can be appreciated by considering the estimate that 5% of adults in the United States are alcoholic and that 30% to 60% of hospitalized individuals are alcoholic.

Effects of an acute overdose. Unless a large amount of concentrated alcohol has been rapidly swallowed on an empty stomach or ingested with another CNS depressant drug, an acute overdose of alcohol commonly causes an individual to pass out before lethal doses can be drunk. However, note that a pint of 100-proof liquor is an L.D.$_{50}$ dose for a small man (see Table 40-6). With rapid drinking of straight liquor, someone can drink enough to die. The greatest danger of acute alcohol intoxication to nonalcoholic individuals is that they may involve themselves or others in traffic accidents (30,000 alcohol-related traffic deaths per year) or that they may fall and injure themselves.

A hangover is common on recovery from an acute alcohol intoxication and includes such symptoms as an upset stomach, thirst, fatigue, headache, depression, anxiety, and generally feeling out of sorts. Many of these symptoms are caused by congeners, the natural by-products of fermentation and aging. Vodka, which is a mixture of pure alcohol and water and contains a few congeners, also produces few hangover symptoms compared to wines and aged spirits, which have higher congener contents. Table 40-7 summarizes drug interactions with alcohol.

Physiologic Changes Associated with Chronic Drinking

Chronic drinking can produce characteristic degenerative changes in the body, as listed in Table 40-8.

Table 40-7   Sources of Drug Interactions with Alcohol

Effect	Interacting drugs	Comments
Increased CNS depression	Barbiturates Meprobamate Hypnotics Antihistamines Narcotic analgesics Monoamine oxidase inhibitors Tricyclic antidepressants Benzodiazepines Chlorpromazine and other sedating phenothiazines	Any drug causing sedation or drowsiness is potentiated by alcohol. Most of these drugs carry warnings not to drive or operate dangerous equipment and stating that the situation worsens if alcohol is ingested. Alcohol can cause coma or death by respiratory depression when combined with CNS depressants even when the dose of either drug is not lethal by itself.
Increased liver metabolism	Barbiturates Phenytoin Tolbutamide Warfarin	When taken over a long period, alcohol induces the liver microsomal enzyme system for drug degradation. This speeds up the metabolism of drugs metabolized by these enzymes so that the effective therapeutic dose must be increased. Alternatively, if an alcoholic person receiving one of these drugs becomes detoxified, the drug dose may have to be lowered.
Gastric and mucosal irritation	Aspirin Nicotine	Aspirin and alcohol act synergistically to irritate the stomach and to cause bleeding. Alcoholic smokers have up to a 15-fold greater incidence of oral cancer.
Hypoglycemia	Insulin	Alcohol acts to lower blood glucose levels independently of insulin and may cause marked hypoglycemia when taken with insulin.
Disulfiram reaction	Disulfiram Sulfonylureas (oral hypoglycemic agents) Nitroglycerin	Disulfiram inhibits the degradation of acetaldehyde, which then accumulates and causes hypotension, GI distress, and headache.
Vasodilation	Guanethidine Nitroglycerin	Alcohol acts centrally to produce vasodilation, which can potentiate the action of these drugs.

These changes are seen after about 10 years of drinking 150 ml of alcohol daily. In addition to these degenerative changes, some alcoholic persons may have blackout spells, periods in which they are awake and functioning but of which they have no memory. Heavy drinking during pregnancy is associated with a 63% incidence of neurologic abnormalities in the offspring. **Fetal alcohol syndrome** is now recognized in the offspring of alcoholic mothers, a syndrome characterized by a flat face with widely spaced, small eyes and mental retardation.

Withdrawal symptoms after chronic drinking

Chronic drinking also leads to withdrawal symptoms when the person stops drinking. The severity of the withdrawal symptoms depends on the individual's drinking history but are most common when a chronic drinker stays intoxicated for 2 or more weeks and then stops drinking. The first symptoms, which appear within a few hours, are tremors and anxiety. As the first stage progresses, bradycardia occurs, the blood pressure increases, and there is heavy sweating, loss of appetite, nausea and vomiting, and insomnia. The second stage of withdrawal is characterized by hallucinations, usually visual, but sometimes involving hearing or feeling things. The patient is still oriented and only mildly confused despite these hallucinations.

Untreated withdrawal. About 10% of untreated patients have seizures within the first 48 hr of withdrawal. **Delirium tremens** is a stage of withdrawal that occurs in about 10% of untreated alcoholic persons 2 to 7 days after the start of withdrawal. Delirium tremens lasts about 2 days, during which time the person is completely disoriented, is extremely agitated, sweats, and has a fever and a changing pulse

Table 40-8   Degenerative Changes Common with Chronic Alcohol Consumption

System	Comments	System	Comments
Brain	Lack of vitamin B_1 (thiamine) common to alcoholic persons produces *Wernicke's disease:* brain lesions manifested as an inability to learn or recall. *Korsakoff's psychosis* describes alcoholic persons who are confused and disoriented as to time or place. Wernicke's disease and Korsakoff's psychosis are considered variations of the same brain disease. Replacement of vitamin B_1 helps reverse symptoms in the early stages but will not restore lost function later.	Heart	Some alcoholic individuals develop an enlarged heart that functions poorly (cardiomyopathy).
		Blood	Because of blood loss and lack of folic acid, alcoholic persons can have both iron deficiency (microcytic) anemia and folate deficiency (macrocytic) anemia. Liver disease may result in clotting factor deficiency. White blood cells and platelets are decreased.
Liver	Chronic drinking produces a fatty liver because in the presence of alcohol, fatty acids are stored in the liver rather than being metabolized. About 75% of alcoholic persons show some cirrhosis after 10 years. In cirrhosis, fibrous tissue replaces liver cells. Severe cases result in liver failure and death. Hepatitis (inflammation of the liver) is also common among alcoholic persons.	Metabolic	Alcoholic persons are often hypoglycemic because alcohol inhibits glucose production by the liver. Since alcohol is converted to a substrate for carbohydrate and fat metabolism, high levels of lipids, lactic acid, uric acid, and ketone bodies may appear in the blood. Plasma magnesium, plasma phosphate, and plasma albumin concentrations are low.
Stomach and GI tract	Alcohol causes gastritis, which leads to ulcers and blood loss. Nonspecific diarrhea is common. Inflammation of the pancreas (pancreatitis) is common.	Skin	The vasodilation caused by alcohol eventually produces a permanent rosy nose and cheeks. Skin ulcers are common.

and blood pressure. The person usually has no memory of delirium tremens.

Treatment of withdrawal. A patient undergoing alcohol withdrawal is usually treated with one of the following benzodiazepines: diazepam, chlordiazepoxide, clorazepate, or oxazepam. This treatment is effective because alcohol is cross-tolerant with the benzodiazepines.

Additional therapy during withdrawal is designed to restore normal metabolic parameters and overcome the thiamin, B_{12}, and folic acid deficiencies. This supportive therapy relieves neurologic symptoms secondary to hypoglycemia, ketosis, and vitamin deficiency.

Aversion therapy with disulfiram. Disulfiram (Antabuse) is prescribed for the detoxified patient who wishes to avoid drinking again (see box). Disulfiram blocks the oxidation of acetaldehyde. The accumulation of acetaldehyde causes unpleasant reactions, which include flushing, throbbing in the head and

neck, throbbing headache, respiratory difficulty, nausea, copious vomiting, sweating, thirst, chest pain, rapid breathing, tachycardia, fainting, weakness, vertigo, blurred vision, and confusion. These effects can be elicited by alcohol for 1 to 2 weeks after disulfiram is discontinued. The reaction lasts from 30 min to 1 to 3 hr. Severe reactions can cause death from cardiovascular collapse or respiratory failure. Because of the severity of the reactions, only well-informed, motivated patients are considered for disulfiram therapy, which is at best a supportive treatment when supplemented by psychiatric therapy. Patients whose drinking problem is lack of moderation after the first drink is taken are considered the best candidates for disulfiram therapy. By itself, disulfiram produces transient effects that usually disappear within 2 weeks such as drowsiness, fatigue, impotence, headache, acne, and a metallic or garliclike aftertaste. Drug interactions with disulfirum are listed in Table 40-9.

PATIENT PROBLEM: ALCOHOL USE AND DISULFIRAM

THE PROBLEM

Disulfiram is prescribed to patients who want to avoid drinking alcohol again. When a patient is taking disulfiram and alcohol is consumed, a serious physiologic reaction occurs. Other drugs also are associated with *disulfiram-like reactions* in combination with alcohol. Examples are furazolidone, metronidazole, chlorpropamide, and the antibiotic moxalactam.

SIGNS AND SYMPTOMS

The combination of alcohol and disulfiram produces flushing, throbbing in the head and neck, throbbing headache, respiratory difficulty, nausea, copious vomiting, sweating, thirst, chest pain, rapid breathing, tachycardia, fainting, weakness, vertigo, blurred vision, and confusion. Severe reactions can cause death.

PATIENT AND FAMILY EDUCATION

Review the signs and symptoms of disulfiram-like reactions. Tell the patient to seek medical help for a severe reaction.

Review sources of alcohol. Obvious sources include ingestion of beer, liquor, or wine. Other dietary sources include sauces that may contain wine, cooking sherry, or liquors; wine vinegars; and some liquid medications such as cough syrups and elixirs. In patients sensitive to this reaction, topical contact with after-shave lotion or colognes, alcohol-containing liniments, or after-bath lotions may produce symptoms. Avoid inhalation of the vapors of any chemical that may contain alcohol such as shellac, varnish, or paint.

Read the labels on food items and medicines. If in doubt about a drug, consult the pharmacist.

Wear a medical identification tag or bracelet indicating that disulfiram is being taken.

Avoid alcohol-containing products for up to 2 weeks after stopping disulfiram or a drug associated with disulfiram-like reactions.

Table 40-9   Drug Interactions with Disulfiram

Drug	Action
Phenytoin (Dilantin), coumarins (oral anti-coagulants)	Potentiated by disulfiram, which inhibits their degradation by the liver microsomal enzymes
Benzodiazepines	Potentiated by disulfiram, which inhibits their plasma clearance
Benzodiazepines and ascorbic acid (vitamin C)	Decreased alcohol-disulfiram reaction by protecting the acetaldehyde-oxidizing enzymes
Tricyclic antidepressants	Increased alcohol-disulfiram reaction by inhibiting the acetaldehyde-oxidizing enzymes
Isoniazid, metronidazole	Can cause neuropsychiatric symptoms by an unknown mechanism in the presence of disulfiram

NURSING IMPLICATIONS SUMMARY

General Guidelines for the Use of the Antianxiety Agents and Sedative-Hypnotics

Drug administration

◆ In the institutional setting, keep side rails up after administering these drugs. Supervise ambulation and smoking. Keep a nightlight on.

◆ Use "sleeping pills" judiciously. Do not deprive patients of needed medication, but use medications as an adjunct to nursing measures such as a backrub, repositioning, a small snack, or a glass of warm milk.

◆ Tactfully assess side effects. Some drugs cause changes in libido or sexual activity. Provide emotional support as appropriate. Consult with the physician about changes in drug or dosage.

◆ Be alert in the outpatient setting to patients who return for prescription refills on an increasingly frequent basis; this may indicate improper use or abuse or lack of knowledge about the hazards of continued use of the drugs. Evaluate patients carefully for possible depression and suicidal tendencies.

Patient and family education

◆ Remind patients to take these drugs only as directed and not to increase the dose or frequency without consulting the physician.

◆ Warn patients to avoid driving or operating hazardous equipment if drowsiness develops. Supervise the play of children.

◆ Warn patients to avoid ingestion of alcohol.

◆ Instruct patients to avoid the use of other drugs that may depress the CNS, unless they are specifically prescribed by the physician. Examples include antiemetics, narcotic analgesics, and antihistamines.

◆ For insomnia, patients should take doses 30 min before bedtime.

◆ Instruct patients that the frequently encountered hangover effect in the morning after use of a sedative-hypnotic is a side effect of the medication and not a sign that the patient needs a larger dose of medication that evening.

◆ Caution patients taking anticonvulsant medication that drowsiness may continue for several days to weeks but should gradually diminish.

◆ Tell patients to inform all health-care providers of all drugs being used, even occasional sleeping pills.

◆ Instruct patients to keep these and all drugs out of the reach of children. Use childproof caps in settings where there are small children. Keep drugs in clearly labeled containers.

◆ Remind patients not to share drugs with friends or relatives.

◆ Refer patients who are having continuing problems with insomnia or anxiety to appropriate resources for counseling or evaluation.

◆ After long-term use, patients may have difficulty discontinuing the medication abruptly. Instruct patients to consult the physician before discontinuing medications.

Benzodiazepines

Drug administration

◆ See the general guidelines.

◆ Monitor blood pressure and pulse, intake and output, and weight. Monitor the respiratory rate, and auscultate breath sounds. Inspect for skin changes.

◆ Menstrual irregularities may develop. Instruct patient to notify the physician. Counsel about contraception as appropriate.

◆ Monitor complete blood count (CBC) and platelets, liver function tests, and blood urea nitrogen (BUN), and serum creatinine levels.

INTRAVENOUS BENZODIAZEPINES

◆ Have a suction machine and equipment for intubation and ventilatory support available.

◆ Keep side rails up.

◆ Monitor respiratory rate and blood pressure. Do not leave patients unattended unless they are sufficiently alert to handle secretions and to call for assistance.

◆ Keep patients on bedrest for 2 to 4 hr after IV doses.

INTRAVENOUS DIAZEPAM

◆ Administer undiluted, at a rate of 5 mg (1 ml) or less over 1 min.

INTRAVENOUS CHLORDIAZEPOXIDE

◆ Dilute each 100 mg with at least 5 ml sterile water for injection. Administer 100 mg diluted over at least 5 min.

INTRAVENOUS LORAZEPAM

◆ Dilute just before administering with an equal volume of compatible IV fluid. Administer at a rate of 2 mg or less over 1 min.

Continued.

INTRAVENOUS MIDAZOLAM

◆ It may be diluted with normal saline or 5% dextrose in water. Rate of administration is often determined by patient response (e.g., 1 mg/4 ml, administered over at least 2 min, until speech is slurred). For conscious sedation, evaluate carefully to avoid overmedication; wait 2 min between increments. Use lower doses in elderly or debilitated patients.

Patient and family education

◆ See the general guidelines.
◆ Instruct patients to report any new side effects.
◆ See Patient Problems: Dry Mouth on p. 166 and Photosensitivity on p. 629.
◆ Tell patients to take doses with meals or a snack to lessen gastric irritation.

Flumazenil

Drug administration

◆ Consult manufacturer's literature for current guidelines.
◆ Monitor vital signs, blood pressure, and level of consciousness. Have a suction machine at the bedside. Keep siderails up. Do not leave the patient unattended.
◆ Administration of this drug to patients who have used benzodiazepines on a chronic basis may precipitate withdrawal symptoms.
◆ Keep the patient and family informed of the patient's condition.

Barbiturates

Drug administration

◆ See the general guidelines.
◆ Monitor blood pressure and pulse, intake and output, and weight. Monitor the respiratory rate, and auscultate breath sounds. Inspect for skin changes.
◆ Monitor CBC, platelet count, and liver function tests.
◆ With IV administration, monitor vital signs and respiratory rate. Have a suction machine and equipment for intubation and ventilatory assistance available. Keep patients on bedrest until stable.

Patient and family education

◆ See the general guidelines.
◆ Instruct patients to report any new side effects.
◆ Take doses with meals or a snack to lessen gastric irritation.

Miscellaneous Agents

◆ See the general guidelines.
◆ Monitor blood pressure and pulse and intake and output.
◆ When used in the doses ordered, side effects are rare.

Disulfiram

◆ See Patient Problem: Disulfiram-like Reactions on p. 614 and review side effects discussed in the text.
◆ Treatment with disulfiram is not a cure for alcoholism and should be used only with other forms of supportive therapy. Assess patients carefully before administering this drug.
◆ Treatment of severe disulfiram reaction may require hospitalization. Instruct the patient's family about the effects of alcohol consumption while the patient is receiving disulfiram.

CHAPTER REVIEW

◆ KEY TERMS

anxiety, p. 599
barbiturates, p. 604
benzodiazepines, p. 599
cross-tolerance, p. 597
delirium tremens, p. 612
drug addiction, p. 597
drug dependence, p. 597
fetal alcohol syndrome, p. 612
hypnotic, p. 595
insomnia, p. 598
REM sleep, p. 597
reticular activating system, p. 596
sedative, p. 595

◆ REVIEW QUESTIONS

1. Define sedative, hypnotic, and antianxiety drugs.
2. What is the reticular activating system, and how is it affected by general CNS depressants?
3. Describe the stages of CNS depression.
4. What is drug dependence?
5. What are withdrawal symptoms? What symptoms would you observe?
6. What is cross-tolerance? What precautions in medications would you observe?
7. Name the stages of sleep, and describe which ones are affected by hypnotics.
8. What is anxiety? What symptoms would you observe?
9. What major advantage do benzodiazepines have over barbiturates?
10. What drug interactions are seen with benzodiazepines? What steps in patient education would you take?
11. Describe the uses of benzodiazepines. For what conditions are these drugs used?
12. Describe the four categories of barbiturates, and list which drugs belong in each category.
13. Describe withdrawal symptoms from barbiturates. What symptoms might you observe?
14. Differentiate between metabolic tolerance and pharmacodynamic tolerance.
15. What are the uses of barbiturates?

16. Are hypnotics more similar to barbiturates or to benzodiazepines?
17. What drug interactions are seen with alcohol?
18. What factors affect alcohol absorption?
19. Describe alcohol metabolism. How does disulfiram interfere with alcohol metabolism?
20. What are the side effects of alcohol ingestion with disulfiram?
21. What physiologic changes are associated with chronic drinking?
22. How is alcohol withdrawal treated? What interventions might you take?

SUGGESTED READING

Sleep and hypnotics

Gillin JC, Byerley WF: The diagnosis and management of insomnia, *N Engl J Med* 322(4):239, 1990.

Shorr RI, Bauwens SF, Landefeld, CS: Failure to limit quantities of benzodiazepine hypnotic drugs for outpatients: placing the elderly at risk, *Am J Med* 89(12):725, 1990.

Anxiety and drug dependence

Beeber LS: Undesirable weight gain and psychotropic medications, *J Psychosoc Nurs Ment Health Serv* 26(10):39, 1988.

Beeber LS: Update on medications for the treatment of anxiety, *J Psychosoc Nurs Ment Health Serv* 27(10):42, 1989.

Johnson JE: Effect of benzodiazepines on older women, *J Community Health Nurse* 5(2):119, 1988.

Karb VB: Midazolam: newcomer to the benzodiazepine family, *J Neurosci Nurse* 21(1):64, 1989.

Murphy EK: Legal considerations in RN monitoring of intravenous sedation, *AORN J* 48(6):1184, 1988.

Roy-Byrne PP, Hommer D: Benzodiazepine withdrawal: overview and implications for the treatment of anxiety, *Am J Med* 84(6):1041, 1988.

Smith DA: New role for prescribing psychotropics in nursing homes, *Geriatrics* 45(2):44, 1990.

Townsend MC: *Drug Guide for Psychiatric Nursing*, Philadelphia, 1990, FA Davis.

Alcohol and alcoholism

Cleary PD and others: Prevalence and recognition of alcohol abuse in a primary care population, *Am J Med* 85(10):466, 1988.

Hayashida M and others: Comparative effectiveness and costs of inpatient and outpatient detoxification of patients with mild-to-moderate alcohol withdrawal syndrome, *N Engl J Med* 320(6):358, 1989.

Stewart-Amidei C: Alcohol and head injury: a nursing perspective, *Crit Care Nurs Q* 10(1):69, 1987.

Valanis B, Yeaworth RC, Mullis MR: Alcohol use among bereaved and nonbereaved older persons, *J Gerontol Nurs* 13(5):26, 1987.

CHAPTER 41

Antipsychotic Drugs

LEARNING OBJECTIVES

After studying this chapter, you should be able to do the following:

♦ Outline the kinds of psychoses discussed.

♦ Distinguish among the five chemical classes of antipsychotic drugs and the three subgroups of the phenothiazines.

♦ Discuss the role of the neurotransmitters dopamine, norepinephrine, and acetylcholine in the actions of the antipsychotics.

♦ Describe the signs and symptoms of extrapyramidal reactions to antipsychotic drugs.

♦ Develop a nursing care plan for a patient receiving one of the antipsychotic drugs discussed.

♦ Develop a care plan for a patient receiving a drug that may cause photosensitivity.

CHAPTER OVERVIEW

♦ One of the remarkable advances in pharmacology in recent decades has been the discovery and application of drugs effective in treating the major mental illnesses: schizophrenia and depression. This chapter discusses the antipsychotic or antischizophrenic drugs, also called *neuroleptic* drugs. **Neuroleptic** refers to the ability of these drugs to cause a general quiescence and a state of psychic indifference to the surroundings.

Nursing Process Overview
ANTIPSYCHOTIC DRUGS
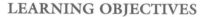
Assessment

Perform a complete physiologic assessment, with a focus on the behavioral component. Assess the patient's emotional affect, ability to interact with others, and ability to initiate appropriate conversation. Assess for abnormal thought processes such as hallucinations or delusions, and observe any unusual mannerisms or conversely, the lack of any outward activity. Evaluate judgment, decision making, and overall thought processes.

Nursing Diagnoses

Altered bowel elimination: constipation secondary to drug side effects

Possible impaired physical mobility related to extrapyramidal side effects of antipsychotic therapy

Management

Patients requiring antipsychotic drug therapy also require psychiatric care, at least during initial drug therapy. Observe patients closely for changes in overall affect and behavior. Monitor vital signs, level of consciousness, blood pressure, and signs of drug toxicity. Serious side effects include extrapyramidal reactions or acute dystonia.

Evaluation

Most patients require continued use of these medications, with brief drug-free periods, for the rest of their lives. Before discharge, verify that the patient or family can explain how to take the medication correctly, what symptoms or side effects should be reported immediately to the physician, what situations indicating overdosage or underdosage should be reported to the physician, and what symptoms of disease exacerbation should be

618

reported to the physician. If other medications are used to treat the underlying condition or side effects of the antipsychotic drugs, ascertain that the patient or family can explain the necessary information about these drugs.

CLINICAL USES OF ANTIPSYCHOTIC DRUGS

The three major uses of **antipsychotic drugs** are to treat psychoses, to prevent vomiting, and to potentiate the action of other central nervous system (CNS) drugs. The individual antipsychotic drugs are described in detail in Table 41-1.

Treatment of Psychoses

Antipsychotic drugs are unique in allowing symptomatic treatment of psychoses. A **psychosis** is a major emotional disorder with an impairment of mental function great enough to prevent the individual from participating in everyday life. The hallmark of a psychosis is the loss of contact with reality. There is no one symptom of a psychosis. Symptoms may include agitation, hostility, combativeness, hyperactivity, delusions, hallucinations, disordered thought and perception, emotional and social withdrawal, paranoid symptoms, and personal neglect. Antipsychotic drugs specifically reduce at least some of these symptoms so that patients can think and function more coherently.

Psychoses account for most of the hospitalizations for mental illness, disabling as many Americans as heart disease and cancer combined.

Functional psychoses

A **functional psychosis** may be an isolated "breakdown" caused by a major traumatic event. This psychosis is usually amenable to treatment with an antipsychotic drug. The acute manic phase of manic-depressive illness is treated with an antipsychotic drug or lithium (see Chapter 42).

Schizophrenia

Schizophrenia is a chronic mental illness with psychotic episodes. Before the advent of the antipsychotic drugs in the 1950s, schizophrenia accounted for most of the patient population in mental hospitals. Today, with continued advances in antipsychotic drug therapy, patients with schizophrenia do not usually require the degree of supervision found in mental hospitals. The current trend is to provide acute initial care in the psychiatric intensive care unit followed by minimum care in community facilities. Antipsychotic drugs do not cure schizophrenia. Treatment is life-

long, although patients may be taken off medication for several weeks or months during a disease remission.

Organic psychoses

An **organic psychosis** results from damage to the brain by infectious diseases, deficiency diseases, lead poisoning, tumors, and injury through trauma or interrupted blood supply such as in cerebrovascular accidents (stroke). Organic psychoses are not treated with antipsychotic drugs as successfully as functional psychoses.

Toxic psychoses

A **toxic psychosis** can arise during withdrawal from alcohol or other drugs. Some toxic psychoses are treated with diazepam, an antianxiety drug, rather than with antipsychotic drugs. Amphetamine can cause a toxic psychosis because it releases dopamine in the CNS, and therefore the blockade of dopamine receptors by antipsychotic drugs provides specific therapy for an amphetamine-induced psychosis.

Antiemetic Use

Several antipsychotic drugs are prescribed to control vomiting. Chlorpromazine, triflupromazine, perphenazine, and prochlorperazine in particular are widely used as antiemetics. Chlorpromazine is also prescribed for intractable hiccups. Because of the numerous side effects of these drugs, their use as antiemetics is restricted to management of postoperative nausea and vomiting, radiation and chemotherapy sickness, nausea and vomiting caused by toxins, and intractable vomiting.

MECHANISMS OF ANTIPSYCHOTIC DRUGS
Chemical Classes

The five chemical classes of antipsychotic drugs are the phenothiazines, the thioxanthenes, the butyrophenones, the dibenzoxazepines, and the dihydroindolones. The latter three classes contribute only four drugs to present clinical use. Ten phenothiazine and two thioxanthene compounds are currently in clinical use as antipsychotic drugs.

Phenothiazines

The largest antipsychotic drug class is the **phenothiazines.** Chlorpromazine was the first phenothiazine introduced in the United States and is still the most widely used drug in this class. Chlorpromazine originally was licensed as an antiemetic drug, later as a drug to potentiate anesthesia, and finally as an antipsychotic drug. The thioxanthenes have a three-ringed main structure that differs by only one atom

Text continued on p. 625.

Table 41-1 Antipsychotic Drugs

Generic name	Trade name	Administration/dosage	Comments
BUTYROPHENONE			
Haloperidol	Haldol* Halperon Paridol† Novoperidol†	Acute psychotic management: ORAL: *Adults and children over 12 years*—1 to 15 mg in divided doses initially, which can be increased gradually up to 100 mg to bring symptoms under control. Dosage is then gradually reduced. Maintenance dose, usually 2 to 8 mg daily. FDA Pregnancy Category C. *Elderly patients and children under 12 years*—0.5 to 1.5 mg daily initially. Dosage increased by 0.5-mg increments if necessary. Usual maintenance dose, 2 to 4 mg daily. INTRAMUSCULAR: *Adults and children over 12 years*—2 to 5 mg every 4 to 8 hr or every hour if acute state requires. Acute symptoms are usually under control in 72 hr, and 15 mg daily is usually sufficient. Chronic schizophrenia: ORAL: *Adults and children over 12 years*—6 to 16 mg in divided doses, gradually increased to achieve control. Doses as high as 100 mg may be necessary to achieve control. Doses then are gradually reduced to achieve maintenance of control, usually 15 to 20 mg daily. *Elderly patients*—0.5 to 1.5 mg initially, increased very gradually. Maintenance dosage, usually 2 to 8 mg daily. Mental retardation with hyperkinesia: ORAL (given after IM treatment as for acute psychoses): *Adults and children over 12 years*—80 to 120 mg daily, gradually reduced to a maintenance dose of about 60 mg daily. *Elderly patients and children under 12 years*—1.5 to 6 mg daily in divided doses; gradually increase dosage up to 15 mg daily for control, then reduce dosage for maintenance. Gilles de la Tourette's syndrome: Initial dosages to achieve control are same as for chronic schizophrenia. Maintenance dosages: *Adults and children over 12 years*—9 mg daily; *Children under 12 years*—1.5 mg daily.	Management of psychotic disorders. Likely to produce extrapyramidal reactions in patients prone to neurologic reactions. In severe cases of hyperkinetic, retarded patients, large doses may bring improvement in social behavior and concentration. Drug of choice for the treatment of Gilles de la Tourette's syndrome. Spectrum of side effects is similar to that of the piperazine phenothiazines: low incidence of sedation and autonomic effects but high incidence of extrapyramidal reactions.
DIBENZOXAZEPINES			
Loxapine succinate	Loxitane Loxapac†	ORAL: *Patients over 16 years*—10 to 25 mg twice daily initially, with dosage increased rapidly over 7 to 10 days to achieve control. Dosage reduced for maintenance to 60 to 100 mg daily; maximum, 250 mg daily. FDA Pregnancy Category C. *Elderly patients*—⅓ to ½ dose just listed.	Effective for schizophrenia and acute psychoses.
Clozapine	Clozaril Leponex	ORAL: *Adults*—Initially, 25 mg 1 to 2 times a day, increasing in increments of 25 to 60 mg/day, as tolerated, to achieve a dose of 300 to 450 mg/day by the end of 2 weeks. Subsequent dosage increments should not exceed 100 mg 1 or 2 times/week.	Atypical antipsychotic, indicated only in the management of severely ill schizophrenic patients failing on other drugs. Monitor for agranulocytosis and seizures.
DIHYDROINDOLONE			
Molindone hydrochloride	Moban	ORAL: *Adults*—15 to 40 mg daily initially, with increased dosage to control symptoms, up to 225 mg daily. Dosage should then be reduced for maintenance. *Elderly patients*—⅓ to ½ adult dose.	Effective for schizophrenia and acute psychoses.

*Available in Canada and United States.
†Available in Canada only.

Table 41-1 Antipsychotic Drugs—cont'd

Generic name	Trade name	Administration/dosage	Comments
PHENOTHIAZINES			
Aliphatic			
Chlorpromazine hydrochloride	Thorazine Chlor-Promanyl† Largactil† Thor-Prom Novo-Chlor-promazine† Various others	Psychiatric outpatients: ORAL: *Adults*—12 to 40 years, average dose 400 to 800 mg daily; over 40 years, a limit of 300 mg daily is suggested. Acutely psychotic, hospitalized patients: INTRAMUSCULAR: *Adults*—25 to 100 mg every 1 to 4 hr until symptoms are controlled. *Elderly or debilitated patients*—10 mg every 6 to 8 hr to control acute symptoms. *Children*—0.5 mg/kg body weight every 6 to 8 hr, gradually increasing dose to a maximum of 40 mg for children under 5 years and 75 mg for those under 12 years. INTRAVENOUS: not recommended because it is highly irritating. Drug must be diluted to at least 1 mg/ml and no more than 1 mg/min given. ORAL: *Adults*—200 to 600 mg daily in divided doses, increased every 2 to 3 days by 100 mg, up to 2 gm if needed. *Elderly or debilitated patients*—⅓ to ½ of adult dose with 20 to 25 mg increments. *Children*—0.5 mg/kg every 4 to 6 hr. To control nausea and vomiting: ORAL: 10 to 25 mg every 4 to 6 hr. INTRAMUSCULAR: 25 mg initially, then 25 to 50 mg every 3 to 4 hr to stop vomiting. Other uses: ORAL: *Adults*—25 to 50 mg 3 or 4 times daily. INTRAMUSCULAR: 25 mg every 3 or 4 hr.	Control of initial acute psychotic episodes is achieved with high doses, which are then tapered to the lowest maintenance dose when the patient's condition stabilizes. Best tolerated by patients under 40 years of age and those hospitalized less than 10 years. Sedation is pronounced at the start of therapy, which may be desired for highly agitated patients. Incidence of hypotension, ophthalmic changes, and dyskinesias is high in older patients. Antiadrenergic and anticholinergic side effects usually diminish after the first week. Not for seizure-prone patients. Severe nausea and vomiting can be controlled by low doses. Other uses include intractable hiccups, tetanus, and acute intermittent porphyria.
Methotrimeprazine hydrochloride	Nozinan Oral Drops† Nozinan Liquid†	ORAL: *Adults*—For psychotic disorders or presurgical sedation: 6 to 25 mg/day in 3 divided doses with meals. Severe psychosis: 50 to 75 mg/day in divided doses with meals. *Children*—0.25 mg/kg body weight/day in 2 or 3 divided doses with meals. Increase gradually as needed, but no more than 40 mg/day in children under 12 years old.	Used as an antipsychotic, analgesic, antianxiety agent, and sedative. For moderate-to-severe pain of bedridden patients; obstetric pain and sedation; anxiety before surgery; and adjunctive therapy in general anesthesia to increase effects of anesthetics.
Methotrimeprazine maleate	Nozinan†	ORAL: *Adults, children*—Same doses as for hydrochloride.	
Methotrimeprazine	Levoprome* Nozinan†	INTRAMUSCULAR: *Adults*—Acute pain: 10 to 20 mg at 4- to 6-hr intervals; Obstetrical pain: 15 to 20 mg, repeat if needed; Postoperative pain: 2.5 to 7.5 mg immediately after surgery, repeated every 3 to 4 hr as needed.	For pain relief.
Promazine hydrochloride	Sparine* Promanyl†	Severely agitated patients: INTRAMUSCULAR: *Adults*—50 to 150 mg initially; if no calming effect in 30 min, additional doses may be given to a total of 300 mg. ORAL: *Adults*—10 to 200 mg every 4 to 6 hr (may also be given IM). ORAL, INTRAMUSCULAR: *Children over 12 years*—10 to 25 mg every 4 to 6 hr.	When the IM route is used, take precautions for postural hypotension. A syrup is available for oral administration; dilute the concentrate in fruit juice or chocolate flavored drinks. Total daily dose for adults should not exceed 1000 mg.

*Available in Canada and United States.
†Available in Canada only.

Continued.

Table 41-1   Antipsychotic Drugs—cont'd

Generic name	Trade name	Administration/dosage	Comments
PHENOTHIAZINES—cont'd			
Aliphatic—cont'd			
Triflupromazine hydrochloride	Vesprin	Psychotic disorders: ORAL: *Adults*—50 to 150 mg daily. *Elderly patients*—20 to 30 mg orally daily. *Children over 2½ years*—0.5 mg/kg body weight, up to 150 mg maximum. INTRAMUSCULAR: *Adults*—50 to 150 mg daily. *Elderly patients*—10 to 75 mg daily. *Children over 2½ years*—0.2 to 0.25 mg/kg up to 10 mg maximum. All daily doses for children should be divided. Nausea and vomiting: INTRAVENOUS: *Adults*—1 mg up to 3 mg. INTRAMUSCULAR: *Adults*—5 to 15 mg every 4 hr up to 60 mg daily. ORAL: *Adults*—20 to 30 mg total daily. ORAL, INTRAMUSCULAR: *Children over 2½ years:* 0.2 mg/kg, to 10 mg in 3 doses daily.	Management of psychotic disorders. Control of nausea and vomiting.
Piperazine‡			
Acetophenazine maleate	Tindal	ORAL: *Adults*—60 mg daily in divided doses that can be increased in 20-mg increments. Optimum level is usually 80 to 120 mg. Occasionally, severe symptoms require 400 to 600 mg. *Elderly patients*—⅓ to ½ adult dose. *Children*—0.8 to 1.6 mg/kg body weight in divided doses. Maximum, 80 mg daily.	Management of psychotic disorders.
Fluphenazine hydrochloride	Moditen† Prolixin Permitil	ORAL: *Adults*—2.5 to 10 mg initially, reduced to 1 to 5 mg daily for maintenance. *Elderly patients*—⅓ to ½ adult dose. INTRAMUSCULAR: *Adults*—1.25 mg increased gradually to 2.5 to 10 mg daily in 3 to 4 doses. *Elderly patients*—⅓ to ½ adult dose.	Most potent of the phenothiazines used for the management of psychotic disorders.
Fluphenazine decanoate	Prolixin Decanoate Modecate†	INTRAMUSCULAR, SUBCUTANEOUS: *Adults under 50 years*—12.5 mg initially, then 25 mg every 2 weeks. Increase by 12.5 mg amounts if needed. Treatment rarely requires more than 100 mg every 2 to 6 weeks.	Long-acting depot forms last at least 2 weeks. Dosage should be stabilized in the hospital, since severe episodes of parkinsonism can appear. Not recommended for elderly patients or patients who have had difficulty with extrapyramidal reactions.
Fluphenazine enanthate	Prolixin Enanthate Moditen Enanthate†		
Perphenazine	Phenazine† Trilafon	ORAL: *Adults*—16 to 64 mg daily in divided doses. *Elderly patients*—⅓ to ½ adult dose. *Children over 12 years*—6 to 12 mg daily. INTRAMUSCULAR: *Adults*—5 to 10 mg initially, then 5 mg every 6 hr with 15 mg maximum daily in ambulatory and 30 mg daily in hospitalized patients. *Elderly patients*—⅓ to ½ adult dose. *Children over 12 years*—lowest adult dose.	For acute psychotic disorders. Lower doses needed when used as an antiemetic.
Prochlorperazine	Compazine	Psychiatric disorders: ORAL: *Adults*—5 to 10 mg 3 to 4 times daily. Raise dosage every 2 to 3 days as required. From 50 to 75 mg daily is common range for mild cases and 100 to 150 mg for severe cases.	More widely used to control severe nausea and vomiting than for psychiatric treatment. Hypotension is seen when given intravenously for surgery.
Prochlorperazine edisylate	Compazine Edisylate		

†Available in Canada only.
‡The piperazine phenothiazines are less sedative in effect and have fewer autonomic side effects than other phenothiazine classes. Extrapyramidal reactions are more common, particularly in large doses in patients over age 40. Piperazine phenothiazines are less likely to produce allergic reactions and do not change ECG tracings.

Table 41-1   Antipsychotic Drugs—cont'd

Generic name	Trade name	Administration/dosage	Comments
PHENOTHIAZINES—cont'd			
Piperazine‡—cont'd			
Prochlorperazine maleate	Compazine Maleate Stemetil†	*Elderly patients*—⅓ to ½ adult dose. *Children over 2 years*—2.5 mg 2 to 3 times daily up to a total dose of 20 to 25 mg. Same dosage used rectally. INTRAMUSCULAR: *Adults*—10 to 20 mg in buttock; repeat every 2 to 4 hr up to 80 mg total. *Elderly patients*—⅓ to ½ adult dose. *Children over 2 years*—0.13 mg/kg body weight initial dose only, then switch to oral. Nausea and vomiting: ORAL: *Adults*—5 to 10 mg 3 or 4 times daily. *Children*—20 to 29 lb, 2.5 mg 1 to 2 times daily; 30 to 39 lb, 2.5 mg 2 to 3 times daily; 40 to 85 lb, 2.5 mg 3 times daily or 5 mg 2 times daily. INTRAMUSCULAR: *Adults*—5 to 10 mg every 3 to 4 hr. *Children*—0.06 mg/lb. RECTAL: *Adults*—25 mg twice daily. *Children*—same as oral dosage.	
Thiopropazate hydrochloride	Dartal†	ORAL: *Adults*—10 mg 3 times/day, adjusting gradually by 10 mg every 3 or 4 days as needed and tolerated. Maintenance dose, 10 to 20 mg 2 to 4 times/day. Reduce the dosage for geriatric, emaciated, or debilitated patients.	To treat psychotic disorders.
Thioproperazine mesylate	Majeptil†	ORAL: *Adults*—Initially, 5 mg/day, adjusted gradually by 5 mg every 2 or 3 days as needed and tolerated. Usual effective dose is 30 to 40 mg/day.	To treat psychotic disorders.
Trifluoperazine	Stelazine Terfluzine† Various others	ORAL: *Adults*—2 to 4 mg daily in divided doses (outpatient), 4 to 10 mg daily (hospitalized). *Elderly or debilitated patients*—⅓ to ½ adult dosage. *Children over 6 years*—1 mg 1 to 2 times daily, gradually raised to maximum of 15 mg. INTRAMUSCULAR: *Adults*—1 to 2 mg every 4 to 6 hr, maximum 10 mg daily. *Elderly or debilitated patients*—⅓ to ½ adult dose. *Children over 6 years*—same as oral dosage.	Management of psychotic disorders.
Piperidine			
Mesoridazine besylate	Serentil*	ORAL: *Adults*—150 mg daily initially. Increased by 50 mg increments until symptoms are controlled. *Elderly patients*—⅓ to ½ adult dose. INTRAMUSCULAR: *Adults and children over 12 years*—25 to 175 mg daily in divided doses (irritating).	Management of psychotic disorders. A metabolite of thioridazine with antiemetic activity and no reported retinopathy.
Pericyazine	Neuleptil†	ORAL: *Adults*—Initially, 5 to 20 mg in the morning and 10 to 40 mg in the evening as needed and tolerated. Maintenance: 2.5 to 15 mg in the morning and 5 to 30 mg in the evening.	To treat psychotic disorders.

*Available in Canada and United States.
†Available in Canada only.
‡The piperazine phenothiazines are less sedative in effect and have fewer autonomic side effects than other phenothiazine classes. Extrapyramidal reactions are more common, particularly in large doses in patients over age 40. Piperazine phenothiazines are less likely to produce allergic reactions and do not change ECG tracings.

Continued.

Table 41-1   Antipsychotic Drugs—cont'd

Generic name	Trade name	Administration/dosage	Comments
PHENOTHIAZINES—cont'd			
Piperidine‡—cont'd			
Pipotiazine palmitate	Piportil L₄†	INTRAMUSCULAR: *Adults*—Initially, 50 to 100 mg, dosage increased in increments of 25 mg every 2 or 3 weeks as needed and tolerated, usually up to a maintenance dose of 75 to 150 mg every 4 weeks.	To treat psychotic disorders.
Thioridazine hydrochloride	Mellaril Novoridazine†	Psychotic disorders: ORAL: *Adults*—50 to 100 mg 3 times daily, increasing up to 800 mg. *Elderly patients*—⅓ to ½ adult dose. *Children over 2 years*—1 mg/kg body weight in divided doses. Depressive neurosis, alcohol withdrawal syndrome, intractable pain, and senility: 10 to 50 mg 2 to 4 times daily.	Management of psychotic disorders. Little antiemetic activity. Safe for patients with epilepsy. Possibly effective in alcohol withdrawal syndrome, intractable pain, and senility. Pronounced sedative and hypotensive side effects initially. One of the least likely of the antipsychotic drugs to cause extrapyramidal reactions because of pronounced anticholinergic action. Photosensitivity has not been reported. Doses over 800 mg daily have produced serious pigmentary retinopathy.
THIOXANTHENES§			
Chlorprothixene	Taractan Tarasan†	ORAL: *Adults and children over 12 years*—75 to 200 mg daily in divided doses. Gradually increase if necessary, with total optimum dose usually being less than 600 mg daily. *Elderly patients*—½ adult dose. INTRAMUSCULAR: *Adults and children over 12 years*—75 to 200 mg daily in divided doses. *Elderly patients*—½ adult dose.	Management of psychotic disorders. Incidence of side effects same as for aliphatic phenothiazines including high sedation, autonomic effects, and low extrapyramidal effects.
Flupenthixol† hydrochloride	Fluanxol†	ORAL: Adults—1 mg 3 times daily initially, increasing by 1 mg every 2 to 3 days as needed. Maintenance dosages: 3 to 6 mg, up to 12 mg maximum daily in divided doses. Elderly patients should be given a lower dose.	Management of psychotic disorders.
Flupenthixol† decanoate	Fluanxol Depot†	INTRAMUSCULAR: *Adults*—initially, 20 to 40 mg every 4 to 10 days. May increase in 20 mg increments.	
Thiothixene	Navane*	ORAL: *Adults and children over 12 years*—6 to 10 mg daily in divided doses. Gradually increase, with the usual optimum dose 20 to 30 mg daily, rarely as high as 60 mg daily. *Elderly patients*—⅓ to ½ adult dose. INTRAMUSCULAR: *Adults and children over 12 years*—4 mg 2 to 4 times daily; gradually increase if necessary to a maximum of 30 mg. *Elderly patients*—⅓ to ½ adult dose.	Management of psychotic disorders. Incidence of side effects same as for piperazine phenothiazines including low incidence of sedation and autonomic effects, and high incidence of extrapyramidal effects.

*Available in Canada and United States.
†Available in Canada only.
§Chemically related to the phenothiazines.

from that of the phenothiazines. The remaining three drug classes, the butyrophenones, the dibenzoxazepines, and the dihydroindolones are chemically different from the phenothiazines and from each other. However, the three classes behave the same pharmacologically with respect to potency and side effects (see Table 41-1).

Subgroups of phenothiazines. The phenothiazines are subdivided into three subgroups based on chemical differences in side groups on the three-ringed main structure. These subgroups are the aliphatic, the piperidine, and the piperazine phenothiazines. The three subgroups differ in potency and in the incidence of key side effects, as summarized in Table 41-2.

Antipsychotic Drugs as Dopamine Receptor Antagonists

Four effects of antipsychotic drugs have been linked to the blockade of dopamine receptors in various parts of the brain. The antipsychotic effect arises from receptor blockade in the limbic system and the antiemetic effect from receptor blockade in the chemoreceptor trigger zone. These effects are used therapeutically. Extrapyramidal effects arise from blockade in the corpus striatum of neurons from the basal ganglia and endocrine effects from blockade in the pituitary gland. These two effects are undesired actions of antipsychotic drugs.

Table 41-2   Antipsychotic Drugs: Drug Class, Potency, and Major Side Effects

| Drug | Equipotent dose | Relative incidence of side effects | | | |
		Sedative effect	Orthostatic hypotension	Anticholinergic effects	Extrapyramidal symptoms
PHENOTHIAZINES					
Aliphatic					
Chlorpromazine	100	High	Moderate	Moderate/high	Moderate
Methotrimeprazine	75	High	High	Moderate	Low/moderate
Promazine	200	Moderate	Moderate	High	Moderate
Triflupromazine	25	High	Moderate	Moderate/high	Moderate/high
Piperidine					
Mesoridazine	50	High	Moderate	Moderate	Low
Pericyazine	10	High	Moderate	High	Moderate
Pipotiazine	100	Low	Low	Low	Low
Thioridazine	100	High	Moderate	Moderate/high	Low
Piperazine					
Acetophenazine	20	Moderate	Low	Low	High
Fluphenazine	2	Low/moderate	Low	Low	High
Perphenazine	8	Low/moderate	Low	Low	High
Prochlorperazine	10	Moderate	Low	Low	High
Thiopropazate	20	Low	Low	Low	High
Thioproperazine	10	Low	Low	Low	High
Trifluoperazine	4	Moderate	Low	Low	High
THIOXANTHENES					
Chlorprothixene	100	High	Moderate/high	Moderate/high	Low/moderate
Thiothixene	4	Low	Low/moderate	Low	Moderate/high
BUTYROPHENONE					
Haloperidol	2	Low	Low	Low	High
DIBENZOXAZEPINE					
Clozapine	75	High	Moderate/high	Moderate/high	Low
Loxapine	10	Moderate	Low/moderate	Low/moderate	Moderate/high
DIHYDROINDOLONE					
Molindone	10	Moderate	Low/moderate	Moderate	Moderate

Dopamine theory of psychosis

Current ideas on the neurochemical origin of psychotic behavior come from an understanding of the action of the antipsychotic drugs. These drugs block receptors in the CNS for the neurotransmitter dopamine. The hypothesis is that too much of this neurotransmitter in the limbic system produces psychotic symptoms. The limbic system is that area of the brain that regulates emotional behavior. Blocking the receptors for dopamine in the limbic system reverses psychotic symptoms.

Extrapyramidal reactions and dopamine deficiency

The antipsychotic drugs also cause the extrapyramidal reactions described in Table 41-3. These extrapyramidal reactions arise from the blockade of dopamine receptors in certain nuclei of the basal ganglia of the brain. This area of the brain is responsible for coordination of movement. A common extrapyramidal reaction is drug-induced parkinsonism. In Parkinson's disease, degeneration of dopamine neurons going to the basal ganglia occurs, resulting in a local deficiency of dopamine (see Chapter 48). Blockade of dopamine receptors in this area of the brain produces the same symptoms as dopamine deficiency.

Emesis and dopamine

Dopamine is the neurotransmitter involved in vomiting (emesis) in the medullary chemoreceptor trigger zone. Antipsychotic drugs are effective in preventing vomiting by blocking these dopamine receptors. As described in Chapter 13, several antipsychotic drugs are commonly used as antiemetic drugs.

Endocrine actions of dopamine

Dopamine inhibits the release of the hormone prolactin by the pituitary gland. Blockade of dopamine leads to hypersecretion of prolactin and secondarily to endocrine disturbances of the reproductive system by mechanisms not yet understood.

Antipsychotic Drugs as Adrenergic and Cholinergic Receptor Antagonists

The phenothiazines and thioxanthenes block receptors for norepinephrine and dopamine. At one time

Table 41-3   Side Effects of Antipsychotic Drugs

Type of effect	Signs and symptoms	Comments
Adrenergic blockade (CNS)	Sedation Postural (orthostatic) hypotension	Usually transient
Cholinergic blockade	Atropine-like effects: dry mouth, blurred vision, constipation, and delayed micturition	Usually transient
Endocrine—dopamine blockade	Males: erection problems Females: menstrual irregularities and unexpected lactation	Usually transient
Extrapyramidal—dopamine blockade	**Acute dystonia:** neck twisting, facial grimacing, abnormal eye movements, and involuntary muscle movements	Most common during the first few days of therapy; usually disappears after brief treatment with antiparkinsonian drugs
	Akathisia: restlessness, difficulty in sitting still, and strong urge to move about	Most common during the first few days of therapy; control with antiparkinsonian drugs or diazepam
	Parkinsonism: motor retardation, masklike face, tremor, rigidity, salivation, and shuffling gait	Most common after the first week of therapy; control with antiparkinsonian drugs
	Tardive dyskinesia: protrusion of tongue, puffing of cheeks, chewing movements, involuntary movements of extremities, and involuntary movements of trunk	Most common when dosage is lowered after prolonged therapy; elderly females at greatest risk; may not be reversible
Allergic reactions	Photosensitivity Cholestatic hepatitis Agranulocytosis	Common Rare

the antipsychotic action was believed to be the blockade of CNS norepinephrine receptors. The finding that the butyrophenone haloperidol blocked only dopamine and not norepinephrine receptors, however, solidified the data implicating the major role of dopamine rather than norepinephrine in psychotic disorders.

CNS effects and adrenergic receptor blockade

Norepinephrine is a neurotransmitter associated with specific neurons in the CNS, just as it is associated with the postganglionic neurons of the sympathetic nervous system. Neurons containing norepinephrine in the reticular activating system of the brain are associated with alertness. The sedative effect of the phenothiazines and the thioxanthenes may result from their blockade of these receptors for norepinephrine. The blockade of norepinephrine receptors in the vasomotor center inhibits peripheral sympathetic tone and causes orthostatic hypotension. The sedative and hypotensive side effects of the phenothiazines and thioxanthenes appear early in therapy. If tolerance does not develop, the dosage can be lowered, or another drug can be tried.

Anticholinergic actions

All the antipsychotic drugs have some anticholinergic action. The atropinelike effects of dry mouth, blurred vision, delayed micturition, and constipation are common side effects. However, a central anticholinergic action is beneficial in controlling some extrapyramidal reactions. Extrapyramidal reactions such as parkinsonian symptoms are believed to reflect a relative lack of dopamine and a relative abundance of acetylcholine in neuronal areas controlling movement coordination (see Chapter 48). Since antipsychotic drugs produce extrapyramidal reactions by blocking the action of dopamine, those drugs that also have substantial ability to block the action of acetylcholine have less tendency to cause extrapyramidal reactions.

PHARMACOLOGY OF ANTIPSYCHOTIC DRUGS

Absorption and Fate

The antipsychotic drugs are administered orally in tablet or syrup form. The syrup form is preferred for patients who hide or do not swallow pills. Many antipsychotic drugs are also available in injectable form. Only fluphenazine is available in two different depot forms for intramuscular (IM) injection, which require administration only every 3 to 6 weeks. Normally, antipsychotic drugs are given in divided daily doses initially and in daily doses when the patient has stabilized. Peak plasma levels of the drug are reached 2 to 3 hr after oral administration. Up to 90% of the drug may be bound to plasma proteins. The drugs are metabolized in the liver and excreted in urine and feces. Excretion is slow, however, and metabolites may be found in urine as long as 6 months after the drug is discontinued. Apparently some metabolites are active. Improvement can last as long as 3 months after medication is halted; whether this reflects remission or presence of persistent active metabolites is unclear.

Antipsychotic effects may not be seen for 7 to 10 days afer the start of therapy, and 4 to 6 weeks are needed to see the full effect of a given dosage regimen. Dosages must be adjusted for individual patients.

Dosage requirement for use as an antiemetic is much smaller than for the antipsychotic effect, and the antiemetic effect is seen within 1 hr of administration.

Extrapyramidal Reactions

The most important side effects of the antipsychotic drugs are extrapyramidal reactions (see Table 41-3). Extrapyramidal reactions are most frequent with the piperazine phenothiazines and least frequent with the aliphatic phenothiazines. The origin of the extrapyramidal reactions is the dopamine blockade in areas of the brain governing motor coordination and movement. Four extrapyramidal syndromes are associated with antipsychotic drugs: acute dystonia, akathisia, pseudoparkinsonism, and tardive dyskinesia. It is important to recognize these bizarre reactions as side effects of drug therapy that require palliative medication or reduction of discontinuance of therapy. Do not treat these reactions as manifestations of the psychotic disease being treated, and do not raise the drug dosage.

Acute dystonia

Acute dystonia is a spasm of muscles of the tongue, face, neck, or back and may mimic seizures. Dystonia is usually seen in the first 5 days of antipsychotic therapy. It may be treated with an antihistaminic or anticholinergic antiparkinsonian drug (see Chapter 48). Injection of one of these drugs usually dramatically relieves the dystonia. Dystonia reactions are most common in patients under 25 years of age and rarely persist after treatment of the acute reaction. Some of the classic reactions seen in dystonia include neck twisting (torticollis), upward gaze paralysis (oculogyric crisis), stereotyped motions of the jaw, and a spasm in which the head and feet create a horseshoe Ω configuration (opisthotonos).

Akathisia

Akathisia is a motor restlessness and may be mistaken for psychotic restlessness or agitation. Akathisia commonly appears after the first few days of therapy, and if not recognized, the antipsychotic drug dosage may again be mistakenly increased to relieve the agitation. Patients experiencing akathisia have difficulty sitting still and may pace about, fidget, or constantly move their legs. Anticholinergic drugs or a muscle relaxant such as diazepam may treat these symptoms. If these treatments are not effective, a different antipsychotic drug may have to be tried. Tolerance does not quickly develop to akathisia, but akathisia disappears when the drug is discontinued.

Pseudoparkinsonism

Pseudoparkinsonism is marked by motor retardation and rigidity. Patients find it difficult to initiate movements or to carry them out. The face resembles a mask because emotions do not register on it. The patient has a shuffling gait and hypersalivates. Tremor is seen in the hands and legs. These parkinsonian symptoms commonly appear after a week of therapy and are treated with antiparkinsonian drugs. Tolerance does not develop to the parkinsonian symptoms. If they cannot be controlled with drug therapy, the antipsychotic drug has to be changed.

Tardive dyskinesia

Tardive dyskinesia is associated with long-term, high-dose antipsychotic therapy. It is most common in elderly females and in patients who have had a stroke. Tardive dyskinesia is the worst of the extrapyramidal reactions, since it cannot be readily treated, is persistent, and may not altogether disappear when drug therapy is discontinued. It usually appears some months after therapy has been started when drug dosage is reduced or discontinued. Tardive dyskinesia may represent the development of receptors that are supersensitive to dopamine after prolonged blockade by the antipsychotic drugs. Thus removing the antipsychotic drug worsens the condition, since dopamine then has ready access to these supersensitive receptors. Antiparkinsonian drugs also worsen the condition, since they either increase dopamine or block the acetylcholine opposing the dopamine. Some common symptoms of tardive dyskinesia are protrusion of the tongue (fly-catcher sign), puffing of the cheeks or the tongue in a cheek (bonbon sign), chewing movements, and involuntary movements of the extremities and trunk. Recent recognition that tardive dyskinesia is a common reaction in up to 50% patients treated for a long time with high doses of antipsychotic drugs has prompted reevaluation of long-term therapy with these drugs. The current choice is to use as low a dose as possible and to put the patient on a "drug holiday" during periods of remission.

Other Side Effects

Several other side effects are associated with antipsychotic drugs (see Table 41-3).

Sedation and postural hypotension

Sedation and postural hypotension are most often seen early in treatment with the aliphatic phenothiazines, the class of phenothiazines with the most prominent adrenergic-blocking activity. These side effects are most likely to be prominent in elderly or debilitated patients. If sedation and hypotension are not severe, the dosage can be reduced and then gradually increased to produce tolerance to these effects. Antipsychotic drugs are not addicting.

Electrocardiographic changes

The aliphatic phenothiazines are also the most likely to produce nonspecific changes in the T wave of the electrocardiogram (ECG). This change has no particular meaning but is undesirable in a patient with concurrent heart disease who is being monitored for ECG changes.

Seizure potential

Antipsychotic drugs must be used with caution in patients with epilepsy, since they can precipitate convulsions. This lowering of the convulsive threshold makes antipsychotic drugs unsuitable to treat drug withdrawal likely to produce seizures such as withdrawal from alcohol, barbiturates, and other sedative-hypnotic drugs.

Endocrine disturbances

The endocrine impairment that results in sexual dysfunction was discussed relative to the dopaminergic-blocking action of the antipsychotic drugs. Females may experience delayed ovulation and menstruation, lack of menstruation (amenorrhea), milk production (galactorrhea), or weight gain. Men may experience impotence, decreased libido, retrograde ejaculation, or moderate breast growth (gynecomastia).

Allergic reactions

Photosensitivity and cholestatic hepatitis occasionally develop during therapy.

Photosensitivity is fairly common and represents an allergic reaction to a metabolite produced not by the body but by reaction with sunlight (see box). The long half-life of the antipsychotic drugs and their metabolites has been discussed. These metabolites accumulate in the skin, where exposure to sun causes chemical changes that can cause skin allergies. Patients taking antipsychotic drugs should not sunbathe, since they risk a painful skin rash. Some patients develop slate-blue patches on their skin. This

---

is an accumulation of drug metabolites, not an allergy, and is not dangerous.

Cholestatic hepatitis can develop with antipsychotic therapy. Jaundice develops when the bile duct becomes blocked by an allergic inflammation caused by metabolites excreted in the bile. It is commonly seen in the first month of therapy with one of the aliphatic phenothiazines. It is normally mild and self-limiting, but if jaundice is detected, the drug should be stopped and an antipsychotic drug from a different chemical class used.

Blood dyscrasias

A blood dyscrasia, the depression of the synthesis of one of the blood elements, occasionally occurs with antipsychotic therapy. Depression of leukocytes is common with antipsychotic therapy but is usually transient and not serious. Agranulocytosis, however, in which leukocytes are no longer produced, is serious and is often fatal. Agranulocytosis is most common within 3 months of the start of therapy. Therefore blood counts should be done early in the therapy. Any sign of fever or sore throat indicates the possible onset of agranulocytosis and should be checked immediately.

Antipsychotic Drugs and Drug Potentiation

Antipsychotic drugs potentiate the action of CNS depressant drugs, including sedative-hypnotic drugs, narcotic analgesics, and anesthetic agents. The potentiation of sedative-hypnotic drugs, including alcohol, is an important drug interaction. The effects of an alcoholic drink or a sleeping pill are greatly exaggerated in patients taking an antipsychotic drug. A toxic overdose of the alcohol or sedative-hypnotic drug therefore becomes possible at a lower dose.

Clinical use is made of the potentiation of narcotic-analgesic drugs by antipsychotic drugs. Terminal cancer patients in chronic pain can be relieved by receiving lower doses of a narcotic-analgesic drug when an antipsychotic drug is also given. This greatly slows the development of tolerance to the narcotics. The antipsychotic drug has the further advantage of controlling the emesis produced by radiation therapy or chemotherapy.

Finally, droperidol, a drug related to the antipsychotic drug haloperidol, is widely used with a narcotic to produce a state of quiescence and indifference to stimuli, which allows bronchoscopy, x-ray studies, burn dressing, and cytoscopy to be performed. Nitrous oxide can be added to this neuroleptic-narcotic combination to produce general anesthesia for surgery, neuroleptanesthesia. The anesthesia results from the synergistic effect of the drugs with nitrous oxide, since nitrous oxide alone is not potent enough to produce surgical anesthesia (see Chapter 45).

General Guidelines for Care of Patients Receiving Antipsychotics

Drug administration

◆ Review common side effects listed in Tables 41-2 and 41-3, since these will be frequently encountered. Assess patients on a regular, ongoing basis for these side effects. Assess thoughtfully: what may appear to be increased agitation may be akathisia, or what may resemble anxiety may be early parkinsonian side effects.

◆ Monitor blood pressure every 4 hr until stable; this may require several days to 2 weeks. Some physicians prefer that blood pressure be monitored with the patient in lying, sitting, and standing positions.

◆ Side effects may make the patient unsteady when ambulating. Supervise ambulation, and assist when appropriate.

◆ Monitor fluid intake and output until patient is stabilized. Weigh the patient weekly. Monitor blood glucose levels.

◆ Contact dermatitis caused by the phenothiazines has been reported. Avoid getting the drugs on the skin, and wash hands carefully after preparing these drugs. If working with these drugs frequently, wear gloves.

◆ Supervise patients carefully to ascertain that medication is swallowed and is not hidden in the mouth to be discarded or stored later. Some antipsychotic drugs are available in syrup, injection, or depot injection forms to ensure that the patient receives the prescribed dose. On an outpatient basis, it may be necessary for a responsible family member to supervise medication taking.

◆ Concentrated oral forms of most antipsychotic drugs are available for institutional use. Dilute dose to at least 60 ml in one of the diluents suggested by the manufacturer.

◆ Monitor patients with a history of seizures carefully, since antipsychotics may alter the seizure threshhold.

◆ For IM injection, choose a large muscle mass. Aspirate before injecting to avoid inadvertent intravenous (IV) administration. Warn patients that drug may cause a burning sensation while being injected. Record and rotate injection sites.

◆ IM injections of nondepot forms of phenothiazines may cause marked hypotension. Keep patients supine for ½ to 1 hr after injection, monitor blood pressure, and supervise ambulation. For rare severe reactions, levarterenol and phenylephrine are the vasoconstrictors of choice; do not use epinephrine.

◆ Read orders and labels carefully. Some drugs are packaged in an aqueous form and an oil-based depot form. Oil-based depot forms are always administered IM, never IV.

◆ When antipsychotics are used as antiemetics, the doses are usually lower. Side effects are milder and include sedation, hypotension, and dry mouth. However, any side effect listed can occur in patients who are extremely sensitive to the drug. When antipsychotic drugs are given as antiemetics with narcotic analgesics, they may potentiate CNS depressive effects of the analgesics, including hypotension and sedation.

◆ The care of the mentally ill is complex and involves the use of many treatment modalities. See texts and articles appropriate to the care of psychiatric patients.

Patient and family education

◆ Review the anticipated benefits and possible side effects of drug therapy with the patient and family. Review extrapyramidal side effects listed in Table 41-3. Since there is no effective treatment for tardive dyskinesia, its appearance should be reported immediately. Fine vermicular (wormlike) movements of the tongue may be the first sign of this side effect. Tell patients and family to report any new signs or symptoms.

◆ See Patient Problems: Dry Mouth on p. 166, Constipation on p. 182, Photosensitivity on p. 629, and Orthostatic Hypotension on p. 234.

◆ Tell patients that several weeks of therapy may be necessary before full benefit can be seen.

◆ Instruct patients to swallow extended-release forms whole; do not crush or chew.

◆ Warn patients to avoid driving or operating hazardous equipment if vision changes or sedation occurs; notify the physician.

◆ Instruct patients to report signs of agranulocytosis including sore throat, fever, and malaise. Tell patients to report signs of liver dysfunction including jaundice, malaise, fever, and right upper quadrant abdominal pain.

◆ These drugs may interfere with the body's ability to regulate temperature. Warn patients to avoid prolonged exposure to extremes of temperature, to allow for frequent cooling-off periods when exercising or in hot environments, and to dress warmly for exposure to the cold.

NURSING IMPLICATIONS SUMMARY—cont'd

◆ Review possible endocrine side effects with patient and family. Assess carefully and tactfully for these side effects. Provide emotional support as appropriate. If endocrine side effects are intolerable, consult the physician for possible drug or dosage change.

◆ Instruct patients to monitor weight (if appropriate to ability and resources). If weight gain is a problem, counsel about low-calorie diets. Refer to a dietitian as needed.

◆ Caution patients to inform all health-care providers of all drugs being taken. Warn patients to avoid over-the-counter drugs unless first approved by the physician.

◆ Caution patients to avoid alcoholic beverages while taking antipsychotics.

◆ Warn diabetic patients that antipsychotics may alter blood glucose levels. Monitor blood glucose levels carefully. Consult the physician about changes in dietary or drug treatment for diabetes.

◆ Tell patients not to discontinue therapy abruptly or without consultation with the physician. Instruct patients to keep these and all drugs out of the reach of children.

◆ The drugs may produce false-positive pregnancy results. Females who suspect they are pregnant should consult the physician. Females may desire to use contraceptive measures while taking these drugs; counsel as appropriate. As always, pregnant or lactating women should avoid all drugs unless first approved by the physician.

◆ If additional drugs are prescribed to treat side effects of antipsychotic agents, review their use and side effects with the patient and family.

Chlorpromazine

Drug administration

◆ See general guidelines above.

INTRAVENOUS ADMINISTRATION

◆ For direct IV push, dilute chlorpromazine in 0.9% sodium chloride to make a dilution of 1 mg/ml. Administer at a rate of 1.0 mg/min in adults or 0.5 mg/min in children. For infusion, further dilute and infuse slowly. Monitor blood pressure. Keep side rails up. Supervise ambulation after dose.

Droperidol

Drug administration

◆ This drug is used as an antiemetic, a preoperative medication, or during anesthesia; see Chapter 45.

◆ IV administration may be given undiluted or may be further diluted. Administer undiluted drug at a rate of 10 mg or less/1 min. Monitor blood pressure. Keep side rails up. Supervise ambulation. Titrate diluted doses to patient response.

Flupenthixol

Drug administration

◆ Read orders and labels carefully. The decanoate form is a depot, in which the drug is suspended in sesame oil. Use a 21-gauge needle. See information on administering oil-based suspensions in Chapter 6.

Fluphenazine

Drug administration

◆ Read orders and labels carefully. The decanoate and enanthate forms are depots, with the drug suspended in sesame oil. Use a dry needle and syringe. A wet needle or syringe causes the drug to turn cloudy. A large-bore needle should be used such as a 21-gauge needle. See information on administering oil-based suspensions in Chapter 6.

Haloperidol

Drug administration

◆ Read orders and labels carefully. The decanoate form is a depot, with the drug suspended in sesame oil. Use a 21-gauge needle. See information on administering oil-based suspensions in Chapter 6.

Perphenazine

Drug administration

INTRAVENOUS ADMINISTRATION

◆ Dilute each 5 mg with 9 ml of normal saline for injection. Administer at a rate of 0.5 mg (1 ml)/1 min. Monitor blood pressure. Keep side rails up. Supervise ambulation.

Continued.

Prochlorperazine

Drug administration

INTRAVENOUS ADMINISTRATION

◆ IV push may be given undiluted. A single dose should not exceed 10 mg. Administer at a rate of 5 mg/ml/min. May also be further diluted and given as an infusion.

Promazine

Drug administration

INTRAVENOUS ADMINISTRATION

◆ May be given undiluted. Administer at a rate of 25 mg/min. Monitor blood pressure. Keep side rails up. Supervise ambulation.

Triflupromazine

Drug administration

INTRAVENOUS ADMINISTRATION

◆ Dilute 10 mg with 9 ml of normal saline for injection. Administer at a rate of 1 mg (1 ml)/ 2 min. Monitor blood pressure. Keep side rails up. Supervise ambulation.

CHAPTER REVIEW

◆ KEY TERMS

acute dystonia, p. 627
akathisia, p. 627
antipsychotic drugs, p. 619
functional psychosis, p. 619
neuroleptic, p. 618
organic psychosis, p. 619
phenothiazines, p. 619
pseudoparkinsonism, p. 628
psychosis, p. 619
schizophrenia, p. 619
tardive dyskinesia, p. 628
toxic psychosis, p. 619

◆ REVIEW QUESTIONS

1. What is the major chemical class of antipsychotic drugs? List the three subclasses.

2. What are the four actions of antipsychotic drugs attributable to blockade of dopaminergic receptors? What symptoms might you see as a result of this blockade?

3. What are two actions of antipsychotic drugs attributable to blockade of receptors for norepinephrine? What symptoms might you see that may be due to this blockade?

4. What are two actions of antipsychotic drugs attributable to blockade of cholinergic receptors? What symptoms might you see that may be due to this blockade?

5. List the four types of extrapyramidal reactions, the key features of each type, and when each type is likely to occur during antipsychotic drug therapy. How can you recognize these reactions?

6. Describe allergic reactions attributed to antipsychotic drugs.

7. For which types of psychoses are antipsychotic drugs generally effective?

8. Name the two clinical uses of antipsychotic drugs other than the treatment of psychoses you might see.

SUGGESTED READING

Baldessarini RJ, Frankenburg FR: Clozapine, a novel antipsychotic agent, *N Engl J Med* 324(11):746, 1991.

Barrett N, Ormiston S, Molyneux V: Clozapine: a new drug for schizophrenia, *J Psychosoc Nurs Ment Health Serv* 28(2):24, 1990.

Beeber LS: Undesirable weight gain and psychotropic medications, *J Psychosoc Nurs Ment Health Serv* 26(10):39, 1988.

Bickal T: A protocol for the diagnosis and treatment of extrapyramidal symptoms of neuroleptic drugs, *Nurse Pract* 12(1):25, 1987.

Dauner A, Blair DT: Akathisia: when treatment creates a problem, *J Psychosoc Nurs Ment Health Serv* 28(10):13, 1990.

Gomez GE, Gomez EA: The special concerns of neuroleptic use in the elderly, *J Psychosoc Nurs Ment Health Serv* 28(1):7, 1990.

Hamilton D: Clozapine: a new antipsychotic drug, *Arch Psychiatr Nurs* IV(4):278, 1990.

Harris E: The antipsychotics, *Am J Nurs* 88:1508, 1988.

Jackson RT, Haynes-Johnson V: Nutritional management of patients undergoing long-term antipsychotic and antidepressant therapies, *Arch Psychiatr Nurs* II(3):146, 1988.

Jeste DV, Krull AJ, Kilbourn K: Tardive dyskinesia: managing a common neuroleptic side effect, *Geriatrics* 45(12):49, 1990.

Masters JC, Spitler R: Neuroleptic malignant syndrome, *J Psychosoc Nurs Ment Health Serv* 24(9):11, 1986.

Michaels RA, Mumford K: Identifying akinesia and akathisia: the relationship between patient's self-report and nurse's assessment, *Arch Psychiatr Nurs* III(2):97, 1989.

Norris AE, Disalver SC, Del Medico VJ: Carbamazepine treatment of psychosis, *J Psychiatr Nurs* 28(12):13, 1990.

Smith DA: New rule for prescribing psychotropics in nursing homes, *Geriatrics* 45(2):44, 1990.

Strome T, Howell T: How antipsychotics affect elders, *Am J Nurs* 91(5):46, 1991.

Townsend MC: *Drug guide for psychiatric nursing*, Philadelphia, 1990, FA Davis.

Vernon GM: Drug-induced and tardive movement disorders, *J Neurosci Nurs* 23(3):183, 1991.

CHAPTER 42

Antidepressant Drugs

LEARNING OBJECTIVES

After studying this chapter, you should be able to do the following:

◆ Briefly describe reactive depression, endogenous depression, and manic-depressive (bipolar) disorder.

◆ Develop a nursing care plan for patients receiving a tricyclic antidepressant, amoxapine, bupropion, fluoxetine, maprotiline, trazodone, a monoamine-oxidase inhibitor, or lithium.

◆ Describe the toxic symptoms of lithium and the corresponding blood level.

◆ Develop a teaching plan for a patient on a tyramine-restricted diet.

CHAPTER OVERVIEW

◆ Drugs covered in this chapter are for severe disturbances of mood, from depression to manic-depressive disorders. Antidepressants, monoamine-oxidase (MAO) inhibitors, and lithium are presented.

Nursing Process Overview

ANTIDEPRESSANTS

Assessment

Antidepressants are used for patients with pronounced, prolonged depression or manic-depressive disease. Perform a thorough physiologic assessment, and assess mental status, focusing on objective signs of depression. Monitor vital signs, weight, and blood pressure.

Possible body image disturbance related to weight gain as a drug side effect
Potential for self-harm
Altered bowel elimination: constipation

Management

Monitor fluid intake and output, weight, and blood pressure. Review serum drug levels if available. Assess the patient's level of consciousness, with attention to excessive sedation. Assess for possible suicidal tendencies. Monitor for side effects of the drugs such as the dry mouth and constipation that may occur with tricyclic antidepressants.

Evaluation

Before discharging a patient for self-management, ascertain that patients or family can explain what drug is being taken, how to take it correctly, the side effects that may occur and those that should be reported immediately to the physician, dietary restrictions associated with the medication being used, and ways in which the success of the drug will be monitored. Verify that patients can explain why follow-up is necessary and when to return for it.

NATURE OF DEPRESSIVE DISORDERS

Depression

Depression is a disorder of mood (affect) that occurs in an estimated 15% to 30% of all adults at some time during their lives. Depression is not a single entity; rather it is a syndrome that can include various symptoms, as outlined in Table 42-1. Depression becomes a medical problem when normal functioning is significantly hampered. Three major categories of depression are recognized: reactive depression, endogenous depression, and manic depressive disorder.

Table 42-1   Symptoms Characteristic of Depression

Parameter	Change
General mood	Low for a week or more
Behavior	Appetite or weight change
	Sleep change; early morning awakening is the most common insomnia; some patients may sleep more than usual, though level of activity is exaggerated or depressed
	Loss of energy
	Loss of interest in activities and/or sex
	Feelings of guilt or self-reproach
	Inability to concentrate
	Thoughts of suicide

Reactive depression, endogenous depression, and manic-depressive disorder

Reactive depression is experienced after some significant loss in life. This depression is usually acute for a couple of weeks and resolves within 3 months. Therapy for reactive depression is to provide emotional support. One of the benzodiazepines, the antianxiety drugs, may be prescribed to relieve anxiety or insomnia if required. An antidepressant drug typically is not needed.

Endogenous depression is depression with no apparent cause. Current views are that endogenous depression is a neurochemical disorder that can be treated with appropriate drug therapy. This concept arose from the observation in the 1950s that reserpine caused depression in patients treated for hypertension. Reserpine depleted the neurotransmitter norepinephrine. About the same time, iproniazid, a drug then used to treat tuberculosis, was found to relieve depression in patients, inhibiting the degradation of norepinephrine by inhibiting the enzyme MAO. These two observations suggested that a deficiency in the brain neurotransmitter norepinephrine is associated with depression. Current evidence favors a biogenic amine theory of depression, in which a deficiency in brain norepinephrine or in another amine neurotransmitter, serotonin, is associated with depression. The two drug classes currently used to treat depression, tricyclic antidepressants and MAO inhibitors, have pharmacologic mechanisms that restore norepinephrine and serotonin in the brain.

Manic-depressive disorder is the third type of depression. The classic manic-depressive patient has a manic period characterized by excessive euphoria, overactivity, a flow of ideas, extreme self-confidence, and little need for sleep, alternating with a period of depression. Lithium is the specific drug treatment for mania.

Depression as a side effect

In addition to these three classes, depression can also be the side effect of some drugs, especially the antihypertensive drugs reserpine, methyldopa, quanethidine, and propranolol. Alcohol and antianxiety drugs often unmask depression by alleviating the anxiety that frequently accompanies depression. Steroids, particularly glucocorticoids and oral contraceptives, can cause depression. Drug-induced depression mimics endogenous depression but is treated by removing the drug or lowering the dose.

DRUGS USED TO TREAT DEPRESSIVE DISORDERS

These drugs are listed in Table 42-2.

Tricyclic Antidepressants
Mechanism of action

The **tricyclic antidepressants** block the reuptake of norepinephrine or serotonin into the presynaptic neurons, as depicted in Figure 42-1. This causes an increase in the synaptic concentration of these neurotransmitters, which is an early effect of the drug. However, clinically no antidepressant response is seen for 2 weeks. Recent research suggests that the tricyclic antidepressants also alter the sensitivity of brain tissue to the action of norepinephrine and serotonin. Since this effect takes 2 weeks to be established, it more closely correlates with the onset of the clinical antidepressant action.

Administration and fate

The tricyclic antidepressants usually are administered orally, although amitriptyline and imipramine are available in injectable forms. Metabolites of the tricyclic antidepressants are active so that an active form of the drug persists despite the drug being well absorbed and readily metabolized by the intestine and liver. The rate of tricyclic metabolism decreases with age, and people over 55 years of age generally are started at half the regular adult dose.

The major side effects of the tricyclic antidepressants are an atropine-like (anticholinergic) effect and sedation. The relative incidence of these side effects among the tricyclics is listed in Table 42-3. Because of these side effects, the drug is usually given before bedtime so that the patient is asleep when the side effects are at their peak. The more sedating tricyclics, amitriptyline and doxepin, are particularly effective

Table 42-2   Antidepressant Drugs

Generic name	Trade name	Administration/dosage	Comments
TRICYCLIC ANTIDEPRESSANTS			
Amitriptyline hydrochloride	Elavil* Endep Levate† Novotrip- tyn†	ORAL: *Adults*—begin with 50 mg at bedtime, increase dosage by 25 to 50 mg if necessary to 150 mg. Alternately, start with 25 mg 3 times daily, increase to 50 mg 3 times daily. Total dosage should not exceed 300 mg daily. Maintenance doses are usually 50 to 100 mg at bed- time. These are outpatient dos- ages; inpatient dosages may be twice as much. FDA Pregnancy Category C. *Adolescents and el- derly*—10 mg 3 times daily plus 20 mg at bedtime (50 mg total) is usually sufficient. INTRAMUSCULAR: 20 to 30 mg 4 times daily.	Bedtime administration is preferred to lessen the discomfort of the se- dation and anticholinergic effects prominent with this drug.
Clomipramine	Anafranil†	ORAL: *Adults*—initially, 25 mg 3 times a day, then up to 200 mg for outpatients, 300 mg for inpa- tients. *Elderly*—20 to 30 mg daily in divided doses.	Used for obsessive-compulsive dis- orders, for blocking panic attacks, and to treat cataplexy associated with narcolepsy.
Desipramine hydrochloride	Norpramin* Pertofrane*	ORAL: *Adults*—begin with 25 mg 3 times daily, increase gradually to a total of 200 mg daily and not more than 300 mg daily; maintenance dosages usually 50 to 200 mg taken at bedtime. *Ad- olescents and elderly*—25 to 50 mg daily; increased to 100 mg in divided doses if necessary.	Sedation and anticholinergic ef- fects are not prominent. Metabo- lite of imipramine.
Doxepin hydro- chloride	Adapin Sinequan* Triadapin†	ORAL: *Adults*—75 mg, increased to 150 mg in divided doses or at bedtime; maintenance dose usu- ally 25 to 150 mg daily and should not exceed 300 mg daily.	Bedtime administration is preferred to lessen the discomfort of the se- dation and anticholinergic effects prominent with this drug. Doxepin is reported to have much less effect on the heart when com- pared to the other tricyclic antide- pressants.
Imipramine hydrochloride Imipramine pamoate	Impril† Janimine Tipramine Tofranil* Tofranil-PM	ORAL: *Adults*—75 mg daily in divided doses or at bedtime. Dose may be increased up to 200 mg daily if required. These are outpatient doses; inpatient doses are ⅓ higher. *Adolescents and elderly*—30 to 40 mg daily, increased to a maximum of 100 mg/day. *Children over 6 years*—for bed-wetting, 25 mg, 1 hr before bedtime; if no re- sponse in 1 week, increase to 50 mg; *over 12 years*—may re- ceive up to 75 mg.	Imipramine is the prototype tri- cyclic antidepressant. Sedative and anticholinergic effects are moder- ate. Can be taken at bedtime.

*Available in Canada and United States.
†Available in Canada only.

Table 42-2   Antidepressant Drugs—cont'd

Generic name	Trade name	Administration/dosage	Comments
TRICYCLIC ANTIDEPRESSANTS—cont'd			
Nortriptyline hydrochloride	Aventyl* Pamelor	ORAL: *Adults*—initially, 40 mg in divided doses or at bedtime; maximum dose 100 to 150 mg daily. *Adolescents and children*—30 to 50 mg daily in divided doses.	A metabolite of amitriptyline. Sedative effect is moderate; anticholinergic effect is mild. Can be taken at bedtime.
Protriptyline hydrochloride	Triptil† Vivactil	ORAL: *Adults*—15 to 40 mg daily divided in 3 to 4 doses; maximum dose 60 mg daily. Increments are added to the morning dose. *Adolescents and elderly*—15 mg daily in 3 doses. No more than 20 mg total.	This is the only tricyclic antidepressant that has little sedative action and can cause insomnia if given at bedtime. Preferred for the patient who has been immobile and sleepy.
Trimipramine maleate	Surmontil	ORAL: *Adults*—75 mg daily increased to 150 mg in divided doses or at bedtime. These are outpatient dosages; inpatient dosages 100 mg daily increased to 200 mg daily with a maximum of 300 mg daily. FDA Pregnancy Category C. *Adolescents and elderly*—50 mg daily, increased to no more than 100 mg daily as required.	Sedation is high, but the anticholinergic effect is moderate.
SECOND-GENERATION ANTIDEPRESSANTS			
Amoxapine	Asendin*	ORAL: *Adults*—75 mg initially, increase to 200 mg daily in divided doses. If no improvement in 3 weeks, increase dosage 50 mg daily every other week to maximum of 400 mg for outpatients, 600 mg for inpatients. FDA Pregnancy Category C.	Related to the tricyclic antidepressants. Low incidence of anticholinergic, sedative, and cardiovascular effects. May be taken at bedtime to lessen daytime sedation or to treat insomnia.
Bupropion	Wellbutrin	ORAL: *Adults*—Initially, 100 mg 2 times/day, the dosage being increased gradually after 3 days of therapy, to 100 mg 3 times/day as needed and tolerated.	A new antidepressant. Seizures may occur at high doses.
Fluoxetine	Prozac	ORAL: *Adults*—initially, 20 mg as a morning dose. May increase by 20 mg if needed after several weeks, adding as a noon dose.	A new antidepressant, chemically unrelated to other antidepressants. A selective blocker of the neuronal uptake of serotonin. Causes insomnia, and depresses the appetite.
Maprotiline	Ludiomil*	ORAL: *Adults*—75 mg, increased to 150 mg daily in divided doses. If no improvement in 3 weeks, increase dosage 50 mg daily every other week to maximum of 300 mg. FDA Pregnancy Category B. *Elderly and adolescents*—⅓ adult dose.	Low incidence of anticholinergic, sedative, and cardiovascular effects. May be taken at bedtime to lessen daytime sedation or to treat insomnia.

*Available in Canada and United States.
†Available in Canada only.

Continued.

Table 42-2   Antidepressant Drugs—cont'd

Generic name	Trade name	Administration/dosage	Comments
SECOND-GENERATION ANTIDEPRESSANTS—cont'd			
Trazodone	Desyrel* Trazon Trialodine	ORAL: *Adults*—75 mg initially, or increased by 50 mg daily every 3 or 4 days to 300 mg if necessary. If no improvement in 3 weeks, increase dosage 50 mg daily every other week to maximum of 300 mg. FDA Pregnancy Category C.	Sedation may be noted. Low incidence of anticholinergic and cardiovascular effects. May be taken at bedtime to lessen daytime sedation or to treat insomnia.
MONOAMINE OXIDASE (MAO) INHIBITORS			
Isocarboxazid	Marplan*	ORAL: *Adults*—20 to 30 mg daily in divided doses; maintenance dose usually 10 to 20 mg daily.	Patient should be instructed in food and drug interactions with MAO inhibitors.
Phenelzine sulfate	Nardil*	ORAL: *Adults*—45 to 75 mg daily in 3 doses or 1 mg/kg body weight in divided doses. Daily dosage should not exceed 90 mg.	Patient should be instructed in food and drug interactions with MAO inhibitors.
Tranylcypromine sulfate	Parnate*	ORAL: *Adults*—20 to 40 mg daily in 2 doses for 2 weeks. Dosage is reduced after a response is obtained. Usually maintenance dose is below 30 mg. Higher doses are not advised for outpatients.	Patient should be instructed in food and drug interactions with MAO inhibitors. Has some psychomotor stimulant activity characteristic of amphetamine.
LITHIUM			
Lithium carbonate	Eskalith Lithane* Lithizine† Lithonate Lithotabs	ORAL: *Adults*—initially 0.6 to 2.1 gm daily divided into 3 doses. Increase or decrease dose by 0.3 gm/day to obtain a blood level of 0.8 to 1.5 mEq/L. FDA Pregnancy Category D.	Blood should not be drawn for determination of lithium levels earlier than 8 hr after the last dose. Levels above 2.0 mEq/L are toxic. Patients should be instructed not to make up a missed dose of lithium.
Lithium citrate	Cibalith-S	Maintenance dose usually 0.9 to 1.2 gm daily in divided doses.	

*Available in Canada and United States.
†Available in Canada only.

in relieving the insomnia of depression when given as a bedtime dose. These drugs do not interfere with the normal sleep pattern described in Chapter 40.

Anticholinergic and sedative side effects are apparent with the first dose of a tricyclic antidepressant, although little lifting of the depression is seen before 2 weeks of therapy. Thus the dose is started at about a third the expected therapeutic dose to allow the patient to develop tolerance to the side effects. The dose is increased to the expected therapeutic dose over the first week. After 2 weeks of drug therapy, the dosage is reviewed in light of side effects and therapeutic response. The final dosage is individualized for the patient. Therapy is discontinued if no response occurs after 1 month. If the patient's depression is relieved, the duration of therapy depends on the severity of the depression being treated. Mild depression might be treated for 2 to 3 months, whereas severe depression might be treated for 1 to 2 years. The drug therapy is then gradually withdrawn. Reappearance of depression is a sign for reinstituting drug therapy. The spectrum of therapy for depression ranges from a few weeks to a lifetime, depending on the severity and recurrence of depression.

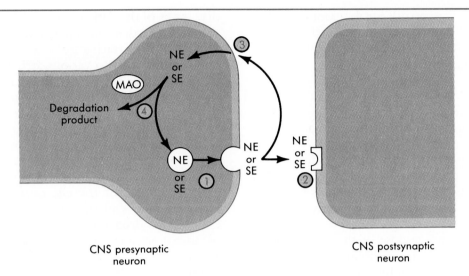

CNS presynaptic
neuron

CNS postsynaptic
neuron

FIGURE 42-1

Depression results from an amine concentration too low to activate sufficient receptors; mania results from overabundance of amine acting at receptor. Biogenic amine theory of depression is applied to actions of antidepressant drugs, tricyclic antidepressants and MAO inhibitors, and to action of lithium, used to treat mania (opposite of depression). *1.* Lithium inhibits release of norepinephrine and serotonin. *2.* Tricyclic antidepressants and MAO inhibitors increase receptor sensitivity to norepinephrine and serotonin. *3.* Tricyclic antidepressants block reuptake of norepinephrine and serotonin. Lithium enhances reuptake of norepinephrine and serotonin. *4.* MAO inhibitors prevent degradation of norepinephrine and serotonin.

Table 42-3   Incidence of Side Effects of Tricyclic Antidepressants*

Drug	Sedative activity	Anticholinergic activity
Amitriptyline	+ + +	+ + +
Desipramine	+	+
Doxepin	+ + +	+ + +
Imipramine	+ +	+ +
Nortriptyline	+	+
Protriptyline	+ /0	+ +
Trimipramine	+ + +	+ +

*Number of + indicates relative activity; + /0 indicates no activity.

Anticholinergic side effects

Anticholinergic side effects include dry mouth, blurred vision, and constipation. Some patients may experience temporary confusion or speech blockage. Patients with glaucoma or those disposed toward glaucoma must have this condition checked when taking tricyclic antidepressants because the anticholinergic effect may worsen this condition. Anticholinergic action also may adversely affect patients with urinary retention or obstruction, particularly elderly ones.

Cardiac effects

Tricyclic antidepressants have three separate pharmacologic actions on the heart: anticholinergic, adrenolytic, and a quinidine-like action. Therefore the final cardiac effect is complex and depends on dosage. The anticholinergic action increases the heart rate. The adrenolytic action prevents the reuptake of norepinephrine into neurons, an action that tends to deplete norepinephrine stores in peripheral neurons. The most common adrenolytic side effect is orthostatic (postural) hypotension. This decrease in blood pressure affects the heart by lowering the workload. The quinidine-like side effects are seen at high concentrations of the tricyclic antidepressants. This decreases heart rate, myocardial contractility, and coronary blood flow. For these reasons, tricyclic antidepressants are contraindicated for patients with a recent myocardial infarction and present special concern for the patient with cardiac disease. Hyperthyroid patients, who are at risk for developing cardiac arrhythmias, have this risk potentiated by the tricyclic antidepressants. Doxepin is a tricyclic antidepressant that has minimum cardiac effects.

Acute toxicity

Tricyclic antidepressants are not addicting, and their abuse potential appears limited. A major problem is their acute toxicity when depressed patients overdose on a tricyclic antidepressant drug in a suicide attempt. Doses of 1 gm of the sedating tricyclics are toxic, and doses of 2 gm are often fatal. Those doses represent only a 5- and 10-fold margin, respectively, over the therapeutic dose.

The toxicity of an overdose of the tricyclic antidepressants is essentially in anticholinergic poisoning. The early symptoms are confusion, inability to concentrate, and perhaps visual hallucinations. More severe signs include delirium, seizures, and coma. Respiration may be depressed. The patient may have a low body temperature early but an elevated body temperature later. The pupils are dilated, the eyeballs are restless, the reflexes are hyperactive, and motor coordination is compromised. Depending on the car-

diac status of the patient and the degree of overdose, the overall cardiac effect may range from quickening of the heart rate (tachycardia) to slowing of the heart rate (bradycardia) to various arrhythmias secondary to an atrioventricular block. Especially serious is the slowing of conduction in the atrioventricular node by the quinidine-like action, which can result in heart block. Sudden death from cardiac arrhythmias may occur several days after an overdose. Physostigmine Antilirium), a peripherally and centrally active anticholinesterase agent, reverses the anticholinergic toxic symptoms of tricyclic overdose. Two mg of physostigmine is administered every 1 to 2 hr as necessary. This drug must be administered frequently because it is short acting, whereas tricyclics are long acting.

Tricyclic antidepressants do not decrease the suicide potential among depressed patients during the early weeks of therapy. Depressed patients with suicidal thoughts are best hospitalized to begin drug therapy rather than being given quantities of drugs that may be used in a suicide attempt. Patients who have attempted or threatened suicide frequently are treated initially with electroconvulsive shock therapy.

Table 42-4   Drug Interactions of Antidepressant Drugs

Drug class	Effect on therapy with a tricyclic antidepressant	Drug class	Effect on therapy with a MAO inhibitor
MAO inhibitors	Hypertensive crisis or high fever	Sympathomimetics* (amphetamine, alpha methyldopa, levodopa, dopamine, tryptophan, epinephrine, and norepinephrine)	Hypertensive crisis
Guanethidine	Antihypertensive effect blocked	Tricyclic antidepressants	Hypertensive crisis
Clonidine	Antihypertensive effect blocked	Alcohol	CNS depression
Anticholinergics	Potentiation of anticholinergic effects	Meperidine	CNS depression
Sympathomimetics	Potentiation of sympathomimetic effects	Sleeping pills	CNS depression
Alcohol	Potentiation of CNS depression	Antihistamines*	CNS depression
Barbiturates	Potentiation of CNS depression; increased metabolism of tricyclic antidepressants	Antihypertensive drugs	Orthostatic hypotension
		Diuretics (particularly thiazides)	Orthostatic hypotension
Benzodiazepines	Potentiation of CNS depression	Insulin	Hypoglycemia
Methylphenidate	Decreased metabolism of tricyclic antidepressants	Oral hypoglycemic drugs	Hypoglycemia

*Preparations frequently containing sympathomimetic or antihistaminic drugs include asthma preparations, cold tablets or capsules, cough medications, nose drops or sprays, sinus preparations, and weight-reducing pills.

Since tricyclic antidepressants can increase the seizure potential, they are not administered concurrently with electroconvulsive shock therapy.

Drug interactions

Table 42-4 lists several drug interactions with the tricyclic antidepressants. The tricyclic antidepressants can potentiate central nervous system (CNS) depression, anticholinergic effects, and sympathomimetic effects. The interaction of guanethidine and a tricyclic antidepressant is classic; the tricyclic antidepressant inhibits the uptake of guanethidine by the neurons so that guanethidine cannot reach its site of action and is therefore ineffective in lowering blood pressure. Clonidine is also blocked from its reuptake site in the CNS by the tricyclic antidepressants.

Specific Tricyclic Antidepressants

Amitriptyline

Amitriptyline (Elavil) is associated with a high incidence of sedation and anticholinergic effects. These properties are more pronounced than with other tricyclic antidepressants and can cause confusion in the older patient. Weight gain sometimes occurs. Amitriptyline has a plasma half-life of 1 to 2 days and is metabolized to nortriptyline, an active tricyclic antidepressant.

Clomipramine

Clomipramine (Anafranil) treats obsessive-compulsive disorder and blocks panic attacks. This drug has a low incidence of sedation but a moderate incidence of anticholinergic and cardiac effects.

Desipramine

Desipramine (Norpramin and Pertofrane) has a low incidence of sedation and anticholinergic effects. It is a metabolite of imipramine and has a plasma half-life of ½ to 3 days.

Doxepin

Doxepin (Adapin and Sinequan) has a high incidence of sedative and anticholinergic side effects. Doxepin does not have the quinidine-like cardiac effect to the degree characteristic of the other tricyclic drugs and therefore is indicated when cardiac function must be considered.

Imipramine

Imipramine (Tofranil) has a moderate degree of sedative and anticholinergic side effects. It is metabolized to desipramine, which is also an active tricyclic antidepressant. Imipramine has a plasma half-life of ½ to 1 day. Imipramine is used to treat enuresis (bedwetting) in older children or adults.

Nortriptyline

Nortriptyline (Aventyl and Pamelor) is moderately sedating and has minimum anticholinergic side effects. It is a metabolite of amitriptyline.

Protriptyline

Protriptyline (Vivactil) is the one tricyclic antidepressant with minimum sedating effect and is therefore most useful in depressed patients who seem physically immobilized by their depression or who sleep excessively. The plasma half-life of protriptyline is 4 to 9 days.

Trimipramine

Trimipramine (Surmontil) is a tricyclic antidepressant with a high incidence of sedation and a moderate incidence of anticholinergic effects.

Second-Generation Antidepressants

New antidepressant drugs have been introduced that are neither tricyclics nor MAO inhibitors. They are regarded as alternatives to tricyclic antidepressants, although their action on norepinephrine and serotonin uptake is not necessarily similar to that of the tricyclics. The new antidepressant drugs have, to a varying degree, a lesser incidence of anticholinergic side effects, less cardiotoxicity, and a faster onset of action than the tricyclics.

Amoxapine

Amoxapine (Asendin) inhibits amine uptake and is a more potent inhibitor of norepinephrine than of serotonin uptake. Chemically related to the tricyclic antidepressants, amoxapine is also a chemical metabolite of the antipsychotic drug loxapine and, as with the antipsychotic drugs, blocks dopamine receptors. Overall, amoxapine treats major depression and relieves anxiety and agitation associated with depression.

Amoxapine has minimum anticholinergic and sedative effects and a lesser incidence of cardiac effects than the tricyclics. Drug interactions are similar to those of the tricyclics.

Bupropion

Bupropion (Wellbutrin) is a new antidepressant that only weakly blocks norepinephrine and serotonin. Bupropion differs from tricyclic antidepressants in having a stimulant rather than a sedative effect. Patients may experience restlessness, agitation, anxiety, and insomnia. Cardiac effects are uncommon.

Fluoxetine

Fluoxetine (Prozac) is a newer antidepressant that blocks the neuronal uptake of serotonin. It is less likely to cause anticholinergic effects such as dry mouth, blurred vision, or constipation. Side effects are more commonly insomnia, nervousness, headache, and nausea. Fluoxetine depresses appetite. It may also treat obsessive-compulsive disorders and alcoholism. There have been reports that fluoxetine may be associated with suicidal ideas in some patients.

Maprotiline

Maprotiline (Ludiomil) is a tetracyclic antidepressant that inhibits norepinephrine but not serotonin uptake. Drug interactions and side effects are similar to those of the tricyclic antidepressants. Incidence of drowsiness, anticholinergic effects, and cardiac effects is less than with amitriptyline or doxepin.

Trazodone

Trazodone (Desyrel) is chemically unrelated to other antidepressant drugs. It inhibits serotonin uptake. Drowsiness is a side effect, but minimum anticholinergic and cardiac effects occur.

MAO Inhibitors

Mechanism of action

The **monoamine-oxidase (MAO) inhibitors** were in use before the tricyclic antidepressants were discovered. MAO inhibitors irreversibly inhibit the enzyme MAO. According to the biogenic amine hypothesis of depression, MAO inhibitors are effective because they prevent the degradation of norepinephrine and serotonin so that the concentration of these CNS neurotransmitters is increased (see Figure 42-1). MAO inhibitors are not as effective as the tricyclic antidepressants in treating common endogenous depression, but they are more effective in treating depressions exhibited as phobias.

Administration and fate

MAO inhibitors are well absorbed orally. They are metabolized in the liver to inactive forms and excreted in urine. Despite this, the onset of action requires 2 to 3 weeks. MAO inhibitors act by irreversible inhibition; removal of enough enzyme to produce clinical effectiveness takes time. Similarly, the effect persists for 2 to 3 weeks after MAO inhibitors have been discontinued, reflecting the time to synthesize adequate MAO.

Sedation and anticholinergic effects are common side effects associated with MAO inhibitors, but these drugs usually are administered in divided doses during the day because of their tendency to cause insomnia if given in the evening. Orthostatic hypotension is sometimes a side effect. At one time, MAO inhibitors were used as antihypertensive drugs. As with the tricyclic antidepressants, MAO inhibitors are not addicting.

Interactions leading to a hypertensive crisis

Several clinically significant problems arise from the interaction of MAO inhibitors with other drugs (see Table 42-4) and certain foods containing tyramine. A hypertensive crisis may be precipitated when a food containing tyramine or a sympathomimetic drug is ingested (see box). Sympathomimetic drugs and tyramine are normally degraded rapidly by MAO of the liver. When MAO is inhibited, tyramine remains undegraded and triggers the release of accumulated norepinephrine, which in turn causes a hypertensive episode. The earliest symptom of such a hypertensive response may be a severe headache. The necessity of avoiding these substances to avert a life-threatening hypertensive crisis is the major limitation of MAO inhibitors. Phentolamine, the alpha-receptor antagonist, may be given to lower blood pressure during a hypertensive crisis.

Acute toxicity

After ingestion of an overdose of a MAO inhibitor, symptoms appear within 12 hr and reflect increased adrenergic activity such as restlessness, anxiety, and insomnia, progressing to include tachycardia and sometimes convulsions. Dizziness and hypotension may occur, whereas some patients have severe headaches and develop high blood pressure. Some patients develop a high fever, which should be reduced with a sponge bath and external cooling. Treatment is supportive to maintain respiration and circulation. Because the effect of the MAO inhibitor is persistent, patients must be watched for at least a week.

DIETARY CONSIDERATION: MAO INHIBITORS AND TYRAMINE

Patients taking MAO inhibitors may experience a hypertensive crisis if they ingest foods containing a large amount of tyramine. Food high in tyramine include:

avocados	papaya products, including
bananas	meat tenderizers
beer	paté
bologna	pickled and kippered her-
canned figs	ring
chocolate	pepperoni
cheese (except cottage	pods or broad beans (fava
cheese)	beans)
cheese-containing food	raisins
(e.g., pizza or macaroni	raw yeast or yeast extracts
and cheese)	salami
liver	sausage
meat extracts (e.g., Marmite	sour cream
and Bovril)	soy sauce
offal	wine and chianti
	yogurt

Specific MAO Inhibitors

Isocarboxazid

Isocarboxazid (Marplan) is not considered as effective as other MAO inhibitors but is prescribed for depressed patients who are unresponsive to tricyclic antidepressants and electroconvulsive shock therapy.

Phenelzine

Phenelzine (Nardil) is the safest MAO inhibitor. Patients with a high level of anxiety who do not respond to a tricyclic antidepressant may respond to phenelzine. Doses must be individualized, since wide variability exists in its metabolism.

Tranylcypromine

Tranylcypromine (Parnate) can have a stimulatory action similar to amphetamine, and the antidepressant activity is seen more rapidly than with other MAO inhibitors.

Lithium for Manic-Depressive Disorder

Mechanism of action

Lithium lowers concentrations of norepinephrine and serotonin by inhibiting their release from and enhancing their reuptake by neurons (see Figure 42-1). These effects, along with the side effects and toxic effect of lithium, are believed to be related to the partial replacement of sodium by lithium in membrane reactions. Lithium is the drug of choice for treating the manic phase of a manic-depressive disorder.

If the patient is severely manic, an antipsychotic drug or electroconvulsive shock therapy may be used initially to subdue behavior. Lithium therapy alone usually reverses mild-to-moderate manic symptoms in 1 to 3 weeks. The duration of lithium therapy depends on the individual. Patients with occasional manic periods may be treated only during those periods. Continuous lithium therapy is indicated for patients in whom lithium reduces the frequency and intensity of their manic-depressive disorder. Evidence shows that lithium may be effective in treating the depression of the manic-depressive disorder and even endogenous depression. However, lithium is approved only for treating acute mania and as prophylaxis for recurrent mania. In research studies, lithium is being tested for its effectiveness in treating various psychiatric and neurologic brain disorders.

Administration and fate

Lithium is administered orally as the carbonate or citrate salt. Since lithium is an element, related in the atomic table to sodium and potassium, it is not metabolized but is excreted by mechanisms similar to those for sodium and potassium. Of the lithium filtered in the kidney, 80% is reabsorbed in the prox-imal tubule, and 20% is excreted in urine. The half-life of lithium in the plasma is 24 hr and is increased to 36 hr in elderly patients, so the relative dose of lithium must be decreased to avoid the cumulation to toxic doses. Other factors that decrease lithium excretion include sodium deficiency, extreme exercise, diarrhea, and postpartum status. Factors that increase lithium excretion include high sodium intake and pregnancy.

Toxicity

The therapeutic index for lithium is relatively small, and at the start of treatment, patients are tested at least weekly to ensure that the plasma level is in the therapeutic range. The therapeutic range is 0.6 to 1.2 mEq/L but as low as 0.2 mEq/L in elderly patients. Common side effects early in therapy include mild nausea, dry mouth, increased thirst, increased urination (polyuria), and fine tremor of the hands. Toxic symptoms begin to appear at 1.5 to 2.0 mEq/L and by 4.0 mEq/L may be fatal. The toxic symptoms are listed in Table 42-5.

Acute lithium toxicity is treated by hastening lithium excretion while maintaining fluid and electrolyte balance. Lithium excretion is increased by administration of an osmotic diuretic such as urea or mannitol. The drugs aminophylline and acetazolamide increase lithium excretion, and one may be given concurrently with the osmotic diuresis. Peritoneal dialysis, or preferably hemodialysis, may be used for severe toxicity or when renal failure occurs.

Contraindications

Lithium therapy is contraindicated in early pregnancy because an increased incidence of congenital malformations in infants of treated mothers has been noted. Secretion of the thyroid hormone thyroxine is inhibited by lithium, and a few patients develop an enlarged thyroid gland and may become hypothyroid. A few patients on lithium therapy develop nephrogenic diabetes insipidus (see Chapter 50), which is reversed when the lithium dose is lowered or discontinued. Paradoxically, administration of a thiazide diuretic may reverse polyuria. A more serious consequence is permanent renal damage (initially without symptoms), which may develop with long-term lithium therapy. The incidence of this damage remains to be evaluated.

Drug interactions

Several drug interactions occur with lithium. Lithium potentiates haloperidol, tricyclic antidepressants, phenothiazines, benzodiazepines, and neuromuscular blocking drugs. Lithium is potentiated by methyldopa, sodium-depleting diuretics, and the phenothiazines.

Table 42-5   Toxic Symptoms of Lithium

Blood level (mEq/L)	Symptoms	Blood level (mEq/L)	Symptoms
Below 1.5	Fine tremor of hands Dry mouth Increased thirst Increased urination Nausea	2.0 to 2.5	Persistent nausea and vomiting Blurred vision Muscle twitching (fasciculations) Hyperactive deep tendon reflexes
1.5 to 2.0	Vomiting Diarrhea Muscle weakness Incoordination (ataxia) Dizziness Confusion Slurred speech	2.5 to 3.0	Myoclonic twitches or movements of an entire limb Choreoathetoid movements Urinary and fecal incontinence
		Above 3.0	Seizures Cardiac arrhythmias Hypotension Peripheral vascular collapse Death

NURSING IMPLICATIONS SUMMARY

General Guidelines for the Use of Antidepressants

Drug administration

◆ The risk of suicide may exist in seriously depressed patients and may persist for several weeks after they begin antidepressant therapy. Some patients who were not suicidal may become so during initial therapy with antidepressants. Assess patients carefully.

◆ Monitor vital signs and weight.

◆ As mood improves, appetite may improve. In addition, some antidepressants contribute to weight gain. If weight gain is significant, counsel patients about weight reduction diets and increased exercise. Provide emotional support as needed. Consult the physician about possible changes in dose or drug.

◆ Many of these drugs alter the seizure threshold. In patients with a history of seizures, pad side rails, and supervise carefully until effects of the medications can be evaluated.

Patient and family education

◆ Tell patients and families that several weeks of therapy may be necessary before full effects of a drug regimen can be evaluated. Some side effects may lessen with continued drug use.

◆ Common side effects are noted in this text, but encourage patients to consult the physician when any new side effects develop.

◆ Teach patients that antidepressants need to be taken as ordered, on a regular basis, even if they begin to feel better. Teach patients to consult the physician before changing the prescribed drug regimen or discontinuing medications.

◆ Warn patients to inform health-care providers of all drugs being taken.

◆ Tell patients to avoid over-the-counter drugs unless first approved by the physician.

◆ Instruct patients to avoid alcohol unless approved in moderation by the physician.

◆ Warn patients to avoid driving or operating hazardous equipment if drowsiness occurs.

◆ Encourage patients and families to stay in touch with the physician and to seek assistance from appropriate health-care personnel including physicians, psychologists, nurses, and therapists.

◆ Remind patients to keep these and all drugs out of the reach of children.

Tricyclic and Second-Generation Antidepressants

Drug administration

◆ See general guidelines.

◆ Monitor vital signs and blood pressure.

◆ Assess for skin changes. Auscultate bowel sounds, and keep a record of stools.

◆ Monitor complete blood count (CBC) and platelet count.

◆ Concentrated solutions are available for some of the antidepressants; consult manufacturer's literature for appropriate diluents.

◆ Supervise patients carefully to ascertain that the medication is swallowed and not hidden in the mouth to be discarded or stored.

◆ Imipramine and other tricyclic antidepressants may be used in the treatment of enuresis in children over 6 years of age. The most frequent side effects are nervousness, sleep disorders, and gastrointestinal (GI) upset, although any side effects listed may occur. Treatment is continued for as short a period as possible to obtain relief, then the dose is tapered. The drug should be taken about 1 hr before bedtime, although early night bed-wetters may have a better response if part of the dose is given in the afternoon and part at bedtime; check with the physician. The treatment of enuresis can be complex. Provide emotional support as needed.

Patient and family education

◆ See general guidelines.

◆ See Patient Problems: Orthostatic Hypotension on p. 234, Dry Mouth on p. 166, Constipation on p. 182, and Photosensitivity on p. 629.

◆ If sedation is a problem, suggest that patients take daily doses at bedtime.

◆ Instruct patients to take doses with meals or a snack to lessen gastric irritation.

◆ Tell diabetic patients to monitor blood glucose levels, since antidepressants may alter them. A change in diet or insulin dose may be necessary.

MAO Inhibitors

Drug administration

◆ See general guidelines.

◆ Monitor vital signs and blood pressure.

◆ Auscultate bowel sounds, and keep a record of stools.

◆ Monitor CBC and platelet count.

◆ Supervise patients carefully to ascertain that the medication is swallowed and not hidden in the mouth to be discarded or stored.

Patient and family education

◆ Review general guidelines.

◆ See Patient Problems: Orthostatic Hypotension on p. 234, Dry Mouth on p. 166, and Constipation on p. 182.

◆ Review dietary restrictions with the patient and family. See Dietary Consideration: Tyramine on p. 642.

◆ Instruct patients to avoid excessive caffeine intake, although small amounts are acceptable.

◆ Tell diabetic patients to monitor blood glucose levels, since antidepressants may alter them. A change in diet or insulin dose may be necessary.

◆ Review drug interactions.

Lithium

Drug administration

◆ See general guidelines.

◆ Monitor vital signs. Inspect for edema.

◆ Assess for symptoms of toxicity (see Table 42-5).

◆ Monitor serum drug levels.

◆ If urinary output is excessive, assess for diabetes insipidus (dilute, high-volume urine with a specific gravity of 1.000 to 1.003).

◆ Supervise patients carefully to ascertain that the medication is swallowed and not hidden in the mouth to be discarded or stored.

Patient and family education

◆ See general guidelines.

◆ Emphasize the importance of returning for follow-up care to have serum drug levels monitored.

◆ Review the signs and symptoms of lithium toxicity, and teach the patient to report them.

◆ Provide emotional support as needed for side effects such as fine hand tremor, polyuria, and metallic taste in the mouth. Remind patients not to discontinue medications without consulting the physician.

◆ Tell patients to take lithium at same time daily. Take doses with meals or a snack to lessen gastric irritation.

◆ See Patient Problem: Dry Mouth on p. 166.

◆ Teach patients to notify the physician if fever or severe or persistent diarrhea or vomiting occurs, since any of these may contribute to electrolyte disturbance, which may contribute to lithium toxicity.

CHAPTER REVIEW

◆ **KEY TERMS**

depression, p. 634
endogenous depression, p. 635
manic-depressive disorder, p. 635
monoamine-oxidase (MAO) inhibitors, p. 642
reactive depression, p. 635
tricyclic antidepressants, p. 635

◆ **REVIEW QUESTIONS**

1. What is the biogenic amine theory of depression?
2. How are the actions of the tricyclic antidepressants, MAO inhibitors, and lithium consistent with the biogenic amine theory of depression?
3. How can drugs cause depression? How would you determine drug-induced depression?
4. What are the major side effects of the tricyclic antidepressants you might see?
5. Describe the acute toxicity of the tricyclic antidepressants. What symptoms might you see?
6. What are the major drug interactions of the tricyclic antidepressants? How should you educate patients?
7. How can a hypertensive crisis be precipitated in a patient taking a MAO inhibitor? What would you teach a patient to help avoid a hypertensive crisis?
8. What common side effects of MAO inhibitors might you see?
9. What symptoms of lithium toxicity might you observe?
10. How do the second-generation antidepressants compare with tricyclic antidepressants?

SUGGESTED READING

Beare PG: Psychotherapeutic drugs: implications in occupational health nursing, *AAOHN J* 35(9):394, 1987.
Beeber LS: Undesirable weight gain and psychotropic medications, *J Psychosoc Nurs Ment Health Serv* 26(10):39, 1988.
Condon EH: Dementia and depression: a devastating pain, *Geriatr Nurs* 10(1):26, 1989.
Glod C, Beeber L: Prozac: pros and cons, *J of Psychosoc Nurs Ment Health Serv* 28(12):33, 1990.
Gold PW, Goodwin FK, Chrousos GP: Clinical and biochemical manifestations of depression, *N Engl J Med* 319(7):413, 1988.
Gomez GE, Gomez, EA: The special concerns of neuroleptic use in the elderly, *J Psychosoc Nurs Ment Health Serv* 28(1):7, 1990.
Harris E: The antidepressants, *Am J Nurs* 88:1512, 1988.
Harris E: Psych drugs: the antidepressants, *Am J Nurs* 88(11):1512, 1988.
Harris E: Lithium: in a class by itself, *Am J Nurs* 89(2):190, 1989.
Jackson RT, Haynes-Johnson V: Nutritional management of patients undergoing long-term antipsychotic and antidepressant therapies, *Arch Psychiatr Nurs* II(3):146, 1988.
McEmany GW: Psychobiological indices of bipolar mood disorder: future trends in nursing care, *Arch Psychiatr Nurs* 4(1):29, 1990.
Porterfield LM: Today's antidepressants, *Adv Clin Care* 5(3):7, 1990.
Schou M: Lithium treatment of manic-depressive illness, *JAMA* 259(12):1834, 1988.
Stewart JT: Diagnosing and treating depression in the hospitalized elderly, *Geriatrics* 46(1):64, 1991.
Townsend MC: *Drug guide for psychiatric nursing*, Philadelphia, 1990, FA Davis.
Valente SM, Saunders JM: Dealing with serious depression in cancer patients, *Nurs 89* 19(2):44, 1989.

CHAPTER 43

Central Nervous System Stimulants

LEARNING OBJECTIVES

After studying this chapter, you should be able to do the following:

◆ Name the appropriate clinical uses of central nervous system stimulants.

◆ Discuss the side effects of these agents.

◆ Develop a nursing care plan for the patient receiving a central nervous system stimulant.

CHAPTER OVERVIEW

◆ The central nervous system (CNS) regulates its level of activity by maintaining excitatory and inhibitory systems. Therefore excessive stimulation of the CNS may be produced by excessive activity of excitatory neurons or by blockade of inhibitory neurons. Many types of chemicals at some dose produce a degree of CNS stimulation by one of these mechanisms. Few of these compounds have legitimate pharmacologic uses. CNS stimulants currently are medically accepted only for the treatment of narcolepsy, attention deficit disorder in children, and obesity. The drugs also are used occasionally as agents to reverse respiratory depression, although they are not generally recommended for these purposes. This chapter examines the mechanism of action of CNS stimulants used in clinical conditions and the properties that make them prominent drugs of abuse.

Nursing Process Overview
CNS STIMULANTS FOR NARCOLEPSY AND ATTENTION DEFICIT DISORDER
Assessment
Obtain a thorough history of the patient's presenting problem. Assess vital signs and weight. In children, assess height. Perform a thorough mental status examination.

Nursing Diagnosis
Possible complication: growth retardation in children

Management
Spend time with the patient or family in identifying reasonable goals of therapy. Monitor the height, weight, and vital signs, and obtain an indication of mental status at periodic intervals. Question the patient about subjective symptoms or problems not evident through observation such as insomnia, agitation, dizziness, headache, and irritability. When children are being treated for attention deficit disorder the parents may be additional sources of information about the response to the drugs.

Evaluation
Before discharge, verify that the patient or family can state why the medication is being used, side effects that may occur, side effects that should cause notification of the physician, any allowable adjustments in dosage that can be made based on side effects (such as giving a nighttime dose at a different time for a child with attention deficit disorder), and any activities or measures that should be used to monitor the effectiveness of the drug in the home such as keeping a weight record.

Table 43-1   CNS Stimulants for Narcolepsy and Attention Deficit Disorder

Generic name	Trade name	Medical use	Administration/dosage	Comments
Amphetamine sulfate (also called racemic or *dl*-amphetamine sulfate)		Narcolepsy	ORAL: *Adults*—5 to 20 mg 1 to 3 times daily. FDA Pregnancy Category C. *Children over 6 years*—2.5 mg twice daily, gradually increased to adult dose if needed.	Dosage is adjusted according to patient's needs and tolerance to side effects on cardiovascular and nervous systems.
		Attention deficit disorder	ORAL: *Children 3 to 6 years*—2.5 mg daily and increase by 2.5 mg increments weekly to achieve desired effect; *6 years and older*—initially 5 mg daily and increase by 5 mg increments weekly to achieve desired effect.	Dosage should be the minimum required for control of symptoms. Long-term continuous use may inhibit growth. Drugs may be withdrawn during less stressful periods such as summer holidays. Schedule II substance.
Dextroamphetamine sulfate	Dexedrine* Oxydess II	Narcolepsy	As for amphetamine sulfate.	As for amphetamine sulfate, except less tendency for cardiovascular toxicity. Schedule II substance (U.S.). Class G (Canada).
		Attention deficit disorder	As for amphetamine sulfate.	
Methamphetamine hydrochloride	Desoxyn	Attention deficit disorder	ORAL: *Children 6 years and older*—5 mg once or twice daily; increase by 5 mg increments weekly to optimum dosage, usually 20 to 25 mg. Extended release tablets are used for maintenance.	Has CNS and cardiovascular toxicity. Schedule II substance.
Methylphenidate hydrochloride	Ritalin*	Attention deficit disorder	ORAL: *Children 6 years and older*—5 mg before breakfast and lunch; increase by 5 to 10 mg at weekly intervals. Maximum daily doses should not exceed 60 mg.	Drug of choice for most children with attention deficit disorder. Schedule II substance (U.S.). Class C (Canada).
		Narcolepsy	ORAL: *Adults*—10 to 60 mg daily divided into 2 or 3 doses.	
Pemoline	Cylert*	Attention deficit disorder	ORAL: *Children 6 years and older*—37.5 mg daily in a single dose; increase weekly by 18.75 mg increments until response is obtained. Do not exceed 112.5 mg daily.	Clinical effects develop over 3 to 4 weeks. Schedule IV substance (U.S.).

*Available in Canada and United States.
†Available in Canada only.

NARCOLEPSY

Narcolepsy is a condition in which patients unexpectedly fall asleep in the middle of normal activity such as while typing, driving a car, or talking. During an attack, patients experience paralysis of the voluntary muscles similar to that of the dream state and may abruptly collapse and fall. Patients with this sleep disorder should be advised to avoid operating cars or dangerous machinery.

The treatment of narcolepsy usually includes the

use of CNS stimulants during active daytime periods. These agents have alerting effects and reduce the sleeping episodes. One class of CNS stimulants used for this purpose is amphetamines (Table 43-1).

The most commonly used CNS stimulant in narcoleptic patients is methylphenidate (see Table 43-1). This drug has been used in combination with imipramine (see Chapter 42). The effect of imipramine on narcolepsy is not produced by the antidepressant effects of the drug. The reversal of narcolepsy is rapid, whereas the antidepressant effects of imipramine develop over a prolonged period.

Although drug therapy may be beneficial for many narcoleptic patients, most also require other therapy such as scheduled daytime naps. Psychologic counseling may help patients to reconcile their living patterns with the constraints imposed by the disease.

ATTENTION DEFICIT DISORDER

Children with **attention deficit disorder** display a variety of symptoms that impair their ability to learn or to maintain appropriate social interactions. These children are excessively active, impulsive, and irritable. Their attention span is very short, and their activity is purposeless. Learning disabilities of various types are frequent in these children. Many children with attention deficit disorder display abnormal electroencephalographic (EEG) patterns and poorer coordination than normal children of the same age. Intelligence is not impaired. Because of the wide range of symptoms produced, this syndrome has been called by many names, including *minimal brain dysfunction, minimal brain damage, hyperkinesis, attention deficit disorder with hyperkinesis,* and *hyperkinetic syndrome with learning disorder.*

Children with attention deficit disorder must receive psychotherapy and counseling, as well as remedial education adjusted to their needs and abilities. Drug therapy to reduce the hyperactive behavior and to lengthen the attention span also may be required. The drugs most effective in controlling this disorder are, paradoxically, CNS stimulants. These agents, which increase agitation and activity in adults, have a calming effect on these children. Amphetamines have been used to control this disorder (see Table 43-1). An equally effective drug with fewer peripheral side effects is methylphenidate (see box). Pemoline is sometimes used but in general is less effective than amphetamines or methylphenidate (see Table 43-1).

Controversy surrounds the diagnosis and treatment of children with attention deficit disorder. Many authorities believe the syndrome is diagnosed more frequently than it exists and suggest that thousands of children may be receiving CNS stimulants unnecessarily. This problem remains to be resolved.

DRUG ABUSE ALERT: METHYLPHENIDATE

THE PROBLEM

Methylphenidate rarely causes toxic psychosis but may cause psychologic drug dependence. Both effects are observed after long-term use of doses in excess of therapeutic doses. The primary patient is obviously most at risk of developing dependence, but health-care personnel must also be alert to the problem among caregivers. For example, adult guardians of children receiving methylphenidate may divert the drug from the child and use it themselves.

SOLUTIONS

◆ Confirm that doses are not being extemporaneously increased by the patient or caregiver
◆ Advise the patient to seek medical advice if drug seems to become less effective after several weeks
◆ See that dosage reduction is gradual so that withdrawal symptoms are minimized

---

Pharmacologic Properties of Specific Agents

Amphetamines

Mechanism of action. **Amphetamines** increase the release and effectiveness of catecholamine neurotransmitters in the brain and in peripheral nerves by several mechanisms. These drugs seem to increase the release of neurotransmitters during normal nervous system activity. In addition, amphetamines block the specific reuptake of catecholamine neurotransmitters into the presynaptic neuron. Because this reuptake system is normally a major mechanism for terminating the action of the neurotransmitters, blockade of the reuptake system produces prolonged and enhanced stimulation of the postsynaptic nerves. Norepinephrine and dopamine are thought to be the catecholamines whose actions are most enhanced by amphetamines.

Amphetamines may affect many sites within the brain. However, many of the clinically observed actions of amphetamines probably are related to activity in two particular regions of the brain, one of which is the reticular activating system. This complex of neurons regulates sensory input to the brain and thus controls the level of arousal. Amphetamines stimulate the reticular activating system, creating increased alertness and sensitivity to stimuli.

The second area of the brain that seems to be especially responsive to amphetamines is in the medial forebrain bundle. This reward, or pleasure, center can be activated by amphetamines. The result to the user is a perception of pleasure unrelated to external stimuli. This stimulation of the pleasure center is thought to be the source of the addictive potential of amphetamines.

Absorpton and fate. Amphetamines for medical uses are given orally. These drugs are well absorbed from the gastrointestinal (GI) tract and produce peak serum concentrations within 2 to 3 hr after ingestion. The half-lives of the various amphetamines in the bloodstream range from 4 to 30 hr. These compounds easily penetrate the blood-brain barrier to produce their CNS effects. Amphetamines are excreted primarily by the kidneys. The rate of excretion is highly dependent on urinary pH. Excretion can be greatly enhanced by acidifying urine.

Toxicity. Amphetamines cause toxic reactions in several organ systems. Unpredictable effects can occur in the GI tract, but vomiting, diarrhea, abdominal cramps, and dry mouth often occur. Anorexia may be produced, but this reaction is caused by the CNS effects of amphetamines.

Most CNS toxicity of amphetamines can be seen as an extension of the effects observed at therapeutic doses. At high doses, amphetamines cause restless behavior, tremor, irritability, talkativeness, insomnia, and mood changes. Excessive aggressiveness, confusion, panic, and increased libido also may occur. More rarely, patients will suffer a syndrome resembling schizophrenia, with delirium or hallucinations. Long-term intoxication with amphetamines frequently causes this schizophrenia-like reaction, sometimes referred to as *toxic psychosis*.

Because of their sympathomimetic effects, amphetamines can cause various reactions in the cardiovascular system. Patients report headache, chilliness, and palpitations. Pallor or facial flushing may be present. Angina and various cardiac arrhythmias can be precipitated. Hypertension or hypotension may be observed at various stages during intoxication. The severely intoxicated patient may die in circulatory collapse.

Amphetamine toxicity differs somewhat, depending on which specific drug is used. Generic amphetamine is a mixture of two forms of amphetamine called d (dextro) and l (levo). The d form of amphetamine stimulates the CNS more effectively than does the l form. Conversely, the l form stimulates the cardiovascular system slightly more effectively than does the d form. Amphetamine, a mixture of d and l forms, causes CNS and cardiovascular toxicity.

The drug sold under the trade name of Dexedrine is dextroamphetamine, the d form of amphetamine. This preparation is more selective for the CNS and does not produce the same degree of cardiovascular toxicity observed with amphetamine. Children receiving amphetamines may suffer growth retardation. This effect can be minimized by giving drug holidays during which drug therapy is suspended.

Drug interactions. Amphetamines interact with several other drugs. Amphetamines block the hypotensive effect of methyldopa and guanethidine. The metabolism of tricyclic antidepressants is blocked by amphetamines, causing these drugs to accumulate unless dosage is reduced. Sympathomimetic drugs can increase the effects of amphetamines. Monoamine-oxidase (MAO) inhibitors also increase catecholamine levels and potentiate the effects of amphetamines.

Methylphenidate

Mechanism of action. Methylphenidate is a mild CNS stimulant. Its exact biochemical mechanism of action is unknown but appears similar to the amphetamines.

Absorption and fate. Methylphenidate is well absorbed orally and is usually prescribed to be given to adults 30 to 45 min before meals. Orally administered methylphenidate is extensively metabolized during the first pass through the liver. The metabolites of methylphenidate are not capable of stimulating the CNS or sympathetic peripheral neurons. Most of the methylphenidate taken orally is excreted in urine as inactive metabolites.

Toxicity. Methylphenidate often causes nervousness and insomnia. Insomnia may be minimized by not administering the drug in the evening. Nervousness is frequently controlled by reducing overall drug dosage. Anorexia, nausea, and abdominal pain may occur with methylphenidate, as with the amphetamines. Cardiovascular effects similar to those produced by amphetamines are also seen.

Methylphenidate can cause allergic reactions in sensitive patients. These reactions may range from mild skin rashes to exfoliative dermatitis and thrombocytopenic purpura.

The drug causes a temporary slowing of growth in prepubertal children. Most children seem to overcome the deficit and ultimately gain normal stature. Slow growth can be minimized by giving the child a drug-free period during therapy.

Drug interactions. Methylphenidate, like the amphetamines, can interact with many other medications. Since methylphenidate causes its effects by release of catecholamines such as norepinephrine, the effects may be greatly increased by MAO inhibitors, sympathomimetic agents, or vasopressors. Methylphenidate also inhibits the metabolism of a variety of drugs, including phenytoin, phenobarbital, primidone, phenylbutazone, imipramine, desipramine, and coumarin anticoagulants. Therefore these drugs must be given at reduced dosages to avoid drug accumulation and excess toxicity when methylphenidate also is being administered. The antihypertensive medication guanethidine is made less effective by methylphenidate, apparently because guanethidine uptake into nerve terminals is blocked.

Pemoline

Mechanism of action. Pemoline stimulates the CNS in a manner similar to that of amphetamines and methylphenidate but lacks the strong sympathomimetic effects of many of those stimulants. The exact biochemical mechanism for the action of pemoline is unknown.

Absorption and fate. Pemoline is well absorbed orally, producing peak serum levels 2 to 4 hr after dosage. The serum half-life for the drug is about 12 hr. Therefore the drug may be given once daily. The kidneys excrete most of the administered pemoline, as unchanged drug and as metabolites.

Although the blood levels reach a plateau within a few days after therapy is begun, the therapeutic effects of pemoline are not immediately evident in hyperkinetic children. Dosage is gradually increased over 2 to 4 weeks after therapy is started. Significant clinical response may not be seen until the third or fourth week.

Toxicity. Pemoline, when used in properly selected children at recommended doses, seldom causes serious toxic reactions. Insomnia often is reported but is a transient reaction in most patients. Pemoline causes anorexia, stomachache, and nausea, which may slow normal weight gain. Children do not seem to suffer permanent growth retardation, but careful records of the child's growth should be maintained to allow assessment during therapy.

Pemoline may produce skin rashes and altered liver function tests. These reversible reactions may be caused by allergy. CNS signs such as irritability, mild depression, dizziness, headache, and hallucinations may be provoked. Tachycardia and agitation usually result with overdosages. Because pemoline may alter dopamine systems within the CNS, signs of dyskinesia should be watched for carefully (see Chapter 41).

Nursing Process Overview
CNS STIMULANTS FOR OBESITY
Assessment

Obesity is a significant health problem in the United States. Obtain a thorough patient assessment, with a focus on vital signs, weight, diet history and usual eating habits, and other existing medical conditions. Establish with the patient reasonable desired weight goals for therapy. Assess mental status.

Nursing Diagnoses

Possible complication: toxic psychosis secondary to drug therapy
Possible complication: addiction or abuse

Management

The goal of therapy with CNS stimulants in treating obesity is to promote weight reduction without producing cardiovascular or mental status effects. Monitor the patient for these side effects, and offer emotional support and information related to control of obesity.

Evaluation

Before discharge, verify that the patient can explain why the medication is being used and how to take it correctly, the hazards of overmedication, side effects that may occur, symptoms that should be reported to the physician, and how abuse of many of these drugs can cause addiction. In addition, check that the patient can explain how to carry out other prescribed measures such as caloric dietary restriction and exercise. Monitor weight and other signs and symptoms as a part of routine follow-up. The CNS stimulants are not used for long-term control of obesity.

ANOREXIANTS

Many CNS stimulants suppress appetite even while stimulating other CNS functions. Because of this effect on appetite, many of these drugs have been used to help control obesity. As a group, these drugs are referred to as ***anorexiants*** or *appetite suppressants* (Table 43-2).

Pharmacology of Specific Agents

Amphetamines were the original CNS stimulants used to control obesity. At the low dosage ranges used in obese patients, tolerance develops to the appetite suppressant properties of amphetamines in 4 to 6 weeks. Long-term use produces many undesirable side effects, including addiction; thus they now are not recommended for use in obesity (see box).

The newer anorexiants listed in Tables 43-2 and 43-3 do not produce the same degree of stimulation of the CNS or cardiovascular systems as amphetamine and its derivatives. However, none of the anorexiants are completely without potentially dangerous systemic side effects.

Some anorexiants resemble the amphetamines in activity and reactions but produce these reactions less frequently and less severely; these include benzphetamine and mazindol. Diethylpropion, unlike other anorexiants, produces little significant cardiovascular stimulation and thus may be used in patients with

Table 43-2 Appetite Suppressants

Generic name	Trade name	Administration/dosage	Comments
Benzphetamine hydrochloride	Didrex	ORAL: *Adults*—25 to 50 mg once daily; may be increased as needed up to 3 doses daily. FDA Pregnancy Category X.	Similar to amphetamine. Schedule III substance.
Diethylpropion hydrochloride	Nobesine† Tenuate* Tepanil	ORAL: *Adults*—25 mg 1 hr before morning, noon, and evening meals and at midevening if needed. Timed-release formulations (75 mg) are taken once daily. FDA Pregnancy Category B.	Safest anorexiant for use in patients with mild cardiovascular disease. Dry mouth and constipation are common reactions. Schedule IV substance (U.S.). Class G (Canada).
Fenfluramine hydrochloride	Ponderal† Pondimin*	ORAL: *Adults*—20 mg 3 times daily before meals. Dosage may be doubled if required. FDA Pregnancy Category C.	Only anorexiant that depresses CNS activity; sedation and depression may occur. Schedule IV substance.
Mazindol	Mazanor Sanorex*	ORAL: *Adults*—doses range from 1 mg daily at breakfast to 1 mg 3 times daily with meals. Minimum dose should be used.	May be used in patients with arteriosclerosis or hyperthyroidism. Schedule IV substance.
Phendimetrazine tartrate	Anorex Bacarate Melfiat Plegine	ORAL: *Adults*—35 mg 2 or 3 times daily taken before meals. Sustained release, 105 mg taken once in the morning.	Stimulates the CNS in the same way as amphetamines. GI distress may occur. Schedule III substance.
Phentermine	Adipex Fastin* Ionamin* Zantryl	ORAL: *Adults*—single dose of 15 to 37.5 mg may be taken 2 hr after breakfast.	Commonly causes insomnia and cardiovascular effects. Schedule IV substance (U.S.). Class G (Canada).
Phenylpropanolamine hydrochloride	Acutrim Dexatrim Diadax Prolamine Unitrol	ORAL: *Adults*—25 mg 3 times daily before meals or 50 to 75 mg of sustained-action formulation once daily at midmorning.	Blood pressure increases occur. These diet preparations should never be used with cold or allergy medications. Nonprescription.

* Available in Canada and United States.
† Available in Canada only.

DRUG ABUSE ALERT: APPETITE SUPPRESSANTS

THE PROBLEM

Many patients experience some level of dependence on the CNS stimulants used as appetite suppressants. Patients may seek them from several physicians rather than follow the advice of a single physician who may limit the use of the drugs to 2 or 3 months. Many appetite suppressants also carry the risk of causing psychotic reactions, as a result of either overdosage or prolonged use.

SOLUTIONS

◆ Warn the patient that the anorectic effect will wear off in 6 to 12 weeks
◆ Warn the patient not to increase dosage to prolong the anorectic effect
◆ Observe for signs of dependence
◆ Offer counseling about healthy dietary limitations and good eating practices

some types of cardiovascular disease. Fenfluramine is unlike the other anorexiant drugs, since it depresses the CNS while suppressing the appetite. Phentermine usually has no effect on mood but, as with the amphetamines, produces cardiovascular stimulation. Phenylpropanolamine mildly suppresses appetite and is included in various nonprescription appetite suppressants, alone or with other agents. Phenylpropanolamine also is often used in nonprescription nasal decongestants (see Chapter 4).

Toxicity and side effects. The use of appetite suppressants in treating obesity is controversial. All the available effective agents carry substantial risks, and many have high abuse potential. Many patients experience some level of dependence on these medications. Fenfluramine may also produce dangerous mental imbalances, although with this drug the danger is depression rather than stimulation of the CNS. Fenfluramine should never be given to a patient with a previous history of depression or suicidal tendencies.

Table 43-3   Systemic Effects of Appetite Suppressants

Generic name	Effects on				
	Mood	Motor activity	Heart rate	Blood pressure	Abuse potential
Benzphetamine	Elevated	May increase	May increase	May increase	High
Diethylpropion	May be elevated	May increase	Unchanged	Unchanged	Relatively low
Fenfluramine	Depressed	Depressed	Usually no change	May increase	Relatively low
Mazindol	May be elevated	May increase	Increased	Usually no change	High
Phendimetrazine	Highly elevated	Increased	Usually no change	Usually no change	High
Phentermine	Usually no change	May increase	Increased	Increased	Relatively low
Phenylpropanolamine	Usually no change	Usually no change	May increase	May increase	Low

Anorexiants cause irritability and insomnia. Sympathetic nervous system effects include dry mouth, blurred vision, heart palpitations, and hypertension. Some of these drugs cause GI distress. The anorexiants have not been proved safe during pregnancy.

Tolerance. Tolerance develops to all the appetite-suppressing drugs in clinical use. Effective weight reduction cannot be maintained by relying on drugs alone to control eating patterns. Persons seeking to lose weight must develop appropriate eating habits and an exercise plan adjusted to their age and physical limitations. Drugs to suppress appetite may help a patient during the initial stages of a weight-reduction program, but these agents are not the key to a successful long-term program. None of these drugs are intended for use in children.

Drug interactions. All the appetite-suppressing agents can interact with many other medications. For example, any sympathomimetic drug may have a much greater effect in patients receiving appetite suppressants, because the appetite-suppressing drugs tend to increase the effectiveness of catecholamines. This precaution should be mentioned to patients, and they should be warned to avoid cold remedies, allergy medications, and nasal decongestants that include sympathomimetic agents.

Blood pressure can be affected by appetite suppressants. Many may directly elevate blood pressure. Phenylpropanolamine is occasionally used clinically for its vasopressor effect. Patients receiving medications to treat high blood pressure should avoid appetite-suppressing drugs.

Nursing Process Overview
CNS STIMULANTS FOR RESPIRATION
Assessment

Complete a thorough patient assessment, focusing on the respiratory system. Auscultate the lungs, check the respiratory rate and depth of respirations, and evaluate the vital capacity. Monitor arterial blood gas levels.

Nursing Diagnoses

Possible complication: increased blood pressure
Altered comfort: nausea and GI discomfort

Management

These drugs are used on a short-term basis. Use an infusion control device or volume control device. Monitor the vital signs, with emphasis on the respiratory system. Keep a suction machine at the bedside. Monitor any serum drug levels if they are being obtained. Assess mental status on a regular basis.

Evaluation

The goal of these drugs is to stimulate the respiratory system so that the patient breaths at a rate and depth approaching normal. These medications are for short-term use in the hospital.

ANALEPTICS

Certain CNS stimulants have generalized effects on the brain stem and spinal cord, as well as on higher

Table 43-4   CNS Stimulants for Respiratory Stimulation

Generic name	Trade name	Administration/dosage	Comments
Aminophylline	Somophyllin Paralon*	ORAL, NASOGASTRIC TUBE: 5 mg/kg initial dose, then 2 mg/kg daily, divided into 2 or 3 doses.	Most commonly used to treat asthma but also used to treat apnea in neonates.
Caffeine (citrated caffeine)		ORAL, NASOGASTRIC TUBE: 10 mg/kg body weight initially, then 2.5 mg/kg daily.	Used in newborn infants.
Doxapram	Dopram*	INTRAVENOUS: *Adults*—0.5 to 2 mg/kg body weight intermittently as needed. For chronic obstructive pulmonary disease, 1 to 2 mg/min infusion for 2 hr.	Rapidly acting drug whose action is over within 12 min. Do not use in newborn infants because of benzyl alcohol content.
Theophylline		ORAL, NASOGASTRIC TUBE: 5 mg/kg body weight initial dose, then 2 mg/kg daily divided into 2 or 3 doses.	Most commonly used to treat asthma but is also used to treat apnea in newborn infants. Effective plasma concentrations range from 5 to 12 μg/ml with toxicity expected above 20 μg/ml.

*Available in Canada and United States.

centers in the brain. These drugs may increase responsiveness to external stimuli and stimulate respiration. As a group, these drugs are referred to as *analeptics* (Table 43-4).

Analeptics have been used primarily to stimulate respiration. The use of these drugs has become less common, because modern techniques of respiratory therapy allow a patient to be adequately ventilated even when the natural reflex is temporarily absent. Respiratory paralysis caused by overdoses of narcotic agents is appropriately treated with specific narcotic antagonists and not with analeptics.

Two properties of the analeptic drugs make them especially hard to control. First, they are nonspecific stimulants of the CNS and may produce unwanted effects in addition to respiratory stimulation. Second, all these drugs at a high enough dose or in a predisposed patient may produce convulsions.

Pharmacology of Specific Agents

Methylxanthines

Methylxanthines include caffeine, aminophylline, and theophylline.

Mechanism of action. Methylxanthines block the destruction of cyclic AMP, the compound that mediates the effects of beta-adrenergic stimulation (see Chapter 10). As a result, these compounds affect many body systems, including the CNS. Caffeine, aminophylline, and theophylline are the forms most often used clinically.

Caffeine may stimulate any level of the CNS, depending on the dose. Mild cortical stimulation is produced by low oral doses such as those available in coffee, tea, and cola or in the nonprescription-alerting medications. At higher doses, caffeine stimulates the medullary centers controlling respiration, vasomotor tone, and vagal tone. Very high doses of caffeine may stimulate the spinal cord and produce generalized convulsions.

Theophylline also acts as a CNS stimulant but exerts more action on the heart than caffeine. Theophylline is most often used clinically to relax bronchial smooth muscle. This action is useful in treating chronic obstructive pulmonary disease and asthma (see Chapter 25). Theophylline has also been used as a respiratory stimulant in newborn infants.

Absorption and fate. Methylxanthines are absorbed from the GI tract. Salt forms of these agents are better absorbed, because the salts are much more soluble in water than are the free alkaloids. The parenteral form of caffeine includes sodium benzoate to maintain solubility of the caffeine.

Caffeine has a half-life in the plasma of about 4 hr. The drug may be partly metabolized in the liver. A portion of a dose appears in urine as the unchanged compound or as metabolites. Aminophylline releases free theophylline in vivo. Theophylline has a half-life in the plasma of 8 to 9 hr in adults.

The metabolism and clearance of methylxanthines may be much lower in neonates than in adults. When these drugs are used in newborn infants, it may be necessary to adjust the dose to allow for the longer persistence of the drugs in the body. Because neonates vary greatly in their ability to metabolize methylxanthines, it may be necessary to measure blood levels of these drugs. Clearance of methylxanthines is also lower in patients with liver disease or congestive heart failure. These patients may also require adjusted doses of methylxanthines.

Toxicity. Methylxanthines frequently irritate the GI mucosa, producing bleeding. Bleeding may occur without other signs or may be accompanied by nausea and vomiting. High concentrations of methylxanthines in the blood can lead to excessive CNS stimulation and convulsions. At ordinary therapeutic concentrations, however, the most common reaction to caffeine is nervousness or jitteriness. Theophylline most commonly increases heart rate (tachycardia).

Doxapram

Mechanism of action. Doxapram stimulates respiration by two mechanisms. At low doses the drug seems to stimulate the peripheral carotid chemoreceptors. This action increases sensitivity to carbon dioxide and thereby increases the impulse to breathe. At slightly higher doses, doxapram stimulates the medullary centers controlling respiration.

Absorption and fate. Doxapram is administered intravenously. The drug is very rapid acting, with effects observed within 1 min after injection. The duration of respiratory stimulation is usually 5 to 12 min. Doxapram may be given repeatedly to sustain a patient throughout a period of respiratory depression.

Toxicity. Doxapram can produce a variety of reactions. Dizziness, apprehension, and disorientation may be reported. Restless, involuntary muscle activity, and increased reflexes are frequently observed. Patients may report a feeling of warmth with flushing, sweating, and increased body temperature. Blood pressure is elevated. Chest pains and cardiac arrhythmias may occur. Extreme agitation, hallucinations, or convulsions usually occur only with overdose, but certain patients may be more susceptible to these reactions. The maximum cumulative dose for doxapram is 3 gm.

Since doxapram increases blood pressure, this drug should not be used in combination with other drugs tending to elevate blood pressure, such as sympathomimetics. Adverse interactions can also occur between doxapram and the inhalation anesthetics that sensitize the heart to catecholamines (e.g., halothane and enflurane). A delay of 10 min or more between the cessation of anesthesia with these drugs and the administration of doxapram is suggested to lessen the possibility of excessive cardiac toxicity.

CNS STIMULANTS AS DRUGS OF ABUSE

CNS stimulants commonly come to the attention of the medical professional as drugs of abuse. The medical uses of these agents are limited. This section discusses the more commonly abused drugs of this class, dealing primarily with the symptoms and sequelae of abuse. The list of drugs covered is necessarily limited. Suggested readings at the end of the chapter give more comprehensive coverage of unofficial or "street" drugs.

Amphetamines

Although the legitimate medical uses of the amphetamines are rather limited, large amounts of amphetamines are still produced. In 1970, the year before amphetamines were put on schedule II, the Department of Justice reported that 38% of the manufactured amphetamines could not be traced and presumably went to illegal markets. Strong restrictions on the manufacture and sale of amphetamines followed, but amphetamine availability seemed to be unimpaired. A Drug Enforcement Administration report in 1976 suggested that amphetamine abuse was increasing and that the source of the drug was largely physicians' prescriptions. Estimates of the extent of amphetamine abuse are obviously filled with uncertainties; however, many experts agree that the most common amphetamine abuser is middle class, gets amphetamines from one or more medical sources, and takes the drugs orally.

Long-term use of low doses of amphetamines can produce psychologic dependence. The drug user may have originally taken the drug intermittently to overcome fatigue or depression. Doses of 5 to 20 mg are effective in the naive user. Persons who take these doses three or four times daily will begin to feel as if they cannot get along without the drug. If the person stops taking the drug, depression ensues. Whether amphetamines produce actual physical withdrawal symptoms is debatable, but this withdrawal depression is sufficiently unpleasant to induce many users to return to amphetamine use.

Heavy use of amphetamines either orally or by injection can lead to severe reactions. Persons taking large doses may begin to show stereotyped behavior consisting of compulsive or repetitive actions. These actions frequently have no useful goal. For example, the user may repeatedly wax one fender of a car or count the pages of a book. Other behavior patterns are less benign. For example, chronic abusers often have the conviction that bugs are crawling under their skin and may mutilate themselves in an attempt to remove them. Some users develop feelings of paranoia and suspicion, feelings that frequently erupt into violent behavior. Many chronic abusers of amphetamines develop toxic, or paranoid, psychosis. This severe reaction involves visual and auditory hallucinations and is frequently mistaken for schizophrenia.

The toxic psychosis of amphetamines is specifically treated with an antipsychotic drug (see Chapter 41).

Cocaine

Cocaine was introduced into medicine as a local anesthetic and is very effective for that purpose. Unfortunately, cocaine is also a stimulant very similar to amphetamine in its mechanism of action and effects on the CNS.

Pure salts of cocaine are difficult to prepare and are consequently very expensive. Until recently, this restriction limited the availability of cocaine. Today, the most commonly used form of cocaine is the free base known as *crack,* which is easy to prepare and inexpensive. It is highly lipid soluble and is quickly absorbed and distributed to the CNS. In this form, cocaine is one of the most addictive substances known.

At moderate doses, cocaine can increase heart rate and blood pressure and produce general CNS stimulation. As with amphetamines, it can produce convulsions if high enough doses are taken. Death by cocaine overdose is relatively rare, but when a fatal overdose is taken, convulsions, cardiovascular collapse, and death may occur within 2 or 3 min of the dose.

Chronic abuse of cocaine produces physical symptoms similar to those produced by amphetamine abuse. Toxic psychosis, stereotyped behavior, and paranoia also are observed.

Caffeine

Caffeine may be the most widely abused drug in the United States, although the effects of this abuse are much less obvious and are usually less devastating than those produced by other abused drugs. Caffeine abuse often takes place unwittingly. Consider the following example:

John has a cup of coffee while dressing in the morning and a second cup at breakfast. At work, John consumes another cup of coffee at the 10:30 AM coffee break. At lunch, John drinks two glasses of iced tea. On afternoon coffee break, John has a chocolate bar and a cola. Before he leaves work, John takes two Excedrin for a headache. At dinner, John drinks two cups of tea. Before bed, John takes two more Excedrin.

Why is John unable to sleep? John cannot sleep because he ingested about 1 gm of caffeine during this typical day.

Most people are aware of the caffeine content of coffee, which ranges from 80 to 150 mg per cup. Less well known is that tea, colas, chocolate, and nonprescription medications such as Excedrin also contain caffeine. In the example given, John took over ½ gm of caffeine in these forms.

Ingestion of more than 500 mg (½ gm) of caffeine daily produces a variety of CNS effects and cardiovascular reactions. Irritability or nervousness is a common complaint, along with sleep disturbances. Patients may report heart palpitations or that their heart is racing. These descriptions may suggest premature ventricular contractions and tachycardia, common symptoms of chronic caffeine toxicity. Diarrhea and GI irritation commonly accompany chronic overdosage with caffeine. Patients complaining of symptoms such as those listed should be questioned about caffeine intake. The person taking the history should ask specifically about individual beverages, foods, and medications that contain caffeine to get an accurate estimate of intake. The caffeine content of common items is presented in Table 43-5.

Psychologic dependence on caffeine may occur. People have great difficulty in omitting the drug from their diets. Nevertheless, patients with peptic ulcer disease should avoid caffeine. Pregnant women may wish to avoid caffeine, since it freely passes to the fetus. Any person who ingests more than 200 mg of caffeine daily should be encouraged to reduce intake to avoid the subtle onset of chronic toxicity.

Table 43-5   Caffeine Content of Commonly Ingested Substances

Substance	Caffeine content
FOODS AND BEVERAGES	
Coffee	
Brewed	80 to 150 mg/5 oz cup
Instant	85 to 100 mg/5 oz cup
Decaffeinated	2 to 4 mg/5 oz cup
Tea, brewed	30 to 75 mg/5 oz cup
Cocoa	5 to 40 mg/5 oz cup
Cola soft drinks*	35 to 60 mg/12 oz bottle or can
NONPRESCRIPTION MEDICATIONS	
Analgesics (Anacin and Vanquish)	32 mg/tablet
Excedrin	65 mg/tablet
COLD MEDICATIONS	
Dristan AF	16.2 mg/tablet
Korigesic	30 mg/tablet
STIMULANTS	
Nodoz	100 mg/tablet
Vivarin	200 mg/tablet

*Many soft drinks other than colas contain caffeine as an additive. The label reveals the presence of caffeine but not the amount.

General Guidelines for Patients Receiving Drugs to Treat Narcolepsy or ADD, or to Suppress Appetite

Drug administration

◆ Assess for CNS side effects; if severe, notify the physician.

◆ In the hospital, pad side rails, and keep them up. Have a suction machine nearby.

◆ Monitor vital signs and blood pressure. Assess mental status.

◆ Monitor behavior. Assess for restlessness, irritability, confusion, insomnia, and mood changes.

◆ Assess for GI symptoms including vomiting, diarrhea, and abdominal cramps.

Patient and family education

◆ Review anticipated benefits and possible side effects of drug therapy. Tell the patient to report any new symptoms.

◆ Tell patients to take these drugs only as directed and not to change dose or frequency without consulting the physician. Point out that these drugs are habit forming.

◆ Remind patients to inform all health-care providers of all drugs being taken. Warn patients to avoid ingesting drugs or foods that also contribute to cardiovascular side effects such as caffeine and caffeine-containing beverages or over-the-counter (OTC) cold preparations containing phenylpropanolamine.

◆ Avoid OTC drugs unless first approved by the phsyician

◆ After long-term use, these drugs should not be discontinued abruptly.

◆ None of these drugs is appropriate to treat general fatigue.

◆ Insomnia may lessen with continued use of a drug, but may be better treated by eliminating the final dose of medication during the day; consult the physician.

◆ See Patient Problems: Dry Mouth on p. 166 and Constipation on p. 182.

◆ Warn diabetic patients to monitor blood glucose levels, since these drugs may alter blood glucose, necessitating a change in diet or insulin.

◆ Warm patients to avoid driving or operating hazardous equipment if nervousness, agitation, or other CNS effects are severe; consult the physician.

◆ Except when specifically prescribed for ADD, these drugs should not be used in children. Keep these and all drugs out of their reach.

◆ These drugs should not be used during pregnancy unless specifically prescribed by the obstetrician. Counsel about contraceptives as needed.

◆ Avoid alcoholic beverages unless approved by the physician.

Drugs to Treat Narcolepsy and Attention Deficit Disorder

Drug administration and patient and family education

◆ See general guidelines.

◆ Weigh the patient 2 or 3 times/week until the effects of the drug can be evaluated. Although not being given for the purpose of weight reduction, most of these drugs will suppress the appetite.

◆ Teach parents to keep careful weight and height records of children.

◆ Reinforce to patients that several weeks of therapy may be necessary until full effect of the drug therapy can be evaluated.

◆ Refer the patient and family for appropriate teaching and counseling for narcolepsy and attention deficit disorder.

Drugs to Suppress Appetite

Drug administration and patient and family education

◆ See general guidelines.

◆ Refer patients for appropriate counseling and instruction on weight-reduction diets. Encourage a regular exercise program.

◆ Tell patients that weight reduction will be greatest during the first few weeks of therapy but will slow after that.

◆ Phenylpropanolamine is also discussed in Chapter 26.

◆ Assess for signs of depression when fenfluramine is used including withdrawal, lack of interest in personal appearance, insomnia, and change in affect.

CNS Stimulants to Stimulate Respiration

Drug administration

◆ Anticipate that seizures may occur. Have a suction machine at the bedside. Keep side rails up, and use padding. Do not leave the patient unattended.

◆ Have oxygen and resuscitation equipment available.

◆ Monitor pulse, blood pressure, and respirations. Monitor ECG tracing.

◆ Monitor temperature.

◆ See manufacturer's literature for specific guidelines about administration of doxapram.

◆ Theophylline is discussed in Chapter 25.

◆ These drugs are rarely used outside of the intensive care setting to stimulate respiration.

CHAPTER REVIEW

◆ KEY TERMS

amphetamines, p. 649

analeptics, p. 654

anorexiants, p. 651

attention deficit disorder, p. 649

narcolepsy, p. 648

◆ REVIEW QUESTIONS

1. What is narcolepsy?
2. How is narcolepsy treated?
3. What is attention deficit disorder? What are some possible signs and symptoms of this problem?
4. How is attention deficit disorder treated?
5. What is the mechanism of action of amphetamines in the CNS?
6. What two brain areas are especially affected by amphetamines?
7. What is the route of administration of amphetamines used in clinical medicine?
8. What toxic reactions are common with amphetamines? How should you assess for these?
9. What other drugs interact with amphetamines?
10. What is the route of elimination of methylphenidate?
11. What toxicity is associated with the use of methylphenidate?
12. How does the action of pemoline differ from that of methylphenidate?
13. How does the duration of action of pemoline differ from that of methylphenidate?
14. How long does it take for full therapeutic effects of pemoline to develop?
15. What toxic reactions are associated with pemoline?
16. Why are CNS stimulants used to treat obesity?
17. How do the nonamphetamine appetite suppressants differ from amphetamines?
18. Which nonamphetamine appetite suppressants produce little cardiovascular stimulation?

19. Which appetite suppressant produces CNS depression?
20. Which appetite suppressant is most often found in OTC obesity medications?
21. What toxic reactions may develop during therapy with the nonamphetamine appetite suppressants?
22. What methylxanthines are sometimes used to stimulate respiration?
23. What reactions are observed to the methylxanthines used to stimulate respiration?
24. How is doxapram administered, and what is its duration of action?
25. What toxicity is observed with doxapram?
26. What is the effect of toxic doses of amphetamines in an amphetamine abuser?
27. How does cocaine differ from amphetamine?
28. What are the effects of chronic overdosage with caffeine?

SUGGESTED READING

Bruera E and others: Narcotics plus methylphenidate (Ritalin) for advanced cancer pain, Am J Nurs 88(11):1555, 1988.

Cerrato PL: Caffeine: how much is too much? *RN* 53(1):77, 1990.

Cohen FL: Narcolepsy: a review of a common, life-long sleep disorder, *J Adv Nurs* 13(5):546, 1988.

Gawin FH: Cocaine addiction: psychology and neurophysiology, *Science* 251:1580, 1991.

Hall WC, Talbert RL, Ereshefsky L: Cocaine abuse and its treatment, *Pharmacotherapy* 10(1):47, 1990.

Noble R: A controlled clinical trial of the cardiovascular and psychological effect of phenylpropanolamine and caffeine, *Drug Intell Clin Pharm* 22(4):296, 1988.

Pfeifer RW, Notari RE: Predicting caffeine plasma concentrations resulting from consumption of food or beverages: a simple method and its origin, *Drug Intell Clin Pharm* 22(12):953, 1988.

Richardson JW, Fredrickson PA, Lin S: Narcolepsy update, *Mayo Clin Proc* 65(7): 991, 1990.

Schneider JR: Should patients with myocardial infarction receive caffeinated coffee? *Focus Crit Care* 15(1):52, 1988.

Smitherman CH: A drug to ease attention deficit-hyperactivity disorder, *MCN* 15(6):362, 1990.

Vandegaer F: Cocaine—the deadliest addiction, *Nurs 89* 19(2):72, 1989.

SECTION X

Drugs to Control Severe Pain or to Produce Anesthesia

Section X discusses drugs that relieve severe acute pain. These drugs have made modern surgery possible. Chapter 44, Narcotic Analgesics (Opioids), focuses on the analgesic uses of opioids for surgery and other conditions in which pain must be controlled. Research has uncovered how opioids mimic natural compounds in the body. Since opioids are a major drug class for illicit use, attention is given to the features of opioid dependence, the role of the specific opioid antagonist naloxone in treating acute opioid overdose, and the role of the long-acting opioid methadone in treating opioid withdrawal. Chapter 45, General Anesthetics, discusses inhalation and intravenous (IV) anesthetics, and combinations of drugs now widely used for balanced anesthesia. Limitations and desirable characteristics of each anesthetic are described. Chapter 46, Local Anesthetics, reviews the surface use of local anesthetics and their use by injection for major surgery.

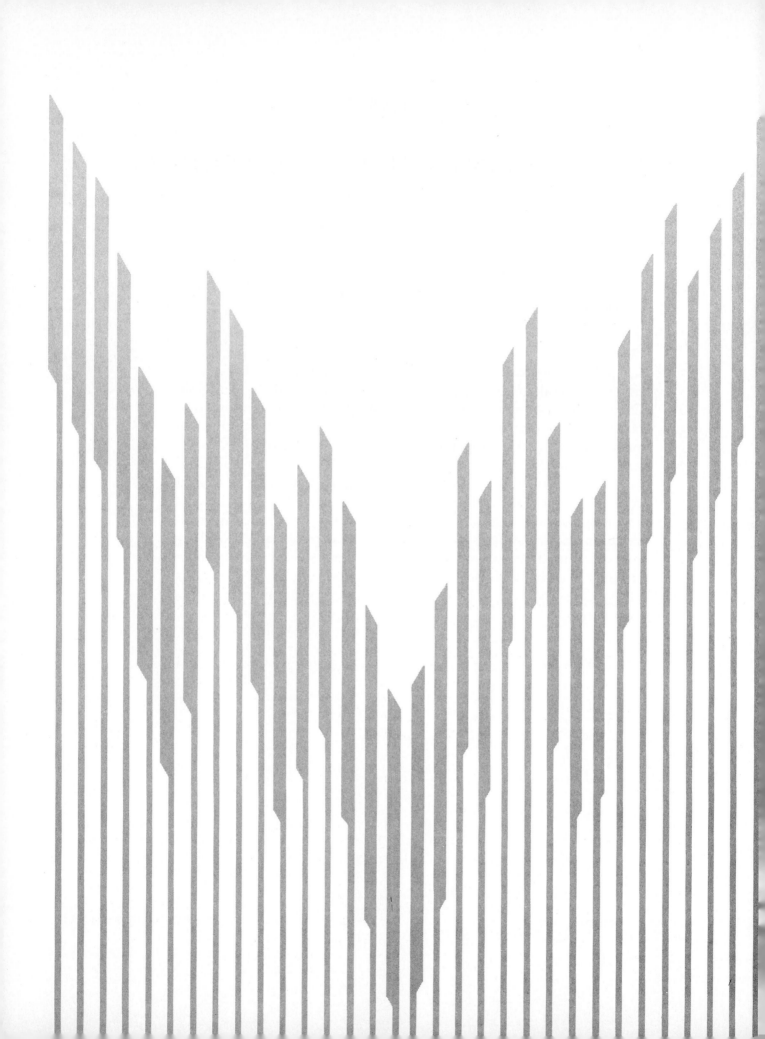

CHAPTER 44

Narcotic Analgesics (Opioids)

LEARNING OBJECTIVES
After studying this chapter, you should be able to do the following:

◆ Explain the action of morphine in the central nervous system and the periphery.

◆ Describe the role of endogenous opioid peptides and the four types of opioid receptors in providing pain relief.

◆ Discuss tolerance and dependence with opioids.

◆ Describe symptoms and treatment of acute opioid toxicity.

◆ Develop a nursing care plan for the patient receiving a narcotic analgesic.

CHAPTER OVERVIEW

◆ Analgesics are drugs that relieve pain. Nonnarcotic analgesics are covered in Chapter 23. This chapter presents the narcotic analgesics (opioids). The nature of pain and its treatment with opioids are described. The pharmacology of morphine, the prototype for the opioids, is reviewed, followed by a discussion of the specific characteristics of clinically used opioids and the narcotic antagonists. The chapter concludes with an examination of the nature and treatment of opioid tolerance and dependence.

Nursing Process Overview

OPIOIDS

Assessment

Assess history, nature, and location of pain. Include objective data on patient's position, facial expression, medical history, vital signs, and age. Perform a brief neurologic examination. Pay close attention to the subjective complaints of pain.

Nursing Diagnoses

Altered bowel elimination: constipation as drug side effect

Altered comfort: nausea and vomiting as drug side effect

Altered thought processes related to drug side effect

Management

Regular use of opioids at identified intervals usually provides better relief of pain than use on a p.r.n. (as needed) basis. No patient who needs medication for pain should be denied it, but augment medication use with nursing care measures to promote comfort, including positioning, distracting, and touching the patient, as well as introducing relaxation techniques. Monitor vital signs, level of consciousness, and frequency of bowel movements; check for nausea and vomiting and urinary retention. Some side effects necessitate discontinuing therapy, decreasing the dose, or using additional kinds of treatments. Have narcotic antagonists available. If antiemetics or other drugs are ordered, monitor side effects; also check compatibilities before administering two or more drugs in the same syringe. Use a microdrip administration set and an infusion monitoring device for constant IV infusion.

Evaluation

Before discharge, verify that patients can explain the name and dose of drugs to be taken, the possible side effects and how to treat them, the signs indicating too large a dose, what to do if the pain worsens, and what drugs to avoid. Determine that patients know to avoid alcohol while these drugs are being taken.

PAIN AND THE USE OF NARCOTIC ANALGESICS

History of Narcotic Analgesics

Analgesics are drugs that relieve pain. Opium has been used to produce analgesia and euphoria throughout history. The word *opium* comes from the Greek *opion,* meaning poppy juice, and the source of morphine today is still the sticky brown gum (opium) collected from the seed pod of *Papaver somniferum,* a variety of poppy. About 10% of the content of opium is morphine. Codeine can also be extracted from opium, although in such small amounts that most medicinal codeine is derived by chemically modifying morphine. Morphine was isolated in 1803 by a German pharmacist and named after Morpheus, the Greek god of sleep. Morphine was the first pure chemical substance that mimicked the pharmacologic effects of the natural product after extraction from the natural product.

Drug dependence as a property of morphine was not realized in the Unites States until the Civil War, when morphine was widely used to treat wounded soldiers, whose addiction subsequently became a significant social problem. Opium and morphine were readily available and were often ingredients of patent medicines. By the late 1800s, attempts were made to modify the structure of morphine to keep the analgesic property but eliminate the addictive potential. The first semisynthetic drug was heroin, but heroin produces drug dependence more readily than morphine. Today, heroin is not a legal drug in the United States or Canada, although it is in other countries. Most narcotic analgesics come under the Controlled Substances Act (United States) or are listed as controlled substances (schedule G) under the Canadian Food and Drugs Act (see Chapter 2).

Morphine is the prototype for the narcotic analgesics, a class of drugs more properly called the **opioids.** Some narcotic analgesics are chemical modifications of morphine. The first purely synthetic morphinelike compound was meperidine (Demerol), which came into clinical use in the 1940s. Because meperidine was not a chemical modification of morphine, widespread belief held that meperidine did not cause drug dependence. Today, meperidine is considered a drug with high abuse potential (schedule II) similar to morphine. The most recent examples of opioids whose abuse potential was not originally recognized are pentazocine (Talwin) and propoxyphene (Darvon), which are now classified as drugs of low abuse potential (schedule IV). The characteristics of opioid dependence and its treatment are discussed later in this chapter.

Overview of Pain

Pain is classified into two major components. Objective pain represents the stimulation of peripheral nerve endings when tissue is damaged. Nonnarcotic analgesics such as aspirin and acetaminophen (Nuprin and Tylenol) act by inhibiting the synthesis of local mediators, the prostaglandins, that are released in damaged tissue to stimulate the nerve endings. In the presence of nonnarcotic analgesics, pain is not felt because the nerves are not stimulated, and the pain message therefore is never delivered to the CNS. Nonnarcotic analgesics are discussed in Chapter 23. Subjective pain represents how a person reacts to pain, usually with fear, anxiety, and withdrawal. The subjective level of pain involves the spinal cord and brain, which collect and process the painful stimuli. The narcotic analgesics blunt this subjective pain, allowing the individual to tolerate pain. With high doses, individuals become unaware of pain and become indifferent to all unpleasant stimuli.

Acute Pain

The major use of opioids is for the short-term treatment of severe, acute pain such as that associated with trauma, surgery, or burns. Opioids are commonly classified by the level of pain they can relieve: severe, severe-to-moderate, and mild pain (Table 44-1). These are not specifically defined categories, however.

The pain of some specific conditions is effectively treated with opioids. These conditions include myocardial infarction, pulmonary edema, labor, preanesthesia and postanesthesia, and sickle-cell crisis. Under some circumstances, pain associated with gastrointestinal (GI) and urinary tract disorders may be treated with an opioid.

In treating actue pain, opioids are administered in sufficient doses to relive pain and at intervals frequent enough to prevent the recurrence of pain. Each patient must be evaluated frequently to determine the need for dosage adjustment. There is little danger of producing drug addiction in treating acute pain because psychologic dependence on opioids is unlikely under most medical circumstances. Most patients are able to discontinue medication with little difficulty. A more common problem is the undermedication of patients in acute pain by health-care providers unduly concerned about causing addiction. The usual 10-mg dose of morphine produces effective analgesia in only two thirds of patients.

Chronic Pain

Opioids treat the chronic pain associated with cancer. Special care must be used to keep the dose as low as possible to prolong the effectiveness of the drug and to keep the patient alert. Nonmedical aspects of pa-

Table 44-1 Comparison of Narcotic Analgesics

Level of pain	Drug	Equivalent analgesic dose (mg) given IM or SC	Time for peak effect (min)	Duration (hr)	Schedule U.S.	Schedule Canada
Severe	Morphine	10	30 to 90	3 to 7	II	N
	Buprenorphine (Buprenex)	0.5	15	4 to 6	V	†
	Dezocine (Dalgan)	10	60 to 120	3 to 6	*	†
	Hydromorphone hydrochloride (Dilaudid)	1.5	30 to 90	4 to 5	II	N
	Levorphanol tartrate (Levo-Dromoran)	2 to 3	60 to 90	5 to 8	II	N
	Methadone (Dolophine)	7.5 to 10	60 to 120	3 to 6	II	N
	Oxymorphone (Numorphan)	1 to 1.5	30 to 90	3 to 6	II	N
Moderate-to-severe	Butorphanol (Stadol)	1.5 to 3.5	30	3 to 4	*	C
	Meperidine (Demerol)	75 to 100	30 to 60	2 to 4	II	N
	Nalbuphine (Nubain)	10	30	3 to 6	*	C
	Oxycodone (Roxicodone)	15	60	3 to 4	II	N
	Pentazocine (Talwin)	40 to 60	30 to 60	2 to 3	IV	N
Mild-to-moderate	Codeine phosphate	120	60 to 90	4 to 6	II	N
	Propoxyphene (Darvon)	180 to 240	60	4 to 6	IV	N

*Not scheduled as a controlled substance.
†Not available.

tient comfort should be considered, including physical, social, mental, and spiritual measures. Often, aspirin, acetaminophen, or nonsteroidal antiinflammatory drugs (NSAIDs) are effective analgesics. The treatment of chronic pain associated with cancer requires an individualized regimen that should be evaluated frequently. If opioids are used, increasing the dosage is usually preferable to increasing the frequency of administration. Since cross-tolerance of opioids is limited, a different opioid may be tried if the one being used must be discontinued because of adverse effects with increased dose.

Anesthesia
Additional uses of opioids include preanesthetic medication and surgical anesthesia. As preanesthetic medication, opioids relieve anxiety and provide sedation so that the patient is not in a fearful state before surgery. More potent analgesics—morphine, meperidine, fentanyl, and hydromorphone—are widely used as components of surgical anesthesia with nitrous oxide. Nitrous oxide by itself is not potent enough for surgical anesthesia but is potentiated by a narcotic analgesic. A muscle relaxant such as tubocurarine is also used. This combination of opioid, nitrous oxide, and muscle relaxant is called *balanced anesthesia* (see Chapter 45). Duration of anesthesia is controlled by the duration of action of the opioid used.

PHARMACOLOGY OF OPIOIDS
The pharmacology of morphine provides the standard for describing and comparing the actions of all opioids.

Biochemical Basis of Opioid Actions
In the early 1970s, scientists demonstrated that specific receptors for opioids exist in the brain, spinal

cord, and gut. These receptors did not recognize any of the known neurotransmitters. This suggested that a previously unknown, naturally occurring substance exists in the brain, spinal cord, and gut that is mimicked by morphine. Such compounds have now been found. So far, three classes of naturally occurring neuropeptides have been characterized. These are **endorphins, enkephalins,** and **dynorphins.**

Beta endorphin is a large peptide derived from the prohormone for adrenocorticotropic hormone (ACTH) and is found in the pituitary gland. The dynorphins are also peptides derived from a larger peptide and found in the pituitary. The enkephalins are pentapeptides (five amino acids) and seem to be neurotransmitters associated with (1) mediation of pain and analgesia; (2) release of growth hormone, prolactin, and vasopressin from the pituitary; (3) modulation of locomotor activity; (4) regulation of mood; and (5) regulation of gut motility.

Four types of opioid receptors have been characterized. The μ (mu) receptor mediates central analgesia, euphoria, respiratory depression, and physical dependence. The μ receptor is associated with classic morphine effects and with endorphins. The κ (kappa) receptor mediates spinal analgesia, miosis, sedation, and appetite regulation. The receptor appears sensitive to opioids with mixed agonist-antagonist activity and to the naturally occurring dynorphins. The δ (delta) receptor is thought to be the primary receptor for the enkephalins and endorphins. The σ (sigma) receptor mediates the dysphoric, hallucinogenic, and cardiac-stimulant effects. The σ receptor appears sensitive to opioid-antagonist activity. The σ receptor may also respond to nonopioid agents such as the hallucinogen phencyclidine. Other opioid receptor types have also been postulated.

These recent discoveries should clarify the nature of analgesia and the development of the opioid type of drug dependence and provide the basis for understanding the role of these opioid peptides in mental disorders, seizure activity, and behavior patterns involving the reward system, eating, and drinking.

With the characterization of opioid receptors, it is clear that opioids such as pentazocine and nalbuphine, which have the least dependence potential, not only have agonistic properties (mimicking effects) but also antagonistic properties (blocking effects). The search for a nonaddicting opioid may depend on finding the drug that has the right combination of agonist-antagonist properties without causing unpleasant side effects.

Actions in the Central Nervous System

Many effects of morphine occur in the central nervous system (CNS).

Analgesia

The analgesia produced by morphine has three characteristics. Morphine raises the threshold for pain perception, making patients less aware of pain. It also reduces anxiety and fear, the emotional reactions to pain. Finally, morphine induces sleep, even in the presence of severe pain.

The biochemical mechanism of pain relief by the opioids is their ability to mimic endogenous compounds, the endorphins, which act at many sites in the brain to modify the perception of and reaction to pain. Support for this concept has come from studies of naloxone (Narcan), which is a specific opioid antagonist. Naloxone blocks the placebo response and reduces the effectiveness of acupuncture anesthesia, processes believed to reflect the activity of endorphins. The interpretation of these effects of naloxone is that naloxone blocks the effect of endorphins, which are released in response to pain to minimize its perception. These studies also provide a biochemical explanation for the effectiveness of the acupuncture technique to reduce pain.

Medullary actions

Morphine affects several medullary centers. The most important is the **respiratory center** which becomes less sensitive to carbon dioxide in the presence of morphine. Tolerance develops to this effect so that individuals who abuse one of the opioids can tolerate doses of opioids that would cause fatal respiratory depression in nondependent individuals. Death from an opioid overdose is frequently caused by respiratory arrest; the victim stops breathing. Similarly, the most important drug interactions with morphine are those arising from a synergistic depression of the respiratory center such as with any of the sedative-hypnotic drugs, antianxiety agents, alcohol, general anesthetics, or phenothiazines. Tolerance does not develop to the respiratory depression produced by these latter drug classes. An individual abusing an opioid and a drug of another class such as alcohol or one of the other sedative-hypnotic drugs can readily succumb to drug-induced respiratory depression.

The **cough center** is the second medullary center depressed by morphine. Morphine seldom is prescribed as a cough suppressant, as is a related drug such as codeine. Cough suppressants (antitussive drugs) are described in Chapter 26. The **chemoreceptor trigger zone** is the third major medullary center affected by morphine. Morphine stimulates this center to produce nausea and vomiting. This is a transient effect, so repeated doses do not usually cause nausea and vomiting. Individuals vary in their sensitivity to this emetic action.

Behavior

The effect of morphine on behavior depends on the mental state of the individual. Euphoria may be experienced if the individual has been in pain or has been fearful and anxious. Therapeutic doses produce minimum sedation, but larger doses cause drowsiness, sleep, or in large doses, coma. A few individuals become excited rather than depressed.

Actions in the Periphery

Gastrointestinal system

Morphine has a profound depressant effect on the GI tract; constipation is a common side effect of morphine administration. Although morphine is not used to treat nonspecific diarrhea, related drugs such as codeine or diphenoxylate are. The common medicinal use of opium historically was to stop diarrhea.

Gastric, biliary, and pancreatic secretions are inhibited by morphine. It treats the pain associated with biliary colic but may exacerbate rather than relieve the pain in some patients, since the biliary tract may go into painful spasms in the presence of morphine.

Urinary retention

Urinary retention is another side effect of morphine. Morphine stimulates the release of vasopressin (an antidiuretic hormone), so more water is absorbed in the kidney tubules, decreasing urine volume. The drug also reduces perception of the need to void.

Cardiovascular effects

Morphine commonly causes hypotension. This may be a result of depression of the vasomotor center in the medulla. In addition, morphine causes histamine release, and histamine is a potent vasodilator. The concurrent administration of a phenothiazine or atropine can intensify the hypotension. In large doses, morphine slows the heart rate.

Ocular effect

A classic effect of morphine is to reduce pupillary size. A pinpoint pupil is one characteristic of a narcotic overdose. However, if the victim is near death, hypoxia causes the release of epinephrine, which dilates the pupil.

Adverse Reactions and Contraindications to Opioids

The common adverse reactions of morphine and the other opioids are those predicted by the pharmacologic actions of morphine, including nausea and vomiting, constipation, urinary retention, itching, and hypotension resulting from histamine release.

Some actions characteristic of morphine are undesirable in certain patients, including the respiratory depression caused by opioids. Patients with impaired respiratory function may be severely compromised by an opioid because their respiratory drive is already impaired. Although in general the opioids relax bronchial smooth muscle, a few patients with asthma experience severe bronchoconstriction and die. These drugs also pass into the milk of a nursing mother and affect the infant.

Patients suffering from a head injury should not be given an opioid, since the decreased respiration increases carbon dioxide retention and carbon dioxide dilates the intracranial blood vessels, worsening the situation. Also, sedative and behavioral effects obscure evaluation of the CNS.

Since opioids can cause hypotension, they must be used cautiously in patients suffering from shock or blood loss, conditions worsened by a hypotensive action.

Acute toxicity

Respiratory depression is the usual cause of death from an acute overdose of an opioid. An overdose is likely to occur in an individual who buys drugs for abuse on the street. Street drugs have unknown purity and concentration, so occasionally drug content is higher than anticipated.

The overdosed individual is stuporous or in a deep sleep and initially is warm, with flushed, wet skin. The next stage is coma, in which respiration is depressed, and as the individual becomes hypoxic (starved for oxygen), the skin becomes cold, clammy, and mottled, and the pupils dilate. Death is then imminent.

CLINICAL USE OF OPIOIDS

The narcotic analgesics currently in use are compared in regards to efficacy, dose, onset, and duration of action in Table 44-1. In addition to these drugs, alfentanil (Alfenta), fentanyl (Sublimaze), and sufentanil (Sufenta) are short-acting narcotic analgesics used primarily in anesthesia.

The major use of the opioids is for the relief of moderate-to-severe pain. These drugs are most effective in relieving the constant dull pain associated with trauma, surgery, heart attack, biliary or ureteral colic, inflammation, or cancer. Isolated, sharp pain is not as effectively relieved by opioids.

Opioids Effective for Relieving Severe Pain

These drugs are presented in Table 44-2.

Morphine

Morphine has already been described as the prototype for the opioids. Chemically, morphine is a base that is positively charged at the pH in the GI tract and

Table 44-2   Narcotic Analgesics

Generic name	Trade name	Administration/dosage	Comments
Buprenorphine hydrochloride	Buprenex	INTRAMUSCULAR: *Adults*—0.3 to 0.6 mg, repeat every 6 to 8 hr as required.	Possesses agonist and antagonist properties. Schedule V substance.
Butorphanol tartrate	Stadol*	INTRAMUSCULAR: *Adults*—1 to 4 mg every 3 to 4 hr. INTRAVENOUS: *Adults*—0.5 to 2 mg every 3 to 4 hr.	Possesses agonist and antagonist properties. Not a scheduled drug.
Codeine sulfate, codeine phosphate		ORAL, INTRAMUSCULAR, SUBCUTANEOUS: *Adults*—30 to 60 mg every 4 to 6 hr. FDA Pregnancy Category C. *Children*—0.5 mg/kg body weight every 4 to 6 hr.	Schedule II substance.
Dezocine	Dalgan	INTRAMUSCULAR, *Adults*—5 to 20 mg every 3 to 6 hr as needed. Maximum daily dose: 120 mg. INTRAVENOUS: *Adults*—2.5 to 10 mg every 2 to 4 hr.	New opoioid with agonist and antagonist properties. Not a scheduled drug.
Hydromorphone hydrochloride	Dilaudid*	ORAL: *Adults*—2 mg every 4 to 6 hr. FDA Pregnancy Category C. INTRAMUSCULAR, SUBCUTANEOUS: *Adults*—1 to 1.5 mg every 4 to 6 hr. May be given by slow IV injection or as a suppository.	Schedule II substance.
Levorphanol tartrate	Levo-Dromoran*	ORAL, SUBCUTANEOUS: *Adults*—2 mg.	Schedule II substance.
Meperidine hydrochloride	Demerol*	ORAL, INTRAMUSCULAR, SUBCUTANEOUS, SLOW INTRAVENOUS: *Adults*—50 to 150 mg every 3 to 4 hr. *Children*—1 to 1.5 mg/kg body weight, maximum 100 mg, every 3 to 4 hr.	Schedule II substance.
Methadone hydrochloride	Dolophine	ORAL, INTRAMUSCULAR, SUBCUTANEOUS: *Adults*—2.5 to 10 mg. For pain relief, repeat every 6 hr.	Used as a replacement drug for opiate dependence or to facilitate withdrawal. Schedule II substance.
Morphine sulfate		ORAL: *Adults*—5 to 15 mg every 4 hr. FDA Pregnancy Category C. INTRAMUSCULAR, SUBCUTANEOUS: *Adults*—5 to 20 mg every 4 hr. *Children* (subcutaneous only)—0.1 to 0.2 mg/kg body weight, maximum 15 mg. INTRAVENOUS: *Adults*—2.5 to 15 mg in 5 ml water, injected over 4 to 5 min. *Children*—0.1 to 0.2 mg/kg.	Not well absorbed orally. Schedule II substance.
Nalbuphine hydrochloride	Nubain*	INTRAMUSCULAR, SUBCUTANEOUS, INTRAVENOUS: *Adults*—10 mg every 3 to 6 hr, maximum single dose 20 mg, and maximum daily dose 160 mg.	Possesses agonist and antagonist properties. Not a scheduled drug.
Oxycodone	Roxicodone Supeudol†	ORAL, *Adults*—5 mg every 3 to 6 hr or 10 mg 3 or 4 times a day as needed. May be increased for severe pain.	Schedule II substance.

*Available in Canada and United States.
†Available in Canada only.

Table 44-2   Narcotic Analgesics—cont'd

Generic name	Trade name	Administration/dosage	Comments
Oxymorphone hydrochloride	Numorphan*	INTRAMUSCULAR, SUBCUTANEOUS: *Adults*—1 to 1.5 mg every 6 hr. INTRAVENOUS: *Adults*—0.5 mg. RECTAL: *Adults*—5 mg every 4 to 6 hr.	Schedule II substance.
Pentazocine hydrochloride	Talwin 50*	ORAL: *Adults*—50 mg every 3 to 4 hr, maximum daily dose 600 mg.	Possesses agonist and antagonist properties. Schedule IV substance.
Pentazocine lactate	Talwin Lactate*	INTRAMUSCULAR, SUBCUTANEOUS, INTRAVENOUS: *Adults*—30 mg every 3 to 4 hr. Subcutaneous route is not recommended, since tissue damage may occur.	
Propoxyphene hydrochloride	Darvon Dolene Novopro-poxen†	ORAL: *Adults*—65 mg every 6 to 8 hr.	Schedule IV substance.
Propoxyphene napsylate	Darvon-N*	ORAL: *Adults*—100 mg every 6 to 8 hr.	Schedule IV substance.

*Available in Canada and United States.
†Available in Canada only.

therefore is not readily abosrbed when taken orally. Since it is readily metabolized within the gut and by the liver, morphine is given by intramuscular (IM) or subcutaneous routes. Elderly patients usually require a smaller dose because they do not metabolize morphine as readily as do younger patients.

Morphine or meperidine treats the pain of an acute myocardial infarction. At analgesic doses, morphine not only relieves the pain but also reduces the anxiety without altering the cardiovascular system. If undue reduction in respiration, heart rate, or blood pressure occurs secondary to morphine administration, it can be reversed by administering naloxone, the narcotic antagonist.

Morphine is the drug of choice in pulmonary edema. The beneficial actions of morphine include relief of anxiety and vasodilation, which reduces the workload of the heart so that it pumps more efficiently. This increased cardiac efficiency relieves the pulmonary edema that arises when the left side of the heart cannot adequately pump the blood being supplied by the pulmonary veins. This inefficiency gives rise to hypertension and edema in the pulmonary system.

Dezocine

Dezocine (Dalgan) is a new, chemically different opioid that relieves pain as effectively as morphine. It is administered by IM or IV routes. Dezocine does not seem to have the dysphoria side effects characteristic of pentazocine. Dezocine does not adversely affect cardiac performance. At higher doses, respiratory depression is not as severe as with morphine.

Hydromorphone

Hydromorphone (Dilaudid) is a semisynthetic derivative of morphine. It is more potent but shorter acting than morphine. Oral doses require more time to become effective but are longer acting than parenteral doses. The actions of hydromorphone are identical to those of morphine.

Oxymorphone

Oxymorphone (Numorphan) is a semisynthetic derivative of morphine that has all the actions of morphine except the antitussive action. Oxymorphone is more potent than morphine but must also be given by injection.

Levorphanol

Levorphanol (Levo-Dromoran) is an opioid that has actions identical to those of morphine. The effective dose is about a fourth that of morphine.

Methadone

Methadone (Dolophine) is an opioid with actions similar to those of morphine. Methadone can be taken orally. Although the onset of action for a single analgesic dose is similar to that for morphine, methadone is highly protein bound and is not readily metabolized. Methadone has a half-life of 25 hr.

Methadone, 40 to 120 mg daily, substitutes for other opioids in drug-dependent individuals and prevents withdrawl symptoms. Methadone currently is used in the treatment of opioid dependence because it is effective orally and only one dose/day is necessary. Also, the long plasma half-life more easily allows the gradual reduction in dose without side effects.

Opioids Effective in Relieving Moderate-to-Severe Pain

These drugs are presented in Table 44-2.

Buprenorphine

Buprenorphine (Buprenex) is an opioid with agonist and antagonist properties. Its abuse potential appears low; it is a schedule V drug in the United States. It is administered intramuscularly. The onset of action is 15 min, and the duration of action is about 6 hr. Buprenorphine is effective for moderate-to-severe pain associated with surgery, cancer, neuralgias, labor, renal colic, or myocardial infarction.

Butorphanol

Butorphanol (Stadol) has agonist and antagonist properties. Its abuse potential appears low, and it is not a scheduled drug in the United States. Administered intramuscularly, butorphanol has an onset of action of 10 to 30 min with a duration of action of about 4 hr. In general, its actions resemble those of morphine, except that butorphanol increases pulmonary arterial pressure and the cardiac workload, making it undesirable for treating the pain of a myocardial infarction.

Hydrocodone

Hydrocodone (Hycodan and Robidone) is a semisynthetic derivative of morphine. In Canada, it is available as a syrup for cough suppression and in tablet form for analgesia or cough suppression. In the United States, hydrocodone is commercially available only in combination with aspirin or acetaminophen.

Meperidine

Meperidine (Demerol) was the first of the synthetic narcotic analgesics. It is shorter acting than morphine and does not have an antitussive effect. Meperidine is widely used for obstetric analgesia. Meperidine is also available in the Unites States as a combination product with acetaminophen.

Nalbuphine

Nalbuphine (Nubain) is a semisynthetic derivative of morphine that has agonist and antagonist properties. The uses and limitations of nalbuphine are primarily those of mederidine or morphine. Nalbuphine may be preferable for treating the pain of a myocardial infarction, since it appears to reduce the oxygen needs of the heart without reducing blood pressure. Nalbuphine is a stronger antagonist than pentazocine, suggesting that the degree of tolerance and drug dependence should be low. However, withdrawal symptoms are seen when nalbuphine is abruptly discontinued, and it causes withdrawal symptoms when administered to an individual already dependent on one of the more common narcotic analgesics.

Oxycodone

Oxycodone (Roxicodone) is a semisynthetic derivative of morphine. It is taken orally. Oxycodone has an onset of action in 10 to 15 min and a duration of action of 3 to 6 hr. In the United States and Canada, oxycodone is also available as a combination product with aspirin or acetaminophen.

Pentazocine

Pentazocine (Talwin) is an opioid with weak antagonist properties. For several years after pentazocine was introduced, it was believed not to produce drug dependence. Pentazocine is now a schedule IV drug, reflecting a low potential for producing drug dependence. Pentazocine causes respiratory depression in the fetus. Unlike morphine, pentazocine increases blood pressure and cardiac work, making it less desirable than morphine for treating the pain of myocardial infarction or pulmonary hypertension. Pentazocine causes dysphoria rather than euphoria. Dysphoria can include nightmares, feelings of depersonalization, and visual hallucinations. Large doses induce seizures. Although there are reports of individuals with drug dependence for pentazocine, its administration to a person dependent on the other narcotic analgesics results in withdrawal symptoms because of its antagonistic properties. In the United States, pentazocine is also available as a combination product with aspirin or acetaminophen.

Opioids Effective in Relieving Mild Pain

These drugs are presented in Table 44-2.

Codeine

Codeine is not administered in doses large enough to be as effective as morphine, since the high dose required to produce an equal degree of analgesia results in a high incidence of side effects. An oral dose of 32 or 65 mg of codeine is equivalent to 2 aspirin tablets (650 mg). At these low doses, codeine seldom produces side effects. At high doses the side effects of codeine are similar to those of morphine. In the United States and Canada, codeine is available as a combination product with acetaminophen or aspirin.

Since codeine causes significant histamine release if given intravenously, codeine is given only intramuscularly or orally. A portion of codeine dose is metabolized to morphine in the liver. Codeine is a schedule II drug is analgesic doses. It is also formulated with the nonnarcotic analgesics for pain relief, and these are usually schedule III drugs. Codeine is an effective cough suppressant at low doses, and it is available for this purpose in dilute solutions as a schedule V drug.

Propoxyphene

Propoxyphene (Darvon), an opioid related to methadone, is not a very potent analgesic. Propoxyphene at a dose of 65 mg is the analgesic equivalent of 2 tablets (650 mg) of aspirin or acetaminophen. Propoxyphene is commonly prescribed in combination with one of the nonnarcotic analgesics. Alone or in combination, propoxyphene is a schedule IV drug. Side effects are not common at analgesic doses. Propoxyphene has low abuse potential but has been implicated as a cause of death when abused in combination with alcohol and other CNS depressant drugs. In the United States, propoxyphene is available as a combination product with acetaminophen or aspirin. In Canada a combination product with aspirin is available.

Narcotic Antagonists

Narcotic antagonists produce few effects when used by themselves under usual circumstances. Their clinical use is to treat an opioid overdose. These narcotic antagonists are presented in Table 44-3.

Naloxone

Naloxone (Narcan) is a pure antagonist for the opioid receptor, making it especially useful in the emergency room. When a comatose patient is brought to the emergency room because of a drug overdose, the first goal is to support respiration and the second is to determine which drug was used. If an opioid is suspected, a specific test is used. Naloxone is administered intravenously, and if the overdose is a result of an opioid, the patient will respond in 2 to 3 min with improved respiration and will return to consciousness. Naloxone displaces the opioid from the receptor but produces no effect of its own. The result is a dramatic reversal of the drug overdose. The patient must still be monitored carefully, however, because naloxone has a short duration of action and its effect may wear off before the overdosed drug has been sufficiently eliminated. If the patient again becomes comatose, naloxone must be given again.

Multiple drug abuse is common, and naloxone only reverses the depression resulting from the narcotic analgesic. It has no effect when the overdose is not caused by a narcotic analgesic.

Naltrexone

Naltrexone (Trexan) is an opioid antagonist. It has little pharmacologic activity but reverses opioid ac-

Table 44-3 Narcotic Antagonists

Generic name	Trade name	Administration/dosage	Comments
Naloxone hydrochloride	Narcan*	INTRAVENOUS, INTRAMUSCULAR, SUBCUTANEOUS: *Adults*—0.4 mg for respiratory depression caused by narcotic overdose. Repeated in a few minutes if necessary, up to 3 doses. For narcotic depression of respiration after surgery: 0.1 to 0.2 mg every few minutes as necessary. FDA Pregnancy Category B. INTRAVENOUS: *Neonates*—0.01 mg/kg body weight.	Pure narcotic antagonist used to reverse respiratory depression from narcotic overdose. Unlike levallorphan, naloxone produces no respiratory depression of its own.
Naltrexone	Trexan	ORAL: *Adults*—initial dose 25 mg. If there are no symptoms of withdrawal, the rest of the daily dose may be given. The usual daily dose is 50 mg, but it may also be administered as 100 mg every other day or 150 mg every third day. FDA Pregnancy Category C.	Adjunctive therapy for drug rehabilitation from opioids. Patients should have completed a withdrawal program and should be free of opioids for 7 to 10 days.

*Available in Canada and United States.

tivity. Naltrexone is orally effective and long acting. It is prescribed for individuals detoxified of opioids. Since naltrexone blocks the effects of opioids, it is used in behavioral therapy to discourage resumption of opioid use. Naltrexone precipitates withdrawal symptoms when administered to an individual addicted to opioids.

OPIOID TOLERANCE AND DEPENDENCE

Drug Tolerance

Drug tolerance occurs when repeated use of a drug results in a lesser response unless the dose is raised. Tolerance develops rapidly to the euphoric effect of the opioids. Individuals abusing narcotic analgesics keep raising the dose to maintain the good feeling associated with the drug. Patients receiving an opioid for severe pain over a limited period may also develop tolerance. Patients are unlikely to become drug dependent because as the pain subsides, so will the need and use of the drug. Tapering the dose of the drug is usually sufficient for a patient to discontinue opioid therapy. However, individuals abusing an opioid to achieve its euphoric effect increase the dose and become drug dependent rapidly. Daily use of one of the opioids can produce drug dependence in 3 weeks. Little or no tolerance develops to the pupillary constriction or to the constipating effect of the opioids.

Drug Dependence

Drug dependence has complex psychologic and social components. In addition to the physical dependence produced by drug tolerance, there is a psychic dependence characterized by a continued desire or craving for the drug. Detoxification of addicted individuals is rarely sufficient to prevent relapse. Medications such as methadone may help in a drug rehabilitation program, but educational and psychosocial interventions are also needed (see box).

Symptoms of withdrawal syndrome

Drug-dependent persons experience distinct physical reactions if the drug is suddenly discontinued. Opioid withdrawal syndrome after the sudden cessation of morphine or heroin use is predictable. The individual has a runny nose (rhinorrhea), gooseflesh (piloerection), tearing (lacrimation), sweating, and yawning 16 hrs after the last dose. The pupils do not react readily to light. Over the next 20 hrs the individual becomes restless, cannot sleep, and experiences muscle twitching. Hot and cold flashes and abdominal cramping occur. By 36 hrs the individual feels nauseous, vomits, and has diarrhea. Withdrawal symptoms are generally the reverse of the drug effects described for the opioids. The body overcompensates when the drug is removed.

DRUG ABUSE ALERT: HEROIN AND OTHER OPIOIDS

BACKGROUND

Heroin and other opioids are abused to achieve euphoria. Heroin is injected intravenously.

PHARMACOLOGY

Heroin is an illegal opioid in the United States and Canada. Side effects include restlessness, vomiting, and drowsiness.

HEALTH HAZARDS

Heroin causes a high degree of physical and psychologic dependence. An overdose produces slow, shallow breathing, clammy skin, convulsions, and coma. Death can result. Withdrawal symptoms include nausea, cramps, chills and sweating, panic, tremors, irritability, and loss of appetite. Repeated injections may lead to infection of heart tissues, skin abscesses, and congested lungs.

Because of needle and syringe sharing, IV drug abuse is associated with a high incidence of transmission of human immunodeficiency virus (HIV) and has become a major risk factor for acquiring acquired immunodeficiency syndrome (AIDS).

Clonidine for withdrawal treatment

Clonidine is an antihypertensive drug that activates central alpha-2 adrenergic receptors (see Chapter 15). This activity reduces sympathetic overactivity. Because of this reduction in centrally mediated sympathetic activity, clonidine is useful in treating opioid withdrawal symptoms, reducing symptoms without producing a withdrawal syndrome.

Methadone for maintenance and detoxification

In the United States the most widely used treatment for addiction to opioids is to substitute methadone, which can be given orally in a daily dose. Since tolerance already has developed to the "kick" from heroin in these individuals, the methadone maintains this tolerance while protecting against withdrawal symptoms. The goal of maintenance is to discourage the individual from continuing to seek drugs and to participate instead in rehabilitation programs. If detoxification (elimination of drug) is the goal, methadone is administered first when withdrawal symptoms appear, and then the dose of methadone gradually is reduced to zero over 1 to 3 weeks. Because methadone has a long half-life in the body, the withdrawal symptoms are not as severe as with morphine or heroin.

NURSING IMPLICATIONS SUMMARY

Narcotic Analgesics

Drug administration

◆ Analgesics, especially narcotic analgesics, constitute one of the most useful classes of medications, since they permit individuals to tolerate short- and long-term pain and thus tolerate surgery and trauma and perhaps to face death more peacefully. Failure of the health care team members to be knowledgable about adequate drug doses, frequency of drug administration, and choice of appropriate medication results in patients receiving inadequate treatment for pain.

◆ Assess patients thoughtfully before administering pain medication. If the decision is made to use a narcotic analgesic, use adequate doses, and administer frequently enough to maintain a therapeutic blood level of medication. Administer medications 30 to 60 min before painful activities such as dressing changes, physical therapy, or whirlpool.

◆ Although narcotic analgesics are useful, they should be used as adjuncts to other nursing measures such as massage, distraction, deep breathing and relaxation exercises, application of heat or cold, or just being there to provide care and comfort. Include effective nursing measures in the care plan, and keep the care plan updated.

◆ Monitor respiratory rate as an indicator of CNS depression. If the rate is less than 12 breaths/min in an adult, withhold additional doses unless ventilatory support is being provided.

◆ Monitor pulse. If bradycardia develops (pulse below 60 beats/min in an adult or 110 beats/min in an infant), withhold the dose, and notify the physician.

◆ Monitor blood pressure. Hypotension is more common in the elderly, the immobilized, and in patients receiving other medications that have hypotension as a side effect; it may also be a sign of sepsis or shock.

◆ Auscultate breath sounds every 2 to 4 hr. Since narcotic analgesics suppress the cough reflex, continue activities to prevent atelectasis and pneumonia such as turning, deep breathing, and incentive spirometry.

◆ Have narcotic antagonists, oxygen, and resuscitation equipment available in settings where narcotic analgesics are administered.

◆ Monitor level of consciousness and mental status. Evaluate findings carefully. For example, restlessness may be due to pain, hypoxia, shock, or an unusual reaction to the analgesic.

◆ Keep side rails up, keep a night light on, supervise ambulation, and discourage smoking.

◆ Monitor intake and output and weight. If nausea and vomiting occur, a switch to another analgesic may be appropriate; consult the physician. If nausea occurs, it may be appropriate to administer an antiemetic concomitantly with the narcotic. The peak effect of many antiemetics occurs at a different time from that of the narcotic; if so, the drugs should be on a different dosing schedule. Also, antiemetics may potentiate CNS depression, but they do not potentiate analgesic effects. Sedation and hypotension may be pronounced.

◆ Assess for urinary retention. It may be more pronounced in elderly patients, the immobilized, and men with preexisting prostatic hypertrophy. Question patients about difficulty in voiding, pain in the bladder area, or sensations of inadequate bladder emptying. Palpate bladder for distention. Suggest patients void before each dose of narcotic.

◆ Although the theoretic possibility of narcotic addiction exists for all patients who receive narcotic analgesics, only a very small percentage of patients do become dependent. Patients who persist in requesting frequent or large doses of pain medication beyond the average time postoperatively should not be automatically characterized as becoming addicted. Pain is a warning signal, and its unexpected persistence should be investigated. If it is suspected that the patient is becoming dependent or addicted, the health-care team should develop an individualized plan to help the patient with the problem.

◆ Some postoperative patients fear requesting any medication for pain because they fear addiction. Reassure patients that the use of narcotics in decreasing amounts over 3 to 5 days will not cause addiction and that recovery will be easier if pain is reduced.

◆ Use of aspirin or acetaminophen along with narcotic analgesics may increase pain relief; consult the physician.

◆ Record carefully the patient's response to pain and the response to narcotic administration.

Continued.

NURSING IMPLICATIONS SUMMARY—cont'd

◆ Check the physician's orders carefully. Observe agency policy regarding expiration date of controlled substances.

◆ In addition to the standard oral, IM, IV, and subcutaneous routes, narcotics may be administered via the intrathecal or intraspinal route, with patient-controlled analgesia (PCA) devices, and with implanted pumps. Become familiar with the equipment in use. Consult current literature for additional information. Review manufacturer's directions and patient instruction information. Ascertain that patients understand the advantages and use of the various routes and equipment being used.

◆ Transdermal dosage forms are now available for some drugs (see Fentanyl, Chapter 45). This route is not appropriate for relief of acute pain. See manufacturer's insert.

◆ Use preservative-free morphine for intrathecal and intraspinal or epidural use.

◆ Dilute doses of meperidine syrup in at least a half-glass of water. When taken undiluted, it may cause temporary mucous membrane anesthesia.

◆ Dilute doses of methadone oral concentrate with water to a volume of at least 90 ml. Dilute dispersible tablets in at least 120 ml of water, orange juice, citrus flavor Tang brand drink, or other acidic fruit beverage. Complete dispersion occurs in about 1 min.

◆ For continuous infusion, use microdrip tubing and an infusion-controlling device to keep the rate of administration steady.

INTRAVENOUS BUTORPHANOL

◆ May be given undiluted. Administer at a rate of 2 mg or less over 3 to 5 min.

INTRAVENOUS DEZOCINE

◆ May be given undiluted. Administer at a rate of 5 mg over 2 to 3 min.

INTRAVENOUS HYDROMORPHONE

◆ Dilute dose with 5 ml of sterile water or normal saline for injection. Administer at a rate of 2 mg or less over 3 to 5 min.

INTRAVENOUS LEVORPHANOL

◆ Dilute dose with 5 ml of sterile water or normal saline for injection. Administer at a rate of 3 mg or less over 4 to 5 min.

INTRAVENOUS MEPERIDINE

◆ Must be diluted. Dilute in at least 5 ml of sterile water or normal saline for injection. Administer dose over 4 to 5 min. For infusion in a narcotic syringe infusor system, dilute each 10 mg in at least 1 ml compatible IV fluid. May also be diluted to 1 mg/ml and given as a constant infusion under the observation of an anesthesiologist.

INTRAVENOUS MORPHINE SULFATE

◆ Dose should be diluted in at least 5 ml of sterile water or normal saline for injection, or other IV solutions. Administer at a rate of 15 mg or less over 4 to 5 min (direct infusion). May also be diluted for infusion.

INTRAVENOUS NALBUPHINE

◆ May be given undiluted. Administer 10 mg or less over 3 to 5 min.

INTRAVENOUS OXYMORPHONE

◆ Dilute dose with 5 ml of sterile water or normal saline for injection. Administer dose over 4 to 5 min.

INTRAVENOUS PENTAZOCINE

◆ May be given undiluted, but dilution is preferable. Dilute each 5 mg with at least 1 ml of sterile water for injection. Administer 5 mg or less over 1 min.

Patient and family education

◆ Review the anticipated benefits and possible side effects of drug therapy. Encourage patients to phone regarding any questions that arise.

◆ Review Patient Problems: Constipation on p. 182 and Orthostatic Hypotension on p. 234.

◆ Patients should take oral doses with milk or a snack to reduce gastric irritation.

◆ Instruct patients to avoid drinking alcoholic beverages while taking narcotic analgesics.

◆ Patients should avoid the use of other medications that may also cause CNS depression such as barbiturates, antiemetics, antihistamines, or tranquilizers, unless first approved by the physician.

◆ Warn patients to avoid driving or operating hazardous equipment if dizzy or drowsy.

NURSING IMPLICATIONS SUMMARY—cont'd

◆ If a combination drug product has been prescribed, review side effects associated with each of the drugs in the combined product.

◆ Remind patients to keep these and all medications out of the reach of children. Accidental overdose with narcotic analgesics in children may quickly lead to death.

Narcotic Antagonists: Naloxone

Drug administration

◆ Monitor blood pressure, pulse, and respiratory rate every 5 min initially, tapering to every 15 min, then every 30 min until stable. Attach acutely ill or comatose patients to electrocardiogram (ECG) monitor. Have a suction machine available.

◆ Auscultate breath sounds. If respiratory symptoms are severe or persistent, notify the physician.

◆ Monitor intake and output; auscultate bowel sounds.

◆ Have drugs, equipment, and personnel available for resuscitation if needed. Do not leave patient unattended until stable.

◆ Continue to monitor the patient closely for several hours after initial treatment, since the effects of the narcotic antagonist may wear off, causing the patient to again display signs of narcotic overdose.

INTRAVENOUS NALOXONE

◆ May be given undiluted or diluted for infusion. Administer at a rate of 0.4 mg over 15 seconds. Infusion is usually titrated to patient response. These drugs are rarely used outside of the acute-care setting.

Narcotic Antagonist: Naltrexone

Drug administration

◆ Assess for CNS effects. It may be difficult to differentiate between effects caused by naltrexone and those caused by the emotional effect of narcotic withdrawal. If insomnia is present, administer doses in the morning.

◆ Obtain baseline measurement of blood pressure, pulse, and ECG tracing, then monitor pulse and blood pressure daily, tapering to monthly if no abnormalities are noted.

◆ Monitor bowel sounds, and keep a record of bowel movements. If abdominal discomfort is severe or persistent, notify the physician.

◆ Monitor respiratory rate, and auscultate breath sounds. If respiratory symptoms are severe or persistent, notify the physician.

◆ Inspect for rash.

◆ Monitor liver function tests.

◆ Naltrexone therapy should not be initiated until the patient has completed detoxification and has been free of opiate drugs for 7 to 10 days.

◆ Before administering oral naltrexone, the patient may be given a naloxone challenge test. In this test a subcutaneous or IV dose of naloxone is administered, and the patient then is observed for signs of opiate withdrawal including nasal stuffiness, rhinorrhea, tearing, sweating, tremor, abdominal cramps, vomiting, goose flesh, and myalgia. If symptoms of withdrawal appear, the patient is not sufficiently drug free to begin naltrexone therapy. The challenge test may be repeated daily until the patient is opiate free.

◆ Monitor patient carefully for at least 1 hr after the first dose of naltrexone for withdrawal symptoms.

◆ Naltrexone should be used only as a component of a medically supervised behavior-modification program designed to help patients maintain an opiod-free state.

Patient and family education

◆ Review with patients the anticipated benefits and possible side effects of therapy. Instruct patients to report unexpected side effects.

◆ Tell patients to take oral doses with meals or a snack to lessen gastric irritation.

◆ Review with patients the need to avoid ingestion of opioids via any route of administration while taking naltrexone. This may include antidiarrhea medications and cough syrups.

◆ Remind patients to inform health-care providers of all medications they are taking, including naltrexone.

◆ Instruct patients to wear a medical identification tag or bracelet indicating the patient is receiving naltrexone.

CHAPTER REVIEW

◆ **KEY TERMS**

chemoreceptor trigger zone, p. 664

cough center, p. 664

drug dependence, p. 670

drug tolerance, p. 670

dynorphins, p. 664

endorphins, p. 664

enkephalins, p. 664

opioids, p. 662

respiratory center, p. 664

◆ **REVIEW QUESTIONS**

1. What are the two components of pain? Which is affected by opioids?

2. Which diseases are associated with chronic pain that the nurse might administer opioids to treat?

3. What are endorphins, enkephalins, and dynorphins? Which actions do enkephalins mediate?

4. What are the three characteristics of the analgesia produced by morphine?

5. What are the three major actions of morphine in the medulla?

6. What actions does morphine have on tissues outside the CNS?

7. What five common adverse reactions to morphine should you monitor?

8. What opioids might you administer to relieve severe pain?

9. What opioids might you administer to relieve moderate-to-severe pain?

10. What opioids are used to relieve mild pain?

11. Which opioids have antagonist and agonist activity?

12. Which opioids are significant in treating pulmonary edema? Pain of a heart attack?

13. Why is naloxone a good drug for treating acute opioid toxicity?

14. Describe withdrawal syndrome for opioids you would observe.

15. What properties of methadone make it useful for maintaining or withdrawing from opioid dependence?

16. What role do opioids have in anesthesia?

SUGGESTED READING

Adams F, and others: Plaques may complicate subcutaneous opioid infusions, *Am J Nurs* 89(1):109, 1989.

Akahoshi MP, Furuike-McLaughlin T, Enriquez NC: Patient controlled analgesia via intrathecal catheter in outpatient oncology patients, *J Intravenous Nurs* 11(5):289, 1988.

Arnold C: Intraspinal analgesia: a new route for an old drug, *J Neurosci Nurs* 21(1):30, 1989.

Blue CL, Purath J: Home care of the epidural analgesic patient: the nurse's role, *Home Healthc Nurse* 7(4):23, 1989.

Eaton JA: Continuous meperidine infusion for postoperative pain, *Orthop Nurs* 7(6):29, 1988.

Eland JM: Pharmacologic management of acute and chronic pediatric pain, *Issues Compr Pediatr Nurs* 11(2/3):93, 1988.

Eland JM: Pain management and comfort, *J Gerontol Nurs* 14(4):10, 1988.

Ferrell BR: Managing pain with long-acting morphine, *Nurs 91* 21(10):34, 1991.

Fifield MY: Relieving constipation and pain in the terminally ill, *Am J Nurs* 91(7):18, 1991.

Gadish HS, Gonzalez JL, Hayes JS: Factors affecting nurses' decisions to administer pediatric pain medication postoperatively, *J Pediatr Nurs* 3(6):383, 1988.

Hansberry JL, Bannick KH, Durkan MJ: Managing chronic pain with a permanent epidural catheter, *Nurs 90* 20(10):52, 1990.

Henrikson ML, Wild LR: A nursing process approach to epidural analgesia, *JOGNN* 17(5):316, 1988.

Hensley JR: Continuous SC morphine for cancer pain, *Am J Nurs* 91(3):98, 1991.

Jones, NH: Creative analgesic dosing in the elderly, *Am J Nurs* 89(10):1285, 1989.

Keller M: Oral morphine solution: effect on pain, confusion, drowsiness, and nausea for the terminally ill patient, *Hospice J* 4(1):55, 1988.

Lindley CM, Dalton JA, Fields SM: Narcotic analgesics: clinical pharmacology and therapeutics, *Cancer Nurs* 13(1):28, 1990.

Litwack K, Lubenow T: Practical points in the management of continuous epidural infusions, *J Post Anesth Nurs* 4(5):327, 1989.

Lloyd G: Opioids in postoperative pain relief, *Prof Nurs* 5(11):582, 1990.

Lloyd G: Opioids: routes of administration, *Prof Nurs* 5(12):634, 1990.

McCaffery M, Beebe A: Giving narcotics for pain: a problem-solver handbook, *Nurs 89* 19(10):161, 1989.

McCaffery M, Ferrell BR: Patient age: does it affect your pain-control decisions, *Nurs 91* 21(9):44, 1991.

McGuire L: Administering analgesics: which drugs are right for your patient, *Nurs 90* 20(4):34, 1990.

McLaughlin-Hagan M: Continuous subcutaneous infusion of narcotics, *J Intravenous Nurs* 13(2):119, 1990.

McNair N: Epidural narcotics for postoperative pain: nursing implications, *J Neurosci Nurs* 22(5):275, 1990.

Mendelson CS: Pain management for ambulatory surgery, *J Post Anesth Nurs* 3(2):109, 1988.

Musgrove DF: Acute postoperative pain: the cause and the care, *J Post Anesth Nurs* 5(5):329, 1990.

Patt R, Jain S: Epidural sufentanil for cancer pain, *Am J Nurs* 90(5):122, 1990.

Pauly-O'Neill S: Children demand (PCA) pain relief, too, *Am J Nurs* 90(5):26, 1990.

Peplin NJ: Intractable pain management with intravenous narcotic administration at home, *J Intravenous Nurs* 12(4):228, 1989.

Poniatowski BC: Continuous subcutaneous infusions for pain control, *J Intravenous Nurs* 14(1):30, 1991.

Porterfield LM: Narcotic analgesics, *Adv Clin Care* 5(4):30, 1990.

Raney JP, Kirk EA: The use of an Ommaya reservoir for administration of morphine sulphate to control pain in select cancer patients, *J Neurosci Nurs* 20(1):23, 1988.

Relieving pain: an analgesic guide. Principles of analgesic use in the treatment of acute pain and chronic cancer pain, *Am J Nurs* 88(6):815, 1988.

Tucker C: Acute pain and substance abuse in surgical patients, *J Neurosci Nurs* 22(6):339, 1990.

Walker M, Wong DL: A battle plan for patients in pain, *Am J Nurs* 91(6):32, 1991.

CHAPTER 45

General Anesthetics

LEARNING OBJECTIVES

After studying this chapter, you should be able to do the following:

◆ Describe characteristics of inhalation anesthetics, intravenous (IV) anesthetics, balanced anesthesia, and neuroleptanesthesia.

◆ Explain minimum alveolar concentration (MAC).

◆ Outline the characteristics of the different agents described in the chapter.

◆ Develop a nursing care plan for the patient receiving a specific general anesthetic agent or a combination of agents.

CHAPTER OVERVIEW

◆ Modern surgery did not begin until the introduction of nitrous oxide, ether, and chloroform as general anesthetics in the late 1800s. The agents used today as general anesthetics include gases (nitrous oxide), volatile liquids (diethyl ether, halothane, methoxyflurane, enflurane, and isoflurane), and IV agents (ketamine and narcotic analgesics). The ultrashort-acting barbiturates, benzodiazepines, and etomidate are used intravenously for induction of anesthesia.

Nursing Process Overview
GENERAL ANESTHESIA
Assessment

Perform a complete physical assessment, with focus on vital signs and respiratory system, laboratory data, and studies specific to known medical problems (e.g., coagulation studies in patients with liver disease or pulmonary function studies in patients with severe chronic obstructive pulmonary disease [COPD]).

Nursing Diagnoses

Altered comfort: nausea and vomiting related to general anesthesia

Ineffective airway clearance: inability to remove airway secretions related to general anesthesia

Management

Delivery of general anesthesia requires knowledge and facility with management of the respiratory and cardiovascular systems, multiple drugs, and the immobilized unconscious patient. For further information, consult appropriate textbooks of nursing, medicine, and anesthesiology.

Evaluation

Perform frequent evaluations of vital signs, respiratory and cardiovascular status, level of consciousness, and ability to handle secretions. Assess degree of postoperative pain, and medicate if appropriate. Assess wound, drainage, intake and output, and other parameters as indicated by the type of surgery performed.

INHALATION ANESTHETICS
Mechanism of Action

General anesthetics act on the central nervous system (CNS) to abolish the perception of pain and the reaction to painful stimuli. They are unusual in their mechanism of action because they do not appear to act by a receptor mechanism. Instead, general anesthetics are believed to alter the lipid structure of cell membranes so that physiologic functions are impaired. The network of neurons making up the CNS is especially vulnerable because alteration of membrane structure interrupts the complex intercommunication necessary for function. The most sensitive system to such alterations is the ascending reticular activating system, the neuronal formation monitoring incoming stimuli and determining what information is to be sent to the brain for processing and response. Consciousness is lost when the ascending reticular activating system ceases to transmit information effectively.

Inhalation anesthetics are gases or volatile liquids administered as gases. The effective concentration of an inhalation anesthetic in the brain does not depend on the solubility of the anesthetic in blood or tissue. Rather, effective concentration depends on the partial pressure of the anesthetic or effective pressure of the gas in the atmosphere. If a constant partial pressure of anesthetic is inhaled, partial pressure in the alveoli rises toward the inhaled level. If the gas is not soluble in blood, little gas is removed by the blood circulating around the alveoli, and the partial pressure of the gas in the blood quickly reaches the inhaled partial pressure. This anesthetic has a rapid onset of action. If the gas is soluble in blood, however, partial pressure of the gas in the alveoli quickly drops, since the gas is being removed more rapidly by the blood than can be replenished by breathing. A long time is required to equilibrate the blood with the gas to where the partial pressure matches that coming into the alveoli. To shorten the time to reach this steady state, anesthesia is induced using a high partial pressure of the gas and then lowering the partial pressure to maintain anesthesia.

Minimum Alveolar Concentration

The potency of an inhalation anesthetic is determined by the **minimum alveolar concentration (MAC)** that produces insensitivity to a skin incision (anesthesia) in 50% of patients. For instance, MAC of 10% is equivalent to a partial pressure of 0.1 atmosphere or 76 mm of mercury at standard conditions (sea level). MAC of 10% means that when air in the alveoli has equilibrated with the body and incoming air, all of which are 10% anesthetic gas, the patient has a 50-50 chance of being unreactive to a skin incision. Surgery is conducted at about 1.4 times the MAC value of the anesthetic chosen.

Distribution and Excretion

The distribution of the anesthetic is determined by the blood flow; thus the brain, liver, and kidneys reach equilibrium first. Excretion of the inhalation anesthetics is largely through the lungs. The anesthetic that is in solution is metabolized by the liver to a variable degree. Certain halogenated hydrocarbons (e.g., enflurane, halothane, and methoxyflurane) are metabolized to products that may damage the liver and kidney.

Emergence is the time during which the patient regains consciousness after the anesthetic has been discontinued. The duration of emergence from the inhaled anesthetics depends on the same factors as induction. The patient's vital signs are carefully monitored in a recovery room, and symptoms of pain or nausea and vomiting much be watched for and treated appropriately.

Specific Agents

Table 45-1 lists specific inhalation anesthetics and their properties.

Diethyl ether

Diethyl ether is a volatile liquid that is flammable and explosive. The MAC is 1.92%. A long time is required for induction and emergence when ether alone is used because it is highly soluble in blood. In addition, ether is unpleasant to inhale because it has a noxious, pungent odor, irritates the respiratory tract, and stimulates secretions. An anticholinergic drug may be administered to minimize these secretions. The explosive hazard and the noxious, pungent odor account for the rare use of ether in modern surgery. Nevertheless, ether is used in areas of the world where sophisticated equipment is unavailable for monitoring the patient. Ether has a wide margin of safety and has few effects on the cardiovascular system, allowing it to be administered without sophisticated control of concentration. Ether produces good analgesia and muscle relaxation, making extra medication unnecessary.

Enflurane

Enflurane (Ethrane) is a halogenated hydrocarbon and a nonflammable liquid. MAC is 1.68%, and induction is fairly rapid. Enflurane is one of the stimulant anesthetics that produce muscle contractions and seizurelike brain wave patterns at high concentrations. Enflurane is usually administered with nitrous oxide to avoid high concentrations, which can cause CNS stimulation and cardiovascular depression. Enflurane causes a decrease in blood pressure resulting from depressed cardiac output and decreased peripheral resistance. Emergence is usually uneventful except for shivering. About 2.5% of enflurane is metabolized to release a low concentration of fluoride ion. The amount of fluoride ion is not harmful, except in patients with preexisting kidney damage.

Halothane

Halothane (Fluothane) is a nonflammable liquid halogenated hydrocarbon and currently is the most widely used volatile liquid anesthetics. MAC is

Table 45-1   Properties of Inhalation Anesthetics

Drug	Physical properties	Onset	MAC	Cardiovascular effects	Muscle relaxation	Elimination	Other properties
Diethyl ether	Flammable liquid	Slow	1.92%	Minimum	Excellent	Lungs	Excellent analgesia. Nausea and vomiting on emergence. Secretions stimulated.
Enflurane (Ethrane)	Nonflammable liquid	Rapid	1.68%	Decreased blood pressure May sensitize heart to catecholamines	Good	Lungs 2% to 5% metabolized by liver	Causes low body temperature, hypothermia and shivering.
Halothane (Fluothane)	Nonflammable liquid	Rapid	0.77%	Decreased blood pressure Sensitizes heart to catecholamines	Fair	Lungs 20% metabolized by liver	Poor analgesia.
Isoflurane (Forane)	Nonflammable liquid	Rapid	1.30%	Minimum	Good	Lungs Little metabolism by liver	Excellent analgesia.
Methoxyflurane (Penthrane)	Nonflammable liquid	Slow	0.16%	Decreased blood pressure	Good	Lungs 70% metabolized by liver	Excellent analgesia.
Nitrous oxide	Nonflammable gas	Very rapid	101%	Minimum	—	Lungs	Widely used with other drugs for anesthesia. Good analgesia.

0.77%, and induction is fairly rapid. Postoperative nausea and vomiting are not problems. Halothane is a direct myocardial depressant and causes a dose-dependent reduction in cardiac output with no change in heart rate, a combination of effects that lowers blood pressure. Halothane also sensitizes the myocardium to exogenously administered catecholamines. This sensitization means that a sympathomimetic drug must be used cautiously during surgery to maintain blood pressure, since sympathomimetic drugs may precipitate arrhythmias. Catecholamines may be used topically such as on the brain or in irrigation of the bladder to stop bleeding. Halothane does not give adequate muscle relaxation; a separate muscle relaxant must be used.

Rarely (1:800,000 patients) halothane is responsible for fatal hepatitis. Current theory is that free radical metabolites, which are very reactive compounds, may be produced by the liver and may damage liver cells.

Isoflurane

Isoflurane (Forane) is a chemical isomer of enflurane, but unlike enflurane, isoflurane is a depressant anesthetic similar to halothane. MAC is 1.3%. Induction is smooth and rapid, and muscle relaxation is adequate. The heart is not sensitized to catecholamines, but the blood pressure falls because of a decrease in the peripheral resistance of blood vessels. Only 0.25% of isoflurane is metabolized. Isoflurane is a more recent anesthetic that many anesthesiologists believe will be widely used in the future.

Methoxyflurane

Methoxyflurane (Penthrane) is a nonflammable liquid halogenated hydrocarbon. It produces analgesia adequate for dentistry and obstetrics. MAC is 0.16%. Methoxyflurane depresses the cardiovascular system but does not sensitize the heart to catecholamines. Methoxyflurane that is not exhaled is metabolized extensively (70%) by the liver to fluoride ion. Prolonged anesthesia with methoxyflurane may result in high-output renal failure because in the presence of the fluoride ion, the kidney loses its concentrating ability so that urine volume is high. This renal failure is usually reversible.

Nitrous oxide

Nitrous oxide is a nonexplosive gas that is widely used. The major limitation of nitrous oxide is that the maximum concentration allowable, 65% to 70% N_2O and 30% to 35% O_2, does not produce surgical anesthesia because MAC is 101%. Nevertheless, nitrous oxide produces good analgesia and is used for this purpose in dental and obstetric procedures. In addition, nitrous oxide is widely used with other anesthetics to produce surgical anesthesia. Its effect is additive with other anesthetics, so a 50% MAC concentration of nitrous oxide and a 50% MAC concentration of another inhalation anesthetic produces surgical anesthesia. In addition, nitrous oxide is widely used as one component of **balanced anesthesia,** in which a narcotic analgesic, a skeletal muscle relaxant, and nitrous oxide are used together to produce surgical anesthesia.

Nitrous oxide has been shown to increase the incidence of spontaneous abortions in females and to decrease spermatogenesis in males who work in operating rooms. Scavenging equipment must now be used in the operating room to remove nitrous oxide. The gas is much more soluble (34 times) than nitrogen in the blood so that pockets of trapped gas in the patient expand as nitrogen leaves and is replaced by larger amounts of nitrous oxide. Locations where trapped gas is common include a blocked middle ear, pneumothorax, loops of intestine, lungs, renal cysts, and in the skull after a pneumoencephalogram. These conditions represent contraindications for nitrous oxide, since the large increases in pressure or volumes that may result after its administration may cause serious damage.

INTRAVENOUS ANESTHETICS

Intravenous anesthetics include the ultrashort-acting barbiturates: thiopental (Pentothal), methohexital (Brevital), and thiamylal sodium (Surital); three benzodiazepines: diazepam (Valium), midazolam (Versed), and flunitrazepam (Rohypnol); and the agents ketamine (Ketaject) and etomidate (Amidate and Hypnomidate). Only ketamine is a true anesthetic, abolishing the perception of and the reaction to pain. The barbiturates and benzodiazepines do not abolish reflex reaction to pain even when they are administered in doses large enough to render the patient unconscious. These drugs are used primarily as induction agents. The advantage of the IV agents is that they are effective seconds after administration.

It may seem paradoxical that an IV anesthetic would be so short acting when it must be metabolized to be excreted. The explanation is that the IV anesthetics are lipid soluble. Initially, they are distributed to the brain, liver, and kidneys, the organs with the largest blood flow, but later the drug is redistributed to body fat and skeletal muscle, which are less well perfused. This redistribution lowers the circulating concentration to that which no longer maintains anesthesia. This redistribution is responsible for the short duration of action. Metabolism of the drug proceeds as the drug passes through the liver.

Table 45-2 lists IV anesthetics.

Barbiturates

Thiopental (Pentothal), methohexital (Brevital), and thiamylal (Surital) are all ultrashort-acting barbiturates used primarily to induce anesthesia. Loss of consciousness occurs within 60 sec of injection. Thiopental or thiamylal is effective as the sole anesthetic for about 15 min. Methohexital is even shorter acting. Barbiturates provide no analgesia and can cause excitement or delirium in the presence of pain in an awake patient. Changes in blood pressure or cardiac output are not common unless the injection is made rapidly. Respiration is markedly depressed, and yawning, coughing, or laryngospasm may occur. Methohexital can cause hiccups.

Solutions of barbiturates should be injected only into veins. Arterial injections can cause inflammation and clotting. The barbiturate solution damages tissue if it leaks around the injection site, and this situation can lead to gangrene.

Benzodiazepines

Diazepam

Diazepam (Valium) is a benzodiazepine used occasionally as an induction agent but more frequently to sedate patients undergoing cardioversion or endoscopic or dental procedures. IV diazepam takes 60 sec to become effective. Sedation, sleep, and amnesia are achieved with little depression of cardiovascular or respiratory functions. Unlike barbiturates, diazepam is metabolized to active products and has a long duration of action (see Chapter 40).

Midazolam

Midazolam (Versed) is a relatively short-acting benzodiazepine used as an IV anesthetic. It should be used only in hospital or ambulatory care settings where respiratory and cardiac functions can be monitored. Midazolam may be administered intravenously or intramuscularly to induce sedation or amnesia.

Table 45-2 Injectable Drugs for Anesthesia

Generic name	Trade name	Administration/dosage	Comments
BARBITURATES			
Methohexital sodium	Brevital Sodium Brietal Sodium†	INTRAVENOUS: *Adults*—for induction, 5 to 12 ml of 1% solution no faster than 1 ml every 5 sec. Maintenance, 2 to 4 ml of 1% solution as required. FDA Pregnancy Category C.	Shortest duration of action (5 to 7 min) of the barbiturates. Some patients develop hiccups after rapid injection. Schedule IV substance.
Thiamylal sodium	Surital*	INTRAVENOUS: *Adults*—for induction, 2 to 4 ml of 2.5% solution every 30 to 40 sec, with maximum dose 3 to 5 mg/kg body weight. Maintenance, 2 to 4 ml of 2.5% solution as required. FDA Pregnancy Category C.	Duration of action about 15 min. Schedule III substance.
Thiopental sodium	Pentothal*	INTRAVENOUS: *Adults*—for induction, 50 to 100 mg (2 to 4 ml) in 2.5% solution every 30 to 40 sec or 3 to 5 mg/kg body weight. Maintenance, 2 to 4 ml of 2.5% solution as required. *Children*—3 to 5 mg/kg as described for adults. FDA Pregnancy Category C.	Duration of action about 15 min. May cause yawning, coughing, or laryngospasm. Schedule III substance.
BENZODIAZEPINES			
Diazepam	Valium*	INTRAVENOUS: *Adults*—0.1 to 0.2 mg/kg body weight to induce sleep, maximum dose 10 to 20 mg. Basal sedation requires only 5 to 30 mg, so 2.5 to 5 mg is injected every 30 sec until light sleep or slurred speech is produced.	Do not mix with other liquids. Local anesthetic may be required for IV injection.
Midazolam	Versed*	INTRAMUSCULAR: *Adults*—for preoperative sedation, 70 to 80 μg/kg, 30 to 60 min before surgery. FDA Pregnancy Category D. *Children*—80 to 200 μg/kg. INTRAVENOUS: *Adults*—for conscious sedation, 2.5 mg administered over 2 min just before the procedure; for general anesthesia, 200 to 350 μg/kg, administered over 5 to 30 sec. *Children*—50 to 200 μg/kg.	Schedule IV substance. Older or debilitated patients should be administered a smaller dose.
MISCELLANEOUS			
Alfentanil	Alfenta*	INTRAVENOUS: *Adults*—for induction of anesthesia, 130 μg/kg body weight. FDA Pregnancy Category C.	Schedule II substance. Potent, short-acting narcotic analgesic. "Lollipop" dosage form is being tested as a presurgical sedative for children. Very short-acting (30 to 45 min) drug.
Droperidol	Inapsine*	INTRAVENOUS: *Adults and children over 2 years*—0.15 mg/kg body weight. Onset: 10 to 15 min. Duration: 3 to 6 hr.	Antipsychotic drug. Used with fentanyl citrate and nitrous oxide to produce neuroleptanesthesia. May cause extrapyramidal symptoms.

*Available in Canada and United States.
†Available in Canada only.

Continued.

Table 45-2   Injectable Drugs for Anesthesia—cont'd

Generic name	Trade name	Administration/dosage	Comments
MISCELLANEOUS—cont'd			
Etomidate	Amidate Hypnomidate	INTRAVENOUS: *Adults and children over 10 years*—for induction, 0.3 mg/kg body weight injected over 30 to 60 sec, may vary between 0.2 and 0.6 mg/kg. FDA Pregnancy Category C.	Nonbarbiturate agent used for induction and sometimes maintenance of anesthesia.
Fentanyl	Duragesic	TRANSDERMAL: *Adults*—Apply to skin of upper torso every 72 hr. Initially, one 2.5-mg transdermal system. For maintenance, dosage may be adjusted every 3 days, according to patient response. Some patients require application every 48 hr.	Patients tolerant to opioids may require higher dosages. First opioid analgesic available in a transdermal system. Not for short-term relief of acute pain.
Fentanyl citrate	Sublimaze*	INTRAVENOUS: *Adults and children over 2 years*—0.002 to 0.003 mg/kg body weight in divided doses over 6 to 8 min. Maintenance, 0.05 to 0.1 mg every 30 to 60 min. Onset: 1 to 2 min. FDA Pregnancy Category C.	Potent, short-acting narcotic analgesic. Used with droperidol and nitrous oxide for neuroleptic anesthesia and with nitrous oxide for balanced anesthesia. Also available in a transdermal patch for chronic pain management (see Chapter 44).
Ketamine	Ketaject Ketalar*	INTRAVENOUS: *Adults and children*—1 to 4.5 mg/kg body weight over 60 sec, ½ of initial dose used for maintenance as needed. INTRAMUSCULAR: *Adults and children*—6.5 to 13 mg/kg body weight, ½ of initial dose for maintenance as needed.	Produces cataleptic anesthesia with good analgesia. Not a scheduled drug.
Propofol	Diprivan*	INTRAVENOUS: *Adults (up to 55 years)*—For induction of anesthesia, increments of approximately 40 mg every 10 sec until adequate anesthesia is achieved. Usual total dose is 2 to 2.5 mg/kg. For maintenance, 25 to 50 mg as required is given by intermittent bolus, or 0.1 to 0.2 mg/kg/min is infused. For elderly, debilitated, or hypovolemic patients, dose is reduced by half.	New IV anesthetic. Rapid onset and recovery. Causes hypotension and respiratory depression.
Sufentanil citrate	Sufenta*	INTRAVENOUS: *Adults*—inital dose is 1 to 8 μg/kg with nitrous oxide and oxygen. Additional doses are 10 to 25 μg/kg. Doses depend on the severity of pain associated with the surgery. *Children over 2 years*—for cardiovascular surgery: 10 to 25 μg/kg with oxygen and a muscular relaxant. Additional doses are 25 to 50 μg (1 to 2 μg/kg). FDA Pregnancy Category C.	Potent, short-acting narcotic analgesic used with nitrous oxide for balanced anesthesia or alone with oxygen and a muscle relaxant.

*Available in Canada and United States.

Other Agents

Etomidate

Etomidate (Amidate and Hypnomidate) is an IV anesthetic for the induction of surgical anesthesia. Etomidate produces minimum cardiovascular or respiratory changes. Since etomidate does not produce analgesia, the short-acting narcotic-analgesic fentanyl citrate also may be infused for total IV anesthesia.

The most frequent side effects of etomidate are pain at the injection site and transient, myoclonic skeletal muscle movements.

Ketamine

Ketamine (Ketaject and Ketalar) is neither a barbiturate nor a benzodiazepine. Unlike those drug classes, ketamine produces a cataleptic anesthesia in which the patient appears to be awake but neither responds to pain nor remembers the procedure. This is sometimes referred to as *dissociative anesthesia*. Ketamine is not a controlled substance and is readily available in emergency rooms. Ketamine is rapidly effective when administered intramuscularly and intravenously. Ketamine alone provides anesthesia for 5 to 10 minutes when given intravenously and for 10 to 20 min when given intramuscularly.

Ketamine enhances muscle tone and increases blood pressure, heart rate, and respiratory secretions. The major side effect is seen in the recovery period, when patients may experience vivid, unpleasant dreams or hallucinations. Adults are more prone than children to these experiences. It may also cause vomiting and shivering. It is chemically related to phencyclidine (PCP), an illicit hallucinogen.

Ketamine should be used cautiously in patients with convulsive disorders, psychosis, mild hypertension, or who are undergoing eye surgery and is contraindicated for patients with coronary artery disease, severe hypertension, cerebrovascular accident (stroke), or treated hypothyroidism.

Propofol

Propofol (Diprivan) is a new IV anesthetic for induction and maintenance of general anesthesia. It is also used with opioids and nitrous oxide in balanced anesthesia. Propofol can cause hypotension, and this is potentiated by opioid analgesics. Propofol is also a respiratory depressant. Recovery from anesthesia is rapid, with minimal psychomotor impairment. The drug is inactivated in the liver.

Narcotic Analgesics and Balanced Anesthesia

The ideal anesthetic would produce analgesia, unconsciousness, muscle relaxation, and reduction of reflex activity. This anesthetic would act promptly and would be rapidly eliminated, remaining unmetabolized and producing no unwanted effects in body tissues. Since no anesthetic has all these desirable properties, several drugs are used in combination to achieve these goals.

For surgical anesthesia, one widely used combination of agents is balanced anesthesia. This combines a narcotic analgesic, nitrous oxide, and a skeletal muscle relaxant. Anesthesia is induced, generally with a short-acting barbiturate or occasionally with diazepam or other agents, and then the narcotic analgesic, nitrous oxide, and skeletal muscle relaxant are administered. Respiration must be controlled, since the narcotic analgesics are potent respiratory depressants, and patients are usually paralyzed by a skeletal muscle relaxant. Nitrous oxide is effective at a 60% concentration because of its synergism with the narcotic analgesic. The skeletal muscle relaxant is necessary because neither the narcotic analgesic nor the nitrous oxide provides the muscular relaxation necessary for surgery. The choice of the narcotic analgesic is determined by the anticipated length of surgery. Alfentanil (Alfenta), fentanyl (Sublimaze), and sufentanil (Sufenta) are short-acting narcotic analgesics primarily used for surgery. Meperidine (Demerol) is widely used for longer surgeries. Morphine is used as an alternate to meperidine, and it is also preferred for cardiac and poor-risk patients.

The advantage of balanced anesthesia is that the cardiovascular system is neither depressed nor sensitized to catecholamines. Respiration is depressed, but controlled ventilation is readily available. The incidence of postoperative nausea, vomiting, and pain is low.

NEUROLEPTANESTHESIA

Neuroleptanesthesia refers to the combination of droperidol (Inapsine), an antipsychotic drug of the butyrophenone class; a narcotic analgesic (usually fentanyl); and nitrous oxide. A skeletal muscle relaxant may be used if needed. A fixed combination of the narcotic analgesic fentanyl and droperidol is available as Innovar. Nitrous oxide produces loss of consciousness, and if it is discontinued, the patient becomes conscious but in an altered state of awareness. Neuroleptanesthesia is useful for elderly and poor-risk patients and for bronchoscopy and carotid arteriography. Innovar alone greatly facilitates intubation in awake patients.

Side effects of neuroleptanalgesia or neuroleptanesthesia are hypotension, a slow heart rate (bradycardia), and respiratory depression. The action of droperidol persists for 3 to 6 hr, whereas the analgesic effect of fentanyl persists of only 30 min. Droperidol has adrenergic-receptor blocking, antifibrillatory, antiemetic, and anticonvulsant actions. About 1% of patients who receive droperidol may have extrapyramidal muscle movements (see Chapter 41) for as long as 12 hr after administration of the drug. These movements may be controlled by administration of atropine or benztropine (see Chapter 48).

NURSING IMPLICATIONS SUMMARY

Drug administration and patient and family education

◆ Techniques of administration of general anesthesia are beyond the scope of this book; for further information consult appropriate textbooks of anesthesia.

◆ Obtain a careful drug history before surgery. Assess for allergic or unusual responses to previous anesthetic agents and for any current medications the patient is taking.

◆ Preoperative medications are an integral part of the planned anesthesia. Administer them as ordered and on time.

◆ To prepare the patient for surgery, teach the patient and family about the surgical procedure and what to expect postoperatively. Have the patient give a return demonstration of any exercises or activities required such as coughing and deep breathing. Provide the patient with an opportunity to ask questions of the anesthesiologist or nurse anesthetist. Schedule a visit to the intensive care unit, if appropriate. Provide emotional support.

Postoperative care

◆ Monitor temperature, pulse, respirations, and blood pressure frequently. With the exception of temperature, this may be every 5 min initially, progressing to every 15 min, then every 30 min and longer. Auscultate lung sounds, and check neurologic status. Do not leave the patient unattended unless the patient can call for assistance and can handle secretions safely.

◆ Keep patients on their sides initially, if possible, to prevent aspiration if vomiting should occur. Keep a suction machine at the bedside, and keep side rails up.

◆ Evaluate patients for pain medication in the immediate postoperative period (first 2 to 4 hr after surgery). Factors to consider include the nature and location of surgery, vital signs, age, weight, level of consciousness, what anesthetic was used, and whether analgesics were administered during surgery. The initial dose of analgesics may be ¼ to ½ the ordered dose of analgesic, but make reductions in dose only after consultation with physician. When Innovar is used, the first dose of postoperative analgesic should be low.

◆ Begin nursing measures to prevent atelectasis and pneumonia as soon as the patient is able. This may include turning and deep breathing, coughing, and other breathing activities.

◆ Effects of anesthesia persist even after patients appear to be alert and awake. If it is necessary to give instructions about activity, diet, or medications, as in the outpatient or day-surgery setting, do so verbally and in writing to the patient, and have at least one family member present.

◆ Do not permit patients in the outpatient setting to drive themselves home if they have received general anesthesia.

◆ Warn patients who have a severe reaction or response to any anesthetic to carry with them the name of the agent. If surgery is ever again needed, teach patients to tell the anesthetist of the previous severe response. Suggest that patients wear a medical identification tag or bracelet indicating the severe reaction.

◆ See the nursing implications summary for narcotic analgesics in Chapter 44. Patients perform needed postoperative activities better if they are adequately medicated for pain.

Ketamine

◆ Ketamine is associated with unpleasant dreams, emergence delirium, irrational behavior, disorientation, and hallucinations. These side effects may be lessened by providing the patient with a quiet wakeup period, perhaps in the quietest corner of the postanesthesia recovery room. Avoid excessive stimulation, although vital signs must be monitored. If psychic effects occur, provide calm reassurance and reorientation. Do not leave the patient unattended. Once the patient is returned to the room, keep it dimly lit, and keep noise and stimulation to a minimum. Inform family members of the probable cause of the behavior, and enlist their aid in patient reorientation and reassurance.

CHAPTER REVIEW

◆ KEY TERMS

balanced anesthesia, p. 678
dissociative anesthesia, p. 681
emergence, p. 676
inhalation anesthetics, p. 676
intravenous anesthetics, p. 678
minimum alveolar concentration (MAC), p. 676
neuroleptanesthesia, p. 681

◆ REVIEW QUESTIONS

1. How are general anesthetics believed to work?
2. What measurement determines the effective concentration of an inhalation anesthetic? How does this differ from the concentration based on total solubility?
3. What is MAC?
4. What factors determine induction and emergence? Outline your responsibilities during the emergence period.
5. Why is diethyl ether seldom used in the United States?
6. Which inhalation anesthetics are halogenated hydrocarbons? What should you monitor in a patient who has received a halogenated hydrocarbon?
7. Which inhalation anesthetics sensitize the heart to catecholamines?
8. Which inhalation anesthetics are metabolized to some degree?
9. Which inhalation anesthetics lower blood pressure during surgery?
10. What factor limits the use of nitrous oxide alone as an anesthetic? How is this limitation overcome?
11. What are the hazards of nitrous oxide to patients and to operating room personnel?
12. Which barbiturates are used as IV induction agents for anesthesia? How is their action effectively terminated?
13. Which benzodiazepines are used as IV induction agents for anesthesia?
14. What is the nature of anesthesia with ketamine? What nursing care activities might be needed with a patient who has received ketamine?
15. What are the properties of an ideal anesthetic?
16. Describe balanced anesthesia.
17. Describe neuroleptanesthesia.

SUGGESTED READING

Biddle C: Adverse reactions to drugs used in anesthesia, *Curr Rev Post Anesth Care Nurses* 10(7):51, 1988.

Karb VB: Midazolam: newcomer to the benzodiazepine family, *J Neurosci Nurs* 32(1):64, 1989.

Kochansky CY, Kochansky SW: Postanesthetic considerations for the patient receiving ketamine, *J Post Anesth Nurs* 3(2):118, 1988.

Lichtiger A: Anesthesia for the geriatric patient, *Curr Rev Recov Room Nurses* 8(21):162, 1987.

Litwack K: Managing postanesthetic emergencies, *Nurs 91* 21(9):49, 1991.

Litwack K: What you need to know about administering preoperative medications, *Nurs 91* 21(8):44, 1991.

CHAPTER 46

Local Anesthetics

LEARNING OBJECTIVES

After studying this chapter, you should be able to do the following:

◆ Describe the mechanism of action of local anesthetics.

◆ Describe side effects and adverse reactions of local anesthetics.

◆ Explain the differences between agents for surface anesthesia and those injected to produce local anesthesia.

◆ Differentiate among infiltration, nerve block, epidural, caudal, and spinal anesthesia.

◆ Develop a nursing care plan for a patient who has received local anesthesia.

CHAPTER OVERVIEW

◆ Local anesthetics reversibly block nerve conduction, leading to loss of sensation and preventing muscle activity. In addition to topical anesthesia, local anesthetics can be infiltrated to various nerve sites, producing anesthesia over a wide area.

◆ Cocaine was the first local anesthetic used clinically, after the observation in the late 1880s that when cocaine was administered orally to patients, their tongues and throats became numb. Its main use as a local anesthetic was to desensitize the cornea to allow local surgery without a general anesthetic. It was quickly recognized that cocaine had a high potential for abuse, and it was replaced by procaine (Novocain) in 1905. Today, lidocaine (Xylocaine), introduced in the 1940s, is the most versatile and widely used local anesthetic. More than 20 local anesthetics are available, but they vary in their suitability for different applications.

Nursing Process Overview
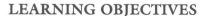
LOCAL ANESTHESIA

Assessment

Assess vital signs and temperature, history of allergies, response to previous surgery, and overall condition.

Nursing Diagnoses

High risk for urinary retention and inability to void
Impaired swallowing and loss of gag reflex secondary to local anesthesia

Management

For minor or brief procedures such as suturing or dental work, careful observation of the patient may be sufficient. For longer procedures or when spinal anesthesia is used, monitor vital signs and other pa-

rameters of patient function. With spinal anesthesia, position the lower extremities carefully. Insert a Foley catheter to allow urinary output. Monitor the level of consciousness. Allergic responses are possible when local anesthetics are used by any route; have epinephrine and equipment for resuscitation available to treat possible anaphylaxis.

Evaluation

All anesthetics require time to wear off, and specific nursing care depends on the area that has been anesthetized. For example, if the throat has been anesthetized for bronchoscopy, evaluate ability to swallow, position patients on the side to reduce the possibility of aspiration, restrict oral intake until patients can swallow, and have a suction machine available at the bedside. After spinal anesthesia, keep patients flat for 12 to 24 hr. Check the position of the lower extremities to prevent pressure areas, and keep patients in bed until sensation returns to the lower extremities. Monitor vital signs and intake and output.

If the patient is still under the effects of the local anesthetic at discharge, verify that the patient can explain any restrictions in activity or diet to be followed until the anesthesia wears off. If analgesic medications are prescribed for use after the anesthesia wears off, the patient should be able to explain their use (see Chapter 44). If a local anesthetic is prescribed for outpatient use, determine that the patient can explain how and with what frequency to use the medication and what to do if it is ineffective.

MECHANISM OF ACTION

Local anesthesia is achieved by drugs that reversibly inhibit nerve conduction. A **local anesthetic** is administered at the desired site of action. The inhibition of nerve conduction persists until the drug diffuses and enters the circulation for subsequent degradation and excretion. All neurons in the area of administration, whether pain, motor, or autonomic, are affected, so in addition to the loss of pain, loss of sensory, motor, and autonomic activities occurs. The size of the nerve fiber determines its sensitivity to local anesthetics; smaller fibers are the most sensitive. Since sensory fibers are smaller than motor fibers, loss of sensation precedes loss of motor activity and, conversely, motor activity is regained before sensory function.

Chemically, most local anesthetics are weak bases, being secondary or tertiary amines. This means that under physiologic conditions most molecules carry a positive charge and are not lipid soluble. However, it is the uncharged form that diffuses across the nerve membrane and then reequilibrates to charged and uncharged forms. Within the neuron the positively charged form blocks nerve conduction. The positively charged form displaces calcium bound to the inner membrane and thus prevents the inward flow of sodium ions. Since the action potential is generated by the influx of sodium ions, the local anesthetic depresses the action potential so that it is not propagated. The resting potential of neurons is not affected by local anesthetics.

SIDE EFFECTS AND ADVERSE REACTIONS

Local anesthetics eventually enter the systemic circulation and can affect other organs, limiting their safety. The relative safety of procaine and chloroprocaine results from their rapid hydrolysis in the plasma by pseudocholinesterases. Other local anesthetics are slowly degraded by the liver and have a longer plasma half-life.

Although cocaine is unique in causing euphoria, all local anesthetics act as central nervous system (CNS) stimulants if absorbed systemically, producing symptoms such as anxiety, tingling (paresthesia), tremors, and ringing in the ears (tinnitus). This CNS stimulation may ultimately result in convulsions. Intravenous (IV) diazepam (Valium) in 2.5-mg increments or small doses of an ultrashort-acting barbiturate such as thiopental (Pentothal), thiamylal (Surital), or methohexital (Brevital) are given to stop these convulsions.

A high plasma concentration of a local anesthetic causes CNS depression, with or without prior symptoms of CNS stimulation. Depression of CNS function is serious, since vasomotor control is lost, and results in profound hypotension, respiratory depression, and coma.

In addition to the CNS effects, direct cardiovascular effects of local anesthetics are important. Local anesthetics cause direct vasodilation, increasing blood flow and favoring removal of the drug. Thus epinephrine is sometimes added to the local anesthetic, since it causes vasoconstriction and prolongs the time the local anesthetic remains at the injection site. Cocaine is unique among the local anesthetics in being a potent vasoconstrictor. Prolonged abuse of cocaine by insufflation (sniffing) can cause loss of nasal septa caused by tissue death after ischemia (insufficient blood flow). Local anesthetics are cardiac depressants. Lidocaine is used to depress cardiac arrhythmias (see Chapter 19).

Local anesthetics that are esters (chloroprocaine, procaine, and tetracaine) can cause an allergic response. Anaphylaxis is rare, and more commonly the topical use of a local anesthetic with an ester bond leads to skin rash (contact dermatitis).

CLINICAL USES

In general, local anesthetics can be divided into those applied topically to provide surface anesthesia and those injected into an area to produce local anesthesia. Only lidocaine (Xylocaine), dibucaine (Nupercaine), and tetracaine (Pontocaine) are used both topically and by injection.

Surface Anesthesia

Those local anesthetics applied as drops, sprays, lotions, creams, or ointments, also called *surface anesthetics,* are listed in Table 46-1. Distinction is made between those drugs safely applied to the eyes, skin, and mucosal areas. Only tetracaine (Pontocaine) is suitable for application to all three sites.

Most drugs for surface anesthesia are effective when applied to the skin. These drugs are poorly soluble, so little systemic absorption occurs when

Table 46-1　Local Anesthetics for Surface Anesthesia

Generic name	Trade name	Eye§	Mucous membranes†	Skin	Comments
Benzocaine	Americaine	0	0	+	Widely used. Included in many nonprescription preparations to relieve sunburn, itching, and mild burns. Long acting and poorly absorbed.
Butacaine	Butyn	0	+	0	For relief of pain from dental appliances.
Butamben	Cetacaine	0	0	+	Nonprescription ointment to relieve itching and burning. Contains benzocaine and tetracaine.
Cocaine hydro-chloride		+	+	0	Schedule II drug. Medically used in ear, nose, and throat procedures when vasoconstriction and shrinking of mucous membranes are desired. Ophthalmic preparations anesthetize cornea and conjunctiva.
Dibucaine hydrochloride	Nupercaine*	0	0	+	Nonprescription skin ointment or cream.
Dyclonine hydrochloride	Dyclone	0	+	+	Suppresses gag reflex and lessens discomfort of genitourinal endoscopy. Precipitated by the iodine of contrast media used in pyelography and should not be used.
Lidocaine Lidocaine hydro-chloride	Xylocaine* Xylocaine hydrochlo-ride*	0 0	+ +	+ +	Widely used for topical anesthesia in ear, nose, and throat procedures; upper digestive tract procedures; and genitourinary procedures. Rapid onset, and intermediate duration. Not irritating, and low incidence of hypersensitivity.
Pramoxine hydrochloride	Tronothane*	0	+‡	+	Nonprescription cream or ointment primarily used to relieve pain of itching, burns, and hemorrhoids.
Proparacaine hydrochloride	Ophthaine*	+	0	0	Applied topically to the eye to anesthetize the cornea and conjunctiva.
Tetracaine hydrochloride	Pontocaine*	+	+	+	Topically, onset is 5 min, and duration is 45 min. Usual topical dose is 20 mg; maximum, 50 mg because of toxicity and slow degradation. Ophthalmic preparations are dilute solutions for instillation.

§ + indicates suitable site for application; 0 indicates site not suitable for application.
†Mucous membranes include the bronchotracheal mucosa and the mucosa of the urethra, rectum, and vagina.
‡Not for application to the bronchotracheal mucosa.
*Available in Canada and United States.

they are applied to the skin to relieve itching or the pain of mild burns. The main potential toxicity of local anesthetics applied to the skin is allergy, usually contact dermatitis. Since several chemical classes are represented by local anesthetics, a drug from a different chemical group can be substituted if an allergy develops.

Mucosal membranes of the nose, mouth, and throat (bronchotracheal mucosa) and of the urethra, rectum, and vagina are highly vascular and allow ready absorption of the local anesthetic into systemic circulation. Application of excessive amounts of local anesthetics to mucosal surfaces is the most common

cause of systemic toxicity with local anesthetics. A local anesthetic is often used to eliminate the gag reflex when inserting an endotracheal tube or to limit the discomfort of endoscopic procedures. The lowest concentration possible of the local anesthetic should be used on mucosal surfaces to avoid systemic toxicity, and the total amount of drug should be recorded and matched against recommended total doses.

Local Anesthetics Administered by Injection

Local anesthetics used by injection are listed in Table 46-2. The potency and the duration of action increase

Table 46-2   Local Anesthetics for Injection

Generic name	Trade name	Local infiltration or nerve block or epidural block‡	Spinal block (subarachnoid)	Duration†	Comments
Bupivacaine hydrochloride	Marcaine*	+	Investigational	Long§	Provides long-acting epidural anesthesia in labor with no reported effects on fetus. Maximum dose, 200 mg.
Chloroprocaine hydrochloride	Nesacaine†	+	Investigational	Short	Little systemic toxicity because of rapid hydrolysis in plasma. No effects reported on fetus after epidural anesthesia in mother. Maximum dose, 800 mg.
Dibucaine	Nupercaine	0	+	Long	The most potent and toxic of the local anesthetics. Onset can take 15 min. Available in heavy (hyperbaric), isobaric, and light (hypobaric) solutions. Total dose, 2.5 to 10 mg, depending on use.
Etidocaine hydrochloride	Duranest	+	0	Long	Highly lipid soluble. Onset for epidural block, 5 min. Profound muscle relaxation is desirable for abdominal surgery but not for labor.
Lidocaine	Xylocaine*	+	+	Intermediate	Widely used local anesthetic. Maximum dose, 300 mg (4.5 mg/kg body weight). Can cause drowsiness, fatigue, and amnesia.
Mepivacaine	Carbocaine*	+	0	Intermediate	Chemically related to lidocaine. Maximum dose, 400 mg (7 mg/kg body weight).
Prilocaine	Citanest*	+	0	Intermediate	Maximum dose, 600 mg (8 mg/kg body weight). Useful for outpatient surgery because of the low incidence of drowsiness or fatigue as side effects. Metabolites can cause methemoglobinemia.
Procaine hydrochloride	Novocain*	+	+	Short	Noted for its safety because of its rapid hydrolysis in plasma. Maximum dose, 600 mg (10 mg/kg body weight). Duration of epidural block is unreliable.
Tetracaine	Pontocaine*	0	+	Long	The most widely used drug for spinal anesthesia. Onset, 5 min. Dose for spinal anesthesia, 2 to 15 mg. Available in hyperbaric, isobaric, and hypobaric solutions.

*+ indicates suitable use; 0 indicates use not suitable.
†Duration without epinephrine: short, 1 hr; intermediate, 2 hr; long, 3 hr (approximations).
*Available in Canada and United States.
§Duration of bupivacaine in nerve block is 6 to 13 hr.

together with the lipid solubility of the drug. The onset of anesthesia is determined by the concentration of drug and the size of the nerve. Before infiltrating an area with a local anesthetic, the syringe should first be aspirated to ensure that a blood vessel has not been entered. This is because the concentration of drug is high and could prove fatal if injected systemically.

The area affected by a local anesthetic depends on how and where it is injected. The anesthesia produced is described by the technique of injection—infiltration, nerve block, epidural, and spinal. These techniques are described with their potential for producing toxic side effects.

Infiltration anesthesia refers to the superficial application of a local anesthetic. To suture a cut or to perform dental procedures, local anesthetic is injected superficially in small amounts to block the small nerves and to numb the area. To work on the scalp or to make an incision in the skin, the anesthetic is infused around the area. Small incisions require a small volume and a low concentration of drug, so little toxicity is associated with these uses. However, systemic toxicity from local anesthetics is frequently seen in the emergency room when large cuts are infiltrated with local anesthetic.

Nerve block anesthesia refers to the injection of a local anesthetic along a nerve before it reaches the surgical site. The volume and concentration of a local anesthetic for a nerve block must be larger than in infiltration anesthesia to penetrate the larger nerve.

The most extensive field of local anesthesia is achieved by applying the local anesthetic around the nerve roots near the spinal cord to produce epidural or spinal anesthesia. As shown in Figure 46-1, the spinal cord proper ends at the lumbar region. The

spinal cord is surrounded by three membranes—first the pia mater, then the arachnoid, and finally the outer membrane, the dura mater. These membranes extend below the spinal cord proper to form a sac in the lumbar and sacral region. The dura mater and arachnoid membranes are close together, and the subarachnoid space is between the arachnoid and pia mater. Cerebrospinal fluid fills the subarachnoid space throughout the spinal cord.

For **epidural anesthesia,** the local anesthetic is administered outside the dura mater (see Figure 46-1) so that the nerve roots are blocked at the point after they emerge from the dura mater. The extent of anesthesia depends on the volume and concentration of local anesthetic used. **Caudal anesthesia** is another form of epidural anesthesia and is achieved by administering the local anesthetic epidurally at the base of the spine (see Figure 46-1). The extent of anesthesia affects only the pelvic region and legs. Caudal anesthesia is used for obstetrics and for surgery on the rectum, anus, and prostate gland.

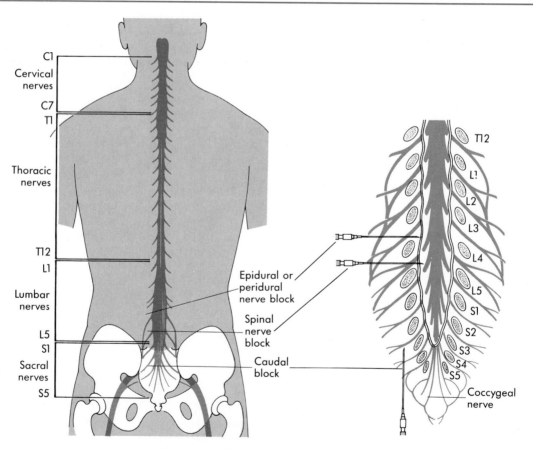

FIGURE 46-1
Sites for injection of local anesthetic to achieve spinal, epidural, and caudal anesthesia.

Spinal anesthesia is achieved by injecting local anesthetic into the subarachnoid space between the arachnoid and pia mater membranes in the lumbar area, usually between the second lumbar and first sacral vertebrae and well below the spinal cord proper. This blocks the nerve roots for the entire lower body. If the solution containing local anesthetic has the same density (isobaric) as cerebrospinal fluid and is administered slowly, it will stay where it is injected and will only slowly diffuse into the rest of the cerebrospinal fluid. The solution of local anesthetic can be made more dense (hyperbaric) by diluting the local anesthetic into 5% dextrose. The solution will then move downward (toward the ground). If the patient is on a tilt bed with feet high and head low, the hyperbaric solution will travel up the spinal cord toward the head and anesthetize more of the body. The solution of local anesthetic also can be diluted with distilled water to be less dense (hypobaric). In patients positioned on the tilt bed, this solution would move to the end of the dura mater and anesthetize only the lower part of the body. Procedures using hypobaric and hyperbaric solutions of local anesthetic require skill in positioning patients. If the level of anesthesia is adjusted to block more of the spinal cord than just the lumbar and sacral regions, there is danger of paralyzing the intercostal and phrenic nerves, thereby paralyzing spontaneous respiration.

If the patient is seated when the local anesthetic is administered as a low spinal anesthetic, only those nerves affecting the parts of the body that would be in contact with a saddle are affected, hence the name *saddle block.* This procedure is used principally in obstetrics for vaginal delivery.

With spinal anesthesia the patient is awake, breathing and cardiovascular function are not immediately affected, and good muscle relaxation is present. These are advantages for patients with heart and lung disease or for elderly persons. However, the sympathetic fibers to the blood vessels are blocked, so vasodilation with hypotension is a frequent side effect of spinal anesthesia. Spinal anesthesia is therefore considered hazardous for abdominal surgery in poor-risk patients because of the potential for sudden vasodilation and hypotension. Spinal anesthesia is widely used in obstetrics, particularly for cesarean sections.

Duration of action

The rate at which local anesthetic is removed from the infiltrated area depends largely on the degree of vascularization. The duration can be increased by 50% to 100% with the inclusion of epinephrine, 1:200,000, or phenylephrine to cause vasoconstriction and thereby restrict systemic absorption. However, epinephrine is contraindicated for infiltration of areas with end arteries (fingers, toes, ears, nose, and penis), since the resultant ischemia may lead to tissue death. Similarly, the addition of a vasoconstrictor is contraindicated in epidural anesthesia in labor because of the potential vasoconstriction of the uterine blood vessels with a resultant decrease in placental circulation. Epinephrine is also contraindicated for patients with severe cardiovascular disease or thyrotoxicosis, in whom cardiac function would be compromised by added vasoconstrictors.

Spinal anesthesia can cause variable hypotension because the neurons controlling vasomotor tone are in the spinal tract. A severe headache may be experienced after spinal anesthesia and may last for hours or days after the anesthetic has worn off. This postspinal headache is believed to reflect a drop in the pressure of the cerebrospinal fluid caused by a leak where the dura mater was penetrated. Incidence of a spinal headache is reduced when patients are kept flat on their backs and instructed not to raise their heads for 12 hr after spinal anesthesia. This minimizes the hydrostatic pressure of the cerebrospinal fluid on the head.

NURSING IMPLICATIONS SUMMARY

Drug administration

◆ Obtain a careful history of previous response to local anesthetics. Remember that "Novocain" is often used by patients to refer to any local anesthetic, regardless of the actual drug.

◆ Monitor the blood pressure and pulse. If epidural, nerve block, or spinal anesthesia is used, monitor respirations. If anesthesia is used during labor and delivery, assess fetal heart tones.

◆ After spinal anesthesia, keep patients flat, usually up to 12 hr. Transfer patients flat from the stretcher to the bed. Use a thin pillow.

◆ Assess patients who have had epidural, nerve block, or spinal anesthesia for ability to void or for a distended bladder. Monitor intake and output. If the patient has not voided in 8 hr after surgery or delivery, notify the physician.

◆ Assist patients who have received epidural, nerve block, or spinal anesthesia when ambulating for the first time.

◆ Position patients carefully in bed after epidural, nerve block, or spinal anesthesia, since they have no sensation to warn of wrinkles, tight sheets, or other skin irritants.

◆ Apply heat or cold to anesthetized area with extreme caution, since patients will be unable to indicate if irritation or burning occurs. If applying heat or cold is necessary, shield the skin well from the heat or cold source, and check patients and the skin surfaces every 5 to 15 min. This applies after oral or dental anesthesia also.

◆ Although serious systemic reactions are rare with local anesthetics, drugs, equipment, and personnel to treat acute allergic reactions should be available in settings where local anesthetics are used.

◆ Patients in the operating or delivery rooms who are receiving local anesthesia may be drowsy from preoperative medications but will usually be alert and able to understand conversation in the room. Keep conversation and noise to a minimum. Avoid discussing other patients, complications, pathology reports, or other inappropriate topics that might alarm the patient.

◆ After bronchoscopy or other procedures in which surface anesthesia may have been applied to the back of the throat, assess the gag reflex and ability to swallow. Do not leave patients unattended until they can safely handle secretions.

Patient and family education

◆ After dental work or injection of anesthetics into tongue, lips, and gums, caution patients to avoid eating or chewing until sensation returns. Patients may inadvertently bite their tongue or cheek.

◆ Tell patients to report any rash or skin irritation occurring as a result of local anesthetic application.

◆ If patients develop an allergic or untoward response to a local anesthetic, instruct them to wear a medical identification tag or bracelet indicating the causative agent.

◆ Instruct patients to use surface anesthetics as instructed and not to increase the frequency of application or to use the preparation on skin surfaces for which it was not designed.

◆ Before discharge, review any limitations the patient may have until the effects of the anesthetic wear off. For example, patients who have had local anesthesia to a joint may be instructed to avoid use of the joint for a certain number of hours or until the anesthesia has worn off.

CHAPTER REVIEW

◆ KEY TERMS

caudal anesthesia, p. 688
epidural anesthesia, p. 688
infiltration anesthesia, p. 687
local anesthetic, p. 685
nerve block anesthesia, p. 688
saddle block, p. 689
spinal anesthesia, p. 689
surface anesthetic, p. 685

◆ REVIEW QUESTIONS

1. What is the mechanism of action of local anesthetics?
2. What property of procaine and chloroprocaine makes them relatively safe?
3. What are toxic effects of systemic absorption of local anesthetics?
4. To what three types of surfaces are local anesthetics applied?
5. Describe the areas of anesthesia achieved by infiltration, nerve block, epidural, and spinal anesthesia.
6. What hazards are associated with spinal anesthesia?
7. How is the duration of local anesthetics prolonged?

SUGGESTED READING

Burden N: Regional anesthesia: what patients and nurses need to know, *RN* 51(5):56, 1988.
Curran MA: Epidural anesthesia: practical considerations, *Curr Rev Nurse Anesth* 10(22):170, 1988.
Komar W: Spinal anaesthesia for the orthopaedic surgical patient, *CONA J* 10(4):6, 1988.
Proposed recommended practices: monitoring the patient receiving local anesthesia, *AORN J* 49(2):623, 1989.

DRUGS TO CONTROL DISORDERS OF CENTRAL MUSCLE CONTROL

Section XI discusses anticonvulsants and drugs to control involuntary muscle movements. Chapter 47, Anticonvulsants, reviews the classification of seizures. The anticonvulsants are presented by drug class but also are referenced for their role in controlling specific seizure patterns. Chapter 48, Central Motor Control: Drugs for Parkinsonism and Centrally Acting Skeletal Muscle Relaxants, covers drugs used to treat disorders of central motor control, in two sections. The first section presents the drug classes used to treat parkinsonism and discusses step therapy to control the symptoms of parkinsonism and the role of these drugs in treating the drug-induced parkinsonian symptoms. The second section presents drugs to control spasticity and drugs acting centrally to relieve local muscle spasms.

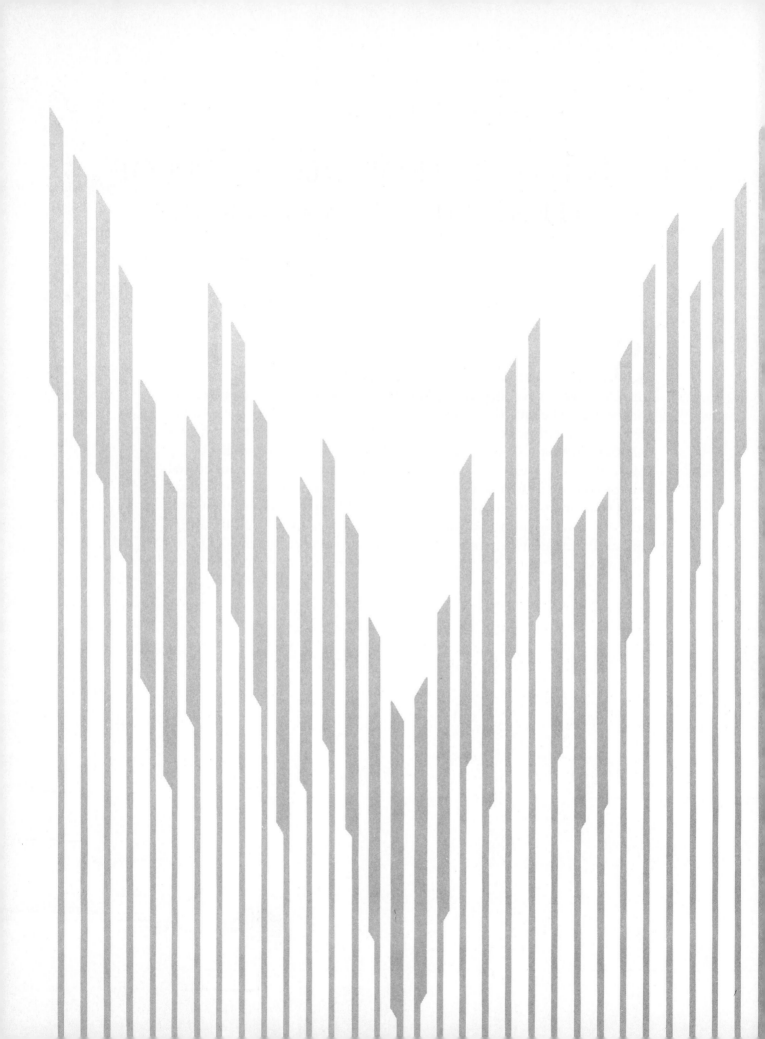

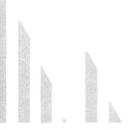

CHAPTER 47

Anticonvulsants

LEARNING OBJECTIVES

After studying this chapter, you should be able to do the following:

◆ Define epilepsy, and describe the characteristics of the following types of seizures: grand mal, petit mal or absence, infantile spasms, myoclonus epilepsy, psychomotor epilepsy, focal seizures, and status epilepticus.

◆ Discuss principles of drug therapy for epilepsy.

◆ Develop a care plan for patients receiving phenobarbital or another barbiturate, phenytoin, ethosuximide or a related drug, trimethadione, diazepam or another benzodiazepine, carbamazepine, and valproic acid or a related drug.

◆ Explain the use of acetazolamide, paraldehyde, and adrenocorticotropic hormone (ACTH) as anticonvulsants.

◆ Develop a teaching plan for a patient receiving drug therapy for control of seizures.

CHAPTER OVERVIEW

◆ Anticonvulsants are used to control seizures. The objective of drug therapy is to control seizures as completely as possible without causing intolerable side effects. Therapy is individualized for the drug or drug combinations used and for their doses.

Nursing Process Overview

ANTICONVULSANTS

Assessment

Most patients using anticonvulsant drugs have had a seizure, and drug treatment is needed on a long-term basis. Obtain a baseline assessment, with special emphasis on areas known to be affected by the drugs to be used. For example, since phenytoin can cause gingival hyperplasia, assess mouth, teeth, and gums at the start of and periodically during therapy.

Nursing Diagnoses

High risk for gingival hyperplasia
Altered comfort: nausea and gastrointestinal distress associated with drug ingestion

Management

Drug dosages are adjusted until seizures are controlled or toxic effects are noted. Monitor the general condition of the patient with an emphasis on known drug side effects. Monitor serum levels of the prescribed drugs if available. If the patient continues to have seizures, observe type, duration, and characteristics of the seizure, and continue nursing measures to prevent injury such as padding side rails or supervising ambulation. Refer the patient to health department, social services, or vocational rehabilitation, if appropriate.

Evaluation

Long-term drug therapy often produces side effects. The health-care team then must decide which side effects cannot be permitted and which can be treated or tolerated. Evaluate the patient regularly through observation, reassess known problem areas (e.g., the mouth with phenytoin therapy), and make appropriate referrals.

Before discharge, verify that the patient or family can name the drugs being taken and how to take them correctly, including dose, time of day, and correct preparation; and can explain side effects that may occur, which need to be reported immediately, how to treat or prevent those that are more likely to occur, and what to do if a dose is missed. Determine that the patient can state the importance of wearing a medical identification tag or bracelet.

EPILEPSY

Epilepsy is a neurologic disorder characterized by a recurrent pattern of abnormal neuronal discharges within the brain, resulting in a sudden loss or disturbance of consciousness, sometimes in association with motor activity, sensory phenomena, or inappropriate behavior. Between 1% and 2% of the population is estimated to have epilepsy. The cause of epilepsy may be unknown (idiopathic) or may be traced to a known brain lesion. In general, epilepsy appearing in childhood or adolescence is likely to be idiopathic, whereas epilepsy appearing in adulthood is likely to relate to a definable cause such as a head injury, cerebrovascular accident (stroke), or brain tumor.

An appropriate choice of drugs, taken on a long-term basis, can control the seizures of epilepsy in about 80% of patients. The choice of drugs depends on a careful diagnosis of the seizure pattern, which ideally is made from the observation of a seizure and the recording of the brain wave pattern with an electroencephalogram (EEG) during the seizure. The diagnosis is critical to the selection of a drug or drugs, since different seizure patterns are controlled by different drugs. Other causes of seizures must be ruled out, since seizures may be secondary to an organic disorder such as a brain tumor, poisoning, fever, hypoglycemia, and hypocalcemia. Overdose of certain drugs such as local anesthetics and ketamine causes seizures. Abrupt withdrawal of some drugs such as the barbiturates and most other sedative-hypnotic drugs, including alcohol, can precipitate seizures.

CATEGORIES OF EPILEPSY

Epilepsy is described most frequently by the classification published by the International League

Table 47-1   International Classification of Seizures

Class	Specific signs and symptoms
Generalized seizures: without focal onset, symmetric on both brain hemispheres. Consciousness is lost unless otherwise indicated.	1. Tonic-clonic seizures (grand mal) 2. Tonic seizures: sustained contraction of a large muscle group 3. Clonic seizures: arrhythmic contractions of parts of the body 4. Absence seizures (petit mal): brief loss of consciousness, 3 spikes/sec on EEG 5. Bilateral massive epileptic myoclonus (consciousness is usually not altered) and isolated clonic jerks 6. Infantile spasms: muscle spasms and bizarre EEG 7. Atonic seizures: loss of postural tone with sagging of the head (head drop) or falling down 8. Akinetic seizures: complete relaxation of all muscles
Partial seizures: focal seizures.	1. Elementary symptoms, consciousness not lost 　a. Motor symptoms (jacksonian). 　b. Sensory (hallucinations—visual, auditory, and taste) or somatosensory (tingling) symptoms 　c. Autonomic symptoms 　d. Compound forms 2. Complex symptoms, consciousness impaired (temporal lobe or psychomotor epilepsy) 　a. Cognitive symptoms: confusion, and memory distorted 　b. Affective symptoms: bizarre behavior 　c. Psychosensory symptoms: automatisms—repetitive, purposeless behaviors
Unilateral seizures: only half of brain involved.	
Unclassified: incomplete data.	

Against Epilepsy in 1970. This classification is presented in Table 47-1. This classification describes the seizure pattern by the area of the brain involved.

Partial and Generalized Seizures

Partial and generalized seizures are the two major categories of epilepsy. These are pictured in Figure 47-1. **Partial seizures** arise from a focal lesion of the brain in which the abnormal discharge of cells involves a limited area. The location of the lesion determines the type of seizure observed—motor, cognitive, behavioral, or sensory. Consciousness is usually not lost, but patients may not remember seizure episodes when cognitive or behavioral function is involved. Focal and psychomotor seizures are examples of partial seizures that are discussed more fully. **Generalized seizures** result from the discharge of cells over both sides of the brain. Grand mal seizures, petit mal seizures, infantile spasms, and myoclonic seizures are examples of generalized seizures which are described more fully.

Tonic-clonic epilepsy

Grand mal or **tonic-clonic epilepsy** involves the contraction of all skeletal muscles. Before the seizure begins, the patient may experience an **aura.** An aura is a sensation peculiar for that patient, which can be a visual disturbance or a certain dizziness or numbness that warns the patient of an impending seizure. The patient then suddenly loses consciousness and may utter a cry as the diaphragm contracts and expels air from the lungs. The seizure consists of sustained (tonic) contractions or intermittent (clonic) contractions of the muscles. The patient may become incon-

tinent. When the contractions cease, the patient regains consciousness. Usually, the patient is confused and drowsy and lapses into prolonged sleep (postictal depression).

Absence epilepsy

Petit mal or **absence epilepsy** occurs mainly in children 4 to 12 years of age. The child suddenly loses consciousness for a few seconds, although body tone is seldom lost, and consciousness is regained with no confusion. The appearance is one of inattention or daydreaming and may be accompanied by slight blinking or hand movements. Attacks usually occur several times a day. The EEG shows a 3/sec spike wave pattern. Absence epilepsy does not generally continue into adulthood, but many patients with absence epilepsy subsequently develop other types of epilepsy, particularly tonic-clonic epilepsy. Thus many physicians treat children prophylactically for tonic-clonic epilepsy in addition to treating absence epilepsy. Some evidence suggests that this prophylactic treatment reduces the incidence of subsequent tonic-clonic epilepsy.

Infantile spasms

Infantile spasms denote a major generalized seizure that occurs in the first year of life. The seizure consists of a sudden, transient, repetitive contraction of the limbs and trunk. A sudden shocklike jerk is accompanied by a sharp cry. The legs are extended, and the arms are brought forward in front of the head. These spasms may occur hundreds of times a day and are believed to originate from a congenital malformation or neonatal injury and to reflect an immature nervous

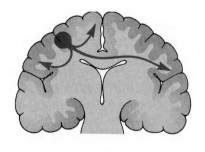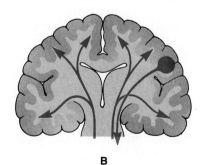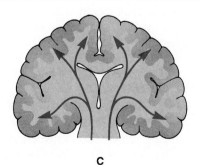

A   B   C

FIGURE 47-1

Schematic representation of how seizures spread. **A,** Focal seizure with spread to adjacent areas. This gives rise to partial seizures. **B,** Focal seizure that gives rise to generalized seizure. **C,** Primary generalized seizure.

system. If the seizures persist after 1 year of age, the seizure pattern changes, usually to a petit mal seizure, a myoclonic seizure, or a head drop seizure in which consciousness is lost for 10 to 15 min, accompanied by a loss of muscle tone in the neck.

Myoclonus epilepsy

Myoclonus epilepsy is a generalized seizure pattern that develops secondary to anoxic brain damage (intentional myoclonus) or as a genetic disorder (progressive myoclonic epilepsy). Intentional myoclonus is a neurologic symptom consisting of sudden involuntary contractions of skeletal muscles, which are aggravated by purposeful activity (hence the term *intentional*) and by visual, auditory, tactile, and emotional activity. Progressive myoclonic epilepsy is a particular form of intentional myoclonus that appears in childhood and becomes progressively worse. When untreated, the genetic disease leads to death after 15 to 20 years.

Psychomotor epilepsy

Temporal lobe or **psychomotor epilepsy** has complex symptoms that include an aura, automatism, and motor seizures, independently or in combination. These seizures usually last about 5 min. The patient remembers the aura but not the automatism or motor seizure. The **automatism** may consist of chewing or swallowing motions, tempermental changes, confusion, feelings of unreality, or unexplained, bizarre behavior. A detailed neurologic examination may be required to differentiate psychomotor epilepsy from psychotic mental illness.

Focal seizures

Focal seizures are not associated with a loss of consciousness. Focal sensory seizures may be visual such as flashes of light; tactile such as a feeling of numbness or tingling; or motor. Focal motor seizures of the jacksonian type begin with clonic seizures of a few muscles on half of the face or in one extremity; the seizures then progresses (march) to include more body musculature (e.g., finger, hand, and arm).

Status epilepticus

Status epilepticus refers to seizures that last 30 min or longer or that are repeated for 30 min or longer and during which consciousness is not regained. Status epilepticus of the generalized tonic-clonic type is a medical emergency. In about 80% of patients, seizures are secondary to a disease, frequently associated with a low blood concentration of calcium or glucose, or secondary to withdrawal from drugs such as the barbiturates or other sedative-hypnotics. The immediate goals are to establish an airway, to stop the seizures, and then to identify their cause.

DRUGS TO CONTROL SEIZURES
General Principles of Drug Therapy for Epilepsy

Several drugs are available for control of epileptic seizures. The drug choice depends on diagnosis of the seizure patterns and on the tolerance and response of the patient to the drug prescribed. Drugs most frequently effective for various seizure patterns are listed in Table 47-2. Table 47-3 lists dosage information for these drugs.

Mechanism of action

The molecular mechanism by which the anticonvulsant drugs act is not understood. In general, these drugs depress the excitability of neurons, particularly those that fire inappropriately to initiate the seizure and thus prevent the spread of seizure discharges. Presumably the mechanisms will be found to modify the ionic movements of sodium, potassium, or calcium across the nerve membrane associated with the action potential or the release or uptake of neurotransmitters.

Because specific mechanisms underlying seizure activity are not understood, development of better drugs for controlling seizures is a matter of screening drugs using animal models that incompletely parallel human seizure disorders.

Drug administration

The drug of choice is started in small doses to allow the patient to develop a tolerance to the drowsiness and motor incoordination (ataxia) associated with most of the anticonvulsant drugs. The exception is phenytoin (Dilantin), initially given in a high loading dose. The dose is increased until the seizures are stopped or until toxic effects of the drug appear. If the drug has been partly effective in controlling seizures, a second drug may be added. If the first drug tried is not effective, the patient is switched to a different one.

Since the most common cause of drug failure is the failure of the patient to take the prescribed drugs, the plasma concentration of drug may be determined before deciding that the drug is ineffective. Patients must be warned not to discontinue medication when the seizures are under control or when the side effects are disturbing. The sudden discontinuance of medication greatly increases the incidence of seizures. Blood and urine analyses often are routinely carried out because many anticonvulsant drugs infrequently produce blood dyscrasias or renal damage.

Many patients with epilepsy require drug therapy throughout their lives to control seizures. However, some patients can discontinue medication. These patients are those reaching adulthood after childhood treatment for absence epilepsy and those patients who

Table 47-2   Drug Choice by Seizure Type

Seizure type	First-choice drugs	Additional drugs for second-choice drugs	Refractory cases
General: tonic-clonic (grand mal)	Carbamazepine Phenytoin Valproic acid	Phenobarbital Primidone	Acetazolamide Bromides, inorganic Ethotoin Mephenytoin Mephobarbital
Partial: cortical focal (including jacksonian)	Carbamazepine Phenytoin	Phenobarbital Primidone Valproic acid	Acetazolamide Clorazepate Ethotoin Mephenytoin Methsuximide Phenacemide
General: absence (petit mal)	Ethosuximide Valproic acid	Clonazepam	Acetazolaminde Clorazepate Methsuximide Phensuximide Paramethadione Trimethadione
General: myoclonus (intentional or progressive)	Valproic acid	Clonazepam	Bromides, inorganic Carbamazepine Clorazepate Methsuximide Phenobarbital Phenytoin
General: infantile spasms	ACTH/corticosteroids	Valproic acid	Clonazepam Nitrazepam
Partial: complex (temporal lobe and psychomotor)	Valproic acid	Clonazepam Phenobarbital Methsuximide	Carbamazepine Phenytoin
Status epilepticus: continuous tonic-clonic	Diazepam Lorazepam	Phenytoin Phenobarbital	Paraldehyde

Table 47-3   Anticonvulsant Drugs

Generic name	Trade name	Administration/dosage	Comments
LONG-ACTING BARBITURATES			
Mephobarbital	Mebaral*	ORAL: *Adults*—400 to 600 mg daily in divided doses. FDA Pregnancy Category D. *Children over 5 years*—32 to 64 mg 3 or 4 times daily; *under 5 years*—16 to 32 mg 3 or 4 times daily.	Metabolized to phenobarbital.
Phenobarbital	Luminal*	ORAL: *Adults*—50 to 100 mg 2 or 3 times daily. FDA Pregnancy Category D. *Children*—15 to 50 mg 2 or 3 times daily.	May begin at twice usual dose for the first 4 days to raise plasma concentration rapidly. Multiple daily doses are to minimize sedation. Effective serum concentration, 15 to 40 µg/ml. In addition to its use for epileptic seizures, phenobarbital is used prophylactically for febrile seizures in children.

Continued.

Table 47-3 Anticonvulsant Drugs—cont'd

Generic name	Trade name	Administration/dosage	Comments
LONG-ACTING BARBITURATES—cont'd			
Phenobarbital—cont'd	Luminal Sodium*	INTRAMUSCULAR, INTRAVENOUS (SLOW): *Adults*—200 to 320 mg, can repeat after 6 hr. INTRAMUSCULAR: *Children*—3 to 5 mg/kg body weight.	For status epilepticus. Sodium salt must be used for injection.
Primidone	Apo-Primidone† Myidone Mysoline*	ORAL: *Adults*—250 mg daily at bedtime or up to 2 gm daily in divided doses. FDA Pregnancy Category D. *Children over 8 years*—as for adults; *under 8 years*—½ adult dosage.	Effective serum concentrations, 5 to 10 µg/ml.
HYDANTOINS			
Ethotoin	Peganone	ORAL: *Adults*—1000 mg daily, increased gradually to 2000 to 3000 mg in 4 to 6 divided doses. *Children*—500 to 1000 mg in divided doses.	
Mephenytoin	Mesantoin*	ORAL: *Adults*—200 to 600 mg daily. *Children*—100 to 400 mg daily.	
Phenytoin	Dilantin*	ORAL: *Adults*—300 mg daily in 3 doses; maintenance dose, 300 to 600 mg daily. *Children*—5 mg/kg body weight daily in 2 or 3 doses; maximum, 300 mg daily.	May be given once a day to improve compliance. Effective serum concentration, 10 to 20 µg/ml. Brand name should be specified because of varying bioavailability.
SUCCINIMIDES			
Ethosuximide	Zarontin*	ORAL: *Adults*—500 mg daily, increased gradually every 4 to 7 days to control seizures. *Children over 6 years*—as for adults; *3 to 6 years*—250 mg daily, increased gradually to control seizures.	Effective serum concentration, 40 to 80 µg/ml.
Methsuximide	Celontin*	ORAL: 300 mg daily for 1 week, increased weekly by 300 mg to control seizures to a maximum dose of 1200 mg daily.	
Phensuximide	Milontin*	ORAL: 500 to 1000 mg 2 or 3 times daily.	
OXAZOLIDINEDIONE			
Trimethadione	Tridione Trimedone†	ORAL: *Adults*—900 mg daily in 3 or 4 doses, can increase by 300 mg daily every 7 days to control seizures; maximum, 2400 mg daily. FDA Pregnancy Category D. *Children*—40 mg/kg body weight daily in 3 or 4 doses.	No longer widely used because of serious side effects and high teratogenic potential. Effective serum concentration of dimethadione (active metabolite), 700 µg/ml or higher.

*Available in Canada and United States.
†Available in Canada only.

Table 47-3   Anticonvulsant Drugs—cont'd

Generic name	Trade name	Administration/dosage	Comments
BENZODIAZEPINES			
Clonazepam	Klonopin Rivotril*	ORAL: *Adults*—1.5 mg daily in 3 doses, increase every 3 days by 0.5 to 1 mg to control seizures; maximum total dose, 20 mg daily. *Infants and children to 10 years*—0.01 to 0.03 mg/kg body weight, increased by 0.25 to 0.5 mg every 3 days to control seizures to maximum dose of 0.2 mg/kg daily.	Effective therapeutic plasma concentrations, 5 to 70 mg/ml.
Diazepam	Valium*	INTRAVENOUS, to terminate status epilepticus: *Adults*—5 to 10 mg (no faster than 5 mg/min, use large vein); can repeat every 10 to 15 min to maximum dose of 30 mg. *Children 30 days to 5 years*—0.2 to 0.5 mg slowly every 2 to 5 min, maximum, 5 mg; *over 5 years*—1 mg slowly every 2 to 5 min; maximum, 10 mg.	See Chapter 40 for use as an antianxiety drug. Rarely used orally as an anticonvulsant agent. Do not mix or dilute into IV fluids.
Lorazepam	Ativan	INTRAVENOUS: *Adults*—4 mg given over 2 min. Maximum dose, 8 mg. *Children*—0.05 to 0.1 mg/kg given over 2 min. Maximum dose, 0.2 mg/kg.	Drug of choice for initial control of status epilepticus. Duration of lorazepam is considerably longer than for diazepam.
MISCELLANEOUS			
Acetazolamide	Acetazolam† Diamox*	ORAL: *Adults and children*—8 to 30 mg/kg body weight in divided doses.	Weak diuretic. Tolerance usually develops.
Adrenocorticotropic hormone (ACTH)		INTRAMUSCULAR: *Infants*—10 units daily, increase by 5 units every 5 days up to 60 units for 6 to 7 weeks.	If ACTH is ineffective, diazepam, 3 mg/lb, is added. If ACTH is effective in 2 weeks, may switch to cortisone, 3 mg/lb, as an alternative to increasing ACTH. Cortisone is brought down by 1 mg/lb over 3 weeks.
Carbamazepine	Epitol-Mazepine† Tegretol* Various others	ORAL: *Adults and children over 12 years*—200 mg twice on day 1, increase by 200 mg daily to control seizures; maximum, 1000 mg (less than 15 years) or 1200 mg (over 15 years). Doses taken every 6 to 8 hr. FDA Pregnancy Category C.	Take medication with meals to avoid GI distress. Effective therapeutic plasma concentrations, 4 to 12 μg/ml.
Paraldehyde		INTRAMUSCULAR, INTRAVENOUS, to terminate status epilepticus: *Adults and children*—0.15 ml/kg body weight. Solution must be diluted. RECTAL: *Children*—0.3 ml/kg diluted 1:1 in olive oil or milk.	Last resort for terminating status epilepticus.

*Available in Canada and United States.
†Available in Canada only.

Continued.

Table 47-3 Anticonvulsant Drugs—cont'd

Generic name	Trade name	Administration/dosage	Comments
MISCELLANEOUS—cont'd			
Valproic acid	Dalpro Depakene*	ORAL: *Adults and children*—15 mg/ kg body weight daily in divided doses. Can be increased by 5 to 10 mg/kg daily every 7 days to control seizures, up to 60 mg/kg daily. FDA Pregnancy Category D.	Effective in controlling myoclonic epilepsy refractory to most other anticonvulsant drugs. Effective serum concentrations reported to be 50 to 100 µg/ml. Also effective for petit mal seizures.
Divalproex	Depakote	ORAL: *Adults*—Initially, 5 to 15 mg/ kg daily; usual maintenance dose is 10 to 20 mg/kg/daily. Children 1 to 12 years—Initially, 10 to 30 mg/ kg/daily. Maintenance dose, 20 to 30 mg/kg/daily.	Combination of the acidic and salt forms of valproic acid. There is a sprinkle form that can be added to food.

*Available in Canada and United States.
†Available in Canada only.

have had several seizure-free years. If the EEG of such a patient appears normal, medication can be gradually discontinued. Seizures recur in 25% to 50% of such patients.

Therapy and pregnancy

Females with epilepsy who want children should be advised that their children carry a two-fold to three-fold greater risk of having congenital defects, particularly when the mother is taking phenytoin (Dilantin) or phenobarbital (Luminal). In the absence of any medication, the fetus is still at greater-than-normal risk because of anoxia during seizures. Pregnancies during which the mother takes trimethadione (Tridione) are associated with an 80% incidence of spontaneous abortions or birth defects. If possible, females taking trimethadione should be switched to ethosuximide (Zarontin) before becoming pregnant.

Long-Acting Barbiturates
Phenobarbital

Phenobarbital (Luminal) has been widely used for 60 years and is a drug of choice to treat grand mal and focal seizures. It is also used to treat withdrawal from barbiturates or alcohol. Phenobarbital is cross-tolerant with alcohol and other barbiturates but requires only once-a-day administration because of its long plasma half-life of 4 days. Because of this long plasma half-life, 14 days are required to reach constant serum concentrations. Phenobarbital is sometimes given intravenously to stop the seizures of status epilepticus, but the degree of respiratory depression can be profound.

The main side effects of the barbiturates are sedation and drowsiness at the beginning of treatment, but tolerance usually develops to these effects. In elderly patients and in children a paradoxical excitement may be seen that impairs learning ability. Phenobarbital increases the incidence of congenital malformations in the fetus but not to the degree associated with phenytoin and trimethadione. Phenobarbital induces liver microsomal enzymes and thus can speed its own metabolism and that of other drugs. Sudden rather than gradual withdrawal of the drug can precipitate convulsions. Barbiturates are contraindicated for patients with the metabolic disorder porphyria and for patients who are depressed and might consider suicide.

Mephobarbital

Mephobarbital (Mebanal) is metabolized by the liver to phenobarbital. Therefore there is no advantage to substituting mephobarbital for phenobarbital.

Primidone

Primidone (Mysoline) is a deoxybarbiturate that is metabolized to phenobarbital and phenylethylmalonamide. Primidone can therefore substitute for phenobarbital to treat grand mal and focal seizures but in addition is effective in treating psychomotor epilepsy.

Hydantoins
Phenytoin

Phenytoin (Dilantin), formerly called diphenylhydantoin, is a drug of choice in controlling grand mal and focal motor epilepsy in adults and is occasionally used in treating psychomotor epilepsy.

Pharmacokinetics. Phenytoin has a plasma half-life of 24 hr, so it takes 4 days to reach steady plasma levels when initiating therapy. To decrease this time, the initial dose is sometimes given as a loading dose at three times the usual daily dose. At serum concentrations much above therapeutic concentrations, the capacity of the liver to metabolize phenytoin is saturated so that plasma concentrations decrease very slowly. Phenytoin is irregularly absorbed from the intestine. Since absorption depends on formulation, it is best to stay with a particular brand of phenytoin.

Phenytoin should not be given intramuscularly or subcutaneously because it is highly irritating and can precipitate in the tissue. The sodium salt can be administered intravenously, but too-rapid administration can produce severe hypotension and cardiac arrest. Sodium phenytoin is administered intravenously to control status epilepticus alone or after IV diazepam has controlled the seizures. IV sodium phenytoin is also used to control some cardiac arrhythmias (see Chapter 19).

Adverse effects. Effective serum concentrations are 10 to 20 μg/ml, and side effects are seen at higher serum concentrations. At greater than 20 μg/ml, involuntary movement of the eyeballs (nystagmus) appears; at greater than 30 μg/ml, ataxia and slurred speech arise. Tremors and nervousness or drowsiness and fatigue may be side effects of higher serum concentrations. However, an acute overdose of phenytoin is seldom fatal. Persistence of these side effects requires reducing the dose or switching to another drug, usually phenobarbital.

About 20% of patients taking phenytoin experience overgrowth of the gums (gingival hyperplasia), which is particularly severe in children. Occasionally, folic acid or vitamin D deficiency can be produced, since phenytoin interferes with the normal metabolism of these compounds. Phenytoin can also cause an allergic rash that can be mistaken for measles or infectious mononucleosis. Phenytoin also worsens acne, which is especially bothersome to teenagers and can increase growth of body hair (hirsutism), which is undesirable in females. There is a higher incidence of congenital malformations in infants of mothers taking phenytoin. These infants are also at risk for hemorrhage and coagulation deficiencies at birth, which can be corrected with vitamin K.

Drug interactions. Important drugs interactions are noted with phenytoin. Phenobarbital can increase the metabolism of phenytoin in some individuals by inducing liver microsomal enzymes, but in others, phenobarbital decreases the rate of drug metabolism of phenytoin by competing with the enzymes for degradation. The oral anticoagulant dicumarol and the anticonvulsant carbamazepine decrease the metabolism of phenytoin by competing with the enzymes for degradation. The anticonvulsant valproic acid displaces bound phenytoin from protein to increase the free concentration of phenytoin while decreasing its total concentration, since more free phenytoin is available for metabolism. Phenytoin enhances the rate of estrogen metabolism, which can decrease the effectiveness of some birth control pills.

Others

Other anticonvulsant drugs related to phenytoin are mephenytoin (Mesantoin) and ethotoin (Peganone). Mephenytoin is associated with a high incidence of agranulocytosis and aplastic anemia. Ethotoin is not widely used, although it does not seem to cause gingival hyperplasia, hirsutism, or ataxia.

Succinimides

Ethosuximide

Ethosuximide (Zarontin) is a drug of choice for controlling petit mal seizures and may be effective in treating myoclonic seizures. The plasma half-life is 30 hr in children and 60 hr in adults. The effective serum concentration is 40 to 80 μg/ml, but serum concentrations of up to 160 μg/ml can be tolerated without excessive toxicity. Side effects include dizziness, drowsiness, and gastrointestinal (GI) irritation. Blood counts are performed routinely because of the occasional occurrence of agranulocytosis. Related drugs are phensuximide (Milontin), which is sometimes effective in treating psychomotor epilepsy, and methsuximide (Celontin).

Oxazolidinediones

Trimethadione

Trimethadione (Tridione) was the first drug effective in controlling absence epilepsy, but it is now a third-choice drug for petit-mal seizures because of the high incidence of serious side effects.

Trimethadione can produce serious allergic dermatitis, kidney and liver damage, agranulocytosis, and aplastic anemia. Blood counts and urinalyses are done routinely with trimethadione therapy. In adults the drug frequently produces an intolerance to light (photophobia). The incidence of spontaneous abortions or congenital anomalies in infants of mothers taking trimethadione is 80%.

The other anticonvulsant of the oxazolidinedione class, paramethadione (Paradione), is no longer used because of its toxicity.

Benzodiazepines

Clonazepam

Clonazepam (Klonopin and Rivotril) is effective in controlling petit mal seizures, myoclonic seizures, and infantile spasms. Tolerance can develop to clonazepam, and seizures recur in about a third of patients. The plasma half-life of clonazepam is 20 to 40 hr. Clonazepam is metabolized in the liver to a compound that probably has little anticonvulsant activity.

Neurologic side effects are commonly seen during therapy with clonazepam and include drowsiness, ataxia, and personality changes. Children may become hyperactive, irritable, aggressive, violent, or disobedient. Slurred speech, tremors, abnormal eye movements, dizziness, and confusion also may be noticed. These effects are dose related and may subside with time or on lowering the dose. Increased salivation and bronchial secretions sometimes occur and create respiratory problems in children.

Diazepam

Diazepam (Valium) administered intravenously, is a drug of choice for terminating the grand-mal seizures of status epilepticus and sometimes is used to terminate the seizures of eclampsia. Oral diazepam occasionally is used with other anticonvulsants to control myoclonic, akinetic, and petit mal seizures. Main side effects are drowsiness, dizziness, and ataxia. Respiratory depression must be watched during IV administration. Overall, diazepam is a safe drug. The major use of diazepam is as an antianxiety drug (see Chapter 40).

Lorazepam

Lorazepam (Ativan) is as effective as diazepam for the initial treatment of status epilepticus. Because lorazepam has a longer duration of action, phenytoin or phenobarbital may then be added for sustained control of seizures. As with diazepam, respiratory depression must be monitored during IV administration.

Miscellaneous Drugs

Acetazolamide

Acetazolamide (Diamox) is used alone or with other drugs in treating absence epilepsy. Mechanism of action is inhibition of the enzyme carbonic anhydrase in the brain, which results in an altered ratio of intracellular to extracellular sodium. Acetazolamide is also a weak diuretic (see Chapter 16). Side effects include loss of appetite, drowsiness, confusion, and tingling. The usefulness of acetazolamide is limited by the frequent development of tolerance to its anticonvulsant action.

Adrenocorticotropic hormone

Adrenocorticotropic hormone (ACTH) is the treatment of choice for infantile spasms. If daily administration for 20 days is effective, the course of treatment is repeated after 2 to 4 weeks, of gluococorticoids (usually prednisone) are given. ACTH stimulates the adrenal cortex to synthesize glucocorticoids (see Chapter 51). The effectiveness of ACTH in treating infantile spasms is related to this endocrine action.

Carbamazepine

Carbamazepine (Tegretol) is particularly effective in controlling the seizures of psychomotor and clonic-tonic epilepsy. Recently, carbamazepine has been shown to control cocaine cravings and may be used to treat cocaine addiction. The plasma half-life is 12 hr, so the drug must be given in divided doses. Carbamazepine is metabolized by the liver, and one of the metabolites has anticonvulsant activity. Absorption from the GI tract is slow; however, this can be improved if the drug is taken at meals.

Carbamazepine is chemically related to the tricyclic antidepressants, and a positive side effect is the increased alertness and improvement of mood in patients. The most frequent side effects are drowsiness, dizziness, ataxia, visual disturbances (particularly double vision), and GI upset. Carbamazepine infrequently causes rashes, liver damage, and bone marrow depression, which require its discontinuance. Blood counts should be made frequently in the early course of treatment and occasionally thereafter.

Drug interactions encountered include decreased plasma concentration in the presence of other anticonvulsants, presumably because the other agents induce drug-metabolizing enzymes in the liver. Propoxyphene napsylate (Darvon-N) dramatically increases plasma concentrations of carbamazepine, probably by competing for metabolizing enzymes.

Paraldehyde

Paraldehyde (Paral) is a sedative-hypnotic drug that is seldom used today because of its objectionable odor and chemical instability on storage. When other drugs are ineffective in terminating status epilepticus, paraldehyde may be tried. An advantage is that administration may be intramuscular (IM), IV, or rectal. When given intravenously, however, it must be diluted and administered slowly not only to avoid producing severe coughing, which can result from bronchopulmonary irritation, but also to avoid irritating the veins, which can result in thrombophlebitis. Use is contraindicated in patients with pulmonary disease, since it aggravates bronchopulmonary disease and in patients with liver disease, since it is metabolized by the liver.

Valproic acid and divalproex sodium

Valproic acid (Depakene) was approved for use as an anticonvulsant in 1978 in response to public pressure. In Europe, valproic acid had been shown to be effective in controlling the seizures of progressive my-oclonus, a particularly disabling type of epilepsy in children for which no effective treatment had been available. In addition, valproic acid is effective in treating petit mal and grand mal seizures. Since the plasma half-life is only 8 to 12 hr, the drug is administered three or four times per day.

Valproic acid is an analogue of the inhibitory central neurotransmitter, gamma-aminobutyric acid (GABA), which inhibits neuronal activity. One mechanism by which valproic acid may act is to increase the concentration of this inhibitory neurotransmitter. Divalproex sodium (Depakote) is a combination of the acid and salt forms of valproic acid.

Side effects. The most frequent side effect seen with valproic acid is GI distress. Sedation is marked at the beginning of treatment unless doses are gradually raised. Overdose has produced coma but with uneventful recovery. The incidence of liver damage among patients taking valproic acid is being examined because of some reports of liver failure.

Drug interactions. Drug interactions with valproic acid include its decreased plasma concentration in the presence of other anticonvulsants that induce liver microsomal enzymes including phenobarbital, primidone, phenytoin, and carbamazepine. Phenytoin also can raise the concentration of free-plasma valproic acid by displacing the fraction bound to plasma proteins.

NURSING IMPLICATIONS SUMMARY

General Guidelines for Anticonvulsant Therapy

Drug administration

◆ Monitor serum drug levels if available.
◆ Assess for side effects. Tactfully question patients about compliance.

Patient and family education

◆ Review with patients the anticipated benefits and possible side effects of drug therapy.
◆ Provide emotional support as patients begin anticonvulsant therapy. Drug side effects are common in the first several months of therapy but often diminish with time. Several months of treatment with a drug or regimen may be needed to determine adequate dosage.
◆ Reinforce to patients the importance of continuing prescribed medications even if they have been seizure-free for an extended period. Stress the need to take drugs as ordered and to avoid abruptly discontinuing prescribed medications, since this may precipitate seizures. Recent evidence suggests that anticonvulsants can be discontinued in some patients who have been seizure-free for a long period. This decision must be made on an individual basis in consultation with the physician.
◆ Counsel patients to learn from the physician what actions to take in the event of a missed dose of drug.

◆ Females of childbearing age may wish to use contraceptives while taking these drugs. If females wish to conceive, counsel them to keep physicians informed so that they can be given current information about drug effects during pregnancy. In addition, remind patients to inform their gynecologist of the anticonvulsants being used. Oral contraceptives are not effective when some of these drugs are taken.
◆ Encourage patients to wear a medical identification tag or bracelet indicating they have a history of seizures. In addition, suggest that they carry in their wallets a card listing current drugs and dosages.
◆ Remind patients to inform all health-care providers of all medications being taken.
◆ Tell patients not to use over-the-counter (OTC) preparations unless approved by the physician.
◆ Warn patients to avoid driving or operating hazardous equipment if drowsiness develops.
◆ Refer patients as needed to local or national agencies, including the local visiting nurse agency, vocational rehabilitation, or the Epilepsy Foundation of America.
◆ Instruct patients to avoid drinking alcoholic beverages unless permitted in small amounts by the physician.
◆ Tell patients not to switch brands of anticonvulsant, since bioavailability may differ between brands; consult the pharmacist and the physician for specific information.

Continued.

NURSING IMPLICATIONS SUMMARY—cont'd

◆ Teach patients using a suspension form to shake the bottle well before pouring each dose. Failure to adequately resuspend the medication may result in inadequate doses when the bottle is nearly full and excessive doses when the bottle is less than half full, since the drug may settle to the bottom of the bottle.

◆ Review the procedure for the prescribed drug form. Usually, swallow capsules whole, without breaking them open. Chewable tablets should be chewed well and not swallowed whole. Enteric-coated forms should be swallowed whole, without crushing or chewing. If in doubt, consult the manufacturer's literature and the pharmacist.

Long-Acting Barbiturates

Drug administration and patient and family education

◆ See general guidelines.
◆ Barbiturates are discussed in Chapter 40.
◆ Phenobarbital is usually effective at a serum concentration of 15 to 40 µg/ml. Primidone is usually effective at a serum concentration of 5 to 12 µg/ml.
◆ Review with families signs of intoxication or overdose including slurred speech, ataxia, and vertigo. If these develop, notify the physician.

INTRAVENOUS PHENOBARBITAL

◆ Dilute sterile powder slowly as directed on the package insert. Drug is also available in solution, which must be diluted. Administer diluted dose at a rate of 1 gr (60 to 65 mg) over 1 min. Monitor vital signs and respiration. Have a suction machine at the bedside, and equipment for intubation and ventilatory support available. Do not leave the patient unattended until the patient is stable and alert.

INTRAMUSCULAR PHENOBARBITAL

◆ Observe for respiratory depression 30 to 60 min after injection. Monitor blood pressure. Supervise ambulation. Keep side rails up.

Hydantoins

Drug administration

◆ See general guidelines.
◆ Therapeutic serum drug level is 10 to 20 µg/ml.

◆ Monitor complete blood count (CBC) and differential, platelet count, liver function tests, and blood glucose level.
◆ Remember that even if used as an anticonvulsant, phenytoin also has cardiovascular effects (see Chapter 19).

INTRAVENOUS PHENYTOIN

◆ Prepare dose with diluent supplied by the manufacturer. Slightly yellow-colored solutions may be used, but discard solutions that are not clear. Do not mix with other drugs or many IV solutions, since precipitation may occur. Flush tubing before and after administration with 0.9% sodium chloride. Administer at a rate of 50 mg or less/min. Monitor blood pressure, and if possible, have patient connected to ECG monitor to monitor cardiac rhythm during and immediately after IV administration. Recent studies have involved dilutions in large volumes of normal saline or lactated Ringer's injection (e.g., 100 mg phenytoin in 50 ml normal saline) to administer phenytoin as an infusion. Use an in-line filter. Consult manufacturer's literature for current recommendations.

Patient and family education

◆ See general guidelines. Review common signs of overdose including ataxia, slurred speech, and nystagmus. Tell the family to report these or any unusual side effects.
◆ Provide emotional support. Acne or hirsutism may be difficult for some patients. Refer patients to a dermatologist as appropriate.
◆ Encourage patients to have regular dental checkups and to have a thorough dental care program that includes flossing, brushing, and rinsing. Even with meticulous oral care, gingival hyperplasia develops in some patients. Provide emotional support.
◆ Instruct patients to take oral doses with meals or a snack to lessen gastric irritation.
◆ Instruct patients to report signs of folic acid deficiency including fatigability, weakness, fainting, and headache.
◆ Encourage ingestion of foods high in vitamin D (see Dietary Consideration: Vitamins on p. 275).
◆ Advise diabetic patients to monitor blood glucose levels, since an adjustment in diet or insulin dose may be necessary.
◆ Tell patients that these drugs may produce a harmless brownish or pinkish discoloration of urine.

NURSING IMPLICATIONS SUMMARY—cont'd

Succinimides

Drug administration

- See general guidelines.
- Monitor CBC and differential, platelet count, and liver function tests.
- Ethosuximide is usually effective at a serum concentration of 40 to 100 μg/ml.

Patient and family education

- See general guidelines.
- Patients should take doses with meals or a snack to lessen gastric irritation.
- Tell patients taking phensuximide that urine may turn red, pink, or red-brown during therapy with this drug; this is harmless.

Trimethadione

Drug administration

- See general guidelines.
- Monitor CBC and differential, platelet count, liver function tests, serum creatinine and blood urea nitrogen (BUN) levels, and urinalysis.

Patient and family education

- See general guidelines.
- Tell patients to report skin rashes or changes immediately. Because side effects are common, encourage patients to stay in close contact with the physician.

Other Drug Groups

- Benzodiazepines are discussed in Chapter 40. Acetazolamide is discussed in Chapter 16. ACTH is discussed in Chapter 51.

Carbamazepine

Drug administration

- See general guidelines.
- Monitor blood pressure and weight.
- Monitor CBC and differential, platelet count, and liver function tests.
- Carbamazepine is usually effective at a serum concentration of 4 to 12 μg/ml.
- This drug may be used to treat tic douloureux (trigeminal neuralgia).

Patient and family education

- See general guidelines.
- See Patient Problems: Photosensitivity on p. 629, Constipation on p. 182, and Dry Mouth on p. 166.

- Tell patients using this medication for trigeminal neuralgia that it is not an analgesic and should not be used for any condition other than that prescribed.
- Tell diabetic patients that this drug may alter urine glucose results. Monitor blood glucose levels.

Paraldehyde

Drug administration

- See general guidelines.
- This drug decomposes readily. Use only fresh, unopened containers, and always check the expiration date beforehand.
- Paraldehyde reacts with some plastics. Use glass containers or syringes to measure and to administer doses.
- The drug imparts a characteristic odor to the patient's breath.
- Paraldehyde is partly excreted via the lungs and may cause coughing and an increase in bronchial secretions. During IV administration, place patients on their sides, and have suction equipment available.
- Consult manufacturer's literature for information about IV and IM administration.
- For rectal instillation, dilute the drug in 2 volumes of olive oil to prevent mucosal irritation. Administer as for a retention enema. Controlling the amount or rate of absorption via this route is difficult.

Patient and family education

- See general guidelines.
- Prepare oral doses in glass or metal containers.
- Dilute oral doses in milk or iced fruit juice to improve taste, to lessen odor, and to reduce gastric irritation.

Valproic Acid and Divalproex Sodium

Drug administration

- See general guidelines.
- Monitor CBC and differential, platelet count, and liver function tests.
- Valproic acid is usually effective at a serum concentration of 40 to 120 μg/ml.

Patient and family education

- See general guidelines.
- See Patient Problem: Constipation on p. 182.

Continued.

NURSING IMPLICATIONS SUMMARY—cont'd

◆ Instruct patients to take oral doses with meals or a snack to lessen gastric irritation.
◆ Patients should take the tablet form whole, without chewing or breaking the tablet.

◆ Tell diabetic patients that this drug may alter urine tests for ketones, giving false-positive results. Monitor blood glucose levels.

CHAPTER REVIEW

◆ **KEY TERMS**

absence epilepsy, p. 697
aura, p. 697
automatism, p. 698
epilepsy, p. 696
focal seizures, p. 698
generalized seizures, p. 697
infantile spasms, p. 697
myoclonus epilepsy, p. 698
partial seizures, p. 697
psychomotor epilepsy, p. 698
status epilepticus, p. 698
tonic-clonic epilepsy, p. 697

◆ **REVIEW QUESTIONS**

1. Define epilepsy, and list some of the known causes. What other conditions can precipitate seizures?
2. Describe grand mal, petit mal, myoclonal, psychomotor, and focal seizures and infantile spasms. List the drug of choice for treating each type of epilepsy.
3. What is status epilepticus, and how is it treated?
4. What considerations need to be made in beginning drug administration to control epilepsy?

5. Which long-acting barbiturates are used in treating epilepsy? What are the side effects?
6. What are the adverse effects and drug interactions of phenytoin?
7. What are the adverse effects of the succinimides?
8. Why is trimethadione no longer widely used to treat petit mal seizures?
9. Which benzodiazepines are used as anticonvulsants? For which seizure types are they effective?
10. What are the uses and side effects of carbamazepine?
11. Why is valproic acid a valuable anticonvulsant?
12. Describe the use of acetazolamide, paraldehyde, and ACTH as anticonvulsants.

SUGGESTED READING

Blake GJ: Carbamazepine for trigeminal neuralgia and pain, *Nurs 91* 21(3):102, 1991.
Engle NS: Phenobarbital for pediatric febrile seizures: risk-benefit update, *MCN* 15(4):257, 1990.
Friedman D: Taking the scare out of caring for seizure patients, *Nurs 88* 18(2):52, 1988.
Gress D: Stopping seizures . . . management of a patient in status epilepticus, *Emerg Med* 22(1):22, 1990.
Noerr B: Phenytoin sodium (Dilantin), *Neonatal Netw* 8(2):63, 1989.
Parks BR Jr: Febrile seizures, *Pediatr Nurs* 14(6):518, 1988.
Seagraves R: Antiepileptic drug therapy for pediatric generalized tonic-clonic seizures, *J Pediatr Health Care* 4(6):314, 1990.

CHAPTER 48

Drugs for Parkinsonism and Centrally Acting Skeletal Muscle Relaxants

---

LEARNING OBJECTIVES

After studying this chapter, you should be able to do the following:

◆ List three classic symptoms of Parkinson's disease, and explain the role of acetylcholine and dopamine in Parkinson's disease.

◆ Develop a care plan for patients receiving anticholinergic drugs, antihistamines, amantadine, bromocriptine, levodopa or carbidopa-levodopa, pergolide, or selegiline to treat Parkinson's disease.

◆ Develop a care plan for patients receiving a centrally acting skeletal muscle relaxant such as diazepam, baclofen, or dantrolene.

◆ Develop a care plan for patients receiving drug therapy for muscle spasms.

CHAPTER OVERVIEW

◆ This chapter covers drug therapy for three types of motor disorders—parkinsonism, muscle spasms, and spasticity. Parkinsonism is a progressive neurologic disorder of the extrapyramidal system caused by the degeneration of the dopaminergic neurons. This results in motor abnormalities. Muscle spasm is an involuntary contraction of a muscle or group of muscles. Spasticity is a common symptom of upper motor neuron lesions. These conditions can be alleviated with appropriate drug therapy.

Nursing Process Overview
DRUGS TO TREAT PARKINSON'S DISEASE

Assessment

Perform a baseline patient assessment, including vital signs, joint movement, amount of tremor, affect and objective signs of the disease, and ability to ambulate and to perform activities of daily living. Because this is often a disease of the elderly, obtain a baseline view of other known health problems such as hypertension, diabetes, and cardiovascular or renal disease.

Nursing Diagnoses

Altered bowel elimination: constipation

High risk for urinary retention

High risk for body image disturbance related to dyskinesia or other drug side effects

Management

Include the patient in the discussion of the goals of therapy. Monitor for subjective and objective improvement and for drug side effects. Improvement in symptoms should outweigh the discomfort of side effects. Some patients find the side effects resulting from a drug are worse than if the disease is untreated, at least at some stages in its progression.

Before discharge, refer the patient to social service, vocational rehabilitation, visiting nurse, and other agencies, if appropriate.

Evaluation

Before discharge and at regular intervals during therapy, ensure patients can explain prescribed drugs and doses; how to take the drugs correctly; the expected goals of therapy; and drug side effects, how to treat them, and when to notify the physician. Verify that

709

patients can explain any necessary dietary or vitamin restrictions.

PARKINSON'S DISEASE

Parkinson's disease is a movement disorder characterized by rigidity, akinesia, and tremor. *Rigidity* means that muscle tone is greatly increased but reflex activity is not. When a limb is passively forced through flexor or extensor movements, the muscular resistance alternately increases and decreases to give a cogwheel effect. *Akinesia* (no motion) refers to the difficulty the patient has in initiating any movement. The face has a masklike, fixed expression devoid of emotion. Early in the course of Parkinson's disease, the difficulty in initiating movement is not as marked and is termed *bradykinesia* (slow motion). The tremor of Parkinson's disease is seen mostly in the limbs at rest and decreases with movement of the limbs.

Role of Acetylcholine and Dopamine

Insight into the neurochemical defect in Parkinson's disease exemplifies our growing knowledge of the role of neurotransmitters in controlling given functions within the central nervous system (CNS). For many years, anticholinergic drugs such as atropine had been used to decrease the tremor characteristics of Parkinson's disease; acetylcholine therefore seemed important in accounting for some symptoms. When the antipsychotic drugs (major tranquilizers) were introduced in the 1950s, symptoms indistinguishable from those of Parkinson's disease began to appear in patients treated with these drugs. It is now known that this is because these drugs block receptors for the CNS neurotransmitter dopamine.

Subsequently, patients with Parkinson's disease were shown to have degeneration of crucial dopaminergic neurons projecting to certain basal ganglia of the extrapyramidal system in the brain. This system is responsible for maintaining motor coordination at the CNS level.

The current understanding of Parkinson's disease is that it represents a deficiency in the neurotransmitter dopamine in certain basal ganglia. Dopamine from these neuronal tracts is believed to exert an inhibitory influence on cholinergic neurons of the extrapyramidal system controlling muscle tone. When dopamine is lacking, muscle tone increases because of the unopposed action of acetylcholine, resulting in muscular rigidity, inhibition of spontaneous movements, and tremor. The lack of dopamine is secondary to a progressive degeneration of specific dopaminergic neurons. This degeneration can be caused by encephalitis, carbon-monoxide poisoning, manganese poisoning, cerebrovascular accident (stroke), or, more commonly, unknown causes. This degeneration cannot be arrested. Drugs alleviate the symptoms for only a few years.

The current rationale for the pharmacologic treatment of Parkinson's disease is to diminish the severity of motor symptoms by blocking the excessive action of acetylcholine or by replenishing the dopamine to return the balance of excitatory acetylcholine action and inhibitory dopamine action toward normal.

Drug-Induced Parkinsonism

Certain drugs also can cause symptoms of Parkinson's disease. Reserpine (Serpasil), which depletes neuronal stores of dopamine and norepinephrine, and the antipsychotic drugs, which block dopamine receptors, are the usual causes of drug-induced parkinsonism. Since symptoms depend on the presence of the drug, lowering the dosage or discontinuing the drug eliminates the symptoms.

Anticholinergic Drugs to Treat Parkinsonism

These drugs are listed in Table 48-1.

Early in the course of Parkinson's disease, an anticholinergic drug is frequently given to lessen rigidity, bradykinesia, and tremor. Atropine and scopolamine, the classic anticholinergic drugs, were used to treat symptoms of Parkinson's disease for many years. Anticholinergic drugs used today are synthetic drugs that are centrally active and produce fewer peripheral side effects. These drugs include procyclidine (Kemadrin), trihexyphenidyl (Tremin and others), benztropine (Cogentin), biperiden (Akineton), and ethopropazine (Parsidol). An anticholinergic drug is also the drug of choice to treat extrapyramidal reactions arising from the antipsychotic drugs including akathisia, acute dystonia, and parkinsonism. Tardive dyskinesia is not reversed by anticholinergic drugs. These extrapyramidal reactions are described in Chapter 41.

Administration and side effects

The dosage of the anticholinergic drugs must be started low and increased gradually to overcome side effects and to individualize the dose. Common side effects of the anticholinergic drugs are dry mouth, constipation, urinary retention, and blurred vision. Common mental effects include impairment of recent memory, confusion, insomnia, and restlessness. Mental effects can become serious, with the development of agitation, disorientation, delirium, paranoid reactions, or hallucinations. Mental problems are more common with elderly patients who have preexisting mental disturbances. Patients who have prior histories of glaucoma, particularly narrow-angle glau-

Table 48-1   Drugs to Treat Parkinsonism

Generic name	Trade name	Administration/dosage	Comments
ANTICHOLINERGICS			
Benztropine mesylate	Cogentin*	ORAL: *Adults*—0.5 to 1 mg at bedtime initially, increased gradually to 4 to 6 mg if required. FDA Pregnancy Category C. For drug-induced extrapyramidal reactions: ORAL, INTRAMUSCULAR, INTRAVENOUS: *Adults*—1 to 4 mg or 2 times daily. For an acute dystonic reaction: ORAL, INTRAVENOUS: *Adults*—2 mg intravenously, then 1 to 2 mg orally twice daily.	To treat Parkinson's disease and drug-induced extrapyramidal reactions. Particularly effective in reversing an acute dystonic reaction to an antipsychotic drug.
Biperiden	Akineton*	ORAL: *Adults*—2 mg 3 times daily; may increase dose up to 20 mg daily if required. FDA Pregnancy Category C. For drug-induced extrapyramidal reactions: ORAL: *Adults*—2 mg 1 to 3 times daily. INTRAMUSCULAR: *Adults*—2 mg repeated as often as every 30 min but no more than 4 doses in 24 hr. *Children*—0.04 mg/kg body weight as often as every 30 min but no more than 4 doses in 24 hr.	To treat Parkinson's disease and drug-induced extrapyramidal reactions.
Ethopropazine	Parsidol Parsitan†	ORAL: *Adults*—50 mg 1 or 2 times daily initially. Mild-to-moderate cases require 100 to 400 mg daily. Severe cases may require 500 to 600 mg daily. FDA Pregnancy Category C.	To treat Parkinson's disease. A phenothiazine with only anticholinergic effects and devoid of antidopaminergic effects.
Procyclidine hydrochloride	Kemadrin* Procyclid†	ORAL: *Adults*—5 mg twice daily, up to 20 to 30 mg daily if required. FDA Pregnancy Category C. For drug-induced extrapyramidal reactions: ORAL: *Adults*—2 to 2.5 mg 3 times daily, increased to 10 to 20 mg daily if required.	To treat Parkinson's disease and drug-induced extrapyramidal reactions.
Trihexyphenidyl hydrochloride	Artane* Trihexy†	ORAL: *Adults*—2 mg 2 or 3 times daily. Increased to 15 to 20 mg daily (usually) or 40 to 50 mg daily (rarely) to control symptoms. FDA Pregnancy Category C. For drug-induced parkinsonism: ORAL: *Adults*—1 mg initially. Subsequent doses increased if symptoms do not decrease. Usual daily dose, 5 to 15 mg.	To treat Parkinson's disease and drug-induced extrapyramidal reactions.
ANTIHISTAMINES			
Diphenhydramine hydrochloride	Benadryl*	ORAL: *Adults*—25 mg 3 times daily, increased to 50 mg 4 times daily if required. For drug-induced extrapyramidal reactions: INTRAMUSCULAR, INTRAVENOUS: *Adults*—10 to 50 mg; maximum, 400 mg daily. *Children*—5 mg/kg body weight intramuscularly daily; maximum 300 mg in 24 hr.	To treat Parkinson's disease and drug-induced extrapyramidal reactions. Marked sedative effects.
Orphenadrine hydrochloride	Disipal*	ORAL: *Adults*—50 mg 3 times daily; up to 250 mg if required.	To treat Parkinson's disease.

*Available in Canada and United States.
†Available in Canada only.

Continued.

Table 48-1 Drugs to Treat Parkinsonism—cont'd

Generic name	Trade name	Administration/dosage	Comments
DRUGS AFFECTING THE AMOUNT OF DOPAMINE IN THE BRAIN			
Amantadine	Symadine Symmetrel*	ORAL: *Adults*—100 mg daily after breakfast for 5 to 7 days. An additional 100 mg may be added after lunch.	Antiviral agent that augments the release of dopamine. Side effects are similar to anticholinergic drugs.
Bromociptine	Parlodel	ORAL: *Adults*—Initially, 1.25 mg twice daily, increased every other week or monthly by 1.25 to 2.5 mg until benefits are achieved or adverse effects become intolerable.	Dopamine agonist. May be added to levodopa or carbidopa-levodopa therapy; occasionally replaces levodopa therapy.
Carbidopa-levodopa	Sinement	ORAL: *Adults*—Initial daily dose should be ¼ the levodopa daily dose. Sinemet should be administered 8 hr. after the last levodopa dose and given in 3 or 4 doses daily. Patients not previously receiving levodopa are started with 10:100 mg (carbidopa:levodopa) 3 times daily, and the dosage is gradually increased as required.	Carbidopa inhibits degradation of dopamine outside the CNS. Levodopa-carbidopa ratio is 10:1.
Levodopa	Dopar Larodopa*	ORAL: *Adults*—initially 300 to 1000 mg daily in 3 to 7 doses during waking hours with food. Increase dosage 100 to 500 mg every 2 to 3 days or more until desired control is achieved. Usually requires 4 to 6 Gm and 6 to 8 weeks to achieve control. After several months to 1 year the dosage may be lowered.	Levodopa is chemical precursor of dopamine.
Pergolide mesylate	Permax	ORAL: *Adults*—Initially, 0.05 mg daily for the first 2 days, increased by 0.1 to 0.15 mg daily at 3-day intervals for 12 days until the antiparkinson effect is optimum or a maximum of 5 mg daily is reached. Can be administered in 3 divided doses daily.	Pergolide has dopaminergic activity.
Selegiline hydrochloride	Eldepryl	ORAL: *Adults*—10 mg/day.	Adjunct for parkinsonian patients who exhibit deterioration in their response to carbidopa-levadopa therapy. Selegiline is also known as *deprenyl*. It inhibits the degradation of dopamine.

*Available in Canada and United States.

coma, or some type of urinary or intestinal obstruction or tachycardia are not good candidates, since anticholinergic drugs can aggravate any of these conditions. Characteristic actions of anticholinergic drugs are discussed in Chapter 9.

Antihistaminic Drugs to Treat Parkinsonism

Antihistaminic drugs that have pronounced anticholinergic effects may be substituted for anticholinergic drugs. The two antihistaminic drugs sometimes used to treat symptoms of parkinsonism are diphenhydramine (Benadryl) and orphenadrine (Disipal) (see Table 48-1). Compared with the anticholinergic drugs, these antihistamines have milder although similar side effects and are less potent. The effectiveness of the antihistamines in treating the symptoms of parkinsonism is attributed to their anticholinergic effect. Antihistamines also have a sedative effect. They are discussed in Chapter 24.

Drugs Affecting the Amount of Dopamine in the Brain

These drugs are listed in Table 48-1.

Amantadine

Amantadine (Symmetrel) is an antiviral agent that also has been found effective in reducing the severity of symptoms of Parkinson's disease when used alone or with an anticholinergic or antihistaminic drug. Amantadine promotes the release of dopamine from the central neurons, an action unrelated to its antiviral action.

Amantadine is often used as a first drug to control the symptoms of parkinsonism. It has the advantages of being effective when administered as a single daily dose and of having few side effects. Side effects seen include dizziness, nervousness, inability to concentrate, ataxia, slurred speech, insomnia, lethargy, blurred vision, dry mouth, gastrointestinal (GI) upset, and rash. Amantadine may also be used with anticholinergic drugs or with levodopa, since it enhances the effectiveness of these other drugs and allows a reduction of their dosage.

Bromocriptine

Bromocriptine (Parlodel) mimics the action of dopamine in the brain. It is an alternative to levodopa when levodopa is contraindicated, is not well tolerated, or does not produce a response. Bromocriptine has a duration of action similar to that of levodopa and may be added to levodopa or carbidopa-levodopa therapy for patients who show symptoms of fluctuating doses such as dystonia and muscle cramps. Doses of bromocriptine must be individualized. Transient dizziness and nausea are common. Hypotension, abdominal pain, blurred vision, double vision, and vasospasm of the fingers and toes in response to cold also occasionally occur.

Carbidopa-levodopa

Carbidopa (Sinemet) inhibits the conversion of levodopa to dopamine. Since carbidopa cannot enter the CNS, only peripheral conversion is inhibited. This means that levodopa is converted to dopamine only in the brain, so the presence of carbidopa lowers the dose of levodopa required by 75%. Since the emetic effects of levodopa reflect peripheral dopamine concentrations, the incidence of nausea and vomiting is reduced greatly with carbidopa-levodopa combination. Carbidopa is available only in a fixed-ratio combination with levodopa.

Levodopa

Mechanism of action. When the drugs just mentioned can no longer adequately relieve the symptoms of Parkinson's disease, levodopa (Dopar and Larodopa) is administered. Levodopa therapy does not stop the progression of Parkinson's disease but relieves the symptoms and dramatically improves ability

to function. Levodopa is the chemical precursor of dopamine, and unlike dopamine, it readily crosses the blood-brain barrier. It is converted to dopamine by the enzyme dopa decarboxylase. About 75% of a dose of levodopa is converted to dopamine in the periphery rather than in the brain, and the high plasma concentration of dopamine is responsible for the nausea and cardiac effects occurring with this therapy.

Administration. Levodopa is taken orally, and the peak effect is seen 1 to 2 hr later. Dosage is adjusted up or down gradually every 2 to 3 days to lessen the incidence of nausea and to avoid precipitating side effects.

Emetic side effects. Dopamine is the neurotransmitter for the chemoreceptor trigger zone of the medulla and thus produces nausea, vomiting, and anorexia. To create tolerance to this emetic action, levodopa therapy must be initiated by starting with low doses that are gradually increased. A snack high in protein also helps to prevent nausea. Antiemetics from the phenothiazine class should not be used, since they block the therapeutic action of dopamine. Trimethobenzamide (Tigan) may be taken early in the morning to control nausea.

Cardiovascular side effects. Another side effect sometimes seen at the start of levodopa therapy is orthostatic hypotension. The mechanism is not known but is believed to be a CNS effect rather than a peripheral effect. This hypotension tends to decrease with time. An increase in heart rate and force of contraction may also be apparent at the start of therapy. These cardiac actions are caused by the direct action of dopamine on the heart. Cardiac arrhythmias may develop and must be controlled by appropriate medication.

Other side effects. Additional side effects of levodopa therapy may be GI effects, including bleeding, difficulty in swallowing, and a burning sensation of the tongue. Respiratory effects such as cough, hoarseness, and disturbed breathing may appear. Because of these side effects, levodopa therapy is used cautiously for patients with a history of heart disease, asthma, emphysema, or peptic ulcer. Problems in urination from incontinence to retention may arise.

Blurred vision or dilated pupils may be caused by levodopa. Levodopa therapy is not considered for patients with narrow-angle glaucoma and only with careful monitoring for patients with chronic (wide-angle) glaucoma. Hepatic, hematopoietic, cardiovascular, and renal function tests are performed periodically on patients receiving long-term levodopa therapy. This is because many laboratory test values are high in patients receiving levodopa therapy, and only careful monitoring can determine whether or not a real problem exists. Hematocrit and white blood cell counts may be lowered by levodopa therapy, but therapy is discontinued only when abnormally low counts are found. Therapy is not initiated in patients with blood disorders.

Additional effects typically noted after the start of levodopa therapy include increased alertness, sense of well-being, and increased libido. These effects are attributed to behavioral roles of dopamine in the brain. Further mental changes may occur with prolonged therapy. Euphoria, restlessness, anxiety, irritability, hyperactivity, insomnia, and vivid dreams frequently occur. Patients occasionally may become paranoid and may experience psychotic episodes or become depressed, with or without suicidal tendencies. These mental changes are usually reversed by lowering the dosage.

Side effects after prolonged therapy. After prolonged therapy with levodopa, abnormal involuntary movements (**dyskinesia**) alternating with a sudden lapse in symptom control (the **"on-off" phenomenon**) may appear. Dyskinesia usually comprises abnormal involuntary movements of the mouth, tongue, face, or neck. Dyskinesia usually appears 1 to 2 hr after the latest dose of levodopa and represents a mild levodopa toxicity. "End-of-dose" akinesia also may occur. This means that the akinesia appears just before a new dose is to be taken and usually can be avoided by increasing frequency of administration.

Pergolide

Pergolide (Permax) has direct dopaminergic action. It is more potent than bromocriptine and has a longer half-life. Overall effectiveness of pergolide with carbidopa-levodopa therapy is similar to bromocriptine. Side effects are similar to those of bromocriptine. The most common reactions are hallucinations, nausea, dry mouth, light-headedness, and dyskinesia.

Selegiline

Selegiline (Eldepryl) (formerly deprenyl) is a newly approved drug that inhibits the enzyme monoamine oxidase B, which degrades dopamine in the brain. Since dopamine is not rapidly degraded in the presence of selegiline, the duration of action and dose of levodopa is reduced. Early morning stiffness and end-of-dose symptoms are decreased. Selegiline is added to levodopa or carbidopa-levodopa therapy.

Centrally Acting Drugs That Control Muscle Tone

The drugs discussed in this section act by central mechanisms to control muscle tone. There are three drugs used to control spasticity, a chronic condition.

Muscle spasm is usually self-limiting. It is more difficult to identify drugs of choice to treat muscle spasm.

Nursing Process Overview
CENTRALLY ACTING SKELETAL MUSCLE RELAXANTS
Assessment

Perform a general assessment with an additional focus on spasticity, including degree of spasticity, aggravating factors, associated pain, and degree to which spasticity interferes with the activities of daily living or the activities that could increase independence. If dantrolene is used, monitor baseline liver function studies.

Nursing Diagnoses

Potential for sexual dysfunction: impotence
High risk for excessive drowsiness and dizziness

Management

During dosage adjustment, monitor the patient for drug effectiveness and side effects. Weeks of therapy may be needed before a lessening of spasticity occurs. These drugs may be used with other therapies, including traction, physical therapy, exercises, bed rest, and application of heat.

Evaluation

Evaluate continuing degree of spasticity. Not all side effects are undesirable, so decisions related to them should be individualized. For example, a patient who is drowsy when receiving short-term diazepam therapy may be better able to tolerate enforced bed rest because of the drowsiness. Before discharge, verify that patients can explain what drugs to take and how to take them correctly; side effects that may occur and which require notification of the physician; how to perform additional therapies such as application of heat and exercises; and when to return for additional help.

CENTRALLY ACTING SKELETAL MUSCLE RELAXANTS
Drugs to Treat Spasticity

Spasticity results from the loss of inhibitory tone in the polysynaptic pathways of the spinal cord so that fine control of motor activity is lost. Since the inhibitory tone is controlled largely by neural pathways from the brain, spasticity is seen in patients in whom these inhibitory pathways have been disrupted

Table 48-2　Centrally Acting Skeletal Muscle Relaxants

Generic name	Trade name	Administration/dosage	Comments
DRUGS TO TREAT SPASTICITY			
Baclofen	Lioresal*	ORAL: *Adults*—Begin with 5 mg 3 times daily. Increase by 5 mg 3 times daily every 3 days as required; maximum, 80 mg.	Diminishes reflex responses by decreasing transmission in the spinal cord.
Dantrolene	Dantrium*	ORAL: *Adults*—25 mg 1 or 2 times daily. Increase to 25 mg 3 to 4 times daily, then 50 to 100 mg 4 times daily as required. Increments are adjusted every 4 to 7 days.	Acts peripherally to inhibit calcium release within the muscle.
Diazepam	Valium*	ORAL: *Adults*—2 to 10 mg 4 times daily. *Children*—0.12 to 0.8 mg/kg body weight daily in 3 or 4 doses. INTRAVENOUS: *Adults*—2 to 10 mg injected no faster than 5 mg (1 ml)/min. Do not mix or dilute with other solutions, drugs, or IV fluids. *Children*—0.04 to 0.2 mg/kg body weight; maximum, 0.6 mg/kg in 8 hr.	Benzodiazepine also used to treat spasticity or muscle spasm.
DRUGS TO TREAT MUSCLE SPASMS			
Carisoprodol	Rela Soma* Various others	ORAL: *Adults*—350 mg 4 times daily.	Related to meprobamate. May cause drowsiness.
Chlorphenesin	Maolate	ORAL: *Adults*—800 mg 3 times daily. Can decrease to 400 mg 4 times daily as improvement is noted.	May cause drowsiness and dizziness.
Chlorzoxazone	Paraflex Parafon Forte DSC	ORAL: *Adults*—250 to 750 mg 3 or 4 times daily. *Children*—20 mg/kg body weight in 3 or 4 divided doses.	May cause drowsiness. Watch for signs of liver damage (rare).
Cyclobenzaprine	Flexeril*	ORAL: *Adults*—10 mg 3 times daily up to a maximum total dose of 60 mg.	Related to tricyclic antidepressants. Does not cause drug dependence, but may cause changes in the liver.
Diazepam	Valium*	Same as for diazepam to treat spasticity.	
Metaxalone	Skelaxin	ORAL: *Adults*—800 mg 3 or 4 times daily.	Monitor patients for development of liver toxicity.
Methocarbamol	Delaxin Robamol Robaxin* Various others	ORAL: *Adults*—1.5 to 2 gm 4 times daily for 2 to 3 days. Decrease to 1 gm 4 times daily for maintenance. INTRAMUSCULAR: *Adults*—500 mg every 8 hr, alternating between the gluteal muscles. INTRAVENOUS: *Adults*—1 to 3 gm daily for a maximum of 3 days. Inject no faster than 300 mg (3 ml)/min.	Not recommended for patients with epilepsy. Do not administer parenterally to patients with impaired renal function because the drug vehicle may worsen kidney function.
Orphenadrine	Flexon Neocyten Norflex* Tega-Flex Various others	ORAL: *Adults*—100 mg twice daily. INTRAMUSCULAR, INTRAVENOUS: *Adults*—60 mg twice daily.	Anticholinergic effects are common side effects. Not for patients with glaucoma, myasthenia gravis, tachycardia, or urinary retention.

*Available in Canada and United States.

through spinal cord injury, strokes, multiple sclerosis, or cerebral palsy. The patient with spasticity has exaggerated reflexes (spinal spasticity) or inappropriate posture (cerebral spasticity). Drugs to treat spasticity are presented in Table 48-2.

Three drugs found to be effective in relieving some cases of spasticity are diazepam (Valium), baclofen (Lioresal), and dantrolene (Dantrium). Diazepam and baclofen are believed to act within the spinal cord to restore some inhibitory tone, but dantrolene is unique in acting within the muscle.

Diazepam

Diazepam (Valium) is a benzodiazepine commonly prescribed as an antianxiety drug (see Chapter 40). Although its action as an antianxiety drug results from depression of the reticular activating system, diazepam also enhances inhibitory descending pathways in the spinal cord governing muscular activity, apparently by enhancing the activity of the inhibitory neurotransmitter gamma-aminobutyric acid (GABA). Diazepam is effective in relieving spasticity associated with spinal cord injury, multiple sclerosis, and cerebral injury and in treating muscle spasms. Relatively high doses are required to relieve muscle hyperactivity, and drowsiness and ataxia may be prominent side effects.

Baclofen

Baclofen (Lioresal) is an analogue of the inhibitory neurotransmitter GABA, and although the effect elicited is that desired of a GABA agonist, this mechanism of action cannot be demonstrated in the laboratory. Baclofen is most effective in relieving spasticity secondary to spinal cord injury and is less effective in relieving spasticity secondary to brain damage. Side effects include drowsiness, ataxia, and occasional GI upset.

Dantrolene

Dantrolene (Dantrium) is not a centrally acting skeletal muscle relaxant but instead affects the muscle directly by interfering with the intracellular release of calcium necessary to initiate contraction. At therapeutic doses, this effect is limited to skeletal muscle and is not seen in the heart or smooth muscle. Dantrolene causes muscular weakness and can worsen the overall condition if the patient already has marginal strength. Dantrolene is most useful for the patient whose spasticity causes pain, discomfort, or limits functional rehabilitation. In addition to the spasticity secondary to spinal cord injury, dantrolene relieves spasticity of stroke, cerebral palsy, or multiple sclerosis, for which the other drugs have limited effectiveness.

The major limitation to the use of dantrolene is liver damage. Baseline liver function studies are done before therapy starts, and regular liver function studies are performed throughout therapy. Dantrolene is discontinued if no relief of spasticity is achieved in 6 weeks.

Muscle Spasms and Their Treatment

Muscle spasms are local muscle contractions initiated by muscle or tendon injury and inflammation. Muscle spasms occur in sprains, bursitis, arthritis, and lower back pain. The primary treatment includes analgesics, antiinflammatory drugs, immobilization of the affected part (if possible), and physical therapy. If relief is not achieved through these means, a centrally acting skeletal muscle relaxant may be added. Although the mechanism postulated for the centrally acting skeletal muscle relaxants is depression of the polysynaptic pathways in the spinal cord modulating muscle tone, drugs used as centrally acting skeletal muscle relaxants are related to various antianxiety drugs. Since anxiety worsens a muscle spasm, treatment of the accompanying anxiety may be the more important mechanism of action.

Centrally acting skeletal muscle relaxants commonly prescribed to treat muscle spasms are listed in Table 48-2 and include carisoprodol (Rela and Soma), chlorphenesin (Maolate), chlorzoxazone (Paraflex), cyclobenzaprine (Flexeril), diazepam (Valium), metaxalone (Skelaxin), methocarbamol (Delaxin and others), and orphenadrine (Norflex and others). With the exception of cyclobenzaprine, these drugs are similar to sedative-hypnotic or antianxiety drugs with respect to side effects, drug interactions, and drug dependence (see Chapter 40); thus short-term rather than long-term therapy is the rule. Cyclobenzaprine is related to the tricyclic antidepressants and does not cause drug dependence or alter sleep patterns.

Drowsiness and dizziness are common side effects of all the centrally acting skeletal muscle relaxants, and they should not be combined with alcohol or other drugs that depress the CNS.

NURSING IMPLICATIONS SUMMARY

General Guidelines for Patients Receiving Drugs to Treat Parkinson's Disease

Patient and family education

◆ Review anticipated benefits and possible side effects of drug therapy.

◆ Teach patients and families that several weeks to months of therapy may be needed in some cases to obtain full benefit of drug therapy. Provide emotional support.

◆ Parkinson's disease is primarily a problem of the elderly. However, if a premenopausal female develops Parkinson's disease, counsel as needed about contraceptives. These drugs should not be used during pregnancy without consulting the physician.

◆ Point out to family that confusion is often a drug side effect in elderly patients and should not be attributed to Parkinson's disease until fully evaluated.

◆ Warn patients not to discontinue these drugs suddenly. Patients should inform all health-care providers of all drugs being taken. They should avoid over-the-counter medications unless approved by the physician.

◆ Counsel patients to avoid the use of alcohol unless permitted in small amounts by the physician.

Other Drug Groups

◆ The anticholinergic drugs are discussed in Chapters 9 and 13.

◆ See Patient Problems: Dry Mouth on p. 166, Constipation on p. 182, and Orthostatic Hypotension on p. 234.

◆ Antihistamines are discussed in Chapter 24.

◆ Phenothiazines are discussed in Chapter 41.

Amantadine

Drug administration

◆ Assess mental status regularly. Be alert to signs of increasing depression including lethargy, apathy, decreased appetite, and loss of interest in personal appearance. Be alert to suicidal tendencies.

◆ Monitor intake and output, daily weight, blood pressure and pulse. Auscultate lung sounds. Inspect for edema and skin changes.

◆ Assess for urinary retention. Suggest patients void before taking drug doses.

◆ Monitor complete blood count (CBC) and differential.

Patient and family education

◆ See the general guidelines.

◆ See Patient Problems: Orthostatic Hypotension on p. 234 and Constipation on p. 182.

◆ Warn patients to avoid driving or operating hazardous equipment if drowsiness or dizziness develops; notify the physician.

◆ Capsules may be opened and contents mixed with a small amount of food or fluid for ease in taking dose, although a liquid preparation is also available.

◆ Tell patients that livedo reticularis (bluish or purplish mottling of the skin) may appear during the first year of therapy and may take several weeks to subside when therapy is discontinued.

Bromocriptine

◆ Bromocriptine is discussed in Chapter 53.

Carbidopa-Levodopa Combination

Drug administration and patient and family education

◆ No specific side effects have been attributed to carbidopa.

◆ Review with patient the information about levodopa.

Levodopa

Drug administration

◆ Monitor neuromuscular, neurologic, and mental status regularly.

◆ Monitor blood pressure and pulse, intake and output, and weight.

◆ Check stools for presence of occult blood. Inspect for skin changes.

◆ Monitor CBC and differential, platelet count, blood urea nitrogen (BUN), and liver function tests.

Patient and family education

◆ See the general guidelines.

◆ See Patient Problems: Constipation on p.182, Orthostatic Hypotension on p. 234, and Dry Mouth on p. 166.

◆ Warn male patients that priapism has been reported; notify the physician if it develops.

◆ Tell the patient that sweat may be darker in color while they take this drug, and urine may be dark, especially if left standing.

Continued.

NURSING IMPLICATIONS SUMMARY—cont'd

◆ Instruct patients to take doses with meals or snack to reduce gastric irritation.

◆ If patients have difficulty swallowing levodopa capsules or tablets, consult the pharmacist about preparing a liquid form.

◆ Tell diabetic patients to monitor blood glucose levels carefully, since tests for urinary glucose and ketone levels may be inaccurate.

◆ There are many side effects of levodopa therapy. Encourage the patient and family to report any new or unexpected findings.

◆ Pyridoxine (vitamin B_6) may reduce the effectiveness of levodopa. Instruct patients not to take any vitamin preparations without consulting the physician. Limit intake of foods high in pyridoxine; see Dietary Consideration: Vitamins on p. 275.

Pergolide

Drug administration

◆ See general guidelines.

◆ Assess for common side effects including hallucinations, nausea, dry mouth, light-headedness, and dyskinesia. See Patient Problem: Dry Mouth on p. 166.

◆ Monitor weight.

◆ Assess patients for worsening symptoms if pergolide and levodopa are administered concurrently.

◆ Monitor the blood pressure. Dosages are increased slowly to lessen the degree of hypotension.

◆ Monitor patients with a history of cardiac arrhythmias carefully when beginning pergolide therapy; increases in atrial premature contractions and sinus tachycardia have been reported.

Selegiline

Drug administration

◆ See Patient Problem: Orthostatic Hypotension on p. 234. Assess for confusion, dizziness, and insomnia.

◆ Instruct patients to avoid driving or operating hazardous equipment if dizziness or syncope develops.

◆ Monitor the blood pressure.

◆ More experience with this drug will bring more information. Instruct patients to report any new signs or symptoms to the physician.

Diazepam

◆ Diazepam is discussed in Chapter 40.

Baclofen

Drug administration

◆ Assess mental status, and monitor regularly.

◆ Monitor blood pressure every 4 hr until stable. Be alert to hypotension when assisting patients to ambulate, especially if they have been immobilized or mostly sedentary before starting drug therapy.

◆ Monitor intake and output and weight. Monitor respiratory rate, auscultate lung sounds, and assess for dyspnea. Inspect for skin changes and edema.

◆ Monitor CBC and urinalysis.

◆ Tactfully question patients regarding impotence. Provide emotional support. Remind patients not to discontinue medications without consulting the physician.

Patient and family education

◆ Teach patients that several days to weeks of therapy may be necessary before improvement is seen. If improvement is not seen in 6 to 8 weeks, the drug is usually withdrawn.

◆ See Patient Problems: Constipation on p. 182 and Dry Mouth on p. 166.

◆ Warn patients to avoid driving or operating hazardous equipment if drowsiness develops.

◆ Caution diabetic patients to monitor blood glucose levels carefully, since an adjustment in diet or insulin may be needed.

◆ Warn patients to avoid the use of alcohol unless permitted in small amounts by the physician.

◆ Remind patients to inform health-care providers of all drugs being taken.

◆ Take dose with meals or a snack to lessen gastric irritation.

Dantrolene

Drug administration

◆ Assess mental status and monitor regularly. Watch for signs of depression including withdrawal, lack of interest in personal appearance, insomnia, anorexia, and weight loss.

◆ Monitor blood pressure and pulse. When used for treatment of malignant hyperthermia, attach patient to cardiac monitor.

◆ Be alert to hypotension when assisting patients to ambulate, especially if patients have been immobilized or primarily sedentary before receiving drug therapy.

◆ Check stools for occult blood.

NURSING IMPLICATIONS SUMMARY—cont'd

◆ Monitor intake and output. Monitor urinalysis, or check urine for blood.

◆ Tactfully assess males regarding difficulty in achieving erection. Provide emotional support. Caution patients not to discontinue medications without consulting the physician.

◆ Auscultate lung sounds, watch for pleural effusion.

◆ Inspect skin for abnormal hair growth or rash.

◆ Monitor CBC and liver function tests.

INTRAVENOUS DANTROLENE

◆ Dilute each 20 mg with 60 ml sterile water for injection that does not contain a bacteriostatic agent. Shake solution until clear. Administer as rapid intravenous IV push. Once reconstituted and diluted, solution must be protected from light and used within 6 hr.

Patient and family education

◆ Review anticipated benefits and possible side effects of drug therapy. Tell patients to notify the physician of any unexpected findings.

◆ See Patient Problems: Constipation on p. 182 and Photosensitivity on p. 629.

◆ Reassure patients that several days to weeks of therapy may be necessary before improvement is seen. If improvement is not seen in 6 to 8 weeks, drug is usually withdrawn.

◆ Warn patients to avoid driving or operating hazardous equipment if dizziness or drowsiness develops.

◆ Warn patients to avoid the use of alcohol unless permitted in small amounts by the physician.

◆ Remind patients to inform all health care providers of all medications being taken.

◆ Instruct patients who develop malignant hyperthermia to wear a medical identification tag or bracelet.

Drugs to Treat Muscle Spasms
Drug administration

◆ Assess for CNS side effects including dizziness, ataxia, and vertigo.

◆ Warn patients that intramuscular (IM) injections may cause a burning sensation at the injection site.

◆ Consult the manufacturer's literature for information about IV administrationn.

◆ For IV administration, keep the patient supine. Keep side rails up. Monitor vital signs. Keep the patient recumbent until blood pressure is stable. Supervise ambulation.

◆ Monitor CBC and differential and liver function tests.

◆ These drugs may cause allergic reactions. Check patients frequently when beginning therapy. Have drugs and equipment available to treat acute allergic reactions in settings where these drugs are administered.

Patient and family education

◆ Review anticipated benefits and possible side effects of drug therapy.

◆ Warn patients to avoid driving or operating hazardous equipment if drowsiness, dizziness, or visual changes develop.

◆ See Patient Problems: Orthostatic Hypotension on p. 234, Dry Mouth on p. 166, and Constipation on p. 182.

◆ Remind patients to use medications only as directed. Inform all health-care providers of all medications being taken.

◆ Warn patients to avoid alcohol unless permitted in small amounts by the physician.

◆ Instruct patients to take oral doses with meals or snack to lessen gastric irritation.

◆ Teach the patient to take the final dose of the day at bedtime.

◆ Warn patients taking chlorzoxazone that urine may turn orange or purple-red while they take drug.

◆ Warn patients taking methocarbamol that urine may turn black, brown, or green while they are taking this drug.

◆ Warn diabetic patients taking metaxalone to monitor blood sugar level carefully. This drug may cause inaccurate results with urine sugar tests.

CHAPTER REVIEW

◆ **KEY TERMS**

akinesia, p. 710

bradykinesia, p. 710

dyskinesia, p. 714

on-off phenomenon, p. 714

muscle spasm, p. 716

Parkinson's disease, p. 710

ridigity, p. 710

spasticity, p. 714

◆ **REVIEW QUESTIONS**

1. Describe the physical characteristics seen in Parkinson's disease.
2. What is the neurochemical defect in Parkinson's disease? How do some drugs mimic this defect?
3. Why are anticholinergic drugs, antihistaminic drugs, and amantadine effective in treating symptoms of parkinsonism? What are major side effects of these drug classes?
4. What is the rationale for administering levodopa to treat the symptoms of parkinsonism? What role does carbidopa play?
5. What are the side effects of levodopa?
6. Define spasticity.
7. How do diazepam, baclofen, and dantrolene reduce spasticity?
8. Describe the origin of muscle spasms.
9. What are the characteristics of the drugs used as centrally acting agents to treat muscle spasms?

SUGGESTED READING

de Roin S, Winters S: Amantadine hydrochloride: current and new uses, *J Neurosci Nurs* 22(5):322, 1990.

Hodges LC, Rapp CG: New drugs for Parkinson's disease, *J Neurosci Nurs* 22(4):254, 1990.

Norris MKG: Action stat! Malignant hyperthermia, *Nurs 90* 20(6):33, 1990.

Vernon GM: Parkinson's disease, *J Neurosci Nurs* 21(5):273, 1989.

SECTION XII

DRUGS AFFECTING THE ENDOCRINE SYSTEM

This section presents the pharmacology of drugs affecting the endocrine system. Chapter 49, Introduction to Endocrinology, defines the terms that must be mastered before the material in the subsequent chapters can be understood. This chapter also describes the concepts involved in treating endocrine diseases or in using hormones in therapy for other diseases. Knowledge of this material promotes understanding of many of the nursing assessments and actions described in later chapters.

Chapters 50 through 55 cover specific endocrine systems. In these chapters the pertinent physiology of the endocrine system is reviewed first. When appropriate, specific endocrine diseases are described so that discussion of the therapy for these diseases becomes more rational. Three classes of agents are described: natural hormones, synthetic forms of hormones, and non-hormonal drugs affecting the endocrine system. The purpose of therapy with each of these agents is clearly defined. Diagnostic tests are also described so that the student may understand the information that must be considered during patient assessment.

Some agents discussed in this section have significant medical uses outside of endocrinology. For example, the synthetic adrenal steroids (see Chapter 51) are widely used as antiinflammatory agents. These drugs are discussed in this section because students find it easier to understand the actions of the synthetic drugs if their similarity to the natural hormones is stressed. For similar reasons the anabolic steroids are considered in this section along with the androgens (see Chapter 54).

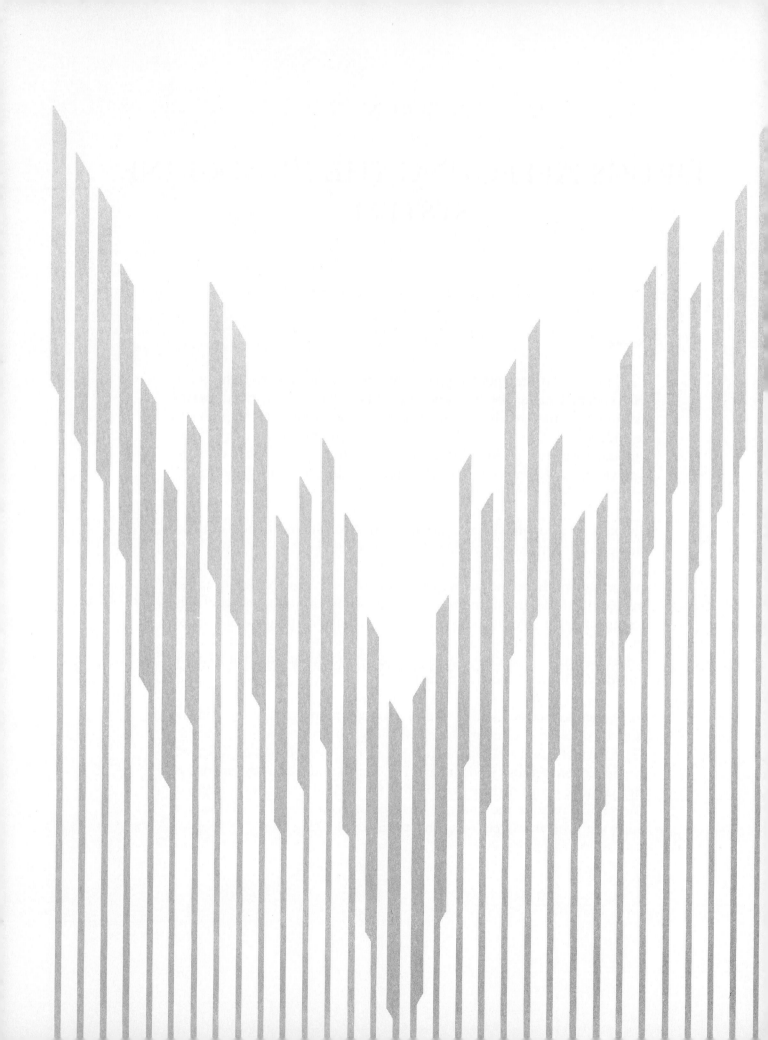

CHAPTER 49

Introduction to Endocrinology

LEARNING OBJECTIVES

After studying this chapter, you should be able to do the following:

◆ Define a hormone.
◆ Name the three uses of hormones in clinical medicine.
◆ Discuss how hormone action is regulated.
◆ Discuss the role of the nurse in hormone therapy.

CHAPTER OVERVIEW

◆ This introduction to endocrinology defines important terms, introduces the classes of hormones, and illustrates the concept of hormonal regulation of body processes. Properties of individual hormones are detailed in subsequent chapters, along with the specific function of each gland and the effects of related drugs.

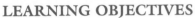

Nursing Process Overview

The specific considerations of endocrine-related drugs are covered in the other chapters of this section. The following presentation illustrates how the general concepts presented in this chapter can guide the nurse through the nursing process.

Assessment

Identify which endocrine organ is involved, and consider what other systems may be affected by the primary condition. For example, pituitary disease may influence multiple organ systems and may require therapy at several levels. It may be necessary to understand the various testing methods used to diagnose the loss of normal endocrine regulation.

Nursing Diagnoses

Possible self-concept disturbance
Knowledge deficit
Possible altered health maintenance

Management

Distinguish between replacement therapy and other forms of endocrine therapy. In replacement therapy the goal is to restore normal levels of a hormone in the patient's body, thereby restoring normal function of the endocrine system. In other types of therapy the goal may be to suppress overfunction of an endocrine tissue, to control the symptoms of excess hormone levels, or to affect a nonendocrine tissue with high levels of hormones. Work with the physician to define the goal of therapy for the patient. Teach the patient about the endocrine condition and the effects of the medications being used.

Evaluation

The nurse must be aware of the expected actions of the endocrine-related drugs and be able to recognize the side effects these agents may produce.

PROPERTIES OF HORMONES

A **hormone** is a substance produced by a particular cell type, which acts on other cells in the body to produce a physiologic or biochemical response. Traditionally, hormones have been considered to be compounds that are synthesized by a specific cell type, are released into the circulation, and act on target tissues elsewhere in the body. An example is thyrotropin (TSH), which is synthesized in the anterior pituitary tissue (adenohypophysis), released into systemic circulation, and taken up by the thyroid gland, there stimulating the production of thyroid hormones (see Chapter 52).

Organs producing hormones that enter systemic circulation are the **endocrine glands**—pancreas, adrenal glands, thyroid gland, parathyroid glands, testes, ovaries, neurohypophysis, and adrenohypophysis. The neurohypophysis and adenohypophysis comprise the pituitary gland, or hypophysis. Those tissues affected by the hormones from the endocrine glands are designated *target tissues*. For example, the target tissue of TSH secreted by the adenohypophysis is the thyroid gland. No other tissue in the body responds to TSH.

Some compounds that have been called *hormones* act strictly locally, producing their effect at or near the site where they are synthesized. Examples of such compounds are acetylcholine, which is synthesized, acts, and is destroyed at the nerve terminal, and prostaglandins, which are formed from membrane fatty acids at the sites of prostaglandin action. Acetylcholine is discussed in Chapter 9, and prostaglandins are considered for their action on the uterus in Chapter 53. These locally acting substances are not discussed further in this chapter.

Hormones may be divided into two classes on the basis of their chemical composition. One class is the steroid hormones, which are derived from cholesterol. This class of hormones includes the hormones of the adrenal gland (cortisol, cortisone, aldosterone, corticosterone, and others) and the hormones of the sex glands (androgens, estrogens, and progestins). Many of these steroid compounds have been synthesized by organic chemists, so their production for medicinal purposes does not depend entirely on isolating them from such natural sources as bovine or porcine adrenal glands obtained as by-products of the meat-packing industry. Some clinically useful steroids are obtained from natural sources, however, because the steroids are present in such high concentrations and are so easily extracted, making the procedure economically feasible. An example of such a preparation is Premarin, a mixture of conjugated estrogens extracted from the urine of pregnant mares. Another useful feature of many, but not all steroid hormones, is that they may be taken orally.

The second class of hormones is formed from amino acids. Two subclasses within this group are amino acid derivatives and proteins. Examples of the first subclass are thyroxine and triiodothyronine, the iodinated tyrosine derivatives produced in the thyroid gland, and the catecholamines, produced in various tissues from the amino acid tyrosine. The second subclass includes peptides and proteins. Peptides and proteins are distinguished arbitrarily by difference in size, with peptides containing fewer amino acids than proteins. Chemically, peptides and proteins are similar in that both are formed by the peptide bond linking carboxyl and amino groups of adjacent amino acids. Examples of peptide hormones are the releasing factors produced in the hypothalamus, including thyrotropin-releasing hormone (TRH), composed of three amino acids; and the neurohypophyseal hormones oxytocin and vasopressin, which are each composed of eight amino acids. Examples of protein hormones within this second subclass include insulin, with 51 amino acids and a molecular weight of 6000; and follicle-stimulating hormone (FSH) with a molecular weight of 41,000.

The active forms of many protein hormones are derived from larger protein molecules called *prohormones*. For example, insulin is originally released as part of a prohormone containing at least 86 amino acids. Cleavage of 35 amino acids from this larger precursor molecule releases active insulin.

The peptide and protein hormones in general are present in very small quantities in natural sources and may be difficult to isolate. For example, insulin, the protein hormone most often used medically, is prepared by pharmaceutical manufacturers in large quantities from bovine or porcine pancreas glands by tedious and expensive extraction procedures. Growth hormone, a protein hormone used to treat a rare endocrine disease, may be extracted from the adenohypophysis, but the only form that is active in human beings is the growth hormone from primate sources. The supply of this hormone therefore was restricted by the limited supply of source material. In the past, growth hormone was obtained postmortem from human adenohyphophysis, but the risk of viral contamination has caused this product to be dropped.

A powerful new method for producing human hormones is based on genetic engineering. Genetic engineering involves taking the genes from one species and inserting them into an unrelated species, thereby creating new characteristics in the recipient. The human genes for insulin, growth hormone, interferons, and other proteins have been inserted into certain bacteria. These altered bacteria then may be grown on a large scale in fermentation tanks and produce large quantities of the human protein. Insulin produced in this way is now sold under the trade name *Humulin*. This human insulin is synthesized by *Escherichia coli* from the human genes artificially inserted into the bacteria. This technique is applicable to a variety of proteins and solves the problem of limited supply of clinically useful proteins. In addition, hormones produced by this technique are less likely to be contaminated with viruses. For this reason, human growth hormone produced by genetically engineered bacteria is now the standard preparation for human use.

The protein and peptide hormones are somewhat

inconvenient for the patient to use. Although thyroxine and triiodothyronine may be taken by mouth, none of the larger peptides and proteins survive the action of digestive juices in the stomach and intestine. Thus peptides and proteins must be administered by injection. Even when given parenterally, these compounds may not be effective because the patient may suffer an allergic, foreign-protein reaction or may develop resistance because of the production of antibodies directed at the foreign protein.

USES OF HORMONES

The hormones discussed in this section are used clinically in one of three ways—as diagnostic agents, in replacement therapy, or as pharmacologic agents.

The most common diagnostic use of hormones is to assess the function of the target organ of the administered hormone. For example, adrenocorticotropin may be administered to test the ability of the adrenal gland to produce steroids. Another adenohypophyseal hormone, thyrotropin, is administered to test the capacity of the thyroid gland to synthesize thyroid hormones.

Replacement therapy is aimed at restoring normal levels of hormones, which, for some reason, a patient's body no longer produces. Physiologic doses are used in an attempt to maintain normal hormone levels without producing toxic effects from hormone excesses. The use of thyroxine to treat hypothyroidism and cortisol to treat Addison's disease (chronic adrenal insufficiency) are examples of replacement therapy. Insulin use in diabetic patients is also an example of replacement therapy.

The use of hormones as pharmacologic agents, with administered doses far in excess of those required to produce physiologic levels, makes use of some function of the compound other than the one seen at physiologic concentrations. For example, adrenal corticosteroids may be given in large doses to suppress inflammatory responses in certain diseases. This antiinflammatory effect is not obvious at physiologic concentrations of the steroid.

REGULATION OF HORMONE ACTION

Hormones are potent agents capable of exerting profound effects on metabolism. It is imperative for healthy functioning of the body that these compounds act only where and when they are needed and that they be present at the proper concentrations. The time of appearance and the concentration of a hormone in the blood may be regulated by controlling its rate of synthesis, release from storage sites, degradation, and clearance from the body. Several hormones are stored after synthesis and are released from storage sites only when the proper stimulus is received. For example, thyroxine and triiodothyronine are stored in complex with thyroglobulin in the thyroid gland. Insulin is stored in granules within the beta cell of the pancreas. In these cases, when the endocrine gland is stimulated to release hormone, the stored hormone is first released. Then, if required, newly synthesized hormone is released into the bloodstream.

Regulation of synthesis and release of many hormones involves the interaction of the central nervous system (CNS) with the endocrine glands. For example, the hypothalamus in the brain controls the hypophysis, which in turn regulates the production of hormones by ovaries, testes, thyroid, and adrenal glands. This system is the negative feedback regulation discussed in Chapter 50.

Hormones disappear from the bloodstream when they are taken up by various organs or when they are degraded by enzymes in the blood. The kidneys are the site of degradation or excretion for several hormones, including most steroids. The kidneys and the liver degrade insulin. Vasopressin, in contrast, is very rapidly destroyed by enzymes in blood. The half-life of vasopressin, (i.e., the time required for half of the injected dose to disappear from the blood) is approximately 15 min. Other hormones persist for much longer periods. For example, thyroxine has a plasma half-life of about 7 days. How rapidly a hormone is lost from the body determines doses and dosage schedules when these hormones are administered. Knowledge of the elimination half-life also helps in dealing with toxic reactions whose duration may be related to the persistence of the compound in the body.

Controlling the location of action of a certain hormone is accomplished in the body in one of two ways. The first localization mechanism is to restrict the distribution of the hormone. Examples are the releasing factors synthesized in the hypothalamus and released into local portal veins carrying the hormones directly to the adenohypophysis and not into the general circulation.

A second mechanism localizes the effect of generally released hormones. These hormones interact with specific receptors, which are found only in their target tissues. The specific receptor is required for hormone activity. For example, progesterone receptors are found primarily in tissues of the female reproductive tract but not in most other organs. Therefore, even though progesterone is released into the general circulation, it acts only on those tissues possessing receptors.

The receptors for hormones may be within cells. For example, steroids and thyroid hormones affect

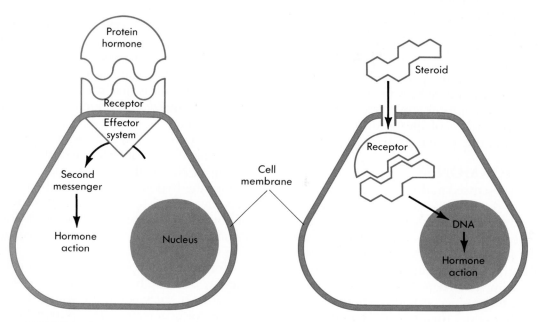

FIGURE 49-1

Sites for hormone receptors. Cell on left illustrates common mechanism for responding to protein hormones, with external receptor interacting through effector system. Cell on right illustrates mechanism shared by steroid hormones and thyroid hormones in which hormone enters cytoplasm, is bound by a receptor, and is carried to the nucleus where effect is produced.

target cells by interacting with intracellular receptors (Figure 49-1). The steroid hormones are bound by soluble receptors, which transport the hormones through the cytoplasm of the cell and into the cell nucleus. The final effect of the hormone is produced by this action within the cell nucleus. Thyroid hormones are transported to the nucleus by nonspecific proteins; in the nucleus the thyroid hormones bind to specific receptors and ultimately alter protein synthesis in the cell.

In contrast to the receptors for steroids and thyroid hormones, receptors for peptide and protein hormones exist on the external surface of cell membranes (see Figure 49-1). The peptide and protein hormones therefore need not enter the cell to become effective. One mechanism by which these externally bound hormones act is by releasing an internal regulator, or second messenger. For example, parathyroid hormone binds to a receptor on the surface of certain kidney cells. This receptor is associated with an enzyme called *adenylate cyclase* so that when parathyroid hormone binds to the receptor, adenylate cyclase is stimulated to release cyclic adenosine monophos-

phate (cyclic AMP) within the cell. Cyclic AMP is the second messenger that alters the internal processes of the cell. Vasopressin acts in a similar way on other cells within the kidney. Not all hormone receptors on the cell surface membrane are linked to adenylate cyclase and cyclic AMP. For example, the multiple metabolic changes produced by insulin within target cells do not depend on cyclic AMP.

The response of a target cell to a hormone depends on the number and availability of hormone receptors. Regulating the number of receptors is therefore another mechanism by which the body can maintain metabolic balance. An example of this type of regulation is found in obese persons with a high food intake. These persons have chronically high insulin concentrations in the bloodstream. To protect itself from the metabolic effects of this high amount of insulin, the body eliminates a certain percentage of the insulin receptors on cells. The loss of insulin receptors, called down-regulation, lowers the responsiveness of the cell to insulin.

Understanding the role of receptors in fulfilling the metabolic role of hormones allows a clearer understanding of endocrine diseases and how they are classified. An endocrine deficiency can arise from a lack of hormone or from a lack of receptors that enables the tissue to respond to the hormone. An example is diabetes insipidus, which may be produced by a lack of antidiuretic hormone (ADH) or by a lack of receptors in the kidney that can respond to ADH. Similarly, diabetes mellitus can be characterized by the lack of insulin in the bloodstream or by high levels of insulin in the bloodstream but lower-than-normal numbers of active insulin receptors on cells.

CHAPTER REVIEW

◆ **KEY TERMS**

endocrine glands, p. 724
hormone, p. 723
prohormones, p. 724
target tissues, p. 724

◆ **REVIEW QUESTIONS**

1. What is a hormone?
2. What is a target tissue?
3. Describe the two major chemical types of hormones.
4. What is a prohormone?
5. Name three ways in which large amounts of hormones may be obtained for clinical use.
6. What are the three primary clinical uses of hormones?
7. Describe how the amount of hormone in the body may be regulated.
8. How may the site of action of a hormone be restricted?
9. In what ways may the actions of hormones be terminated?
10. What is a releasing factor?
11. What are the two main types of hormone receptors? How do these receptors differ in the way they interact with hormones?
12. Describe the two general types of endocrine deficiency diseases.

SUGGESTED READING

Anthony CP, Thibodeau GA: *Textbook of anatomy and physiology,* ed 13, St Louis, 1991, Mosby–Year Book.
Fredholm, BB: Diversity in receptor signalling: cellular individuality and the search for selective drugs, *J Intern Med* 229:391, 1991.
Wahli W, Martinez E: Superfamily of steroid nuclear receptors: positive and negative regulators of gene expression, *FASEB J* 5:2243, 1991.

CHAPTER 50

Drugs Affecting the Pituitary Gland

LEARNING OBJECTIVES

After studying this chapter, you should be able to do the following:

- Identify the two parts of the pituitary gland.
- Describe the function of the two hormones of the neurohypophysis.
- Describe the function of the gonadotropic hormones.
- Identify the source and use of growth hormones.
- Develop a nursing care plan for the patient receiving drug therapy for diabetes insipidus, for growth hormone deficiency, or to suppress excessive release of growth hormone.

CHAPTER OVERVIEW

- The pituitary gland, or hypophysis, lies in the sella turcica, a bony cavity at the base of the brain. Although the gland weighs less than 1 gm, it is the primary regulator of the endocrine system, controlling normal growth and regulating water balance.
- The pituitary gland is divided into two portions with very different tissue compositions and embryologic origins. These two regions are the anterior pituitary, or adenohypophysis, and the posterior pituitary, or neurohypophysis. The structure and function of each of these tissues, the function and regulation of the various hormones produced, and the pathologic states resulting from abnormalities in hormone production are considered in this chapter.

Nursing Process Overview

PITUITARY THERAPY

Assessment

In most cases, patients with pituitary hormone problems have had chronic excesses or deficiencies of the hormones before the diagnosis is made. Perform a thorough examination to obtain baseline data, paying particular attention to subjective and objective changes that the patient may indicate have occurred over an extended period.

Nursing Diagnoses

Knowledge deficit

Fluid volume excess related to excessive dose of vasopressin

Management

Monitor the patient for expected drug side effects. Before discharge, begin the teaching and emotional support needed to help the patient move to self-management.

Evaluation

Before discharge, ascertain that the patient can explain why the prescribed drugs are necessary, how to administer them correctly, signs of overdosage or underdosage, and side effects that might occur and which ones should be reported immediately. If a patient does not have a medical identification tag or bracelet before leaving the hospital, state the need to obtain one.

NEUROHYPOPHYSIS

The *posterior pituitary,* or **neurohypophysis,** is composed of nerve fibers embryologically derived from the hypothalamus. Close contact between the central nervous system (CNS) and the neurohypophysis is maintained by the nerve fibers that run from the hypothalamus through the hypophyseal stalk to the neurohypophysis (Figure 50-1). Two octapeptide hormones closely related in structure are released by the neurohypophysis. These are antidiuretic hormone

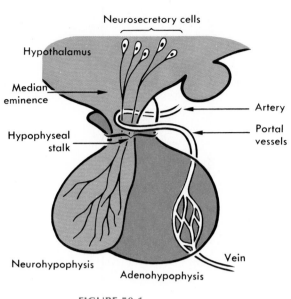

FIGURE 50-1
Anatomy of pituitary gland.

and oxytocin. They are synthesized in the hypothalamus and are transported in secretion granules down the axons running between the hypothalamus and the neurohypophysis. The granules accumulate at the nerve fiber terminals and are stored in the neurohypophysis, where their release into the systemic circulation is regulated by nerve impulses originating in the hypothalamus. Damage to the hypophyseal stalk impairs transport of the secretory granules to the neurohypophysis and interferes with appropriate release of the hormones into the circulation.

Neurohypophyseal Hormones

Antidiuretic hormone

Mechanism of action. Antidiuretic hormone **(ADH),** also called *vasopressin,* has as its primary target tissue the renal tubular epithelium (Table 50-1). ADH increases the permeability of certain sections of the renal tubule to water, allowing water to be reabsorbed from the tubule and returned to the bloodstream. This is the mechanism by which healthy kidneys concentrate urine.

In addition to regulating water balance by acting on the renal tubular epithelium, ADH also modulates CNS activity. CNS effects of ADH may influence affective behavior, memory, thermoregulation, and the function of the anterior pituitary. ADH is not yet used clinically for these CNS effects.

Regulation of secretion. Secretion of ADH is regulated mainly in response to plasma osmolarity, the concentration of solute molecules that increase osmotic pressure (see Chapter 17). In dehydration the effective osmotic pressure of blood increases. The osmoreceptors of the hypothalamus respond to this change by stimulating the neurohypophysis to secrete ADH, which in turn causes the kidney to conserve body water and to prevent or slow further dehydration. This recovery from dehydration is aided further by concomitant stimulation of the thirst center, leading to increased intake of fluids. Reduction in the effective plasma volume caused by hemorrhage or reduced cardiac output stimulates ADH release and promotes antidiuresis.

In addition to these physiologic controls, certain drugs also may influence ADH secretion. Acetylcholine, nicotine, morphine, barbiturates, and bradykinin cause release of ADH in healthy subjects. Ethanol and phenytoin may promote diuresis by inhibiting ADH release.

Effects of ADH deficiency. When ADH is markedly reduced or absent because of destruction of the hypothalamic region responsible for its synthesis or because of separation of the hypophyseal stalk above the median eminence (see Figure 50-1), urinary concentration is impossible, and large volumes of dilute, sugar-free urine are produced. This condition is called *diabetes insipidus* and is not to be confused with the disease diabetes mellitus, which arises from the inability to use blood glucose or to release insulin.

Diabetes insipidus is not a life-threatening condition unless severe electrolyte imbalances develop. As long as the patient has a fully functional thirst center and can balance the excessive fluid losses with high

Table 50-1   Neurohypophyseal Hormones

Descriptive name	Other names	Target tissues	Target tissue response
Antidiuretic hormone	ADH Vasopressin	Renal tubule epithelium Smooth muscle in blood vessels Smooth muscle of GI tract	Increased water permeability Vasoconstriction Contraction, increasing GI motility
Oxytocin	—	Uterine smooth muscle Breast myoepithelium	Increased uterine contractions Milk letdown

Table 50-2 Drugs to Treat Diabetes Insipidus

Generic name	Trade name	Drug class	Administration	Properties	Uses	Side effects
Desmopressin acetate	DDAVP* Stimate	Synthetic derivative of vasopressin	Nasal or parenteral	Peptide with longer serum half-life than vasopressin; increases renal reabsorption of water	Replacement therapy	Mild vasoconstriction; mild smooth muscle contraction; FDA Pregnancy Category B
Lypressin	Diapid	Synthetic derivative of vasopressin	Nasal	Peptide with short serum half-life; increases renal reabsorption of water	Replacement therapy	Difficulty breathing because drug accidentally inhaled; smooth muscle contraction
Posterior pituitary extract	Pituitrin*	Neurohypophyseal hormone	Parenteral	Peptide with short serum half-life; contains ADH and oxytocin (see Chapter 53)	Rarely used	Vasoconstriction; smooth muscle contraction; FDA Pregnancy Category C
Vasopressin	Pitressin* Pressynt	Neurohypophyseal hormone	Parenteral	Peptide with short serum half-life; increases renal reabsorption of water	Short-term maintenance of unconscious patient with diabetes insipidus; to stimulate peristalsis	Vasoconstriction; smooth muscle contraction stimulates GI motility
Vasopressin tannate in oil	Pitressin Tannate in oil*	Neurohypophyseal hormone	IM depot	Preparation slowly absorbed; increases renal reabsorption of water	Replacement therapy	Vasoconstriction; smooth muscle contraction
Chlorothiazide	Diuril	Thiazide diuretic	Oral	Mild sodium and water depletion lowers water delivery to collecting ducts in kidneys	Control of diuresis in diabetes insipidus	Hyponatremia; hypokalemia
Chlorpropamide	Diabinese*	Sulfonylurea hypoglycemic agent	Oral	Increases release of ADH from posterior pituitary and increases ADH action in kidney	Control of diuresis in diabetes insipidus	Hypoglycemia; FDA Pregnancy Category C
Clofibrate	Atromid S* Claripex†	Hypolipidemic agent	Oral	Increases release of ADH from posterior pituitary	Control of diuresis in diabetes insipidus; rarely used	Nausea, weakness, and muscle cramps; increased risk of cardiovascular disease
Carbamazepine	Tegretol*	Anticonvulsant	Oral	Increases release of ADH from posterior pituitary	Control of diuresis in diabetes insipidus	Dizziness, confusion, and drowsiness; water retention; hyponatremia

*Available in Canada and United States.
†Available in Canada only.

fluid intakes, severe imbalances do not occur frequently. When a person is unconscious and unable to take in adequate fluids, however, severe dehydration may set in before the condition is noticed. Thus, following traumatic head injuries or surgery to the hypothalamic region of the brain, it is critically important for health-care personnel to monitor urinary specific gravity and blood sodium levels, along with fluid intake and urinary volumes, to detect excessive diuresis and resultant dehydration.

In many patients with trauma to the hypothalamus or the hypophyseal stalk the resultant diabetes insipidus may be transitory. In patients whose condition is chronic, reversal of symptoms can be achieved by replacement therapy with a form of ADH or by therapy with pharmacologic agents that relieve the symptoms of the disease.

ADH replacement therapy. Because ADH is a peptide hormone, it cannot be administered orally, and all replacement therapy with ADH involves the administration of the hormone parenterally or intranasally (Table 50-2).

Vasopressin (Pitressin), an aqueous preparation of purified ADH, is not routinely used because the half-life of ADH in the blood is short. This preparation is injected intramuscularly or subcutaneously two or three times daily for short-term management of patients. The duration of action of vasopressin may be extended by slowing absorption. Lypressin, a synthetic form of ADH that is sprayed onto the mucous membranes of the nasal passages, is usually administered four times daily. Posterior pituitary extract was used in the past, but it tended to irritate nasal passages and to produce unwanted effects caused by proteins other than ADH that were present in the extract.

Desmopressin acetate (DDAVP) administered intranasally is the drug of choice in replacement therapy for chronic diabetes insipidus. DDAVP is a chemically altered form of vasopressin, differing from the natural hormone by having a long serum half-life, a more potent antidiuretic effect, and less pressor activity. It is administered only once or twice daily, unlike other ADH preparations. Side effects caused by the pressor action of vasopressin are also less problematic with this vasopressin derivative.

Long-term control of diabetes insipidus also may be achieved with vasopressin tannate in peanut oil, which is given as an intramuscular (IM) depot injection. Patients have reported normal concentration of urine for up to 48 hr after injection of this preparation. Patients should be warned not to repeat the injection until the diuresis recurs. Since the introduction of lypressin and desmopressin acetate for intranasal administration, the use of vasopressin tannate in oil has declined. Although the intranasal drugs are not as long acting, they are more convenient to administer than vasopressin tannate. Many patients report difficulty in getting consistent dosages with vasopressin tannate in oil because of problems in achieving completely homogeneous suspensions of the drug in the oily vehicle.

ADH has been used as a pressor agent but now is not recommended for that use. Its vasoconstrictor action prevents its safe use for patients with vascular or coronary artery disease. Even small doses may cause difficulty to a patient prone to angina attacks. Occasionally, this vasoconstrictor action is used to help control massive gastrointestinal (GI) bleeding, especially from esophageal varices.

ADH can also promote activity of the smooth muscle of the intestinal tract. During routine therapy of diabetes insipidus the action of ADH on intestinal smooth muscle may result in nausea, belching, and cramps.

Other drugs to treat diabetes insipidus. Agents other than ADH preparations have been used to treat diabetes insipidus (see Table 50-2). Paradoxically, thiazide diuretics (see Chapter 16) are effective in some cases, especially when combined with one of the other oral agents listed in this section. The effectiveness of the thiazide diuretics apparently is based on their blockade of electrolyte reabsorption, resulting initially in increased sodium and water excretion. The kidney responds to this change by reabsorbing more water by mechanisms that do not depend on ADH. Moderate salt restriction enhances the action of these drugs in many patients. Dosages of the thiazides used to treat diabetes insipidus are the same as those used for other indications (see Chapter 16). The most common side effect is potassium depletion, which in extreme cases may induce cardiac arrhythmias and impair neuromuscular functions and the normal functions of the GI tract and kidney. Although any thiazide might be selected for use in diabetes insipidus, chlorothiazide is listed in Table 50-2 as the representative drug for the class.

Chlorpropamide, a sulfonylurea used as an oral hypoglycemic agent to treat diabetes mellitus (see Chapter 55), is also used at comparable doses for diabetes insipidus. Alone or with a thiazide diuretic, chlorpropamide is usually effective in reducing urine volumes. The major potential toxicity is hypoglycemia. When chlorpropamide is used to treat diabetes insipidus, the action sought is a direct sensitization of the kidney to vasopressin so that lower-than-normal levels of vasopressin cause nearly normal water reabsorption. It apparently is not effective in patients who produce no vasopressin. Evidence suggests chlorpropamide may also stimulate the pituitary to release vasopressin.

Clofibrate, an oral agent used to reduce serum triglyceride levels (see Chapter 21), may also be effective in treating diabetes insipidus and may be used alone or in combination with a thiazide diuretic. It may produce nausea or rarely muscle cramps and weakness. Clofibrate increases the release of ADH from the posterior pituitary. The dose of clofibrate used for diabetes insipidus is the same as for the lipid-lowering effect.

Carbamazepine is an anticonvulsant that occasionally has been used to control diabetes insipidus. Its action is similar to that of clofibrate; both drugs cause release of ADH from the posterior pituitary. The potentially severe side effects of carbamazepine limit its usefulness in diabetes insipidus. Various CNS effects may be seen and often necessitate cessation of therapy. Blood dyscrasias also may occur.

The form of diabetes insipidus covered in the previous paragraphs is called *central diabetes insipidus* because it arises from a lack of secretion of ADH from the neurohypophysis. The symptoms of diabetes insipidus may also arise if the neurohypophysis is producing normal amounts of ADH, but the kidney is unresponsive or responds poorly to ADH. This syndrome, called **nephrogenic diabetes insipidus,** may be treated by the thiazide diuretics but is resistant to therapy by ADH. Although nephrogenic diabetes insipidus may arise as a genetic disease, it also may be induced by drugs that impair the ability of the kidney to react to ADH. Drugs such as lithium used in treating mental disease (see Chapter 42) and demeclocycline, a tetracycline antibiotic (see Chapter 32), can induce nephrogenic diabetes insipidus by this mechanism.

The **syndrome of inappropriate ADH (SIADH)** secretion is a rare condition in which patients show symptoms of water intoxication including hyponatremia, or low sodium levels in the blood (see Chapter 17), and low serum osmolality. Despite these conditions, the kidneys continue to excrete sodium. The symptoms of SIADH are caused by the release of more ADH than is appropriate, based on the normal osmotic regulatory signals. In most patients with SIADH, the excess ADH is released by a tumor such as a bronchogenic carcinoma. Other less common causes of SIADH are CNS disorders, including head injuries or infections, and extreme physical stress such as after surgery or extreme emotional stress. A variety of drugs occasionally may trigger SIADH, including carbamazepine, chlorpropamide, clofibrate, cyclophosphamide, narcotics, nicotine, thiazide diuretics, and vincristine.

Treatment of SIADH usually is aimed directly at removing the cause of the condition such as removing the tumor or discontinuing the drug thought to precipitate the disorder. Fluid restriction, infusion of hypotonic saline, and diuretics all may help control the fluid and electrolyte imbalances associated with SIADH. If the cause of excessive ADH cannot be completely removed, symptoms may be relieved by administering drugs that render the kidneys less sensitive to ADH. Demeclocycline is preferred, although lithium is effective in some patients. Demeclocycline and lithium may induce nephrogenic diabetes insipidus in persons with normal ADH levels.

Oxytocin

The second hormone released by the neurohypophysis is **oxytocin.** The major target organs of this octapeptide hormone are breast myoepithelium and the smooth muscle of the uterus, especially during the second and third stages of labor. Oxytocin is discussed in detail in Chapter 53. Briefly, oxytocin speeds delivery by promoting uterine contractions during the final stages of labor when the cervix is fully dilated. A second important function of oxytocin is to cause milk ejection by stimulating contraction of the myoepithelium of the alveoli of the breast.

The regulation of oxytocin release is a particularly good example of the close interaction of the CNS with pituitary function. Suckling by the infant induces afferent nerve impulses from the breast to the brain, which causes more oxytocin to be synthesized and stored hormone to be released. A similar reflex loop may operate in parturition when dilation of the cervix is thought to stimulate synthesis and release of oxytocin.

No specific syndrome resulting from abnormalities in oxytocin function has been described.

ADENOHYPOPHYSIS

The anterior pituitary, or **adenohypophysis,** constitutes approximately 75% by weight of the pituitary gland and is regarded as the master gland of the entire endocrine system. The adenohypophysis secretes several peptide hormones, most of which directly stimulate secretion by the adrenal glands, the thyroid gland, and the reproductive organs (Table 50-3).

The adenohypophysis synthesizes several peptide hormones in addition to the clinically important ones shown in Table 50-3. Melanocyte-stimulating hormone (MSH) is released in response to corticotropin-releasing factor (CRF), the factor that controls ACTH.

Lipotropin (beta LPH) is a weak stimulator of lipolysis, but this action is probably not the main function of the peptide. Fragments of lipotropin are identical to beta endorphin and metenkephalin, endogenous opioids released not only in the pituitary but also in several sites in the brain. The endorphin

Table 50-3 Physiologic Action of Adenohypophyseal Hormones

Descriptive name	Other names	Hypothalamic-releasing factor	Target tissue	Target tissue response
Adrenocorticotropic hormone	ACTH Corticotropin	Corticotropin-releasing factor (CRF)	Adrenal cortex Pigment cells of skin	Increased steroid synthesis Increased pigmentation
Follicle-stimulating hormone	FSH	Gonadotropin-releasing hormone (GnRH); FSH-releasing hormone (FRH and FSH-RH)	Ovary Seminiferous tubules	Increased estrogen production Maturation
Growth hormone	GH Somatotropin Somatropin STH	Somatotropin or growth hormone—releasing factor (SRF or GRF); somatostatin or somatotropin-release inhibitory factor (SRIF)	Whole body	Increased anabolism, cell size, and cell numbers
Luteinizing hormone or interstitial cell–stimulating hormone	ICSH LH	Gonadotropin-releasing hormone (GnRH); luteinizing hormone–releasing factor or hormone (LRF, LRH, LHRF, and LHRH)	Ovary Leydig cells	Ovulation; formation of corpus luteum Increased androgen synthesis
Prolactin	LTH Luteotropic hormone	Prolactin-inhibiting factor (PIF); prolactin-releasing factor (PRF)	Breast	Milk formation
Thyroid-stimulating hormone	Thyrotropin TSH	Thyrotropin-releasing hormone or factor (TRH and TRF)	Thyroid gland	Increased T_3 and T_4 synthesis

and enkephalin peptides may be neurotransmitters in the hypothalamus, aiding in regulation of pituitary function, body temperature, and cardiovascular function (see Chapter 44).

The protein called *pro-opiomelanocortin* (POMC) is a precursor molecule that may be broken down by the various cell types found in the adenohypophysis to ACTH, MSH, beta lipotropin, or beta endorphin. Although POMC, MSH, and lipotropin have no obvious clinical applications to date, synthetic derivatives of the endogenous opioids are being widely studied as potential analgesic agents.

Although the adenohypophysis is true secretory tissue that synthesizes and releases its hormones, control of those secretions lies in the brain. Small polypeptides, called *neurohormones,* are synthesized in the median eminence of the hypothalamus and are released into the portal venous system (see Figure 50-1) that carries them directly to the adenohypophysis. In the adenohypophysis, these neurohormones, which may be releasing or inhibitory hormones, act on the specific target cell to stimulate or to inhibit synthesis and release of the proper hormone.

Adenohypophyseal Hormones

Growth hormone

Mechanism of action. **Growth hormone** regulates the length of the long bones of the skeleton, which determine adult stature. In addition, the hormone is a potent anabolic agent that causes many tissues to increase cell size and numbers. This anabolic action results from changes produced in protein, carbohydrate, and fat metabolism. The hormone increases the rate of amino acid transport into cells and elevates the cellular rate of protein synthesis. Growth hormone also antagonizes the action of insulin, which tends to decrease glucose uptake and carbohydrate use, thus elevating liver glycogen and blood glucose levels. Finally, growth hormone increases the mobilization of fats for energy, which leads to a rise in blood levels of free fatty acids.

Many of the actions of growth hormone are mediated by peptides called **somatomedins.** Growth hormone stimulates production of somatomedins by the liver. The somatomedins then act on various body tissues to change metabolism. Somatomedins also have been called *insulin-like growth factors;* in addition to stimulating growth of the skeleton, these peptides may have insulin-like actions on other tissues.

Regulation of secretion. The secretion of growth hormone is regulated by two factors from the hypothalamus, one stimulating and one inhibiting release. The releasing factor is a protein containing about 40 amino acids. The inhibitory factor is a smaller, 14–amino-acid peptide called *somatostatin.* In addition to regulating growth hormone release, somatostatin may also influence thyroid-stimulating hormone (TSH) and adrenocorticotropic hormone (ACTH) release from the pituitary gland. Somatostatin is found in other tissues such as gut and pancreas (see Chapter 55) and may play different regulatory roles in those tissues.

Growth hormone deficiency. Damage to the hypophysis may cause it to produce insufficient quantities of hypophyseal hormones, a condition called *panhypopituitarism*. Adults suffering from this syndrome may require replacement therapy with thyroid hormones, adrenal steroids, and appropriate sex steroids. Children with panhypopituitarism may also suffer growth stunting because of a lack of growth hormone.

True pituitary dwarfism can be treated successfully with growth hormone preparations. Of the many forms of growth stunting, only that form caused by growth hormone deficiency is appropriately treated with growth hormone. The standard preparations for therapy are prepared by recombinant DNA techniques. Somatotropin, recombinant has the same amino acid sequence as the natural hormone found in the human hypophysis. Somatrem is a recombinant-derived form that has one more amino acid than natural growth hormone. Children or adolescents with pituitary dwarfism who receive growth hormone typically show an immediate increase in growth and may increase 1 foot or more in height over several years of treatment. Ultimately, resistance to the protein develops, and growth tapers off.

Growth hormone should not be used in adolescents whose epiphyses have sealed because stimulation of further natural growth is unlikely. These preparations should not be used to enhance size or bulk in healthy young athletes because the risks outweigh the minimal benefits.

Many actions of growth hormone antagonize those of insulin, and in predisposed individuals, prolonged treatment with growth hormone may precipitate diabetes mellitus. Thus patients receiving growth hormone are monitored to detect elevated blood glucose levels or altered glucose tolerance. In adults with established diabetes, destruction of the hypophysis with loss of growth hormone reduces their insulin requirement.

Excess growth hormone. Acromegaly and gigantism are produced by excess growth hormone, but the age of onset causes marked differences in the manifestations of the disease. Excessive growth hormone from an early age produces the rare condition of gigantism. Growth rates of 3½ inches/year have been reported. One pituitary giant on record was 8 feet 11 inches tall.

If the onset of excessive growth hormone production is delayed until after puberty (i.e., after the plates of the long bones have joined and normal skeletal growth has halted), acromegaly results. In this condition, only those tissues still able to grow and expand respond to growth hormone, resulting in malproportions. Typically, the bones of the fingers flare at the end, and the fingers thicken to produce a spatula-like appearance. Bones and cartilage of the face also grow and thicken, producing coarse features and a massive lower jaw.

Both gigantism and acromegaly usually are caused by pituitary neoplasms, which secrete excessive amounts of growth hormone. Consequently, therapy is designed to destroy or to remove the tumor. Successful treatment results in the arrest of the progressive symptoms of the disease but does not erase the existing deformations. When removal or destruction

Table 50-4   Growth Hormone and Related Drugs

Generic name	Trade name	Description	Clinical use
Bromocriptine mesylate	Parlodel*	Bromocriptine is related to ergot alkaloids used as oxytocics.	Suppresses release of growth hormone and prolactin (see Chapter 53)
Octreotide	Sandostatin*	Octreotide is an analogue of somatostatin.	Suppresses release of growth hormone, insulin, and glucagon; also slows intestinal transit time
Somatrem	Protropin*	Synthetic somatropin differs by one amino acid from the natural hormone.	Replacement therapy for pituitary dwarfism
Somatropin, recombinant	Humatrope*	Somatropin produced by recombinant technology is chemically identical to natural hormone.	Replacement therapy for pituitary dwarfism

*Available in Canada and United States.

of the tumor is not possible or is only partially successful, the drug bromocriptine may inhibit release of growth hormone from the hypophysis. Octreotide, an analogue of somatostatin, can also help suppress excessive release of growth hormone (Table 50-4).

Gonadotropic Hormones

Mechanism of action

The gonadotropic hormones of the adenohypophysis are follicle-stimulating hormone (FSH), luteinizing hormone (LH), and prolactin. FSH and LH regulate maturation and function of the male and female sexual organs. In women, prolactin stimulates milk formation in the estrogen- and progestin-primed breast.

In the maturing male, FSH causes the seminiferous tubules to mature. LH, which is sometimes called *interstitial cell-stimulating hormone* in the male, increases the number of testicular interstitial cells and stimulates their secretion of androgens. These androgens are the male steroid hormones that complete the maturation process, leading to the production of viable sperm and to the development of the secondary male sexual characteristics.

In the maturing female, FSH and LH are produced in greater quantities at puberty and stimulate ovarian estrogen production. Estrogens, the female steroid hormones, cause the female secondary sex characteristics to develop.

Regulation of gonadotropin secretion in adult females. In addition to their role in development, FSH and LH control the menstrual cycle in the mature female (Figure 50-2). The regulation of this function involves the hypothalamus, the adenohypophysis, the ovaries, and the endometrium, or uterine lining. The first event in the cycle is a rise in the concentration of FSH in the blood. In response, in the ovary, one of the hundreds of primordial follicles begins to develop. As the follicle matures under the influence of FSH, it begins to produce increasing amounts of estrogens, which greatly increase the adenohypophyseal secretion of LH. The surge of LH at midcycle is the primary trigger for ovulation, the release of the ovum from the mature follicle.

In the second half of the menstrual cycle, LH causes the follicle from which the ovum was released to develop into a thickened, secretory tissue called *corpus luteum*. The corpus luteum secretes large quantities of progesterone, another female steroid hormone. By day 21 of the cycle, the large quantities of circulating estrogen and progesterone inhibit secretion of FSH and LH from the adenohypophysis (see Figure 50-2), and the corpus luteum begins to involute. Steroid hormone production falls rapidly as the corpus luteum fails and brings about the final stage in the cycle, the collapse of the endometrial lining.

During menses the entire inner surface of the uterus is denuded, and the endometrium rapidly collapses to about 65% of its former thickness. About 70 ml of blood and serum is lost along with necrotic and dissolving tissue during a typical menstrual period. Normally, this blood does not clot because of the presence of fibrinolysin in the fluid. Fibrinolysin is an enzyme that digests the fibrin matrix on which blood clots form. Despite the seemingly favorable environment for bacterial growth, the uterus during menstruation is resistant to infection. A contributing factor to this resistance is the presence of many leukocytes in the menstrual fluid.

Effects of gonadotropin deficiency. Alterations in hypophyseal or ovarian function can upset the finely balanced interaction of these tissues. Throughout childhood, pituitary secretion of FSH and LH is low, and circulating sex steroid concentrations are also low. At puberty the adenohypophysis greatly increases its secretion of FSH and LH. If this increase does not occur, sexual development does not take place, because androgen, estrogen, and progesterone production are not induced.

Gonadotropin-releasing hormone (GnRH) may help diagnose the cause of failure of sexual development (see Chapter 53). FSH may be used clinically to help reverse female infertility (see Chapter 53). For long-term replacement therapy in patients with hypogonadism, the androgens and estrogens are usually used (see Chapters 53 and 54).

Adrenocorticotropic Hormone

Mechanism of action

When ACTH is released by the adenohypophysis, it stimulates the adrenal cortex to synthesize and to release cortisol, a major adrenocortical steroid hormone, as well as other glucocorticoids and minor amounts of sex steroids (see Chapter 51).

Regulation of secretion. Cortisol blood levels are monitored by the hypothalamus, which adjusts the rate of release of corticotropin-releasing factor (CRF) into the hypophyseal portal venous system to the adenohypophysis, thereby controlling the systemic levels of ACTH. When cortisol levels become too high, the hypothalamus reduces CRF release. The adenohypophysis, lacking appropriate stimulation, reduces ACTH production, and blood levels of ACTH fall. The adrenocortical production of cortisol then falls because of the lowered ACTH levels. Blood levels of the adrenal steroid thus are prevented from exceeding an upper limit. Conversely, when cortisol levels in the blood fall too low, the hypothalamus normally prevents a dangerously low level from developing. CRF is released in large amounts into the hypophyseal portal venous system; in response the

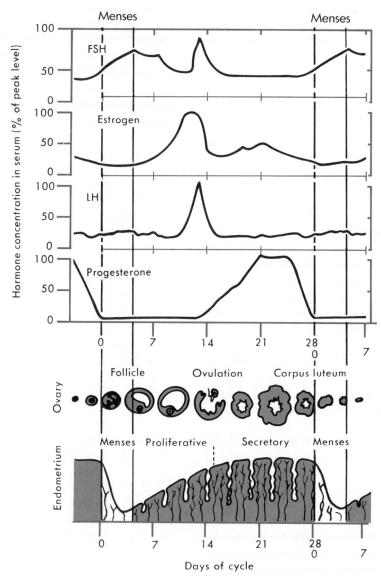

FIGURE 50-2

Pituitary regulation of menstrual cycle. Changes in circulating hormone levels are correlated with ovarian follicle and endometrial alterations.

adenohypophysis releases ACTH, and in response to ACTH the adrenal cortex elevates cortisol production. This intricate regulatory sequence is an example of a negative feedback loop, a regulatory mechanism in which the end product of a reaction sequence inhibits the operation of the sequence, thereby keeping the concentration of the product between certain limits (Figure 50-3).

Thyroid-Stimulating Hormone

Negative feedback regulation applies not only to the adrenal cortex and the ovary but also to the thyroid gland (see Figure 50-3). TSH is discussed in Chapter 52.

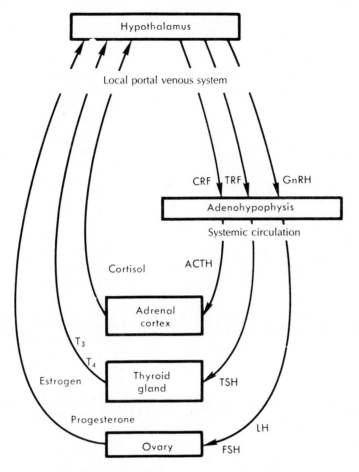

FIGURE 50-3

Regulation of hormone synthesis by negative feedback loops. Each *arrow* indicates a hormone, its source, and its target tissue. Hypothalamic synthesis of individual releasing factors is suppressed by high blood concentrations of the appropriate final hormone. For example, cortisol suppresses CRF synthesis and release, thereby blocking further cortisol synthesis. Other loops are similarly regulated.

NURSING IMPLICATIONS SUMMARY

Care of the Patient with Diabetes Insipidus

Drug administration

◆ Monitor fluid intake and output, serum sodium levels, and urine specific gravity. Diabetes insipidus is characterized by dilute urine, in large volume, with output often exceeding input, and with urine specific gravity of 1.000 to 1.003. This condition is often diagnosed initially by an alert nurse.

◆ Uncontrolled diabetes mellitus may be associated with excessive urine production. Monitor urine and blood glucose levels and urine-specific gravity to help differentiate the two.

◆ Monitor blood pressure. Monitor serum electrolyte level.

◆ Read orders carefully. Vasopressin and vasopressin tannate in oil are different and have different requirements for administration.

◆ See p. 87 for a discussion of administration of oil-based IM preparations.

INTRAVENOUS DESMOPRESSIN ACETATE

◆ May be given undiluted in diabetes insipidus. Administer a single dose over 1 min. Monitor blood pressure and pulse. This drug may also be administered intravenously in patients with hemophilia A and von Willebrand's disease. For these conditions, it is diluted and is administered as an infusion. Consult manufacturer's literature.

Patient and family education

◆ Review with patients the anticipated benefits and possible side effects of drug therapy.

◆ If appropriate, teach the patient to measure urine output at home. Most patients will not need to do this, since they can usually tell when urine output is increasing and another dose of medication is needed.

◆ In preparing a patient for discharge with a drug for nasal administration, review the manufacturer's instructions. Have the patient give a return demonstration.

◆ Teach patients that a severe cold, nasal surgery, or anything that interferes with their ability to sniff may necessitate a temporary switch to an injectable drug, and they should contact the physician.

◆ If GI distress develops, it may indicate too high a dose. If GI distress is severe or persistent, notify the physician.

◆ Generally, if more than two sprays/nostril of a drug are needed, it is better to increase the frequency of dosage rather than the number of sprays for each dose.

◆ If a dose is missed, take the dose as soon as it is remembered, unless within a few hours of the next dose, in which case the patient should take a dose but omit the next scheduled dose. Do not double up for missed doses. Reinforce to patients the need to consult the physician for questions about doses.

◆ Refer patient to a community-based nursing agency for follow-up as appropriate.

◆ Teach patients with diabetes insipidus to wear a medical identification tag or bracelet indicating their diagnosis.

◆ Avoid ingestion of alcohol unless permitted in small amounts by the physician.

◆ Chlorothiazide and other thiazide diuretics are discussed in Chapter 16.

◆ Chlorpropamide is discussed in Chapter 55.

◆ Clofibrate is discussed in Chapter 21.

◆ Carbamazepine is discussed in Chapter 47.

◆ Oxytocin and bromocriptine are discussed in Chapter 53.

Somatrem and Somatropin

Drug administration

◆ Monitor weight and height.

◆ Monitor blood glucose levels.

◆ Encourage patients to return for regular follow-up.

◆ Warn patients that pain and swelling at the injection site may occur.

Patient and family education

◆ Review anticipated benefits and possible side effects of drug therapy. Warn patients to take drug only as ordered and not to increase dose unless directed to do so by the physician.

◆ Warn diabetic patients to monitor blood glucose levels carefully, since changes in diet or insulin may be necessary.

◆ Consult with the physician, then teach family to monitor and record patient's weight, height, and other parameters regularly.

NURSING IMPLICATIONS SUMMARY—cont'd

Octreotide

Drug administration

◆ Monitor blood glucose levels.
◆ Preferred sites for subcutaneous administration include the hip, thigh, or abdomen. Rotate sites.
◆ Assess for GI symptoms including abdominal pain, diarrhea, and nausea and vomiting.

Patient and family education

◆ Review administration technique.
◆ Take doses between meals and at bedtime to help avoid GI symptoms.
◆ Warn diabetic patients to monitor blood glucose levels carefully, since changes in diet or insulin may be necessary.

Panhypopituitarism

◆ The patient who loses all or nearly all pituitary function from trauma, surgery, or disease must be treated with replacement hormonal therapy to survive. Treatment with exogenous forms of cortisol usually substitutes for ACTH loss. Thyroid hormones usually replace TSH. Growth hormone is not usually replaced, except in children. ADH may or may not be replaced exogenously. The gonadotropic hormones are rarely used in replacement therapy. Estrogens and androgens are used as needed for cosmetic and comfort purposes. In the female, it is difficult to recreate the monthly cyclic surges of these hormones, so this may not be attempted unless requested by the patient; she is usually sterile. Oxytocin is not replaced unless the woman has been able to conceive and the hormone would be needed during labor and delivery. For information about individual hormones, see Chapters 51 to 55.
◆ Teach patients requiring hormonal replacement therapy to wear a medical identification tag or bracelet.

CHAPTER REVIEW

◆ KEY TERMS

adenohypophysis, p. 732
antidiuretic hormone (ADH), p. 729
diabetes insipidus, p. 729
growth hormone, p. 733
nephrogenic diabetes insipidus, p. 732
neurohypophysis, p. 728
oxytocin, p. 732
somatomedins, p. 733
syndrome of inappropriate ADH (SIADH), p. 732

◆ REVIEW QUESTIONS

1. What are the two divisions of the pituitary gland, or hypophysis?
2. What is the nature of neurohypophyseal tissue?
3. What hormones are released by the neurohypophysis?
4. Where are the hormones released by the neurohypophysis synthesized?
5. What is the target tissue of antidiuretic hormone (ADH)?
6. What is the mechanism of action of ADH?
7. What physiologic conditions stimulate the release of ADH?
8. What is diabetes insipidus? How should you assess for this?
9. What two types of therapy may be used to treat diabetes insipidus?
10. Compare and contrast the route of administration and duration of action of vasopressin and vasopressin tannate in oil.
11. What advantage does desmopressin acetate (DDAVP) have over other vasopressin preparations?
12. What are the side effects associated with vasopressin?
13. What is the mechanism of action by which thiazide diuretics control diuresis in diabetes insipidus?
14. What is the mechanism of action of chlorpropamide and clofibrate in treating diabetes insipidus?
15. What are the target tissues of oxytocin?

16. How is the secretion of oxytocin controlled?

17. What hormones are secreted by the adenohypophysis?

18. Where are the hormones secreted by the adenohypophysis synthesized?

19. What are the target tissues of growth hormone?

20. What are the anabolic effects of growth hormone?

21. What are the antiinsulin effects of growth hormone? What would the manifestations of this be in the patient?

22. What are somatomedins?

23. What is the effect of growth hormone deficiency?

24. How is growth hormone deficiency treated?

25. What is the effect of excess growth hormone?

26. What are the gonadotropic hormones?

27. What are the target tissues of follicle-stimulating hormone (FSH)?

28. What are the target tissues of luteinizing hormone (LH)?

29. What are the target tissues of prolactin?

30. What roles do FSH and LH play in causing the development and release of a mature ovum from the ovary?

31. What are the effects of gonadotropin deficiency?

32. What is the target tissue for adrenocorticotropic hormone (ACTH)?

33. How is the concentration of ACTH in the blood regulated?

SUGGESTED READING

Anthony CP, Thibodeau GA: *The endocrine system.* In *Textbook of anatomy and physiology,* ed 13, St. Louis, 1991, Mosby–Year Book.

Council on Scientific Affairs: Drug abuse in athletes. Anabolic steroids and human growth hormone, *JAMA* 259(11):1703, 1988.

Filicori M, Flamigni C: GnRH agonists and antagonists: current clinical status, *Drugs* 35:63, 1988.

Hartshorn J, Hartshorn E: Pharmacology update: vasopressin in the treatment of diabetes insipidus, *J Neurosci Nurs* 20(1):58, 1988.

Howrie DL: Growth hormone for the treatment of growth failure in children, *Clin Pharm* 6(4):283, 1987.

Lechan RM: Neuroendocrinology of pituitary hormone regulation, *Endocrinol Metab Clin North Amer* 16(3):475, 1987.

Patterson LM, Noroian EL: Diabetes insipidus versus syndrome of inappropriate antidiuretic hormone, *DCCN* 8(4):226, 1989.

Press M: Growth hormone and metabolism, *Diabetes Metab Rev* 4(4):391, 1988.

Salva KM and others: DDAVP in the treatment of bleeding disorders, *Pharmacotherapy* 8(2):94, 1988.

Yucha C, Suddaby P: David could have died of thirst, yet he never felt thirsty, *Nurs 91* 21(7):42, 1991.

CHAPTER 51

Drugs Affecting the Adrenal Gland

LEARNING OBJECTIVES

After reading this chapter, you should be able to do the following:

- Describe the two types of hormones produced in the adrenal glands.
- Describe the use of adrenocorticoids as replacement therapy.
- Compare cortisol or cortisone with betamethasone or dexamethasone relative to their antiinflammatory and mineralocorticoid activity.
- Describe side effects observed with pharmacologic doses of adrenocorticoids.
- Develop a nursing care plan for a patient receiving an adrenocorticoid.

CHAPTER OVERVIEW

◆ The human adrenal gland is divided into two distinct functional units, the adrenal medulla and the adrenal cortex. These regions of the gland differ in embryologic origin, type of cells composing the tissue, and hormones produced. The structure and function of these regions of the adrenal gland, the regulation of synthesis of the various hormones produced, and the pathologic states arising from abnormalities in hormone production are discussed in this chapter. The widespread clinical uses of several of these hormones and their derivatives in diagnosis and therapy are also considered.

Nursing Process Overview
DRUGS AFFECTING THE ADRENAL GLAND

Assessment

Perform a complete patient assessment. Monitor temperature, pulse, respiration, blood pressure, and weight, and check the blood and urine for glucose. Observe the body and skin carefully, noting color and character of the skin, distribution of body mass (fat and muscles), the presence of bruises or petechiae, and the condition of hair and nails. Determine the time of onset of these problems if appropriate.

Nursing Diagnoses

Body image disturbance
Possible complication: electrolyte abnormalities
Possible complication: fragile bones resulting in increased susceptibility to fractures

Management

Adrenocortical steroids are one of the most frequently used groups of drugs and may be prescribed as a temporary adjunct to treatment, even if hormonal insufficiency has not been demonstrated. Monitor the blood pressure, weight, serum electrolyte levels, and sugar concentration in the blood and urine. Remember that wound healing may be slowed, infection may be masked, and improvement in appetite and sense of well-being may be due to drug therapy. Drug-induced diabetes may require treatment with insulin. In planning for discharge, determine with the physician the discharge dose and schedule of drugs, and begin teaching the patient.

Evaluation

Before discharge, ascertain that the patient can explain why the drug has been prescribed, the desired goals of therapy, how to take the drug correctly (e.g., daily or alternate-day therapy), and side effects that may occur. The patient should be able to explain additional therapies needed because of the drug such as antacid therapy or dietary restrictions such as a low sodium diet. Ensure that the patient can explain special circumstances requiring notification of the physician such as nausea and vomiting preventing taking the drug, illnesses that might necessitate a dosage increase, or effects of the drug on other medical problems (e.g., diabetes requiring an increase in insulin dose). Patients must know not to discontinue or decrease the dose without physician approval and, if receiving long-term therapy, to obtain and wear a medical identification tag or bracelet. Finally, verify that the patient can explain if any parameters should be monitored at home such as weight, blood pressure, or blood glucose concentration.

ADRENAL CORTEX

The adrenal cortex is composed of lipid-rich secretory tissue embryologically derived from the coelomic epithelium. Three distinct layers within the cortex may be distinguished on the basis of histology. These regions differ not only in cellular arrangement but also in the major steroid hormone produced and in the regulation of steroid synthesis (Figure 51-1).

Adrenal Steroids   *↳preserve Na⁺*

Mineralocorticoids

The outer layer, or zona glomerulosa, is the site of conversion of the precursor cholesterol to the **mineralocorticoids**. These steroids act on the kidney, causing retention of sodium and associated water and promoting potassium loss.

Regulation of mineralocorticoid synthesis is primarily through the **renin-angiotensin system** (Figure 51-2). The regulatory trigger for this feedback system is in the kidney, where lowered blood sodium levels or lowered intravascular volume causes the release of renin into the bloodstream. Renin is an enzyme, which in the bloodstream converts angiotensinogen, a protein from the liver, to angiotensin I. Another enzyme found in the blood and the lungs rapidly converts angiotensin I to angiotensin II. Angiotensin II in turn stimulates the adrenocortical zona glomerulosa to secrete the mineralocorticoids, especially aldosterone. The result of this regulatory loop is that the mineralocorticoids released into the bloodstream slow the further loss of sodium and water through the kidneys. When sodium and water retention exceeds certain limits, the plasma volume expands, and renin release decreases. When the concentration of renin falls, production of angiotensin II slows, aldosterone secretion by the adrenal gland

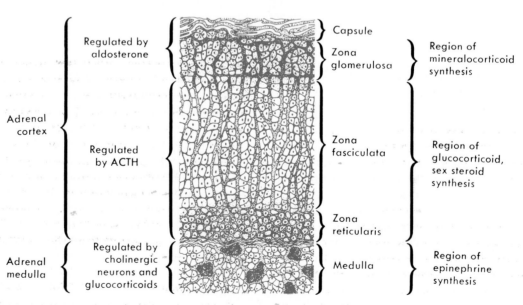

FIGURE 51-1

Regions of adrenal gland. Each histologically distinguishable zone of adrenal gland synthesizes specific hormones and is controlled by specific regulators. Medulla forms center of adrenal gland and is thicker than shown in cross-section.

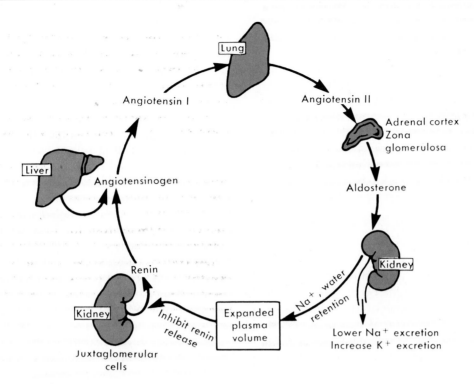

FIGURE 51-2

Negative feedback loop regulating mineralocorticoid synthesis and release. Kidney is key to regulating synthesis and release of aldosterone, the primary natural mineralocorticoid. Renin is released from juxtaglomerular cells of kidney to set cascade in motion, and the kidney is ultimate target of aldosterone. Expanded plasma volume, which results when the kidney retains sodium ion (Na$^+$) and water, is regulator that halts renin release.

falls, and the kidneys begin to rid the body of accumulated sodium.

Glucocorticoids

The inner two layers of the adrenal cortex convert cholesterol to the **glucocorticoids** and the sex steroids, primarily androgens and progestins. The synthesis of these steroids is regulated by the hypophysis and the hypothalamus via the negative feedback loop described in Chapter 50. Cortisol is the major glucocorticoid produced, and it is also the key to regulation of steroid synthesis in the zona fasciculata and zona reticularis. Low levels of cortisol in the blood stimulate and high levels suppress total steroid synthesis by respectively raising and lowering adrenocorticotropic hormone (ACTH) release from the hypophysis.

Glucocorticoid action. The glucocorticoids produce potent and varied effects on metabolism. The primary metabolic effect is stimulation of gluconeogenesis (the formation of new glucose) by actions on the liver and peripheral tissues. In striated muscle, glucocorticoids mobilize amino acids from muscle protein. The result is an increase in circulating levels of amino acids and an overall depletion of muscle protein, which ultimately is expressed as a negative nitrogen balance (more nitrogen is excreted than is absorbed in the diet). In the liver, glucocorticoids increase the activities of enzymes that convert amino acids to glucose. Much of this excess glucose is then stored in the liver as glycogen. In addition, amino acids are the ultimate source of precursors for fat synthesis, which is also increased in the presence of glucocorticoids.

Glucocorticoids have many direct actions in the body. They maintain water diuresis by antagonizing the effects of antidiuretic hormone in the kidney, lower the threshold for electrical excitation in the brain, and reduce the amount of new bone synthesis. In addition, the glucocorticoids affect the immune system by suppressing the activity of lymphoid tissue and by reducing the numbers of circulating lymphocytes. These steroids also reduce inflammatory processes by impairing synthesis of prostaglandins and related compounds, an action that has several useful therapeutic applications.

In addition to the direct effects, glucocorticoids have permissive activities that allow the body to deal successfully with stress or trauma. For example, cortisol sensitizes the arterioles to norepinephrine, allowing the catecholamine to increase blood pressure. In the liver, cortisol must be present before epinephrine and glucagon can stimulate hydrolysis (breakdown) of liver glycogen to glucose, releasing the sugar as an energy source for peripheral muscle.

Abnormalities of Adrenal Hormone Production

Adrenal insufficiency

Failure of the adrenal cortex is life-threatening. If the failure is sudden, which might occur after adrenal injury or thrombosis, death may occur within hours. Early symptoms of **acute adrenal insufficiency** include confusion, restlessness, and nausea and vomiting. Circulatory collapse, deep shock, and death may follow rapidly.

If synthesis of glucocorticoids is reduced but not halted, patients may not be in immediate danger, in the absence of stress or trauma, but they may still suffer from inadequate amounts of the glucocorticoids. This chronic primary adrenal insufficiency is called *Addison's disease*. Symptoms include weakness, weight loss, dehydration, hypotension, hypoglycemia, and anemia. Most patients with Addison's disease also display increased skin pigmentation. This unusual or excessive tanning is caused by a direct effect on melanin-containing skin cells by the chronic excess of ACTH, which is secreted by the hypophysis in response to the elevated corticotropin-releasing factor (CRF) induced by chronically low blood levels of cortisol.

Symptoms similar to those of Addison's disease are produced when the adenohypophysis is diseased or destroyed and no longer produces adequate ACTH. Without ACTH, the zona reticularis and zona fasciculata do not synthesize cortisol, and over time, these adrenal tissues atrophy. This condition is called *secondary adrenal insufficiency*. One characteristic that often visibly distinguishes these patients from those with Addison's disease is the absence of excessive pigmentation. In secondary adrenal insufficiency the hypophysis does not release large quantities of ACTH, and the skin is not darkened.

Excessive glucocorticoids

Overproduction of cortisol, a condition called *Cushing's syndrome,* may be induced by a variety of fac-

tors. Some patients have high cortisol production from tumors of the adrenal cortex, which may synthesize massive amounts of the steroid. Other patients have high cortisol synthesis because of increased ACTH release into the bloodstream, which keeps the zona fasciculata and zona reticularis maximally stimulated to produce the glucocorticoids. Excess ACTH usually comes from a tumor of the hypophysis, but occasionally the ACTH comes from some unusual source such as a lung tumor, which would not ordinarily be expected to synthesize ACTH. Most often, however, Cushing's syndrome is caused by administration of glucocorticoids.

The symptoms of Cushing's syndrome can be predicted from the metabolic actions of cortisol. Certain fat stores, especially those on the face and shoulders, are increased as a result of cortisol stimulation of fat synthesis. The extremities may be weak and in more advanced cases may be thin because of the muscle-wasting effects of the hormone. The skin is fragile and easily bruised as a result of protein breakdown in that tissue. Examination of the skin on the trunk may reveal striae, or stretch marks, over areas where fat deposition is most pronounced. Many patients also have superficial fungal infections of the skin, related in part to the fragility of the skin and to the reduced host immune response caused by the excess steroid. Bone thinning occurs because of changes in calcium metabolism; compression fractures of the spine may occur relatively easily. Diabetes may be precipitated from the increased insulin demand caused by excess cortisol. Hypertension is very common in these patients, and atherosclerosis may occur. Mood changes are also common and may be extreme. Psychosis may be precipitated.

Hyperaldosteronism

Certain tumors of the adrenal gland produce excessive amounts of aldosterone, or less often, one of the other mineralococorticoids. In these patients, two types of symptoms appear, those associated with hypertension and those associated with hypokalemia (low blood potassium concentration). Hypertension is produced by the sodium and water retention arising from excess aldosterone acting on the kidneys, whereas the muscle weakness associated with hypokalemia is a result of the potassium-wasting action of the steroid in the kidneys. Treatment ultimately involves surgical removal of the tumor.

Secondary sexual abnormalities

The sex steroids produced in the adrenal cortex are of minor importance in normal circumstances, the output of the adrenal glands being small compared with that of the gonads. Under certain conditions, however, sex steroid overproduction in the adrenal glands may produce a devastating endocrine imbalance. For example, a female with an androgen-producing tumor of the adrenal gland may undergo masculinization, including suppression of the menstrual cycle and development of secondary male sex characteristics. A male with an estrogen-producing tumor may develop breast tenderness and enlargement with loss of libido. A child may show precocious sexual development.

Pharmacology of Adrenal Steroids and Related Compounds

Actions

Three major activities of the adrenal steroids are metabolic effects on carbohydrate, protein, and fat metabolism; antiinflammatory and immunosuppressive activity; and sodium-retaining activity associated with potassium loss. The first two are classified as glucocorticoid actions and the third as a mineralocorticoid action.

The natural adrenal steroids, cortisol, cortisone, and corticosterone, possess glucocorticoid and mineralocorticoid activity, although one action usually predominates. Treatment with one of these natural compounds therefore produces multiple effects. For example, cortisol in the high doses required for antiinflammatory action changes metabolism, as expected from a glucocorticoid, but also produces excessive sodium retention and potassium loss, a mineralocorticoid effect.

Synthetic glucocorticoids have been designed that are essentially free of mineralocorticoid activity. These drugs include betamethasone, dexamethasone, methylprednisolone, paramethasone, and triamcinolone (Table 51-1). These synthetic glucocorticoids

Table 51-1 Activity of Natural and Synthetic Adrenal Steroids Used Systemically

Generic name	Drug class	Activity relative to hydrocortisone		Major use	Major toxicity
		Antiinflammatory	Sodium-retaining		
Betamethasone	Glucocorticoid (synthetic)	25.0	0	As for hydrocortisone	Overdosage causes hydrocortisone-like effects on fat, protein and carbohydrate metabolism but little sodium retention
Cortisone	Glucocorticoid (natural)	0.8	0.9	Antiinflammatory agent	As for hydrocortisone
Dexamethasone	Glucocorticoid (synthetic)	30.0	0	As for hydrocortisone	As for betamethasone
Fludrocortisone	Mineralocorticoid (synthetic)	About 1.0	About 100	For replacement therapy in adrenal insufficiency; for therapy in adrenal disease causing salt loss	Overdosage produces symptoms of excess salt and water retention with potassium loss
Hydrocortisone (also called cortisol)	Glucocorticoid (natural)	1.0	1.0	For replacement therapy in adrenal insufficiency; as an antiinflammatory agent in a variety of nonendocrine diseases	Overdosage produces symptoms of Cushing's disease; abrupt withdrawal produces symptoms of adrenal insufficiency
Methylprednisolone	Glucocorticoid (synthetic)	5.0	0	As for hydrocortisone	As for betamethasone
Paramethasone	Glucocorticoid (synthetic)	10.0	0	As for cortisone	As for betamethasone
Prednisolone	Glucocorticoid (synthetic)	4.0	0.8	As for hydrocortisone	As for hydrocortisone
Prednisone	Glucocorticoid (synthetic)	3.5	0.8	As for hydrocortisone	As for hydrocortisone
Triamcinolone	Glucocorticoid (synthetic)	5.0	0	As for hydrocortisone	As for betamethasone; has high muscle-wasting activity

have the additional advantage of producing antiinflammatory effects at lower doses than the naturally occurring glucocorticoids.

Duration and mechanism of action

The durations of action of the various adrenal steroids are listed in Table 51-2. For this class of drugs, the duration of action is not the same as the plasma half-life of the drug. The duration of action refers to the length of time adrenal suppression is detectable after a single steroid dose. For example, prednisone suppresses adrenal function up to 36 hr after a single dose, but the plasma half-life is only about 2½ hr. This discrepancy may be explained in part by the mechanism of action of the steroid hormones. To produce their effects, the steroids must pass through the membranes of target cells, bind to soluble receptors in the cell cytoplasm, and be transported to the cell nucleus (see Chapter 49). Once in the nucleus the steroid induces changes in ribonucleic acid (RNA) and protein synthesis, which ultimately may be expressed as some change in the function of the target cell. A considerable time lag may occur between the uptake of the steroid into the cell and the appearance of the effect in the target cell. Further time may elapse before the effect is terminated and the steroid is destroyed.

Preparations

Adrenal steroids used clinically are summarized in Tables 51-2 and 51-3. The chemical form of the steroid determines the pharmacokinetics of the preparation. In their naturally occurring forms, most glucocorticoids are relatively insoluble in water. Because these drugs form suspensions but not true solutions in water, preparations are not suitable for intravenous (IV) administration, although they may be injected into tissues (see Table 51-2). In contrast, sodium phosphate and sodium succinate derivatives of several glucocorticoids are quite water soluble. This IV administration of an adrenal steroid preparation requires sodium phosphates of cortisol (hydrocortisone), betamethasone, dexamethasone, and prednisolone or sodium succinates of cortisol and methylprednisolone. No other forms of these drugs should be administered intravenously.

Administered intramuscularly as suspensions, many glucocorticoids are dissolved and absorbed slowly from the injection site, producing a relatively long duration of action (see Table 51-2). For many glucocorticoids the acetate ester is an insoluble, slowly absorbed form that yields a prolonged duration of action. Preparations that combine sodium phosphate and acetate esters have a rapid onset and a prolonged effect; the highly soluble sodium phosphate yields rapid action, whereas the poorly soluble acetate form remains at the site as a depot to release the active agent slowly.

Topical steroid preparations are used primarily to control various dermatologic conditions (see Table 51-3). Since the steroids are applied directly to the skin, a therapeutic dose may be achieved at the site where action is desired. Since the total dose of steroid is small and the drugs are not well absorbed through the skin, systemic actions are usually avoided. Absorption of a significant dose is possible with chronic, heavy application to wide areas of the skin or with rectal applications, also considered a topical route.

Certain steroid forms have been promoted primarily because of specific enhancement of topical activity. For example, betamethasone valerate is much more active topically than is betamethasone. Likewise, the acetonide derivative of triamcinolone is superior to the parent compound as a topical agent.

The ophthalmic preparations are forms for topical application to the eye. Relatively high doses of steroids may be achieved in the eye, ordinarily with low absorption into systemic circulation. With chronic high doses, some drug may pass into the body and may cause toxic effects. Toxicity is also possible in the eye. Certain patients with a genetic predisposition toward glaucoma show increased intraocular pressure after using an ophthalmic steroid preparation. For most patients the intraocular pressure returns to normal when the drug is discontinued, but a few patients have developed glaucoma that did not respond to medication and required surgery. Another common adverse reaction to steroids is secondary eye infection. These infections are commonly viral or fungal and may be dormant conditions, which are activated when host defenses are suppressed by steroids. The use of steroids in injured eyes may allow a new infection to develop.

Adrenal steroids are currently being used as topical agents to control asthma (see Table 51-3). By administering the drugs as aerosols, delivery is directed to affected tissues in the lung without the necessity of high systemic doses.

Nasal steroids are usually administered to control rhinitis, allergies, or nasal polyps (see Table 51-3). Steroids are appropriate in those allergic patients who do not benefit from decongestants and antihistamines.

Adrenal suppression

Patients should not be abruptly withdrawn from long-term systemic steroid therapy. All adrenal steroids suppress the normal function of the hypothalamus, adenohypophysis, and adrenal glands. If exogenous steroids are withdrawn suddenly, patients

Table 51-2 Glucocorticoids and Mineralocorticoids Used Systemically

Generic name	Trade names*	Route†	Onset	Duration
Betamethasone	Celestone	PO	1 hr	3 days
Betamethasone sodium phosphate	Selestoject	IV, IM	Rapid	Short
Betamethasone acetate/sodium phosphate	Celestone soluspan	IM, IA, IL, IS, ST	1 to 3 hr	1 to 2 weeks
Cortisone acetate	Cortone acetate	PO IM	Rapid Slow	1 to 1½ days >2 days
Dexamethasone	Decadron	PO	1 hr	3 days
Dexamethasone acetate	Dalalone LA	IM IA, ST, IL	<8 hr Slow	6 days 1 to 3 weeks
Dexamethasone sodium phosphate	Decadrol	IV, IM IA, IS, IL, ST	Rapid Slow	Short 3 to 21 days
Fludrocortisone acetate	Florinef	PO	Intermed.	Intermed.
Hydrocortisone	Cortef Cortenema	PO IM Rectal	<1 hr <4 hr 3 to 5 days	1½ days Days
Hydrocortisone acetate	Hydrocortone acetate	IA, IS, IB, IL, ST	<24 hr	3 to 28 days
Hydrocortisone cypionate	Cortifoam Cortef	Rectal PO	5 to 7 days 1 hr	1 to 2 days
Hydrocortisone sodium phosphate	Hydrocortone phosphate	IV, IM	Rapid	Short
Hydrocortisone sodium succinate	Solu-Cortef	IV, IM	Rapid	Variable
Methylprednisolone	Medrol	PO	<1 hr	1½ days
Methylprednisolone acetate	Depo-Medrol	IM IA, IL, ST	6 to 48 hr Slow	1 to 4 weeks 1 to 5 weeks
Methylprednisolone sodium succinate	Solu-Medrol	IV, IM	Rapid	Intermed.
Paramethasone acetate	Haldrone	PO	<1 hr	2 days
Prednisolone	Prelone	PO	<1 hr	1½ days
Prednisolone acetate	Predicort	IM	Slow	
Prednisolone acetate/sodium phosphate	Generic	IM, IB, IS, IA, ST	Slow	3 to 28 days
Prednisolone sodium phosphate	Predicort RP	IV, IM IA, IL, ST	<1 hr Slow	Short 3 to 21 days
Prednisolone tebutate	Predalone TBA	IA, IL, ST	1 to 2 days	1 to 3 weeks
Prednisone	Meticorten	PO	<2 hr	1½ days
Triamcinolone	Aristocort	PO	<2 hr	2 days

*Representative trade names are given.
†Abbreviations: IA, intraarticular; IB, intrabursal; IL, intralesional; IM, intramuscular; IS, intrasynovial; IV, intravenous; PO, oral; ST, soft tissue. *Continued.*

Table 51-2 Clinical Summary of Glucocorticoids and Mineralocorticoids Used Systemically—cont'd

Generic name	Trade names*	Route†	Onset	Duration
Triamcinolone acetonide	Kenalog	IM	1 to 2 days	1 to 6 weeks
		IB, IA, IS, IL, ST	Slow	Weeks
Triamcinolone diacetate	Kenacort	PO	<2 hr	Intermed
	Aristocort forte	IM	Slow	4 to 28 days
		IL	Slow	1 to 2 weeks
		IA, IS, ST	Slow	1 to 8 weeks
Triamcinolone hexacetonide	Aristospan	IA, IL	Slow	3 to 4 weeks

*Representative trade names are given.
†Abbreviations: IA, intraarticular; IB, intrabursal; IL, intralesional; IM, intramuscular; IS, intrasynovial; IV, intravenous; PO, oral; ST, soft tissue.

Table 51-3 Corticosteroids Preparations for Nonsystemic Use

Use	Preparations	Trade names*	Comments
ANTIASTHMATIC			
Inhalation aerosol	Beclomethasone dipropionate	Beclovent, Vanceril	
	Dexamethasone sodium phosphate	Decadron Respihaler	
	Flunisolide	AeroBid	FDA Pregnancy Category C
	Triamcinolone acetonide	Azmacort	FDA Pregnancy Category D
DENTAL			
Paste and pellets	Betamethasone sodium phosphate	Betnesol	
	Hydrocortisone acetate	Orabase-HCA	FDA Pregnancy Category C
	Triamcinolone acetonide	Oracort	
DERMATOLOGIC			
Topical creams, gels, ointments, lotions, and sprays	Alclometasone	Aclovate	FDA Pregnancy Category C
	Amcinonide	Cyclocort	FDA Pregnancy Category C
	Beclomethasone	Propaderm	FDA Pregnancy Category C
	Betamethasone benzoate	Uticort	FDA Pregnancy Category C
	Betamethasone dipropionate	Alphatrex	FDA Pregnancy Category C
	Betamethasone valerate	Valisone	FDA Pregnancy Category C
	Clobetasol propionate	Dermovate	FDA Pregnancy Category C
	Clocortolone pivalate	Cloderm	FDA Pregnancy Category C
	Desonide	Tridesilon	FDA Pregnancy Category C
	Desoximetasone	Topicort	FDA Pregnancy Category C
	Dexamethasone	Decaderm	FDA Pregnancy Category C
	Dexamethasone sodium phosphate	Decadron	FDA Pregnancy Category C
	Diflorasone diacetate	Florone	FDA Pregnancy Category C
	Diflucortolone	Nerisone	FDA Pregnancy Category C
	Flumethasone	Locacorten	FDA Pregnancy Category C
	Fluocinolone acetonide	Synalar	FDA Pregnancy Category C
	Fluocinonide	Lidex	FDA Pregnancy Category C
	Flurandrenolide	Cordran	FDA Pregnancy Category C
	Halcinonide	Halog	FDA Pregnancy Category C
	Hydrocortisone	Hytone	FDA Pregnancy Category C
	Hydrocortisone acetate	Cortaid	FDA Pregnancy Category C
	Methylprednisolone acetate	Medrol	FDA Pregnancy Category C
	Mometasone furoate	Elocon	FDA Pregnancy Category C
	Triamcinolone acetonide	Kenalog	FDA Pregnancy Category C

*Representative trade names.

Table 51-3   Corticosteroids Preparations for Nonsystemic Use—cont'd

Use	Preparations	Trade names*	Comments
NASAL			
Aerosols and solutions	Beclomethasone dipropionate	Beconase, Vancenase	FDA Pregnancy Category C
	Dexamethasone sodium phosphate	Decadron turbinaire	FDA Pregnancy Category C
	Flunisolide	Nasalide, Rhinalar	
OPHTHALMIC-OTIC			
Solutions, suspensions, and ointments	Betamethasone sodium phosphate	Betnesol	
	Dexamethasone	Maxidex	FDA Pregnancy Category C
	Dexamethasone sodium phosphate	Decadron	FDA Pregnancy Category C
	Fluorometholone	FML	FDA Pregnancy Category C
	Hydrocortisone	Cortamed	FDA Pregnancy Category C
	Medrysone	HMS liquifilm	FDA Pregnancy Category C
	Prednisolone acetate	Ocu-Pred-A	FDA Pregnancy Category C
	Prednisolone sodium phosphate	Ocu-Pred	FDA Pregnancy Category C
RECTAL			
Ointments and suppositories	Hydrocortisone	Proctocort	
	Hydrocortisone acetate	Anusol-HC	

may die of acute adrenal insufficiency because their own adrenal glands cannot immediately produce the required steroids. This type of reaction is most likely in patients receiving relatively high doses for long periods. It may require 6 to 9 months for the natural negative feedback loop that regulates adrenal steroid synthesis to regain normal function after long-term steroid therapy, apparently because atrophy of the tissues occurs to some extent. Schedules for gradual withdrawal from steroids are available and must be followed faithfully, with dosage adjusted only to relieve symptoms of adrenal insufficiency if they develop during withdrawal.

To minimize hypothalamic-pituitary-adrenal suppression during long-term therapy with a glucocorticoid, many physicians prefer an alternate-day treatment schedule once an effective dosage has been established. The patient is given a single, large dose of the steroid in the early morning of the treatment day. This regimen mimics the normal daily cycle, in which glucocorticoid levels are high in the morning and decrease throughout the day. On the next day, no drug is given. The intermediate-acting steroids normally used in this regimen suppress the hypothalamic-pituitary-adrenal system for only about 12 to 36 hr (see Table 51-2). Therefore on the day no drug is given the normal regulatory mechanisms recover, and the patient's adrenal gland produces glucocorticoids. Most patients complain of some discomfort on the drug-free day, but these complaints must be weighed against the benefits of maintaining adrenal function. Not all diseases are adequately controlled by this regimen, so frequent assessment is necessary.

Drug-induced Cushing's syndrome

In all the steroid derivatives produced so far, increased antiinflammatory action also has been associated with increases in the metabolic effects characteristic of glucocorticoids. Therefore any of the compounds with glucocorticoid activity, if given in high enough doses, will produce Cushing's syndrome. This toxicity is one of the most common reactions seen with glucocorticoid therapy (see Table 51-1). Most endocrinologists see many more patients with Cushing's syndrome produced by drugs than any other form of the disease. For these patients the steroid dose should be reduced, if allowed by the severity of the condition being treated. Even when the condition being treated is not life-threatening, dose reduction may be difficult because many patients tolerate the symptoms of steroid overdose better than the symptoms of the inflammatory disease being treated, although the drug overdose may be medically more dangerous.

Toxic reactions

Toxic reactions to antiinflammatory doses of the glucocorticoids resemble the symptoms of naturally occurring Cushing's syndrome but are not identical. For example, peptic ulcer is a rather common finding in a patient receiving high doses of steroids but is relatively rare in Cushing's syndrome that is not drug

Table 51-4 Toxic Reactions to Long-Term Glucocorticoid Therapy

Toxic reaction	Cause	Comments
Impaired glucose tolerance or hyperglycemia	Gluconeogenic action of glucocorticoids	If diabetes develops, it is usually mild and reversible.
Fat deposition on trunk of body increased, as are plasma triglyceride levels	Stimulation of lipid synthesis by glucocorticoids	Changes in lipid metabolism produce classic Cushing-type signs of moon face and truncal obesity.
Muscle weakness or wasting	Stimulation of protein breakdown by glucocorticoids	This side effect is more pronounced with fluoride derivatives of glucocorticoids, such as triamcinolone.
Peptic ulcer or intestinal perforation	Direct irritation or protein-wasting effects of glucocorticoids	Steroids may induce these conditions, or they may mask the symptoms and allow the condition to progress to a serious stage before diagnosis.
Pancreatitis	Not known, but may involve effects on lipid metabolism	Glucocorticoids may mask symptoms of disease in early stages.
Growth inhibition	Glucocorticoid inhibition of growth hormone action	Glucocorticoids should be given with caution to children; doses below those producing growth inhibition should be used if possible.
Mood changes or psychoses	Not known	All patients receiving glucocorticoids should be observed closely for altered mood or behavior, especially those with a past history of this type of disorder.
Osteoporosis or bone fractures	Glucocorticoids alter several aspects of calcium metabolism that increase bone resorption	This side effect is noted especially in patients with arthritis, in postmenopausal women, or in persons with low calcium intake.
Sodium retention and potassium loss	Mineralocorticoid activity associated with some glucocorticoids	Newer, synthetic glucocorticoids minimize these effects.
Increased susceptibility to infection	Glucocorticoid inhibition of immune system	Infections are more difficult to eradicate in these patients, even with good antibiotic therapy.
Glaucoma	Glucocorticoids interfere with normal aqueous outflow from the eye and elevate intraocular pressure	The risk is especially great in genetically predisposed or diabetic patients.
Cataracts	Not known	Topical or systemic therapy has been implicated.

induced. Other common symptoms of glucocorticoid toxicity are listed in Table 51-4. These reactions occur after long-term administration of glucocorticoids. Large doses given for a short time to control acute allergic responses or other acute conditions are not usually associated with any significant signs of toxicity. For these purposes a large dose might be given on day 1, with the dose halved for each of the succeeding 3 or 4 days and then stopped before toxic reactions develop.

Drug interactions

The effect of many drugs are altered in patients receiving glucocorticoids. Steroids may increase excretion of salicylates by the kidneys and may necessitate increasing salicylate dosage in a patient receiving both drugs. In other instances, glucocorticoids may directly affect the action of a drug. Certain coumarin anticoagulants are less effective when steroids are present. In some cases, drugs may have an unexpected effect in patients receiving glucocorticoids. For example, a safe level of anesthetic given to produce general anesthesia may cause dangerous hypotension in a patient receiving long-term steroid therapy because the adrenal cortex is suppressed.

One of the most common drug interactions involves liver metabolism of drugs. Steroids, barbiturates, phenytoin, and many other drugs are all inactivated by the same liver microsomal enzyme system. These enzymes can be induced (i.e., more enzymes may be formed when certain drugs are chronically available in the bloodstream). Enzyme induction speeds up drug metabolism, not only for the drug that induced the enzymes but also for any other drug metabolized by these enzymes. For example, phenobarbital may exacerbate asthma being treated with glucocorticoids by increasing the destruction of the steroid in the liver. The same effect may be seen if an asthmatic patient who is receiving long-term steroid therapy has an asthmatic crisis. Ordinarily a dose of 100 mg of hydrocortisone treats an acute asthma attack. In the patient who has been receiving long-term therapy with glucocorticoids, however, 300 to 1000 mg of hydrocortisone may be required to achieve the same effect, again presumably because of the increased ability of the liver to destroy the hormone.

Clinical uses

The adrenal steroids are used clinically (1) at physiologic doses in replacement therapy for endocrine diseases such as pituitary deficiency or adrenal hypofunction or (2) at pharmacologic doses in the therapy of various nonendocrine diseases.

Replacement therapy. Examples of replacement therapy include the use of cortisol to treat Addison's disease or secondary adrenal insufficiency. When used in replacement therapy, doses of adrenal steroids are relatively low because they are intended only to replace amounts of the hormone normally present. Since the normal daily production of cortisol is about 15 to 25 mg, the daily replacement dose would be designed to achieve approximately the level of activity produced by that amount of cortisol. Table 51-1 shows the relationship of the activities of the various agents to the activity of cortisol. Wide variations in dosage exist because stress and other factors affect the steroid requirement. Each patient's dosage must be adjusted to needs and monitored to ensure continued success of the therapy. Although usual replacement doses slightly exceed normal daily production of steroids, these doses would not be expected to cause Cushing's syndrome.

Successful treatment of adrenal insufficiency frequently is obtained simply with cortisol (hydrocortisone) or cortisone, natural glucocorticoids with sufficient mineralocorticoid activity to maintain sodium balance in many individuals. Other patients may require additional supplementation with a drug such as fludrocortisone, an orally absorbed mineralocorticoid.

Antiinflammatory therapy. In pharmacologic doses the antiinflammatory action of the glucocorticoids is the primary action sought. The level of steroid at the site of action must be much higher than normally would be found at that site to achieve the antiinflammatory effect. In some cases, this goal may be achieved by topical or local application of the steroid; in other cases the steroids must be administered systemically (see Table 51-4).

Other uses. Steroids in one form or another have been used to treat many conditions. Evaluating these treatments is frequently difficult and requires large-scale clinical testing with careful comparison of the results for treated patients with those of untreated or placebo-treated individuals. Table 51-5 lists 30 nonendocrine diseases in which glucocorticoid therapy is effective, based on an FDA evaluation of information supplied by the National Academy of Sciences and the National Research Council. Not all forms of these diseases respond to steroids, but the drugs may prove useful to most patients at some stage of their disease. Specific notes concerning the treatment regimen used are also included in Table 51-5. Table 51-6 lists the same information for diseases in which glucocorticoid therapy has not been rigorously proved to be effective. Nevertheless, the glucocorticoids are frequently used clinically to treat these conditions.

Compounds Used in Diagnosing Adrenal Disorders

Adrenocorticotropic hormone

Adrenocorticotropic hormone (ACTH and corticotropin) is discussed in Chapter 50 as part of the natural feedback regulatory cycle controlling adrenal function. ACTH directly stimulates the adrenal cortex to synthesize adrenal steroids. This action can be used diagnostically to distinguish between Addison's disease and secondary adrenal insufficiency resulting from pituitary dysfunction (Table 51-7). Normal adrenal glands respond to ACTH by synthesizing and releasing cortisol into the bloodstream, where it may be measured. In Addison's disease the adrenal gland cannot respond to ACTH, and no excess cortisol is produced. In patients who have low pituitary function the adrenal gland may be suppressed and may respond less rapidly to ACTH than would a normal gland.

In the past, ACTH has been used to treat adrenal insufficiency or other diseases responding to gluco-

Table 51-5   Nonendocrine Conditions Effectively Treated with Glucocorticoids†

Condition	Treatment regimen	Rationale
ALLERGIC STATES		
Bronchial asthma Serum sickness	Systemic steroids control acute episodes that are unresponsive to conventional therapy.	Glucocorticoids block histamine-induced and other inflammatory responses. In asthma, glucocorticoids may enhance effects of sympathomimetic agents.
Contact dermatitis	Topical therapy is used as required. Systemic therapy is rarely justified.	
COLLAGEN DISEASES		
Acute rheumatic carditis Systemic lupus erythematosus	Systemic steroids control acute episodes or lower doses for maintenance. Topical steroids control dermatologic manifestations of lupus erythematosus.	Glucocorticoids antagonize autoimmune responses, causing tissue damage in these diseases.
DERMATOLOGIC DISEASES		
Mycosis fungoides Pemphigus Seborrheic dermatitis Severe erythema multiforme Severe psoriasis	Topical therapy is used as needed. Some skin lesions may require injection at the site. Systemic therapy may be used when symptoms are widespread or especially severe.	Glucocorticoids have antiinflammatory and antimitotic actions that control symptoms.
EDEMATOUS STATES		
Cerebral edema Nephrotic syndrome	Systemic steroids for short periods to control acute episodes; used with other treatment.	Therapy empiric.
HEMATOLOGIC DISORDERS		
Autoimmune hemolytic anemia Thrombocytopenia	Systemic steroids are used in large doses for acute disease; lower doses to maintain remission.	Glucocorticoids antagonize autoimmune processes, destroying blood cells.
NEOPLASTIC DISEASES		
Leukemias Lymphomas	Systemic steroids along with other antineoplastic agents produce remissions and palliation of symptoms.	Glucocorticoids have antilymphocytic action, which aids in destroying tumors of these tissues.
JOINT INFLAMMATION		
Bursitis, nonrheumatic	Injection into joint usually preferred.	Antiinflammatory effect provides symptomatic relief.
OPHTHALMIC DISEASES		
Allergic conjunctivitis Chorioretinitis Iritis and iridocyclitis Keratitis	Superficial conditions may be treated with steroids applied directly to the eye. Diseases of the internal structures of the eye may require systemic therapy.	Glucocorticoid antiinflammatory action reduces permanent eye damage and controls acute symptoms.
RHEUMATIC DISORDERS		
Acute and subacute bursitis Acute gouty arthritis Acute nonspecific tenosynovitis Ankylosing spondylitis Psoriatic arthritis Rheumatoid arthritis	Intraarticular injection may be required for selected cases. Modest oral doses minimize side effects while providing relief for many patients.	Glucocorticoid inhibition of inflammatory and autoimmune processes relieves symptoms of disease.
RESPIRATORY DISEASES		
Pulmonary tuberculosis Symptomatic sarcoidosis	Systemic steroids may give symptomatic relief to certain patients.	Glucocorticoid antiinflammatory action may relieve symptoms of disease, but no long-term benefit is demonstrable.

†FDA designation

Table 51-6 Nonendocrine Conditions Treated With Glucocorticoids†

Condition	Treatment regimen
ALLERGIC STATES	
Urticaria	Systemic steroids used when disease is not adequately controlled by conventional methods
DENTAL CONDITIONS	
Postoperative inflammatory reactions	Local application
EDEMATOUS STATES	
Cirrhosis of the liver with ascites	Systemic steroids used with diuretics
Congestive heart failure	
GASTROINTESTINAL DISEASES	
Intractable sprue	Systemic steroids may aid in short-term recovery but do not change the long-term prognosis
Regional enteritis	
Ulcerative colitis	
RESPIRATORY DISEASES	
Interstitial pulmonary fibrosis	Systemic steroids used with other therapy or after other therapy has failed
Pulmonary emphysema with bronchial edema	

†Designated as "probably effective" by the FDA for these indications.

corticoids. The rationale for this therapy was that adrenal function was maintained and that a natural balance of steroids was produced. In practice, however, ACTH therapy was not as reliable or convenient as steroid therapy. ACTH must be injected because it is a peptide, whereas oral glucocorticoids are available. In addition, the response of the adrenal gland to ACTH was not easily predictable, making dosage adjustment unreliable. Finally, many patients developed antibodies to ACTH, and as a result, they became unresponsive to it. For these reasons and others, ACTH is no longer widely used in therapy.

Dexamethasone

The highly potent synthetic glucocorticoid dexamethasone also is used diagnostically to test steroid suppression of cortisol synthesis. Relatively small doses of dexamethasone administered over 2 days inhibit cortisol production in a healthy person and, to a lesser extent, in a person with pituitary-induced Cushing's syndrome. Ordinarily, tumor production of cortisol is unaffected.

Metyrapone

Metyrapone (Metopirone) blocks cortisol synthesis in the adrenal gland and may be used to test the ability of the hypophysis to increase ACTH release. Before the test is run, it should be demonstrated that the patient's adrenal glands respond to ACTH. While metyrapone is being administered, cortisol synthesis falls dramatically. In healthy persons the fall in blood

Table 51-7 Agents Used in Diagnosing Adrenal Gland Dysfunction

Generic name	Trade name	Administration/dosage	Comments
Corticotropin	Acthar*	INTRAMUSCULAR, SUBCUTANEOUS: 20 units 4 times daily. INTRAVENOUS: 10 to 25 USP units in 500 ml of dextrose infused over 8 hr. *Children*—1.6 USP units/kg body weight daily.	Used to determine if the adrenal gland can respond to normal regulation. Side effects are those expected of adrenal steroids and allergic reactions. FDA Pregnancy Category C.
	Cortrophin Zinc HP Acthar Gel	INTRAMUSCULAR REPOSITORY: 40 to 80 units every 24 to 72 hr.	This longer-acting form may be preferred for therapy.
Cosyntropin	Cortrosyn*	INTRAMUSCULAR, INTRAVENOUS: *Adults*—0.25 mg single dose. *Children under 2 years*—0.125 mg single dose.	Synthetic form of ACTH used for diagnostic purposes only. Less allergenic than ACTH. FDA Pregnancy Category C.
Metyrapone	Metopirone*	ORAL: *Adults*—750 mg every 4 hr for 6 doses. *Children*—15 mg/kg every 4 hr for 6 doses.	Used to determine if ACTH levels rise appropriately when the adrenal gland lowers cortisol production. Metyrapone blocks cortisol production, leading to cortisol precursors in urine if ACTH is present. Drug may induce acute adrenal insufficiency in some patients. FDA Pregnancy Category C.

*Available in Canada and United States.

cortisol level stimulates the hypothalamus and in turn the hypophysis, with the result that ACTH is released into the bloodstream. Under the influence of ACTH, early steps in steroid synthesis proceed, but metyrapone prevents cortisol from being formed in normal amounts. Therefore the steroid precursors accumulate and are excreted in urine. If no precursors accumulate under these conditions, it is concluded that the hypophysis failed to produce ACTH. If the metyrapone test is administered to a person with adrenalin sufficiency, a danger exists of precipitating an adrenal crisis, because in these patients metyrapone may stop cortisol synthesis.

ADRENAL MEDULLA

The adrenal medulla arises from neuroectodermal tissue during embryonic life and remains closely associated with the autonomic nervous system at maturity. The cells (pheochromocytes or chromaffin cells) can synthesize catecholamines by the same series of reactions found in nerve terminals and can release catecholamines into the bloodstream in response to sympathetic cholinergic presynaptic neurons. One major difference between the synthetic pathways is that nerve terminals form norepinephrine as the final product, whereas the adrenal medulla converts norepinephrine to epinephrine. The enzyme for this final conversion is induced by adrenal steroids, indicating that the anatomic proximity of the disparate tissues of the cortex and medulla may have functional importance.

The hormones of the adrenal medulla are not essential to survival, but they are useful in adapting to stress. Epinephrine produces widespread effects throughout the body, mediated by the beta- and alpha-adrenergic receptors. The actions of epinephrine are discussed in Chapter 10, and the clinical uses of epinephrine are discussed in Chapter 14.

NURSING IMPLICATIONS SUMMARY

Glucocorticoids

Drug administration

◆ See Table 51-4 for a list of toxic reactions associated with long-term glucocorticoid therapy.
◆ Assess mental status and neurologic function.
◆ Assess for signs of depression including lack of interest in personal appearance, withdrawal, insomnia, and anorexia.
◆ Monitor blood pressure, pulse, and weight. Auscultate lung and heart sounds.
◆ Check stools for presence of occult blood.
◆ Monitor complete blood count (CBC) and differential and serum electrolytes and blood glucose.
◆ Use care in moving and positioning immobilized patients on long-term therapy to prevent fractures and bruising. Pad side rails as appropriate.
◆ Glucocorticoids are given via many routes (see Tables 51-2 and 51-3). Read labels carefully. Ascertain that the preparation can be given via the ordered route.
◆ Wear gloves to apply topical preparations.

INTRAVENOUS BETAMETHASONE SODIUM PHOSPHATE

◆ May be given undiluted or diluted. Administer undiluted dose over at least 1 min.

INTRAVENOUS DEXAMETHASONE SODIUM PHOSPHATE

◆ May be given undiluted. Administer 15 mg or less over 1 min.

INTRAVENOUS HYDROCORTISONE SODIUM PHOSPHATE

◆ May be given undiluted. Always use a separate syringe. Administer 25 mg or less over 1 min.

INTRAVENOUS HYDROCORTISONE SODIUM SUCCINATE

◆ Reconstitute as directed on label of vial. Administer direct IV at a rate of 500 mg or less over 1 min.

INTRAVENOUS METHYLPREDNISOLONE SODIUM SUCCINATE

◆ Reconstitute as directed on label of vial. Administer direct IV at a rate of 500 mg or less over 1 min or longer.

INTRAVENOUS PREDNISOLONE SODIUM PHOSPHATE

◆ May be given undiluted at a rate of 10 mg or less over 1 min.

NURSING IMPLICATIONS SUMMARY—cont'd

Patient and family education

◆ Review anticipated benefits and possible side effects of drug therapy. With short-term use (over 7 to 10 days), side effects may be minimal if noticeable. With chronic use, some side effects will usually develop. Tell patients to report any new side effects.

◆ Take oral doses with meals or a snack to lessen gastric irritation. Some physicians prescribe antacids or other drugs prophylactically to lessen the risk of ulceration.

◆ See Patient Problem: Constipation on p. 182.

◆ If weight gain is excessive, counsel about weight reduction diets; consult the physician about a change in glucocorticoid or dose. Other dietary modifications may include decreasing sodium intake and increasing potassium intake. See Dietary Considerations: Potassium Sources on p. 252 and Sodium on p. 233. Encourage patients to increase protein intake.

◆ Warn diabetic patients to monitor blood glucose levels carefully, since glucocorticoids increase blood glucose levels. A change in diet or insulin may be necessary.

◆ Notify the physician if tarry stools develop or "coffee ground" emesis occurs.

◆ Avoid rough activities if skin becomes fragile and easily bruised.

◆ Warn patients on long-term therapy to take doses every day as ordered, even if they are sick. Failure to take ordered doses, even for a few days, may result in adrenocortical insufficiency in susceptible patients.

◆ Remind patients to inform all health-care providers of all medications being used. Do not take any medications unless approved by the physician.

◆ Warn patients not to increase or decrease dose without consulting the physician.

◆ Teach patients not to have immunizations while taking glucocorticoids unless approved by the physician.

◆ Tell patients to avoid skin testing unless approved by the physician.

◆ Encourage patients on long-term therapy to wear a medical identification tag or bracelet indicating that glucocorticoids are being used.

◆ Menstrual difficulties may develop with long-term therapy. Instruct women to keep a record of menstrual periods. Counsel about contraceptive methods as appropriate. Warn patients to notify the physician if pregnancy is suspected.

◆ Large doses of glucocorticoids increase susceptibility to infection and mask the symptoms of infection. Warn patients about this side effect. Instruct patients to notify the physician of fever, cough, sore throat, malaise, and injuries that do not heal. Instruct patients to avoid contact with individuals with active infections.

◆ Review the drug and route of administration prescribed for the patient. Review manufacturer's instruction for administration. Ascertain that the patient can administer the ordered drug correctly; see Chapter 6.

◆ Remind patients not to share medications with others. Remind patients to keep all medications out of the reach of children.

Mineralocorticoids

Drug administration

◆ All glucocorticoids also have mineralocorticoid activity but in varying amounts; see Table 51-1.

◆ Monitor weight, blood pressure, and pulse. Auscultate lung and heart sounds.

◆ Monitor serum electrolyte level.

◆ For a discussion of subcutaneous implantation of drugs, see Chapter 54.

◆ For a discussion of intramuscular (IM) injection of oil-based medications, see Chapter 6.

Patient and family education

◆ Review anticipated benefits and possible side effects of drug therapy.

◆ Counsel about sodium restriction and increasing potassium intake as needed. See Dietary Considerations: Potassium Sources on p. 252 and Sodium on p. 233.

◆ Encourage the patient to wear a medical identification tag or bracelet.

◆ Remind patients to inform all health-care providers of all drugs being used.

CHAPTER REVIEW

◆ KEY TERMS

acute adrenal insufficiency, p. 744
Addison's disease, p. 744
Cushing's syndrome, p. 744
glucocorticoids, p. 743
mineralocorticoids, p. 742
renin-angiotensin system, p. 742
secondary adrenal insufficiency, p. 744

◆ REVIEW QUESTIONS

1. What are the two functional units of the adrenal gland?
2. What are mineralocorticoids?
3. In which part of the adrenal cortex are mineralocorticoids synthesized?
4. What hormones regulate mineralocorticoid synthesis?
5. Where are glucocorticoids synthesized?
6. What are the main effects of glucocorticoids on metabolism?
7. What is the result of untreated acute adrenal insufficiency?
8. What is Addison's disease? How would you assess for this?
9. What is secondary adrenal insufficiency?
10. What is Cushing's syndrome?
11. What are the symptoms of Cushing's syndrome? How would you assess these?
12. What is the effect of overproduction of mineralocorticoids?

13. What are the three major activities or actions of adrenal steroids?
14. What is the effect of chronic overdosage with glucocorticoids? What signs and symptoms would you assess?
15. Why should steroid therapy not be stopped suddenly in a patient who has been receiving long-term therapy?
16. What are the advantages and disadvantages of alternate-day therapy?
17. What are the two major clinical uses of adrenal steroids?
18. What is the aim of replacement therapy in treating adrenal insufficiency?
19. Which mineralocorticoids are available for clinical use?
20. Which are the water-soluble glucocorticoid preparations, and when are they preferred over the suspensions?
21. Which steroids are particularly effective as topical agents?
22. What drug interactions commonly occur with adrenal steroids?
23. How is ACTH used in diagnosis?
24. Why is ACTH not commonly used in replacement therapy?
25. What hormone is released by the adrenal medulla?

SUGGESTED READING

Ianuzzi LP: Oral steroids in rheumatoid arthritis: helpful but not remittive, *Postgrad Med* 82(5):295, 1987.
Johnson CE: Aerosol corticosteroids for the treatment of asthma, *Drug Intell Clin Pharm* 21(10):784, 1987.

CHAPTER 52

Drugs Affecting the Thyroid and Parathyroid Glands

LEARNING OBJECTIVES

After studying this chapter, you should be able to do the following:

- Discuss the rationale for therapy of hypothyroidism.
- Describe the classes of drugs used for hypothyroidism.
- Discuss the rationale for therapy of hyperthyroidism.
- Describe the classes of drugs used for hyperthyroidism.
- Develop a nursing care plan for the patient receiving drug therapy for hypothyroidism or hyperthyroidism.

CHAPTER OVERVIEW

◆ The thyroid gland is a richly vascularized, horseshoe-shaped structure lying across the trachea in the region of the larynx (Figure 52-1). The gland contains at least two cell types differing in function and embryologic origin. These are the follicular cells, derived from endoderm at the base of the tongue, and the parafollicular cells, derived from ultimobranchial bodies. A third endocrine tissue closely associated with the thyroid is found in the parathyroid glands. These small bodies normally lie behind the lobes of the thyroid but rarely may be found within the thyroid. The function of each of these tissues, the hormones produced, and the medications commonly used in diagnosing and treating disease states associated with deficient or excessive thyroid or parathyroid function are described in this chapter.

Nursing Process Overview

THYROID THERAPY

Assessment

The nursing process in diseases of the thyroid gland is the same, whether the problem is hyperthyroidism or hypothyroidism. In most cases the original problem develops insidiously. Obtain a complete assessment of the patient, including temperature, pulse, respiration, blood pressure, weight, history of weight changes, level of energy, mood, subjective feeling, and response to temperature. Check the height of children. Question family members to determine onset of symptoms. Check thyroid function test results and blood glucose levels.

Nursing Diagnoses

Body image disturbance

Activity intolerance related to fatigue secondary to excessive metabolic rate

Management

Monitor the temperature, pulse, respiration, blood pressure, weight, height of children, and blood glucose level. Question about the subjective response to therapy. If weight reduction is an additional goal of therapy, teach about diet, or refer as needed. If radioactive iodine is used, follow hospital procedures for the handling of radioactive materials.

Evaluation

Before discharge, check that patients can explain the action of the drug and how to take the prescribed dose. Other parameters the patient should monitor and record at home include pulse, weight, and height. Explain the side effects that may occur and what to

757

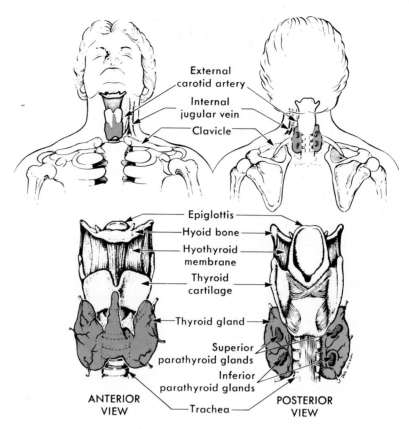

FIGURE 52-1
Anatomic location of thyroid and parathyroid glands.

do about them, adjustments needed in the treatment of other medical problems (e.g., changes in insulin or anticoagulant doses), the need for continuing the medication, and the need to wear an identification tag or bracelet. With radioactive iodine, the patient will not be on long-term drug therapy but should be able to explain what symptoms should be reported to the physician.

THYROID GLAND
Follicular Cells

The function of the **follicular cells** of the thyroid is to regulate the basal metabolic rate (BMR), mainly by altering oxidative processes in target tissues. The iodine-containing hormones, thyroxine (T_4) and tri-iodothyronine (T_3), released by the follicular cells into the general circulation, establish the metabolic rates for most body tissues. Regulation of thyroid

hormone levels in the blood is accomplished in part by the negative feedback system described in Chapter 50. Thyroid-stimulating hormone (TSH) from the anterior pituitary (adenohypophysis) stimulates each of the steps in thyroid hormone synthesis described in the next section.

Synthesis of Thyroid Hormones

The first step in synthesizing the iodine-containing thyroid hormones is iodine uptake by the follicular cell (Figure 52-2). Because iodide ion levels in the bloodstream are relatively low, the follicular cell must concentrate iodine to carry out the synthetic reactions required. In the normal human body the concentration of iodide ion in the thyroid is 30 to 40 times that found in plasma. In the second step in thyroid hormone synthesis, iodide ion activation is catalyzed by the peroxidase enzyme formed in follicular cells. This activation step takes place on the surface of the

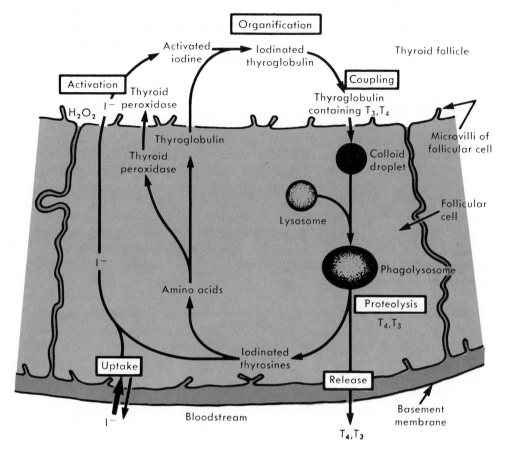

FIGURE 52-2

Synthesis of T_3 and T_4 by follicular cells within the thyroid gland. A single follicular cell is depicted. Cell base is in close contact with blood, and cell apex is in contact with colloid. These cells surround areas of colloid to form thyroid follicles. Parafollicular cells of thyroid gland do not directly contact colloid.

microvilli, which protrude into the colloid filling the thyroid follicle.

Once activated, iodine may be attached to thyroglobulin in a process called *organification*. Thyroglobulin, a large protein synthesized in the follicular cell and extruded into the follicle, is the major protein component of colloid. Most iodine atoms are attached to tyrosine molecules contained within the peptide chains of thyroglobulin. The tyrosine may contain one (3-monoiodotyrosine, or MIT) or two (3,5-diiodotyrosine, or DIT) atoms of iodine.

After iodination, some tyrosine molecules may undergo a coupling reaction in which two molecules of DIT combine to produce one molecule of thyroglobulin-bound T_4. Coupling may also occur between one molecule each of DIT and MIT to yield one molecule of T_3. These coupling reactions are also believed to be catalyzed by the perioxidase enzyme from the follicular cell.

Thyroglobulin serves primarily as a storage depot for thyroid hormones and the precursors MIT and DIT. In healthy persons, each molecule of thyroglobulin contains about six molecules of MIT, five molecules of DIT, and two molecules of T_4. Less T_3 is stored. A single molecule of T_3 occurs in about one out of three molecules of thyroglobulin within the follicles. Normal thyroids thus contain a 30-day supply of T_3 and T_4 and a 20-day supply of iodine stored as MIT and DIT.

When release of thyroid hormones is required, TSH stimulates the microvilli of the follicular cells to move droplets of colloid into the cell. Once inside the cell, the colloid droplets fuse with lysosomes to form vesicles called *phagolysosomes*. The low pH and the protein-digesting enzymes from the lysosomes allow digestion (proteolysis) of the thyroglobulin to amino acids. During proteolysis, T_3, T_4, MIT, and DIT are released into the cell. T_3 and T_4 are transported to the cell surface and are released into the bloodstream. In contast, MIT and DIT are retained within the cell, and the iodine they contain is reclaimed for use in new hormone synthesis. Patients who lack the salvage pathway lose excessive iodide ion in urine and ultimately fail to produce sufficient thyroid hormones. This syndrome is a rare cause of hypothyroidism.

The thyroid gland normally releases 70 to 90 μg of T_4 daily but only 1 to 6 μg T_3. Most T_3 is formed in peripheral tissues from T_4.

Disposition of Thyroid Hormones

Once in the blood, thyroid hormones are rapidly and almost completely bound to plasma proteins. Most of the hormones are bound to a special alpha globulin called *thyroid-binding globulin* (TBG). A less important carrier is prealbumin. Very little thyroid hormone is bound to plasma albumin in normal persons because the thyroid hormones are so tightly bound to TBG. However, the amount of thyroid hormone that may be bound to TBG is limited. TBG can bind about 2.5 times more hormone than it ordinarily carries. When that limit is reached, the excess hormone is bound to albumin and prealbumin. These proteins are less avid carriers than TBG but have nearly unlimited capacity for hormones.

The relative distribution of T_3 and T_4 differs within the body. T_4 is much more abundant than T_3 in the thyroid and in blood. However, T_3 is less tightly bound to plasma proteins than T_4. More importantly, because T_4 is rapidly converted to T_3 in most tissues, the most abundant form of thyroid hormone in target cells is T_3. T_3 is also the primary thyroid hormone that binds to nuclear receptors, setting off the metabolic events characteristic of thyroid action. For these reasons, T_3 may be considered to be the most important thyroid hormone.

T_3 and T_4 are metabolized by the liver to glucuronide and sulfate derivatives, which then are eliminated in bile. No significant reuptake of the hormones occurs from the gut. Other hormone destruction occurs in the target tissues, where the hormones are deiodinated and transformed to inactive products.

HYPOTHYROIDISM

Hypothyroidism occurs whenever the production of thyroid hormones is insufficient to meet the body's demands. Mild hormone deficiencies produce minimum disease with vague symptoms, sometimes making the condition difficult to diagnose. Untreated patients may ultimately develop characteristic signs and symptoms related to the slowing of metabolic rates and changes in the central nervous system (CNS) (Table 52-1). The severe form of the disease is called *myxedema*.

Hypothyroidism may develop in the fetus when a pregnant woman receives antithyroid drugs. However, the most common cause of hypothyroidism in newborns is an embryologic or genetic defect that arrests thyroid development or prevents its function. A child lacking adequate thyroid function during fetal development may appear nearly normal at birth, since much of fetal development can proceed without fetal thyroid hormones. If the disease is not detected very soon after birth, however, irreversible brain damage and associated physical signs develop. Congenital hypothyroidism is called *cretinism*.

Hypothyroidism that develops after the neonatal period but before puberty is called juvenile hypothyroidism. The most prominent early sign of juvenile hypothyroidism is growth stunting. If not appropriately treated, juvenile hypothyroid patients suffer not only arrested growth but also other signs and symptoms associated with adult forms of the disease.

Diagnosis

Hypothyroidism is diagnosed by the judicious use of a combination of the thyroid function tests summarized in Table 52-2. An understanding of these tests requires knowledge of normal thyroid physiology and an understanding of the negative feedback regulation of the thyroid (see Chapter 50).

In **primary hypothyroidism** the thyroid gland is defective; in most patients the reason for this is unknown, although in some a specific disease or chemical exposure may be responsible. The diagnosis of primary hypothyroidism requires establishing that a patient has lower-than-normal thyroid hormone levels and elevated levels of TSH in the bloodstream. Of the many tests available, TSH determinations are the most widely used. Free thyroxine (FT_4) levels are lower than normal in 80% to 90% of hypothyroid patients tested. Serum T_4 or T_3 uptake may also be measured, although each of these tests may be affected by conditions unrelated to thyroid disease that change the serum concentration of TBG (see Table 52-2).

The thyroidal uptake of iodine is also lowered in hypothyroidism. However, this test is seldom useful in diagnosing the disease, since thyroidal uptake is affected by intake of iodine, whether as part of the diet or as a constituent of medications. The patient may not be aware that iodine is being taken. For example, potassium iodide, used an an expectorant, is a constituent of several prescription cough medicines.

Table 52-1   Thyroid Disorders

Condition	Symptoms	Physical appearance
Hypothyroidism, adult on-set (also called *myxedema* and *Gull's disease*)	Diminished vigor and muscle weakness Reduced mental acuity Emotional changes, especially depression Slow relaxation of deep tendon reflexes Muscle cramps Constipation Decreased appetite Abnormal menses in females Slow pulse and enlarged heart Tendency to gain weight Lowered basal metabolic rate	Puffy face and eyes Thin, coarse hair and eyebrows Dry, scaly, cold, and slightly yellow skin Enlarged tongue Slow, husky speech Dull or slow-witted appearance
Hypothyroidism, congenital (cretinism)		
At birth	Absence of distal femoral and proximal tibial epiphyses Slowed brain development	Essentially normal Slightly longer and heavier than normal
At 3 months with no treatment	Lethargy Feeding difficulty Constipation Neonatal jaundice, persistant Respiratory distress Hoarse cry Intermittent cyanosis	Enlarged tongue Puffy face and thick neck Poor muscle tone Depressed nasal bridge with broad, flat nose Distended abdomen Umbilical hernia Short legs
Hyperthyroidism (also called *thyrotoxicosis* or *Graves' disease*)	Cardiac arrhythmia Enlarged thyroid gland Rapid pulse rate Increased basal metabolic rate Muscle weakness and wasting Fine tremor Heat intolerance Weight loss in most patients	Restlessness or nervousness Abrupt actions and speech Warm, moist palms Loosening of fingernails from nail beds Bulging eyes with sclera visible all around iris White, unpigmented patches on the skin (vitiligo)

Although primary hypothyroidism is the most common, other forms of hypothyroidism do occur. If the hypophysis fails to release adequate TSH, insufficient thyroid hormone is synthesized, and **secondary hypothyroidism** develops. Occasionally a patient with damage to the hypothalamus fails to produce thyrotropin-releasing hormone (TRH), which is required to stimulate TSH production in the pituitary (see Chapter 50); this is called *tertiary hypothyroidism.*

Secondary and tertiary hypothyroidism may be distinguished from primary hypothyroidism by measuring TSH. Whereas in primary hypothyroidism TSH is elevated by the natural action of the negative feedback system attempting to elevate thyroid hormone levels, TSH levels are low or undetectable in the other two forms of hypothyroidism. If the TSH assay is not available, a TSH test may be performed in which injected TSH is expected to stimulate T_4

formation and release in secondary or tertiary hypothyroidism but not in primary hypothyroidism (see Table 52-2).

Secondary and tertiary hypothyroidism may be distinguished from each other by the protirelin (TRH) test, which measures the ability of the hypophysis to respond to its normal regulatory hormone (see Table 52-2). If TSH rises after TRH administration, the implication is that the hypothalamus is defective, and both the anterohypophysis and the thyroid would be capable of normal function if properly stimulated.

Replacement Therapy

Treatment of hypothyroidism requires replacement therapy with the thyroid hormones. The goal of therapy is to produce the euthyroid state (normal thyroid hormone levels). Several preparations containing natural or synthetic forms of the hormones are available (Table 52-3). Selecting one of these oral agents is

Table 52-2   Tests to Evaluate Thyroid Function

Test	Procedure	Diagnostic use	Normal values	Comments
Serum T_4	Total serum T_4 is measured by competitive protein binding test or radioimmunoassay.	To distinguish hyperthyroid or hypothyroid conditions from euthyroid state.	5 to 12 μg/100 ml serum	Conditions that elevate TBG levels (e.g., pregnancy or estrogen administration) also elevate total serum T_4 levels. Lowered TBG levels in cirrhosis or nephrotic syndrome also lower total serum T_4 levels. In both cases, free hormone levels are usually normal, and patients are functionally euthyroid.
Free thyroxine (FT_4)	FT_4 is measured by radioimmunoassay or equilibrium dialysis.	To distinguish hyperthyroid or hypothyroid conditions from euthyroid state.	1 to 2.5 ng/100 ml	Normal values may vary greatly from laboratory to laboratory.
T_3 uptake (T_3U) or resin T_3 uptake (RT_3U)	Test measures the degree of saturation of patient's TBG with endogenous thyroid hormones.	To distinguish hyperthyroid or hypothyroid conditions from euthyroid state.	25% to 45%, or 0.82 to 1.35 when expressed as a ratio of T_3U to normal	Hyperthyroidism elevates ratio; hypothyroidism lowers ratio. Levels of TBG and T_4 in the blood affect the test more than do T_3 values.
Serum T_3	Total serum T_3 is measured by specific radioimmunoassay.	To distinguish hyperthyroid conditions from euthyroid state.	0.08 to 0.20 μg/100 ml	Test is not useful in hypothyroidism, since T_3 may be more abundant than T_4.
Serum TSH	Serum TSH is measured by specific radioimmunoassay.	To distinguish hypothyroid conditions from euthyroid state; to distinguish primary from secondary hypothyroidism.	0.5 to 5 μU/ml	Primary hypothyroidism shows elevated TSH levels; secondary hypothyroidism caused by pituitary failure shows little or no TSH.
Protirelin test (TRH test)	Synthetic TRH (500 μg) is given intravenously, causing a peak release of TSH 30 min later in patients with normal pituitary glands.	To distinguish hypothyroidism caused by pituitary failure from other forms of hypothyroidism.	Peak levels of TSH seen in normal patients are 5 to 35 μU/ml serum.	No rise is usually observed in serum TSH level in hyperthyroid patients.
Thyroid uptake of radioiodine	Radioactivity in the thyroid is measured 4, 6, and 24 hr after administration of tracer dose of radioactive iodine.	To distinguish hyperthyroid and hypothyroid conditions from euthyroid state.	Normal glands take up 10% to 35% of tracer dose in 24 hr.	This test may be affected by dietary intake of iodine, by administration of iodine-containing medications, or by use of antithyroid drugs.
TSH test	Bovine TSH is given intramuscularly after which serum T_3 and T_4 or radioiodine uptake is measured.	To distinguish primary from secondary hypothyroidism.	Normal thyroids respond by increasing iodine uptake and T_4 release.	This test is rarely used when TSH levels are to be measured.
Thyroid suppression tests	T_3 (75 μg) is given daily for 7 days. Radioiodine uptake by thyroid gland is measured before and after test.	To distinguish hyperthyroid conditions from euthyroid state.	Uptake is 50% or less of the pretest uptake.	This test may be dangerous for elderly patients, weakened patients, or patients with heart disease.

Table 52-3 Drugs to Diagnose or Treat Hypothyroidism

Generic name	Trade name	Administration/dosage	Properties	Comments
NATURAL THYROID HORMONES				
Thyroglobulin	Proloid*	ORAL: *Adults*—32 to 160 mg daily for maintenance. Initial doses are small and are gradually increased to maintenance levels. FDA Pregnancy Category A.	Contains T_3, T_4, and other iodine-containing compounds.	Replacement therapy for hypothyroidism. Overdose produces the same symptoms as seen with thyroid U.S.P.
Thyroid U.S.P.		ORAL: *Adults*—60 to 120 mg daily is usual for maintenance. Initial doses 15 mg daily. Double the dose every 2 weeks until effective maintenance dose is reached. FDA Pregnancy Category A.	Impure mixture of thyroid components that includes T_3 and T_4.	Replacement therapy for hypothyroidism. Overdose produces symptoms of hyperthyroidism. Too large a dose at onset of therapy may cause vascular occlusion, especially in patients with arteriosclerosis.
SYNTHETIC THYROID HORMONES				
Levothyroxine sodium	Eltroxin† Levothroid Synthroid*	ORAL: *Adults*—75 to 125 µg daily for maintenance. Initial doses are small and are gradually increased to maintenance levels. *Children over 1 year*—2 to 6 µg/kg body weight daily. INTRAVENOUS: *Adults*—Up to 0.5 mg daily. FDA Pregnancy Category A.	Chemically pure form of T_4.	Replacement therapy for hypothyroidism. IV form for myxedemic coma. Peak effect occurs 9 days after start of therapy.
Liothyronine sodium	Cytomel*	ORAL: *Adults*—25 to 100 µg daily for maintenance. Initial doses should be low and gradually increased to maintenance levels. FDA Pregnancy Category A.	Chemically pure form of T_3.	Replacement therapy for hypothyroidism. Peak effect occurs in 2 days. Not for cretinism because T_3 may not cross the blood-brain barrier as well as T_4.
Liotrix	Euthroid Thyrolar*	ORAL: *Adults*—30 µg T_4 with 7.5 µg T_3, or 25 µg T_4 with 6.25 µg T_3. Doses may be gradually increased as needed. FDA Pregnancy Category A.	Chemically pure T_4 and T_3 combined in a 4:1 ratio.	Replacement therapy for hypothyroidism.
ADENOHYPOPHYSEAL HORMONES				
Protirelin (thyrotropin-releasing hormone, TRH)	Relefact TRH* Thypinone	INTRAVENOUS: *Adults*—500 µg. *Children*—7 µg/kg.	Synthetic preparation of natural hypothalamic tripeptide hormone.	Diagnostic agent (see Table 52-2). May transiently produce nausea, flushing, changes in blood pressure, and an urge to urinate.
Thyrotropin (TSH)	Thytropar*	INTRAMUSCULAR, SUBCUTANEOUS: 10 IU once or twice daily. FDA Pregnancy Category C.	Extract of bovine antero hypophysis contains natural peptide, TSH.	Diagnostic agent (see Table 52-2). Releases thyroid hormones that may precipitate adrenal crisis in patients with secondary adrenal insufficiency. May also cause cardiovascular symptoms.

*Available in Canada and United States.
†Available in Canada only.

largely a matter of preference for the physician. The only appropriate clinical use of these thyroid hormones is to treat thyroid deficiency. They should never be used in weight loss programs.

Thyroid U.S.P.

Thyroid U.S.P. is a defatted extract of whole thyroid glands. It contains T_4 and T_3 in the natural ratio of 2.5:1. The iodine content of these preparations is regulated by law in the United States. Although thyroid hormone activity is not directly standardized in these products, many physicians have found them to be quite constant in potency, especially when fresh, dry preparations are compared. Considerable potency may be lost on long storage or if the powder becomes moist.

Thyroglobulin

Thyroglobulin is also prepared from whole thyroid glands and, as with thyroid extracts, contains T_4 and T_3 in the ratio of 2.5:1. This preparation is more expensive than thyroid U.S.P. Some physicians prefer thyroglobulin because it is standardized directly for thyroid hormone activity rather than for total iodine content.

Levothyroxine sodium

Levothyroxine sodium is a pure synthetic form of the natural thyroid hormone thyroxine, or T_4. It therefore has the properties of T_4, including high affinity for serum proteins, long half-life in the bloodstream, and conversion to T_3 by peripheral tissues.

Liothyronine sodium

Liothyronine sodium is a pure synthetic form of the natural thyroid hormone triiodothyronine, or T_3. It therefore has the properties of T_3 including shorter half-life in the bloodstream than T_4, greater potency than T_4, and conversion to inactive products in peripheral tissues. In addition, T_3 seems to be absorbed better from the gut than T_4.

Liotrix

Liotrix is a thyroid preparation that contains both pure synthetic T_4 and T_3 in the ratio of 4:1. This mixture was designed to produce normal thyroid function tests when therapy was adequate. In contrast, if T_3 is given alone, a patient may be clinically euthyroid. Since T_3 is not converted to T_4, however, any diagnostic test based on T_4 likely gives low values. In theory, mixtures containing 4:1 ratios of T_4 to T_3 bring T_3, T_4, and protein-bound iodine (PBI) all within normal range during therapy. No firm evidence shows that this treatment has any clinically apparent advantage to the patient over the use of T_4.

Potency of agents used to treat hypothyroidism. One obvious difference among the preparations just discussed is their relative potencies. In terms of biologic activity, 60 mg of thyroid U.S.P. = 60 mg thyroglobulin = 1 mg or less of levothyroxine = 0.025 mg of liothyronine = liotrix tablets containing 0.06 mg T_4 + 0.015 mg T_3 or 0.05 mg T_4 + 0.0125 mg T_3. A wide range of tablet sizes is available in each of these preparations, so a dosage may be adjusted easily to the patient's particular need.

Absorption, distribution, and excretion. The protein-binding properties of the thyroid hormones explain some clinically important differences between these agents. T_4, being more highly protein bound, leaves the bloodstream more slowly than does T_3. Therefore the onset of action for T_4 is about 2 days, whereas T_3 effect may be expected within 6 hr of administration (Figure 52-3). Moreover, T_4, which is bound to plasma protein, is less available for elimination, excretion, or tissue biotransformation than is T_3. Thus T_4 persists longer in the body than T_3. The effects of a single equimolar dose (same number of molecules) of T_3 and T_4 are shown in Figure 52-3, in which the basal metabolic rate (BMR) was followed as an indicator of thyroid hormone action in these hypothyroid subjects. When patients are switched from T_4 to T_3, or vice versa, these different time courses must be considered. For example, a patient being switched from a preparation containing primarily T_4 to T_3 alone might suffer from excessive thyroid hormone action if started immediately on full T_3 doses after T_4 administration is terminated. Therefore patients are given small doses of T_3 after T_4 is stopped, and the dose of T_3 is gradually raised as necessary to maintain the euthyroid state.

In a newly diagnosed hypothyroid patient, thyroid medications are started at very low doses and are increased at varying intervals until the euthyroid state is achieved. Thyroid U.S.P. and levothyroxine doses are doubled roughly every 2 weeks, but liothyronine doses are doubled weekly until adequate control is achieved. These gradually increasing doses are justified, since a sudden return to adequate thyroid hormone levels produces acute stress on several body systems. One common and dangerous example observed occasionally even with low doses is the production of angina pectoris, coronary occlusion, or stroke in elderly or predisposed patients. Another difficulty may be a relative adrenal insufficiency, which arises primarily in patients with inadequate hypophysis function who suffer secondary hypothyroidism and secondary adrenal insufficiency. If thyroid hormone therapy is started in these patients without also restoring adequate glucocorticoid levels, they may suffer a dangerous adrenal crisis.

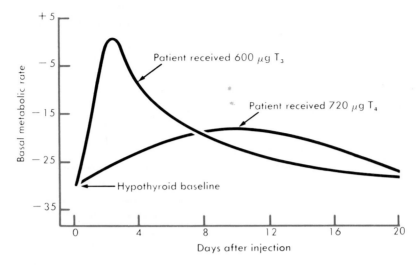

FIGURE 52-3

Time-course of thyroid hormone effects. Patient in each test received single oral dose of medication indicated. Doses T_3 and T_4 administered are equimolar (equal number of molecules).

Severe hypothyroidism may ultimately result in myxedemic coma. In this state, patients possess most of the clinical features of hypothyroidism, including low body temperature as a result of the profoundly lowered metabolic rate, depressed CNS, and hypoventilation (see Table 52-1). Patients at this stage of the disease must be treated aggressively with thyroid hormones, glucocorticoids, and other supportive measures. Since rapid replacement with thyroid hormones is necessary, some physicians prefer to use the more rapidly acting T_3. However T_3 is not readily available commercially in an injectable form. Since T_3 is rapidly absorbed from the gastrointestinal (GI) tract, T_3 tablets may be crushed and administered through a nasogastric tube. Alternatively, some physicians prefer to use the commercially available T_4 injection form that is administered intravenously.

Catecholamines must sometimes be used to combat the shocklike symptoms found in myxedemic coma. Patients so treated are especially at risk for cardiac arrhythmias, since catecholamines and thyroid hormones may cause this dangerous consequence.

Elimination of the thyroid hormones used in replacement therapy is the same as for the normal hormones, the major routes being biliary excretion and tissue metabolism of the compounds.

HYPERTHYROIDISM

Hyperthyroidism occurs whenever excess thyroid hormones are released into the circulation. The dis-

ease may range from very mild forms displaying few of the symptoms shown in Table 52-1 to a severe condition called *thyroid storm* in which death may result from an uncontrolled rise in body temperature and vascular collapse. Increased thyroid hormone production may result from hyperfunction of the entire gland or from the excessive output of one or more small nodules within the thyroid. A rare cause of hyperthyroidism is excess TSH, either from the pituitary gland (hypophysis) or from a tumor.

Several terms describe various forms of hyperthyroidism. Basically, hyperthyroidism may occur with or without thyroid nodules. The disease without nodules is the most common form and is referred to as toxic diffuse goiter, thyrotoxicosis, or *Graves disease* (or rarely Basedow's or Parry's disease). Many patients with this disease display exophthalmos (bulging eyes). Since many patients also have enlarged thyroid glands, another common name for this condition is *exophthalmic goiter*. Toxic nodular goiter produces the same general symptoms as Graves' disease, except that eye symptoms are rare in the nodular form.

Hyperthyroidism is rare in children and is most common in adults in the third or fourth decade of life. Women are affected much more frequently than men, but the reasons for which are not clear. Also, Graves' disease seems to be precipitated in women by puberty, pregnancy, or menopause. Subacute thyroiditis can produce a reversible form of hyperthyroidism. This condition seems to appear sometime after recovery from viral diseases and may be caused by the infectious process.

Diagnosis of Hyperthyroidism

Hyperthyroidism is characterized by elevated serum T_4, serum T_3, free T_4, and free T_3 levels in most patients. Thus diagnostic tests that directly measure one of these parameters (serum T_4 and serum T_3 testing) are most often used. The T_3 resin uptake test also may be used because hyperthyroidism increases the degree of TBG saturation with thyroid hormones. Radioactive iodine uptake also may be measured and is useful in distinguishing between various forms of hyperthyroidism. These diagnostic tests form part of a larger clinical picture. Much information is gained by determining the size of the thyroid by palpation, presence or absence of nodules in the thyroid, and the results of a thyroid scan to measure the pattern of radioactive iodine concentration in the gland.

Diagnosis of Graves' disease has been aided by the realization that the disease has an immunologic basis. In this condition the thyroid is chronically overstimulated by a group of immunoglobulins that supplant TSH as the regulator of thyroid function. These immunoglobulins are found in the sera of nearly all patients who have Graves' disease, and the amounts of the immunoglobulins correlate with the severity of the hyperthyroidism observed.

Drug Therapy

Hyperthyroidism most often is controlled with drugs or radioactive iodine. The drugs fall into two main classes, those that control the symptoms of hyperthyroidism and those that lower the production of T_3 and T_4 by the thyroid.

Propranolol

Propranolol, a drug previously discussed as a beta-adrenergic blocking agent (see Chapters 10 and 15), represents the class of drugs that controls symptoms of hyperthyroidism but produces no significant long-term change in thyroid hormone levels. Propranolol is effective because it alters the response of peripheral tissues to the high circulating levels of thyroid hormones. Blockade of the beta receptors reduces the symptoms of palpitation, tremor, sweating, proximal muscle weakness, mental agitation, and cardiac arrhythmias. One advantage of propranolol therapy is that clinical improvement is seen rapidly. With many other drugs, relief of symptoms may be greatly delayed. Propranolol or other blockers of beta-adrenergic receptors may be used to prepare a hyperthyroid patient for surgery.

Thioamides

The thioamides represent the class of drugs that inhibits the synthesis of thyroid hormones. Although the exact mechanism of action of these compounds is not agreed on, they inhibit each step in synthesis except iodine uptake (see Figure 52-2), and they are thought to inhibit preferentially the peroxidase-catalyzed reactions (coupling and organification). Since these compounds are primarily enzyme inhibitors, they do not directly destroy thyroid tissue but only prevent its excessive action.

Thioamide action on the thyroid gland is immediate, and reduced hormone synthesis can be demonstrated within hours. Observable clinical response to the drugs, however, does not appear for days or weeks, the period required for stored thyroid hormones to be depleted. Patients may be maintained on a thioamide for months, provided the hyperthyroidism is well controlled during that time. Usually, after about 1 year, the thioamide is withdrawn and thyroid function is reevaluated. Many patients remain euthyroid after the thioamides are discontinued. For this 15% to 50% of patients treated, no further therapy may ever be required.

Thioamides are absorbed rapidly after oral administration and are concentrated in the thyroid. The drugs are also distributed to other tissues and cross the placenta to enter the fetus. Thioamides appear in the milk of nursing mothers, and they are metabolized and excreted in urine.

Two thioamides, methimazole and propylthiouracil, currently are used in the United States (Table 52-4). These drugs differ primarily in potency and in the incidence of toxic reactions. Propylthiouracil also inhibits the conversion of T_4 to T_3 in peripheral tissues.

Iodine

Iodine is the oldest of the antithyroid preparations currently in use. Although iodine is the required starting material for synthesis of thyroid hormones, high concentrations of iodine suppress continued uptake of iodine and synthesis of thyroid hormones in the thyroid gland. Suppression of hormone synthesis is by no means complete with iodine administration, and many patients return to the hyperthyroid state even with continued high doses. Iodine is seldom used today for long-term suppression of a hyperactive thyroid gland. The most common current use of iodine is to prepare a hyperthyroid patient for surgery. Iodine not only suppresses thyroid function but also reduces vascularization of the gland, thus reducing surgical risk. Iodine pretreatment is especially important for hyperthyroid patients who have received thioamide therapy because those drugs increase vas-

Table 52-4 Drugs Used to Treat Hyperthyroidism

Generic name	Trade name	Administration/dosage	Properties	Comments
THIOAMIDES				
Propylthiouracil (PTU)	Generic Propyl-Thyracil†	ORAL: *Adults*—50 to 300 mg daily in 3 doses. Initially 300 to 600 mg daily is given in 3 or 4 doses. FDA Pregnancy Category D. *Children over 10 years*—half the adult dose. *Children 6 to 10 years*—one-quarter the adult dose.	Inhibits thyroid hormone synthesis but not release. Inhibits conversion of T_4 to T_3 by peripheral tissues.	Used to lower thyroid hormone levels. Clinical improvement of hyperthyroid state is delayed. Agranulocytosis may occur in 1.4% of patients during first 2 months of therapy; skin rashes occur in roughly 3% of patients. Mild leukopenia occurs in 10% of patients.
Methimazole	Tapazole*	ORAL: *Adults*—5 to 30 mg daily in one or 2 doses. Initially 30 to 60 mg daily is given in 1 or 2 doses for severe hyperthyroidism. FDA Pregnancy Category D. *Children 6 to 10 years*—0.4 mg/kg body weight daily in 1 or 2 doses.	Inhibits thyroid hormone synthesis but not release.	Used to lower thyroid hormone levels. Clinical improvement of hyperthyroid state is delayed. Agranulocytosis, leukopenia, and skin rashes as for PTU may occur; more likely to cause vasculitis.
BETA-ADRENERGIC BLOCKER				
Propranolol hydrochloride	Inderal*	ORAL: *Adults*—40 to 240 mg daily in divided doses. INTRAVENOUS: *Adults*—5 mg or less administered at 1 mg/min or more slowly.	Controls symptoms of hyperthyroidism but does not lower T_3 and T_4 release from the thyroid.	Controls palpitations, tremor, sweating, proximal muscle weakness, and cardiac symptoms of hyperthyroidism by competitively blocking beta-adrenergic receptors. Bronchospasm may occur in asthmatic patients; may precipitate heart failure in patients with heart function maintained by sympathetic tone.
IODINE				
Potassium iodide	Pima Thyro-Block†	ORAL: *Adults*—250 mg 3 times daily as presurgical medication. INTRAVENOUS: *Adults*—250 to 500 mg daily for thyrotoxic crisis.	Produces short-term inhibition of thyroid hormone synthesis by direct action on the thyroid.	Used as presurgical medication to reduce the size of the thyroid gland. Used with thioamide and propranolol for hyperthyroid crisis. May produce iodism.
RADIOACTIVE IODINE				
¹³¹I as NaI		ORAL: *Adults*—4 to 10 mCi (148 to 370 megabecquerels) as a single dose for Graves' disease. For thyroid carcinoma, single doses of up to 150 mCi (5.5 gigabecquerels) may be used. Smaller doses are used for diagnostic purposes (see Table 52-2).	These radionuclides are concentrated in the thyroid and release radiation, which destroys thyroid tissue.	Used to destroy thyroid tissue without surgery for control of Graves' disease or thyroid carcinoma. Hypothyroidism ultimately develops in most patients.

*Available in Canada and United States.
†Available in Canada only.

Table 52-5   Miscellaneous Antithyroid Agents

Compound	Use or occurrence	Action on the thyroid
Aminosalicylates	Antituberculosis therapy	Hypothyroidism and goiter may occur with long-term use.
Aminotriazole	Herbicide (food contaminant)	Suppresses thyroid function.
Amiodarone	Antiarrhythmic	Complex action on thyroid metabolism. Thyroid hormone concentrations are commonly altered; up to 10% of patients suffer hypothyroidism; 1 to 3% of patients develop hyperthyroidism.
Dimercaprol	To treat heavy metal poisoning	May block iodine uptake into thyroid.
Goitrin	Found in plants of the mustard family and in turnips	Chronically high intake may cause goiter.
Iocetamic acid, Iodipamide, iohexol, Iopamidol, iopanoic acid, Iophendylate, iothalamate, Ioxaglate, ipodate	Radiopaque contrast agents used as aids in diagnostic imaging	These organic iodine compounds block iodine uptake by thyroid.
Lithium	Antimanic	Goiter and hypothyroidism may be induced, especially in the elderly.
Phenylbutazone	Nonsteroidal antiinflammatory	May block iodine uptake by thyroid.
Sulfonamides	Antibacterial agents	Goiter may rarely be produced.

cularization of the thyroid gland. In addition, iodine may be used as part of emergency therapy for hyperthyroid crisis. In this situation, iodine is administered intravenously after a thioamide has been given.

Radioactive iodine

Radioactive iodine is used to treat hyperthyroidism and in diagnosis. Therapy depends on the ability of the radioactive iodine to be concentrated in the thyroid gland, where it then destroys surrounding tissue by emitting low-energy radiation. Iodine doses are small. The use of radioactive iodine allows the thyroid to be functionally destroyed without resorting to surgery. Nearly all patients treated with radioactive iodine ultimately become hypothyroid and require treatment with thyroid hormones. The incidence of hypothyroidism is about 10% of treated patients during the first year after therapy and about 3%/year thereafter. Because of the likelihood of hypothyroidism, patients should be urged to return periodically for thyroid evaluation.

Other antithyroid compounds

Thyroid function can be influenced by many different chemicals, including some that are used in medicine. Table 52-5 summarizes the effects of some of these compounds.

DIETARY CONSIDERATION: CALCIUM

Calcium is important for growth and maintenance of healthy bones and for its role in nerve and muscle function and blood clotting. Some medical conditions contribute to hypocalcemia (low blood calcium levels) including hypoparathyroidism, kidney disease, massive cellulitis, burns, and peritonitis. An extremely low level of calcium can result in tetany, a medical emergency, which is treated with intravenous (IV) calcium. Milder cases of hypocalcemia may be treated in part by having the patient increase dietary intake of calcium. Good dietary sources of calcium include the following:

◆ blackstrap molasses
◆ calcium-fortified orange juice
◆ cheese
◆ clams
◆ dark-green leafy vegetables (e.g., kale and spinach)
◆ ice cream
◆ milk products
◆ oysters
◆ salmon
◆ sardines
◆ tofu, if made with calcium carbonate
◆ yogurt

PARAFOLLICULAR CELLS

The **parafollicular cells,** which constitute about 10% to 20% of total thyroid cells, synthesize the peptide hormone called *calcitonin.* In animals, calcitonin is thought to prevent blood calcium levels from exceeding the normal range after meals; its physiologic role in humans has not been resolved. Nevertheless, calcitonin does have demonstrable effects when administered exogenously. Calcitonin prevents the loss of calcium from bone, augments the urinary excretion of calcium and phosphate, and blocks the absorption of calcium from the small intestine (see box).

Calcitonin has been used therapeutically to treat Paget's disease, in which excessive bone resorption leads to thinned and fragile bones. One preparation often used clinically is a synthetic form of salmon calcitonin (Table 52-6), the most potent of the naturally occurring forms of the hormone. The dose is

Table 52-6 Agents That Alter Calcium Metabolism

Generic name	Trade name	Administration/dosage	Clinical use
Calcitonin-human	Cibacalcin	SUBCUTANEOUS: *Adults*—initially 0.5 mg daily, then reduced by lowering frequency of dosing or using 0.25 mg daily. FDA Pregnancy Category C.	To control Paget's disease (excessive bone remodeling).
Calcitonin-salmon	Calcimar*	INTRAMUSCULAR, SUBCUTANEOUS: *Adults*—100 units daily or higher if required. FDA Pregnancy Category C.	To lower hypercalcemia in hyperparathyroidism or vitamin D intoxication. To control Paget's disease.
Etidronate	Didronel*	ORAL: *Adults*—5 mg/kg daily for up to 6 months. FDA Pregnancy Category B. INTRAVENOUS: *Adults*—7.5 mg/kg daily for 3 days. FDA Pregnancy Category C.	To control Paget's disease. Hypercalcemia following cancer chemotherapy. Not effective for hypercalcemia caused by hyperparathyroidism.
Parathyroid hormone		INTRAVENOUS: *Adults*—200 units.	Diagnosis of pseudohypoparathyroidism. (Not currently available commercially.)
Vitamin D Calcifediol	Calderol	ORAL: *Adults*—50 μg daily or 100 μg on alternate days. FDA Pregnancy Category C. *Children*—20 to 50 μg daily.	Treatment of metabolic bone disease in patients on dialysis for chronic renal failure.
Calcitriol	Rocaltrol* Calcijex	ORAL: *Adults*—0.25 to 3 μg daily. INTRAVENOUS: *Adults*—0.5 μg three times weekly. FDA Pregnancy Category C.	Treatment of rickets and pseudohypoparathyroidism.
Dihydrotachysterol	Hytakerol*	ORAL: *Adults*—doses range from 0.1 to 2.5 mg daily, as needed to maintain normal serum calcium concentration. FDA Pregnancy Category C.	Treatment of hypoparathyroidism and postoperative tetany.
Ergocalciferol	Calciferol* Deltalin Drisdol* Ostoforte†	ORAL: *Adults*—400 units daily is normal replacement dose; therapy for rickets may require 50,000 to 500,000 units daily.	Treatment of rickets.

*Available in Canada and United States.
†Available in Canada only.

50 to 100 units given intramuscularly or subcutaneously. Some patients suffer nausea and vomiting, facial flushing, and occasional inflammatory reactions at the injection site. Since the hormone is a peptide and is administered in a gelatin solution, allergic reactions may occur. A synthetic form of human calcitonin is available (see Table 52-6). This form is less likely to cause allergic reactions than is salmon calcitonin.

Nursing Process Overview
PARATHYROID THERAPY
Assessment

Disorders involving only the parathyroid glands are unusual. Hypoparathyroidism is seen most often in patients who have had accidental removal or destruction of the parathyroid glands during thyroid surgery or other surgical procedures. Symptoms of hypoparathyroidism include paresthesia, muscle spasms, tetany, and convulsions. Hypoparathyroidism is seen most often with tumors of the parathyroid gland. Perform a total patient assessment, and monitor vital signs and serum calcium levels.

Nursing Diagnoses

Possible complication: hypercalcemia

Management

The plan of therapy is to return serum calcium levels to the normal range and to treat any underlying condition. Monitor vital signs, measure serum calcium levels, and check for progression or regression of any symptoms discovered during the initial assessment. If calcitonin is prescribed for outpatient use, instruct the patient in the correct procedure for subcutaneous drug administration.

Evaluation

Before discharge, verify that the patient can explain how and why to take the prescribed drugs, demonstrate any special administration techniques, and explain what symptoms should warrant notification of the physician. The patient should understand the need to wear a medical identification tag or bracelet.

PARATHYROID GLANDS
Actions of Parathyroid Hormone

The parathyroid glands synthesize parathyroid hormone, a peptide whose major function is to maintain blood calcium levels above the critical threshold required for body function. In many ways, parathyroid hormone acts opposite to calcitonin. For example,

parathyroid hormone increases reabsorption of calcium from bones, lowers renal excretion of calcium, and, along with vitamin D, increases calcium absorption from the intestine. The overall interaction of parathyroid hormone, calcitonin, and vitamin D allows the body to maintain blood calcium levels within a very narrow margin. Close control of calcium levels is required because very small changes in blood calcium levels can profoundly alter many cellular functions.

Hyperparathyroidism

Hyperparathyroidism (excess parathyroid hormone) usually arises from excess secretion of parathyroid hormone from a tumor. Many patients with this condition show decreases in bone calcification as a result of the action of parathyroid hormone. High amounts of calcium are excreted by these patients, and renal stones are common. No specific inhibitors of parathyroid release are available for clinical use; thus therapy consists primarily of surgery to remove the source of excess parathyroid hormone synthesis. Calcitonin may temporarily control hypercalcemia in hyperparathyroidism.

Hypercalcemia resulting from cancer chemotherapy may be controlled with etidronate, a synthetic analogue of inorganic pyrophosphate. Etidronate is not effective in hyperparathyroidism.

Hypoparathyroidism

Hypoparathyroidism (insufficient parathyroid hormone) usually results after thyroid or parathyroid surgery, but idiopathic (unknown cause) forms of the disease exist. Whatever the cause, hypoparathyroidism is associated with hypocalcemia. This electrolyte imbalance produces symptoms such as paresthesia, muscle spasms, tetany, and convulsions. In theory, parathyroid hormone could be used to raise blood calcium levels in conditions in which blood levels are abnormally low; however, administration of one of the forms of vitamin D with or without calcium is the preferred treatment.

Several forms of vitamin D are available for clinical use. Vitamin D_3, or cholecalciferol, is normally formed in the skin by irradiation of 7-dehydrocholesterol. Vitamin D_3 is therapeutically equivalent to vitamin D_2, or ergocalciferol. Both drugs are available in orally administered forms suitable for convenient, long-term therapy. Calcitriol (1,25-dihydroxycholecalciferol) is the most active vitamin D derivative and is the final active metabolite of the vitamin. Although very effective, this drug form is expensive. Since adequate treatment is possible for most conditions with other forms of the vitamin, calcitriol is reserved for those rare patients who respond only to this drug form.

In pseudohypoparathyroidism the kidney, bone, and intestine do not respond normally to parathyroid hormone. Parathyroid hormone is occasionally used to diagnose this condition. Some patients respond to calcitriol.

Pharmacology of Vitamin D

Vitamin D, a lipid-soluble substance, is adequately absorbed after oral administration. It is transported in blood by a specific alpha globulin. Depending on what form of the vitamin is administered, various biotransformations are possible. The liver converts vitamin D_3 to more active 25-hydroxyvitamin D_3. The kidney converts 25-hydroxyvitamin D_3 to calcitriol, the most active metabolite of the vitamin. Most vitamin D metabolites are excreted in bile. Excess or deficiency of vitamin D produces symptoms that are primarily those expected with high or low blood calcium concentrations.

NURSING IMPLICATIONS SUMMARY

Natural and Synthetic Thyroid Hormones

Drug administration

- The side effects of these drugs are essentially the same as the symptoms of hyperthyroidism; see Table 52-1
- Assess for headache, insomnia, nervousness, and tremor.
- Monitor blood pressure and pulse. If pulse is greater than 100 beats/minute in an adult, withhold the dose, and notify the physician.
- Monitor the ECG before starting therapy and at regular intervals.
- Monitor weight. Assess for edema, pallor, and fatigue.

INTRAVENOUS LEVOTHYROXINE

- Dilute with diluent provided. Administer at a rate of 0.1 mg or less over 1 min.
- Monitor thyroid function tests.

Patient and family education

- Review anticipated benefits and possible side effects of drug therapy.
- Tell patients that several weeks to months of therapy may be needed before full benefit is seen. Encourage patients to return for regular follow-up and blood tests.
- Take doses in the morning to avoid nighttime insomnia.
- Warn diabetic patients to monitor blood glucose levels carefully, since an adjustment in diet or insulin dose may be needed.
- Encourage patients to wear a medical identification tag or bracelet stating that thyroid medication is used regularly.
- Teach patients not to switch brands of medication without consulting the physician or the pharmacist.
- Instruct women to keep a record of menstrual periods, since menstrual irregularities may occur.

- Remind patients to inform all health-care providers of all drugs being used. Regular use of thyroid replacement hormones may contribute to interactions with other drugs.

Methimazole and Propylthiouracil

Drug administration

- Overdose would produce clinical hypothyroidism; see Table 52-1.
- Assess for tingling of fingers and toes. Monitor weight. Inspect patients for skin changes or hair loss.
- Monitor complete blood count (CBC) and differential and thyroid and liver function tests.

Patient and family education

- Review anticipated benefits and possible side effects of drug therapy. Side effects may not appear for days to weeks after beginning therapy; remind patients to report any new side effects.
- Instruct patients to report signs of agranulocytosis such as fever, chills, sore throat, and unexplained bleeding or bruising.
- Take doses with meals or a snack to lessen gastric irritation.
- Patients may take doses without meals, but however doses are taken, they should be taken the same way each time, either always with meals or always on an empty stomach.
- Encourage patients to return as instructed for follow-up.
- Remind patients to inform all health-care providers of all drugs being used.
- If more than one dose/day is prescribed, it is best to space doses evenly throughout the day. Work with the patient to develop a satisfactory dosing schedule.

Continued.

NURSING IMPLICATIONS SUMMARY—cont'd

Iodine

Drug administration and patient and family education

- Dilute oral iodine solution well in juice, milk, or beverage choice. The solutions may stain teeth; take with a straw.
- Signs of iodism (excessive iodine) include metallic taste in the mouth, sneezing, swollen and tender thyroid gland, vomiting, and bloody diarrhea. Concomitant excessive use of over-the-counter (OTC) preparations containing iodine (e.g., asthma or cough preparations) may contribute to iodism.
- Consult the manufacturer's literature for information about IV iodine.

Radioactive Iodine

Drug administration and patient and family education

- The radiation dose of radioactive iodine is not high, but those preparing or administering the preparation should be careful to avoid spilling the mixture on themselves or on countertops. Wear rubber gloves. Follow agency protocol for handling radioactive substances.
- Side effects are rare but include soreness over the thyroid gland and, in rare cases, difficulty in swallowing and breathing because of gland enlargement. Eventually, many patients who take radioactive iodine will become hypothyroid.

Calcitonin

Drug administration

- Monitor weight. If vomiting or diarrhea occurs, monitor intake and output.
- Warn patients that flushing may occur.
- Before the first dose of calcitonin-salmon, a test dose may be ordered to check for allergic response. Consult manufacturer's literature. Have drugs, equipment, and personnel available to treat acute allergic reactions in settings where calcitonin-salmon is used.
- Assess for hypercalcemia or hypocalcemia (see Table 17-1).
- Monitor serum electrolyte levels.

Patient and family education

- Review anticipated benefits and possible side effects of drug therapy.

- Encourage patients to return for regular follow-up visits. For home administration, teach patient to administer the drug subcutaneously. Review injection technique, and have patients give a return demonstration.
- Store calcitonin-salmon in the refrigerator. Store calcitonin-human at a temperature below 77°F, but do not refrigerate.
- Refer to patient to a community-based nursing care agency as needed.
- Tell patients that taking ordered doses in the evening may minimize flushing.
- Encourage patients on long-term therapy to wear a medical identification tag or bracelet indicating that calcitonin is being taken regularly.
- A low-calcium diet may be prescribed. Review Dietary Consideration: Calcium on p. 768 for food items which should be used in limited amounts when trying to restrict calcium intake. Refer to a dietitian as needed.

Etidronate

Drug administration

- Assess for bone pain, which may occur in patients with Paget's disease.
- Monitor serum electrolyte levels. Assess for signs of hypocalcemia (see Table 17-1).
- Monitor serum creatinine and blood urea nitrogen (BUN) levels.
- For IV etidronate, dilute in 250 ml or more of normal saline. Infuse 250 ml over at least 2 hr.

Patient and family education

- Review anticipated benefits and possible side effects of drug therapy.
- Provide emotional support. Weeks to months of therapy may be required to obtain maximum drug effect. Remind patients not to discontinue therapy without consulting the physician.
- Instruct patients to take doses with black coffee, tea, fruit juice, or water, on an empty stomach, at least 2 hr before or after food.
- Notify patients not to take doses within 2 hr of ingesting milk or milk products, antacids, mineral supplements, or medicines high in calcium, magnesium, iron, or alumninum.
- Take a dietary history. Patients should continue following a well-balanced diet with adequate but not excessive amounts of calcium and vitamin D.

Vitamin D Preparations

Drug administration

- The side effects are essentially those of hypercalcemia and are a result of overdosage. They include ataxia, fatigue, irritability, seizures, somnolence, tinnitus, hypertension, GI distress or constipation, and hypotonia in infants. Other symptoms of overdose include headache, increased thirst, metallic taste in the mouth, nausea or vomiting, and fatigue.
- Assess for CNS effects. Ongoing assessment is important, since some symptoms such as fatigue may be difficult to distinguish from those accompanying renal failure or chronic disease.
- Monitor blood pressure and pulse. Monitor intake and output.
- Monitor serum calcium levels and urinalysis.

Patient and family education

- Review anticipated benefits and possible side effects of drug therapy. Encourage patients to notify the physician if any new side effects occur.
- Remind patients not to increase or decrease dose without consulting the physician.
- Warn patients to avoid OTC preparations that contain calcium, phosphorus, or vitamin D unless approved by the physician.
- Warn patients to avoid driving or operating hazardous equipment if fatigue, somnolence, vertigo, or weakness occurs.
- Remind patients to inform all health-care providers of all drugs being used. Avoid using any medications not previously approved by the physician.
- Avoid antacids containing magnesium.
- Avoid excessive amounts of substances containing vitamin D (see Dietary Consideration: Vitamins on p. 275).

CHAPTER REVIEW

◆ KEY TERMS

◆ REVIEW QUESTIONS

1. What is the function of the follicular cells of the thyroid gland?
2. What hormones are produced by the follicular cells of the thyroid gland?
3. What is the function of thyroid-stimulating hormone (TSH), and where is it produced?
4. What are the steps in thyroid hormone synthesis?
5. How much T_3 and T_4 is stored in the thyroid gland?
6. What is the function of thyroglobulin?
7. How are the thyroid hormones transported in the bloodstream?
8. How are the thyroid hormones eliminated?
9. Which of the thyroid hormones is found most abundantly in target cells?
10. What are the characteristic signs of hypothyroidism? How should you assess for these?
11. In primary hypothyroidism, how do the blood concentrations of TSH and thyroid hormones differ from normal?
12. What is the difference between secondary hypothyroidism and tertiary hypothyroidism?
13. What is the treatment for all forms of hypothyroidism?
14. Which of the available preparations of thyroid hormones is the most potent?
15. How do T_3 and T_4 differ in onset and duration of action?
16. What side effects may occur with replacement therapy of thyroid hormones? How should you assess for these?

17. Which thyroid hormone is available as an injectable preparation?
18. Why would the administration of T_3 by nasogastric tube sometimes be preferred over injection of T_4 in the treatment of myxedema coma?
19. How does Graves' disease differ from subacute thyroiditis?
20. What general classes of drugs are used to treat hyperthyroidism?
21. To what class of drugs does propranolol belong, and why is it useful in treating hyperthyroidism?
22. What is the mechanism of action of the thioamides?
23. How are the thioamides distributed in the body?
24. How may radioactive iodine be used in the treatment of hyperthyroidism?
25. What is the function of the parafollicular cells of the thyroid?
26. What are the metabolic effects of calcitonin?
27. What forms of calcitonin are used to treat Paget's disease? How do they differ?
28. How may etidronate be used clinically?
29. What is the function of the parathyroid glands?
30. What are the metabolic effects of parathyroid hormone?
31. What are the symptoms of hypoparathyroidism? How should you assess for these?
32. How is hypoparathyroidism treated?
33. Which of the metabolites of vitamin D is the most active?
34. What is the metabolic function of vitamin D?
35. What is the fate of vitamin D in the body?

SUGGESTED READING

Calloway C: When the problem involves magnesium, calcium or phosphate, *RN* 50(5):30, 1987.

Griffiths EC: Clinical applications of thyrotrophin-releasing hormone, *Clin Sci* 73(5):449, 1987.

Lockhart JS, Griffin CW: Action stat! Tetany, *Nurs 88* 18(8):33, 1988.

Mahon SM: Symptoms as clues to calcium levels, *Am J Nurs* 87(3):354, 1987.

McMillan JY: Preventing myxedema coma in the hypothyroid patient, *DCCN* 7(3):136, 1988.

O'Neil JR: Action stat! Thyroid crisis, *Nursing 87* 17(11):33, 1987.

Oppenheimer JH and others: Advances in our understanding of thyroid hormone action at the cellular level, *Endocr Rev* 8(3):288, 1987.

Samuels HH and others: Regulation of gene expression by thyroid hormone, *J Clin Invest* 81(4):957, 1988.

Sarsany SL: Thyroid storm, *RN* 51(7):46, 1988.

Waters HF, Stuckey PA: Oncology alert for the home care nurse: hypercalcemia, *Home Healthc Nurse* 6(1):32, 1988.

Yeaomans AC: Assessment and management of hypothyroidism, *Nurse Pract* 15(11):8, 1990.

CHAPTER 53

Drugs Acting on the Female Reproductive System

LEARNING OBJECTIVES

After studying this chapter, you should be able to do the following:

- Describe the clinical utility of estrogens, progestins, and combinations of these agents.
- Discuss the drugs that can increase female fertility.
- Compare the actions and uses of the three classes of oxytocic drugs.
- Develop a nursing care plan for a patient receiving a drug discussed in this chapter.

CHAPTER OVERVIEW

◆ Female reproductive function depends on a complex, intricately regulated interaction of endocrine tissues. The negative feedback loop regulating the menstrual cycle involves the hypothalamus, the anterohypophysis, and the ovaries (see Chapter 50). Actions of the natural female hormones, clinical uses of synthetic and natural drugs affecting the female reproductive system, endocrine control of pregnancy, and drugs used during childbirth and the postpartum period are discussed in this chapter.

Nursing Process Overview

DRUGS AFFECTING THE FEMALE REPRODUCTIVE SYSTEM

Assessment

Drugs acting on the female reproductive system provide replacement therapy, cause or inhibit ovulation and conception, aid in pregnancy or labor, and treat hormonally sensitive tumors. Obtain a complete patient assessment, focusing on the problem being addressed by the drug. Monitor the temperature, pulse, respiration, blood pressure, weight, description of the menstrual cycle, assessment of breasts (male and female), and condition of skin. In the pregnant female, take a history of previous pregnancies and deliveries, and assess the fetus (e.g., fetal heart tones and position).

Nursing Diagnoses

Possible complication: vascular disorders
Self-concept disturbance: acne and weight gain related to drug therapy

Management

Because of controversies surrounding the use of some of these drugs, the patient should be fully informed of possible side effects and benefits before therapy is

started. Continue to monitor the pulse, blood pressure, and weight. Explain patient activities needed in detail to help ensure success. For example, activities such as using alternative birth control measures during the first month of birth control pill therapy, keeping temperature charts to monitor possible ovulation, and saving urine specimens to measure hormone or drug excretion need thorough explanations. With oxytocics, monitor the mother and fetus closely, and use an intravenous (IV) infusion monitoring device. Monitor calcium levels in the patient being treated for cancer.

Evaluation

Before discharge, verify that the patient can explain why and how to take the drug, possible side effects that might occur, which side effects require immediate medical attention, and the risks associated with therapy.

HORMONES INVOLVED IN FEMALE REPRODUCTION

Sources of Hormones

The major hormones involved in developing and maintaining female reproductive capacity include examples of all the chemical classes of hormones. The hypothalamus supplies gonadotropin-releasing hormone (GnRH), a peptide that acts directly on the anterohypophysis, stimulating synthesis and release of follicle-stimulating hormone (FSH) and luteinizing hormone (LH). In addition, the central nervous system (CNS) neurotransmitter dopamine is the inhibitory factor that regulates the release of prolactin from the anterohypophysis. FSH, LH, and prolactin are the major gonadotropins. These hormones each have a different primary target tissue. FSH stimulates the ovarian cells, which form the follicle and nurture the maturing ovum. Under the influence of FSH, these cells synthesize the potent steroid estrogen known as *estradiol*. LH acts primarily on the mature follicle to cause release of the ovum. Prolactin stimulates breast tissue to promote milk production. Prolactin also may affect the ovary, but details of how the hormone acts in this tissue are lacking.

The major steroid hormones regulating female reproduction are estrogens and progestins. **Estrogens** are compounds that stimulate female reproductive tissues; **progestins** are compounds that specifically stimulate the uterine lining. Estrogens are produced primarily in the FSH-stimulated cells of the ovarian follicle. Progesterone, the most important progestin, is synthesized in the cells remaining in the follicle after the expulsion of the ovum. This tissue is called the corpus luteum.

All the steroids produced in the ovary are derived from cholesterol. Progestins are formed first and are the precursors of androgens. Androgens, the steroid hormones capable of producing masculinization, are primarily precursors of estrogen synthesis in females. Androstenedione is the androgen precursor of estrone, a circulating estrogen formed mostly in peripheral tissues and not in the ovary. Estradiol, the most abundant circulating estrogen, is formed in the ovary.

Hormones Affecting Development of the Female Reproductive System

At birth the ovary is already in an advanced stage of development and contains between 2 and 4 million oocytes, cells that will form ova. The primordial follicles containing oocytes are not quiescent during the prepubertal years but undergo a process called *atresia* in which oocytes are destroyed and follicles are resorbed. At **menarche,** when menstrual cycles begin during puberty, an estimated 400,000 oocytes remain. Even after ovulation is initiated, atresia continues and is responsible for the destruction of more than 99% of the follicles present in the ovary.

As puberty begins the immature ovaries are stimulated by increasing amounts of pituitary gonadotropins. As a result, estrogen synthesis is promoted, and estrogen levels in the blood rise. The primary function of estrogens during early puberty is to promote

development of the reproductive system. The uterus and fallopian tubes enlarge to adult proportions. The vagina enlarges, and the vaginal epithelium thickens and strengthens. In the breasts, estrogen promotes proliferation of stromal tissue, as well as ductile tissue, which is responsible for the production of milk needed by the suckling infant.

The secondary sexual characteristics also depend on estrogens. These hormones promote increased deposition of fat, especially in the breasts and hips. Without estrogens, the typical contours of the female body do not develop.

Estrogens are also involved in regulating the start and the stop of the growth spurt that is characteristic of puberty. Along with other hormones, estrogen causes retention of calcium and phosphorus and thereby promotes bone growth. Estrogens also induce closure of the epiphyses. When this closure occurs, no further increase in height occurs.

Hormones Affecting Ovulation

Ovulation requires proper functioning of the hypothalamus, anterohypophysis, and ovaries in the negative feedback loop described in Chapter 50. FSH and LH are required to act on the developing follicle before a mature ovum may be released to begin its journey down the fallopian tube to the uterus. Estrogen synthesis is required for its action on the follicle and for its ability to trigger the midcycle surge of LH from the anterohypophysis.

Hormones Affecting Endometrial Function

The uterus is composed of smooth muscle (myometrium) and glandular epithelium (endometrium). The endometrium, which nourishes and supports the ovum during development, is controlled primarily by estrogens and progestins. Estrogens promote proliferation of the endometrium during the first half of the menstrual cycle before ovulation occurs. Progesterone, which is formed in the corpus luteum of the ovary during the second half of the menstrual cycle, acts on the endometrium and the myometrium. Progesterone reduces myometrial activity, preventing muscular contractions, and promotes development of the secretory capacity of endometrium. Actions on these two tissues aid in establishing the environment in which the fertilized ovum may implant successfully and begin development. Once implantation of the ovum has occurred, progesterone continues to alter the endometrium, ultimately changing the tissue so that a second implantation becomes impossible.

Hormones in Pregnancy

Pregnancy requires that a mature ovum be released from the ovary at the appropriate time, that the ovum be fertilized successfully within about 2 days of its release, and that the ovum be able to implant within the endometrium and to draw nourishment to support the early stages of development. The most important hormone during these first days and weeks of pregnancy is progesterone. Without adequate progesterone, the endometrium is sloughed and the fertilized ovum is lost. Luteal progesterone is produced for about the first 10 weeks of pregnancy. Control of progesterone synthesis is exercised by cells of the fetus, which develop into the placenta. A few days after implantation of the ovum in the endometrium, these fetal cells begin to produce a hormone called *human chorionic gonadotropin (HCG),* which takes over control of the corpus luteum and maintains its production of progesterone. By the fifth week of pregnancy the placenta has developed to where it begins to synthesize progesterone directly. Placental progesterone production increases during the remainder of the pregnancy, whereas progesterone production in the corpus luteum virtually disappears.

The continuing high progesterone levels during pregnancy are thought to aid in maintaining the pregnancy by suppressing myometrial contractions. At the end of pregnancy, progesterone levels begin to decrease, allowing the uterus to begin to produce **prostaglandins.** Prostaglandins, which are hormones formed from fatty acids within cell membranes, are capable of stimulating powerful uterine contractions. Although the exact role of prostaglandins in normal childbirth is not yet established, contractions produced by prostaglandins are sufficiently strong to bring about the expulsion of the fetus from the uterus.

Oxytocin, a hormone produced by the neurohypophysis, is also capable of inducing uterine contractions. The uterus increases its sensitivity to oxytocin at term and during the puerperium (period immediately after birth). Oxytocin also acts on breast tissue, where it stimulates the myoepithelium of the breast and promotes milk letdown. Suckling by the infant sets off a reflex action in which oxytocin release is stimulated. The CNS controls this process; the sight of the infant is sufficient in some women to induce oxytocin release and milk letdown. Oxytocin action is responsible for the improved uterine muscle tone in nursing mothers and for the more rapid return of the uterus to the pregravid size in these women.

AGENTS AFFECTING FEMALE SEXUAL FUNCTION

Many conditions of the female reproductive tract for which women seek medical aid may be treated successfully by replacement therapy. The most common conditions are those that arise as a result of estrogen deficiency. A lack of estrogen during puberty prevents normal growth and sexual development; menarche

may not occur. This endocrine malfunction is one of several abnormalities that may be responsible for amenorrhea (no menstrual cycles). After menopause the gradual decline in estrogen levels may cause symptoms including vasomotor symptoms (hot flashes and sweating), osteoporosis (bone loss), and atrophy of vaginal and urethral tissue.

Other medical problems of the female reproductive system cannot be ascribed definitely to a specific hormone deficiency. Nevertheless, many of these conditions respond to hormones used for some pharmacologic action rather than as replacement therapy. The rationale for therapy for these conditions is listed in Table 53-1.

Estrogen doses used in the clinical setting vary depending on the condition being treated. When used in replacement therapy, estrogen doses tend to be low. Higher doses treat conditions such as advanced breast cancer. A drug handbook or the pharmacist should be consulted for the dose of a specific preparation in a specific condition.

Estrogens

Absorption and excretion. Estrogens of various types are available in the United States (Table 53-2). The two naturally occurring steroid estrogens used in the clinical setting are estradiol and estrone. As steroids, these compounds are not water soluble, but they are soluble in oil. With estradiol, slower absorption and longer duration of action may be achieved by using the cypionate or the valerate ester of the natural steroid. Estradiol is absorbed orally if the drug crystals are reduced to particles 1 to 3 μm in diameter.

Estrone is not well absorbed orally in its natural form but may be used orally if it is converted to the piperazine sulfate. Estrone is also the major component of various estrogen mixtures described as *esterified or conjugated estrogens.* These mixtures, which are isolated from sources such as urine of pregnant mares, are relatively cheap and are effective for many purposes, and all can be taken orally, making them a convenient drug form for many patients.

Synthetic estrogens such as ethinyl estradiol are also available. Ethinyl estradiol is more potent than naturally occurring estrogens. This drug used orally has a relatively short duration of action but persists in the body longer than any of the natural estrogens.

Nonsteroidal estrogens are all oral agents. The best known of these drugs is diethylstilbestrol (DES). DES, which was discovered in 1938, was once widely used to prevent spontaneous abortions. The children who were in utero at the time of DES treatment may have suffered from the drug effects. As adults, female offspring have an increased incidence of vaginal adenosis and adenocarcinoma; male offspring may be more prone to develop epididymal cysts. DES is still

Table 53-1 Pharmacologic Therapy of Dysfunctions of the Female Reproductive System

Clinical condition	Treatment	Rationale
Hypogonadism	Cyclic estrogen-progestin or menotropins	Estrogens are required to promote secondary sex characteristics. Other hormonal support may be required for full fertility.
Amenorrhea	Bromocriptine or gonadorelin	Drugs are effective only for specific types of conditions producing amenorrhea.
Menopause		
Vasomotor symptoms	Estrogens	Hot flashes and sweating are relieved by estrogens.
Osteoporosis	Estrogens	Loss of calcium may be halted temporarily but not reversed.
Atrophy of vaginal and urethral tissue	Estrogens	Estrogen support is needed to maintain tissue tone.
Dysfunctional uterine bleeding	Estrogen and progestin	Combination stops bleeding; drug withdrawal induces endometrial sloughing.
Luteal phase defect (infertility)	Progestins	Infertility resulting from inadequate synthesis of progesterone from the corpus luteum may be treated by progestin early in pregnancy.
Postpartum breast engorgement	Bromocriptine	Blocks prolactin synthesis, thus removing a major stimulus for milk formation.
Metastatic breast carcinoma	Estrogens, androgens, or progestins	Tumors show differing sensitivities to these hormones.
Metastatic endometrial carcinoma	Progestins	Natural suppressive effect of progestins on the endometrium is retained in some of these tumors.
Galactorrhea	Bromocriptine	Drug suppresses prolactin release, thereby preventing the excessive stimulation of breast secretory tissue.
Dysmenorrhea	Oral contraceptives or prostaglandin inhibitors	Suppression of ovulation gives relief to many but not all patients. Drugs such as ibuprofen, indomethacin, mefenamic acid, naproxen, and ketoprofen relieve symptoms by preventing excessive production of prostaglandins.
Pelvic endometriosis	Estrogen and progestin Danazol	Suppresses proliferation of endometrial tissue. Inhibits gonadotropins, thus preventing proliferation of endometrial tissue.
Anovulation (infertility)	Bromocriptine, clomiphene citrate, menotropins, HCG, gonadorelin, or urofollitropin	Ovulatory failure may be corrected by use of agents that promote gonadotropin release (clomiphene) or supply them directly (menotropins). HCG acts as LH to trigger release of the ovum.
Premenstrual tension	Ergotamine, diuretics, or antianxiety agents	Therapy is empiric and is often ineffective.

Table 53-2   Estrogens

Generic name	Trade name	Chemical form	Administration‡
Chlorotrianisene	TACE*	Nonsteroid	Capsules for oral use, primarily for prostatic carcinoma
Dienestrol	Dienestrol*	Nonsteroid	Vaginal cream
Diethylstibestrol (DES)	Stilphostrol Honvol†	Nonsteroid di-phosphate	Tablets for oral use or solution for injection; used primarily as anti-neoplastic agent
Estradiol	Estrace*	—	Tablets for oral use; cream for vaginal application
	Estraderm	—	Transdermal system
	Depo-Estradiol Cypionate Depogen DuraEstrin	Cypionate	Oil (cottonseed, with chlorobu-tanol as preservative) solution for IM injection
	Delestrogen* Femogex†	Valerate	Oil (sesame or castor) solution for IM injection
Estrogens, conjugated	Premarin* Progens	Sulfate esters	Tablets for oral use, solution for injection, or vaginal cream
Estrogens, esterified	Estratab Menest	Sulfate ester, pri-marily estrone	Tablets for oral use
Estrone	Theelin Unigen	—	Aqueous suspension in parabens and benzyl alcohol for IM injec-tion
	Oestrilin†		Intravaginal cream and supposito-ries
Estropipate (piperazine estrone sulfate)	Ogen*	Estrone pipera-zine sulfate	Tablets for oral use or vaginal cream
Ethinyl estradiol	Estinyl*	—	Tablets for oral use
Quinestrol	Estrovis	—	Tablets for oral use

*Available in Canada and United States.
†Available in Canada only.
‡All estrogens are considered FDA Pregnancy Category X.

available for clinical use and has been used as estrogen replacement therapy or for any other use for which estrogens are approved.

Natural estrogens do not persist long in the body because they are rapidly metabolized by the liver and excreted by the kidney. Ethinyl estradiol is less rapidly metabolized and is therefore longer acting than nat-ural estrogens. Nonsteroidal estrogens are not me-tabolized rapidly and also persist longer than natural ones.

Toxicity. Side effects of estrogens include over-reactions of certain reproductive tissues to the hor-mones. Breast tenderness is reported by many women receiving estrogens. Estrogens stimulate the endo-metrium to proliferate, and some evidence suggests that estrogens may increase the risk of endometrial cancer. No firm evidence shows that estrogens in-crease the risk of breast cancer.

Estrogens are frequently associated with acute ad-verse reactions such as nausea and vomiting, anorexia, and mild diarrhea. Malaise, depression, or excessive irritability are also related to estrogen therapy in some women. Estrogens promote salt and water retention and may therefore produce edema in some patients. Atherosclerosis is a definite risk for patients receiving estrogens, especially if they have other high-risk fac-

Table 53-3 Estrogens in Fixed Combinations with Androgens

Estrogens	Trade name	Androgens	Administration
Conjugated estrogens	Premarin with methyltestos-terone*	Methyltestosterone	Tablets for oral use
Diethylstilbestrol (DES)	Tylosterone	Methyltestosterone	Tablets for oral use
Esterified estrogens	Estratest	Methyltestosterone	Tablets for oral use
Estradiol benzoate Estradiol dienanthate	Climacteron†	Testosterone enanthate	For deep IM injection
Estradiol cypionate	Depo-Testadiol Duratestrin	Testosterone cypionate	Oil solution for IM injection
Estradiol valerate	Deladumone Estrand†	Testosterone enanthate	Oil solution for IM injection
Ethinyl estradiol	Halodrin	Fluoxymesterone	Tablets for oral use

For other fixed combinations of estrogens and progestins, see Table 53-6.
*Available in Canada and United States.
†Available in Canada only.

tors such as smoking. Hypertension has been associated with estrogen use.

Uses. Estrogens may be used as replacement therapy or in pharmacologic doses for a variety of dysfunctions of the female reproductive tract.

Estrogens are also available in fixed combinations with androgens for use in controlling vasomotor symptoms in menopause (Table 53-3). To a certain degree, these combinations violate pharmacologic principles. The main objection to fixed combinations is that dosage adjustment for best effectiveness of both drugs becomes impossible in some patients. For example, some women may be extremely sensitive to the androgen in a fixed estrogen-androgen combination. To reduce the androgen level, it would be necessary to administer less of the medication, but this would also reduce the estrogen dose. The overall result may be that the effectiveness of one of the drugs is lost or diminished.

The most important estrogen combinations are those with progestins, which are discussed in the section on oral contraceptive drugs. These combinations are available with so many different ratios of estrogen to progestin that adjustment for individual patient needs is possible.

Progestins

Absorption and excretion. Progestins available for medical use include the natural steroid hormone progesterone and synthetic derivatives of that compound (Table 53-4). Although progesterone is not useful orally, many derivatives are administered conveniently and effectively by that route. Injections of progesterone are painful and may produce local inflammation. Progesterone and other progestins are rapidly metabolized by the liver and are eliminated in urine.

Toxicity. Adverse reactions to progestins may involve several organ systems other than reproductive organs. Some of these reactions are similar to those seen with estrogens including edema, breast tenderness and swelling, gastrointestinal (GI) disturbances, depression, and weight change. Other reactions include changes in menstrual blood flow, midcycle spotting or breakthrough bleeding, cholestatic jaundice, and rashes. Many progestins have some androgenic activity and may cause masculinization of female fetuses. Patients with a history of thromboembolic disorders or thrombophlebitis should not be treated with progestins.

Uses. Progestins are used clinically for their effects on the endometrium. High doses suppress bleeding of the endometrium, and withdrawal induces sloughing of the tissue. Lower doses of progestins induce changes in the endometrium and cervical mucus that prevent pregnancy. This use of progestins is discussed in the section on contraceptive agents.

AGENTS THAT RESTORE FERTILITY

Loss of fertility in a female may occur for many reasons. Therapy depends in part on evaluating the cause of infertility. In some females the hypophysis and the

Table 53-4　Progestins Used Clinically (see Table 53-6)

Generic/trade name	Chemical form	Administration
Hydroxyprogesterone (Duralutin and Gesterol L.A.)	Caproate	Oil solution for IM injection; action persists 9 to 17 days. FDA Pregnancy Category D.
Medroxyprogesterone (Depo-Provera*)	Acetate	Aqueous suspension for IM injection.
(Provera*)	Acetate	Tablets for oral use.
Megestrol (Megace*)	Acetate	Tablets for oral use in treating endometrial carcinoma.
Norethindrone (Micronor and Norlutin)	—	Tablets for oral use. FDA Pregnancy Category X.
(Norlutate)	Acetate	Tablets for oral use. FDA Pregnancy Category X.
Progesterone (Femotrone)	—	Aqueous suspension or oil solution for IM injection. FDA Pregnancy Category D.

*Available in Canada and United States.
†Available in Canada only.

Table 53-5　Fertility Agents

Generic name	Trade	Classification	Mechanism of action	Administration/dosage
Bromocriptine mesylate	Parlodel*	Inhibitor of prolactin release	Lowers high levels of prolactin, which interfere with pituitary or ovarian function.	ORAL: 1.25 to 2.5 mg once daily initially, then 2.5 mg 2 or 3 times daily.
Clomiphene citrate	Clomid* Serophene	Nonsteroid	Stimulates ovulation, probably by hypothalamic mechanisms.	ORAL: 50 mg daily on days 5 through 10 of the menstrual cycle.
Gonadorelin	Factrel*	Synthetic GnRH	Stimulates release of LH and FSH from the anterohypophysis.	INTRAVENOUS, SUBCUTANEOUS: 100 μg once for diagnosis or repeated for infertility. FDA Pregnancy Category B.
Gonadotropin chorionic	Follutein Pregnyl	Placental hormone related to LH	Stimulates ovulation by an action resembling that of LH.	INTRAMUSCULAR: 5000 to 10,000 units once in an appropriately primed patient. FDA Pregnancy Category C.
Menotropins	Pergonal*	Human urinary menopausal gonadotropins	FSH and LH in the preparation stimulate the ovaries.	INTRAMUSCULAR: 75 units each of FSH and LH daily for 9 to 12 days.
Urofollitropin	Metrodin*	Human urinary menopausal FSH	FSH stimulates the ovaries.	INTRAMUSCULAR: 150 units daily. FDA Pregnancy Category X.

*Available in Canada and United States.

ovary seem normal, but the proper stimulus to activate follicular development is not transmitted. For these females, clomiphene citrate may be effective (Table 53-5). This drug seems to activate the hypophysis by hypothalamic mechanisms, and ovarian stimulation is thus achieved. Stimulation of several follicles may be induced by clomiphene, and multiple births have occurred.

In females whose hypophysis cannot supply sufficient gonadotropins to properly stimulate the ovary, infertility also may occur. For these women, menotropins may be prescribed. This mixture of compounds extracted from urine of postmenopausal females contains FSH and LH in approximately equal amounts. When LH action alone is required, HCG may be prescribed. HCG is chemically related to LH and possesses many of the same physiologic actions, including the ability to stimulate ovulation.

Bromocriptine mesylate is a chemical relative of the ergot alkaloids, which are used as oxytocic agents. Bromocriptine is clinically useful because it can inhibit prolactin secretion. Bromocriptine is approved in the United States to control **galactorrhea** (spontaneous milk production) caused by excessive prolactin secretion, usually from functional tumors. **Amenorrhea** (no menstrual cycles) and infertility also are produced when prolactin secretion is excessive. Bromocriptine suppression of prolactin secretion reverses these symptoms, and fertility becomes possible.

CONTRACEPTIVE AGENTS
Oral Contraceptives

Reversible sterility induced by pharmacologic agents has been possible since the late 1950s, when the oral contraceptive agents became available. These agents contain a combination of estrogen and a progestin or a progestin alone (Table 53-6). The effectiveness of oral contraceptives is very high. Most reports give estimates of less than 1 failure/200 woman years of use for the combined estrogen-progestin agents. This pregnancy rate is in contrast to rates of 1 failure/25 to 50 woman years for mechanical devices such as intrauterine devices (IUDs), diaphragms, and condoms. The first contraceptive agents contained relatively high amounts of estrogens, but the agents available today have lower estrogen content. These lower estrogen combinations are usually as effective as the older agents and may be associated with a lower incidence of side effects (Table 53-7).

Estrogen-progestin combinations suppress ovulation. In addition, these drugs induce changes in the cervical mucus, which makes it difficult for sperm to enter the uterus. Changes also occur in the endometrium that make implantation difficult even if fertilization occurs. The preparations containing progestins alone alter the cervical mucus and the endometrium as the combination products do, but they do not always suppress ovulation. The effectiveness of agents containing only progestins is less than that of the combined preparations.

To achieve contraception and to simulate the normal menstrual cycle, the oral contraceptives usually are taken for 21 consecutive days. The increased estrogen and progestin levels produced suppress the hypothalamus and the hypophysis so that no LH is released at the time when ovulation would normally occur. This is the mechanism by which ovulation is suppressed. During the 7 days when hormones are not administered, the endometrium involutes and sloughs off, primarily as a result of loss of progestin activity. This withdrawal period prevents excessive proliferation of the endometrium.

The progestins in oral contraceptives are synthetic derivatives of natural compounds. Progesterone, a natural progestin, is used in an IUD. This device (Progestasert) is not to be confused with the more common IUDs that contain no hormonal agents. The progesterone-releasing IUD was developed to administer the fertility-controlling drug directly to the target tissue. The very small amounts of progesterone released are retained within the reproductive tract rather than being systemically absorbed. The effectiveness of this device depends on the purely mechanical effects of the IUD and on the pharmacologic effects of progesterone.

Toxicity. Side effects produced by oral contraceptives may come from the estrogen or the progestin component. Side effects caused by estrogens may include nausea, bloating, breast fullness, edema, hypertension, and cervical discharge. Patients who report these symptoms may be tried on a preparation with low estrogen such as Loestrin 1/20 or Lo/Ovral. Side effects associated with progestins include hair loss, hirsutism, oily scalp, acne, increased appetite and weight gain, tiredness and depression, breast regression, and reduced menstrual blood flow. All oral contraceptives fall into FDA Pregnancy Category X.

Oral contraceptives are among the most widely used drugs today. Throughout the world, 50 million or more females rely on these agents for prevention of pregnancy. Oral contraceptives are highly effective, but questions about the safety of these agents have been raised. In particular the incidence of unexpected serious or fatal medical conditions has been studied in the relatively healthy females who receive oral contraceptives. Risk of certain serious medical conditions is now shown to be increased in oral contraceptive users when they are compared with similar females

Table 53-6 Oral Contraceptives

Progestin	Estrogen	Progestin : estrogen ratio	Trade name
Ethynodiol diacetate	Ethinyl estradiol	1.0 mg : 50 μg 1.0 mg : 35 μg	Demulen 1/50* Demulen 1/35
Levonorgestrel	Ethinyl estradiol	0.15 mg : 30 μg 0.05 mg : 30 μg (6 tablets), and 0.075 mg : 40 μg (5 tablets), and 0.125 mg : 30 μg (10 tablets)	Nordette and Levien Triphasil† and Tri-Levlen†
Norethindrone	None	0.35 mg	Micronor*, Norlutin, and Nor-QD
Norethindrone acetate	Ethinyl estradiol	2.5 mg : 50 μg 1.5 mg : 30 μg 1.0 mg : 50 μg 1.0 mg : 20 μg	Norlestrin 2.5/50* Loestrin 1.5/30* Norlestrin 1/50* Loestrin 1/20
Norethindrone	Ethinyl estradiol	1.0 mg : 50 μg 1.0 mg : 35 μg 0.5 mg : 35 μg 0.4 mg : 35 μg 0.5 mg : 35 μg (10 tablets), and 1.0 mg : 35 μg (11 tablets) 0.5 mg : 35 μg (7 tablets), and 0.75 mg : 35 μg (7 tablets), and 1.0 mg : 35 μg (7 tablets) 0.5 mg : 35 μg (7 tablets), and 1.0 mg : 35 μg (9 tablets), and 0.5 mg : 35 μg (5 tablets)	Ovcon-50 Genora 1/35, N.E.E. 1/35, Nelova 1/35, Norcept-E, Norethin 1/35, Norinyl 1 + 35, and Ortho-Novum 1/35 Brevicon*, Modicon, and Nelova 0.5/35E Ovcon-35 Nelova 10/11‡ and Ortho-Novum 10/11‡ Ortho-Novum 7/7/7§ Tri-Norinyl¶
Norethindrone	Mestranol	1.0 mg : 50 μg	Norinyl 1 +50, Genora 1/50, Nelova 1/50, Norethin 1/50, and Ortho-Novum 1/50
Norethynodrel	Mestranol	9.85 mg : 150 μg 5.0 mg : 75 μg	Enovid 10 mg Enovid 5 mg
Norgestrel	Ethinyl estradiol	0.5 mg : 50 μg 0.3 mg : 30 μg	Ovral* Lo/Ovral
Norgestrel	None	0.075 mg	Ovrette

All oral contraceptives are FDA Pregnancy Category X.
*Available in Canada and United States.
†Triphasic preparation—0.05 mg : 30 μg pills are taken the first 6 days of the cycle, 0.075 mg : 40 μg pills the next 5 days, and 0.125 mg : 30 μg pills the next 10 days of the cycle, followed by a week of no medication or placebo.
‡Biphasic preparation—0.5 mg : 35 μg pills are taken the first 10 days of the cycle, and 1.0 mg : 35 μg pills the next 11 days of the cycle, followed by a week of no medication or placebo.
§Triphasic preparation—0.5 mg : 35 μg pills are taken the first 7 days of the cycle, 0.75 mg : 35 μg pills the next 7 days, and 1.0 mg : 35 μg the next 7 days, followed by a week of no medication or placebo.
¶Triphasic preparation—0.5 mg : 35 μg pills are taken the first 7 days of the cycle, 1.0 mg : 35 μg pills the next 9 days, and 0.5 mg : 35 μg pills the next 5 days of the cycle, followed by a week of no medication or placebo.

Table 53-7   Oral Contraceptives: Adverse Reactions

Adverse reaction	Relation to oral contraceptives	Comments
Thromboembolytic diseases	Risk increased 2- to 7-fold in users over nonusers. Incidence about 100:100,000 woman years; fatalities 2:100,000 woman years.*	Obesity, family history of thromboembolytic disorders, immobility, or group A blood type may increase risk. Group O blood type females have lower risk. Directly related to estrogen dosage.
Thrombotic stroke	Risk increased 3.1- to 6-fold. Incidence about 25:100,000 woman years; fatalities 0.5:100,000 woman years.*	Hypertension increases risk.
Hemorrhagic stroke	Risk increased at least 2-fold. Incidence about 10:100,000 woman years.*	Hypertension and heavy smoking are strong risk factors.
Myocardial infarction	Risk increased about 2-fold over nonusers when estrogen doses exceed 50 μg daily.	Synergistic increase in risk if oral contraceptives are used by smokers.
Hypertension	Between 1% and 5% of patients show an increase in blood pressure. Clinical hypertension is more rare.	Risk is increased by age, obesity, and parity.
Gallbladder disease	Risk increased an estimated 2-fold*	Risk may be related to duration of use.
Liver disease	Up to 50% of patients show altered liver function. Incidence 10:100,000 woman years for jaundice. Tumors are rare.	Reversible. Dangerous for patients with preexisting liver disease (hepatitis or cholestasis). Liver tumors may be related specifically to mestranol.
Carbohydrate metabolism	Many patients show reduced glucose tolerance.	Important only in prediabetic females who may become insulin-dependent. Related to dose and potency of progestin.
Lipid metabolism	Many patients have increased serum triglyceride levels.	Reversible effect; relationship to coronary artery disease in these patients is unknown.
Chloasma	3% to 4% of patients treated.	Increased sensitivity to sunlight also occurs. Reversible.
Headaches	Variable reports with no clear conclusion.	Chronic headache may presage stroke.
Visual disturbances	Have been associated with use of oral contraceptives.	Temporary blindness, blind spots, and changes in field of vision have been reported.
Emotional state disturbances	Variable reports with no clear conclusion.	No evidence that oral contraceptives significantly increase depression.
Endometrial cancer	No increased risk when combined estrogen-progestin agents used.	Risk is increased by estrogens alone but is reduced by progestins. Some studies suggest protection.
Cervical cancer	No relationship established.	Frequency of coitus and number of sexual partners more important risk factors.
Breast cancer	No relationship established.	Benign breast tumors are improved.
Permanent infertility	No relationship established.	Most patients quickly return to fertility when oral contraceptives are discontinued.
Outcome of later pregnancies	No increased risk to mother or fetus has been demonstrated.	Data are for pregnancies begun after oral contraceptives have been discontinued.

*Risk may be less with the lower dose estrogen products currently in use.

who do not take these drugs (see Table 53-7).

As with any medication, oral contraceptives must be considered in terms of the risk-to-benefit ratio. Of first importance may be how much value the patient places on almost complete protection against unwanted pregnancy. Females who desire this high level of control should then consider the safety factors of the medication. Many of the dangerous complications (e.g., cerebrovascular accident (stroke) and thromboembolytic diseases) are rare even among oral contraceptives users. The risk of these complications is greater than the risk among nonusers of oral contraceptives but much lower than the risk of these complications during pregnancy. Females should also consider the other predisposing risk factors such as smoking, obesity, and hypertension. The combination of oral contraceptives with these conditions leads to unacceptable risk for many patients. All females receiving oral contraceptives should be urged to stop smoking.

Some medical conditions are improved or the symptoms are ameliorated by oral contraceptives. Many patients report a reduction in menstrual disorders and especially in dysmenorrhea. Menstrual blood flow usually is reduced, and anemia is prevented or lessened in many females. Benign breast tumors are improved in a time-dependent fashion by oral contraceptive therapy.

Current medical information suggests that oral contraceptives are safe in relatively young females in whom other risk factors are minimized. Females with a history of hypertension or thromboembolytic disease probably should not receive the drugs. Females who elect to receive oral contraceptives should receive thorough physical examinations yearly. The dose of estrogen and progestin should be the lowest dose that achieves contraception and prevents unwanted side effects such as breakthrough bleeding.

Careful history taking may reveal symptoms that the patient has not linked to oral contraceptive use. Migraine headaches, dizziness, and visual disturbances frequently are not related by the patient to oral contraceptive use and may not be mentioned spontaneously. Breakthrough bleeding, excessive cervical mucus formation, breast tenderness, and other changes in the reproductive tract usually are quickly connected to oral contraceptive use by the patient. These symptoms may be more annoying than serious. Severe headaches or visual disturbances are often early signs of impending stroke and may be sufficient cause to discontinue the medications.

Contraceptive Implants
When long-term pharmacologic contraceptive protection is desired, systemic absorption can be achieved without the need for daily oral dosing. Because most forms of the steroid hormones such as estrogens and progestins are relatively insoluble in water, they are slowly absorbed from tissue sites when injected. This property can be used to advantage by confining the drugs to insoluble polymers that can then be implanted under the skin. Small amounts of drug are continuously released over very long periods of time. One example of such an application is the contraceptive Norplant (Figure 53-1). Six slender capsules each containing 36 mg of the synthetic progestin levonorgestrel are implanted subdermally. This application affords contraceptive protection for up to 5 years.

DRUGS USED DURING CHILDBIRTH AND POSTPARTUM CARE
Physiology of Childbirth
To understand the pharmacologic management of labor and delivery, an understanding of the physiologic processes involved is necessary. During stage I of parturition, uterine contractions begin to increase in frequency and intensity, and the cervix begins to dilate. In stage II, uterine contractions occur at the rate of about 1 every 2 min. The cervix is fully dilated, and uterine contractions bring about the delivery of the infant. During stage III of labor, frequency of the contractions decreases, and the placenta separates from the uterus and is expelled. Uterine contractions continue for hours to days, with the frequency and intensity of the contractions diminishing with time.

When contractions occur during labor and delivery, the myometrium compresses the major blood vessels supplying oxygen to the fetus. The result is that during a contraction, the fetus is relatively anoxic. When the uterus relaxes between contractions, this condition is quickly rectified. If the uterus is overstimulated and fails to relax sufficiently between contractions, the result may be prolonged fetal anoxia that may harm the fetus. Induction of labor with one of the oxytocic drugs carries with it the risk of producing this condition. Therefore all patients in whom labor is being induced should receive continuous care, and fetal monitoring should be done when possible. Oxytocin is the drug of choice to induce or stimulate labor because it seems to allow the uterus to relax between contractions. The ergot alkaloids and other oxytocic drugs tend to increase the overall tone of the myometrium and the strength of contractions and therefore carry a greater risk of producing fetal anoxia.

Uterine contractions that occur after delivery have two beneficial effects on the mother. First, they are responsible for expulsion of the afterbirth and produce a general cleansing of the uterus. Second, these

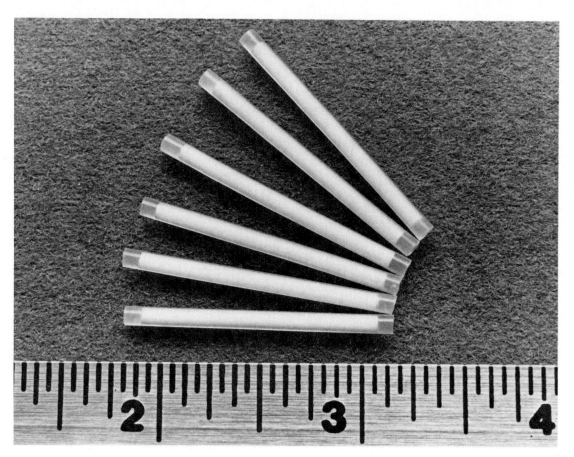

FIGURE 53-1
New contraceptive implant form Norplant.

contractions aid in controlling postpartum bleeding by clamping the vessels that were ruptured by the birth process. If bleeding is a problem at this stage, the physician may use one of the agents with a longer and more continuous action such as one of the ergot alkaloids. The ergot alkaloid preparations are also the only oxytocic drugs that may be effectively administered orally.

Oxytocic Drugs

Oxytocic drugs induce contraction of the myometrium (Table 53-8). The drug class is named for the natural neurohypophyseal hormone oxytocin. The uterus is relatively insensitive to the action of oxytocin until labor has started. No clear role of oxytocin in regulating unassisted, normal labor has been established.

Another class of natural hormones, the prostaglandins, is involved in regulating myometrial activity. These derivatives of fatty acids are rapidly formed in their target tissues and are very rapidly degraded without persisting in the bloodstream for any appreciable time. In the uterus, these hormones induce very powerful myometrial contractions. Recent research has suggested that prostaglandins, especially the E and F series (PGE_2 and $PGF_{2\alpha}$), may play a role in natural induction of labor. Prostaglandin levels rise in the amniotic fluid and other pelvic reproductive tissues as term approaches. This increasing concentration of prostaglandins has been suggested to be the stimulus causing Braxton-Hicks contractions, the mild myometrial contractions occurring during the final few weeks of pregnancy.

Although prostaglandins have been investigated for use in the induction of labor, these drugs elevate uterine muscle tone and may be dangerous to the fetus. The drugs are potent stimulators of the myometrium and have been successfully used to induce abortion during the second trimester when the uterus is resistant to oxytocin. Systemic side effects of these

Table 53-8 Oxytocic Drugs

Generic name	Trade name	Administration/dosage	Medical use	Adverse effects
Oxytocin	Pitocin Syntocinon*	INTRAVENOUS: 1 to 2 mU/min, gradually increased up to about 10 mU/min.	Induction or stimulation of labor.	Stimulates uterine contraction, but allows relaxation between contractions. Fetal or maternal cardiac arrhythmias, acute hypertension, nausea, and water intoxication may occur. Overdose may produce uterine hypertonicity with fetal or maternal injury.
		INTRAVENOUS: 10 U infused at 20 to 40 mU/min. INTRAMUSCULAR: 3 to 10 U (0.3 to 1 ml) postpartum.	Control of uterine atony or bleeding.	Same as above.
	Syntocinon*	NASAL: 1 spray of 40 U/ml solution before nursing.	Aids in breast feeding by stimulating milk let-down.	Also causes nasal vasoconstriction. Onset of action is within 2 or 3 min; duration of action is short.
ERGOT ALKALOIDS				
Ergonovine maleate	Ergotrate maleate*	ORAL: 0.2 to 0.4 mg 2 to 4 times daily for 2 days. INTRAVENOUS, INTRAMUSCULAR: 0.2 mg repeated at 2 or 4 hr, up to maximum of 5 doses.	Control of postpartum bleeding.	May cause nausea and vomiting. Hypertensive episodes are especially likely when vasopressors or spinal anesthesia is also used.
Methylergonovine maleate	Methergine	ORAL: 0.2 to 0.4 mg 2 to 4 times daily for 2 days. INTRAMUSCULAR, INTRAVENOUS: 0.2 mg repeated at 2 or 4 hr, up to maximum of 5 doses.	Same as for ergonovine maleate.	May cause nausea and vomiting, transient hypertension, headache, dizziness, palpitation, or chest pain.
PROSTAGLANDINS				
Carboprost tromethamine	Hemabate Prostin/15 M	INTRAMUSCULAR: 250 µg initially, repeated every 1½ to 3½ hr as needed. FDA Pregnancy Category C.	Abortion in second trimester; control of post partum bleeding.	Vomiting and diarrhea are common; fever also is observed in about 12% of patients.
Dinoprost tromethamine	Prostin F2 Alpha†	INTRAUTERINE: 40 mg slowly infused. Second dose of 10 to 40 mg may be given 24 hr later if needed.	Abortion in second trimester.	Nausea and vomiting are common. Vasomotor disturbances and chest pain are possible.
Dinoprostone	Prostin E2	VAGINAL: 20 mg suppositories inserted every 3 to 5 hr until abortion ensues.	Abortion in second trimester.	GI symptoms are common; cardiovascular symptoms are possible.

*Available in Canada and United States.
†Available in Canada only.

drugs can be serious, and the most comfortable and safest route of administration may well be transabdominal instillation into the amniotic fluid. Administered in this fashion, the drug stays primarily within the uterus and persists in action for hours.

Compounds other than oxytocin and prostaglandins have been discovered to be powerful oxytocics. Among the most clinically useful of these drugs are the ergot alkaloid derivatives (see Table 53-8). The ergot alkaloids are produced by fungal contaminants of rye and other cereal grains. These fungal products have been known as poisons since the Middle Ages, when it was noted that people who ate grain contaminated with this fungus suffered from dry gangrene. This extreme reaction is caused by the potent vasoconstrictive effect of the ergot alkaloids. Blood flow to the limbs may be reduced so severely that the tissues die, and the limbs eventually fall away with little or no bleeding. In addition, pregnant women who ate the affected grain entered an abrupt and devastating labor that expelled fetuses at any stage of development. Today it is not this crude mixture of ergot alkaloids that is useful in the clinic but rather derivatives of the compounds.

Uterine Relaxants

Specific uterine relaxation in cases of hypertonicity or premature labor is not yet possible. Nevertheless, several types of compounds produce uterine relaxation along with other reactions. For example, premature labor is sometimes treated with agents that stimulate beta-2–adrenergic receptors, since stimulation of these receptors in the uterus causes relaxation of the myometrium. Agonists of beta-2–adrenergic receptors cause side effects throughout the body, however, as a result of beta-adrenergic receptor stimulation in other tissues.

The best beta-2–adrenergic agonist for use in halting premature labor is ritodrine. This agent effectively relaxes the myometrium but also affects the peripheral vasculature and other tissues. The heart is sensitive to stimulation by ritodrine, suggesting that the drug is also an agonist with some activity on beta-1–ad-

renergic receptors. Ritodrine usually is administered intravenously when premature labor begins. When contractions have been controlled for 12 to 24 hr, the patient may be started on oral ritodrine, and the intravenous (IV) infusion may be discontinued. The major side effects noted with this drug have been heart palpitations, nausea and vomiting, trembling, flushing, and headache. These effects appear transient and rarely cause termination of therapy. Patients should be observed for undue tachycardia or signs of cardiac distress. The fetal heart may also be stimulated by ritodrine. Ritodrine increases the workload of the mother's heart and is contraindicated in patients with preexisting cardiac disease. The primary indication for ritodrine is to halt spontaneous labor when it appears after the twentieth week of pregnancy and before the thirty-sixth week. Spontaneous labor beginning before the twentieth week frequently is associated with a defective fetus and is usually not interrupted.

CNS depressants may halt premature labor. Ethanol, which is an inhibitor of oxytocin release and a CNS depressant, has been used to halt premature labor. The levels required to relax the uterus are sufficient to produce acute alcohol intoxication. Controlled clinical trials have suggested ritodrine is more effective and less toxic.

General anesthetics may also relax the uterus. Enflurane and halothane are the preferred agents. In addition to CNS effects, these agents may act directly on the myometrium and may also slow catecholamine release from the adrenal gland, thus reducing endogenous stimulators of myometrial activity.

Progesterone is the natural steroidal compound that normally functions as a uterine relaxant. The use of this compound or one of the other progestins is not recommended in cases of uterine hypertonicity during delivery, since the hormone may not reach the uterus in sufficient quantities to relax the uterus quickly and effectively. Use of progesterone during earlier stages of pregnancy may cause undesirable effects on the developing fetus.

NURSING IMPLICATIONS SUMMARY

Estrogens, Progestins, or Combinations, Including Oral Contraceptives

Drug administration

◆ Monitor blood pressure, pulse, and weight. Assess for skin changes.

◆ Instruct patients to report leg pain, sudden onset of chest pain, shortness of breath, coughing up of blood, dizziness, changes in vision or speech, or weakness or numbness of an arm or leg, since these may indicate pulmonary embolism or other thromboembolic problems.

◆ Assess for signs of depression including withdrawal, insomnia, anorexia, and lack of interest in personal appearance.

◆ Assess tactfully for changes in libido. Patients may be reluctant to discuss this problem.

◆ Patients with metastatic bone cancer who are started on hormonal therapy may develop severe hypercalcemia. Monitor serum electrolyte levels (see Table 17-1)

◆ Monitor complete blood count (CBC) and liver function tests.

◆ For a discussion of intramuscular (IM) administration of oil-based suspension, see Chapter 6.

◆ For a discussion of subcutaneous implantation, see Chapter 54.

Patient and family education

◆ Review anticipated benefits and possible side effects of drug therapy. Review Table 53-7. Tell patients to notify the physician if any new side effects develop.

◆ Counsel or refer patients as needed about stopping smoking, losing weight to achieve desirable weight, and modifying diet to decrease cholesterol and triglycerides.

◆ Warn diabetic patients to monitor blood glucose levels carefully, since these drugs may alter glucose levels.

◆ Tell patients to take doses with meals or a snack to lessen nausea. This side effect usually lessens with continued use. Patients should try taking the dose at bedtime rather than in the morning.

◆ Warn patients to avoid driving or operating hazardous equipment if visual changes occur; notify the physician.

◆ Instruct females to report any vaginal bleeding or menstrual irregularities. Notify the physician immediately if pregnancy is suspected.

◆ Remind patients to inform all health-care providers of all medications being used. It may take several months for these drugs to be completely eliminated, even when the patient has stopped using them, so the patient should be reminded to inform health-care providers for up to several months after therapy has stopped.

◆ Remind patients to take drugs only as ordered and not to increase or decrease the dose without consultation with the physician. Overdose can occur even with vaginal creams when they are used excessively. Also, tell women using vaginal creams not to use them as a vaginal lubricant during intercourse, since this may lead to absorption by the male partner.

◆ Typical instructions for missed doses include the following: if a single contraceptive tablet is missed, take the missed dose as soon as remembered. If two consecutive doses are missed, the patient should double up on each of the next two doses, then resume the regular schedule but use additional contraceptive measures until she completes that cycle. If three or more consecutive doses are missed, the patient should stop the pills for 7 days after the first missed dose, then begin a new cycle of pill use. In addition, the patient should take further contraceptive measures from the time the missed tablets are noticed until 7 days after the new course of therapy is started. Some physicians may give different instructions, and some products may carry different instructions; see the manufacturer's leaflet. Encourage the patient to call the physician or nurse with specific questions.

Continued.

◆ Many drugs interfere with effectiveness of birth control pills. Teach patients to ask the physician or pharmacist about this possibility whenever a new medication is being used.

◆ For transdermal application, review with the patient the instruction leaflet provided by the manufacturer.

◆ If a woman discontinues oral contraceptives to become pregnant, it is recommended that she use an alternative form of birth control for 2 months after stopping the pills to ensure more complete excretion of the hormonal agents before conceiving and thus reducing the potential effects of the medications on the fetus.

◆ Teach patients how to do a breast self-examination, and encourage them to perform this monthly.

◆ Patients taking estrogens may develop brown areas on the skin. See Patient Problem: Photosensitivity on p. 629.

◆ Tell patients taking birth control pills that the drugs work best when used regularly. Keep an additional month's supply on hand, and avoid running out of pills.

◆ Remind patients to keep all medications out of the reach of children.

General Guidelines: Fertility Agents

Patient and family education

◆ Teach patients as indicated to keep a record of basal body temperature, consistency of vaginal mucus, and 24-hr urine specimen as prescribed by the physician.

◆ Make certain patients understand the best time of the month to have intercourse to attempt to get pregnant based on the drugs being used.

◆ Provide emotional support. Treatment of infertility problems may be prolonged and discouraging.

◆ Encourage patients to return as directed for blood tests, sonograms, examinations, additional medications, and other therapies as prescribed.

◆ Remind patients to keep all drugs out of the reach of children.

◆ If pregnancy is suspected, notify the physician, since these drugs should usually not be continued during pregnancy.

Bromocriptine

Drug administration

◆ Assess mental status. Assess for signs of depression including lack of interest in personal appearance, withdrawal, anorexia, and insomnia.

◆ Monitor pulse and blood pressure. Check stools and emesis for occult blood.

Patient and family education

◆ Review anticipated benefits and possible side effects of drug therapy. Tell the patient to report any new side effects.

◆ See Patient Problems: Constipation on p. 182, Dry Mouth on p. 166, and Orthostatic Hypotension on p. 234.

◆ When used to treat Parkinson's disease, full benefit of this drug may not be seen for several weeks. Provide emotional support. See Chapter 48.

◆ See the general guidelines for infertility.

◆ Take doses with meals or a snack to lessen gastric irritation. Warn patients to avoid driving or operating hazardous equipment if drowsiness develops.

◆ Avoid drinking alcoholic beverages unless permitted by the physician.

◆ Depending on the patient's age and reason for taking bromocriptine, counsel about methods of birth control as appropriate.

Clomiphene Citrate

Drug administration and patient and family education

◆ Review the anticipated benefits and possible side effects of drug therapy. Common side effects include breast discomfort, headache, heavy menstrual periods, and nausea or vomiting. Encourage patients to notify the physician if any unexplained side effects develop.

◆ Typical instructions for taking this drug are to count the first day of the menstrual cycle as day 1. Begin clomiphene in the dose ordered on day 5, and continue daily until the prescribed number of doses is completed. Review instructions with the patient, and check to see that she understands the dosing schedule. The drug may also be prescribed for men; review the physician's prescription with the patient.

NURSING IMPLICATIONS SUMMARY—cont'd

◆ Warn patients to avoid driving or operating hazardous equipment if changes in vision occur; notify the physician.

◆ See the general guidelines for infertility.

Gonadorelin

◆ Except for allergic reaction, usually after multiple doses, no serious side effects have been reported with this drug. Warn patients that itching may occur at the injection site. Consult the manufacturer's literature. See the general guidelines for infertility.

Gonadotropin, Chorionic

Drug administration and patient and family education

◆ Review the anticipated benefits and possible side effects of drug therapy. Remind patients to notify the physician if any unexpected side effects develop or if any side effects are severe or persistent.

◆ In females, common side effects include breast enlargement, headache, irritability, edema, fatigue, depression, or stomach or pelvic pain.

◆ This drug may be used to treat cryptorchidism, if no anatomic obstruction is present. Notify the physician if acne, enlargement of the penis or testes, growth of pubic hair, or rapid increase in height develops.

◆ Warn patients to avoid driving or operating hazardous equipment if excessive fatigue or visual changes occur; notify the physician.

◆ See the general guidelines for infertility.

Menotropins

Drug administration and patient and family education

◆ Review anticipated benefits and possible side effects of drug therapy. Tell the patient to report any new, severe, or persistent side effects.

◆ This drug is often administered with chorionic gonadotropin. Side effects are often related to excessive ovarian stimulation and include abdominal discomfort, nausea and vomiting, diarrhea, increased weight, and hypertension.

◆ The drug may also be administered to men. It may cause breast enlargement.

◆ See the general guidelines for infertility.

Urofollitropin

Drug administration and patient and family education

◆ Review anticipated benefits and possible side effects of drug therapy. Tell the patient to report any new, severe, or persistent side effects.

◆ Common side effects include bloating, pelvic pain, nausea and vomiting, and breast tenderness.

◆ See the general guidelines for drugs for infertility.

Danazol

Drug administration

◆ This drug may be used to treat endometriosis, fibrocystic breast disease, hereditary angioedema, and hematologic disorders including idiopathic thrombocytopenic purpura (ITP). It has weak androgenic and anabolic properties (see Chapter 54).

◆ Assess for weight gain. Inspect for acne, edema of dependent areas, and hirsutism. Monitor blood pressure.

Patient and family education

◆ Review anticipated benefits and possible side effects of drug therapy. Encourage patients to notify the physician if any unexpected side effects develop. Common side effects in females include reduction in breast size, hirsutism, weight gain, deepening of voice, and emotional lability. Side effects caused by the androgenic properties of the drug may be less noticeable in male patients.

◆ Tell patients to notify the physician if pregnancy is suspected.

◆ Tell female patients that menstrual periods may diminish or cease while on this drug (depending on dose). They should keep a record of menstrual periods.

◆ Side effects are dose related but may be intolerable to some patients. Remind patients to take drugs as ordered for best effects and not to discontinue therapy without consulting the physician.

◆ Warn diabetic patients to monitor blood glucose levels carefully while taking this drug; a change in diet or insulin dose may be needed.

Continued.

Oxytocin

Drug administration

◆ See Table 53-8. Monitor level of consciousness, weight, and intake and output. Monitor blood pressure and pulse. Auscultate lung and heart sounds.

◆ Monitor fetal heart sounds; notify the physician of significant changes in rate or rhythm; follow agency protocol.

◆ Monitor serum electrolyte levels, CBC and platelet count.

◆ Do not leave patient unattended when IV oxytocin is being used.

◆ Monitor vaginal bleeding.

◆ Have drugs, equipment, and personnel available to treat acute allergic reactions in settings where oxytocin is administered.

◆ For IV use, dilute as ordered or according to agency protocol. Use a microdrip infusion set and an infusion monitoring device. Measure dose according to physician order and patient response.

Patient and family education

◆ Review anticipated benefits and possible side effects of drug therapy. Instruct the patient to call for assistance if any new side effects develop.

◆ For intranasal spray, instruct patients to sit upright to use spray; for nose drops, tell the patient to tilt head back to administer drops. When intranasal use is prescribed to promote milk ejection, review with the mother other actions that may also aid in milk ejection such as relaxing, massaging breasts, staying well hydrated, getting enough sleep, and cuddling the infant before trying to nurse.

Ergot Alkaloids

Drug administration

◆ See Table 53-8. Monitor level of consciousness, weight, and intake and output. Monitor blood pressure and pulse. Auscultate lung and heart sounds.

◆ Monitor serum electrolyte level, CBC and platelet count.

◆ Monitor vaginal bleeding.

◆ Have drugs, equipment, and personnel available to treat acute allergic reactions in settings where ergot alkaloids are administered.

◆ For IV use, drug may be administered undiluted. Administer at a rate of 0.2 mg or less over 1 min.

◆ Read labels carefully; do not confuse ergotamine with ergonovine.

Patient and family education

◆ Review anticipated benefits and possible side effects of drug therapy. Instruct the patient to call for assistance if any new side effects develop.

◆ Avoid smoking while using ergot alkaloids.

Prostaglandins

Drug administration

◆ See Table 53-8. Monitor level of consciousness, weight, and intake and output. Monitor blood pressure, pulse, and temperature. Auscultate lung and heart sounds.

◆ Keep side rails up. Have a suction machine available.

◆ Monitor serum electrolyte level, CBC, and platelet count.

◆ Monitor vaginal bleeding. Palpate fundus at regular intervals.

◆ GI symptoms are common; antidiarrheal and antiemetic medications may be ordered concomitantly or prophylactically.

◆ Monitor intake and output.

Patient and family education

◆ Review with patients the anticipated benefits and possible side effects of drug therapy. Instruct patients to call if any unexpected side effects develop.

◆ Provide emotional support. Refer for counseling if appropriate.

Ritodrine

Drug administration

◆ Review information about beta-2—adrenergic receptors in Chapter 10.

◆ Monitor blood pressure and pulse, uterine contractions, and fetal heart tones. Assess patient and fetus every 5 min when initiating IV therapy, every 15 to 30 min when the patient is stable, and every 4 hr when the patient is taking oral maintenance doses (or according to agency protocol). Fetal monitoring may be indicated.

◆ For IV administration, use a minidrip infusion set and an infusion control device.

◆ Stay calm. Provide reassurance to the mother as possible. The drug may increase the subjective sense of anxiety and may cause tachycardia, tightness in the chest, tremor, and other symptoms.

Patient and family education

◆ Review anticipated benefits and possible side effects of drug therapy.

◆ Review with the patient the limits of activity.

◆ Tell the patient to notify the physician if labor begins again, membranes rupture, or contractions increase in frequency or duration.

CHAPTER REVIEW

◆ KEY TERMS

amenorrhea, p. 782

estrogens, p. 776

galactorrhea, p. 782

human chorionic gonadotropin (HCG), p. 777

menarche, p. 776

oxytocin, p. 777

progestins, p. 776

prostaglandins, p. 777

◆ REVIEW QUESTIONS

1. What are the gonadotropic hormones?
2. How are the synthesis and release of FSH, LH, and prolactin regulated?
3. What are the major steroid hormones affecting the female reproductive tract?
4. What are the functions of estrogens during puberty?
5. What hormones regulate ovulation?
6. What effect do estrogens have on the endometrium in the adult female?
7. What effects does progesterone have on the endometrium and myometrium?
8. What is the function of progesterone in pregnancy?
9. What is the role of HCG in pregnancy?
10. How do the steroidal estrogens differ from the nonsteroidal estrogens in duration of action and route of excretion from the body?
11. What side effects and toxic reactions are seen with the chronic use of estrogens? How should you assess for these?
12. What side effects are characteristic of pharmacologic use of progestins?
13. What is the mechanism of action of clomiphene citrate, and what is its medical use?
14. What hormones are contained within menotropins?
15. What is the mechanism of action of bromocriptine, and how is it currently used?
16. What is the mechanism of action of gonadorelin, and what is its medical use?
17. What is the mechanism of action of urofollitropin, and what is its medical use?
18. What agents are used to produce pharmacologic contraception?
19. What is the mechanism of action of the oral contraceptive agents?
20. What side effects occur with use of the oral contraceptives? What should you teach about these side effects?
21. How do oxytocin and prostaglandins differ in their ability to stimulate uterine contractions?
22. What are the ergot alkaloids?
23. How does the administration and effect of the ergot alkaloids differ from that of oxytocin?
24. What is the mechanism of action of ritodrine?

SUGGESTED READING

Franklin M: Recently approved and experimental methods of contraception, *J Nurse Midwife* 35(6):365, 1990.

McKeon VA: Estrogen replacement therapy: current guidelines for education and counseling, *J Gerontol Nurs* 16(10):6, 1990.

Mishell DR: Update on oral contraceptives, *Drug Therapy* 19(4):118, 1989.

Monier M, Laird M: Contraceptives: a look at the future, *Am J Nurs* 89(4):496, 1989.

Nelson L: Clomiphene citrate for infertility, *Drug Therapy* 19(1):65, 1989.

Nevin MM: Dormant danger of DES, *Can Nurse* 84(3):16, 1988.

Orshan SA: The pill, the patient, and you, *RN* 31(7):49, 1988.

Osteosporosis: estrogen connection clearer, *Am J Nurs* 88(1):13, 1988.

Sherrod RA: Coping with infertility: a personal perspective turned professional, *MCN* 13(3):191, 1988.

CHAPTER 54

Drugs Acting on the Male Reproductive System

LEARNING OBJECTIVES
After studying this chapter, you should be able to do the following:
- Describe the uses of androgens.
- Describe the uses and abuses of anabolic steroids.
- Develop a nursing care plan for the patient receiving androgens

CHAPTER OVERVIEW
◆ The major reproductive hormones in men are **androgens.** These steroids are synthesized primarily in the testes and to a lesser extent in the adrenal glands. Within the testes the status of interstitial or Leydig cells and the seminiferous tubular cells is most important for determining male sexual potential. Leydig cells synthesize testosterone, the primary masculinizing steroid hormone. The seminiferous tubules contain the germ cells that in the adult male produce functional sperm. The endocrine control of male sexual development and function, the actions of natural male hormones, and the clinical uses of synthetic and natural drugs acting on the male reproductive system are discussed in this chapter.

Nursing Process Overview
DRUGS AND THE MALE REPRODUCTIVE SYSTEM
Assessment
Perform a complete patient assessment before initiating drug therapy. Assess the vital signs, blood pressure, weight, serum calcium level, height, and glucose content of urine and blood. Focus part of the assessment on the presenting problem. For example, in treatment of reduced androgen production, an assessment of the secondary sexual characteristics should be included. In the patient receiving androgen therapy for its anabolic effects, assess nutritional needs, level of mobility, and intake and output.

Nursing Diagnoses
Body image disturbance: acne secondary to androgen therapy
Body image disturbance: masculinization of females secondary to androgen therapy

Management
Monitor the vital signs and other data mentioned in assessment. Review possible and probable side effects. Refer patients receiving steroids for their anabolic effects to the hospital or community dietitian.

Evaluation
Before discharge, verify that the patient can explain how and why to take the drugs, anticipated side effects, side effects that require immediate notification of the physician (e.g., symptoms of hypercalcemia in the cancer patient), how to treat side effects that may be troublesome but are not serious, and what parameters should be measured regularly at home to monitor the effectiveness of the drug.

PITUITARY REGULATION OF REPRODUCTIVE POTENTIAL IN THE MALE
In the adult male, sexual function depends on the proper interaction of the hypothalamus, adenohy-

pophysis, and the testes. Regulation of testicular function is by a negative feedback loop similar to others previously mentioned. The primary hormones in this cycle are testosterone from the testes; interstitial cell-stimulating hormone (ICSH), also called *luteinizing hormone (LH)*; follicle-stimulating hormone (FSH) from the adenohypophysis; and gonadotropin-releasing hormone (GnRH; see Chapter 50) from the hypothalamus. When testosterone levels in the blood are low, GnRH is released from the hypothalamus to enter the adenohypophysis through the portal venous system. Under the influence of GnRH, ICSH and FSH are released from the hypophysis into the general circulation, where they may act on testicular tissues.

The action of these regulatory hormones is slightly different during the three stages of life in which they act. During fetal development, Leydig cells develop in the embryonic testes as a result of stimulation with the maternal hormone, human chorionic gonadotropin (HCG). These embryonic cells produce the small amounts of testosterone necessary for the development of the male external genitalia; without testosterone, genetically male infants are born with female genitalia. After birth, Leydig cells regress, since the stimulus of HCG is no longer available.

The second period of life when these regulatory processes are most important is puberty. In childhood, very low concentrations of gonadotropins are found in the blood. With the onset of puberty the hypophysis begins to synthesize and release greater quantities of ICSH and FSH. The target organ for ICSH in the male is the Leydig cell, where ICSH stimulates testosterone production. FSH acts directly on the cells of the seminiferous tubule and associated cells to prepare that tissue for spermatogenesis. This process cannot be completed unless testosterone from the Leydig cells is also present. With FSH and testosterone acting on the seminiferous tubules, mature sperm can be produced. Testosterone acts not only within the testes but also throughout the body at this stage of life. These actions are discussed in the next section.

The third period of life to be considered is sexual maturity. During this time, ICSH is important in the maintenance of sexual function because it is still required for the synthesis of testosterone, which maintains spermatogenesis.

A third hormone of the anterohypophysis involved in male sexual function is prolactin. The mechanisms by which prolactin release in males is regulated are not completely understood. However, men with pituitary tumors that secrete large quantities of prolactin often have decreased libidos and low concentrations of ICSH, FSH, and testosterone in their blood-

stream. Prolactin seems to suppress synthesis and release of ICSH and FSH from the hypophysis and may directly interfere with the actions of these hormones on the testes.

ANDROGENS
Testosterone and Other Naturally Occurring Steroids

The major steroid affecting male sexual function is **testosterone.** This hormone is synthesized in the Leydig cells and in the adrenal cortex. Testosterone is a potent androgen, a substance that stimulates growth of the organs of the male reproductive tract. Testosterone is responsible for the enlargement and maturation of the penis, scrotum, seminal vesicles, prostate gland, and other accessory tissues of the male reproductive tract. These actions constitute the primary sexual effects on the male.

Testosterone is also responsible for the development of secondary sexual characteristics. The increased testosterone level during puberty stimulates growth of facial and pubic hair and hair on chest and armpits. Sustained levels of testosterone trigger the onset of baldness in genetically predisposed males. The other dramatic changes that occur in the pubertal male are also related to the increased testosterone levels and include lowering of the voice caused by thickening of the vocal cords, stimulation of sebaceous glands, and stimulation of the libido. Psychologists working with primates other than humans have related aggression to high testosterone levels.

In addition to these primary and secondary sexual effects, testosterone also has profound effects on metabolism. Androgens are anabolic; (i.e., they stimulate synthetic rather than degradative processes). Testosterone increases nitrogen retention, protein formation, and overall metabolic rate. This anabolic action is responsible for the increase in muscle mass associated with puberty and the distribution of this mass in the male pattern. In addition, calcium is retained, and the size and strength of bone are enhanced. Blood-forming cells are also affected so that more red blood cells may be formed.

Although testosterone is the major circulating androgen in human males, it is not the only metabolically important androgen. Evidence shows that testosterone is transformed within many target cells to dihydrotestosterone, which is a more potent androgen than testosterone. Small amounts of another androgen, androstenedione, may also affect various tissues of the body.

Testosterone and androstenedione are close chemical relatives of the estrogens, steroid hormones that have feminizing effects. Some tissues in the brain, breasts, and testes, can convert androgens to estro-

Table 54-1 Androgens

Generic name	Trade name	Administration/dosage	Duration of action	Adverse reactions
NATURAL HORMONE				
Testosterone	Andro Andronaq Histerone Malogen† Testaqua	INTRAMUSCULAR: *Adults*—aqueous suspension for IM use only. Doses range from 10 to 100 mg. FDA Pregnancy Category X.	Relatively short. Doses must be repeated 2 or 3 times/week.	Masculinization in females. Precocious sexual development and premature closure of the epiphyses in children. Excessive sexual stimulation (short-term) or inhibition of testicular function (long-term) in males.
TESTOSTERONE ESTERS				
Testosterone cypionate	Andronaq-LA Duratest	INTRAMUSCULAR: *Adults*—oil solution for deep injection into gluteal muscle, 100 to 400 mg. FDA Pregnancy Category X.	3 to 4 weeks.	Same as for testosterone.
Testosterone enanthate	Delatestryl* Durathate	INTRAMUSCULAR: *Adults*—oil solution for deep injection into gluteal muscle, 50 to 400 mg. FDA Pregnancy Category X.	2 to 4 weeks.	Same as for testosterone.
Testosterone propionate	Testex Malogen†	INTRAMUSCULAR: *Adults*—oil suspension for IM use only. Doses range from 25 to 100 mg. FDA Pregnancy Category X.	Relatively short. Doses must be repeated 2 or 3 times/week.	Same as for testosterone.
ORAL ANDROGENS				
Fluoxymesterone	Halotestin* Ora-Testryl	ORAL: *Adults*—5 to 20 mg daily (male), and 10 to 40 mg daily (female). FDA Pregnancy Category X.	Short. Doses must be repeated daily.	Same as for testosterone. Nausea and vomiting, diarrhea, and peptic ulcerlike symptoms. May increase sensitivity to anticoagulants. Hepatotoxicity, including jaundice.
Methyltestosterone	Android Metandren* Oreton Testred	ORAL: *Adults*—tablets or capsules, 10 to 50 mg daily (male), and 50 to 200 mg daily (female). FDA Pregnancy Category X.	Short. Doses must be repeated daily.	Same as for testosterone. Nausea and vomiting, diarrhea, peptic ulcer-like symptoms. May increase sensitivity to anticoagulants. Hepatotoxicity, including jaundice.
BUCCAL AGENTS				
Methyltestosterone	Android-Muquets Metandren Oreton	ORAL: *Adults*—tablets for buccal administration, 5 to 25 mg daily (male), and 25 to 100 mg daily (female). FDA Pregnancy Category X.	Short. Doses must be repeated daily.	Same as for testosterone. May increase sensitivity to anticoagulants. Hepatotoxicity, including jaundice.

*Available in Canada and United States.
†Available in Canada only.

gens. Low estrogen concentrations therefore are found in the blood of healthy adult males. These estrogens have no obvious influence on healthy men, but under certain circumstances, estrogen concentrations may increase and produce pathologic signs such as breast development.

Replacement Therapy

Androgenic drugs are primarily used in replacement therapy for patients who have reduced endogenous androgen production. For some patients the loss of androgens occurs early and prevents the normal changes of puberty. Androgen loss after puberty may cause a loss in libido or sexual desire or may cause mild feminizing tendencies. Aging males produce less testosterone than younger men and may suffer loss of sexual drive. Some older men suffer more severe symptoms suggestive of a male climacteric, or male menopause. These conditions and others related to specific malfunctions of the male sexual organs may be treated with testosterone or one of the other androgenic compounds (Table 54-1). For these patients with reduced natural testosterone production, this treatment constitutes replacement therapy.

Certain forms of impotence and feminization do not respond well to replacement therapy with androgenic steroids. One type of patient unresponsive to androgens has very high blood levels of prolactin. Prolactin may interfere with the production and function of ICSH and FSH, lowering testosterone production. Bromocriptine, a drug that blocks prolactin synthesis, lowers prolactin levels, increases testosterone and ICSH and FSH levels, and restores sexual potency in some patients. Bromocriptine is also used to control galactorrhea and to restore fertility in females (see Chapter 53).

Testosterone in its natural form is not water soluble and therefore is used as an aqueous suspension suitable only for intramuscular (IM) injection (see Table 54-1). In this form the drug has a short duration of action and produces somewhat erratic clinical responses. Testosterone can be absorbed from the gastrointestinal (GI) tract; however, this route of administration does not produce clinically useful testosterone concentrations in the bloodstream because the steroid absorbed from the intestine passes directly into the portal circulation and enters the liver before it circulates to the rest of the body. The liver can inactivate testosterone rapidly by forming less active metabolites or by converting the steroid to a glucuronide or sulfated derivatives.

Testosterone esters are much more useful than testosterone for producing sustained androgenic effects. Two preparations commonly used clinically are testosterone enanthate and testosterone cypionate (see Table 54-1). Both are supplied as suspensions in oil; when injected intramuscularly, they are slowly absorbed and therefore are effective for 3 to 4 weeks. This increased convenience for the patient is at the cost of less flexibility in control. Another testosterone ester, testosterone propionate, has a short duration of action more similar to that of testosterone.

Orally absorbed androgens have been developed, including methyltestosterone and fluoxymesterone. These compounds are effective orally because they are resistant to the action of liver enzymes that degrade testosterone. Unfortunately, these compounds also are associated with liver toxicity of various types, including cholestatic jaundice.

Tablets of methyltestosterone are available for buccal administration. Absorption through the mucous membranes of the mouth may be more effective than oral administration because buccally absorbed materials do not directly enter portal circulation and therefore are circulated to the rest of the body before they enter the liver (see Chapter 1).

Androgens have been used for various conditions in females such as relief of dysmenorrhea, menopausal symptoms, and postpartum breast engorgement, but other agents now are preferred (see Chapter 53). Androgens are still indicated for treatment of certain advanced breast carcinomas (see Chapter 39). The high doses used for this purpose exceed those required for replacement therapy and may be expected to cause masculinization (see Table 54-1).

Danazol, a weak androgen, is used to suppress LH and FSH release from the hypophysis and to block steriodogenesis in the gonads and adrenals. It also relieves the tenderness of fibrocystic breast disease and controls endometriosis (see Chapter 53). It is also useful in treating angioedema.

ANABOLIC STEROIDS

In addition to androgenic properties the natural male steroids also possess anabolic properties that may be useful in certain clinical situations (Table 54-2). For example, these drugs may be used to treat conditions for which increased nitrogen retention and protein formation are desirable. Accordingly, these drugs may alleviate the catabolic state produced by severe trauma. Patients who have suffered extensive burns or surgery may benefit from the action of the **anabolic steroids.** Anabolic hormone effects on red blood cell formation make these drugs valuable in the treatment of certain forms of anemia.

Although a few anabolic compounds have relatively low androgenic potency, all anabolic steroids possess androgenic properties to some degree. These androgenic effects may be indistinguishable in healthy males, but they may become obvious when

Table 54-2 Anabolic Steroids

Generic name	Trade name	Administration/dosage	Major clinical uses
Nandrolone decanoate	Deca-Durabolin* Kabolin	INTRAMUSCULAR: *Adults*—oil solution for deep IM injection, 50 to 200 mg. Repeat doses every 3 to 4 weeks. *Children*—25 to 50 mg. Repeat doses every 3 to 4 weeks. FDA Pregnancy Category X.	Refractory anemias
Nandrolone phenpropionate	Androlone Durabolin*	INTRAMUSCULAR: *Adults*—oil solution for deep IM injection, 50 to 100 mg. Repeat doses every 1 to 4 weeks. FDA Pregnancy Category X.	Metastatic breast cancer.
Oxandrolone	Anavar	ORAL: *Adults*—tablets, 5 to 10 mg daily in 2 to 4 doses. *Children*—0.25 mg/kg body weight intermittently. FDA Pregnancy Category X.	To produce weight gain after severe trauma.
Oxymetholone	Anadrol Anapolon†	ORAL: *Adults*—tablets, 1 to 5 mg/kg body weight/day up to 100 mg total daily dose. FDA Pregnancy Category X.	Anemias.
Stanozolol	Winstrol*	ORAL: *Adults*—tablets, 2 mg 3 times daily for initial therapy. Reduce dose when response allows. *Children*—1 mg twice daily with meals, only during an attack. FDA Pregnancy Category X.	Hereditary angioedema.

*Available in Canada and United States.
†Available in Canada only.

the compounds are used to treat women or children. Patients receiving these compounds may develop increased libido. Males may develop priapism (continuous erection). Females should be especially watched for androgen-induced changes such as inappropriate hair development, voice changes, or personality alterations. Children should be watched closely for precocious sexual development. These compounds, while promoting bone growth in children, also promote fusion of the epiphyses, which permanently halts skeletal growth. Therefore full adult height may be diminished, although a growth spurt may be attained when the drugs are first given. For this reason and because of the effects on sexual development, these drugs are less than ideal for therapy in children.

Anabolic steroids are inappropriate for use in athletes seeking to increase bone or muscle mass. In healthy young males the anabolic effects are minimal, but the side effects can be serious (altered liver function, reduced gonadotropin levels, lowered testosterone synthesis, and depressed spermatogenesis). In healthy young females, bone and muscle mass may be increased more dramatically but at the cost of virilization and menstrual disturbances.

NURSING IMPLICATIONS SUMMARY

Androgens

Drug administration

- Assess mental status and neurologic function.
- Assess for signs of depression including insomnia, lack of appetite, loss of interest in personal appearance, and withdrawal.
- Monitor weight, pulse, and blood pressure. Assess for edema and skin changes. Auscultate lung and heart sounds.
- Monitor complete blood count (CBC) and differential, serum electrolyte level, and liver function tests.
- Assess for signs of liver dysfunction including right upper quadrant abdominal pain, malaise, fever, jaundice, and pruritus.
- Assess for hypercalcemia (see Table 17-1).
- When prescribed for children, review the proposed long-term treatment plan. Therapy for children is often intermittent to allow drug-free periods to permit normal bone growth. The child's progress may be monitored with regular x-ray studies of wrists and hands to monitor bone maturation. Monitor weight and height.
- For a discussion of IM administration of oil-based suspensions, see Chapter 6.
- Pellets for subcutaneous implantation can be inserted surgically or with a specially designed injector. Either procedure can be done easily in the physician's office; aseptic technique must be used. Usual sites of insertion are the infrascapular area or along the posterior axillary line. Two or more pellets may be inserted at one time, although not necessarily into the same subcutaneous pouch. The drugs will be absorbed slowly from the pellets for up to 4 to 6 months. Sloughing of the pellets can occur; instruct patients to notify the physician. Sloughing often indicates placement too superficially or lack of aseptic technique. Because the dose of subcutaneous pellets cannot be regulated easily, proper dosage is determined by oral medication before a switch is made to the subcutaneous route. For additional information, see the information supplied by the manufacturer.
- For buccal tablets, instruct patients to place tablets in the mouth between the upper or lower gum and the cheek and to allow the tablet to dissolve. While the tablet is in place, the patient should refrain from eating, drinking, chewing, or smoking. Instruct patients to rotate sites with each administration. Remind patients to maintain a program of good regular oral hygiene and to report any oral irritation to the physician.

Patient and family education

- Review anticipated benefits and possible side effects of drug therapy. Tell patients to report any new side effects.
- Assess patients tactfully for side effects such as decreased ejaculatory volume, amenorrhea, menstrual irregularities, virilization of females, and clitoral enlargement. Children may experience premature virilization. Patients may be reluctant to discuss these problems, or children may not know how to do so. Provide emotional support. Remind patients to take drugs as ordered for best effects and not to stop taking the drug without notifying the physician.
- Instruct patients to notify the physician if priapism develops.
- Tell patients to take oral doses with meals or a snack to lessen gastric irritation.
- Warn diabetic patients to monitor blood glucose levels frequently for the first 2 weeks of therapy and after androgen therapy is completed, since a change in insulin dose or diet may be needed.

Continued.

NURSING IMPLICATIONS SUMMARY—cont'd

Anabolic Steroids

Drug administration

◆ Assess mental status. Assess for signs of depression including lack of interest in personal appearance, insomnia, loss of appetite, and withdrawal.

◆ Monitor weight, blood pressure, and pulse. Assess for of edema and skin changes.

◆ Monitor CBC and differential and liver function tests.

Patient and family education

◆ Review anticipated benefits and possible side effects of the drug therapy. Tell patients to take drugs only as ordered and not to share drugs with others. Anabolic steroids should not be used to change body size or function for athletic purposes.

◆ Take oral doses with meals or a snack to lessen gastric irritation. If GI symptoms are severe or persistent, notify the physician.

◆ Assess tactfully for changes such as hirsutism and virilization in females or gynecomastia or decreased libido in males. Provide emotional support as needed. Remind patients to take medications as ordered for best effects and not to stop medications without notifying the physician.

◆ Notify the physician if priapism develops.

◆ Warn diabetic patients to monitor blood glucose levels carefully when starting or ending therapy with steroids, since an adjustment in insulin dose or diet may be necessary.

◆ Patients who have been burned, traumatized, or immobilized should be informed that the effectiveness of anabolic steroids may be enhanced by concomitant use of a diet high in calories and protein. Continue regular physical therapy to help reduce bone demineralization.

CHAPTER REVIEW

◆ **KEY TERMS**

◆ **REVIEW QUESTIONS**

1. Which three organs produce hormones that affect male sexual development and function?

2. What is the function of GnRH in the adult male?

3. What is the function of ICSH in the adult male?

4. What is the function of FSH in the adult male?

5. What is the function of testosterone during fetal development in males?

6. What is the primary natural androgenic steroid?

7. What effect does testosterone have on metabolism? How should you assess for this?

8. What is the most common clinical use of androgen steroids?

9. Why is testosterone not administered by the oral route?

10. What advantages do testosterone esters such as testosterone enanthate have over testosterone for long-term replacement therapy of androgen deficiency?

11. What two androgenic steroids are well absorbed orally?

12. What disadvantages do the orally administered androgenic steroids possess compared with other androgenic agents?

13. What is the advantage of administering testosterone by the buccal route rather than by the oral route? What are teaching points associated with this route of administration?

14. What is the major effect of the anabolic steroids?

15. What side effect is frequently associated with anabolic steroids?

SUGGESTED READING

Anthony CP, Thibodeau, GA: *The male reproductive system.* In *Textbook of anatomy and physiology*, ed 13, St Louis, 1991, Mosby–Year Book.

Council on Scientific Affairs: Drug abuse in athletes. Anabolic steroids and human growth hormone, *JAMA* 259(11):1703, 1988.

Yelverton GA: Anabolic steroids, *Pediatr Nurs* 15(1):63, 1989.

CHAPTER 55

Drugs to Treat Diabetes Mellitus

LEARNING OBJECTIVES

After studying this chapter, you should be able to do the following:

- Discuss the difference between insulin-dependent and noninsulin-dependent diabetes mellitus.
- Explain the advantages of the different forms of insulin.
- Explain the clinical uses of sulfonylureas.
- Develop a nursing care plan for the patient with diabetes.
- Develop a teaching plan for the patient with diabetes.

CHAPTER OVERVIEW

- Within the pancreas, an exocrine gland that supplies digestive juices to the small intestine, lie discrete clusters of cells with different functions from those of most pancreatic cells. These cell clusters, called the *islets of Langerhans,* contain several types of endocrine cells. Three of these cell types release peptide hormones that affect glucose metabolism. Alpha (A) cells synthesize and release the peptide hormone glucagon, beta (B) cells synthesize and release insulin, and D cells synthesize somatostatin. This chapter includes an examination of the function of the islet cells, a description of diabetes mellitus, and a description of the drugs used in the diagnosis and control of that disease.

Nursing Process Overview

DIABETES MELLITUS

Assessment

Diabetes occurs in all age groups. Baseline assessment data include all the usual assessment data, with emphasis on the vital signs, weight, blood glucose and urine glucose concentrations, and any signs indicating possible long-term effects such as the development of ulcers on the lower extremities. Assess the condition of skin and nails, and note the presence of any unusual signs or symptoms.

Nursing Diagnoses

Possible complication: hypoglycemia
Knowledge deficit

Management

In relation to drug therapy, monitor blood glucose, and examine other appropriate laboratory work such as electrolytes or arterial blood gas levels. Begin plan-

ning for discharge as soon as the patient is diagnosed. Teach the patient about the medications that have been prescribed and their method of administration and how to test blood glucose. Refer patients as appropriate to the hospital or community dietitian, the local visiting nurse association, and the local diabetes association.

Evaluation

Before discharge, verify that the patient can explain why the drugs are prescribed and can demonstrate how to administer insulin or other medications correctly. Be certain the patient can explain the symptoms of hyperglycemia and hypoglycemia and how to treat them and other prescribed aspects of care such as foot care, dietary restrictions, and any limitations in activity that have been prescribed. Check that the patient can demonstrate how to test for blood glucose level and can state what to do based on the information obtained from this test.

NORMAL HORMONAL REGULATION OF METABOLISM

Glucose Metabolism

One of the rules of metabolic regulation is that the body seldom relies on a single mechanism to control an important physiologic function. This rule applies especially to the processes by which the body regulates glucose use. The primary hormone regulating glucose metabolism is **insulin,** a peptide hormone synthesized in the B cells of the pancreas. Insulin stimulates glucose uptake in fat and muscle cells and the conversion in the liver of glucose to the storage carbohydrate glycogen.

Insulin does not work alone, however, and its metabolic actions must always be considered in relation to the actions of other hormones. For example, the elevated blood glucose level after a meal stimulates insulin release from the pancreas. Blood glucose level is thereby lowered because insulin stimulates the burning of glucose for energy in fat and muscle cells and the storage of glucose in the liver. As blood glucose levels fall in response to insulin, glucagon release from the A cells of the pancreas is stimulated. Glucagon in many ways directly opposes the action of insulin in glucose metabolism. Glucagon stimulates the liver to break down glycogen and amino acids so that glucose is released into the blood. Glucagon also inhibits the uptake of glucose by muscle and fat cells. By balancing the action of these hormones, the body protects itself from high blood glucose (hyperglycemia) and low blood glucose (hypoglycemia).

Even the concept of metabolic balance achieved with two antagonistic hormones does not adequately describe glucose regulation. For example, somatostatin (see Chapter 49) released from D cells inhibits release of insulin and glucagon from islet cells. Other hormones antagonize the peripheral effects of insulin. Cortisol, an adrenocortical glucocorticoid, and epinephrine, a catecholamine from the adrenal medulla, which are elevated during stress, antagonize the actions of insulin in muscle or fat cells (Table 55-1). The overall action of these two hormones is to increase blood glucose levels. Growth hormone (see Chapter 50) also increases blood glucose, primarily by lowering glucose uptake in muscle cells.

Fat and Protein Metabolism

Although insulin is most frequently considered as a regulator of glucose metabolism, it is also important in regulating fat and protein metabolism. Insulin directly stimulates the synthesis of storage lipid within

Table 55-1   Metabolic Actions of Insulin and Insulin-Opposing Hormones

Tissue and metabolic process	Insulin	Glucagon	Epinephrine	Cortisol	Growth hormone
LIVER					
Glycogen formation	Increase	Decrease	Decrease	Increase	—
Glucose formation from amino acids	Decrease	Increase	—	Increase	Decrease
Glucose formation from glycogen	Decrease	Increase	Increase	—	—
SKELETAL MUSCLE					
Glucose uptake or use	Increase	Decrease	Decrease	Decrease	Decrease
Amino acid uptake	Increase	—	—	—	Increase
Protein synthesis	Increase	Decrease	—	Decrease	Increase
Glucose release from glycogen	Decrease	Increase	Increase	—	—
FAT CELLS					
Synthesis of storage lipid	Increase	Decrease	Decrease	Decrease	Decrease
Release of free fatty acids from stored lipid	Decrease	Increase	Increase	Increase	Increase
BLOOD					
Glucose level	Decrease	Increase	Increase	Increase	Increase
Free fatty acid level	Decrease	Increase	Increase	Increase	Increase

the fat cell, blocks the breakdown and release of stored lipid, and promotes protein synthesis by stimulating amino acid uptake and by directly stimulating protein synthetic processes.

As in carbohydrate metabolism, the action of insulin in regulating fat and protein metabolism is opposed by other hormones (see Table 55-1). For example, epinephrine, glucagon, cortisol, and growth hormone all stimulate fat breakdown in fat cells, thereby directly opposing the action of insulin in that tissue. These hormones therefore tend to raise the blood content of free fatty acids and other breakdown products of lipids. In addition, glucagon and cortisol block protein synthesis in direct opposition to insulin action. Growth hormone differs from the other insulin-opposing hormones in that growth hormone directly stimulates protein synthesis in many body tissues. An understanding of this delicate balance of hormonal actions is important to appreciate the origin of some of the metabolic derangements that occur in diabetes mellitus.

DIABETES MELLITUS
Types and Causes

In **diabetes mellitus,** insulin action is lost. If all insulin production ceases, the disease is referred to as *insulin-dependent diabetes mellitus (IDDM).* Other terms for this form are *type I* or *juvenile-onset* diabetes. If insulin production continues but is insufficient to meet the body's demands, the disease is referred to as *noninsulin-dependent diabetes mellitus (NIDDM),* also called *type II* or *adult-onset* diabetes; most diabetic persons have this type. As the names imply, diabetes characterized by absence of insulin production is primarily a disease of the young, although it may occur later in life. NIDDM is usually a disease of persons who are over 40 years of age or obese. Diabetes in these patients may involve insulin resistance; insulin concentrations in the blood may be normal, but the target tissues are unresponsive to insulin.

The exact cause of diabetes mellitus has not been established, but several factors may contribute to its development. Heredity may play a role in some types of diabetes, especially NIDDM, but it has never been proved that heredity alone determines who will or will not develop the disease. For example, in older individuals a clear link exists between obesity and NIDDM.

Viral infections have been implicated in IDDM, partly through epidemiologic evidence linking viral epidemics to unexpected increases in new cases of IDDM. Viruses can produce diabetes in laboratory animals, and at least one case is now on record in which viruses were isolated from the pancreas of a child who died during the acute onset of diabetes mellitus. The viruses from this child produced diabetes in experimental animals.

Metabolic Derangements

Significant metabolic derangements occur when insulin action is lost. Without insulin, less glucose is used in muscle and fat cells, and more glucose is released into the circulation by the liver. Muscle cells, starved for energy sources, break down protein and release amino acids into the bloodstream. The liver converts a portion of these amino acids into glucose and returns it to the bloodstream. These processes contribute to the persistent elevated levels of glucose in the blood. When glucose levels in the blood exceed a certain threshold (about 160 mg/dl), glucose begins to appear in urine.

The most common early symptoms of diabetes mellitus result directly from osmotic and metabolic changes. Patients frequently first note a feeling of constant fatigue, since energy production in body cells is impaired. An increased frequency of urination (polyuria), often first noticed at night, occurs because of the excess glucose in urine that produces an osmotic diuresis (i.e., more water must be excreted to carry out the high concentration of glucose). As urine output increases, most patients develop excessive thirst (polydipsia), which results from the body's efforts to maintain normal hydration despite excessive fluid losses through the kidney. Some patients develop perineal infections, made likely by the presence of glucose in urine.

The alterations in metabolism produced by insulin deficiency and the relative excess of catabolic hormones (catecholamines and steroids) ultimately result in greater-than-normal protein and fat breakdown. The protein is metabolized to amino acids and then to glucose, whereas the fats are converted to free fatty acids and then to ketone bodies that are released into the circulation. These excess breakdown products may cause the patient to become ketotic or acidotic. Ketoacidosis is a serious acute complication of diabetes mellitus, and ketoacidotic coma is associated with mortalities of 3% to 30%. Mortality is highest when treatment is delayed. Ketoacidosis is primarily seen in patients with IDDM who have little or no endogenous insulin production. These patients are sometimes called *ketosis-prone diabetics.* Patients with NIDDM who produce enough insulin to suppress lipid breakdown are resistant to ketosis.

Any diabetic person may become comatose as a result of dehydration. As the plasma becomes hyperosmolar (higher solute concentration than normal for blood), water is pulled from body tissues, and severe water and electrolyte imbalances occur. Patients in this type of hyperosmolar coma tend to be older and to have an even higher mortality rate than the patients in ketoacidotic coma.

Long-Term Complications

Pathologic changes in blood vessels, nerves, and kidneys occur in diabetic patients. Blood vessel defects are observed in the retina, where hemorrhages may destroy sight. Other vessels may be similarly affected, although those changes are not so easily observed in the early stages of the disease. At later stages, circulation to the limbs may be grossly impaired. Pathologic changes also occur in the kidney, at first affecting glomerular filtration rate, then progressing to glomerulosclerosis with thickening of the capillary basement membranes. Nephrotic syndrome with protein loss through the kidney and frank kidney failure are late complications of diabetes. Nerve function is impaired so that late in the disease there may be loss of feeling in the limbs or other parts of the body. Sexual impotence is common among diabetic men.

Evidence from research laboratories suggests that many of the late pathologic changes may be delayed or reduced in severity by strict control of the blood sugar level from the earliest possible time after the appearance of diabetes. Clinical studies have not yet proved or disproved a relationship between the degree of diabetes control and the development of long-term complications in human patients. A 10-year prospective study (Diabetes Control and Complications Trial) sponsored by the National Institutes of Health may provide definitive answers.

Diagnosis

Diabetes mellitus is diagnosed by applying one of the following procedures.

Fasting blood sugar (FBS) is determined by obtaining 1 to 3 ml of blood from an individual after a 12-hr fast and measuring the glucose content by any of several methods approved for use in clinical laboratories. Most conveniently, the blood is taken in the early morning. The range of normal fasting plasma sugar values is 60 to 100 mg/dl for venous blood. A value above 140 mg/dl in a truly fasting individual suggests the diagnosis of diabetes mellitus.

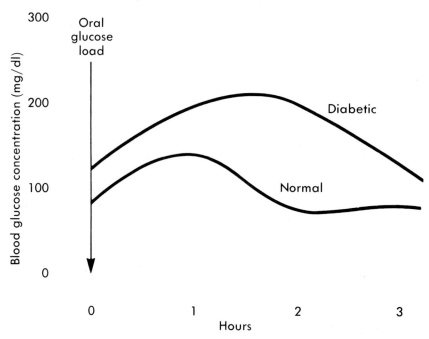

FIGURE 55-1

Typical oral glucose tolerance tests for normal and diabetic patients. Test is performed preferably in ambulatory patients in morning before breaking overnight fast. Oral glucose load is about 75 gm given in solution. Blood is drawn at appropriate intervals (before glucose and 60, 90, 120, and 180 min after) and is analyzed for glucose concentration.

Values between 100 and 140 mg/dl may require further patient evaluation.

Glucose in urine **(glucosuria)** is conveniently tested in screening programs with commercially available pretreated test strips (Dextrostix), which develop a particular color when exposed to urine containing glucose. Glucose does not routinely appear in urine of nondiabetic persons because a blood sugar level of about 160 mg/dl is required before healthy kidneys allow glucose to spill into urine. Some diabetic persons spill glucose into urine at lower blood glucose concentrations, possibly as a result of impaired renal function.

The *oral glucose tolerance test (OGTT)* detects not only persons who are overtly diabetic but also those who may progress to clinical diabetes. The test consists of administering 50 to 100 gm of glucose orally. Blood samples are then taken at hourly or 30-min intervals, and the glucose levels in the plasma are compared with the value obtained from a sample taken immediately before the glucose was administered. In a healthy person, plasma glucose levels rise in response to this acute glucose load and immediately trigger the release of insulin from the B cells of the pancreas. As a result of the circulating insulin, glucose levels begin to fall within about 1 hr after the glucose load is administered and return to normal within 2 hr (Figure 55-1). In contrast, plasma glucose levels of the diabetic person fall more slowly than those of the healthy person because insulin is not released to aid in disposition of the glucose load. Plasma glucose levels in diabetic persons remain over 200 mg/dl of plasma 2 hr after the glucose load.

Treatment

Insulin therapy
Mechanism of action. Insulin is used to treat diabetes when presumably no functional B cells are left in the islets to respond to glucose levels. Such treatment constitutes replacement therapy. The administered insulin restores the ability of cells to use glucose as an energy source and corrects many associated metabolic derangements.

Absorption and fate. Insulin must be administered by injection because it is a protein and therefore would be digested and destroyed in the gastrointestinal (GI) tract. In its natural form, insulin is relatively soluble in water and is rather quickly absorbed from subcutaneous injection sites. This property is reflected in the pharmacologic behavior of regular insulin for injection (Table 55-2), which is rapidly absorbed, has its peak effect within 2 to 4 hr, and is no longer active after approximately 8 hr. The longer-acting insulin preparations are prepared by crystallizing insulin in the presence of zinc to form slowly dissolving crystals or in the presence of protein (protamine) to form slowly dissolving complexes. These preparations differ from regular insulin and from each other in onset and duration of action primarily because of differences in absorption from the injection site.

The health-care professional must be familiar with the properties of the major insulin products. With these various insulin forms, control can be adjusted to fit the lifestyle and metabolic demands of individual patients. Diabetic persons must become proficient not only in the techniques of storing, preparing, and injecting their insulin, but they also must be taught the proper testing procedures. Moreover, they must understand the onset and duration of action of the insulin preparations they are receiving to avoid complications.

As an example of the many patterns of dosage that may be used successfully, consider the following hypothetical case.

A person with IDDM who has been maintained on a single dose of lente insulin before breakfast each morning has started to show hyperglycemia by the next morning. To overcome this problem, the physician splits the insulin dose, giving 80% of the daily dose in the morning and the remainder before supper. The rationale for this therapy is simple. Lente insulin injected at around 7 AM reaches its peak effect around dinner time (see Table 55-2). The small dose administered before supper helps to protect the patient from developing hyperglycemia overnight.

Many individualized schemes for insulin dosage may be devised. Nevertheless, in all cases the principle is the same; doses of insulin must be timed so that the patient is protected from hyperglycemia at any time and from hypoglycemia during peak periods of insulin action.

Side effects. Insulin therapy is associated with two major acute side effects. If therapy is inadequate, the person may go into a coma resulting from the uncontrolled metabolic derangements. The blood sugar concentration is high, and ketoacidosis or hyperosmolar coma may result. If inadvertent insulin overdosage occurs or if a patient does not eat or overexercises, the patient may lapse into coma resulting from a hypoglycemic reaction. It is critical for the health-care professional to be able to differentiate between these conditions. The distinguishing symptoms are outlined in Table 55-3. Treatment of hypoglycemia consists of elevating blood glucose levels by oral administration of sugar in conscious patients or by glucagon injection or glucose intravenous (IV) infusion in unconscious patients. Treatment of diabetic coma requires insulin administration to lower blood sugar concentration and to reduce ketone body formation.

Table 55-2   Insulin Preparations

Generic name	Classification	Description	Pharmacokinetics		
			Onset	Peak	Duration
Insulin injection	Rapid acting	Clear solution containing no zinc or modifying agents; IV or subcutaneous injection.	Within 1 hr	2 to 4 hr	6 to 8 hr
Prompt insulin zinc suspension	Rapid acting	Cloudy suspension of amorphous insulin precipitated with zinc to slow absorption; subcutaneous only.	1 to 2 hr	4 to 7 hr	12 to 16 hr
Isophane insulin suspension	Intermediate acting	Cloudy suspension of insulin complexed with protamine to slow absorption; subcutaneous only.	2 to 4 hr	10 to 16 hr	18 to 30 hr
Insulin zinc suspension	Intermediate acting	Cloudy suspension containing 30% semilente insulin and 70% ultralente insulin; subcutaneous only.	1 to 2 hr	10 to 16 hr	18 to 30 hr
Protamine zinc insulin suspension	Long acting	Cloudy when well mixed; suspension of insulin complexed with more protamine than NPH insulin; subcutaneous only.	6 to 8 hr	14 to 24 hr	24 to 36 hr or longer
Extended insulin zinc suspension	Long acting	Cloudy when well mixed; large complexes of insulin with zinc to slow absorption; no protein modifiers; subcutaneous only.	5 to 8 hr	16 to 24 hr	24 to 36 hr or longer

Allergic reactions to insulin may occur. Local allergic reactions usually do not require treatment. Systemic allergic responses to insulin are more rare. Severe allergic reactions usually may be prevented in a sensitive patient by using a more highly purified insulin preparation (single component insulin) or by using insulin derived from a different source (see next section). For example, a patient sensitive to the standard preparations containing porcine and bovine insulin may be able to take more purified forms without allergic symptoms.

Many patients receiving insulin therapy have insulin antibodies in their blood. These antibodies may contribute to insulin resistance in some patients.

Insulin may also provoke subcutaneous fat near injection sites to atrophy. This lipoatrophy leads to the formation of hollows or depressions in the skin. Careful rotation of injection sites minimizes this ef-

fect. Lipoatrophy may be less common with the highly purified insulin preparations.

Forms of insulin. Three types of insulin are available in the United States—bovine, porcine, and human. Bovine and porcine insulin are obtained from the pancreas of animals slaughtered for food. Many commonly used preparations are mixtures of bovine and porcine insulin that also may contain proinsulin as a contaminant (Table 55-4). Highly purified insulins with a much lower level of proinsulin contamination are available.

Human insulin comes from two sources. Semisynthetic human insulin is prepared by converting porcine insulin to the human form by chemically changing the one differing amino acid. Human insulin is also produced by recombinant deoxyribonucleic acid (DNA) techniques; human genes for insulin are inserted into bacteria, which then produce large

Table 55-3   Differential Diagnosis of Diabetic Coma and Hypoglycemic Reactions

Clinical data	Diabetic coma	Hypoglycemic reactions
Symptoms	Thirst Abdominal pain Nausea and vomiting Headache Constipation Shortness of breath (Kussmaul breathing)	Nervousness Hunger Sweating Weakness Stupor Convulsions
Signs	Facial flushing Air hunger Soft eyeballs Normal or absent reflexes Acetone breath	Pallor Shallow respiration Normal eyeballs Babinski reflex may be seen
Urine glucose	Positive	Negative or low
Urine acetone	Positive	Negative
Blood glucose	High (above 250 mg/dl)	Low (below 60 mg/dl)
Blood CO_2	Low	Normal
Precipitating factors	Untreated diabetes Infection or disease appearing in a previously controlled diabetic patient High degree of emotional or psychologic stress	Insulin overdosage Skipping meals Excessive exercise before meals
History	Onset of symptoms usually occurs over a period of days.	Onset of symptoms is related to the type of medication used; regular insulin overdose produces symptoms more rapidly than the longer-acting insulins or oral agents.

amounts of the protein to be processed and purified.

The hypoglycemic actions of the various forms of insulin are similar; however, the various preparations differ slightly in pharmacokinetics and side effects. For example, human insulin preparations have a slightly shorter duration of action than corresponding porcine preparations. Dosages may need slight adjustment when switching from one preparation to another. Human insulin and purified porcine insulin are less antigenic than the other types available. Patients may be switched to one of these forms to help control allergic side effects associated with insulin therapy.

Oral hypoglycemic agents

Mechanism of action. The oral hypoglycemic agents used in the United States and Canada are **sulfonylureas.** These drugs are useful only for patients who produce some insulin on their own (i.e., patients with NIDDM). Clinical studies of patients with NIDDM have shown that many have low, normal, or even above-normal insulin levels in their blood. The cells of many of these patients, however, are resistant to the action of insulin. Insulin action there-

fore is lost not because insulin is missing, but because target cells fail to respond normally.

Sulfonylureas stimulate insulin release from the pancreas. The newer ones such as glyburide and glipizide also may diminish hepatic glucose production and may directly increase tissue responsiveness to insulin. These actions tend to diminish fasting plasma glucose concentrations and to improve glucose use by fat and muscle cells. The effectiveness of sulfonylureas in obese patients with NIDDM is enhanced by caloric restriction and weight loss. This dietary manipulation also tends to increase the responsiveness of target cells to insulin.

Absorption and fate. Sulfonylureas are well absorbed orally and tend to bind well to serum proteins. The sulfonylureas differ from one another primarily in onset and duration of action (Table 55-5). The onset and duration of action of these drugs is strongly influenced by their metabolic fate in the body. For example, tolbutamide is relatively short acting because it is quickly converted in the body to an inactive product. In contrast, acetohexamide and tolazamide must be converted in the body to active products before they become effective. Hence they are inter-

Table 55-4   Insulin Preparations

Generic name	Trade name	Source	Concentration (units/ml)
Insulin injection	Regular Iletin I	Beef/pork mixture	40 or 100
	Regular Insulin	Pork	100
	Regular Purified Beef Iletin II	Beef, purified	100
	Regular Purified Pork Insulin, and Velosulin	Pork, purified	100
	Regular Purified Pork Iletin II	Pork, purified	100 or 500
	Novolin R and Velosulin Human	Semisynthetic human	100
	Humulin R	Human, recombinant DNA	100
	Humulin BR	Human, recombinant DNA (buffered)	100
Prompt insulin zinc suspension	Semilente Iletin I	Beef/pork mixture	40 or 100
	Semilente Insulin	Beef	100
	Semilente Purified Pork Insulin	Pork, purified	100
Isophane insulin suspension (NPH)	NPH Iletin I	Beef/pork mixture	40 or 100
	NPH Insulin	Beef	100
	NPH Purified Beef Iletin II	Beef, purified	100
	NPH Purified Pork Iletin II, NPH Purified Pork Insulin, and NPH Insulatard	Pork, purified	100
	Humulin N	Human, recombinant DNA	100
	Novolin N and Insulatard NPH Human	Semisynthetic human	100
	Mixtard	Pork, purified (70% NPH, 30% regular insulin)	100
	Mixtard Human and Novolin 70/30	Semisynthetic human (70% NPH, 30% regular insulin)	100
	Humulin 70/30	Human, recombinant DNA (70% NPH, 30% regular insulin)	100
Insulin zinc suspension	Lente Iletin I	Beef/pork mixture	40 or 100
	Lente Insulin	Beef	100
	Lente Purified Beef Iletin II	Beef, purified	100
	Lente Purified Pork Iletin II and Lente Purified Pork Insulin	Pork, purified	100
	Novolin L	Semisynthetic human	100
	Humulin L	Human, recombinant DNA	100
Protamine zinc insulin suspension	Protamine Zinc Iletin I	Beef/pork mixture	40 or 100
	Protamine Zinc Purified Beef Iletin II	Beef, purified	100
	Protamine Zinc Purified Pork Iletin II	Pork, purified	100
Extended insulin zinc suspension	Ultralente Iletin I	Beef/pork mixture	40 or 100
	Ultralente Insulin	Beef	100
	Ultralente Purified Beef Insulin	Beef, purified	100
	Ultralente Humulin U	Human, recombinant DNA	100

Table 55-5 Oral Antidiabetic Agents

Generic name	Trade name	Dosage range	Duration of action	Metabolic fate
Acetohexamide	Dimelor† Dymelor	0.25 to 1.5 gm daily, single or divided dose. FDA Pregnancy Category C.	12 to 24 hr	Converted by liver to an active metabolite, which appears in blood later and stays longer than the parent compound. Active metabolite excreted via the kidney.
Chlorpropamide	Diabinese* Glucamide	0.1 to 0.75 gm daily, single dose. FDA Pregnancy Category C.	Up to 60 hr	Metabolized; excreted through the kidney.
Glipizide	Glucotrol	2.5 to 40 mg daily. Doses greater than 15 mg should be divided. FDA Pregnancy Category C.	12 to 24 hr	Completely absorbed from GI tract. Extensively bound to plasma protein. Metabolized by liver to inactive metabolites. Excreted in urine.
Glyburide	Diabeta* Micronase	1.25 to 20 mg daily. FDA Pregnancy Category B.	16 to 24 hr	Metabolized by liver, with metabolites eliminated in bile and in urine.
Tolazamide	Tolinase	0.1 to 0.75 gm daily; single dose for lower range, divided dose for higher range. FDA Pregnancy Category C.	12 to 24 hr	Slowly absorbed from GI tract. Converted by liver to several mildly active metabolites, which are excreted via kidney.
Tolbutamide	Orinase*	0.5 to 3 gm daily, divided doses. FDA Pregnancy Category C.	6 to 12 hr	Metabolized in liver to an inactive compound.

*Available in Canada and United States.
†Available in Canada only.

mediate in action. Chlorpropamide is the longest-acting member of the class and is tightly bound to plasma protein. This drug is metabolized and excreted in urine.

The two newest sulfonylureas are glyburide and glipizide. Glyburide is extensively metabolized, with the products excreted primarily in bile and secondarily in urine. Glipizide is also converted to inactive metabolites by the liver, but excretion is primarily via the kidney. Both are many times more potent than other sulfonylureas. For example, 5 mg of glyburide or glipizide has an effect equivalent to that of 250 mg of chlorpropamide or tolazamide. At the doses used in patients, clinical effects are similar.

Side effects. Side effects of sulfonylurea therapy include GI distress and neurologic symptoms such as muscle weakness and paresthesias. Liver function tests may be altered, and mild hematopoietic toxicity may be seen in some patients. Frank allergy to the drugs occurs in some patients, with skin reactions being more common than the more dangerous forms of allergic response. The incidence of these types of reactions is reported to be less than 5% of patients treated.

Hypoglycemia is a danger with sulfonylureas and may be caused by drug overdose, drug interaction, altered drug metabolism, or the patient failing to eat. Sulfonylureas should not be used when renal or liver function is inadequate; normal function of those organs is required for metabolism and elimination of the sulfonylureas (see Table 55-5). Elderly patients also occasionally show excessive hypoglycemic reactions to these drugs.

The use of sulfonylureas in the treatment of diabetes mellitus is controversial. Some clinical studies suggest that treatment with sulfonylureas is no more effective than dietary therapy alone. Other studies have suggested that the toxicity of the sulfonylureas is higher than previously expected.

Of special concern is the apparent increase in risk of death from cardiovascular disease in patients receiving a sulfonylurea in the large-scale study conducted by the University Group Diabetes Program (UGDP). Although these questions are far from resolved, some treatment centers avoid the use of sulfonylureas and control mild NIDDM with diet and exercise alone or, if necessary, combine diet and exercise with low doses of insulin. Even when the sulfonylureas are used, careful attention to the diet is required for best results.

Drug interactions. The sulfonylureas are implicated in certain drug interactions that can have serious consequences to the patient. The major interactions occur with ethyl alcohol, phenylbutazone, sulfonamides, salicylates, phenothiazines, and thiazides.

Patients receiving sulfonylureas should routinely avoid alcohol. Several interactions between alcohol and sulfonylureas are possible. Some patients receiving sulfonylureas develop a "disulfiram reaction" when they ingest alcohol. The most striking symptoms of this reaction are unpleasant flushing and severe headache. Other patients on sulfonylureas become hypoglycemic when they ingest alcohol, probably because ethanol is a hypoglycemic agent in some people.

Hypoglycemia can result when one of several drugs is given to a patient taking sulfonylureas, most importantly the antiinflammatory agents, phenylbutazone and salicylates, and sulfonamide antibiotics. These three drugs are all tightly bound to plasma protein and may displace sulfonylureas, which tend to be highly bound to serum protein. Thus blood concentrations of free sulfonylurea are elevated. Since the free drug is the active form, the result is an enhancement of the hypoglycemic effect of the sulfonylurea. In addition to this mechanism, phenylbutazone may block excretion of the active metabolite of acetohexamide, an action that also tends to increase hypoglycemia. Sulfonamides may inhibit the metabolic breakdown of tolbutamide and thereby may enhance its hypoglycemic action.

Phenothiazines such as chlorpromazine may impair the effectiveness of sulfonylureas. Chlorpromazine inhibits the release of insulin from B cells in the pancreas and elevates adrenal production of epinephrine, a hormone that can raise blood glucose levels (see Table 55-1). These actions of chlorpromazine directly antagonize the hypoglycemic action of sulfonylureas.

Thiazide diuretics possess hyperglycemic activity in addition to their diuretic actions; thus they may impair diabetes control with sulfonylureas.

Diet therapy

Mechanism of action. Obesity, or more specifically excessive caloric intake, tends to reduce the number of insulin receptors. An understanding of this disease mechanism helps in appreciating the rationale for dietary control of diabetes. Reduced caloric intake allows the insulin receptors to increase and makes the available insulin more effective. Dietary restriction may lower insulin requirements in obese diabetic persons and in many cases may be the only form of therapy required. The effectiveness of sulfonylureas in obese patients with NIDDM is enhanced by caloric restriction and weight loss.

Careful dietary control is important for all diabetic persons. Successful long-term treatment of the condition frequently involves counseling by a dietitian and supportive follow-up for the rest of the patient's life.

General Guidelines

Patient and family education

◆ Teach patients and families the signs and symptoms of hyperglycemia and hypoglycemia (see Table 55-2).

◆ The development of hypoglycemia may relate to the time insulin or oral agent was taken (see Tables 55-2 and 55-5). If possible, obtain a blood glucose level. Whether or not a blood glucose level is obtained, treat by administering a fast-acting carbohydrate such as ½ cup fruit juice, ½ cup cola drink (not diet forms), ½ cup regular gelatin dessert, 4 cubes or 2 packets of sugar, 2 squares of graham crackers, or 2 to 3 pieces of hard candy. Instruct patients to carry hard candy or other sources of carbohydrate with them at all times. Glucagon may be used if the patient is unconscious. Teach family members how to use this, and instruct the patient to have glucagon always available.

◆ If hypoglycemia is severe, repeated, or occurs without explanation, consult the physician.

◆ Teach or refer patients as needed to a dietitian about appropriate dietary restrictions. Losing weight to desirable body weight is helpful in controlling diabetes.

◆ Encourage participation in a regular exercise program.

◆ Review foot care and other aspects of personal hygiene to prevent infection.

◆ Teach patients how to test blood glucose level. Review methods of testing and frequency, and supervise the patient performing the test activity for accuracy. If a urine test method is being used, point out to the patient that some drugs may cause urine test results to be inaccurate. Teach the patient to ask the physician and pharmacist if there is a possibility of drug-urine test interaction whenever new drugs are prescribed.

◆ Refer patients as appropriate to the health department or other community-based nursing care agencies for follow-up.

◆ Refer patients to the American Diabetes Association or local support groups for additional information and resources; examples of such resources include syringes adapted for the visually impaired, information booklets, automatic insulin injectors, and cookbooks.

◆ Encourage patients with diabetes to wear a medical identification tag or bracelet.

◆ Instruct patients to avoid drinking alcoholic beverages.

◆ Teach patients to avoid smoking. Patients who begin or stop smoking may require an adjustment in diet or drug.

◆ Warn patients to inform all health-care providers about the diabetes and the type of drug used to control it.

◆ Avoid taking any drug unless first approved by the physician. Many drugs cause changes in blood glucose level. Teach patients to monitor blood and/or urine glucose level carefully when starting or stopping a new medication.

◆ The specific regimen prescribed for any patient is based on many factors, including age, type of diabetes, severity of diabetes, weight, resources available, philosophy of the health-care team, and other medical problems the patient may have. Although general guidelines are noted in this text, consult fundamentals of nursing texts and other printed resources as needed.

◆ Caution female patients to consult the physician before attempting to conceive, since management of diabetes may be modified during pregnancy. A diabetic female who becomes pregnant should notify the physician immediately.

Insulin

Drug administration

◆ Local allergic reactions involving itching, redness, swelling, or stinging at the injection site are usually transient and are not uncommon. Anaphylaxis is very rare. Insulin resistance occasionally involves antibodies to insulin. It may not be possible to eliminate local allergic reactions. Supervise insulin administration technique, since scrupulous attention to technique may lessen local irritation. Record and rotate sites on a systematic basis so that accessible sites are not overused (see Chapter 6). Prepare dose of insulin as ordered, and let it warm to room temperature. Cleanse the injection site carefully, and allow skin surface to dry completely. Pinch skin between thumb and fingers of one hand, and insert needle into the "pocket" between the subcutaneous fat and muscle; a 45° to 90° angle can be used, depending on the amount of subcutaneous fat and the length of the needle. Inject the insulin, and withdraw the needle. Apply moderate pressure to the site but do not rub. Disposable syringes are designed for one-time use but are sometimes reused. As they are reused, the needle point becomes duller. If irritation is a problem, the patient may want to use a new needle or syringe more often.

Continued.

NURSING IMPLICATIONS SUMMARY—cont'd

- If local irritation is severe or persistent, consult the physician about a change in type of insulin.
- Systemic reactions are rare and may be due to the animal source of the insulin (bovine, porcine, or mixed bovine-porcine). Treat symptomatically, and notify the physician.
- Use regular insulin for patients on "sliding scale" management.
- Consult with the physician about diabetes management when patients are permitted nothing by mouth (NPO) in preparation for surgery or are otherwise unable to maintain usual dietary intake.
- For IV use, only regular insulin can be used. Insulin adsorbs to bags, tubing, and other items made of polyvinyl chloride (PVC). For continuous infusion, flushing the system with the diluted insulin mixture (e.g., 100 units regular insulin in 500 ml normal saline) before connecting it to the patient may decrease the amount of insulin lost to adsorption to the PVC. Measure the rate of infusion to the patient response, blood glucose levels, and ordered rate of drop of blood glucose level. Also monitor serum electrolyte level, especially potassium.
- Only regular insulin is used in insulin pumps. Review the manufacturer's instruction sheet with the patient.
- Observe agency policies regarding insulin administration. For example, many hospitals require that insulin doses be checked by two licensed nurses before administration.

Patient and family education

- Review the general guidelines and the information about injection.
- Teach patients that only syringes marked for units of insulin should be used with insulin. There are special syringes available for doses less than 50 U. Review carefully with the patient the need to obtain the correct concentration and type of insulin and correct syringe.
- To mix insulins, always draw up the regular (unmodified) insulin first, then the other insulin that is ordered. If two modified insulins are to be drawn up together, either can be drawn up first, but the patient should establish a pattern and always draw the same one up first.
- Some mixtures of insulin in a syringe must be administered within a few minutes of drawing them up, although others are stable for longer periods. Consult the physician or pharmacist.
- Regular insulin is clear, and modified insulins are cloudy. Do not use discolored insulins or ones that appear grainy. Warm and resuspend insulins by rotating the vials between the hands; avoid vigorous shaking.
- Generally, insulin injected into the abdomen is absorbed the fastest, insulin in the arm is absorbed more slowly, and insulin is absorbed slowest when injected in the thigh. However, several things may influence this. For example, a diabetic patient who jogs has faster absorption from the thigh when jogging and using the thigh muscles. Consider the daily habits of the patient in working out an appropriate plan for diabetes management.
- Insulin can be safely kept at room temperature for up to 1 month. Insulin kept at room temperature for longer than 1 month should be discarded. Insulin may be stored in the refrigerator for longer than 1 month. Do not freeze insulin. Check the expiration date.
- Teach the patient that when illness occurs it is important to maintain fluid intake. Consult the physician about specific guidelines for insulin dose and diet when the patient is sick. Remind the patient to contact the physician whenever a question occurs about management.

Representative Common Drug Interactions

Drugs or drug classes interacting	Mechanism/result of interaction	Text references/comments
Acetaminophen and alcohol (ethanol)	Chronic alcohol abuse and high doses of acetaminophen damage the liver. Additive effects of these agents may be fatal.	Chapter 23. This interaction is most important for alcoholics with liver damage from chronic alcohol ingestion.
Acetaminophen and chloramphenicol	Acetaminophen may increase the elimination half-life of chloramphenicol. As a result, chloramphenicol may accumulate, increasing the risk of dose-dependent bone marrow suppression.	Chapters 23 and 32. This interaction can usually be avoided by selecting an alternative agent for one of the drugs.

Alcohol (ethanol) and barbiturates or chloral hydrate (sedative-hypnotics)	CNS depression caused by alcohol may greatly enhance the action of other depressant drugs, leading to severely impaired motor activity, unconsciousness, respiratory depression, and death as dose increases.	Chapter 40. In addition to sedative-hypnotics, many other classes of drugs may produce this interaction:
		    Antihistamines producing marked sedation alone, e.g., diphenhydramine or chlorpheniramine (Chapter 24)
		    Benzodiazepines, especially diazepam (Chapter 40)
		    Meprobamate (Chapter 40)
		    Opioids such as morphine and codeine (Chapter 44)
		    Phenothiazines, especially chlorpromazine (Chapter 41)
		    Phenylbutazone (Chapter 23)
		    Propoxyphene (Chapter 23)
		    Tricyclic antidepressants, especially amitriptyline (Chapter 42)

Alcohol (ethanol) and disulfiram	Disulfiram blocks metabolism of ethanol, leading to accumulation of toxic metabolites. Symptoms are flushing, hypotension, headache, nausea, and difficulty in breathing. Some sensitive persons experience more serious cardiovascular reactions.	Chapter 40. This very striking interaction with ethanol is observed with several drugs other than disulfiram:
		    Cefamandole, cefoperazone, and moxalactam (Chapter 30)
		    Chlorpropamide, a sulfonylurea (Chapter 55)
		    Procarbazine (Chapter 39)
		    Metronidazole (Chapter 38)

Continued.

Drugs or drug classes interacting	Mechanism/result of interaction	Text references/comments
Allopurinol and cyclophosphamide or mercaptopurine (cytotoxic anticancer drugs)	Allopurinol is chemically related to cytotoxic nucleotide analogues and may have additive effects with other cytotoxic agents. The result is excessive toxicity as if from an overdose of the anticancer drug.	Chapters 23 and 39. Allopurinol is often administered to cancer patients to prevent excess uric acid formation. Doses of the anticancer agents may need to be reduced when allopurinol is added.
Allopurinol and dicumarol or warfarin (anticoagulants)	Allopurinol may interfere with the metabolism of the anticoagulants by enzyme systems in the liver. As a result, the anticoagulants accumulate and may cause dangerous bleeding episodes.	Chapters 20 and 23. Only a few patients may show this serious interaction, but all patients receiving both drugs should be carefully watched for excessive action of the anticoagulant.
Aspirin (salicylates) and antacids	Antacids may promote excretion of salicylates by alkalinizing urine. Antacids such as sodium bicarbonate or magnesium aluminum hydroxide can reduce salicylate concentrations in the blood to subtherapeutic levels.	Chapter 23. This interaction is most important for those patients receiving high doses of salicylates for extended periods.
Aspirin (salicylates) and dicumarol or warfarin (anticoagulants)	Aspirin interferes with platelet aggregation and thus has anticoagulant activity even at low doses. The additive effects of aspirin with other potent anticoagulants may cause serious bleeding, a reaction intensified by the tendency of aspirin to cause GI bleeding.	Chapters 20 and 23. This interaction is most important for patients regularly receiving anticoagulants who begin taking aspirin regularly.

Aspirin (salicylates) and GI irritants	Salicylates induce GI bleeding, which may worsen the effects of other irritant drugs. Glucocorticoids may mask the symptoms of ulceration and may allow perforation or hemorrhage to occur before the condition is noticed.	Chapter 23. Several drugs may irritate the GI mucosa enough to cause bleeding or even ulceration:
		    Alcohol (Chapter 40)
		    Glucocorticoids (Chapter 51)
		    Phenylbutazone (Chapter 23)

Aspirin (salicylates) and probenecid or sulfinpyrazone (uricosuric agents)	The ability of both drugs to promote uric acid excretion is diminished when the drugs are combined.	Chapter 23. Patients should not receive aspirin and probenecid or sulfinpyrazone concurrently.
Chloramphenicol and phenytoin	Chloramphenicol inhibits enzymes in the liver that metabolize phenytoin. As a result, phenytoin elimination may be impaired, and the drug may accumulate to toxic levels.	Chapters 47 and 32. During short-term therapy with chloramphenicol, patients receiving phenytoin should be carefully monitored to prevent toxicity. Some physicians prefer to choose an alternative antibiotic, if possible.

Chlordiazepoxide, diazepam, flurazepam, lorazepam (benzodiazepines), and CNS depressants	CNS depression produced by benzodiazepines is additive with that of other drugs. The result may be dangerous, and potentially fatal, CNS depression.	Chapter 40. Benzodiazepines may cause this interaction with these drugs:
		    Alcohol (Chapter 40)
		    Antihistamines (Chapter 24)
		    Antipsychotic drugs (Chapter 41)
		    Barbiturates (Chapter 40)
		    Opiate analgesics (Chapter 44)
		    Tricyclic antidepressants (Chapter 42)

Chlorthalidone, ethacrynic acid, furosemide, or thiazides (potassium-depleting diuretics) and corticosteroids	Both corticosteroids and diuretics can cause potassium loss from the body over time.	Chapters 16 and 51. Potassium supplements may be required to prevent severe depletion.

Drugs or drug classes interacting	Mechanism/result of interaction	Text references/comments
Cimetidine and chlordiazepoxide or diazepam (benzodiazepines)	Cimetidine seems to inhibit the liver enzymes that degrade diazepam and chlordiazepoxide. Patients taking cimetidine who then receive one of these benzodiazepines might be expected to accumulate the benzodiazepine and show excessive drowsiness, ataxia, and other signs of benzodiazepine overdose.	Chapter 40. This interaction does not occur with oxazepam or lorazepam because these benzodiazepines are not metabolized by the liver in the same way as diazepam and chlordiazepoxide. Patients should be warned about driving or carrying out other hazardous tasks when receiving cimetidine and diazepam or chlordiazepoxide.
Cimetidine and dicumarol or warfarin (anticoagulants)	Cimetidine inhibits liver enzymes that metabolize many of the anticoagulants. Therefore cimetidine causes accumulation of the anticoagulants, increasing the risk of overdose and bleeding.	Chapters 13 and 20. This interaction makes careful monitoring of prothrombin times necessary when stabilization has been achieved with the patient taking an anticoagulant, and cimetidine is then added.
Cimetidine and phenytoin	Cimetidine may inhibit the liver enzymes that metabolize phenytoin, leading to phenytoin accumulation and intoxication.	Chapters 13 and 47. Symptoms of phenytoin intoxication are often mild, but additive bone marrow depression with cimetidine is also possible. Phenytoin blood levels may need monitoring.
Cimetidine and propranolol (beta-adrenergic receptor blocker)	Cimetidine inhibits liver enzymes that may metabolize many beta-adrenergic blocking agents. Propranolol concentrations are elevated when cimetidine is also administered; dangerous bradycardia has resulted.	Chapters 13 and 14. In addition to propranolol, other similarly metabolized beta-adrenergic blocking agents may be involved.
Cimetidine and theophylline	Cimetidine inhibits the enzymes in the liver that metabolize theophylline, causing accumulation and theophylline toxicity.	Chapters 13 and 25. This interaction may require that theophylline levels be monitored during cimetidine therapy to prevent theophylline toxicity.
Clofibrate and dicumarol or warfarin (anticoagulants)	Clofibrate greatly enhances the anticoagulant activity of warfarin and dicumarol by displacing the anticoagulants from plasma-binding proteins and possibly by other mechanisms.	Chapters 20 and 21. Doses of the anticoagulants may need to be reduced significantly to avoid dangerous overdosage and bleeding.
Dicumarol and chlorpropamide or tolbutamide (sulfonylureas)	Metabolism of the sulfonylureas may be reduced. The drugs may also compete for plasma protein-binding sites. Both actions tend to increase blood concentrations of active sulfonylurea. The most commonly reported result is an acute hypoglycemic reaction.	Chapters 20 and 55. This interaction may be controlled by using a different anticoagulant or by carefully monitoring blood concentrations of the drugs.
Digoxin (digitalis glycoside) and chlorthalidone, ethacrynic acid, furosemide, or thiazides (potassium-depleting diuretics)	Since hypokalemia increases the likelihood of digitalis toxicity, concurrent use of digitalis preparations and one of the potassium-depleting diuretics may lead to dangerous cardiac arrhythmias.	Chapters 16 and 18. This interaction may be overcome by using a potassium supplement.
Digoxin (digitalis glycoside) and quinidine or quinine	Quinidine and its chemical relative quinine slow renal excretion of digoxin, which may double serum concentrations of digoxin and lead to digoxin toxicity.	Chapters 18 and 19. These drugs should be used together only if serum concentrations of digoxin can be carefully monitored.

Continued.

Drugs or drug classes interacting	Mechanism/result of interaction	Text references/comments
Doxycycline and phenobarbital	Barbiturates can induce enzymes in the liver that may aid in eliminating doxycycline from the body. As a result, doxycycline metabolism may increase, and inadequate concentrations of the antibiotic may appear in the blood.	Chapters 40 and 32. Other tetracyclines are eliminated by renal mechanisms to a greater degree and are therefore less likely to produce this interaction.
Erythromycin and theophylline	Patients receiving high doses of theophylline may accumulate toxic concentrations of theophylline when erythromycin is added. The mechanism is unknown.	Chapters 25 and 31. This interaction seems most important for patients receiving high doses, but all patients receiving both drugs should be watched closely for theophylline toxicity.
Furosemide and phenytoin	The diuretic activity of a fixed dose of furosemide may be drastically reduced in a patient receiving phenytoin. The mechanism is not understood.	Chapters 16 and 47. Increased doses of furosemide may be required to maintain control of symptoms.
Gentamicin and ethacrynic acid or furosemide (loop diuretics)	The loop diuretics and the aminoglycoside antibiotics are capable of impairing balance and causing hearing loss. When given together, especially in high doses, the risk of ototoxicity seems to be greater.	Chapters 16 and 33. Although this interaction is best documented with gentamicin, it is also a possibility with other aminoglycosides (amikacin, kanamycin, neomycin, netilmicin, streptomycin, and tobramycin).
Indomethacin and propranolol or thiazides (antihypertensives)	Indomethacin elevates blood pressure and interferes with the adequate control of hypertension by a variety of drugs.	Chapters 15 and 23. Blood pressure control needs to be carefully monitored in hypertensive patients given indomethacin.
Levodopa and chlordiazepoxide or diazepam (benzodiazepines)	Some patients receiving both drugs lose the antiparkinsonian action of levodopa. The mechanism of this interaction is not known.	Chapters 40 and 48. Patients receiving both drugs should be closely observed to ensure that parkinsonian symptoms are being adequately controlled.
Methyldopa and levodopa	These drugs may enhance the effects of each other by unknown mechanisms. Side effects of levodopa may also worsen.	Chapters 15 and 48. Doses of either or both drugs may need to be reduced.
Methyldopa and lithium carbonate	Lithium tends to accumulate in the blood of patients receiving methyldopa. The brain may also be sensitized to the effects of lithium.	Chapters 15 and 42. Serum concentrations of lithium may need monitoring in patients receiving methyldopa.
Methyltestosterone or methandrostenolone (anabolic steroids) and dicumarol or warfarin (anticoagulants)	Anabolic steroids may enhance the anticoagulant effects of warfarin or dicumarol, possibly by effects on metabolism. Increased risk of bleeding may occur.	Chapters 20 and 51. This interaction should be expected and the dose of anticoagulant reduced accordingly.
Oral contraceptives and barbiturates, phenytoin, or primidone (anticonvulsants)	The anticonvulsants may induce liver enzymes that degrade the steroid components of oral contraceptives. The result may be unexpected pregnancy.	Chapters 47 and 53. Breakthrough bleeding may signal contraceptive failure. Mechanical contraception may be required, although some women may be protected with different doses of oral contraceptives.
Oral contraceptives and rifampin	Rifampin may induce enzymes in the liver that metabolize the steroid components of progestin-only or combined estrogen-progestin oral contraceptives. The result may be unexpected pregnancy.	Chapters 53 and 35. Other antibiotics may also increase the failure rate of oral contraceptives: Penicillins, especially ampicillin (Chapter 30) Tetracyclines, such as oxytetracycline (Chapter 32)

Drugs or drug classes interacting	Mechanism/result of interaction	Text references/comments
Phenobarbital and dicumarol or warfarin (anticoagulants)	Barbiturates can induce enzymes in the liver that metabolize the anticoagulants. As a result, the effect of the anticoagulant is reduced or lost.	Chapters 20 and 40. Many physicians would prefer to avoid the interaction by substituting another drug for the barbiturate.
Phenobarbital and sodium valproate	Sodium valproate increases the serum concentrations of phenobarbital by an unknown mechanism. As a result, excessive sedation can occur.	Chapter 47. When these drugs are combined to treat epilepsy, doses of phenobarbital may need to be reduced.
Phenylbutazone and acetohexamide, chlorpropamide, glyburide, or tolbutamide (hypoglycemic agents)	Phenylbutazone may lower excretion, metabolism, and protein binding of the hypoglycemic agents. These actions may result in accumulation of the hypoglycemic agents and may trigger an acute hypoglycemic reaction.	Chapters 23 and 55. The same effect may be produced by oxyphenbutazone, a metabolite of phenylbutazone.
Phenylbutazone and dicumarol or warfarin (anticoagulants)	Phenylbutazone and its metabolite oxyphenbutazone can displace the anticoagulants from plasma protein-binding sites and may also interfere with metabolism of the anticoagulants. These actions greatly enhance the anticoagulant activity of fixed doses of dicumarol or warfarin and may cause dangerous bleeding.	Chapters 20 and 23. This interaction is so well documented and potentially so serious that many physicians choose not to use these drugs together.
Phenytoin and dicumarol or warfarin (anticoagulants)	Phenytoin toxicity may be enhanced, and anticoagulant drug effect may be either diminished or enhanced as a result of multiple interacting effects on metabolism.	Chapters 20 and 47. The possibility of this interaction requires that the clinical effects of both drugs be carefully monitored during therapy.
Phenytoin and disulfiram	Disulfiram may inhibit enzymes in the liver that metabolize phenytoin. As a result, phenytoin may accumulate to toxic levels.	Chapters 40 and 47. This interaction would normally be avoided by withholding disulfiram or possibly by substituting a different anticonvulsant.
Phenytoin and folic acid	Folic acid deficiency can occur in patients regularly receiving anticonvulsants. Attempts to supplement with folic acid may hasten the metabolic clearance of the anticonvulsants. The result is lower blood concentrations of the anticonvulsant with the danger of loss of seizure control.	Chapter 47. This interaction may also occur between folic acid and primidone.
Phenytoin and isoniazid	Isoniazid inhibits the enzymes in the liver that metabolize phenytoin. As a result, serum concentrations of phenytoin can rise to dangerous levels.	Chapters 47 and 35. Patients receiving both drugs should be carefully monitored for accumulation of phenytoin. Slow acetylators of isoniazid are more at risk of this interaction than are fast acetylators.
Phenytoin and phenylbutazone	Phenylbutazone displaces phenytoin from plasma protein-binding sites and inhibits the metabolism of phenytoin by enzymes in the liver. Both actions tend to increase the serum concentration of active phenytoin. Serious accumulation and toxicity can result.	Chapters 23 and 47. Phenytoin dosage may need to be reduced to avoid toxicity when both drugs are administered. Oxyphenbutazone, a metabolite of phenylbutazone, is presumed to behave similarly to the parent drug.

Continued.

Drugs or drug classes interacting	Mechanism/result of interaction	Text references/comments
Phenytoin and sulfamethoxazole (sulfonamides)	Sulfonamides can interfere with enzyme systems in the liver that metabolize phenytoin. As a result, phenytoin may accumulate to dangerous levels.	Chapters 47 and 34. This interaction is best documented with sulfamethoxazole and the preparation of sulfamethoxazole combined with trimethoprim. The interaction is best avoided by selecting an alternative antibiotic. If a sulfonamide must be used, care should be taken to monitor phenytoin blood levels.
Propoxyphene and carbamazepine	Propoxyphene raises serum levels of carbamazepine by unknown mechanisms. The result may be excessive carbamazepine toxicity.	Chapters 44 and 47. This interaction is often avoided by substituting a different analgesic for propoxyphene.
Propranolol and epinephrine	Beta-adrenergic blocking drugs such as propranolol, which block beta-1 and beta-2 receptors, prevent beta-adrenergic stimulation of the heart by direct-acting sympathomimetics. With epinephrine the remaining unopposed alpha-adrenergic effects may drastically slow the heart.	Chapters 14 and 18. This interaction is more likely with the nonselective beta-adrenergic blocking drugs.
Propranolol and insulin or sulfonylureas (hypoglycemic agents)	Propranolol may increase the frequency of serious hypoglycemic reactions and may mask the tachycardia that often warns of impending hypoglycemia.	Chapters 14, 19, and 55. Diabetic patients receiving any nonselective beta-adrenergic blocking drug should be warned of the increased risk of insidious onset of hypoglycemia.
Propranolol and verapamil	These drugs depress contractility of the heart by independent mechanisms. When the drugs are given together, depression of cardiac function may be severe.	Chapters 14 and 19. Propranolol is not usually combined with verapamil. Other beta-adrenergic blockers may show the same interaction.
Quinidine and barbiturates, phenytoin, or primidone (anticonvulsants)	The anticonvulsants may increase enzymes in the liver that metabolize quinidine. Therefore quinidine is rapidly removed from the body and the antiarrhythmic effect may be lost.	Chapters 19 and 47. This interaction is especially dangerous during the periods when the anticonvulsant is started or withdrawn from a patient who has been stabilized on a set dose of quinidine.
Rifampin and digitoxin (digitalis glycoside)	Rifampin induces drug-metabolizing enzymes in the liver, thereby increasing elimination of digitoxin. As a result, the serum concentration of digitoxin falls, with concurrent loss of digitalis action.	Chapters 18 and 35. This interaction requires that patients receiving both drugs be carefully watched for signs that the digitalis effect is being lost.
Theophylline and ephedrine	When used together to treat asthma, these drugs are no more effective than theophylline alone but seem to produce additive toxicity. The mechanism is unknown.	Chapter 25. This combination offers no advantage and the potential for disadvantages. Therefore the direct combination should be avoided.
Thiazide diuretics or chlorthalidone and insulin or sulfonylureas (hypoglycemic agents)	Thiazide and related diuretics raise blood glucose concentrations, which may impair diabetes control.	Chapters 16 and 55. These drugs can be used together so long as the dose of the hypoglycemic agent is adjusted to maintain diabetes control.
Thiazide diuretics or chlorthalidone and lithium carbonate	Lithium concentrations in the blood are raised by the concurrent use of thiazide or related diuretics. Dangerous accumulation of lithium may result over a long period.	Chapters 16 and 42. Lithium levels in the blood must be carefully monitored if thiazides or related diuretics must also be administered.

Drugs or drug classes interacting	Mechanism/result of interaction	Text references/comments
Thyroid hormones and dicumarol or warfarin (anticoagulants)	Thyroid hormones seem to increase the rate of breakdown of blood factors. The anticoagulants inhibit synthesis of the factors. Combining the drugs results in a marked anticoagulant effect that may lead to dangerous bleeding episodes.	Chapters 20 and 52. Close monitoring is necessary when the dose of anticoagulant is adjusted in a patient receiving thyroid hormones or when thyroid hormone therapy is added in a patient previously stabilized on a dose of anticoagulant.
Tolbutamide and chloramphenicol or rifampin	Chloramphenicol and rifampin inhibit enzymes in the liver that metabolize tolbutamide. As a result, tolbutamide accumulates, and acute hypoglycemia may occur.	Chapters 55, 32, and 35. Many physicians prefer to avoid the interaction when possible by substituting another antibiotic. Chlorpropamide and possibly other sulfonylureas may behave similarly to tolbutamide.
Warfarin and barbiturates, griseofulvin, or rifampin	Barbiturates, rifampin, and possibly griseofulvin may induce enzymes in the liver that metabolize warfarin. As a result, warfarin is eliminated more rapidly, and adequate anticoagulation may be lost.	Chapters 20, 40, 35, and 36. Warfarin doses may be increased to offset the effects of increased metabolism, but there is risk of bleeding if the inducing drugs are suddenly withdrawn.
Warfarin and metronidazole or sulfamethoxazole/trimethoprim	Metronidazole inhibits the enzymes in the liver that metabolize warfarin, whereas sulfamethoxazole/trimethoprim may have other effects. Both antimicrobial preparations markedly enhance the anticoagulant activity of warfarin.	Chapters 20, 34, and 38. This interaction should be expected when warfarin is combined with either antimicrobial agent. Doses of warfarin should be reduced to prevent dangerous bleeding episodes.
Warfarin and sulindac	Sulindac in some way enhances the anticoagulant activity of warfarin and possibly other anticoagulants. Bleeding may result.	Chapters 20 and 23. For some patients, reducing the dosage of warfarin may control the interaction. Other patients may require discontinuation of the sulindac.

Disorders Index*

*(i) = illustration
  (t) = table

823

Comprehensive Index*

A

ABBOKINASE (*urokinase*), 323(t), 324
Abbreviations, pharmaceutical, 104(t)
Abdominal distension, atropine and, 161
ABDV regimen, 580(t)
ABIPLATIN (*cisplatin*), 562(t)
Abscess, amebic disease and, 537
Absence epilepsy, 697
absorbable gelatin film, 325, 326(t)
absorbable gelatin sponge, 325, 326(t)
Absorption of drug, 6-9, 11
Abuse, drug; *see* Drug abuse
acebutolol
   action potential effects of, 299(t)
   for angina, 208(t)
   as antiarrhythmic drug, 302(t)
   for hypertension, 227(t), 233
acetaminophen
   as analgesic-antipyretic drug, 358, 359(t)
   antidote for, 69(t)
   drug interactions with, 815(t)
   education about, 372-373
   effects of, 51
ACETAZOLAM (*acetazolamide*)
   as anticonvulsant, 701(t)
   as diuretic, 259, 259(t)
   for glaucoma, 157(t)
acetazolamide, 160, 704
   administration of, 263
   as anticonvulsant, 701(t)
   as diuretic, 259, 259(t)
   for glaucoma, 157(t)
acetbutolol, 135(t)
   as antiarrhythmic drug, 300(t), 307
acetohexamide, 809(t)
   drug interactions with, 819(t)
Acetone odor, poisons causing, 65(t)
acetophenazine, 622(t)
   side effects of, 625(t)
Acetylation of drug, 22
Acetylator, isoniazid and, 506
Acetylcholine
   myasthenia gravis and, 141-142
   as neurotransmitter, 117, 118(i), 119
   Parkinson's disease and, 710
   poisoning and, 70
   role of, 121
Acetylcholinesterase inhibitor, 125
   myasthenia gravis and, 142-145

acetylcysteine
   as antidote, 69(t)
   as mucolytic, 413(t)
ACHOMYCIN (*tetracycline hydrochloride*), 476(t)
Acid
   amino
      hormones formed from, 724
      infusion of, 282
      in total parenteral nutrition, 274-275
   bile, 338
   hydrochloric, 169
   stomach
      drug absorption and, 8
      ulcers and, 169, 170-171(t), 171-173
   tetrahydrofolic, 492, 493(i)
   vanillylmandelic, 119
Acid urine, 360
Acidification of urine, 71
Acidity, drug absorption and, 8
Acidosis
   metabolic, 271
   respiratory, 271
Acinar cell, 411
Acne
   over-the-counter drugs for, 56-57
   tetracyclines for, 478
Acquired immunity, 419
Acquired immunodeficiency syndrome, 424, 527
   clinical drug trials and, 31
   drugs for, 529
   immunotoxins and, 436
   Pneumocystis carinii pneumonia in, 539
Acromegaly, 734
ACTA-CHAR (*activated charcoal*), 67(t)
ACTH; *see* Adrenocorticotropic hormone
ACTHAR (*corticotropin*), 753(t)
ACTI-B$_{12}$ (*vitamin B$_{12}$*), 348(t)
ACTIDIL (*triprolidine hydrochloride*), 385(t)
Action potential, cardiac, 286, 287(i), 297-298
ACTIVASE (*alteplase*), 323, 324
activated charcoal, 67, 73
Active ingredients, 24-25
Acute glaucoma, 158
ACUTRIM (*phenylpropanolamine hydrochloride*), 652(t)
acyclovir, 529, 530(t), 533
ADALAT (*nifedipine*), 209(t), 211
ADAPIN (*doxepin*), 636(t), 641
ADD; *see* Attention deficit disorder
Addiction, 597
Addison's disease, 744
ADENOCARD (*adenosine*), 302(t)
Adenohypophyseal hormone, 763(t)
Adenohypophysis, 732-737

---

*Generic drugs are in lower case italics.
  Trade names are in small caps.
  (i) = illustration
  (t) = table

Guide to Special Features